For Instructors

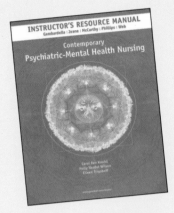

Instructor's Resource Manual

ISBN: 0-13-062309-1

This manual contains a wealth of material to help faculty plan and manage the Mental Health nursing course. It includes chapter overviews, detailed lecture suggestions and outlines, learning objectives, a complete test bank, answers to the textbook critical thinking exercises, teaching tips, and more for each chapter. The IRM also guides faculty how to assign and use the text-specific Companion Website, www.prenhall.com/kneisl, and the free student CD-ROM that accompany the textbook.

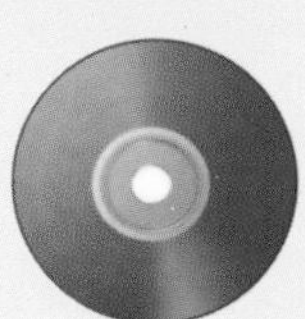

Instructor's Resource CD-ROM

ISBN: 0-13-062300-8

This cross-platform CD-ROM provides illustrations in PowerPoint from the textbook for use in classroom lectures. It also contains the Test-Gen electronic test bank, answers to the textbook critical thinking exercises, a printed version of the IRM, and animations and videos from the Student CD-ROM and Companion Website. This supplement is available to faculty free upon adoption of the textbook.

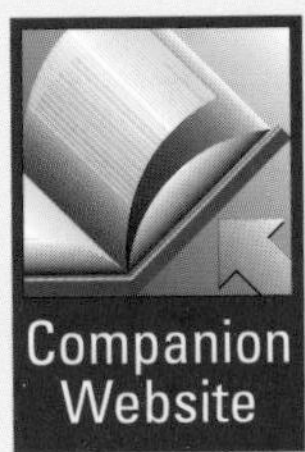

Companion Website Syllabus Manager www.prenhall.com/kneisl

Faculty adopting this textbook have free access to the online Syllabus Manager on the Companion Website, www.prenhall.com/kneisl. Syllabus Manager offers a whole host of features that facilitate the students' use of the Companion Website, and allows faculty to post syllabi and course information online for their students. For more information or a demonstration of Syllabus Manager, please contact a Prentice Hall Sales Representative.

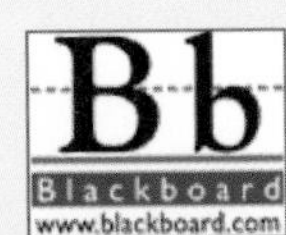

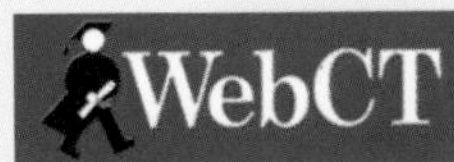

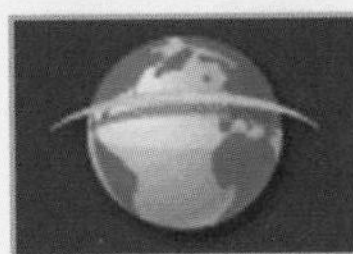

Online Course Management Systems

Also available are online companions available for schools using course management systems. The online course management solutions feature interactive modules, electronic test bank, PowerPoint images, animations and video clips, and more. For more information about adopting an online course management system to accompany **Contemporary Psychiatric-Mental Health Nursing**, please contact your Prentice Hall Health Sales Representative or go to the appropriate website below:

Blackboard: http://cms.prenhall.com/blackboard/index.html
WebCT: http://cms.prenhall.com/webct/index.html
CourseCompass: http://cms.prenhall.com/coursecompass/

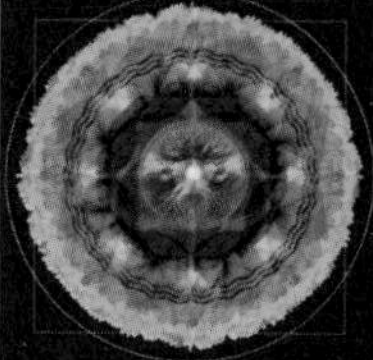

BRIEF CONTENTS

atric–Mental Health Nursing

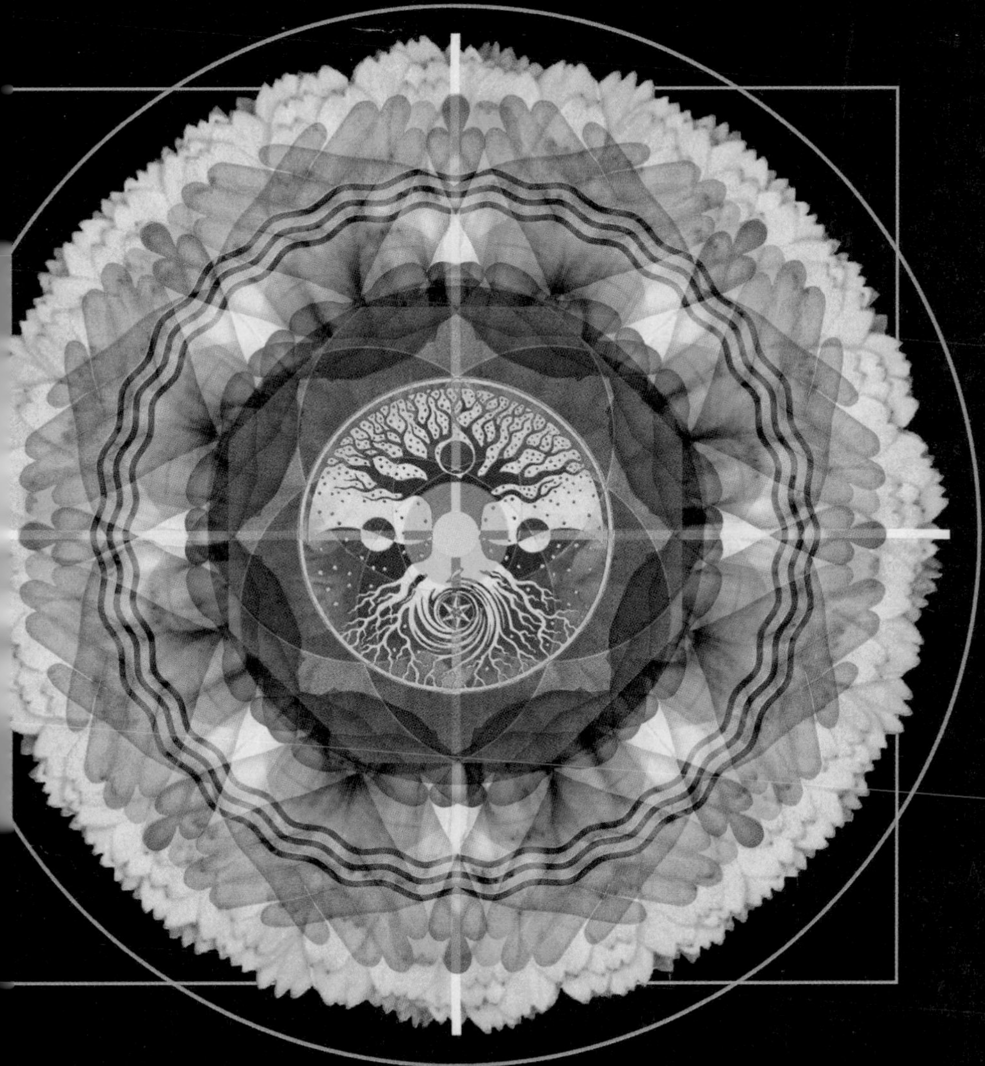

Carol Ren Kneisl, RN, MS, APRN, DABFN
Holly Skodol Wilson, BSN, MSN, PhD
Eileen Trigoboff, RN, APRN/PMH-BC, DNS, DABFN

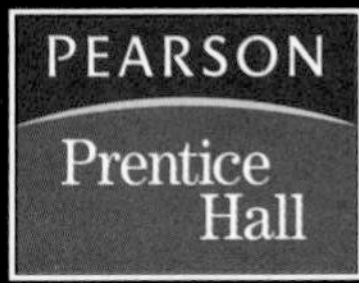

Upper Saddle River, New Jersey 07458

Library of Congress Cataloging-in-Publication Data

Kneisl, Carol Ren
Contemporary psychiatric-mental health nursing / by Carol Ren Kneisl, Holly Skodol Wilson, Eileen Trigoboff.—1st ed.
p. ; cm.
Includes bibliographical references.
ISBN 0-13-041582-0
1. Psychiatric nursing. I. Wilson, Holly Skodol. II. Trigoboff, Eileen. III. Title.
[DNLM: 1. Mental Disorders—nursing. 2. Psychiatric Nursing. WY 160 K68c 2004]
RC440.K646 2004
610.73'68–dc21 2002044547

Notice: Care has been taken to confirm the accuracy of the information presented in this book. The authors, editors, and the publisher, however, cannot accept any responsibility for errors or omissions or for consequences from application of the information in this book and make no warranty, express or implied, with respect to its contents.

The authors and the publisher have exerted every effort to ensure that drug selections and dosages set forth in this text are in accord with current recommendations and practice at time of publication. However, in view of ongoing research, changes in government regulations, and the constant flow of information relating to drug therapy and drug reactions, the reader is urged to check the package inserts of all drugs for any change in indications of dosage and for added warnings and precautions. This is particularly important when the recommended agent is a new and/or infrequently employed drug.

The authors and publisher disclaim all responsibility for any liability, loss, injury, or damage incurred as a consequence, directly or indirectly, of the use and application of any of the contents of this volume.

Publisher: *Julie Levin Alexander*
Assistant to Publisher: *Regina Bruno*
Editor-in-Chief: *Maura Connor*
Managing Development Editor: *Marilyn Meserve*
Development Editor: *Elisabeth Garofalo*
Media Development Editor: *John J. Jordan*
Assistant Editor: *Yesenia Kopperman*
Editorial Assistant: *Sladjana Repic*
Director of Production and Manufacturing: *Bruce Johnson*
Managing Production Editor: *Patrick Walsh*
Production Liaison: *Danielle Newhouse*
Production Editor: *Linda Begley, Rainbow Graphics*
Manufacturing Buyer: *Pat Brown*
Design Director: *Cheryl Asherman*
Design Coordinator: *Maria Guglielmo*
Interior Designer: *Amanda Kavanagh*
Cover Designer: *Mary Siener*
Cover and Interior Illustration: *The Great Mother by Cynthia Cunningham Baxter*
Electronic Art Creation: *ElectraGraphics*
Manager of Media Production: *Amy Peltier*
New Media Project Manager: *Stephen Hartner*
New Media Production: *Eclectic Multimedia*
Marketing Manager: *Nicole Benson*
Marketing Assistant: *Janet Ryerson*
Channel Marketing Manager: *Rachele Triano*
Composition: *Rainbow Graphics*
Cover printer: *Lehigh Press*
Printer/Binder: *Von Hoffmann/St. Louis*

Pearson Education LTD.
Pearson Education Australia PTY, Limited
Pearson Education Singapore, Pte. Ltd
Pearson Education North Asia Ltd
Pearson Education, Canada, Ltd
Pearson Educación de Mexico, S.A. de C.V.
Pearson Education–Japan
Pearson Education Malaysia, Pte. Ltd
Pearson Education, Upper Saddle River, New Jersey

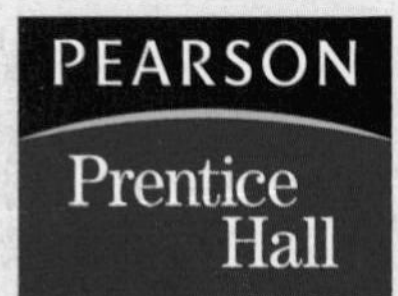

10 9 8 7 6 5 4
ISBN 0-13-041582-0

CONTENTS

CHAPTER 3. Evidence-Based Practice in Psychiatric–Mental Health Nursing 42

CHAPTER 4. Psychobiology 57

CHAPTER 5. Stress, Anxiety, and Coping 80

UNIT III. Clients with Mental Disorders 233

CHAPTER 12. Cognitive Disorders 234

CHAPTER 13. Substance-Related Disorders 260

PREFACE

Millions of people worldwide suffer from mental health disorders. In fact, five of the leading causes of disability in the world today are psychiatric in nature. Psychiatric–mental health nursing is a specialized area that employs a wide range of explanatory theories and research on human behavior as its science and the purposeful use of self as its art. Understanding people who are searching for meaning through interaction in complex times demands the most authoritative and contemporary knowledge and clinical competence. It is through the power of knowledge and clinical competence that psychiatric–mental health nurses can help clients from diverse cultures to live with uncertainty, unfamiliarity and unpredictability and to pursue creative healing on psychobiologic and spiritual levels. Our goal for this textbook, *Contemporary Psychiatric–Mental Health Nursing,* and its companion supplements is to provide students and practicing psychiatric–mental health nurses with the most up-to-date, evidence-based, culturally competent, authoritative, comprehensive resource available and to present it in an accessible, clinically relevant, and professional format.

UNDERLYING THEMES

Throughout this textbook, we as authors try to remain true to values of humanism, interactionism, cultural competence, the relevance of meaning, and the importance of empathy and empowerment in the nurse–client relationship. We believe that psychiatric–mental health nursing is concerned with the quality of human life and its relationship to optimal psychobiologic health, feelings of self-worth, personal integrity, self-fulfillment, spirituality, and creative expression. The psychiatric–mental health nurse's scope of practice is broad enough to include issues such as alienation, identity crises, sudden life changes, and troubled family relationships. It may involve issues of poverty and affluence, cross-cultural disparities in access to health care, and the human experiences of birth, death, and loss. Psychiatric–mental health nursing is concerned with sustaining and enhancing the mental health of both the individual and the group, while its practice locale is often found in the community.

In exploring the theme of global mental health, each unit of this book opens with compelling photographs and stories of individuals from around the world who face a variety of mental health issues. By presenting the readers with this global perspective, we hope to promote awareness of the relevance of those same global issues in our own culturally diverse society.

Along these lines, we selected a Mandela to represent the essence of this book. *Mandela* is the Sanskrit word for circle and symbolizes wholeness or organization around a unifying center. The goal of this book is to explore science, art, and spirituality as a path toward our shared vision of global mental health. It is a synthesis of elements important to a holistic view. The Mandela used throughout this book and on its cover is entitled *The Great Mother,* created by Cynthia Cunningham Baxter. It consists of hands and a mother tree, which is consistent with nursing's goals of care, compassion, and comfort.

CONTEMPORARY TRENDS

The themes, ideas, knowledge, tools, and organization of this textbook were expressly designed for psychiatric–mental health nursing students and clinicians who are committed to developing the habits of mind, responsibility, and practice that will make a difference in view of contemporary trends. Specifically, this text prepares students to tailor and humanize interventions for traditional as well as "new" psychiatric–mental health clients often encountered in forensic settings, homeless shelters, and in other community-based and rehabilitation-oriented settings.

Furthermore, because advances in neuroscience and the study of the human genome are redefining our conception of the basis for mental disorders, a solid grounding in psychobiology is threaded throughout the book. Brain imaging assessment and concise yet comprehensive information on the expanding array of psychopharmacologic treatment is yet another strong emphasis. We recognize that psychiatric–mental health clients are racially and culturally diverse and include growing numbers of mentally ill elders, children, adolescents, and people with coexisting substance use disorders or comorbidities with other chronic illnesses such as HIV/AIDS. Therefore, we devote separate chapters to each of the above topics. We feel confident in entitling this book *Contemporary Psychiatric–Mental Health Nursing* because of its explicit links to contemporary trends in our field.

ORGANIZATION

The detailed table of contents at the beginning of the book makes its clear organization easy to follow. The book is divided into five parts. Unit I clusters six chapters that provide comprehensive coverage of the theoretic basis for psychiatric–mental health nursing. In Unit II, we address topics traditionally associated with psychiatric–mental health nursing, such as using the nursing process, therapeutic communication, assessment, advocacy and client rights, and creating a therapeutic environment. Unit III focuses on caring for clients with specific DSM-IV-TR mental disorders. First, we outline the defining characteristics of each disorder, then we cover the biopsychosocial theories necessary to understand them, and finally we apply the nursing process to caring for clients with these disorders. Unit IV shifts the focus to vulnerable populations that require comfort and care from psychiatric–mental health nurses. These populations include people at risk for self-destructive behavior, abuse, or violence; psychiatric–mental health clients with HIV/AIDS; and specific age groups. Unit V of the book provides authoritative coverage of nursing intervention strategies and desired outcomes, including a wide range of modalities, from individual, group, and family interventions to psychopharmacology and complementary and alternative healing practices. Throughout the book, experts contributed their knowledge and skills on all the topics covered.

FEATURES

The following noteworthy features weave together the threads of research, theory, and practice into a comprehensive and contemporary fabric of knowledge and competencies essential to psychiatric–mental health nursing. The content and processes are clearly applicable to the care of identified psychiatric–mental health clients, yet they are also relevant when integrated into the care of all those with whom we interact as professional nurses.

- *Using Research Evidence.* In addition to a full chapter devoted to evidence-based psychiatric–mental health nursing practice (Chapter 3), each chapter includes a clinical vignette illustrating how research evidence shapes the plan of care for a particular client.
- *Case-Based Critical Thinking Challenges.* Because critical thinking skills are essential to evidence-based practice, a Critical Thinking Challenge begins each chapter, challenging readers to analyze a case scenario that is related to the chapter topic. The discussion points for the critical thinking challenge appear in the Instructor's Resource Manual accompanying this text.
- *Caring for the Spirit.* These boxes reinforce the belief in the interconnection of mind, body, and spirit. They appear throughout the book and are designed to promote the understanding of the client's essence, meaning, and purpose in life, as well as the nurse's role in supporting spirituality.
- *Culture and Family Awareness* icons throughout the book call the reader's attention to content that bears on the importance of developing cultural competence and the value of including the family as partners in psychiatric–mental health care.
- *Medication* icons throughout identify sections of the text that discuss psychopharmacology.
- *Case Studies and Nursing Care Plans* are found in each of the clinical chapters. These plans use NANDA, NOC, and NIC nomenclature and illustrate linkages among them when caring for clients diagnosed with specific mental disorders according to the DSM-IV-TR.
- *Assessment Guidelines, Intervention Guidelines, Client–Family Teaching* boxes all present clinically relevant strategies in a succinct, user-friendly format. Assessment Guidelines contain lists of assessment points. Intervention Guidelines list specific nursing intervention strategies along with their rationales. Client–Family Teaching boxes provide specific client-oriented information that contains sample language a nurse can use when working with clients.
- *Nursing Self-Awareness.* Appearing throughout the book, these boxes engage the reader in a process of introspection and self-questioning that is essential to the therapeutic use of self.
- *Rx Communication.* Each of the clinical chapters focuses on clients within a particular psychiatric diagnostic category and includes a specially designed box to offer sample dialogues of *what a nurse can say* in response to clients. In addition, we provide the rationale for at least two different but helpful alternatives. This feature is designed to provide students with a beginning repertoire of communication interventions useful when interacting with psychiatric–mental health clients.
- *Case Management, Community-Based Care, and Home Care.* Each of the psychiatric disorders chapters and vulnerable populations chapters includes specific information that reflects the fact that the setting for much of psychiatric nursing practice today is found in the community rather than in the hospital.
- *MediaLink* and *EXPLORE MediaLink.* At the beginning of each chapter, a MediaLink box lists specific content, animations and videos, NCLEX review questions, tools, and other interactive exercises that appear on the accompanying Student CD-ROM and the Companion Website. Special MediaLink tabs appear in the margins throughout the chapter that refer the student to the topics and activities on the media supplements. Finally, at the end of each chapter, EXPLORE MediaLink sections encourage students to use the CD-ROM and the Companion Website to apply what they have learned from the text in case studies and care plans, to practice NCLEX questions, and to use additional resources. The purpose of the MediaLink feature is to further enhance the student experience, build upon knowledge gained from the textbook, prepare students for the NCLEX, and foster critical thinking.
- *Focus Questions* provide the reader with guidance for actively reading the chapter and getting the most out of it.
- *Key Terms* alert the reader to the vocabulary used in the chapter and are available in the Audio Glossary found on the Student CD-ROM or the Companion Website.
- *Cross-References* pinpoint specific content linked to supporting chapters when more depth is required. The icon refers the reader to content in other sections of the book.
- *References.* Each chapter includes a bibliography of the most up-to-date resources on the topic. WebLinks throughout guide the reader to online information which can be accessed via the Companion Website at www.prenhall.com/kneisl.

COMPREHENSIVE TEACHING AND LEARNING PACKAGE

The following supplements were developed to support *Contemporary Psychiatric–Mental Health Nursing* and enhance both the student and instructor experiences in this course:

- *Student CD-ROM.* This CD-ROM is packaged *free* with the textbook. It provides an interactive study program that allows students to practice answering NCLEX-style questions with rationales for right and wrong answers. It also contains an Audio Glossary, animations and video clips, and a link to the Companion Website (an Internet connection is required).
- *Companion Website* www.prenhall.com/kneisl. This *free* online study guide is designed to help students apply the

concepts presented in the book. Each chapter-specific module features objectives, Audio Glossary, chapter summary for lecture notes, NCLEX Review questions, case studies, care plan activities, class discussion questions, WebLinks, and Nursing Tools, such as Standards of Psychiatric–Mental Health Nursing Practice, and more. Faculty adopting this textbook have *free* access to the online Syllabus Manager feature of the Companion Website. Syllabus Manager offers a whole host of features that facilitate the students' use of the Companion Website, and allows faculty to post syllabi and course information online for their students. For more information or a demonstration of Syllabus Manager, please contact a Prentice Hall Sales Representative.

- *Clinical Companion for Psychiatric–Mental Health Nursing.* This clinical companion serves as a portable, quick reference to psychiatric–mental health nursing. Topics include DSM-IV-TR classifications, common diagnostic studies, over 20 clinical applications for mental health disorders, medications, and much more. This handbook will allow students to bring the information they learn from class into any clinical setting.
- *Instructor's Resource Manual.* This manual contains a wealth of material to help faculty plan and manage the Mental Health Nursing course. It includes chapter overviews, detailed lecture suggestions and outlines, learning objectives, discussion points, a complete test bank, answers to the textbook critical thinking exercises, teaching tips, and more for each chapter. The IRM also guides faculty on how to assign and use the text-specific Companion Website, www.prenhall.com/kneisl, and the free student CD-ROM that accompany the textbook.
- *Instructor's Resource CD-ROM.* This cross-platform CD-ROM provides illustrations and text slides in PowerPoint for use in classroom lectures. It also contains an electronic test bank, answers to the textbook critical thinking challenges, and animations and videos from the Student CD-ROM. This supplement is available to faculty free upon adoption of the textbook.
- *Online Course Management Systems.* Also available are Blackboard, WebCt, and CourseCompass online companions available for schools using course management systems. The online course management solutions feature interactive modules, electronic test banks, PowerPoint slides including images and discussion points, animations and video clips, and more. For more information about adopting an online course management system to accompany *Contemporary Psychiatric–Mental Health Nursing,* please contact your Prentice Hall Health Sales Representative or go online to www.prenhall.com/demo.

THE TEXTBOOK AS A MAP, A COMPASS, AND AN INSPIRATION

Psychiatric–mental health nursing is poised at a crossroads. We are challenged to bring complex thinking to a complex world if we are to actualize our contribution to global mental health—the vision to which this text is dedicated. This book has been crafted to provide you with the best possible evidence generated in research to help you achieve your goal of excellence in practice. It offers a fully integrated bio/psycho/social perspective rather than relying on any single theory or ideology. It encourages you to become personally, professionally, and spiritually willing to muster the courage and hope necessary to forge proactive steps in our future and to make a commitment to work globally in a contemporary landscape and mindscape.

We have the opportunity to forge a new synthesis of professional wisdom in face of tough mind–body–spirit problems and needs. We need to face the new millennium's critical transitions with intelligence, stamina, wit, creativity, skill, and moral courage. Global mental health can become a shared emergent vision constructed in a way that is respectful of the rich diversity of the citizens of our contemporary world. We created this book to provide you with a map, a compass, and the inspiration to succeed in your current work. We hope that it encourages you to become a participant and leader in facing the broader challenges ahead of us.

Carol Ren Kneisl
Holly Skodol Wilson
Eileen Trigoboff

ACKNOWLEDGMENTS

This book draws deeply from many wells. A diverse group of students, colleagues, and clients provided encouragement and opportunities to put into practice what we teach. Each has had a significant and lasting impact on this text.

We are especially grateful to Maura Connor, Editor-in-Chief at Prentice Hall. This text is a testament to her vision, optimism, and energy.

The stance of mind and heart of our Developmental Editor, Elisabeth Garofalo, protected the consistency of this text throughout the challenges. She is not only skilled, she is authentic.

We could not have asked for a better team than the one at Prentice Hall. They have been a steady source of encouragement and support and contributed in countless ways. The design team, Cheryl Asherman and Maria Guglielmo, made the cover and the text distinctive, beautiful, and accessible. Sladjana Repic, Editorial Assistant, coordinated the myriad tasks that go into producing a book of this size. She was steady, as well as gracious. Marilyn Meserve, Senior Managing Editor, provided guidance and support to do whatever was needed to help us get the job done. Danielle Newhouse, Production Liaison, shepherded this project through the production process with her usual capable, practical, "can-do" style. Every project needs a great facilitator and for us Patrick Walsh, Managing Production Editor, filled this role. Yesenia Kopperman, Assistant Editor, managed and developed our supplement package.

Linda Begley, Rhonda Peters, Susan Cooper, and Edgar Bowery at Rainbow Graphics made sure that each and every page looked its best. They are topnotch in their field. Robert Starnes at ElectraGraphics drafted the illustrations that so ably enhance the content.

Thanks also to Kay Hanks, RN and Ruby Anthony of East Louisiana Mental Health System and Sue Joffee, Buffalo Psychiatric Center, Buffalo, New York for the historical photographs.

A talented group of contributors—friends and colleagues—generously shared the power of their collective wisdom and clinical expertise in several chapters:

Kay K. Chitty, RN, EdD
Adjunct Professor, College of Nursing
Medical University of South Carolina
Charleston, South Carolina

Judith Coram, RN, MSN
Clinical Faculty, University of Washington
Seattle, Washington
Adjunct Faculty, University of Colorado
Colorado Springs, Colorado

Carol Bradley-Corpuel, RN, CS, MSN
Clinical Adjunct Faculty, Orvis School of Nursing
University of Nevada-Reno
Psychiatric Clinical Nurse Specialist
Saint Mary's Regional Medical Center
Reno, Nevada

Sue C. DeLaune, RN, MN, BC
Adjunct Faculty, Loyola University
New Orleans, Louisiana
President & Education Director
SDeLaune Consulting, Mandeville, Louisiana
Education Consultant to Nursing
New Orleans Adolescent Hospital

Karen Lee Fontaine, RN, MSN, AASECT
Professor, Purdue University-Calumet
Hammond, Indiana

Gloria Kuhlman RN, DNSc
Professor of Nursing, Ohlone College
Fremont, California
Clinical Nurse Specialist,
Veterans Administration Medical Center
Palo Alto, California

Pamela Marcus, RN, APRN/PMH-BC
Adjunct Clinical Faculty, Prince George's Community College
Clinical Director,
Crisis Response System, Affiliated Sante Group
Private Practice, Upper Marlboro, Maryland

Beth Moscato, RN, PhD, CNS
Research Assistant Professor,
Department of Social & Preventive Medicine
School of Medicine and Biomedical Sciences,
University of Buffalo
Buffalo, New York

Kimberly Pelish, RN, MSN
Certified Adult Nurse Practitioner
Emergency Department Case Management Team
at San Francisco General Hospital
UCSF Department of Psychosocial Medicine
San Francisco, California

Bethany J. Phoenix, RN, PhD, CNS
Assistant Clinical Professor,
Department of Community Health Systems
School of Nursing, University of California
San Francisco, California

Elizabeth A. Riley RN, MS, NPP
Director of Nursing and Adult Services
Four Winds Hospital
Private Practice
Saratoga Springs, New York

Marlene Reimer RN, PhD, CNN(C)
Professor, Faculty of Nursing
University of Calgary,
Alberta, Canada

Sandra J. Weiss, PhD, DNSc, RN, FAAN
Professor, Department of Community Health Systems
University of California
San Francisco, California

Several reviewers read and critiqued drafts. Thank you for your generosity in sharing your insightful comments with us.

Carla Abel-Zieg, MS, RN, CS, ARNP
Assistant Professor, Creighton University, Omaha, Nebraska

Jan V. R. Belcher, RN, PhD, CS
Associate Professor, Wright State University, Dayton, Ohio

Barbara Mathews Blanton, MSN, RN, CARN
Clinical Instructor, Texas Woman's University, Dallas, Texas

Kathleen C. Buchheit, EdD, RN
Professor, Morningside College, Sioux City, Iowa

Karma Castleberry, RN, CS, PhD
Professor, Radford University, Radford, Virginia

Jeanneane L. Cline, RN, MS, CS, CHTP, LMFT, LCDC
Clinical Instructor, University of Texas-Arlington, Arlington, Texas

Patricia R. Dean, RN, MSN
Associate Professor, Florida State University, Tallahassee, Florida

Lourdes A. D. de la Cruz, MHSc, MScCHN
Professor, Sheridan College, Mississauga, Ontario

Sharon D. Dettenrieder, MSN, RN
Department Chair and Professor, Hartwick College, Oneonta, New York

Marilyn S. Fetter, PhD, RN, CS
Assistant Professor, Villanova University, Villanova, Pennsylvania

Brian Fonnesbeck, RNC, MN
Associate Professor, Lewis Clark State College, Lewiston, Idaho

Tamara George, RN, PhD
Associate Professor, Hope College, Holland, Michigan

Rebecca Crews Gruener, MS
Associate Professor, Louisiana State University, Alexandria, Louisiana

Patricia Becker Hentz, EdD, RN, CS
Associate Professor, University of Southern Maine, Portland, Maine

Mary K. Kane, CRNP, CS-P
Assistant Professor, Salisbury University, Salisbury, Maryland

Dianne Kinsey, RN, MSN, EdD
Professor, Cedar Crest College, Allentown, Pennsylvania

Nancy L. Kostin, RN, MSN
Assistant Professor, Madonna University, Livonia, Michigan

Virginia Lester, RN, MSN, CNS
Assistant Professor, Angelo State University, San Angelo, Texas

Pam Lindsey, MS, RN
Interim Undergraduate Program Director, Mennonite College of Nursing at Illinois State University, Normal, Illinois

Joan C. Masters, MA, MBA, RN
Assistant Professor, Bellarmine University, Louisville, Kentucky

Maryellen McBride, MN, ARNP, CARN
Assistant Professor, Washburn University, Topeka, Kansas

Yvonne D. McKoy, RN, CS, PhD, DABFN
Professor, Xavier University, Cincinnati, Ohio

Elizabeth Ann Moseley, MN, RN
Instructor, Henderson State University, Arkadelphia, Arkansas

Cynthia A. Pearson, MSN, RN, CS
Faculty Instructor, University of Delaware, Newark, Delaware

Ona Z. Riggin, EdD, ARNP
Emeritus Distinguished Professor, University of South Florida, Tampa, Florida

Jana Saunders, RN, PhD
Assistant Professor, Medical College of Georgia, Athens, Georgia

Sharon Schmidt, MS, RN, CS, CRADC, PMHNP, Psy.D
Assistant Professor/Psychiatric Mental Health Nurse Practitioner, Oregon Health Science University, LaGrande, Oregon

Margaret L. Trimpey, RN, MSN
Faculty, University of Tennessee at Chattanooga, Chattanooga, Tennessee

Kathleen Tusaie, PhD, RNCS
Assistant Professor, University of Akron, Akron, Ohio

A. Kim Van Wagoner, RN, MSN, MA, PhDCand.
Chair of Nursing, Brigham Young University, Rexburg, Idaho

Barbara Jones Warren, PhD, RN, CNS, CS
Associate Professor, Ohio State University, Worthington, Ohio

Carolyn White, RN, MSN, CRNP
Clinical Assistant Professor, University of South Alabama, Mobile, Alabama

Celia E. Wills, BSN, MS, PhD, RN
Associate Professor, Michigan State University, East Lansing, Michigan

Fatma A. Youssef, DNSc., MPH, RN
Professor, Marymount University, Arlington, Virginia

We wish to acknowledge the writers who developed the content for the supplements that accompany this textbook.

Susan C. Bobek, RN, PhD
Associate Professor, College of Nursing, University of North Alabama
Florence, Alabama
Companion Website

Jane Bostick, PhD, RN
Assistant Professor of Clinical Nursing Sinclair School of Nursing, University of Missouri-Columbia
Companion Website

Lourdes A. D. de la Cruz, MHSc, MScCHN
Professor of Nursing, Sheridan College Brampton, Ontario, Canada
Student CD-ROM

Lucille C. Gambardella, PhD, RN, CS, APN-BC
Chairperson and Professor, Division of Nursing
Wesley College, Dover, Delaware
Instructor's Resource Manual and Instructor's Resource CD-ROM

Jere Hammer, RN, MSN
Department Chair, Austin Community College Austin, Texas
Companion Website

Nelda Jeane, RNC, MSN, CNS
Associate Professor of Nursing, Louisiana State University
Alexandria, Louisiana
Instructor's Resource Manual and Instructor's Resource CD-ROM

Patricia A. McCarthy, PhD, RN, CS
Chairperson and Professor, Youngstown State University
Youngstown, Ohio
Instructor's Resource Manual and Instructor's Resource CD-ROM

Sharon L. Phillips, DNSc, CNS, RN
Associate Professor, Youngstown State University
Youngstown, Ohio
Instructor's Resource Manual and Instructor's Resource CD-ROM

Eileen Trigoboff, RN, APRN/PMH-BC, DNS, DABFN
Clinical Nurse Specialist, Buffalo Psychiatric Center
Buffalo, New York
Companion Website

Kim Webb, RN, MN
Chairperson, Division of Nursing
Northern Oklahoma College, Tonkawa, Oklahoma
Instructor's Resource Manual and Instructor's Resource CD-ROM

ABOUT THE AUTHORS

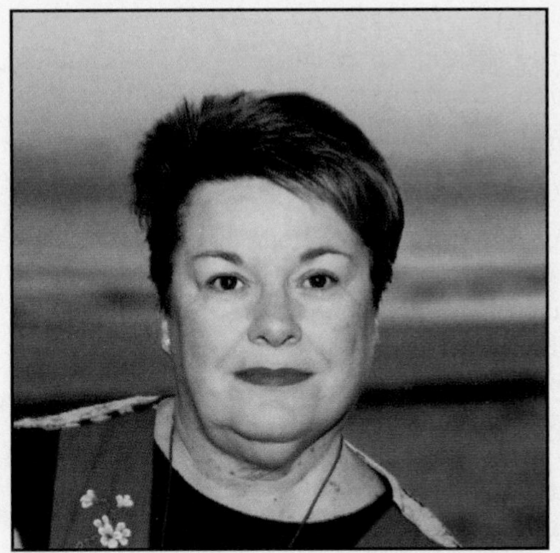

Carol Ren Kneisl, RN, MS, APRN, DABFN, has had a variety of psychiatric–mental health nursing experiences as a Clinical Nurse Specialist in Adult Psychiatry–Mental Health. She has taught psychiatric–mental health nursing in a diploma school, a baccalaureate program, and a master's program that prepared clinical specialists in psychiatric–mental health nursing. She has been a staff nurse, a nurse manager, and a nursing supervisor, and has supervised the group therapy of clinical nurse specialists and psychiatry medical residents.

Carol is also a nurse entrepreneur. She is the President of Nursing Transitions, a corporation that provides continuing education for psychiatric–mental health and corrections/forensic nurses. Her company sponsored the first national nursing conference focused on AIDS. She is a national and international speaker and consults with nurses and mental health and forensic agencies on topics such as group therapy, stress management, self-awareness issues and strategies, implementation of client rights, competency to stand trial, and negligence and malpractice in psychiatric–mental health nursing.

Carol has authored or contributed to 18 nursing textbooks and several nursing journals. She has been an associate editor of a psychiatric nursing review journal and has served on several editorial boards. She is a Diplomate in the American College of Forensic Examiners, Board of Forensic Nurse Examiners (DABFN). Carol was among the first nurses in the country to develop clinical specialist certification in conjunction with nurses from New York and New Jersey. Their work formed the basis for the national certification granted through the American Nurses Credentialing Center of the American Nurses Association.

She is a graduate of one of the oldest diploma schools in the country, the Millard Fillmore Hospital School of Nursing in Buffalo, New York, from which she received the Alumna of the Century award on the occasion of the school's 100-year anniversary. Carol has a BS in nursing from the University of Buffalo and an MS as a Clinical Nurse Specialist in psychiatric nursing from the University of California at San Francisco, and holds a certificate in community mental health administration from the State University of New York at Buffalo.

Carol is a docent of the Pensacola Museum of Art and the mother of two adult children—a daughter who is a right-brained artist and a son who is a left-brained mathematician. She writes and consults from her home on the beach in Orange Beach, Alabama.

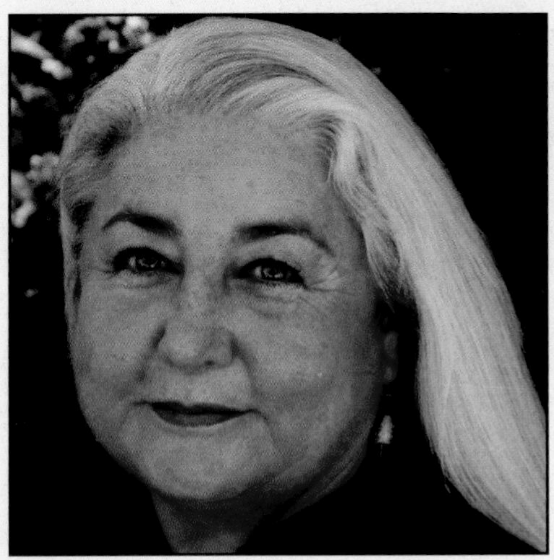

Holly Skodol Wilson, BSN, MSN, PhD, is a Professor Emerita in the Department of Community Health Systems at the University of California, San Francisco School of Nursing. Her most recent funded research focused on Quality of Life Assessment for ethnically diverse HIV-infected persons and symptom management and medication adherence among HIV/AIDS patients. She has taught psychiatric–mental health nursing assessment and qualitative research methods across all programs at UCSF since 1969. Dr. Wilson earned her BSN from Duke University, where she subsequently received the distinguished alumnae award, her MSN in psychiatric nursing at Case-Western Reserve University and her PhD in the Sociology of Psychiatry and Education at the University of California, Berkeley.

Dr. Wilson has published over 80 scientific and scholarly articles in the professional literature and is author, co-author and contributor to 18 books, foremost among them are her award-winning Psychiatric Nursing and Nursing Research texts. She has also served on the editorial boards of numerous peer-reviewed nursing journals. Dr. Wilson is a national and international speaker and consultant on topics including psychiatric assessment, qualitative clinical research and nursing education. She was among the few nurses selected as a Kellogg National Leadership Fellow and has presented papers or served as visiting Professor throughout Asia, New Zealand, Australia, Kenya, Israel, Egypt, Scandinavia, South America, Puerto Rico, and Canada, as well as the United States. She was elected a fellow in the American Academy of Nursing in 1979, and has served as a Distinguished Lecturer for Sigma Theta Tau.

Holly is the single mother of three adult daughters and enjoys her young grandchildren, who live near her home in Mill Valley, California. When not writing, consulting, teaching, and traveling, Holly is a nature enthusiast and a fan of film and the arts.

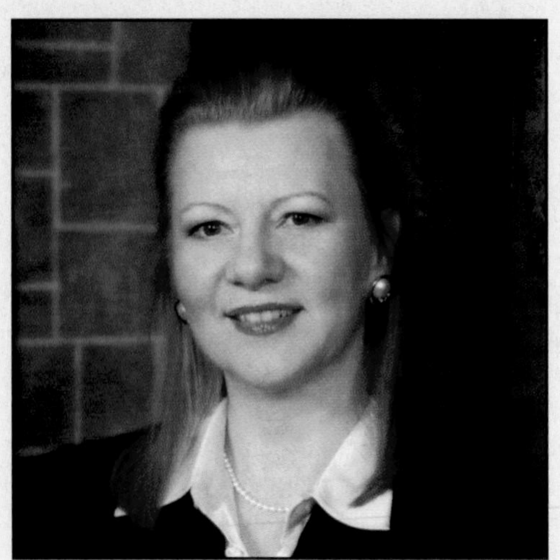

Eileen Trigoboff, RN, APRN/PMH-BC, DNS, DABFN, is a Clinical Nurse Specialist with a specialty in Adult Psychiatry–Mental Health in a private psychotherapy practice in Western New York. An important part of her practice is the national and international interdisciplinary supervision of, and consultation with, other mental health and health care professionals. She has a position as a Clinical Nurse Specialist in psychiatry at the Buffalo Psychiatric Center in Buffalo, New York. Dr. Trigoboff is the Chair of the Institutional Review Board at the facility that reviews, modifies, and supervises all scientific research in health-related issues conducted in a large part of New York State under the Office of Mental Health's auspices. She has taught associate degree, bachelor's degree, and graduate-level nursing students on all aspects of the nursing process, research methodologies, statistics, and pharmacology. Dr. Trigoboff has also been the Nurse of Distinction, an honor awarded to outstanding nurse clinicians.

Dr. Trigoboff earned her BSN, her MS as a Clinical Nurse Specialist in psychiatric nursing, and her Doctorate in Nursing Science (DNS) in psychiatric nursing from the State University of New York at Buffalo. Dr. Trigoboff received a National Institutes of Mental Health Individual National Research Service Award Pre-Doctoral Research Fellowship for her dissertation research on medication teaching and psychopharmacology. Her research interests span nursing interventions from the use of the Nurses' Observation Scale for Inpatient Evaluations (NOSIE) for assault predictions with seriously and persistently mentally ill clients to the effectiveness of a relaxation audiotape program on psychiatric inpatients. She is a member of the Sigma Theta Tau International Honor Society for Nursing and is a Diplomate in the American College of Forensic Examiners, Board of Forensic Nurse Examiners (DABFN). Dr. Trigoboff is author, co-author, and contributor to 12 books and numerous journal articles. She has presented internationally on a wide variety of clinical, research, and professional topics to health care, governmental, and corporate organizations. She continues to be an international speaker and consultant on topics including professional issues, assessment, psychopathologies, and interventions. She also serves on the editorial boards of several professional journals. She is active in community service venues, including clinical settings and family support groups. She also serves as a computer systems consultant to facilities in her local area and belongs to numerous professional nursing organizations.

Eileen enjoys her devoted clinical psychologist husband, her interesting relationship with her Congo African Grey parrot, a large and loving family, good friends, international travel, reading, and gardening.

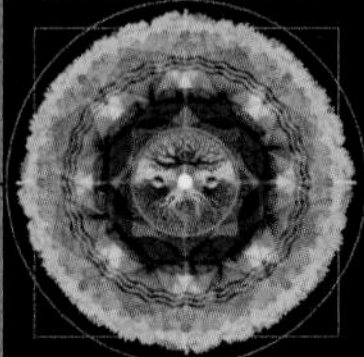

A GUIDE TO

Contemporary Psychiatric-Mental Health Nursing

Focus Questions

Focus Questions stimulate thought by identifying essential concepts and key issues addressed in the chapter.

Key Terms

Key terms are identified in bold, blue type and are defined in the audio glossary on the accompanying Student CD-ROM and the Companion Website.

MediaLink

The MediaLink at the beginning of each chapter lists additional specific content, animations, video tutorials, NCLEX review items, assessment tools, and other interactive exercises that appear on the accompanying Student CD-ROM and the Companion Website (www.prenhall.com/kneisl).

Chapter Outline

Chapter outlines pinpoint the main issues discussed throughout the chapter.

Critical Thinking Challenge

The Critical Thinking Challenge begins each chapter and includes a brief, case-based scenario that will challenge readers to analyze an issue, or an assertion related to the chapter topic. Questions that follow stimulate critical thinking. Analysis and discussion points for the Critical Thinking Challenge appear in the Instructor's Resource Manual.

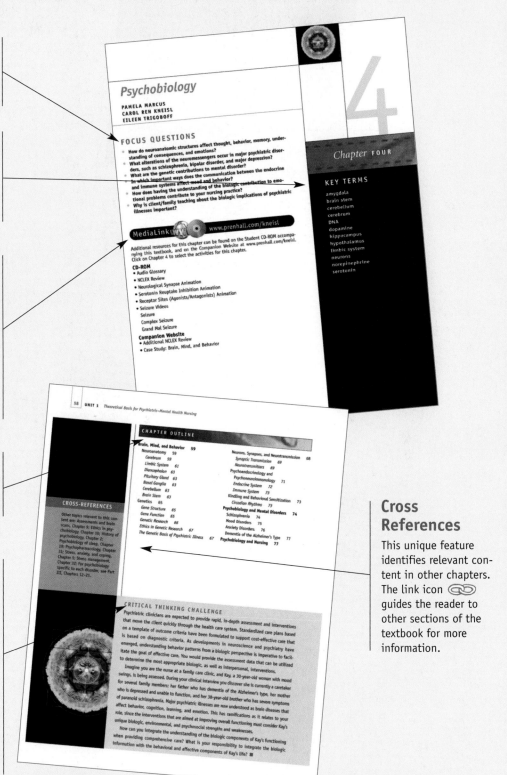

Cross References

This unique feature identifies relevant content in other chapters. The link icon guides the reader to other sections of the textbook for more information.

4

Psychobiology

PAMELA MARCUS
CAROL REN KNEISL
EILEEN TRIGOBOFF

Chapter FOUR

FOCUS QUESTIONS

- How do neuroanatomic structures affect thought, behavior, memory, understanding of consequences, and emotions?
- What alterations of the neuromessengers occur in major psychiatric disorders, such as schizophrenia, bipolar disorder, and major depression?
- What are the genetic contributions to mental disorder?
- In which important ways does the communication between the endocrine and immune systems affect mood and behavior?
- How does having the understanding of the biologic contribution to emotional problems contribute to your nursing practice?
- Why is client/family teaching about the biologic implications of psychiatric illnesses important?

KEY TERMS

amygdala
brain stem
cerebellum
cerebrum
DNA
dopamine
hippocampus
hypothalamus
limbic system
neurons
norepinephrine
serotonin

MediaLink www.prenhall.com/kneisl

Additional resources for this chapter can be found on the Student CD-ROM accompanying this textbook, and on the Companion Website at www.prenhall.com/kneisl. Click on Chapter 4 to select the activities for this chapter.

CD-ROM
- Audio Glossary
- NCLEX Review
- Neurological Synapse Animation
- Serotonin Reuptake Inhibition Animation
- Receptor Sites (Agonists/Antagonists) Animation
- Seizure Videos
  - Seizure
  - Complex Seizure
  - Grand Mal Seizure

Companion Website
- Additional NCLEX Review
- Case Study: Brain, Mind, and Behavior

CHAPTER OUTLINE

CROSS-REFERENCES

Other topics relevant to this content are: Assessments and brain scans, Chapter 9; Ethics in psychobiology, Chapter 10; History of psychobiology, Chapter 2; Psychobiology of sleep, Chapter 19; Psychopharmacology, Chapter 31; Stress, anxiety, and coping, Chapter 5; Stress management, Chapter 32; For psychobiology specific to each disorder, see Part III, Chapters 12–21.

CRITICAL THINKING CHALLENGE

Psychiatric clinicians are expected to provide rapid, in-depth assessment and interventions that move the client quickly through the health care system. Standardized care plans based on a template of outcome criteria have been formulated to support cost-effective care that is based on diagnostic criteria. As developments in neuroscience and psychiatry have emerged, understanding behavior patterns from a biologic perspective is imperative to facilitate the goal of effective care. You would provide the assessment data that can be utilized to determine the most appropriate biologic, as well as interpersonal, interventions.

Imagine you are the nurse at a family care clinic, and Kay, a 30-year-old woman with mood swings, is being assessed. During your clinical interview you discover she is currently a caretaker for several family members: her father who has dementia of the Alzheimer's type, her mother who is depressed and unable to function, and her 38-year-old brother who has severe symptoms of paranoid schizophrenia. Major psychiatric illnesses are now understood as brain diseases that affect behavior, cognition, learning, and emotion. This has ramifications as it relates to your role, since the interventions that are aimed at improving overall functioning must consider Kay's unique biologic, environmental, and psychosocial strengths and weaknesses.

How can you integrate the understanding of the biologic components of Kay's functioning when providing comprehensive care? What is your responsibility to integrate the biologic information with the behavioral and affective components of Kay's life? ■

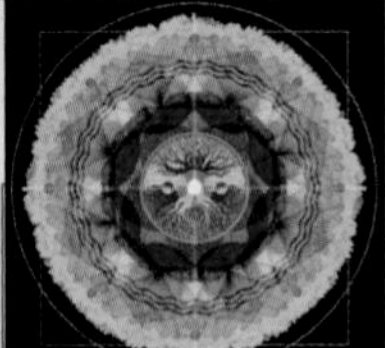

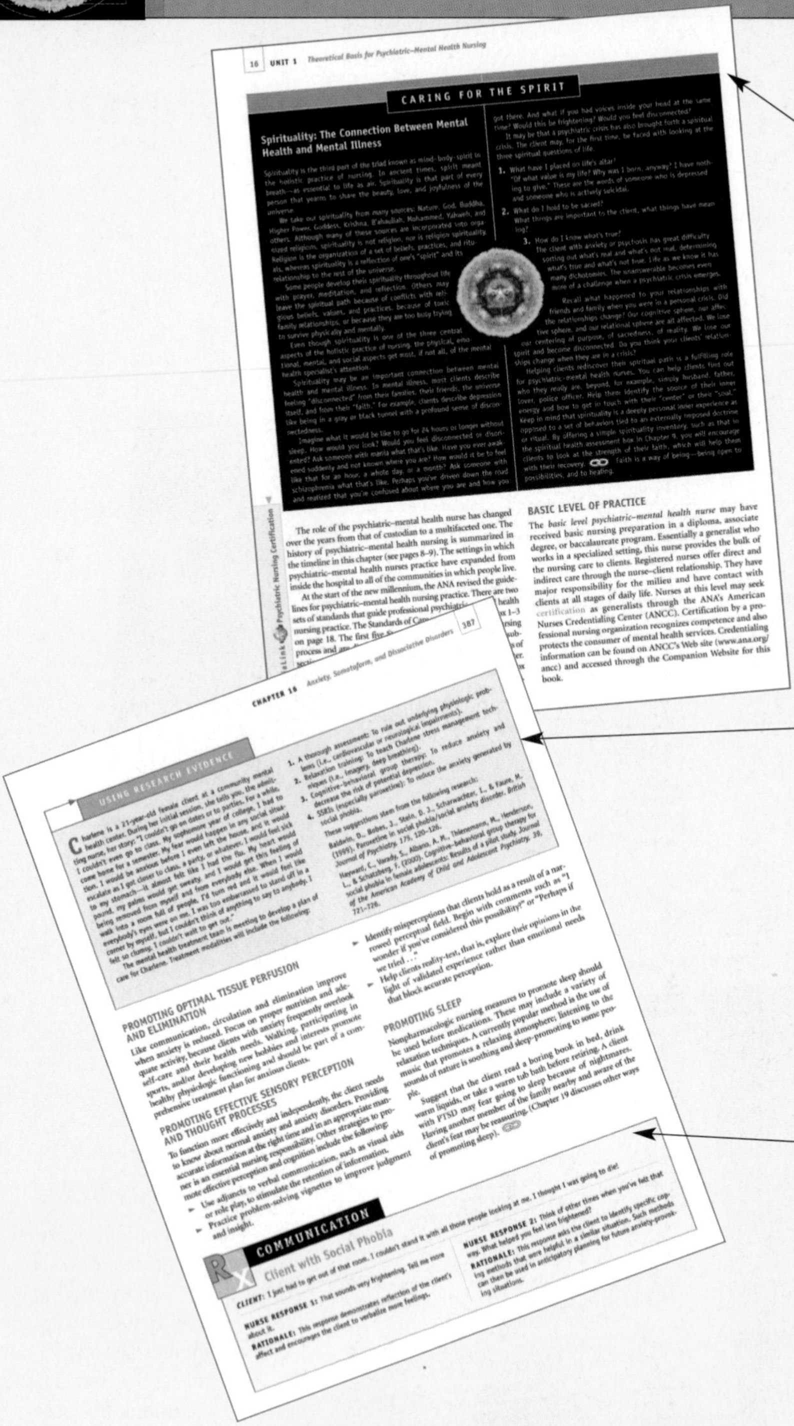

Caring for the Spirit

The belief in the inter-connection of mind, body, and spirit is reinforced in the Caring for the Spirit features. These encourage the reader to support not only the client's but also one's own spirituality.

Using Research Evidence

Evidence-based nursing practice is encouraged in this feature, which is found in every chapter. A brief clinical scenario and suggested nursing interventions are linked to one or more current research citations.

Rx Communication

This feature provides verbatim examples of possible responses to a client and the rationales for at least two different helpful alternatives to illustrate how the reader can apply therapeutic communication principles.

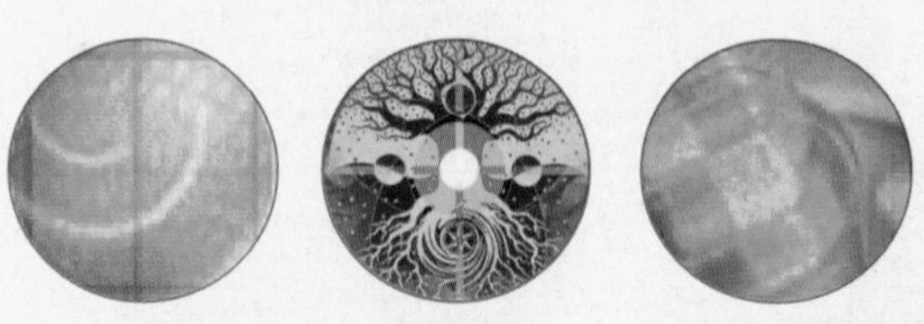

Culture, Family, and Medication Icons

Special icons call attention to content that develops cultural competence, includes the family as partners in psychiatric-mental health care, or relates to psychopharmacology.

Culture

Family

Medication

Clinical Examples

Several clinical examples are found in each chapter. They enliven the chapter by providing brief client scenarios and applying them to chapter topics.

Client/Family Teaching

This feature provides specific, client-oriented information designed to teach clients and family members strategies for managing symptoms of illness, preventing illness, or maintaining mental health.

Case Study and Care Plan

Case studies are detailed clinical scenarios linked to nursing care plans for clients with mental disorders. They are found in all of the chapters in Unit III entitled "Clients with Mental Disorders."

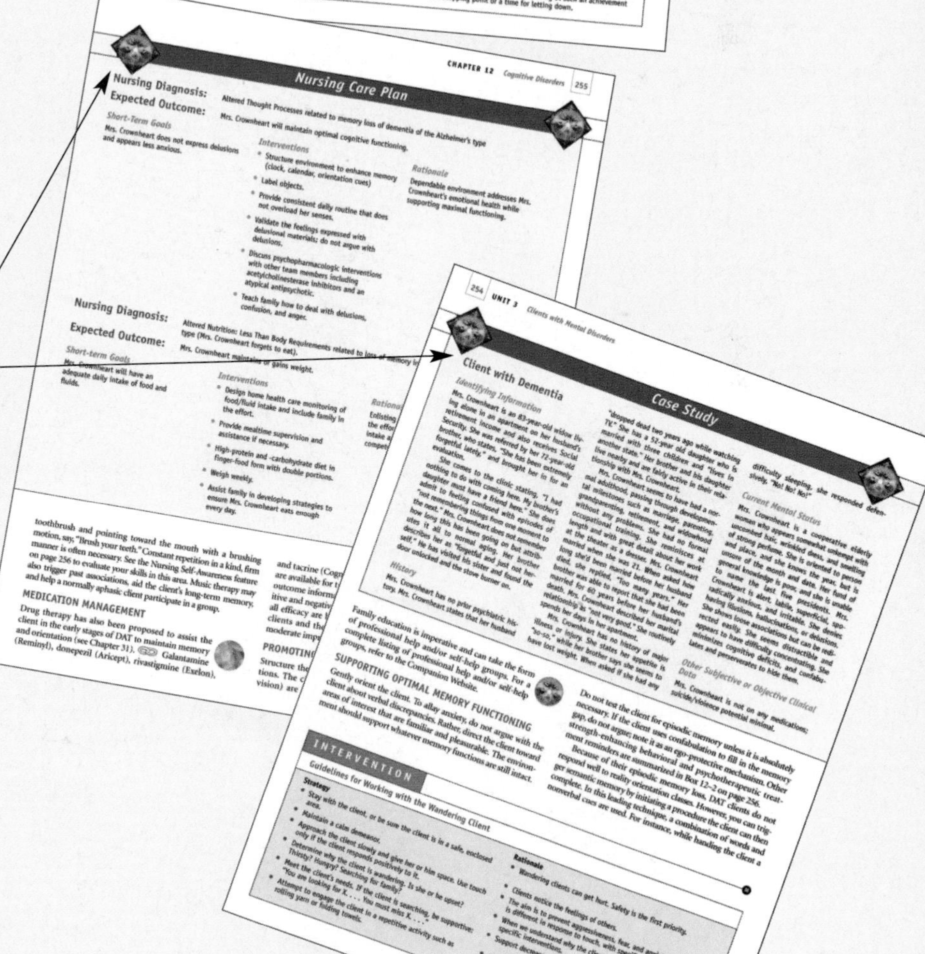

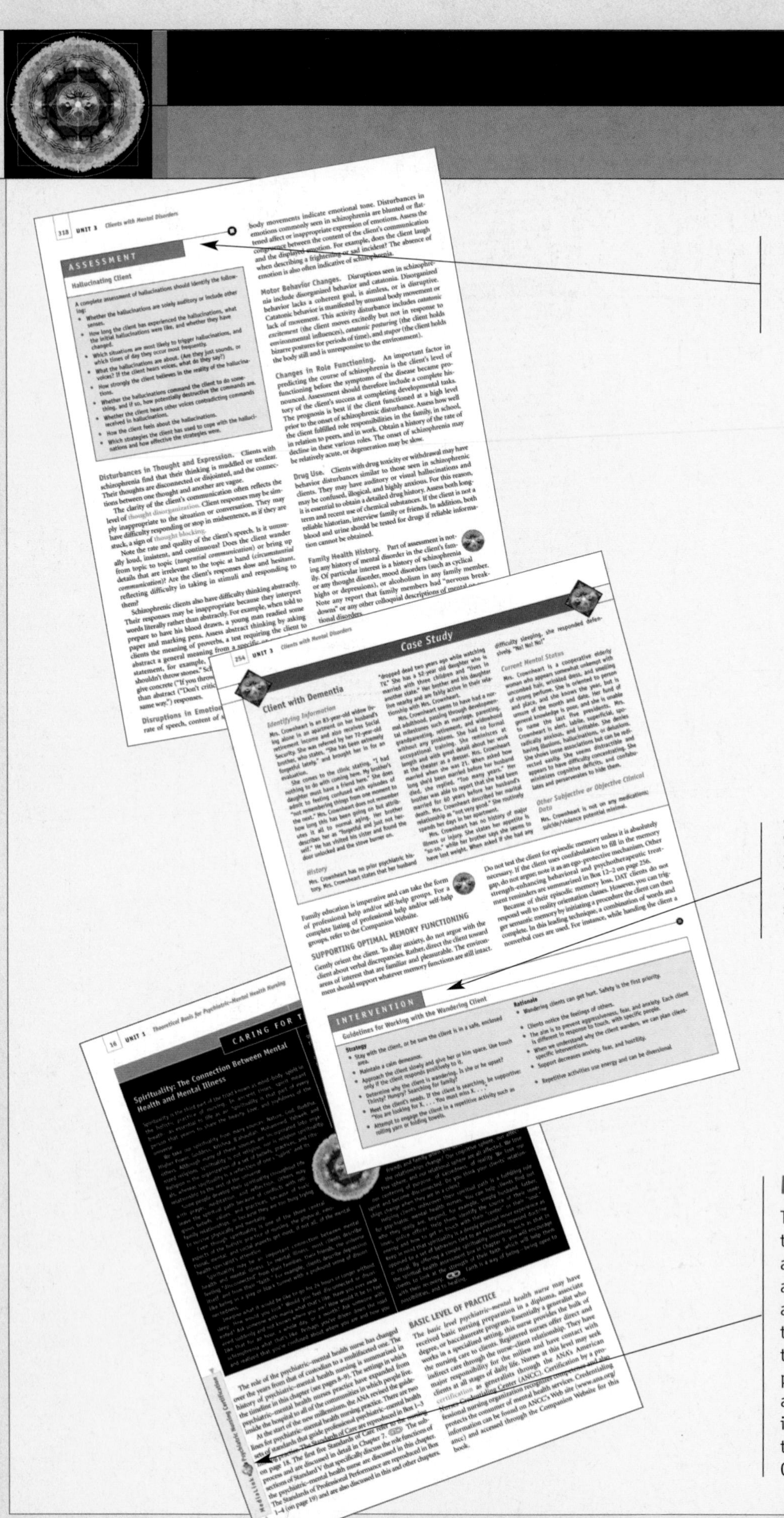

Assessment Boxes

Assessment boxes include the data specific to identifying client problems, motivations, strengths, and resources.

Intervention Boxes

Intervention boxes are designed as a bulleted list of nursing intervention strategies with accompanying rationales.

MediaLink Tabs

Throughout this text, the authors refer the reader to additional resources, animations or videos, and interactive applications on the Student CD-ROM and Companion Website accompanying this book. Readers will find MediaLink tabs in the margin of the page to prompt the student to the specific applications and resources. An icon indicates whether the activity is on the Student CD-ROM or the Companion Website.

DSM-IV-TR Classification

This book includes the most current diagnostic criteria from the APA 2000 *Diagnostic and Statistical Manual of Mental Disorders (DSM-IV-TR)* in each of the disorders chapters in Unit III.

Nursing Self-Awareness

Found in every chapter, this special feature engages the reader in a process of introspection and self-inquiry.

EXPLORE MediaLink

Found at the end of each chapter, EXPLORE MediaLink encourages readers to use the CD-ROM and the Companion Website to apply what they have learned from the text in case studies, practice NCLEX questions, and other additional resources.

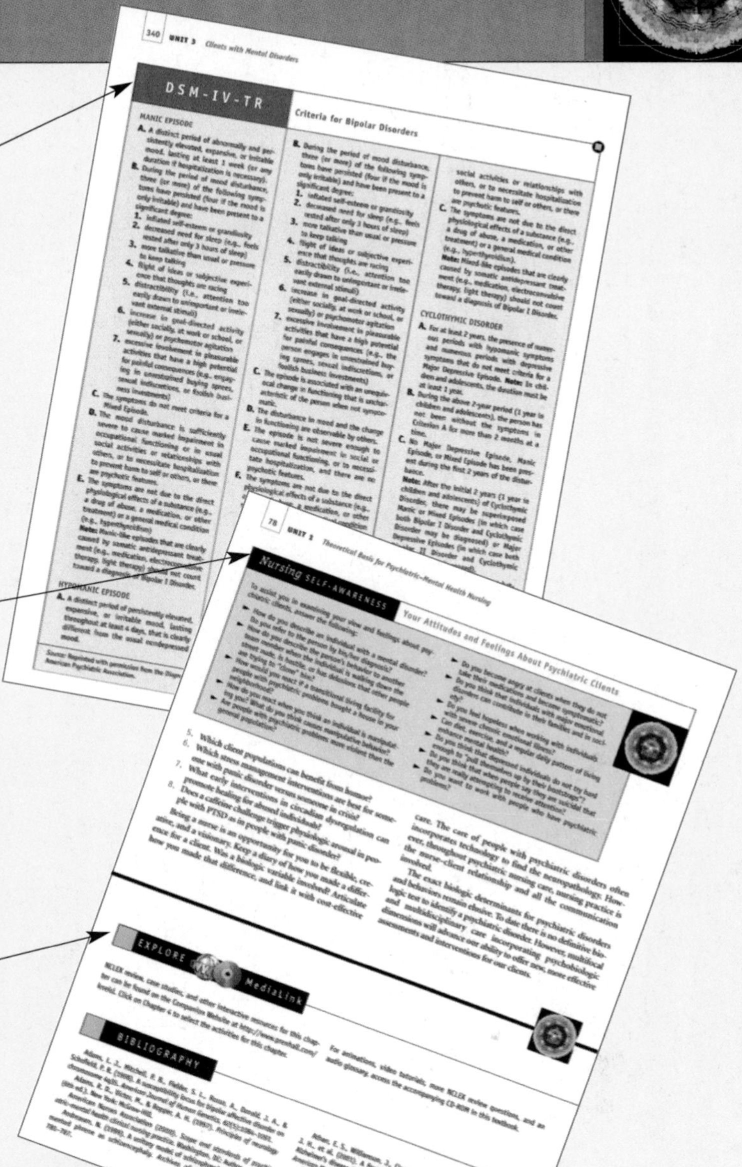

Additional Media Resources:

Animation and Video Tutorials—On the Student CD-ROM, the student will find animations and video clips illustrating difficult concepts or exhibiting examples of client behaviors.

NCLEX Reviews—Both the Student CD-ROM and the free Companion Website offer the student an abundance of NCLEX review questions for each chapter of the book. The questions provide comprehensive rationales, as well as identify how the questions correlate to the NCLEX test plan.

Care Plan Activities—Each clinical chapter on the Companion Website provides the student with a case scenario and asks the student to develop a care plan for the client. Students can e-mail these care plans to instructors as homework assignments.

Case Studies—For each chapter on the Companion Website, the student can review a client scenario and answer several critical thinking questions related to that client's care. Students can e-mail their responses to the case studies to instructors as homework assignments.

Learning from Clients—On the Companion Website, this module appears in the chapters for specific disorders. In this module, the student will watch video clips of client interviews, and will have the opportunity to respond to questions about the client's behavior and nursing care. Students can e-mail their responses to instructors as homework assignments.

SPECIAL FEATURES

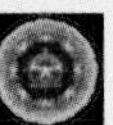 Nursing Self-Awareness

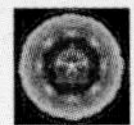 Using Research Evidence

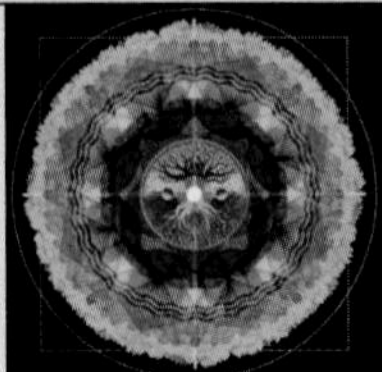

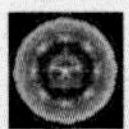 Caring for the Spirit

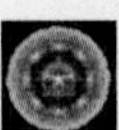 Client/Family Teaching

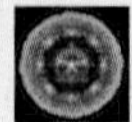 DSM-IV-TR Diagnostic Criteria

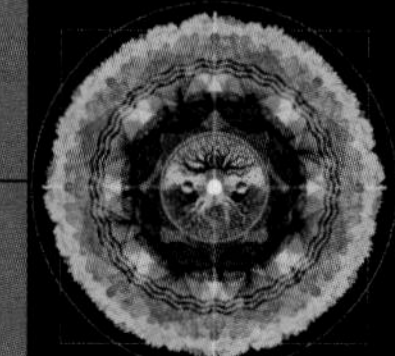

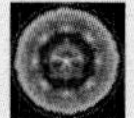

Rx Communication

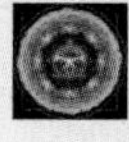

Case Study and Nursing Care Plan

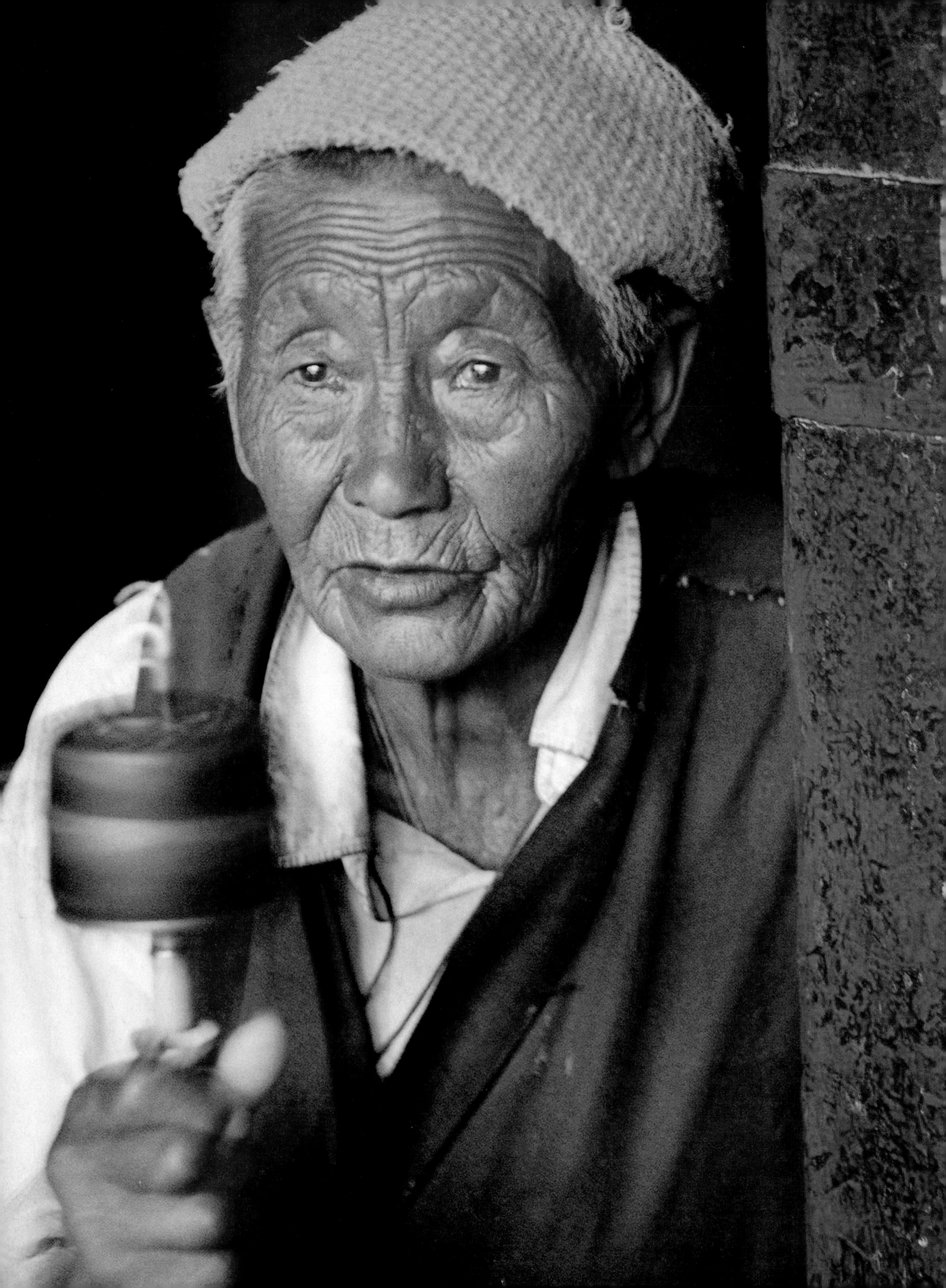

UNIT *One*

Theoretical Basis for Psychiatric–Mental Health Nursing

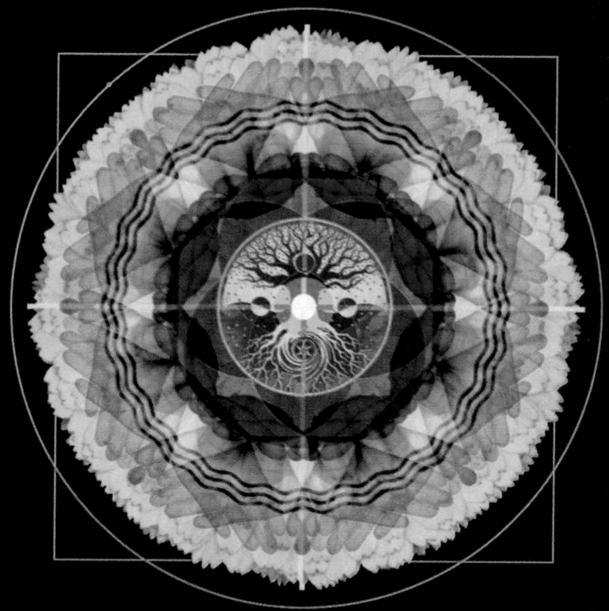

Pasang, a woman in her late 70s, lives near the top of the world in Gyantse, Tibet. Spinning a prayer wheel helps her move into a trance-like state to cope with fearfulness and to pray. She tells us that her fear began in middle age when all her brothers were killed in a local war. Chaos, crisis, and emotional distress occur in every corner of the world and remind us of our responsibility to make a difference in world mental health issues. Millions of people worldwide suffer from psychiatric disorders. Five of the leading causes of disability in the world—the global burden of disease—are mental health conditions. This unit offers a starting point for a Global Mental Health Imperative. You will learn about psychiatric–mental health nursing roles, philosophy, theory, research, and cultural competence essential to participating in a powerful international initiative to correct cultural inequities and promote quality of life for people like Pasang.

Source: Keren Su/Getty Images, Inc.—Taxi

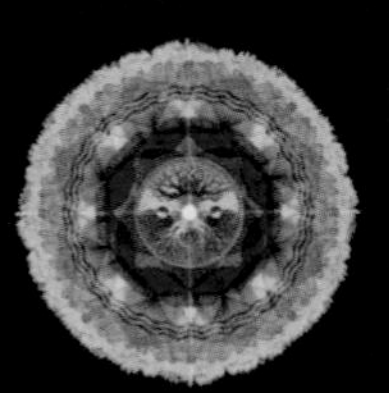

1

The Psychiatric–Mental Health Nurse's Personal Integration and Professional Role

CAROL REN KNEISL
HOLLY SKODOL WILSON

Chapter ONE

KEY TERMS

advanced practice registered nurse (APRN)
aggressive behavior
assertive behavior
burnout
certification
deviance
empathy
nonassertive behavior
psychiatric–mental health nursing
self-awareness
spirituality

FOCUS QUESTIONS

- How does the concept of personal integration relate to the self and to psychiatric nursing practice?
- What are the qualities that enable psychiatric–mental health nurses to practice the use of self artfully in therapeutic relationships?
- Why do psychiatric–mental health nurses use empathy in their clinical practice?
- In what specific ways do the American Nurses Association (ANA) Scope and Standards of Psychiatric–Mental Health Nursing Practice guide the delivery of contemporary psychiatric–mental health nursing?
- What are the differences and similarities among the roles of the psychiatric–mental health nurse and other members of the mental health team?
- Which factors influence the success with which the mental health team achieves collaboration among itself and with clients and their significant others?

MediaLink www.prenhall.com/kneisl

Additional resources for this chapter can be found on the Student CD-ROM accompanying this textbook, and on the Companion Website at *www.prenhall.com/kneisl*. Click on Chapter 1 to select the activities for this chapter.

CD-ROM
- Audio Glossary
- NCLEX Review

Companion Website
- Additional NCLEX Review
- Case Study: Your Professional Role

CHAPTER OUTLINE

CROSS REFERENCES

Other topics relevant to this content are: Anxiety and coping, Chapter 5; Client rights, Chapter 10; Code of ethics for nurses, Chapter 10; Nurses' role in milieu therapy, Chapter 11; Nurses' role in one-to-one relationships, Chapter 28; Nurses' role in groups and families, Chapter 29; Relaxation and stress management techniques, Chapter 32.

CRITICAL THINKING CHALLENGE

You find your psychiatric–mental health nursing clinical experience professionally challenging, intellectually stimulating, and personally rewarding. You are considering becoming a psychiatric nurse upon graduation and have discussed your feelings with a classmate; with your neighbor, a critical care nurse; and with your primary care physician.

Your classmate says you won't be a real nurse and that you'll forget all the skills you learned in school. Your neighbor, a critical care nurse, thinks you'll be bored as a psychiatric–mental health nurse. The high drama, split-second decisions, and high-tech atmosphere of the critical care unit is, she says, the setting where a good student like you would be the happiest and could make the greatest contribution. Your primary care physician suggests that you should be cautious. With the explosion in psychobiologic research and the discovery of more effective psychopharmacologic agents, she thinks it will be likely that in a few years there will be no need for psychiatric–mental health nurses and you'll be out of a job.

What do you think? ■

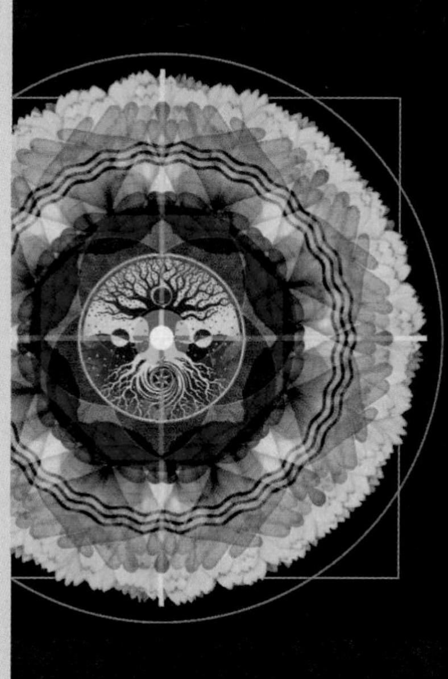

The value of self-knowledge is a recurring theme in both the popular and the professional literature. Libraries are stocked with volumes dealing with the undiscovered self, the expansion of human awareness, spirituality and the care of the soul, strategies for self-realization, and the like. A common thread in all these is the idea that the quality and nature of a person's relationship with others are strongly influenced by the person's self-view. Consider the following comments made by students in their psychiatric nursing clinical experience:

CLINICAL EXAMPLE

I just can't take it. . . . I feel myself getting confused about who is the crazy one. There's such a fine line. Sometimes I think I'll be a patient here.

I hated psych—it just didn't seem like nursing to me. I really like to keep busy. When you change someone's dressing, you really feel like you've helped them. Here it's all so uncertain.

All I kept thinking about was that a lot of the patients had done really weird things. This one guy had lived in an apartment with his dead mother's body for three months before they brought him in. Another had tried to shoot the governor. I never felt safe even turning my back on them.

This chapter explores some dimensions of self-knowledge through an examination of the concepts of personal integration and professional role. First, we will examine recurring problems that pertain to the nurse's identity and some strategies for coping with them. Second, we will discuss the clinical roles, the clinical scope, and the clinical standards of contemporary psychiatric–mental health nursing practice at both the basic and advanced levels. Reading the History of Psychiatric Nursing timeline in this chapter (■ Figure 1–1) (pages 8 and 9) will help you to appreciate the history of psychiatric nursing and the traditions from which it continues to develop. Our goal is to enhance the nurse's interactions with psychiatric clients.

Personal Integration

Many students and practitioners faced with relating to people whose behavior they view as offensive, frightening, curious, or socially inappropriate find that their personal attitudes, expectations, myths, and values make it difficult for them to fulfill their professional roles. This was the case in the following example:

CLINICAL EXAMPLE

Penny, a baccalaureate nursing student, had selected a clinical placement at a substance abuse clinic in the community. Despite her initial interest, she developed a pattern of absences from the clinic. When her faculty adviser discussed this observation with her, Penny blurted out that, much to her surprise, she was unable to assist with the group meetings for pregnant heroin addicts. The thought of addicting babies before their births—babies who would ultimately suffer because of their mothers' self-indulgence—horrified Penny. She found herself judging their choices constantly and avoiding interaction with them. "I feel like they should be shot instead of given all this free support and sympathy."

For many nurses, confrontation with **deviance** (behavior outside the social norm of a specific group; should not be construed to mean negative behavior) reinforces a personal sense of stability. Others are threatened by such confrontation.

CLINICAL EXAMPLE

One psychiatric nurse, in recalling her childhood experiences with community deviants, commented on the intense and sometimes morbid excitement that she and her friends found in taunting "Crazy Helen" to run out on her porch and shout incoherently at the neighborhood children or in telling bizarre stories about a grotesque old man called "Nutty Nick," who walked along a road late at night laughing and talking to himself.

The interest these characters held for the children, along with "Vince-the-Window-Peeper" and "Red-the-Bum," was reawakened in her as she approached her first psychiatric nursing experience. It was all very frightening, yet seductive and stimulating at the same time. The nursing students gossiped about the bizarre histories of their assigned clients as if to reaffirm their separateness from them—their sense of being normal and okay.

Dealing with people whose personal integration is fragmented, dissolving, divided, or alienated puts the nurse's own identity on the line as well. To respond with both compassion and the critical distance necessary to be effective, psychiatric professionals must confront their own identity; separate it from another's identity, which may indeed be dissolving; and finally integrate different values and behaviors comfortably in the therapeutic relationships they develop with clients.

This personal quality is called *detached concern*—the ability to distance oneself in order to help others. It is an essential quality not only in avoiding *burnout*, a problem discussed later in this chapter, but also in using appropriate *assertiveness* when collaborating with colleagues, and in maintaining *empathic abilities* in highly stressful situations.

In the conventional focus on the client, the nurse is regarded as the caregiver, the provider of services, the counselor or therapist. Little attention is paid to the stresses psychiatric nurses experience in attempting to relate fully to clients while maintaining their own personal integration.

CREATING A COMMON GROUND

Nurses often find that encounters with psychiatric clients are distancing experiences. The nurses become acutely aware of their difference and separateness from clients. They reaffirm their own subjective view of reality and rationalize their actions to keep these actions consistent with their sense of self as healthy, normal people.

Because people are constantly building and protecting their own self-images, they try to get others to see their image of themselves. However, it is impossible to see another's self-image or world view exactly as that person experiences it. Despite this fact, psychiatry has traditionally attempted to get certain people, labeled *crazy*, to assume the perspective of certain other people, called *therapists.*

A more acceptable alternative seems to lie in the creation of some common ground, a mutually understood, negotiated reality. Even to this common ground the nurse and the client bring their own conceptions, feelings, and attitudes toward and images of each other and themselves. In many instances, the nurse's image of the client—how the nurse expects the client to act or feel—is not the same as the client's self-image. This is confusing to both client and nurse and hinders the establishment of therapeutic relationships and effective communication.

FEELINGS: THE AFFECTIVE SELF

The ultimate effectiveness of efforts to relate to and communicate with others depends on how well people know themselves and develop the ability to be sensitive to and care about others. Self-awareness and caring seem to go hand in hand. At the root of social interaction is people's ability to understand and care about each other's attitudes and feelings. Because each human being is unique, this ability called *empathizing* is a difficult and challenging task. (Empathy is discussed in greater detail later in this chapter.) One way to develop this ability is to practice it. Learning to be aware of one's responses to expression of feelings from another person is a starting point.

CLINICAL EXAMPLE

Josh is a middle-aged man who sought out nursing as a career. Although he is highly proficient in technical skills and charming and engaging in relationships with most clients, he discovers a surprising intolerance for some of the tears, complaints, and self-preoccupation of depressed clients. He finds himself responding with admonitions to stop it, to bite the bullet, to grow up. He personally has seldom allowed himself to experience his own sadnesses but jokingly characterizes himself as a firm believer in repression and denial. The need to empathize with people unable to control their feelings evoked such discomfort that he found himself unable to work with such clients.

Self-Awareness of Feelings

Feelings are like icebergs: Only the tips stick up into consciousness, and the deeper parts are submerged (■ Figure 1–2 on page 10). One such feeling is fear. The conscious part may be experienced as dislike, avoidance, or reluctance. At a deeper level, the feeling is reported as anxiety. Even deeper, the person may acknowledge, "I feel scared." Deeper yet, the person may experience genuine panic. Such an iceberg may well explain Josh's attitude toward tearful, depressed clients. His annoyance, irritation, sarcasm, and disdain may represent the tip of the iceberg of Josh's fear of depression.

The iceberg comparison also applies to other feelings, such as love, hurt, and guilt. A person feeling love may be aware only of a liking or attraction for another. Beneath the tip of that iceberg are feelings of warmth and affection. Deeper are feelings of love, and at the deepest level may be feelings of fusion or ecstasy.

Problems with Submerged Feelings

One characteristic of icebergs of feeling is that at the tip the feelings lose their experiential quality and become translated into impulses to act. For example, a person with submerged guilt may express it by frequent worrying and explaining and may be completely unaware of the underlying feelings. The behavior is the only outward manifestation.

People lose touch with their feelings over time as they shape their sense of self. They hear such messages as "boys don't cry" or "girls are too sensitive" and incorporate these injunctions into their emerging self-system, especially into the "me" or "self for others." Not being sufficiently aware of one's feelings has several disadvantages:

- What people don't know *can* hurt them. Repressed feelings may reappear in behaviors that are difficult to alter. For example, hidden anger may emerge in migraine headaches or the use of sarcasm. (See also the Caring for the Spirit feature in Chapter 5.)
- People who are not aware of their feelings find it difficult to make decisions. It is hard to tell a "should" from a wish. Without some awareness of their real wants, they may have trouble saying no or requesting something they need. They are more likely to rely on others—experts, authorities, rules and regulations, and so forth—for guidance.
- People who, like Josh, are "out of touch with" or unaware of their feelings may find it difficult to be really close to and empathic toward others. Intimacy and empathy demand the expression of here-and-now feelings, whether positive or negative.

Most people realize the value of thinking clearly. They understand that it is a learned ability and takes practice. Feeling clearly (authentically) can also be practiced and learned.

Dominant Emotional Themes

Nurses need to explore the dominant emotional themes in their personalities. If they find that they respond to many situations with the same feelings, they are probably narrowing their range of potential feelings.

MediaLink Case Study: Your Professional Role

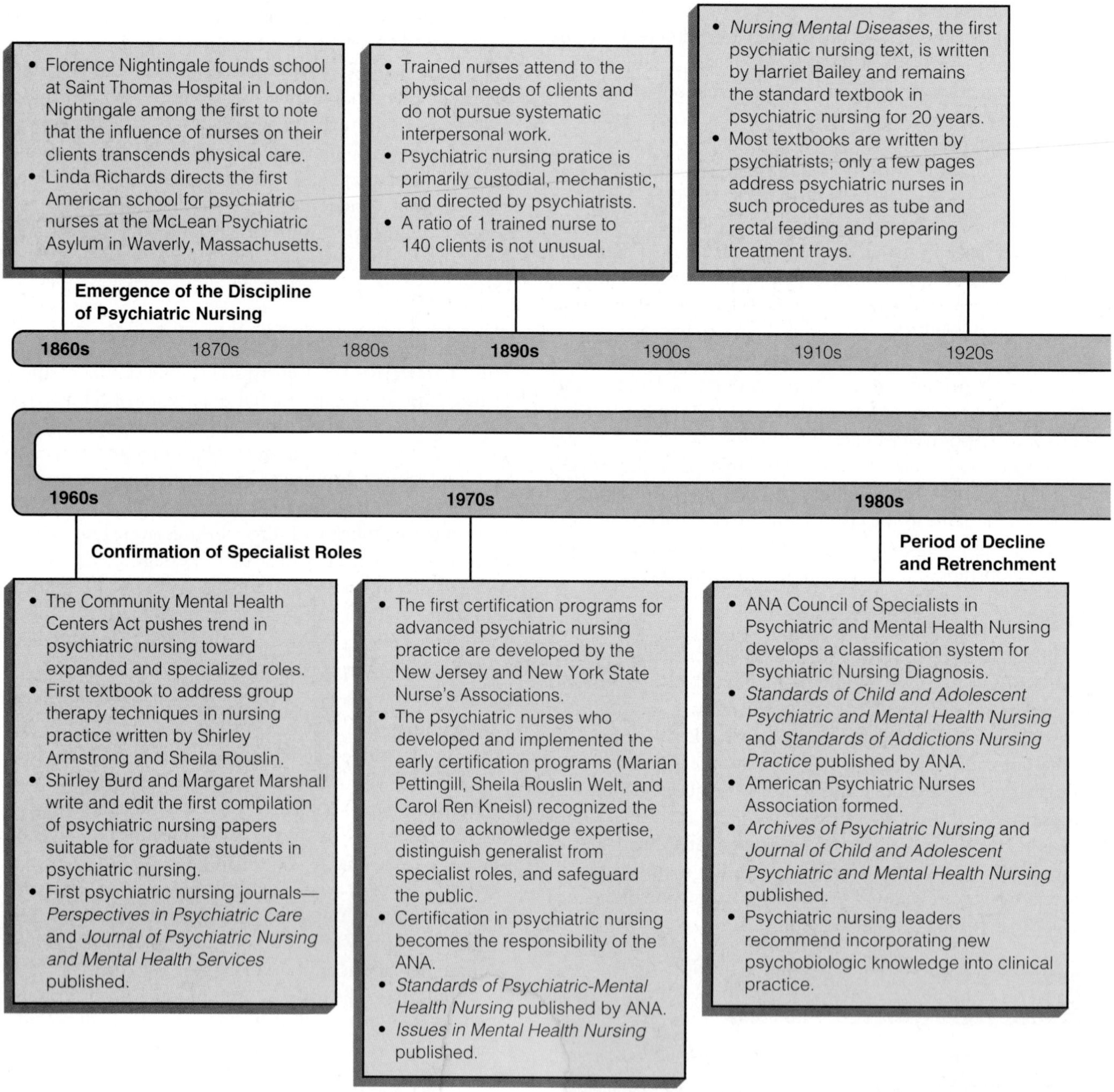

1860s — Emergence of the Discipline of Psychiatric Nursing

- Florence Nightingale founds school at Saint Thomas Hospital in London. Nightingale among the first to note that the influence of nurses on their clients transcends physical care.
- Linda Richards directs the first American school for psychiatric nurses at the McLean Psychiatric Asylum in Waverly, Massachusetts.

1870s

1880s

1890s

- Trained nurses attend to the physical needs of clients and do not pursue systematic interpersonal work.
- Psychiatric nursing pratice is primarily custodial, mechanistic, and directed by psychiatrists.
- A ratio of 1 trained nurse to 140 clients is not unusual.

1900s

1910s

1920s

- *Nursing Mental Diseases*, the first psychiatric nursing text, is written by Harriet Bailey and remains the standard textbook in psychiatric nursing for 20 years.
- Most textbooks are written by psychiatrists; only a few pages address psychiatric nurses in such procedures as tube and rectal feeding and preparing treatment trays.

1960s — Confirmation of Specialist Roles

- The Community Mental Health Centers Act pushes trend in psychiatric nursing toward expanded and specialized roles.
- First textbook to address group therapy techniques in nursing practice written by Shirley Armstrong and Sheila Rouslin.
- Shirley Burd and Margaret Marshall write and edit the first compilation of psychiatric nursing papers suitable for graduate students in psychiatric nursing.
- First psychiatric nursing journals—*Perspectives in Psychiatric Care* and *Journal of Psychiatric Nursing and Mental Health Services* published.

1970s

- The first certification programs for advanced psychiatric nursing practice are developed by the New Jersey and New York State Nurse's Associations.
- The psychiatric nurses who developed and implemented the early certification programs (Marian Pettingill, Sheila Rouslin Welt, and Carol Ren Kneisl) recognized the need to acknowledge expertise, distinguish generalist from specialist roles, and safeguard the public.
- Certification in psychiatric nursing becomes the responsibility of the ANA.
- *Standards of Psychiatric-Mental Health Nursing* published by ANA.
- *Issues in Mental Health Nursing* published.

1980s — Period of Decline and Retrenchment

- ANA Council of Specialists in Psychiatric and Mental Health Nursing develops a classification system for Psychiatric Nursing Diagnosis.
- *Standards of Child and Adolescent Psychiatric and Mental Health Nursing* and *Standards of Addictions Nursing Practice* published by ANA.
- American Psychiatric Nurses Association formed.
- *Archives of Psychiatric Nursing* and *Journal of Child and Adolescent Psychiatric and Mental Health Nursing* published.
- Psychiatric nursing leaders recommend incorporating new psychobiologic knowledge into clinical practice.

FIGURE 1–1 ■ *The History of Psychiatric Nursing*

CLINICAL EXAMPLE

Whatever the occasion, Marge used it to be tired or bored. Fatigue and chronically depressed states were routine for her. Holidays, vacations, dinner engagements all evoked the same predictable response.

Joan was afraid of everything. When she met her brother at the plane, her first question was, "Aren't you afraid of flying?" She was afraid driving home from the airport. The prospect of starting back to school scared her.

1930s — Movement of Psychiatric Nursing into the Mainstream of Nursing

- National League for Nursing Education recommends that psychiatric nursing content and clinical experience be part of the curriculum in all basic nursing programs.
- Psychiatric nursing activities continue to be custodial nursing care, including housekeeping tasks and keeping the keys to locked wards, cabinets, and even toilet tissue containers.

1940s

- New medical surgical procedures (deep sleep therapy, insulin shock therapy, psychosurgery, and electroshock therapy) promote the role of psychiatric nurses as participants in psychiatric treatment.
- Nursing leaders recommend elimination of single-focus schools marking the beginning of the mainstreaming of psychiatric nursing.
- National Institute of Mental Health (NIMH) established; National Mental Health Act helps develop psychotherapeutic roles for nurses.

1950s — Confirmation of Psychiatric Nursing as a Specialty

- Hildegard Peplau emphasizes psychodynamic concepts and counseling techniques; Gwen Tudor Will demonstrates nursing interventions with a sociopsychiatric base.
- Frances Sleeper advocates psychiatric nurses as psychotherapists.
- First doctoral program in nursing is based on June Mellow's system of psychiatric nursing therapy.
- National League for Nursing introduces the concept of psychiatric nurse specialist; first NIMH grants to integrate mental health concepts into nursing curriculum.

1990s — Decade of the Brain

- Several psychiatric nurses appointed to President Clinton's task force on health care reform.
- *Standards of Psychiatric Consultation Liaison Nursing* published by ANA.
- Revised *Standards of Psychiatric- Mental Health Clinical Nursing Practice* published by ANA.
- *Psychopharmacology Guidelines for Psychiatric-Mental Health Nurses,* intended to increase knowledge of psychopharmacology and improve patient care, published by ANA.
- *Journal of the American Psychiatric Nurses Association* published.
- Psychiatric nursing leaders urge nurses to use the challenging circumstances posed by burgeoning information, reduced funding, and health care reform to clarify nursing's unique contribution to mental health care.

2000s — Beginning of a New Millennium

- American Nurses Association, in collaboration with the American Psychiatric Nurses Association and the International Society of Psychiatric- Mental Health Nurses publishes the revised *Scope and Standards of Psychiatric-Mental Health Nursing Practice.*
- An increase in the numbers and types of alternative and nontraditional treatment settings provide new opportunities for psychiatric-mental health nurses to provide mental health care in primary care environments as well as in psychiatric settings.
- As knowledge continues to explode in psychobiology, genetics, and human behavior, psychiatric nursing leaders focus on the need to integrate the biological, psychological, social, spiritual, and environmental realms of the human experience into mental health services while remaining centered in the nursing domain with it's focus on caring.

People who feel the same way in a variety of situations may be missing a lot of what is happening in those situations. They perceive only what will fit a narrowed range of feelings. Becoming aware of limited emotional themes is a way to begin to widen the range of feelings.

Acceptance of Disapproved Feelings

Most people have been taught to block off an awareness and expression of certain feelings. Children are taught that being rude or ungrateful or cranky is rarely acceptable. To retain love

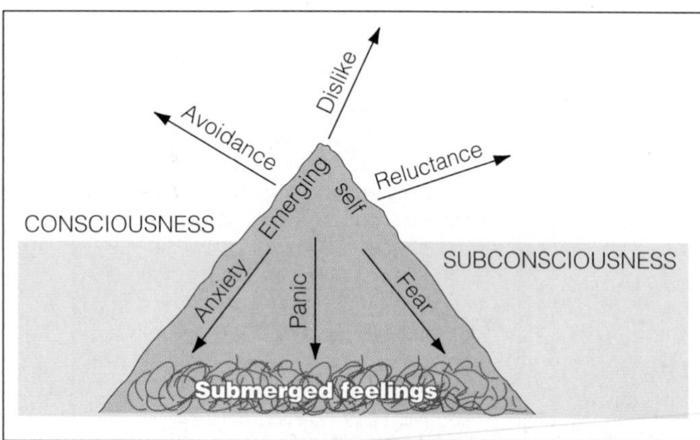

FIGURE 1–2 ■ *Self-awareness of feelings. Superficial feelings are visible; deeper feelings are submerged.*

and approval, they usually comply, not by stopping the feelings but by acting as if they didn't have them. Nursing students often get similar messages from teachers. It is not acceptable to find a client repulsive, to dislike someone who is sick and dependent, or to express anger at or criticism of the teacher. Positive feelings of attraction and love may also seem unacceptable. Failure to recognize these feelings can interfere with interactions.

Recognizing and accepting their own feelings make nurses less vulnerable to other people's ideas about how they should feel. Nurses often feel guilty when they don't feel what others imply they should feel. Nurses who can allow themselves the right to their own feelings can also allow clients the right to have and express theirs.

BELIEFS AND VALUES

Beliefs and values take three major forms:

1. Rational beliefs are beliefs that are supported by available evidence.
2. Blind belief is belief in the absence of evidence.
3. Irrational belief is belief held despite available evidence to the contrary.

Dogmatic belief (opinions or beliefs held as if they were based on the highest authority) includes both blind and irrational belief. Dogmatically held beliefs are not based on personal experience. Operating on the basis of dogmatically held beliefs often causes nurses to distort their personal experiences of the world to fit their preconceptions. The following are examples of some strongly held beliefs about behaviors that are labeled "mental illness":

- Most clients in mental hospitals are dangerous.
- People who seek counseling are mentally disordered.
- If parents loved their children more, there would be fewer mental disorders.
- When a person has a worry, it is best not to think about it.
- Many people become mentally disordered just to avoid the problems of life.
- People would not become mentally disordered if they avoided bad thoughts.
- Anyone who is in a hospital for a mental disorder should not be allowed to vote.
- To become a psychiatric client is to become a failure in life.
- One of the main causes of mental disorders is a lack of moral strength.

Most research on strongly held beliefs indicates that people usually know more about the things they believe than about those they don't believe. By staying ignorant about anything they don't already agree with, they can avoid changing. This posture cuts off personal growth and learning that could be derived from the unknown. Obviously, clients are better served by nurses who are aware of their own dogmatically held beliefs and then challenge those beliefs.

Attitudes and Opinions

A feeling is a transitory experience. A feeling held over a period of time is called an attitude. An attitude linked to an idea or belief becomes an opinion. An opinion, then, involves both thinking and feeling. Research in this area has shown that people are more comfortable when their beliefs are consistent with their attitudes. People do several things to keep their attitudes and beliefs consistent:

- They repress any belief or attitude that seems inconsistent.
- They distract their awareness from conflict either physically (such as by leaving the room) or psychologically (such as by daydreaming).
- They distort their perceptions to fit an existing attitude or belief.

Similar maneuvers take place to keep actions consistent with attitudes or beliefs.

Arriving at Values

Every day, each person meets life situations that call for thought, opinion forming, decision making, and action. At every turn in their personal and professional lives, nurses are faced with choices. Their choices are based on the values they hold, but often those values are not really clear. People actively value something to the degree that they are willing to put energy into doing something about it. Their values are shown in their interests, preferences, decisions, and actions.

CLINICAL EXAMPLE

In talking with colleagues, Susan, a psychiatric–mental health nurse, claims to value interacting with clients more than doing paperwork. Yet a quick assessment of how she spends her time—all excuses taken into account—reveals that she acts on other values.

Mel, a nurse working in a state hospital unit for profoundly developmentally disabled children, claims that he believes these clients are human beings, despite their uncommunicative, immobile forms.

USING RESEARCH EVIDENCE

Your nursing instructor at the homeless shelter mental health clinic to which you and three other classmates have been assigned has planned a clinical conference for the next morning. She has asked you and your classmates to bring with you the nursing care plans that the four of you submitted to her. In the nursing care plans that you and your classmates have written she has circled terms—dangerous, manipulative, defiant, noncompliant, incompetent, incorrigible junkie—that were used to describe residents of the homeless shelter. She has asked you to read two articles before tomorrow, to review your nursing care plans, and to consider the following: Does the use of these terms indicate an underlying negative attitude toward persons with mental disorder or substance dependence; which of these terms are judgmental; which of these terms are demeaning; what do these terms say about the values you and your classmates hold? She has also asked you to reevaluate your homeless shelter clients and to use terms that are neither pejorative nor labeling. The research evidence on which she has based her directions to you can be found in the following articles:

Clauden, G., & Long, A. (2000). Communication is the essence of nursing care. *British Journal of Nursing, 9*(15), 979–984.

Pescosolido, B. A., Monahan, J., Link, B. G., Stueve, A., & Kikuzawa, S. (1999). The public's view of the competence, dangerousness, and need for legal coercion of persons with mental health problems. *American Journal of Public Health, 89*, 1339–1346.

He demonstrates this value in the hours he spends trying to communicate his presence and concern for them, using acupressure and touch performed slowly and with genuine feeling.

The distinction in the above examples is between *cognitive* and *active values.* Susan verbally subscribes to values but fails to act on them. These are cognitive values. Mel's actions demonstrate that he gives more than lip service to the idea of the dignity of all living beings. He follows active values.

Taking Care of the Self

Knowing who they are is just a beginning for nurses. Taking care of others requires that nurses respect and care for themselves. Assertiveness, the need for solitude, maintaining physical health, attending to cues of personal stress and avoiding burnout, are actions crucial to preserving the nurse's personal integration.

ASSERTIVENESS

Have you ever had difficulty expressing yourself in a staff meeting? Did you find yourself feeling hopeless, resentful, angry? Were you wishing you had the courage to speak up? Hoping someone else would?

Are you intimidated by the high-pressure tactics of supervisors, physicians, teachers? Do you remain silent but seething? Do you speak up but sound defensive? Do you say yes when you mean no?

Have you ever needed to give someone counseling? Did you avoid the problem, hoping things would change? Did you find yourself beating around the bush? Or did you find yourself being overly harsh when you finally gave the correction?

These questions are from a manual written specifically to help nurses cope with on-the-job stressors by using assertiveness techniques to express themselves more effectively (Muff, 1984, pp. 239–240). Often people are either so timid that they do not get what they want or so aggressive and belligerent that they offend and alienate others. **Assertive behavior** is asking for what one wants or acting to get it in a way that respects other people. It is midway between **nonassertive behavior** (timid holding back) and **aggressive behavior** (inconsiderate, offensive aggression).

Compare the nonassertive, aggressive, and assertive behaviors listed in ■ Table 1–1 to see which descriptions best characterize your behavior with others. Fortunately, old behaviors can be unlearned, and new behaviors can be learned.

TABLE 1–1 Comparison of Nonassertive, Aggressive, and Assertive Behaviors

Nonassertive	Aggressive	Assertive
"I'm not angry (but I am scared)!"	"I'm not scared (but I am angry)!"	"I'm both angry and scared!"
"I always do everything wrong."	"They always do everything wrong."	"Neither one of us are perfect, and there's nothing wrong with that."
"I'll try to make it (but I don't intend to because I'm resentful of your demands)."	"You must be crazy if you think I'll be there. Who do you think you are?"	"We should spend some time together and talk about our relationship."
"I never achieve my goals."	"The only way I can achieve my goals is by forcing others to agree with my way of thinking."	"I almost always achieve the goals I set for myself."

Nursing SELF-AWARENESS

Recognizing Your Rights

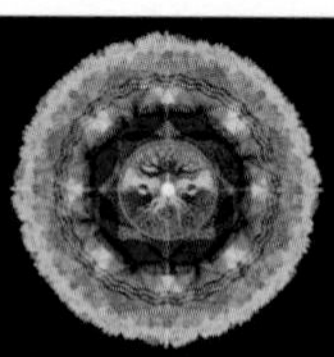

Thoughtfully consider the list below. While it was originally designed to help women health care professionals recognize their rights (Chenevert 1994), it is applicable to health care professionals of both sexes:

- You have the right to be treated with respect.
- You have the right to a reasonable workload.
- You have the right to an equitable wage.
- You have the right to determine your own priorities.
- You have the right to ask for what you want.
- You have the right to refuse without making excuses or feeling guilty.
- You have the right to make mistakes and be responsible for them.
- You have the right to give and receive information as a professional.
- You have the right to act in the best interest of the client.
- You have the right to be human.

Remembering that you have rights is not enough; you must assert them.

Source: Reprinted with permission from Elsevier Science.

Nurses need to recognize their rights as nurses before they can assume responsibility for asserting them. Review the Nursing Self-Awareness feature in terms of the behavioral descriptions in Table 1–1 and develop a personal plan for adopting a wider range of assertive behaviors in your professional life.

SOLITUDE

Most people need time alone to assimilate what has happened in time spent with other people. They also need it for relief from responding to the demands of others. Aloneness need not mean physical distance. People can be alone in a crowded library. The crucial factors are that they are making no demands on others and that no one is making demands on them. After a sanctioned time away, most people return refreshed to their relationships, work, and usual circumstances. Planning for time alone is highly preferable to reaching a breaking point and then aggressively and irresponsibly running away from others.

PERSONAL PHYSICAL HEALTH

An important way of taking care of oneself is to provide for the physical health of the body. A proper diet, adequate rest, and exercise rejuvenate and restore the body. All these activities potentially make nurses more alive and better able to share themselves with their clients.

ATTENDING TO INTERNAL STRESS SIGNALS

Nursing students encountering emotionally disturbed clients commonly begin seeing in themselves all the "symptoms" about which they are learning. This perception is probably due more to heightened awareness of and attention to emotional aspects of their lives than to anything else. However, it is important for nurses to learn to recognize and respond to their own genuine stress signals. All people have times in their lives when they feel a little "crazy." They may become very upset at small disturbances or see things out of proportion to their ultimate importance. These feelings are significant warning signals that the person is not coping adequately with stress.

"Crazy" times can be important turning points in people's lives. They are strong messages that change is needed. It is foolish to ignore these messages. In their daily lives, nurses are often tempted to handle their own symptoms of stress by suppressing them with tranquilizers or other drugs. They could serve themselves better by really experiencing their feelings and attending to what the signals are saying. Help in managing stress creatively is the subject of Chapter 32. Using the complementary/alternative therapies recommended in Chapter 32 will help nurses to gain control of their lives and ease tension before it becomes unmanageable.

Pain and suffering are sources of some of the most intensely experienced stresses in life. Events such as the death of loved ones, divorce, illness, separation from loved ones, and failure are all part of the cycle of life's experience. Being told that they deserve it, or that they really don't have it so bad and therefore have no right to feel the way they feel, does not help people cope with pain and suffering. People want to continue what *was* instead of living with what *is*. They need to find ways of handling their suffering without being destroyed by it. Some people need to replace what they have lost with something similar. Others need to explore a new dimension in their lives. Classmates, friends, and family members can be great sources of support. Being able to both give and receive support strengthens the individual.

According to an old Buddhist teaching, a third of people's suffering is inevitable but they themselves create the rest of it. Realizing that pain and hardship are part of what it is to be a human being makes the pain a bit gentler. It is important to attend to genuine feelings about the loss or prospective loss. The alternative to experiencing pain is to live on the surface, out of touch with the joyful experiences in life as well as the painful ones. A more life-enhancing approach is to experience all aspects of life.

BURNOUT

CLINICAL EXAMPLE

After hours, days, and months of listening to other people's problems, something inside you can go dead and you don't care anymore. That's when you'd rather sit at the desk and do the paperwork than be out talking to clients on the floor.

This nurse verbalizes one of the possible consequences of working intensely with troubled people. Burnout is the name given this phenomenon, and it happens to poverty lawyers, social workers, clinical psychologists, childcare workers, prison personnel, and others who struggle to retain both their objectivity and their concern for the people with whom they work. **Burnout** is a condition in which health care professionals lose their concern and feeling for their clients and come to treat them in detached or even dehumanized ways. It is an attempt to cope, by distancing oneself, with the stresses of intense interpersonal work. It hurts not only clients but also psychiatric professionals, in that they become ineffective and dissatisfied.

In many cases, burning out involves not only thinking in derogatory terms about clients but also believing that somehow they deserve any problem they have. Benner and Wrubel (1989) caution us not to make the mistake of thinking that caring is the cause of burnout and thus try to prevent the "disease" of burnout by protecting oneself from caring. According to them, the sickness is the loss of caring, and the return of caring is the recovery.

There is little doubt that burnout plays a major role in the poor delivery of psychiatric care. It is also a key factor in low staff morale, absenteeism, and high job turnover.

Cues to Burnout

Cues to burnout can be found in the language used to describe clients. Burnout victims may refer to their clients as "crocks," "vegetables," "wackos," and so forth, or they may become highly analytic and abstract: "That's just a manifestation of his primary process thinking." Another cue is lack of involvement with clients. Some nurses "hide" in the nurses' station or staff conference room to avoid interacting. Some openly reject bids for human contact. "Going by the book" rather than considering the unique factors in a situation is a way of minimizing personal involvement with the client. By rigidly applying the rules, the nurse can avoid thinking about the client's specific problems. Burnout can transform an original and creative nurse into a mechanical bureaucrat. Another cue to burnout is joking put-downs, which makes their work seem less frightening and overwhelming.

CLINICAL EXAMPLE

When the nurse is asked where Mr. G is, she laughingly reports that he's taking a shower in preparation for his MMPI test. Everyone in the nurses' station breaks up in gales of laughter.

In a discharge conference, the psychiatrist says he'd like to discharge E, a young male client with a history of violent outbursts. The nurse replies, "With or without baseball bat?" and everyone chuckles.

Reducing Burnout

Most research indicates that the causes of professional burnout are rooted not in the permanent psychologic characteristics of individuals but rather in the social context of their work. Most nurses usually expect the presence of negative conditions: large client loads, time pressures, and daily confrontation with suffering, pain, and death. It is the absence of positive factors—a sense of significance, rewarding interpersonal relationships, the appreciation of others, challenge, and variety—that is most distressing. The strategies listed in Box 1–1 can be used to reduce and modify the occurrence of burnout.

Qualities of Effective Psychiatric–Mental Health Nursing

According to the American Nurses Association (ANA), **psychiatric–mental health nursing** is the diagnosis and treatment of human responses to actual or potential mental health problems. It is a specialized area of nursing practice that employs the wide range of explanatory theories of, and research on, human behavior as its science and the purposeful use of self as its art. Interventions include the continuous and comprehensive primary mental health care services necessary for the promotion of optimal mental health, the prevention of mental illness, health maintenance, management of, and referral for, mental and physical health problems, the diagnosis and treatment of mental disorders and their long-term effects, and rehabilitation (2000, pp. 10–11). Self-awareness, empathy, and moral integrity all enable psychiatric nurses to practice the use of self artfully in therapeutic relationships. Some characteristics of artful therapeutic practice are respect for the client, availability, spontaneity, hope, acceptance, sensitivity, vision, accountability, advocacy, spirituality, and empathy.

BOX 1–1 Strategies to Reduce and Modify the Occurrence of Burnout

- Request a lower staff–client ratio. You can then give more attention to each client and have time to focus on the positive, nonproblematic aspects of the client's life.
- Recognize that no one is perfect. Your clients deserve the best care you can provide; it may not always be perfect care, and it isn't 24-hours-a-day, 7-days-a-week care.
- Take all sanctioned breaks rather than guilt-provoking escapes from the work situation.
- Talk over your problems to get advice and support when you need it.
- Express, analyze, and share your feelings about burning out. This lets you get things off your chest and gives you the chance to get constructive feedback from others and perhaps a new perspective as well.
- Understand your own motivations in pursuing a psychiatric–mental health nursing career and recognize your expectations for work with clients. Deal with your clients' problems, not your own.
- Attend to your own internal stress signals.
- Pursue happiness and satisfaction in your personal life through family, friends, social or spiritual organizations, and hobbies and recreational interests.

RESPECT FOR THE CLIENT

The behavior of many psychiatric clients demonstrates their loss of self-respect. Some may appear dirty and disheveled. Others may plead, beg, or cry. Still others may try to do physical harm to themselves or others. A relationship in which they experience a sense of dignity and receive messages of respect is of inestimable value. You can convey respect in relationships with clients by:

- Taking the time and energy to listen.
- Taking care not to invalidate clients' experience of their world with comments such as "It's not so bad," "Don't be that way," "Time heals all wounds," or "Keep a stiff upper lip."
- Giving clients as much privacy as possible during examinations and treatments or when they are upset.
- Minimizing experiences that humiliate clients and strip them of identity, thus allowing them to make as many of their own choices and be in control of as much of their own lives as possible.
- Being honest with clients about medicines, privileges, length of stay, and so on, even when the truth may be difficult to handle.

AVAILABILITY

Of all the members of the mental health team, the nurse has the richest opportunity to be available to clients when needed. Because they are with clients on a relatively constant basis, nurses have the responsibility for:

- Creating a nurturing, healing milieu.
- Assisting suffering clients to meet their basic human needs.
- Collecting and conveying crucial data about clients that will influence decisions around them.

SPONTANEITY

Many nurses have come to believe that therapeutic relationships with psychiatric clients require them to be stiff, stilted robots uttering clichés from a list of unnatural-sounding communication "techniques." Nurses who are comfortable with themselves, aware of therapeutic goals, and flexible about using a repertoire of possible interventions for any particular clinical problem find that being natural and spontaneous, while keeping therapeutic goals uppermost in their minds, is their most effective "technique." Clients experience such nurses as authentic. Each nurse is unique and necessarily brings a different personal style to practice. We have different ways of putting the words together to convey to clients that we accept and care about them. Sometimes we say it with nonverbal behavior: keeping promises, being on time, touching, and staying with a client who needs someone. We need to trust our own natural styles, combined with sound communication principles such as those discussed in Chapter 8, in working toward therapeutic goals.

HOPE

Effective psychiatric nursing practice is characterized by hope and optimism that all clients, no matter how debilitated, have the capacity for growth and change. Even clients whose most marked attributes are chronicity and deterioration can be helped to some optimal level of well-being by a nurse who believes in their possibilities and is willing to search for some strengths to build on. In one day treatment center, a client joined in a partnership with a creative nurse to assist less able clients toward self-care. It is not unusual in such a situation for the healing to become a source of help to the healer–client.

ACCEPTANCE

There is a distinction between acceptance and approval. Acceptance means refraining from judging and rejecting a client who may behave in a way the nurse dislikes. Therapeutic work requires that clients be able to examine, explore, and understand their coping mechanisms without feeling the need to cover up or disguise them to avoid negative judgments or punishments. Nurses who tell clients what they should say or do or feel deny these clients the acceptance they need to explore their problems.

SENSITIVITY

Genuine interest and concern provide the basis for a therapeutic alliance. Clients recognize the falseness of memorized phrases and assumed postures. You convey general interest and concern by trying to understand the client's perspective, working with the client on mutually formulated goals, and persisting even when break-throughs and improvements are subtle and slow instead of dramatic and quick.

VISION

Because psychiatric–mental health nurses focus their work on enhancing the quality of life for all human beings, they must come to terms with a personal and professional vision of what quality means. Some conditions of life associated with high quality are influence or power, freedom, accountability, self-determinism, openness to gratifying experience, action, mastery, a sense of purpose or meaning, privacy, hope, stability, nonviolence, and intimacy.

ACCOUNTABILITY

According to Peplau (1980), the need for personal accountability—professional integrity—is greater in psychiatric practice than in any other type of health care. Clients in mental health settings are usually more vulnerable and defenseless than clients in other health care settings, particularly because their conditions hinder their thinking processes and their relationships with others. Psychiatric–mental health nurses are accountable for the nature of the effort they make on behalf of clients and answerable to clients for the quality of their efforts. As Peplau puts it, "Personal accountability is an attitude—a quality of the heart and mind of those professionals who are competent and determined that every psychiatric patient will have the best problem-resolving assistance possible" (1980, p. 133).

Psychiatric–mental health nurses are accountable to themselves, their peers, their profession, and the public in the following ways:

- Accountability to self involves bringing personal behavior under conscious control so that the nurse becomes the person-as-nurse she or he wants to be.
- Accountability to peers involves engaging in peer review with nurse colleagues to give and receive feedback intended to improve the quality of care.
- Accountability to the profession involves clarifying the role of the psychiatric nurse, keeping current with changes in the field, and encouraging self-regulation to protect the public and enhance the quality of care.
- Accountability to the public requires keeping abreast of knowledge in the field, becoming credentialed according to level of competence, applying the ANA standards of psychiatric–mental health nursing practice, and protecting the rights of clients and their families.

ADVOCACY

Throughout history, psychiatric–mental health nurses have been ardent supporters of a neglected, ignored, and forgotten population—the mentally ill. In the twenty-first century, there is a need for new energy and political activism. In this era of health care reform, there is an especially important concern—ensuring that the needs and the rights of mentally disordered people are not over-looked or ignored while the explosion of knowledge in science and technology revolutionizes how nurses practice mental health care.

A newly energized political activism calls for nurses to speak out publicly for the health, welfare, and safety of their clients; to take steps to protect their rights; to write articles for the popular press; to lobby their congressional representatives on behalf of better mental health for all people; and to run for political office. The power that such a large group of citizen nurses could wield on behalf of their clients would be awesome.

SPIRITUALITY

Spirituality, the search for meaning in life and a belief in a higher power, is at the core of each person's existence. Spirituality varies in strength from person to person. Some people already have a meaningful philosophy of life. Others, on a spiritual journey, search for life's meaning and purpose. Still others experience hopelessness, despair, and spiritual distress.

Some of your clients will have maladaptive behavior that involves religiosity. (To differentiate between religiosity and spirituality, see the Caring for the Spirit feature on page 16.) They may attempt to resolve internal conflicts or conflicts with others through religious rituals or practices. For such clients, their spirituality becomes a central focus in their treatment.

Helping clients in their search for meaning and purpose is possible when nurses have beliefs that sustain them rather than beliefs that are sources of conflict (Taylor, 2002). You must meet your own spiritual needs satisfactorily before you can have a meaningful relationship with your clients.

To help you on your journey of spiritual growth, contemplate these questions:

1. What gives the greatest meaning or purpose to your life?
2. How do you express your spirituality or your philosophy of life?
3. How does God/Higher Power/Ultimate Other/The Transcendent function in your personal life?
4. What kinds of confusion or doubt do you have about your religious beliefs?
5. What do you do to show love for yourself?
6. What brings you joy and peace in your life?
7. How do you heal your spirit?
8. What art, music, or literature nurtures your spirit?
9. How does your spirituality affect your experience as a nurse?

Answering these questions, eventually fully, and asking yourself how you can change your situation will make you a spiritual activist for yourself and for your clients.

EMPATHY

Comprehension of and ability to use the process of empathy give the nurse one strategy for responding to the feelings of aloneness often experienced by people who are psychiatric clients. Perhaps the most important function of empathic understanding is to help the psychiatric mental health nurse give the client the very precious feeling of being understood and cared about.

Empathy is a pervasive phenomenon in the life experience of all people. **Empathy** can be defined as the ability to feel what others feel and respond to and understand the experience of others on their terms. A nurse who empathizes with a client momentarily abandons the personal self and relives the emotions and responses of someone else. People in everyday life tend to empathize most with those to whom they feel closest. In psychiatric practice, nurses must seek to empathize with those from whom they feel most separate or whose closeness threatens the nurses' own sense of integration.

The capacity for empathy relies on personal integration. A firm sense of self is necessary for a person to be a good empathizer. As people continue to interact with others, they learn to be sensitive to others without losing their own integration.

CRITICAL THINKING

The ability to think critically is crucial for psychiatric–mental health nurses. A critical thinker analyzes information before drawing conclusions about it. It is purposeful, reasonable, reflective thinking that drives problem solving and decision making and aims to make judgments based on evidence (Alfaro-LeFebre, 2001). To encourage you to think critically, we have provided critical thinking challenges at the beginning of every chapter. To develop effective, critical thinking habits, implement the strategies that are suggested in Box 1–2 on page 17.

Professional Role

A central concern of psychiatric–mental health nurses continues to be rehumanizing psychiatric care in a technologic society. It requires a judicious blending of "high touch" with "high tech"—a person-to-person human experience.

CARING FOR THE SPIRIT

Spirituality: The Connection Between Mental Health and Mental Illness

Spirituality is the third part of the triad known as mind–body–spirit in the holistic practice of nursing. In ancient times, spirit meant breath—as essential to life as air. Spirituality is that part of every person that yearns to share the beauty, love, and joyfulness of the universe.

We take our spirituality from many sources: Nature, God, Buddha, Higher Power, Goddess, Krishna, B'ahaullah, Mohammed, Yahweh, and others. Although many of these sources are incorporated into organized religions, spirituality is not religion, nor is religion spirituality. Religion is the organization of a set of beliefs, practices, and rituals, whereas spirituality is a reflection of one's "spirit" and its relationship to the rest of the universe.

Some people develop their spirituality throughout life with prayer, meditation, and reflection. Others may leave the spiritual path because of conflicts with religious beliefs, values, and practices, because of toxic family relationships, or because they are too busy trying to survive physically and mentally.

Even though spirituality is one of the three central aspects of the holistic practice of nursing, the physical, emotional, mental, and social aspects get most, if not all, of the mental health specialist's attention.

Spirituality may be an important connection between mental health and mental illness. In mental illness, most clients describe feeling "disconnected" from their families, their friends, the universe itself, and from their "faith." For example, clients describe depression like being in a gray or black tunnel with a profound sense of disconnectedness.

Imagine what it would be like to go for 24 hours or longer without sleep. How would you look? Would you feel disconnected or disoriented? Ask someone with mania what that's like. Have you ever awakened suddenly and not known where you are? How would it be to feel like that for an hour, a whole day, or a month? Ask someone with schizophrenia what that's like. Perhaps you've driven down the road and realized that you're confused about where you are and how you got there. And what if you had voices inside your head at the same time? Would this be frightening? Would you feel disconnected?

It may be that a psychiatric crisis has also brought forth a spiritual crisis. The client may, for the first time, be faced with looking at the three spiritual questions of life.

1. What have I placed on life's altar?
   "Of what value is my life? Why was I born, anyway? I have nothing to give." These are the words of someone who is depressed and someone who is actively suicidal.
2. What do I hold to be sacred?
   What things are important to the client, what things have meaning?
3. How do I know what's true?
   The client with anxiety or psychosis has great difficulty sorting out what's real and what's not real, determining what's true and what's not true. Life as we know it has many dichotomies. The unanswerable becomes even more of a challenge when a psychiatric crisis emerges.

Recall what happened to your relationships with friends and family when you were in a personal crisis. Did the relationships change? Our cognitive sphere, our affective sphere, and our relational sphere are all affected. We lose our centering of purpose, of sacredness, of reality. We lose our spirit and become disconnected. Do you think your clients' relationships change when they are in a crisis?

Helping clients rediscover their spiritual path is a fulfilling role for psychiatric–mental health nurses. You can help clients find out who they *really* are, beyond, for example, simply husband, father, lover, police officer. Help them identify the source of their inner energy and how to get in touch with their "center" or their "soul." Keep in mind that spirituality is a deeply personal inner experience as opposed to a set of behaviors tied to an externally imposed doctrine or ritual. By offering a simple spirituality inventory, such as that in the spiritual health assessment box in Chapter 9, you will encourage clients to look at the strength of their faith, which will help them with their recovery. Faith is a way of being—being open to possibilities, and to healing.

The role of the psychiatric–mental health nurse has changed over the years from that of custodian to a multifaceted one. The history of psychiatric–mental health nursing is summarized in the timeline in this chapter (see pages 8–9). The settings in which psychiatric–mental health nurses practice have expanded from inside the hospital to all of the communities in which people live.

At the start of the new millennium, the ANA revised the guidelines for psychiatric–mental health nursing practice. There are two sets of standards that guide professional psychiatric–mental health nursing practice. The Standards of Care are reproduced in Box 1–3 on page 18. The first five Standards of Care refer to the nursing process and are discussed in detail in Chapter 7. The subsections of Standard V that specifically discuss the role functions of the psychiatric–mental health nurse are discussed in this chapter. The Standards of Professional Performance are reproduced in Box 1–4 (on page 19) and are also discussed in this and other chapters.

MediaLink Psychiatric Nursing Certification

BASIC LEVEL OF PRACTICE

The *basic level psychiatric–mental health nurse* may have received basic nursing preparation in a diploma, associate degree, or baccalaureate program. Essentially a generalist who works in a specialized setting, this nurse provides the bulk of the nursing care to clients. Registered nurses offer direct and indirect care through the nurse–client relationship. They have major responsibility for the milieu and have contact with clients at all stages of daily life. Nurses at this level may seek **certification** as generalists through the ANA's American Nurses Credentialing Center (ANCC). Certification by a professional nursing organization recognizes competence and also protects the consumer of mental health services. Credentialing information can be found on ANCC's Web site (www.ana.org/ancc) and accessed through the Companion Website for this book.

BOX 1–2 Strategies That Promote Critical Thinking

- Anticipate questions others might ask, such as "What will my supervisor or instructor want to know?" *This helps identify a wider scope of questions that must be answered to gain relevant information.*
- Ask "What if" questions like "What if something goes wrong?" or "What if we try?" *This helps you be proactive and creative.*
- Look for flaws in your thinking. Ask questions like, "What's missing?", "Have I recognized my biases?", and "How could this be made better?" *This helps you evaluate your thinking and make improvements.*
- Ask someone else to look for flaws in your thinking. *You're usually too close to your own work to be objective; others bring a fresh eye and may bring new ideas and perspectives.*
- Develop "good habits of inquiry" (habits that aid in the search for the truth, like always keeping an open mind, verifying information, and taking enough time). *These habits can make critical thinking more automatic.*
- Develop interpersonal skills, such as conflict resolution and getting along with those who have different communication styles. *If you don't have good interpersonal skills, you're unlikely to get the help or information you need to think critically.*
- Replace "I don't know" and "I'm not sure" with "I'll try." *This demonstrates you have the ability to find answers and mobilizes you to locate resources.*
- Turn errors into learning opportunities. *We all make mistakes: They're stepping stones to maturity and new ideas. If you aren't making mistakes, maybe you're not trying hard enough.*

Nurses who work at the basic level, according to the American Nurses Association (2000), perform the following functions:

- Counseling clients in improving or regaining their previous coping abilities, fostering mental health, and preventing mental illness and disability (Standard Va). Criteria that you can use to judge that this standard has been met are:
  1. Counseling promotes the patient's personal and social integration.
  2. Counseling reinforces healthy behaviors and interaction patterns, and helps the client modify or discontinue unhealthy ones.
  3. The documentation of counseling interventions, including communication and interviewing techniques, problem-solving activities, crisis intervention, stress management, support groups, relaxation techniques, assertiveness training, substance abuse counseling, conflict resolution, and behavior modification, is completed.
- Providing, structuring, and maintaining a therapeutic environment in collaboration with the client and other health care clinicians (Standard Vb). Criteria that you can use to judge that this standard has been met are:
  1. The client is familiarized with the physical environment, the schedule of activities, and the norms and rules that govern behavior and activities of daily living, as applicable.
  2. Current knowledge of the effects of the environment on the client is used to guide nursing actions and provide a safe environment.
  3. The therapeutic environment is designed to make use of the physical environment, social structures, culture, and other available resources.
  4. Therapeutic communication among clients and staff supports an effective milieu.
  5. Specific activities are selected that meet the client's physical and mental health needs.
  6. Limits of any kind (e.g., restriction of privileges, restraint, seclusion, time-out) are used in a humane manner, are the least restrictive necessary, and are employed only as needed to ensure the safety of the patient and of others.
  7. The client is given information about the need for limits and the conditions necessary for removal of the restriction, as appropriate.
- Structuring interventions around the client's activities of daily living to foster self-care and mental and physical well-being (Standard Vc). Criteria that you can use to judge that this standard has been met are:
  1. The self-care activities chosen are appropriate for the client's physical and mental status as well as age, developmental level, gender, social orientation, ethnic/social background, and education.
  2. The self-care interventions assist the client in assuming responsibility for activities of daily living, including maintaining a medication regimen, engaging in health-promoting behaviors, and seeking therapeutic interventions when appropriate.
  3. Self-care interventions are aimed at maintaining and improving the client's functional status and quality of life.
- Using knowledge of psychobiologic interventions and applying related clinical skills to restore the client's health and prevent further disability (Standard Vd). Criteria that you can use to judge that this standard has been met are:
  1. Current research findings are applied to guide nursing actions related to psychopharmacology, other psychobiological therapies, and complementary therapies.
  2. Psychopharmacologic agents' intended actions, untoward or interactive effects, and therapeutic doses are monitored, as are blood levels, vital signs, and laboratory values where appropriate.
  3. Nursing interventions are directed toward alleviating untoward effects of psychobiological interventions, when possible.
  4. Nursing observations about the client's response to psychobiological interventions are communicated to other health clinicians.
- Assisting clients in achieving satisfying, productive, and healthy patterns of living by providing health teaching (Standard Ve). Criteria that you can use to judge that this standard has been met are:
  1. Health teaching is based on principles of learning.
  2. Health teaching occurs on an individual basis or within a group context, depending on the information content and client's ability.

BOX 1–3 ANA Standards of Psychiatric–Mental Health Nursing Practice

Standards of Care

Standard I. Assessment

The psychiatric–mental health nurse collects patient health data.

Standard II. Diagnosis

The psychiatric–mental health nurse analyzes the assessment data in determining diagnoses.

Standard III. Outcome Identification

The psychiatric–mental health nurse identifies expected outcomes individualized to the patient.

Standard IV. Planning

The psychiatric–mental health nurse develops a plan of care that is negotiated among the patient, nurse, family, and health care team and prescribes evidence-based interventions to attain expected outcomes.

Standard V. Implementation

The psychiatric–mental health nurse implements the interventions identified in the plan of care.

Standard Va. Counseling

The psychiatric–mental health nurse uses counseling interventions to assist patients in improving or regaining their previous coping abilities, fostering mental health, and preventing mental illness and disability.

Standard Vb. Milieu Therapy

The psychiatric–mental health nurse provides, structures, and maintains a therapeutic environment in collaboration with the patient and other health care clinicians.

Standard Vc. Promotion of Self-Care Activities

The psychiatric–mental health nurse structures interventions around the patient's activities of daily living to foster self-care and mental and physical well-being.

Standard Vd. Psychobiological Interventions

The psychiatric–mental health nurse uses knowledge of psychobiological interventions and applies clinical skills to restore the patient's health and prevent further disability.

Standard Ve. Health Teaching

The psychiatric–mental health nurse, through health teaching, assists patients in achieving satisfying, productive, and healthy patterns of living.

Standard Vf. Case Management

The psychiatric–mental health nurse provides case management to coordinate comprehensive health services and to ensure continuity of care.

Standard Vg. Health Promotion and Health Maintenance

The psychiatric–mental health nurse employs strategies and interventions to promote and maintain health and prevent mental illness.

The following advanced practice interventions (Vh–Vj) may be performed only by the APRN-PMH.

Standard Vh. Psychotherapy

The APRN-PMH uses individual, group, and family psychotherapy, and other therapeutic treatments to assist patients in preventing mental illness and disability, treating mental health disorders, and improving mental health status and functional abilities.

Standard Vi. Prescriptive Authority and Treatment

The APRN-PMH uses prescriptive authority, procedures, and treatments in accordance with state and federal laws and regulations, to treat symptoms of psychiatric illness and improve functional health status.

Standard Vj. Consultation

The APRN-PMH provides consultation to enhance the abilities of other clinicians to provide services for patients and effect change in the system.

Standard VI. Evaluation

The psychiatric–mental health nurse evaluates the patient's progress in attaining expected outcomes.

Source: Reprinted with permission from American Nurses Association, American Psychiatric Nurses Association, International Society of Psychiatric–Mental Health Nurses, *Scope and Standards of Psychiatric–Mental Health Nursing Practice,* © 2000 American Nurses Publishing, American Nurses Foundation/American Nurses Association, Washington, DC.

3. Health teaching for the client includes information about coping, interpersonal relations, mental health problems, mental disorders, social skills, and treatments and their effects on daily living, as well as information pertinent to physical status or developmental needs.
4. Constructive feedback and positive rewards reinforce the client's learning.
5. Practice sessions, homework assignments, and experiential learning are used as needed.
6. Health teaching provides opportunities for the client and significant others to question, discuss, and explore their thoughts and feelings about past, current, and projected use of therapies to make informed choices.

► Providing case management to coordinate comprehensive health services and to ensure continuity of care (Standard Vf). Criteria that you can use to judge that this standard has been met are:

1. Case management services are based on a comprehensive approach to the client's physical, mental, emotional, and social health problems and resource availability.
2. Case management services are provided in terms of the client's needs, resources, and the accessibility, availability, quality, and cost-effectiveness of care.
3. Health-related services and more specialized care are negotiated on behalf of the client with the appropriate agencies and providers as needed.

BOX 1–4 **ANA Standards of Professional Performance**

Standard I. Quality of Care

The psychiatric–mental health nurse systematically evaluates the quality of care and effectiveness of psychiatric–mental health nursing practice.

Standard II. Performance Appraisal

The psychiatric–mental health nurse evaluates one's own psychiatric–mental health nursing practice in relation to professional practice standards and relevant statutes and regulations.

Standard III. Education

The psychiatric–mental health nurse acquires and maintains current knowledge in nursing practice.

Standard IV. Collegiality

The psychiatric–mental health nurse interacts with and contributes to the professional development of peers, health care clinicians, and others, as colleagues.

Standard V. Ethics

The psychiatric–mental health nurse's assessments, actions, and recommendations on behalf of patients are determined and implemented in an ethical manner.

Standard VI. Collaboration

The psychiatric–mental health nurse collaborates with the patient, significant others, and health care clinicians in providing care.

Standard VII. Research

The psychiatric–mental health nurse contributes to nursing and mental health through the use of research methods and findings.

Standard VIII. Resource Utilization

The psychiatric–mental health nurse considers factors related to safety, effectiveness, and cost in planning and delivering patient care.

Source: Reprinted with permission from American Nurses Association, American Psychiatric Nurses Association, International Society of Psychiatric–Mental Health Nurses, *Scope and Standards of Psychiatric–Mental Health Nursing Practice,* © 2000 American Nurses Publishing, American Nurses Foundation/American Nurses Association, Washington, DC.

4. Relationships with agencies and providers are maintained throughout the client's use of the health care services to ensure continuity of care.

- Employing strategies and interventions that promote and maintain health and prevent mental illness (Standard Vg). Criteria that you can use to judge that this standard has been met are:
  1. Health promotion and disease prevention strategies are based on knowledge of health beliefs, practices, evidence-based findings, and epidemiological principles, along with the social, cultural, and political issues that affect mental health in an identified community.
  2. Health promotion and disease prevention interventions are designed for clients identified as being at risk for mental health problems.
  3. Consumer alliances and consumer participation are sought, as appropriate, in identifying mental health problems in the community and planning, implementing, and evaluating programs to address those problems.
  4. Community resources are identified to assist consumers in using prevention and mental health care services appropriately.
  5. Research findings are utilized to promote health and prevent mental illness.
- Performing intake screening and evaluation including physical and psychosocial assessments, planning for care, recognizing the need for additional clinical data, and referring the client for more specialized testing and evaluation.
- Providing crisis intervention, stabilization, and direct counseling services to persons in crisis as individual needs arise, or as members of crisis teams.
- Focusing on psychiatric rehabilitation and improving an individual's quality of life by facilitating symptom management and by promoting relapse prevention.
- Responding to the mental health needs of individuals, families, or groups in social environments that are integral parts of people's daily lives—homes, schools, and work sites—and in a range of intermediate- and long-term care settings that exist for the treatment and support of those with severe and persistent mental disorders (these settings are discussed in greater detail in Chapter 11).
- Promoting access to mental health care through telehealth, that is, using various electronic means of communication (telephone consultation, faxing, computers, electronic mail, image transmission, interactive video sessions) to establish and maintain a therapeutic relationship with a client.
- Functioning as an advocate by joining consumer and professional groups to reduce the stigma associated with mental disorder, lobbying on behalf of better mental health and psychiatric care, becoming politically active at the local, state, and federal level, and running for public office.
- Mobilizing community action and community resources to ameliorate the sociocultural factors that adversely affect mental health through participation on community planning boards, and with advisory groups and other key people.

ADVANCED LEVEL OF PRACTICE

According to the ANA (2000), the **advanced practice registered nurse** in psychiatric–mental health (APRN-PMH) is a licensed registered nurse who is educationally prepared as a clinical nurse specialist or a nurse practitioner at the master's or doctorate degree level in the specialty of psychiatric–mental health nursing. Advanced practice psychiatric–mental health nurses may also seek certification at the advanced level through ANCC. They may use the initials CS (certified specialist). The advanced-level certification is a means of protecting consumers. *In addition to the basic-level role functions,* the APRN-PMH carries out the following advanced level role functions. The first three compose Standard Vh–Vj of the ANA Standards of Care (2000) reproduced in Box 1–3:

- Providing psychotherapy to clients through all generally accepted methods of brief or long-term therapy, specifically including individual therapy (e.g., insight therapy, behavioral therapy, goal- or solution-oriented therapy, relationship therapy, cognitive therapy, and play and other expressive therapies), group therapy, couple/marital therapy, and family therapy. Criteria that you can use to judge that this standard has been met are:
  1. The therapeutic contract with the client is structured to include:
     a. Purpose, goals, and expected outcomes.
     b. Time, place, and frequency of therapy.
     c. Participants involved in therapy.
     d. Confidentiality.
     e. Availability and means of contacting therapist.
     f. Responsibilities of both client and therapist.
     g. Fees and payment schedule.
  2. Knowledge of personality theory, growth and development, psychology, neurobiology, psychopathology, social systems, small-group and family dynamics, stress and adaptation, and theories related to selected therapeutic methods is used, based on the client's needs.
  3. Therapeutic principles are used to understand and interpret the client's emotions, thoughts, and behaviors.
  4. The client is helped to deal constructively with thoughts, emotions, and behaviors.
  5. Increasing responsibility and independence are fostered in the client to reinforce healthy behaviors and interactions.
  6. In the client's absence, provision for care is arranged.
  7. When it is determined that the provision of some aspect of physical care required by the client would impair the therapist–client relationship, referral for that care is made to another clinician.
- Prescription of pharmacological agents and the ordering and interpretation of diagnostic and laboratory testing according to applicable state and federal regulations. Criteria that you can use to judge that this standard has been met are:
  1. Psychiatric treatment interventions and procedures are prescribed according to the client's mental health care needs and are evidence-based.
  2. Procedures are used as needed in the delivery of comprehensive care.
  3. Psychopharmacological agents are prescribed based on a knowledge of psychopathology, neurobiology, physiology, expected therapeutic actions, anticipated side effects, and courses of action, for unintended or toxic effects.
  4. Pharmacological agents are prescribed based on clinical indicators of the client's status, including the results of diagnostic and laboratory tests, as appropriate.
  5. Intended effects and potential adverse effects of pharmacological and nonpharmacological treatments are monitored and treated as necessary.
  6. Information about intended effects, potential adverse effects of the proposed prescription, and other treatment options, including no treatment, is provided to the client.
  7. Informed consent is obtained for treatment.
- Serving as a consultant–liaison in nonpsychiatric health care arenas such as hospitals, extended care facilities, rehabilitation centers, and outpatient clinics to provide mental health specialist consultation or direct care psychiatric–mental health nursing services. Criteria that you can use to judge that this standard has been met are:
  1. Consultation activities are based on models of consultation, systems principles, communication and interviewing techniques, problem-solving skills, change theories, and other theories as indicated.
  2. Consultation is initiated at the request of the consultee.
  3. A working alliance, based on mutual respect and role responsibilities, is established with the client or consultee.
  4. Consultation recommendations are communicated in terms that facilitate understanding and involve the consultee in decision-making.
  5. Implementation of the system change or plan of care remains the consultee's responsibility.
- Assisting other psychiatric–mental health clinicians and clinician-trainees by providing clinical supervision to further develop their clinical practice skills, meet the standard for ongoing peer consultation, and provide essential peer supervision.

Source: Reprinted with permission from American Nurses Association, American Psychiatric Nurses Association, International Society of Psychiatric–Mental Health Nurses, *Scope and Standards of Psychiatric–Mental Health Nursing Practice,* © 2000 American Nurses Publishing, American Nurses Foundation/American Nurses Association, Washington, DC.

The Mental Health Team

The psychiatric–mental health nurse is an integral and important part of the mental health team. Of all the disciplines involved in mental health care, nursing is the one most likely to have an overall view of the client's situation.

Role definitions that were traditionally assigned to specific disciplines have become increasingly blurred. Psychiatric–mental health nurses, social workers, and psychologists, among others, have more direct influence than ever before. Roles are less specifically defined, and in many community settings, mental health professionals take on whichever functions they do best.

The descriptions in ■ Table 1–2 of the education and functions of mental health team members reflect more traditional distinctions. Keep in mind that many of the functions are now shared across disciplines when the team member has been

TABLE 1–2 The Mental Health Team

Team Member	Education/Preparation	Role
Psychiatric–mental health nurse	A registered nurse with specialized preparation in psychiatric–mental health nursing; level of expertise depends on education, which may include up to the doctoral level.	Responsible for the nursing care of mental health clients; has major responsibility for the milieu.
Psychiatrist	A medical physician whose specialty is mental disorders; has completed an approved psychiatric residency.	Responsible for diagnosis and treatment of persons with mental disorders.
Clinical psychologist	A psychologist specially educated and trained in mental health; certification requires completion of an approved doctoral program and a clinical internship.	Performs psychotherapy; plans and implements programs of behavior modification; selects, administers, and interprets psychological tests.
Psychiatric social worker	A graduate of a master's program in social work with an emphasis in mental health; may have a doctoral degree.	Helps clients and their families cope more effectively; identifies appropriate community resources; may perform counseling and psychotherapy.
Occupational therapist	Prepared in occupational therapy at the baccalaureate or master's level with a specialty in mental health care.	Uses manual and creative techniques to elicit desired interpersonal and intrapsychic responses; teaches self-help activities, helps clients prepare to seek employment.
Recreational therapist	May be prepared at informal or formal levels in university physical education and health education programs.	Plans and guides recreational activities to provide socialization, healthful recreation, and desirable interpersonal and intrapsychic experiences.
Creative arts therapist	May be prepared at informal or formal levels in colleges and universities.	Uses art, music, dance, and literature to facilitate interpersonal experiences and increase social responses and self-esteem.

appropriately educated for the task and when laws and regulations permit the sharing of functions.

Collaborating on the Mental Health Team

Psychiatric–mental health nurses, whether practicing in institutions or in private practice settings, must plan and share with others to deliver maximum mental health services to clients. The purpose of collaboration is to make the best use of the different abilities of mental health team members so that the client receives the most effective service available. Relationship problems among mental health team members must be worked through to avoid distorting the team's efforts on behalf of the client.

COOPERATION VERSUS COMPETITION

The key to working together on a problem with a common purpose is cooperation rather than competition. Working together in cooperation ensures movement toward the common goal, whereas inappropriate competition hinders goal achievement and may be destructive to the competing individuals.

Most of our present understanding of cooperative and competitive behavior has come from the efforts of game theorists, who have researched player behavior. According to game theorists, players can be identified and placed in categories as follows:

- Maximizers—those interested only in their own gain.
- Rivalists—those interested only in defeating their partners.
- Cooperators—those interested in helping both themselves and their partners.

Maximizers and rivalists jeopardize the client's welfare because they put themselves first and the client last. Rivalists direct their energies toward being "one up" through put-downs of others. They are concerned not with the client but with the process of winning. Cooperators are interested in helping both themselves and their colleagues to aid the client. Participants who actively recognize the importance of each individual member of the mental health team can influence maximizers and rivalists to become cooperators.

Effective collaboration is based on respect for the position from which another participant acts. Our values and our culture direct our beliefs and the climate in which we operate. Knowing this, we can become aware of the values and culture of others, and, in turn, respect them. For a full discussion of culture and what it means to be culturally competent, refer to Chapter 6.

Unfortunately, the process of socialization into a profession may make it difficult for a person to respect, accept, and trust the position of another. As students become committed to a profession through the process of socialization, they tend to view members of other disciplines with suspicion.

Administrative and peer support creates an atmosphere in which nurses are free to share their knowledge, skills, and evolving ideas. Such support increases creativity, depth, and perspective in nursing. Self-exploration and self-assessment, through reading and dialogue with other nurses and mental health team members, can help nurses embrace a spirit of cooperation.

ENGAGING THE CLIENT IN COLLABORATION

Include clients and their significant others in the collaborative process of the mental health team whenever possible. Clients' participation in their own health care assures nurses that their clients are informed consumers of mental health services.

Clients can also be invited to participate in case conferences. These conferences often have an important place in the functioning of mental health agencies and may have a number of purposes. Encourage clients to participate in case conferences that involve collaboration among several agencies or several mental health care workers moving toward similar goals.

Consult the client about the information to be shared with other members of the mental health team. It is not always easy for the nurse to determine exactly how much to share and with whom. When the boundaries of confidentiality are not clear, confer with the supervisor or a colleague to determine what should be shared. Decisions should take into consideration what agreement exists between nurse and client about sharing information and how the person or agency receiving information will use that information in the client's best interest. Refer to Chapter 10 for a thorough discussion of client rights as they relate to confidentiality.

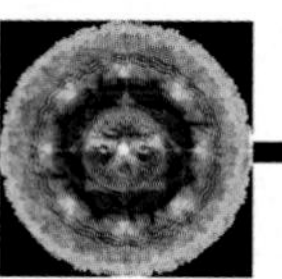

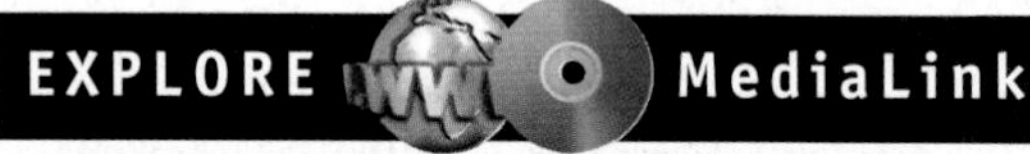

EXPLORE MediaLink

NCLEX review, case studies, and other interactive resources for this chapter can be found on the Companion Website at http://www.prenhall.com/kneisl. Click on Chapter 1 to select the activities for this chapter.

For animations, video tutorials, more NCLEX review questions, and an audio glossary, access the accompanying CD-ROM in this textbook.

BIBLIOGRAPHY

Alfaro-LeFevre, R. (2001, March). Improving your ability to think critically. *Nursing Spectrum*, 25–30.

American Nurses Association (1995). *Nursing's social policy statement*. Washington, DC: Author.

American Nurses Association (2000). *Scope and standards of psychiatric–mental health nursing practice*. Washington, DC: Author.

Barker, P. (1999). *The philosophy and practice of psychiatric nursing*. Edinburgh: Churchill Livingstone.

Benner, P., & Wrubel, J. (Eds.) (1986). Coping with caregiving. In *The primacy of caring: Stress and coping in health and illness* (pp. 365–406). Menlo Park, CA: Addison-Wesley.

Bodger, C. (1999). *Smart guide to relieving stress*. New York: John Wiley & Sons.

Chenevert, M. (1994). *STAT: Special techniques in assertiveness training for women in the health professions* (4th ed.). St. Louis: Mosby.

Clarke, L. (1999). *Challenging ideas in psychiatric nursing*. London: Routledge.

Clauden, G., & Long, A. (2000). Communication is the essence of nursing care. *British Journal of Nursing, 9*(15), 979–984.

Cohen, J. I. (2000). Stress and mental health: A biobehavioral perspective. *Issues in Mental Health Nursing, 21*, 185–202.

Flaskerud, J. H., & Wuerker, A. K. (1999). Mental health nursing in the 21st century. *Issues in Mental Health Nursing, 20*, 5–17.

Forchuk, C., Westwell, J., Martin, M-L., Bamber-Azzapardi, W., Kosterewa-Tolman, D., & Hux, M. (2000). The developing nurse–client relationship: Nurses' perspectives. *Journal of the American Psychiatric Nurses Association, 6*, 3–10.

Keltner, N. L., Folks, D. G., Palmer, C. A., & Powers, R. E. (1998). *Psychobiological Foundations of Psychiatric Care*. St. Louis: Mosby.

Lipkin, G. B., & Cohen, R. G. (Eds.) (1998). Looking at the health worker. In *Effective approaches to patient's behavior* (5th ed.) (pp. 16–25). New York: Springer.

Lipkin, G. B., & Cohen, R. G. (Eds.) (1998). Looking at the patient. In *Effective approaches to patient's behavior* (5th ed.) (pp. 16–25). New York: Springer.

McBride, A. (1996). Psychiatric–mental health nursing in the 21st century. In A. McBride, & J. Austin, (Eds.), *Psychiatric–mental health nursing: Integrating the behavioral and biological sciences*. Philadelphia: Saunders.

Mohr, W., & Noone, M. (1997). Deconstructing progress notes in psychiatric settings. *Archives of Psychiatric Nursing, 11*, 325–329.

Muff, J. (1984). Balancing communication. In: E. E. M. Smythe (Ed.), *Surviving nursing*. Menlo Park, CA: Addison-Wesley.

Palmer-Erbs, V. K., & Anthony, W. A. (1995). Incorporating psychiatric rehabilitation principles into psychiatric–mental health nursing practice: An opportunity to develop a full partnership among nurses, consumers, and families. *Journal of Psychosocial Nursing and Mental Health Services, 33*, 36–44.

Peplau, H. E. (1980). The psychiatric nurse—accountable? To whom? For what? *Perspectives in Psychiatric Care, 18*(3), 128–134.

Pescosolido, B. A., Monahan, J., Link, B. G., Stueve, A., & Kikuzawa, S. (1999). The public's view of the competence, dangerousness, and need for legal coercion of persons with mental health problems. *American Journal of Public Health, 89*, 1339–1346.

Reck, R. R., & Long, B. G. (2000). *The win-win negotiator: How to negotiate favorable agreements that last*. New York: Pocket Books.

Smoyak, S. A., & Skiba-King, W. (1998). Historical influences on today's education and practice. In: A. Burgess (Ed.), *Advanced practice psychiatric nursing* (pp. 15–26). Stamford, CT: Appleton-Lange.

Spector, R. E. (2000). *Cultural diversity in health and illness* (5th ed.). Upper Saddle River, NJ: Prentice Hall.

Taylor, E. J. (2002). *Spiritual care*. Upper Saddle River, NJ: Prentice Hall.

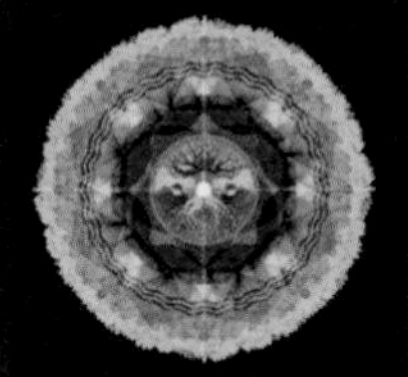

Philosophy and Theories for Interdisciplinary Psychiatric Care

HOLLY SKODOL WILSON

2

Chapter TWO

FOCUS QUESTIONS

- What are the major ideas of interactionism?
- What are the major principles of humanism?
- What has been the influence of the knowledge explosion in psychobiology?
- How do the premises of human interactionism and psychobiology relate to psychiatric–mental health nursing?
- What are the assumptions and key ideas of medical–psychobiologic, psychoanalytic, behaviorist, social–interpersonal, and nursing theories?
- Can you discuss the implications each theory has for psychiatric–mental health nursing?

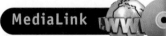

www.prenhall.com/kneisl

Additional resources for this chapter can be found on the Student CD-ROM accompanying this textbook, and on the Companion Website at *www.prenhall.com/kneisl*. Click on Chapter 2 to select the activities for this chapter.

CD-ROM
- Audio Glossary
- NCLEX Review

Companion Website
- Additional NCLEX Review
- Case Study: Theories for Psychiatric Care

KEY TERMS

conditioned response
conditioning
conscious
defense mechanism
ego
general systems theory
holistic
humanism
id
interpersonal theory
mental disorder
negative reinforcement
nursing theory
operant conditioning
positive reinforcement
preconscious
primary prevention
psychoanalysis
psychoanalytic theory
psychobiology
reflected appraisals
reinforcement
self-system
shaping
symbolic interactionism
superego
token economy
unconscious

CHAPTER OUTLINE

CROSS REFERENCES

Other topics relevant to this content are: Cognitive and behavioral interventions, Chapter 30; Contemporary roles of psychiatric–mental health nurses, Chapter 1; Cultural competence in psychiatric–mental health nursing, Chapter 6; Defense mechanisms, Chapter 5; Evidence-based practice, Chapter 3; Psychobiology, Chapter 4.

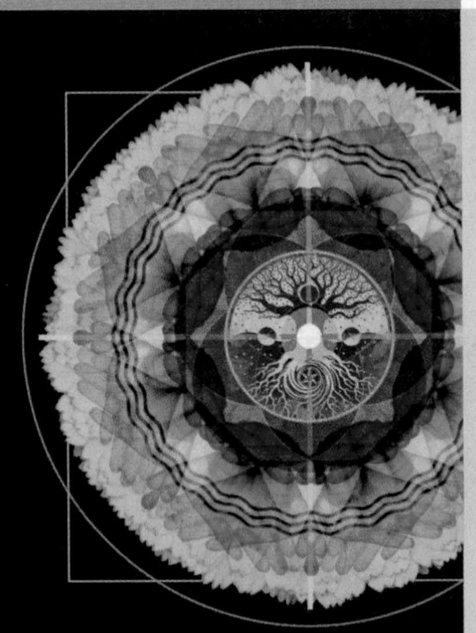

CRITICAL THINKING CHALLENGE

Sonia Jones, a 38-year-old musician, comes to the psychiatric clinic complaining of depression, anxiety, and fear about her increasing use of methamphetamines (speed) and alcohol. Sonia's reason for seeking help to is get clean and sober. Some members of the treatment team, however, cite a randomized clinical trial and psychobiologic theory that support treating the depression prior to addressing Sonia's coexisting addictive disease. Your own clinical wisdom and past experience convince you that both conditions must be addressed simultaneously.

When you don't have established theory or clear research findings to guide your clinical decisions, how important are clinical preferences and clinical wisdom? Do you think they constitute evidence on which to base practice? ■

To practice psychiatric–mental health nursing humanistically, nurses must devote themselves to understanding what makes people human, how they express their joy of living, their sadness, their desire to love, their hopes for growth. Understanding these phenomena becomes even more crucial when psychiatric nurses must explain how the joy of living suddenly turns to the desire to die, how love of self and others turns to violence and hate, how the hope for growth turns to withdrawal and despair, and how alterations in the brain relate to these human experiences.

This chapter introduces you to a holistic philosophy that includes humanism, interactionism, and the knowledge explosion in **psychobiology**. In this chapter, we also compare the basic assumptions and implications for practice in the dominant theories for interdisciplinary psychiatric care. These are:

- Medical–psychobiologic theory
- Psychoanalytic theory
- Behaviorist theory
- Social–interpersonal theories
- Nursing theories

Clinicians choose one or a combination of these theories in determining what information to assess about clients, what intervention outcomes and approaches to recommend, and what ultimate evaluation criteria to set. Your approach to understanding psychiatric clients is influenced by your philosophy. Theories, on the other hand, provide the conceptual tools to formulate that understanding and to interpret clinical data.

Humanistic Interactionism and Psychobiology: The Mind–Body–Spirit Connection

The classic psychiatric and psychologic approaches have described and classified signs and symptoms of *illness*, then accounted for it by individual psychologic dynamics such as character disorder, weak ego, or failed defense mechanisms. The basis for this text is a new synthesis of psychosocial and psychobiologic knowledge required for practice in the twenty-first century.

SCOPE OF PSYCHIATRIC–MENTAL HEALTH NURSING PRACTICE

All nurses are concerned with the quality of human life and its relationship to health. The psychiatric nurse is especially concerned with the relationship between the individual's optimal psychobiologic health and feelings of self-worth, personal integrity, self-fulfillment, and creative expression. Just as important are the satisfying of basic living needs, comfortable relationships with others, and the recognition of human rights. These elements collectively define mental health. The psychiatric nurse's scope of practice is broad enough to include issues such as alienation, identity crises, sudden life changes, and troubled family interactions. It may deal with poverty and affluence, the experiences of birth and death, the loss of significant others, or the loss of body parts. It is concerned with sustaining and enhancing the individual and the group. Yet it also must address basic life issues of eating, sleeping, grooming, and hygiene shared by psychiatric clients.

This broad-ranging, humanistic, interactional, and psychobiologic view of the scope of psychiatric–mental health nursing is dramatically different from the exclusively medical or behavioral science orientation of the last 50 years.

One major study and two important reports provide direction for our mental health practice in the twenty-first century. The *Global Burden of Disease* study demonstrated that 5 of the top 10 causes of disability worldwide were psychiatric disorders—depression (ranked number one), schizophrenia, bipolar disorder, alcohol abuse, and obsessive–compulsive disorder (Murray & Lopez, 1996). The report by the United States Department of Health and Human Services (USDHHS, 2002), *Healthy People 2010*, identified the major public health problems in the United States and determined specific mental health objectives to be achieved by the end of this decade. These mental health objectives are listed in Box 2–1.

The second important report was the United States Surgeon General's report on mental health and mental illness (USDHHS, 1999). This report underscored the importance of under-

BOX 2–1 Healthy People 2010 Mental Health Objectives

- Reduce the suicide rate.
- Reduce the rate of suicide attempts by adolescents.
- Reduce the proportion of homeless adults who have serious mental illness (SMI).
- Increase the proportion of persons with SMI who are employed.
- Reduce the relapse rates for persons with eating disorders including anorexia nervosa and bulimia nervosa.
- Increase the number of persons seen in primary health care who receive mental health screening and assessment.
- Increase the proportion of children with mental health problems who receive treatment.
- Increase the proportion of juvenile justice facilities that screen new admissions for mental health problems.
- Increase the proportion of adults with mental disorders who receive treatment.
- Increase the proportion of persons with co-occurring substance abuse and mental disorders who receive treatment for both disorders.
- Increase the proportion of local governments with community-based jail diversion programs for adults with SMI.
- Increase the number of states and the District of Columbia that track consumers' satisfaction with the mental health services they receive.
- Increase the number of states, territories, and the District of Columbia with an operational mental health plan that addresses cultural competence.
- Increase the number of states, territories, and the District of Columbia with an operational mental health plan that addresses mental health crisis interventions, ongoing screening, and treatment services for elderly persons.
- Increase the proportion of worksites employing 50 or more persons that provide programs to prevent or reduce employee stress.

Source: Department of Health and Human Services. (2002). *Healthy people 2010.* Retrieved August 20, 2002, from the World Wide Web, http://www.healthypeople.gov.

MediaLink Healthy People 2010

standing that mental disorders are "real" illnesses, that people should be educated to seek help for symptoms of mental disorder, and that we have an obligation to provide safe and effective treatment for all citizens by improving the delivery of mental health care services. All three developments emphasize the importance of promoting and maintaining mental health and improving mental health delivery systems around the world.

These data can be found on the United States Department of Health and Human Services Web site (www.dhhs.gov; www.healthypeople.gov), through a direct resource link on the Companion Website of this book.

DEFINING THE CONCEPT OF MENTAL DISORDER

We believe that concepts such as "mental disorder" and "mental health" are interactional and derive their meaning not only from changes in brain structure and biochemistry but also from the definitions given to certain behavior by certain people. We advocate looking at the social conditions under which someone is called "mentally ill." We view mental illness and mental health as outgrowths of intra- and interpersonal processes.

Determining that someone is mentally ill is often a matter of judgment, even when brain chemicals are altered. The appropriateness of behavior depends on whether it is judged plausible or not according to a set of social, ethical, and legal rules that define the limits of appropriate behavior and reality. For example, if a man on a street corner says he is Napoleon, people will not believe him and will consider his statement symptomatic or disturbed. If a man at a masquerade party says he is Napoleon, people reach a different conclusion. Alterations in brain biochemistry may be present in both social contexts.

With the preceding as philosophic background, we support the concept of **mental disorder** as defined by the American Psychiatric Association's *Diagnostic and Statistical Manual of Mental Disorders (DSM-IV-TR):*

> A clinically significant behavioral or psychological syndrome or pattern that occurs in an individual that is typically associated with either a painful symptom (distress) or impairment in one or more important areas of functioning (disability) or with a significantly increased risk of suffering, death, pain, or loss of freedom. In addition, this syndrome or pattern must not be merely an expectable and culturally sanctioned response to a particular event, for example, the death of a loved one. . . . Neither deviant behavior (e.g., political, religious, or sexual) nor conflicts that are primarily between the individual and society are mental disorders unless the deviance or conflict is a symptom of dysfunction in the individual as described above (APA, 2000, p. xxxi).

Psychiatric–mental health nurses are concerned with the care of clients who have identified mental disorders. However, our concerns extend to the wide range of human responses to mental distress, disability, and disorder. For example, an addicted parent may not only suffer from shame, unemployment, and abusive outbursts of anger but may also lose a sense of purpose and meaning, and experience a disturbed self-concept and spiritual distress. These responses have detrimental effects on the health of children, partners, and other significant people in the person's life.

Like many concepts in the human sciences, the concept of mental disorder lacks a definition that covers all situations. Faced with such a diverse array of human problems, the psychiatric–mental health nurse is challenged to synthesize a holistic philosophy for practice that can be the basis for care. See ■ Figure 2–1 (pages 28–29) for the shifting approaches to mental disorder throughout history.

BASIC PREMISES OF INTERACTIONISM

One central idea in the approach we advocate has come to be known as **symbolic interactionism,** a term introduced by Herbert Blumer (1969) to describe an approach to the study of human conduct. It is based on three philosophic premises:

1. Human beings act toward things (other people, events) on the basis of the meaning that the things have for them. Life experiences may have different meanings for different people.
2. The meaning of things in a person's life is derived from the social interactions that person has with others. We learn meanings during our experiences with others.
3. People handle and modify the meanings of the things they encounter through an interpretive process. They come to their own conclusions.

Implications for Psychiatric–Mental Health Nursing Practice

The First Premise: Different Meanings for Different People. We believe that all behavior has meaning. The psychiatric nurse must be wary of interventions that ignore, discount, or discredit the meaning an experience has for the client in favor of the nurse's own definition of the situation. Thus, nurses must develop skill in observing, interpreting, and responding to the client's lived experiences in the hope of arriving at a common ground of negotiated meanings and authentic communication.

The Second Premise: Meanings Arise in One's Social World. We believe meanings arise in the *process* of interaction with others. It is essential, therefore, that psychiatric nurses take into account the social and cultural environment of each client. A holistic assessment of a client accounts for the interaction patterns in that person's social world.

A shaved head, tattoos, baggy denim pants worn low on the hips, and a woolen cap, which appear deviant in a milieu of business suit–wearing bankers and executives, may represent rather close adherence to dress and demeanor codes of some street gang subcultures.

Similarly, it is within interpersonal interaction that clients can learn new definitions for life situations and new repertoires for action. This is the heart of the psychiatric nurse's therapeutic and caring role. The sensitive, intelligent, and humanistic use of self within interpersonal relationships is a key part of the psychiatric–mental health nurse's skill. Nurses have a particular potential for helping clients redefine their experiences in more satisfying ways, learn new patterns of coping with stress, and generally enhance the quality of their lives and social worlds. Such is the essence of psychiatric–mental health nursing.

The Third Premise: Meaning Is a Basis for Behavior. We believe that people handle situations in terms of what they consider vitally important about the situation. To understand clients' actions, the psychiatric–mental health nurse must identify the meanings those actions have for them.

Nurses need to keep this premise in mind when responding to an expression of human distress. A nurse may say, "I wouldn't worry about it," or "Don't feel that way," "You are reacting inappropriately," or "It's not so bad." Such clichés are not usually helpful, not because they are inherently "untherapeutic" but because in voicing them the nurse invalidates the basic premise that people interpret the world in their own way to act in a specific situation.

Interactionism offers psychiatric–mental health nursing a perspective of human beings as having purpose and control over their lives, even if they have altered brain structure and chemistry and stressful environments. Interactionism as interpreted here provides the premise for a philosophy of caring with a strong humanistic cast. Interactionism acknowledges the interaction of psychology, psychobiology, and sociocultural contexts.

BASIC PREMISES OF HUMANISM

One of the purposes of this chapter is to specify a philosophic basis for subsequent chapters. The three premises of interactionism provide us with a partial orientation. A theory of life centered on human beings, termed **humanism**, adds to the philosophic perspective.

The central concept of humanism is that the chief end of human life is to work for well-being within the limitations of life in today's world. Humanism is a philosophy of service to benefit humanity through reason, science, and democracy.

The humanistic perspective has the following eight central propositions:

1. The human being's mind is indivisibly connected with the body.
2. Human beings have the power or potential to solve their own problems.
3. Human beings, while influenced by the past, possess freedom of creative choice and action and are, within certain limits, masters of their own destinies.
4. Human values are grounded in life experiences and relationships, and our highest goal must be the happiness, freedom, and growth of all people.
5. Individuals attain well-being and a high quality of life by harmoniously combining personal satisfactions with activities that contribute to the welfare of the community.
6. We should develop art and awareness of beauty so that the aesthetic experience becomes a pervasive reality in people's lives.
7. We should apply reason, science, and democratic procedures in all areas of life.
8. We must continually examine our basic convictions, including those of humanism.

See Lamont's classic book (1967) for an elaboration of these propositions.

Implications for Psychiatric–Mental Health Nursing Practice

As a philosophy underlying psychiatric–mental health nursing practice, humanism means devotion to the interests of human beings wherever they live and whatever their status or culture. It reaffirms the spirit of compassion and caring toward others. It is a constructive philosophy that wholeheartedly affirms the joys, beauty, and values of human living.

The subsequent chapters in this text attempt to show how these basic premises can be put to use in psychiatric–mental health nursing practice. Some fundamental concepts are described briefly in the following sections.

A Holistic View of the Mind–Body Relationship. Our humanistic interactional view is that physical and mental factors are interrelated and that a change in one may result in a change in another. For example, anger may result in increased blood pressure. An invading organism, a decrease in a neurotransmitter, or a structural change in the body can alter thought processes. Low self-esteem can result in hunched shoulders and severe skeletal muscle contractures.

The implications for psychiatric–mental health nursing are clear. Healing and caring must be approached **holistically**. The psychiatric–mental health nurse deals with the biologic aspects of a primarily psychologic or emotional pattern and the psychologic or emotional aspects of biologic experiences.

CLINICAL EXAMPLE

Kate S., a prominent television personality who wants to remain anonymous, is hospitalized for a severe eating disorder on an integrated medical/psychiatric unit, and you are assigned to provide her care. She weighs under 90 pounds for her 5′ 7″ frame, is dehydrated, malnourished, and obsessed with getting back to work and looking good in an industry that expects bone-thin women anchors for the news.

As a nurse educated to recognize both her physical and her psychosocial needs, you are challenged to formulate a holistic, integrated care plan.

Psychiatric–mental health nursing care can be given not only in mental health care settings but also in general health care settings and may be directed toward clients whose immediate problems are primarily physical. This text will guide you with the requiste knowledge

An Expanded Role for Nurses. The humanistic interactional perspective on mental disorders implies an expanded role for psychiatric–mental health nurses. We believe that psychi-

Era of Magico-Religious Explanations
• Mental and physical suffering not differentiated.
•"Spirits of torment" acting outside the body are responsible for ills.
• No distinctions made between medicine, magic, and religion.
• Primitive healers address spirits by appeal, prayer, bribery, intimidation, appeasement, punishment.
• Healing methods include exorcism, magical ritual, incantation.

Preliterate Times

Era of Organic Explanations
• Hippocrates (460-370bc) rejects demonology and proposes that psychiatric illnesses caused by imbalances in "body humors:" blood, black bile, yellow bile, and phlegm.
• Psychiatric suffering comes within the realm of medical practice.
• Imbalances in body humors often corrected by bloodletting.

Early Civilization

Era of Alienation
• Return to the magic, mysticism, and demonology of preliterate times.
• Madness viewed as dramatic encounter with secret powers and influenced by the moon (lunacy).
• Malleus Maleficarum (The Witches' Hammer) by Dominican monks Johann Sprenger and Heinrich Kraemer published 1487 rationalized mental illness in terms of magical explanation.
• Violent insane shackled in prisons or sent to sea "in search of reason."

The Medieval Period

Early 20th Century

Era of Psychoanalysis
• Emil Kraepelin (1856–1926) creates system of distinct disease entities and differentiates bipolar disorder from schizophrenia.
• Sigmund Freud (1856–1939) explains human behavior in psychological terms and demonstrates that behavior can be changed through psychoanalysis.

Mid-20th Century

Era of Ideologic Expansion
• From the mid-1940s to the mid-1950s, a strong rift between biologic orientation and dynamic orientation develops.
• By the early 1950s several drugs for the treatment of mental disorder were in common use.
• In 1946 the National Institute of Mental Health (NIMH) opened for research, training, and provision of preventive, therapeutic, and rehabilitative psychiatric services.
• Harry Stack Sullivan (1892–1949) developed the interpersonal theory of psychiatry.
• By 1960 family therapy had become both a diagnostic tool and a mode of treatment.
• Erik Erikson formulated his psychosocial theory of development.
• Psychotropic drugs help staff members manage large numbers of clients in crowded conditions.
• Group therapy and short-term therapy recognized as options to costly long-term therapy or hospitalization.
• Milieu therapy developed by Maxwell Jones in England.

Late 20th Century

Deinstitutionalization and the Community Mental Health Movement
• In 1961the Joint Communication on Mental Illness and Health presented Action for Mental Health to Congress calling for a shift from institutional to community-based care, more equitable distribution of mental health services, preventive services, consumer participation in planning and delivery of mental health workers, education of more mental health professionals, public support for research, shared federal, state, local funding for construction and operation of community mental health centers.
• Congress passed the Mental Retardation Facilities and Community Mental Health Centers Construction Act.
• Between 1955 and 1975 the number of resident clients in state mental hospitals decreased nearly 66 percent.
• The Community Mental Health Systems Act of 1980 authorized funding of community mental health centers, services to high-risk populations, ambulatory mental health care centers, rape research and services, but was repealed in 1981 and replaced by the Omnibus Budget Reconciliation Act, placing mental health programs into an alcohol, drug abuse, and mental health services block grant.

FIGURE 2–1 ■ *A schematic of the history of psychiatry.*

The Renaissance

Era of Confinement
- In 1656 Hôpital Générale in Paris founded to confine the mad, poor, and various deviants.
- The "insane" have no recourse to appeal.
- Madness not linked to medicine; could only be mastered by discipline and brutality.
- Radical physicians like Johann Weyer (1515–1588) believed that "those illnesses whose origins are attributed to witches come from natural causes."

Late 18th and Early 19th Centuries

Era of Moral Treatment
- Physicians classify symptoms of mental disorders without understanding the sources of mental suffering.
- In 1794 Philippe Pinel (1745–1826) treated inmates in the French institutions Bicetre and Salpetriere with humanity and was thus considered mad.
- In England, William Tuke (1732–1822) focused on "moral treatment" in a humane milieu called the York Retreat.
- In America, Benjamin Rush (1746–1813) focused on humanitarianism and moral treatment at the Pennsylvania Hospital.

Late 19th and Early 20th Centuries

Era of Public Mental Hospitals
- Dorthea L. Dix (1802–1887) founds or enlarges over 30 mental hospitals.
- Moral treatment replaced by custodial care.
- Clifford Beers (1876–1943) published his book describing his own intense suffering and mental anguish, leading to the development of preventative psychiatry and the formation of child guidance clinics.

The 1990s

The Decade of the Brain
- The primary innovation of the 1990s is the "biologic revolution:" collaboration of science and technology to expand concepts of mental disorder proposed by psychological, behavioral, and psychoanalytic theories.
- A report by the National Advisory Health Council calls the gains made in research-based knowledge about the epidemiology, diagnosis, treatment, and prevention of major mental illnesses a "quantum leap in understanding the brain."
- Client advocacy groups welcome psychiatry's shift toward psychosocial rehabilitation for client self-care.
- The National Alliance for the Mentally Ill (NAMI), establishes a separate research foundation to study the biologic basis of major mental illness.

The New Millennium

Era of Health Care Reform
- Reform of psychiatric care has decreased length of hospital stays and increased client acuity.
- The advancing explosion in neuroscience has reshaped our conception of the bases of mental disorders.
- Innovations in technology have informed diagnostic practices such as brain imaging.
- The array of psychopharmacologic treatments available continues to expand.
- Populations of psychiatric clients include growing numbers of mentally ill elders, more people with coexisting substance use disorders, more comorbidities with chronic illnesses including HIV/AIDS, and expanding racial and cultural diversity.
- A yearning for spirituality has been reawakened in clients as well as health care providers.
- The study of genomes and the biology of the brain touch ethical, moral, and political nerves.

atric nurses should be prepared to work for change within social and political systems. Psychiatric–mental health nursing can no longer be limited to client-oriented activities designed exclusively to control symptoms and increase the capability of individuals to adjust satisfactorily to the existing social condition. Instead, psychiatric–mental health nursing must be involved in social goals that advance health holistically. Because psychiatric–mental health nursing has political consequences, it is essential that nurses begin to develop a philosophic and ethical framework to guide and evaluate the political outcome of therapeutic intervention.

Negotiation and Advocacy. In this book, the model for intervention and change is one of negotiation and advocacy. The responsibility for change remains with the person who seeks psychiatric help or consultation. Clients are held accountable for their own behavior. They are not the passive recipients of care given by psychiatric professionals. Instead, they are empowered in the process of developing new perspectives and encouraged to weigh alternatives and make self-directed choices. They and their families are educated about their disorder and their medications.

BASIC PREMISES OF PSYCHOBIOLOGY

The last decades have seen major breakthroughs in knowledge about the brain, the mind, the spirit, and behavior. This knowledge explosion has been termed **psychobiology**. Research has generated new understanding of how genetics, immunology, biorhythms, brain structure, and brain biochemistry influence mental disorders. New imaging techniques make it possible to view what has never been seen before. New drugs to correct biochemical imbalances in the brain are being prescribed. Researchers are exploring such psychobiologic interventions as exposure to bright light and white noise, and the restriction of nutrients and nonnutrients believed to affect behavior.

Implications for Psychiatric–Mental Health Nursing Practice

Some authorities argue that psychiatric–mental health nurses should continue to focus on the human aspects of care as psychiatry moves toward "remedicalization." They fear that by embracing the biologic sciences we will diminish the art of psychiatric–mental health nursing. Others, ourselves included, contend that, to bring a contemporary holistic perspective to psychiatric–mental health nursing care, we must integrate the rapidly accumulating knowledge in psychobiology. We do not give up our humanistic, psychosocial, and interactional premises simply because we recognize the value of the breakthroughs being made in psychobiology. Instead, as we redefine the traditional art of psychiatric–mental health nursing care and caring in the new millennium, our practice and research must integrate "high tech" and "high touch," nature and nurture, the biologic sciences and the behavioral sciences.

Theories for Interdisciplinary Psychiatric Care

Dominant social attitudes and philosophic viewpoints have influenced the understanding and approaches to mental disorder throughout history, and concepts that may be considered modern may have roots in earlier eras (see ■ Figure 2–1).

MEDICAL–PSYCHOBIOLOGIC THEORY

The medical–psychobiologic model in psychiatry originated in the era of classification. The classification of mental disturbances brought the emotional and behavioral aspects of people into the domain of the medical doctor. During this period, the systematic observation, naming, and classification of symptoms were emphasized. Emil Kraepelin's monumental descriptive diagnostic classification system is acknowledged as the first comprehensive medical model. It included the notions that the cause of mental illness was organic, that it was located in the central nervous system, that the disease followed a predictable course, and that treatment should be based on accurate diagnosis. Contemporary research findings in the field of psychobiology lend support to some of these early ideas but advance them and make them specific in important ways.

Assumptions and Key Ideas

Medical–psychobiologic theories view emotional and behavioral disturbances like any physical disease. Thus, abnormal behavior is directly attributable to a disease process, a lesion, a neuropathologic condition, a toxin introduced from outside the body, or (most recently) a biochemical abnormality of neurotransmitters and enzymes. The medical–psychobiologic position can be summarized as follows:

- The individual suffering from emotional disturbances is sick and has an illness or defect.
- The illness can, at least presumably, be located in some part of the body (usually the brain's limbic system and the central nervous system's synapse receptor sites). Factors related to mental disorders include excesses or deficiencies of certain brain neurotransmitters, alterations in the body's biologic rhythms, including the sleep-wake cycle; and genetic predispositions.
- The illness has characteristic structural, biochemical, and mental symptoms that can be diagnosed, classified, and labeled.
- Mental diseases run a characteristic course and have a particular prognosis for recovery.
- Mental disorders respond to physical or somatic treatments, including drugs, chemicals, hormones, diet, or surgery.
- Psychobiologic explanations of mental disorders can reduce the stigma often associated with them, and can discourage claims that mental disorders result from a lack of willpower or moral character.

Implications for Psychiatric–Mental Health Nursing Practice

Nurses who were first involved in the care of psychiatric clients were primarily responsible for the client's physical well-being. Their responsibilities included administering drugs prescribed by the physician and caring for clients undergoing treatments such as insulin shock, electroshock therapy, or hydrotherapy.

Psychobiologic theories are the conceptual basis for the continued use of biologic therapies in the care of psychiatric clients, the hospital as the setting for care, research into the genetic transmission of mental illness, research on biochemical and metabolic variables among diagnosed psychiatric clients, and dominance of the medical doctor—the psychiatrist—in the mental health team. As long as psychiatric clients are admitted to and reimbursed for care according to medical diagnoses, knowledge of this framework is crucial. Furthermore, as long as psychobiologic knowledge expands, psychiatric–mental health nurses are responsible for translating that knowledge into care practices that recognize the biologic factors related to mental disorders. Chapter 4 of this text provides an authoritative source of such contemporary psychobiologic knowledge. Advances in psychobiologic theory and research are also integrated throughout specific disorders and interventions chapters.

PSYCHOANALYTIC THEORY

Psychoanalytic theory is usually credited to the Viennese physician Sigmund Freud (1962b). Freud believed that all psychologic and emotional events, however obscure, were understandable. For the meanings behind behavior, he looked to childhood experiences that he believed caused adult neuroses. Psychoanalytic therapy consists of clarifying the meaning of events, feelings, and behavior and thereby gaining insight about them. Freud's work shifted the focus of psychiatry from classification to a dynamic view of mental phenomena.

Assumptions and Key Ideas

The basic principles of psychoanalytic theory are discussed below.

Psychic Determinism. Psychic determinism states that no human behavior is accidental. Each psychic event is determined by the ones that preceded it. Events in people's mental lives that seem random or unrelated to what went before are only apparently so. Thus, psychoanalysts never dismiss any mental phenomenon as meaningless or accidental. They always search for what caused it, why it happened. For example, people commonly forget or misplace things. They usually view this as just an accident. Psychoanalysts seek to demonstrate that the accident was caused by a wish or intent of the person involved. Psychoanalysts also view dreams as subject to the principle of psychic determinism, each dream and each image in each dream bearing some relationship to the rest of the dreamer's life.

Role of the Unconscious. Significant unconscious mental processes occur frequently in normal as well as abnormal mental functioning. These processes are called simply the *unconscious*. Much of what goes on in people's minds is unknown to them, and this accounts for the apparent discontinuities in their mental life. If the unconscious motivation of some behavioral symptoms is discovered, the apparent discontinuities disappear, and the cause becomes clear.

Psychoanalysis. The most powerful and reliable method for studying the unconscious is the technique that Freud evolved over several years called **psychoanalysis.** The basic logic behind psychoanalysis is as follows:

1. The client underwent a *traumatic experience* that stirred up intense and painful emotion.
2. The traumatic experience represented to the client some ideas that were incompatible with the dominant ideas constituting the ego. Thus, the client experienced a *neurotic conflict*.
3. The incompatible idea and the neurotic conflict associated with it force the ego to bring into action **defense mechanisms.** Chapter 5 describes in detail common defense mechanisms.
4. Therapy is directed toward resolving the conflict by uncovering its roots in the unconscious. If the client is able to release the repressed feelings associated with the conflict, the symptoms disappear.

Strategies used in psychoanalysis are hypnosis, the interpretation of dreams, and free association, in which the client is encouraged to express every idea that comes to mind—no matter how insignificant, irrelevant, shameful, or embarrassing—ignoring all self-censorship and suspending all judgment.

Topography of the Mind. Freud classified mental activities as levels of awareness in the mind; according to a body of thought now referred to as *topographic theory*. Any mental event that occurred outside of conscious awareness represented the **unconscious** region. Mental events that could be brought into conscious awareness through an act of attention were said to be **preconscious.** Those that occurred in conscious awareness were regarded as the **conscious** surface of the mind. This topographic model, although still used to classify mental events in terms of the quality and degree of awareness, has been supplanted by the structural model.

Structure of the Mind. With the publication of *The Ego and the Id* in 1923, Freud abandoned the topographic model of the mind for the *structural model* (1962a). The structural model of the mind contends that there are three distinct entities: the id, the ego, and the superego. The **id** is a completely unorganized reservoir of energy derived from drives and instincts. The **ego** controls action and perception, controls contact with reality, and, through the defense mechanisms, inhibits primary instinctual drives. One of its fundamental functions is also the capacity for developing mutually satisfying relationships with others. The **superego** is concerned with moral behavior. Frequently, the superego allies itself with the ego against the id, imposing demands in the form of conscience or guilt feelings. The id in a child operates according to what Freud called the *pleasure principle:* the tendency to seek pleasure and avoid pain. This is not always possible, so the demands of the pleasure principle have to be modified by the *reality principle.* The reality principle is a learned ego function by which people develop the capacity to delay the immediate release of tension or achievement of pleasure. The relationship between Freud's levels of awareness and his concepts of id, superego, and ego is often depicted as an iceberg (see ■ Figure 2–2). Using this image, the id is completely below the water's surface and the superego partially below and partially above the surface. In comparison to the superego, the ego is more fully above the surface in the realm of conscious awareness.

Drives. Freud believed that psychic energy was derived from drives. He used the word cathexis to refer to the attachment of psychic energy to a person or a thing. The greater the cathexis, the greater the psychologic importance of the person or object. Freud accounted for the instinctual aspects of a person's mental life by assuming the existence of two drives, the *sexual drive* and the *aggressive drive*. The former gives rise to the erotic component of mental activity, and the latter gives rise to the destructive component. The sexual drive came to be known as the *libido.* ■ Table 2–1 presents the stages of psychosexual development according to Freud.

Erikson's Eight Stages of Man. Freud's stages of personality development were called stages of psychosexual development because of the shifting emphasis of sources of pleasure or gratification. Erik Erikson, a neo-Freudian, also formulated a developmental theory of personality that attempted to take into account not just biologic instincts but also cultural and interpersonal tasks that have to be accomplished in order to move forward developmentally (■ Table 2–2). Erikson's developmental theory is also considered more optimistic than Freud's because he believed that clients in therapy could return to a developmental task that had not been accomplished and relearn it (Erikson, 1963).

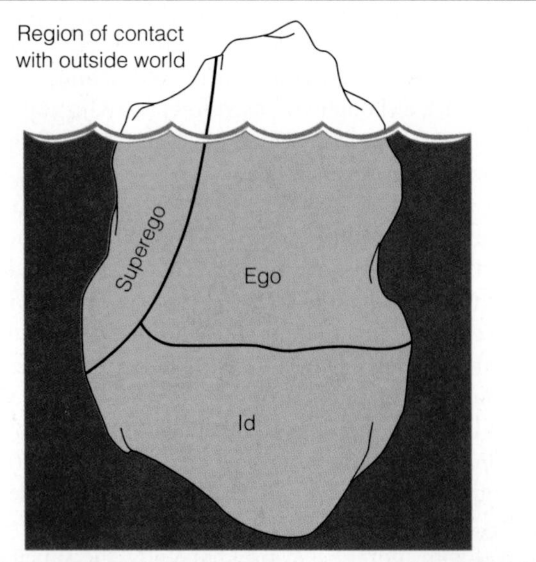

FIGURE 2–2 ■ *The relationship between levels of awareness components of the mental personality depicted as an iceberg.*

Implications for Psychiatric–Mental Health Nursing Practice

Psychoanalytic theory has historically provided a very limited treatment role for the nurse. Psychoanalytic clients are usually seen in the analyst's office as private clients. With the emergence of psychoanalytically oriented settings such as Chestnut Lodge in Rockville, Maryland, nurses became somewhat more involved, sharing at least in the psychoanalytic language, concepts, and speculations about client dynamics and personality development.

BEHAVIORIST THEORY

Behaviorist theory in psychiatry has its roots in psychology and neurophysiology. To the behaviorist, symptoms associated with neuroses and psychoses are clusters of learned behaviors that persist because they are somehow rewarding to the individual. One of the most important contributions to this framework was made by Pavlov (1849–1936), who in 1902 discovered a phenomenon he called the **conditioned response** in a famous experiment with a dog and a bell. The basic principle of the conditioned response is this:

1. A response is a reaction to a stimulus.
2. If a new and different stimulus is presented with or just before the original stimulating event, the same response reaction can be obtained.
3. Eventually the new stimulus can replace the original one, so that the response occurs in reaction to the new stimulus alone.

The conditioned or learned response is viewed as the basic unit of all learning, the unit on which more complex behavioral patterns are constructed. Such construction occurs through a process called **reinforcement,** in which behaviors are rewarded and persist. Pavlov's theories have continued into the present and are valued for their simplicity, concreteness, and objectivity. Some behaviorists see them as the key to understanding and controlling the whole range of undesirable human behavior.

Assumptions and Key Ideas

The fundamental premises of behaviorist theory are as follows:

- Human beings are merely complex animals. The difference between humans and other animals is one of degree and not kind. Thus the use of animal experience as an analog to human experience is clearly justifiable.
- The self in humans is the sum or repository of past conditionings or simply the behavioral repertoire. Therapists can know clients only by the clients' behavior.
- Behavior is the way in which an animal acts. It can be observed, described, and recorded.
- There is no autonomous person. People are what they do and what they are reinforced for doing by conditions in their environment.
- The self is a structure of stimulus–response chains or hierarchies of habit. It is possible to know and predict conditions under which behavior will occur.

TABLE 2–1 Freud's Psychosexual Stages

Stage	Age Span	Task	Key Concept
Oral	0–18 months	Satisfaction and anxiety management from oral activity	Oral activity gives pleasure and is a source for learning
Anal	18 months–3 years	Learning muscle control for toilet training	Delayed gratification and rule internalization
Phallic	3–6 years	Gender identification and genital awareness	Repression of attraction to the opposite-sex parent, leading to same-sex identification
Latency	6–12 years	Repression of sexuality	Oedipal conflict resolved with a shift to other interests and friends
Genital	12 years–young adult	Channeling sexuality into relationships with members of the opposite sex	Reemerging sexuality to motivate behavior

- The symptoms of a mental disorder are, in fact, the substance of that person's troubles. There is no hidden motive, no underlying cause, no internal pathogenic process. There is only the symptom or the behavior, and the aim of behaviorist therapy is to change the behavior.
- The classification of mental illness is meaningful only to provide legal labels. It provides little or no assistance in prescribing a treatment program.
- People can control others whether others want to be controlled or not. Control is neither good nor bad in and of itself.
- The therapist determines what behavior should be changed and what plan should be followed. Change is effected by identifying events in the client's life that have been critical stimuli for the behavior and then arranging interventions for *extinguishing* those behaviors. A changed way of acting precedes a changed way of thinking, according to behaviorist theory.

Both Joseph Wolpe (1956) and B. F. Skinner (1971) are associated with psychiatric treatment approaches that represent one form of **conditioning** and reflect the above assumptions. Wolpe

TABLE 2–2 Erikson's Eight Developmental Stages

Age	Stage of Development	Task/Area of Resolution	Concepts/Basic Attitudes
Birth–18 months	Infancy	Trust versus mistrust	Ability to trust others and a sense of one's own trustworthiness; a sense of hope; withdrawal and estrangement
18 months–3 years	Early childhood	Autonomy versus shame and doubt	Self-control without loss of self-esteem; ability to cooperate and to express oneself; compulsive self-restraint or compliance; defiance, willfulness
3–5 years	Late childhood	Initiative versus guilt	Realistic sense of purpose; some ability to evaluate one's own behavior; self-denial and self-restriction
6–12 years	School age	Industry versus inferiority	Realization of competence, perseverance; feeling that one will never be "any good," withdrawal from school and peers
12–20 years	Adolescence	Identity versus role diffusion	Coherent sense of self; plans to actualize one's abilities; feelings of confusion, indecisiveness, possibly antisocial behavior
18–25 years	Young adulthood	Intimacy versus isolation	Capacity for love as mutual devotion; commitment to work and relationships; impersonal relationships, prejudice
25–65 years	Adulthood	Generativity versus stagnation	Creativity, productivity, concern for others; self-indulgence, impoverishment of self
65 years to death	Old age	Integrity versus despair	Acceptance of the worth and uniqueness of one's life; sense of loss, contempt for others

Source: From *Identity and the Life Cycle* by Erik H. Erikson. Copyright 1980 by W. W. Norton & Company, Inc. Copyright © 1959 by International Universities Press, Inc. Used by permission of W. W. Norton & Company, Inc.

defined *neurotic behavior* as unadaptive behavior acquired in anxiety-generating situations. He based his therapeutic method on the introduction of a response that inhibits anxiety when situations occur that ordinarily evoke anxiety. Relaxation, for example, was considered incompatible with anxiety and, therefore, effective in inhibiting it. Thus, Wolpe would direct his intervention to a counterconditioning technique, usually putting the client under hypnosis and using various techniques for gradual *desensitization.* For example, a man afraid of dying might gradually attempt to overcome his anxiety at seeing a coffin, attending a funeral, and so on, by trying to relax in these situations.

Skinner's approach, called **operant conditioning,** emphasizes discovering why the behavioral response was elicited in the first place and what actively reinforces it. The key concept in operant conditioning is reinforcement. Skinner originally used the term **positive reinforcement** to describe an event that increases the probability that the response will recur—a reward for behavior. A **negative reinforcement** was defined as an event likely to decrease the possibility of recurrence because it penalizes the behavior.

Other contemporary behaviorists have redefined Skinner's original terms and introduced some new ones. Positive reinforcement is still an environmental event that rewards and thus increases the probability of a behavioral response. Negative reinforcement can mean removal of an adverse stimulus (such as an electric shock to animals or the restriction of people's privileges) to increase the likelihood of a behavior's recurrence. *Positive punishment,* in contrast, is the introduction of aversive stimuli to decrease the likelihood of the recurrence of a behavior. *Negative punishment* removes something that has been a prior reinforcer, thus again decreasing the likelihood of such behaviors as smoking, drug abuse, truancy, temper outbursts, and abuse. ■ Table 2–3 lists examples of each of these behaviorist concepts.

The term for an intervention designed to change a client's behavior is **shaping.** It is a procedure of manipulating reinforcement to bring the person closer to the desired behavior. There are, according to Skinner, times in a client's life when responses are accidentally reinforced by a coincidental pairing of response and reinforcement. This accidental pairing may play a role in the development of phobias (irrational fears) and other distressing and/or dysfunctional behaviors.

Implications for Psychiatric–Mental Health Nursing Practice

Most psychiatric–mental health nurses acknowledge that the application of principles of behavior modification to clients is quite complex. The use of this approach raises issues of control, responsibility for behavior, and the morality of using negative or punitive stimuli in a therapeutic context, to name only a few. Therapists who successfully resolve such basic philosophic issues have designed and implemented successful behavior-modification plans with disturbed, overtly aggressive children, developmentally disabled clients, and violently self-destructive people.

In many institutional environments, clients follow prescribed schedules for daily living that include a **token economy.** Clients are rewarded for desired behavior by token reinforcers, such as food, candy, and verbal approval. The movement toward community-based psychiatric treatment has made plain some of the shortcomings and economic realities of therapies aimed toward resolving everyone's intrapsychic conflicts. The movement has instead attempted to replace maladaptive behavior with behavior that allows people to function effectively within their natural environment. When parents or others in the client's environment are taught to implement the behavior change procedures, therapy moves away from the artificial situation of the therapist's office into the client's total environment. It no longer requires the presence of highly trained, often expensive experts and thus makes treatment more affordable.

Psychiatric–mental health nurses have had a special role in teaching behaviorist principles to people with little training so that they can act as change agents. Nonprofessional staff on psychiatric wards can be taught the effective use of behaviorist principles to eliminate chronic, maladaptive behavior. Hyperactive children or children with borderline intelligence can be treated in the home by their parents when nurses teach the parents to use approaches such as frequency counts on specific behaviors to be modified, time-outs (short periods of isolation) for undesired behavior, and the bestowal of attention, praise, and affectionate physical contact as rewards.

SOCIAL–INTERPERSONAL THEORIES

Social–interpersonal theories of psychiatry grew out of a general dissatisfaction with approaches that account for mental ill-

TABLE 2–3 Examples of Behaviorist Concepts

Concept	Purpose	Example
Positive reinforcer	Increase recurrence of the behavior through reward	Leave of absence from the hospital, percontract with the client
Negative reinforcer	Increase recurrence of the behavior by removing aversive consequences	Removal of restrictions on phone calls or visitors, per contract with client
Positive punishment	Decrease the behavior by adding aversive consequences	Quiet time
Negative punishment	Decrease the behavior by withdrawing a reinforcer or reward	Withdrawal of privileges, such as recreational outings in a residential milieu

ness in terms of either intrapersonal mechanisms (the symptoms of a disease) or individual personality dynamics such as anxiety, ego strength, and libido. Advocates of this perspective assert that other theories neglect the crucial social processes and cultural variation involved in the development, identification, and resolution of disturbed human responses.

Assumptions and Key Ideas

Three separate but philosophically congruent schools of thought contribute to social–interpersonal theories. These are the labeling theory, the interpersonal–psychiatric, and the general systems approaches. The assumptions and key ideas of each are discussed below.

Labeling Theory. The *labeling theory* approach is summarized partially by sociologist Kai Erikson (1962): "Deviance is not a property inherent in certain forms of behavior; it is a property conferred upon these forms by audiences which directly or indirectly witness them." Thus, mental illness is a *label* applied to certain behaviors that violate the rules of conduct imposed by others.

Interpersonal–Psychiatric Theory. Psychiatrists Adolf Meyer (1948–1952) and Harry Stack Sullivan (1953) made significant contributions to social–interpersonal theory in the first half of the twentieth century. Sullivan trained with William Alanson White and Adolf Meyer rather than Freud. He is viewed as the least reductionist of psychiatric theorists and emphasizes modes of interaction as the real focus of psychiatric inquiry. Sullivan became the theoretic and ideologic leader of the interpersonal school of psychiatry often associated with the William Alanson White Foundation.

One concept that plays a crucial role in the organization of behavior, according to Sullivan, is the **self-system** or *self-dynamism.* The self-system provides tools that enable people to deal with the tasks of avoiding anxiety and establishing security. The self is a construct built from the child's experience. It is made up of **reflected appraisals** the person learns in contact with significant others. The self develops in the process of seeking physical satisfaction of bodily needs and security. To feel secure, the self essentially requires feelings of approval and prestige as protection against anxiety. Rewarding appraisals from others yield what Sullivan calls the *good-me* aspect of the self. Anxiety-producing appraisals result in the *bad-me.* The *not-me* exists normally in dreams and in aspects of experience that are poorly understood and later experienced as dread, horror, and loathing among mentally disordered people. In summary, Sullivan emphasizes the pervasive interaction between the organism and the environment.

Sullivan emphasizes the developmental tasks of the personality (■ Table 2–4). Nonetheless, Sullivan has little to say about the impact on behavior of specific variations in the social or cultural scene. Like Sullivan, other advocates of the interpersonal school of psychiatry, such as Karen Horney (1950) and Erich Fromm (1941), stress the general climate in the immediate family. Alfred Adler (1971), however, attempts to understand more of the social and cultural conditions influencing behavior. The interpersonal school of psychiatry in general focuses less on social context than the labeling theory perspective and takes a developmental–interpersonal view of the self. The *self-actualization* and hierarchy of needs theories of Abraham Maslow (1962) belong squarely in this school (■ Figure 2–3).

General Systems Theory. **General systems theory,** when applied to living systems (people), provides a conceptual framework for integrating the biologic and social sciences with the physical sciences. In psychiatry, it offers a resolution of the mind–body dichotomy, an integration of biologic and social approaches to the nature of human beings, and an approach to psychopathology, diagnosis, and therapy. Karl Menninger (1963) views normal personality functioning and psychopathology in terms of general systems theory. His work addresses four major issues:

TABLE 2–4 Sullivan's Stages of Interpersonal Development

Age	Stage	Task/Key Concept
Birth–18 months (to appearance of speech)	Infancy	Experiences anxiety in interaction with mother figure; learns to use maternal tenderness to gain security and avoid anxiety
18 months–6 years (from first speech to need for playmates)	Childhood	Learns to delay gratification in response to interpersonal demands; uses language and action to avoid anxiety
6–9 years	Juvenile	Develops peer relationships and uses environment outside the family to shape self
9–12 years	Preadolescence	Develops a caring relationship with same-sex peer, chum relationship
12–14 years	Early adolescence	Develops interest in opposite-sex relationships
14–21 years	Late adolescence	Has satisfying relationships; directs sexual impulses
21 years +	Adulthood	Establishes a love relationship

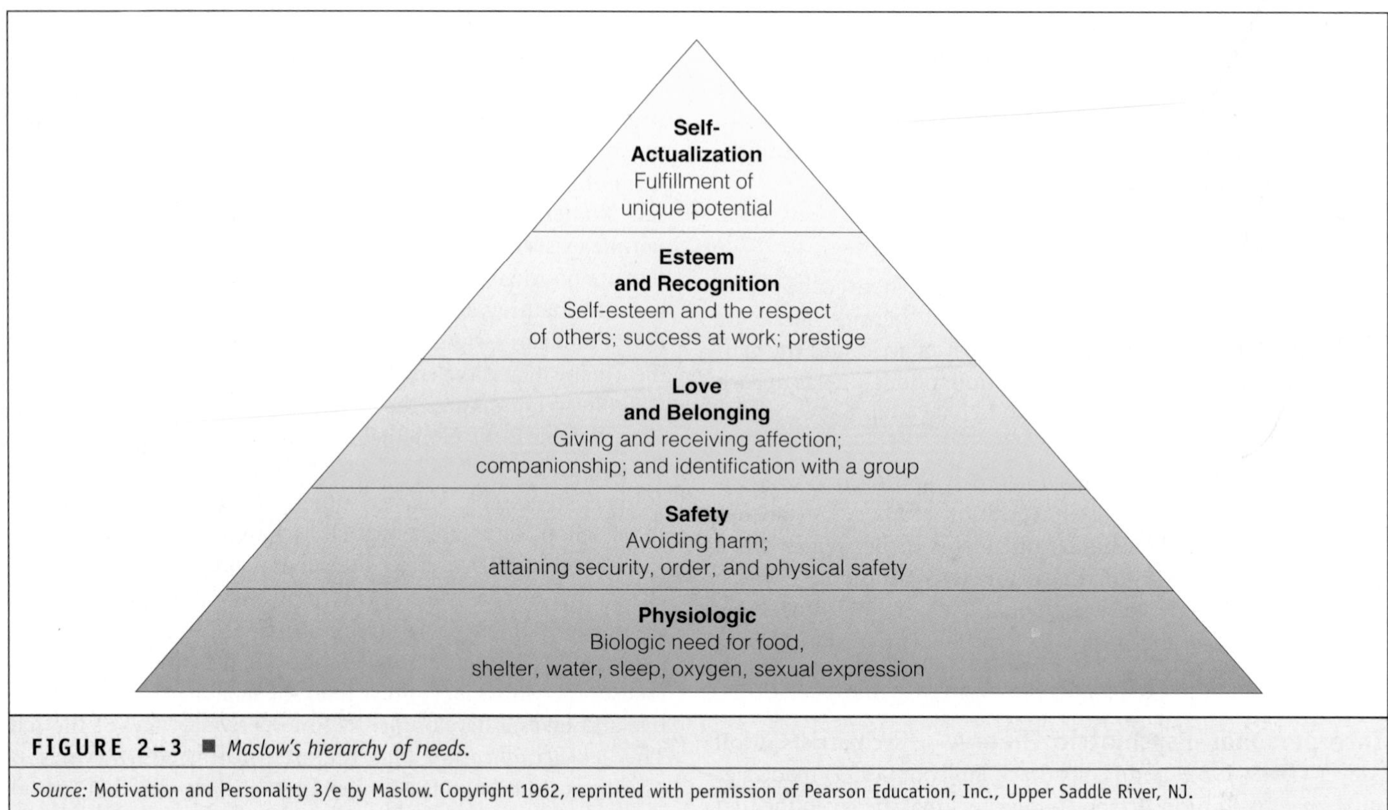

FIGURE 2–3 ■ *Maslow's hierarchy of needs.*

Source: Motivation and Personality 3/e by Maslow. Copyright 1962, reprinted with permission of Pearson Education, Inc., Upper Saddle River, NJ.

1. Adjustment or individual–environment interaction.
2. The organization of living systems.
3. Psychologic regulation and control, known as *ego theory* in psychoanalysis.
4. Motivation, which is often called *instinct* or *drive* in the psychoanalytic framework.

A salient point of Menninger's theory is the idea of *homeostasis* (equilibrium). He asserts that the greater the threat or stress on a system, the greater the number of system components involved in coping with or adapting to it. Therefore, pathology can exist at various levels, from the cell and organ level to the group and community level. An example of the former might be the behavioral changes that follow cellular alterations due to addictive drugs, to a blood clot, or to a tumor. Examples of pathology at the group level include family violence. At the community level, overpopulation, pollution, homelessness, and poverty are instances of pathology. In general systems theory, all represent abnormalities or stresses on matter–energy processes and would be included within the domain of psychiatric professionals.

In Menninger's view, a system's well-being depends on the amount of stress on it and the effectiveness of its coping mechanisms. He asserts that "mental illness" is an impairment of self-regulation in which comfort, growth, and production are surrendered for the sake of survival at the best level possible but at the sacrifice of emergency coping devices. Therapists using the general systems approach emphasize current conflicts, restoration of impaired systems of functioning, and subsequent reintegration of the restored function into future coping strategies.

Implications for Psychiatric–Mental Health Nursing Practice

Social–interpersonal theories give independent and collaborative psychiatric–mental health nursing clear theoretic direction and support. Nursing roles are associated with shifts in the delivery of psychiatric services variously termed *case management, social psychiatry, community psychiatry, psychoeducation*, and *milieu therapy.* All are associated with efforts to provide psychiatric services more efficiently to large groups of people, particularly those previously neglected, and attempts to counteract the debilitating effects of long-term institutionalization. All are also associated with a movement to address the client's social context in providing psychiatric care. According to these orientations, all social, psychologic, and biologic activity, including research developments in psychobiology, affecting the mental health of the population is important to professionals in community psychiatry. Therapeutic interventions may include programs for social change, political involvement, community organization, social planning, family support groups, and education about medications, symptom management, and family environment. Many implications for practice can be derived from this theoretic model:

- Clients are approached in a holistic way, reflecting the interrelationship and interaction between the biophysical, psychologic, and socioeconomic–cultural dimensions of human life. This increases the number of factors the nurse must assess when caring for a client.

- Because of the increased number and diversity of variables to be considered, graduate and undergraduate content in psychiatric–mental health nursing education must be revised. Curricula must include concepts, theories, and research findings to support extended thinking about mental health, culture, social systems, ethnicity, deviant behavior, social support, psychobiology, and the human condition. These new content areas drawn from the social and natural sciences must then be integrated with conventional psychiatric–mental health nursing content to form an internal coherent knowledge base.
- Definitions of the client must include the concept of the client system. A family, a couple, an aggregate, or even a community may collectively constitute the client.
- Intervention strategies include **primary prevention** achieved through psychoeducation, social change, and research.
- Therapy focuses on helping troubled people gain a useful perspective on their lifestyle and social environment and develop coping skills and resources, rather than on exclusively repressing and controlling their symptoms.
- The psychiatric–mental health nurse must be prepared to function as an autonomous member of the mental health team and to assume more responsibilities. There is a shift away from the dominance of the physician in decision making and toward diffusion of roles. Practitioners' roles are based less on background discipline than on availability and interest in helping the client. For example, a cadre of mental health professionals who could become chronic care experts is sorely needed, particularly those who can synthesize psychobiologic knowledge with psychosocial rehabilitation skills and psychoeducation.

Once clients are viewed as becoming dysfunctional in the context of unhealthy or problem-filled interpersonal relationships, establishing healthy, constructive interpersonal relationships becomes important in their care. Psychiatric nurses can apply concepts of milieu therapy, primary prevention, social psychiatry, community psychiatry, and psychobiologic interventions to implement this fundamental idea. The following case example is an illustration:

CLINICAL EXAMPLE

Mrs. Seminara is a 67-year-old, upper-middle-class woman in good physical health. She has become increasingly untidy, forgetful, reclusive, sad, and suspicious since the death of her aggressive, bank president husband from a heart attack six months ago. She recently sold the large house where she had lived for the past 45 years and moved into a two-bedroom apartment in a nearby town. Because of apartment rules, she was unable to take her 12-year-old cat. She sold the house because her husband had told his lawyers that she should do so. (He had made all the family decisions while he lived.) Mrs. Seminara has taken to skipping meals except for candy bars because she must rely on a friend to drive her to the grocery store. (Her husband never felt she needed to learn to drive.) Her younger sister (age 59), seeking advice about Mrs. Seminara's behavior, phoned the community mental health center at the suggestion of the family physician.

The social–interpersonal psychiatric–mental health nurse assessing this situation would tend not to view Mrs. Seminara's symptoms as psychologic conflicts reflecting her ambivalence toward her dead husband or as manifestations of a mental disorder, such as major, single-episode depression. Instead, the nurse would focus on the way Mrs. Seminara is functioning in her current interpersonal situation and her holistic human responses to it. In this analysis, the nurse does not view Mrs. Seminara as "diseased" and therefore in exclusive need of a somatic treatment such as medication. Instead, treatment consists of helping Mrs. Seminara develop strategies for coping with her new situation and satisfying her needs. The nurse would seek out the younger sister and other family members in an attempt to enhance Mrs. Seminara's social support network. Efforts may be directed toward mobilizing other environmental forces (including the nurse) to provide company, stimulation, and proper nutrition for Mrs. Seminara, since the absence of all three contributes to her symptoms and discomfort. The clinical situation would undoubtedly reinforce the psychiatric nurse's political efforts to point out the potential consequences of lifelong passive dependence of some adult women. The nurse may also become involved in community organizations working for better services for older clients. ■ Table 2–5 on page 38 presents a comparison of the traditional theories upon which psychiatric–mental health nurses base their plans of care.

Nursing's Theoretic Heritage

The concept of nursing as primarily technologic has been replaced by the idea that nursing is theory-based. Still, nursing remains more divergent than convergent when it comes to identifying the theories to be applied. Most authorities concur that *theoretic pluralism*—the simultaneous refinement and testing of numerous contenders for **nursing theory**—is highly appropriate for the present phase in nursing's scientific and intellectual history. Let's briefly examine a few of the best-known nursing theorists and identify the concepts and principles most relevant to psychiatric–mental health nursing. Most of these theorists accept the focal concepts for nursing as *people, nursing, health*, and *society*.

PEPLAU

Hildegard Peplau published her nursing theory in the classic book *Interpersonal Relations in Nursing* (1952). She defined nursing as a significant therapeutic interpersonal process, and the core concepts of her theory were the four phases of the nurse–client relationship:

TABLE 2–5 Major Features of Traditional Psychiatric Theories Compared

Theory	Assessment Base	Problem Statement	Goal	Dominant Interventions
Medical–psychobiologic	Individual client symptoms	Disease	Symptom management; cure	Psychopharmacology and other biologic therapies
Psychoanalytic	Intrapsychic; unconscious	Conflict	Insight	Psychoanalysis
Behaviorist	Behavior	Learning deficit	Behavior change	Behavior modification or conditioning
Social-interpersonal	Interactions between individual and social contexts	Interpersonal dysfunction	Enhanced awareness and quality of interpersonal interactions	Group, family, and milieu therapies

1. Orientation
2. Identification
3. Exploitation (or working)
4. Resolution

Some say that these phases are ancestors of the phases of the nursing process. Psychiatric–mental health nurses continue to use Peplau's theory to understand and guide decisions in the one-to-one therapeutic relationship. Refer to Chapter 28 for details on individual counseling.

OREM

Dorothea Orem's (1971) theory of self-care was originally introduced around 1959 and identified 10 universal self-care requisites, divided into 6 categories that encompass both physical and psychosocial human needs. Orem also introduced a second order of concepts originally called health deviation self-care demands to refer to care required in the event of illness, injury, or disease. Nursing, a second key component of her scheme, was divided into compensatory, partially compensatory, and supportive–educational systems of care that could be matched to the client's assessed level of self-care functioning in each area. This theory firmly established the notion of a goal of self-care as integral to the discipline of nursing's perspective on the meaning of health (Orem, 1995). Orem's theory is particularly well adapted to meeting nursing care needs of the severely and chronically mentally ill.

ROGERS

Martha Rogers (1970) drew on knowledge from anthropology, sociology, religion, philosophy, mythology, and general systems theory to define nursing as a holistic science of unitary human beings. Rogers' key nursing principles, called the principles of homeodynamics, view human beings holistically. Changes in life processes are irreversible, nonrepeatable, and rhythmic and indicate patterns of increasing complexity and organization. Most of her concepts have counterparts in general systems theory, but she has added the notions of life processes, change, and human–environmental interaction to the concepts central to nursing. Rogers' work gives psychiatric–mental health nurses a mandate to use holistic principles as a guide to practice and to consider human being and environment interactions and change.

ROY

Sister Callista Roy's (1976) adaptation theory views people as constantly faced with the need to adapt to focal, contextual, and residual stimuli. She identifies four modes of human adapting: *physiologic needs, self-concept, role function,* and *interdependence.* Obviously, these adaptive modes again include physiologic, psychologic, and social aspects of people. The notion of coping or adapting to stimuli again relates nursing to people in interaction with their environment. Recent versions of Roy's adaptation theory have incorporated humanistic assumptions about the dignity of human beings and the role of nurses in promoting integrity (Roy & Andrews, 1999).

ORLANDO

Ida Jean Orlando's theory (1961) grew out of dissatisfaction with the possibility that nursing care was governed by organizational rules rather than attention to client needs. She emphasized the importance of deliberative nursing action based on the meanings that are validated between the nurse and client.

WIEDENBACH

Ernestine Wiedenbach (1964) was influenced by the work of Orlando. Her theory was also developed around the client's need for help and validation of such need through client perceptions. She was particularly interested in problems of discomfort and the nurse's role in observing, assessing, exploring, and validating feelings, thoughts, and fears.

TRAVELBEE

Joyce Travelbee is another nurse theorist who, along with Orlando and Weidenbach, focuses on the meaning in nurse–client interactions. Travelbee (1966) explains in detail the concepts of sympathy, rapport, and suffering and emphasizes the importance of communication and stages of nurse–client relationships. Her view of humanity, uniqueness, existential encounters, and nursing is highly congruent with values in psychiatric–mental health nursing.

Nursing Theory's Contemporary Directions

Each of the early nursing theorists has revisited her original formulation to move closer to psychiatric–mental health nursing values of humanism, interactionism, cultural competence, the relevance of meaning and the importance of empathy and empowerment in the nurse–client relationship. The late Joyce Travelbee, discussed in the preceding section; Josephine Paterson and Loretta Zderad; and Jean Watson are theorists whose existential origins and subsequent conceptualizations are particularly congruent with the philosophy of psychiatric–mental health nursing advocated in this text.

PATERSON AND ZDERAD

Paterson and Zderad's 1976 book was republished in 1988, reflecting the contemporary nature of their original ideas. They were a decade ahead of their time in rejecting a mechanistic cause and effect view of nursing science and urged instead that observations of the experience of nurses in practice should be the basis of any useful nursing theory. Their theory portrays nursing as a lived dialogue that incorporates an intersubjective transaction in which both nurse and client are present in the experience in an existential way that includes mutuality and intimacy. Their theory relies heavily on existential philosophers and emphasizes the freedom of human choice and responsibility for one's actions. It is a highly abstract theory with a major focus on the process of interaction (or dialogue) between nurse and client.

WATSON

Jean Watson's theory of human caring was influenced by Jungian psychology, feminist theory, and Maslow's psychologic concept of self-actualization (Watson, 1988). Caring–healing within Watson's framework is based on values such as kindness, concern, and love of self and others and involves what she terms as *carative* factors: a humanistic–altruistic value system, faith–hope, and sensitivity of self and others. Her theory emphasizes sensitivity to self and values clarification regarding personal and cultural beliefs that might pose barriers to transpersonal caring. Establishing a helping–trusting human care relationship is pivotal to Watson's theory. She credits much of her thinking on therapeutic relationships and communication to the work of Carl Rogers, identifying congruency, empathy, and warmth as foundational to a caring relationship that conveys authenticity and genuineness and facilitates the client's expression of emotions. In her most recent work, Watson also develops the notion of spiritual environment and the interconnectedness of all things including the connection between healing and the ecology of the earth (Watson, 1999).

BENNER

Patricia Benner (1983, 1996, 1999), part philosopher, part theorist, has added to nursing's understanding of the language of caring. Her ideas have been generated by observing and interviewing nurses engaged in clinical practice. Her goal has been to disclose the nature of clinical wisdom, particularly around caring and comforting practices. She argues for the importance of forming nurse–client relationships, teaching and coaching, and bearing witness to the illness experience.

Implications for Psychiatric–Mental Health Nursing Practice

The **interpersonal theory** of psychiatric–mental health nursing originated by Hildegard Peplau (1952) remains the nursing theory that has shaped psychiatric–mental health nursing most directly. Influenced by American psychiatrist Harry Stack Sullivan and learning theorist Carl Rogers, Peplau conceptualized the one-to-one nurse–client relationship as the situation in which clients can accomplish developmental tasks such as learning to trust or learning to collaborate and practice healthy communication and behaviors. More contemporary nurse theorists, however, have also laid the foundation for concepts that are central to psychiatric–mental health nursing practice. Nursing theorists have:

USING RESEARCH EVIDENCE

Anile M is a 21-year-old native of New Delhi, India. She was brought to the United States after a devastating earthquake destroyed her entire family and her family's home. She is living with an uncle who married an American in a large, urban East Coast city. Her American relatives stay with her in the outpatient psychiatric clinic because she has severe nightmares, refuses to eat, and cries most of the day. Her psychiatric diagnosis is posttraumatic stress disorder, and she is started on appropriate medications. As her psychiatric–mental health nurse and case manager, you formulate a nursing care plan that addresses the following considerations.

1. Anile is not only suffering symptoms of posttraumatic stress disorder but she is engaged in the process of multiple transitions. To understand the transitions fully, it will be necessary to uncover and describe the effects and the meanings of the changes involved.
2. Providing a culturally competent clinician with whom she can feel and stay connected is cited as an important condition for a positive transition experience.
3. The client's confidence, coping and mastery of new skills, and behaviors needed to manage the new situation and environment influence healthy completion of a transition. You deliberately include client teaching to support Anile in interpreting her symptoms, making decisions, taking action, accessing resources, and negotiating with the U.S. health care system.

Your plan of care is based on both theory and research, summarized in the following journal article:

Meleis, A., Sawyer, L. M., Messias, D. K. H., & Schumacher, K. (2000). Experiencing transitions: An emerging middle-range theory. *Advances in Nursing Science, 23*(1), 12–28.

- Differentiated nursing from medicine with emphases on caring and comforting rather than curing.
- Placed the importance of interpreting meaning at the center of their theories.
- Focused on interaction between the nurse and the client.
- Advocated humanistic and existential values of client dignity and nurse authenticity as crucial to quality of care.

A review of nursing theories indicates some clear differences in emphasis and perspective and some intriguing similarities. From these theories the parameters of our discipline emerge. Such parameters provide the beginnings for directing practice, focusing nursing research, and providing a framework of concepts integral to the preparation of professional students. For points of critique of nursing theories, see A. I. Meleis's authoritative book, *Theoretical Nursing* (1997).

Approaches associated with two or more different theories are often used in combination. For example, bizarre, self-destructive behavior may be controlled with medications so that the client is more available for group or individual therapy. Such a combined or eclectic approach demands that you be capable of functioning according to all theories of care, depending on which is best for the client and best fits the resources and limitations of the situation. If you give adequate consideration to the theoretic framework of your psychiatric–mental health nursing, you will foster practice-oriented research and clinical judgments that can be articulated and taught to others. Research is a tool for developing psychiatric–mental health nursing theory that synthesizes the most useful elements of these theories.

Nursing SELF-AWARENESS

Choosing a Theory

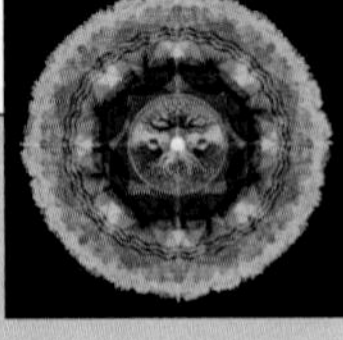

Psychiatric–mental health nurses use one or a combination of the theories presented in this chapter to interpret the meaning of client behavior and to apply the nursing process to their practice. In clinical work the selection of theories for practice may be influenced by a variety of factors. Ask yourself these questions:

1. What theory do you rely on to interpret the meaning of client behaviors?
2. What theory most accurately conceptualizes the client outcomes and interventions you use?
3. How has your education influenced your choice of theories?
4. How does the service setting (including the recording and payment systems) influence your choice of theories?
5. How does the need to be efficient and practical influence your choice of theories?
6. How do attributes such as the race, ethnicity, age, gender, and social class of clients influence your choice of theories?

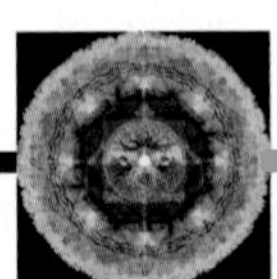

EXPLORE MediaLink

NCLEX review, case studies, and other interactive resources for this chapter can be found on the Companion Website at http://www.prenhall.com/kneisl. Click on Chapter 2 to select the activities for this chapter.

For animations, video tutorials, more NCLEX review questions, and an audio glossary, access the accompanying CD-ROM in this textbook.

BIBLIOGRAPHY

Adler, A. (1971). *The practice and theory of individual psychology.* New York: Humanities Press. Trans.

American Psychiatric Association (2000). *Diagnostic and statistical manual of mental disorders* (4th ed., Text Revision) (DSM-IV-TR). Washington, DC: Author.

Benner, P. (1983). Uncovering the knowledge embedded in clinical practice. *Image: Journal of Nursing Scholarship 15*(2), 36–41.

Benner, P. (1996). *Expertise in nursing practice: Caring, clinical judgment and ethics.* New York: Springer.

Benner, P. (1999). *Clinical wisdom and interventions in critical care: A thinking-in-action approach.* Philadelphia: Saunders.

Blumer, H. (1969). *Symbolic interaction: Perspective and method.* New York: Prentice Hall.

Erikson, E. (1963). *Childhood and society* (2nd ed.). New York: Norton.

Erikson, K. (1962). Notes on the sociology of deviance. *Social Problems, 9,* 308.

Freud, S. (1962a). *The ego and the id.* New York: Norton.

Freud, S. (1962b). *The standard edition of the complete psychological works of Sigmund Freud* (24 vols). New York: Hogarth Press.

Fromm, E. (1941, Winter). *Escape from freedom.* New York: Irvington.

Henderson, V. (1966). *The nature of nursing.* New York: Macmillan.

Horney, K. (1950). *Neurosis and human growth.* New York: Norton.

King, I. M. (1971). *Toward a theory of nursing: General concepts of human behavior.* New York: Norton.

Lamont, C. (1967). *The philosophy of humanism.* New York: Frederick Ungar.

Maslow, A. (1962). *Toward a psychology of being.* New York: Van Nostrand.

Meleis, A., Sawyer, L. M., Messias, D. K. H., & Schumacher, K. (2000). Experiencing transitions: An emerging middle-range theory. *Advances in Nursing Science, 23*(1), 12–28.

Menninger, K. (1963). *The vital balance.* New York: Viking Press.

Meyer, A. (1948–52). *Collected papers of Adolf Meyer, 1–4.* Baltimore: Johns Hopkins University Press.

Murray, C. J., & Lopez, A. D. (1996). Evidence-based health policy: Lessons from the Global Burden of Disease Study. *Science, 274*, 740–761.

Orem, D. E. (1971). *Nursing: Concepts of practice.* New York: McGraw-Hill.

Orem, D. E. (1995). *Nursing: Concepts of practice* (5th ed.). New York: McGraw-Hill.

Orlando, I. (1961). *The dynamic nurse–patient relationship.* New York: G. P. Putnam's Sons.

Patterson, J. G., & Zderad, L. T. (1988). *Humanistic nursing* (Publication No. 41-2218). New York: National League for Nursing.

Peplau, H. E. (1952). *Interpersonal relations in nursing.* New York: Putnam.

Rogers, M. E. (1970). *The theoretical basis in nursing.* New York: F. A. Davis.

Roy, C. (1976). *Introduction to nursing: An adaptation model.* New York: Prentice Hall.

Roy, C., & Andrews, H. A. (1991). *The Roy Adaptation Model: The definitive statement.* Norwalk, CT: Appleton & Lange.

Skinner, B. F. (1971). *Beyond freedom and dignity.* New York: Prentice Hall.

Travelbee, J. (1966). *Interpersonal aspects of nursing.* Philadelphia: Davis.

U.S. Department of Health and Human Services (1999). *Mental health: A report of the surgeon general.* Rockville, MD: National Institute of Mental Health.

U.S. Department of Health and Human Services (2002). *Healthy people 2010.* Retrieved August 20, 2002, from the World Wide Web, http://www.healthypeople.gov.

Watson, J. (1988). New dimensions in human caring theory. *Nursing Science Quarterly, 1*(4), 175–181.

Watson, J. (1999). *Postmodern nursing and beyond.* New York: Churchill Livingstone.

Wiedenbach, E. (1964). *Clinical nursing: A helping art.* New York: Springer.

Wolpe, J. (1956). Learning versus lesions as the basis of neurotic behavior. *American Journal of Psychiatry, 112*, 923–931.

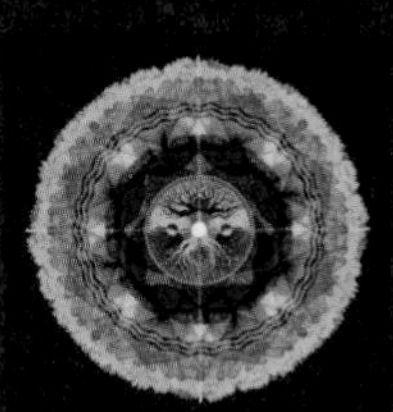

3

Chapter THREE

Evidence-Based Practice in Psychiatric–Mental Health Nursing

HOLLY SKODOL WILSON

KEY TERMS

best practices
clinical algorithms
critical pathways
ethnography
evidence-based practice
practice guidelines
randomized clinical trials

FOCUS QUESTIONS

- **What is the meaning of "evidence-based" psychiatric–mental health nursing practice?**
- **How have contemporary conditions in the psychiatric–mental health environment created a mandate for evidence-based practice?**
- **Why is the ability to think critically essential to evidence-based practice?**
- **What steps are involved in developing a system of evidence-based psychiatric nursing care?**
- **How do you find the best evidence?**
- **How do you evaluate evidence you find?**

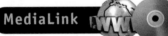

MediaLink 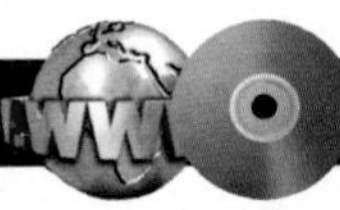 www.prenhall.com/kneisl

Additional resources for this chapter can be found on the Student CD-ROM accompanying this textbook, and on the Companion Website at www.prenhall.com/kneisl. Click on Chapter 3 to select the activities for this chapter.

CD-ROM
- Audio Glossary
- NCLEX Review

Companion Website
- Additional NCLEX Review
- Case Study: Evaluating Evidence

CHAPTER OUTLINE

Cross References

Other topics relevant to this content are: Assessment documentation, Chapter 9; Client rights regarding research, Chapter 10; Ethics, Chapter 10; Liability and the psychiatric nurse, Chapter 10; Outcome measurement, Chapter 7; Practice guidelines for psychiatric–mental health nursing, Chapter 1; Strategies that promote critical thinking, Chapter 1

CRITICAL THINKING CHALLENGE

You work in the "Dual Diagnosis" Unit of a community hospital in Southern California, where more and more clients are being referred after drug offenses. Even though you are a new graduate, expectations associated with your professional role, as well as the contemporary nursing shortage, require you to assume major leadership responsibilities for shaping psychiatric–mental health nursing practice on your unit. You are asked to change the system of psychiatric–mental health nursing to "evidence-based practice." What does this term mean, and how do you intend to accomplish this mandate? What support will you need from nursing management? Do you agree that the "gold standard" for care must be randomized clinical trials conducted in traditional research designed to test hypotheses? What is the place of critical thinking, clinical wisdom, and client preference in the context of evidence-based practice? How will a narrow vision of evidence-based practice limit and constrain your staff's ability to individualize care? ■

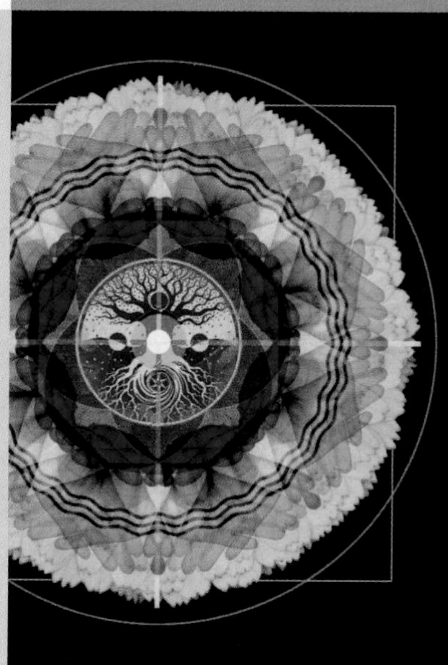

Every nurse in our field of psychiatric–mental health has always cared enough to believe that whatever we did or taught to other nurses could ultimately be helpful to clients. We embraced the potential to give a battered woman support as she stands strong in a court of law; we have helped estranged families reconcile; we have cared enough to provide comfort and hope to addicts withdrawing in a jail. We have taught the chronically mentally ill living skills so they could wash their own clothes and shop for their own food. We have invited dancers and musicians into geropsychiatric settings to provide stimulation and enhance quality of life. We have been present to consult about what psychotropic medicines are safe to give to a dehydrated homeless person in the emergency room. We have led groups in which grieving parents feel free to express their feelings and established therapeutic relationships with individuals who must struggle through crises. We have brought what a psychiatric–mental health nurse colleague from Puerto Rico calls "grace" to our clients. We are now faced with the challenge of documenting, measuring, and supporting with evidence the outcomes of what we have done and whether it works or fails. Conditions in the contemporary mental health care environment demand that our caring be linked with accountability for client outcomes as well as cost containment. We must, to the extent possible, base psychiatric–mental health nursing on sound, convincing evidence.

In this textbook you will find a perspective of what evidence-based practice means and how to engage in it. Each chapter presents: (a) a clinically situated case example in which existing research can help guide decisions for care (e.g., Using Research Evidence feature); (b) a critical thinking challenge that prompts you to improve your critical thinking skills; (c) a bibliography of current and selected classic references that offers you the most contemporary resources about what is known; (d) information, examples, strategies, interventions, and summaries of the best evidence currently available presented in boxes, figures, tables, the text itself, and online using our Web site that links to other online resources.

Experts in psychiatric–mental health nursing agree that we do not at present have sufficient evidence from traditional science to guide all our practices, nor should we always rely on it. ■ Figure 3–1 illustrates the steps of traditional science in which hypotheses are tested by conducting controlled experiments to reach a conclusion about a scientific question. This textbook reminds you that nursing is as much an art of caring and comfort as a science. Yet, this chapter will guide you through the process of finding, evaluating, and using evidence on which to base your best practices.

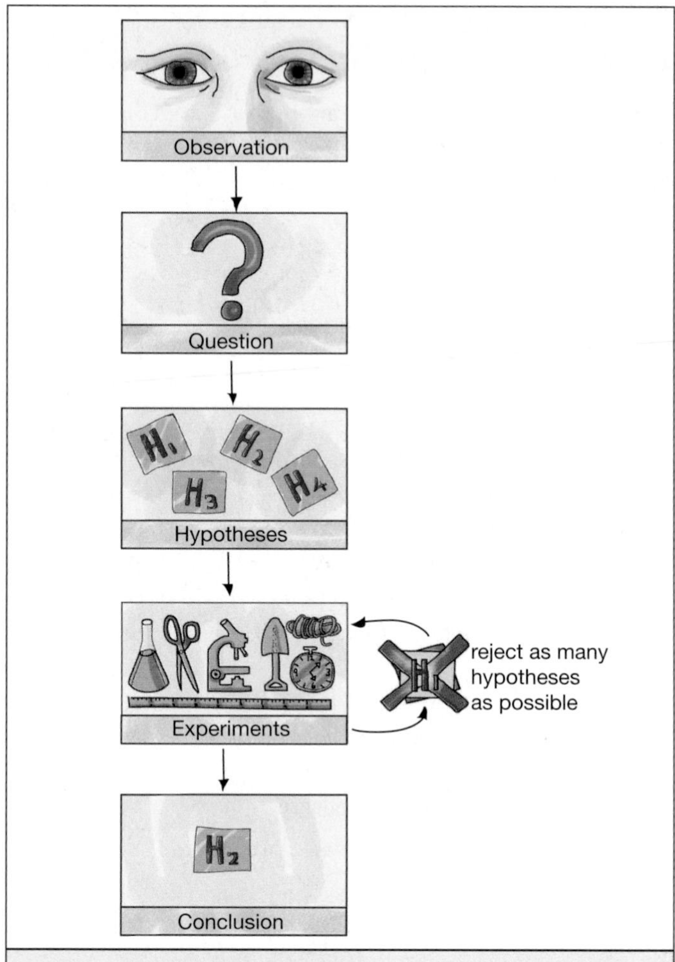

FIGURE 3–1 ■ *The traditional scientific method for testing hypotheses to answer questions.*

Source: Krogh, D. (2000). *Biology: A guide to the natural world* (p. 5). Upper Saddle River, NJ: Prentice Hall.

Contemporary Conditions Mandating Evidence-Based Practice

Health care reform in the twenty-first century has had a profound effect on the way in which psychiatric care is delivered in many countries throughout the world. The length of hospital stays has decreased while client acuity has increased. A knowledge explosion in the neurosciences has reshaped our conception of the bases of mental disorder. Innovations in technology have broadened diagnostic practices including sophisticated brain imaging. The array of psychopharmacologic treatments available is ever expanding. The study of stem cells and genome research holds promise for disease cures, yet both inspire continuing ethical debate. The yearning for spirituality has been reawakened in clients as well as in psychiatric–mental health nurses. A global economy is transforming the way mental health care is provided to diverse populations and particularly the way that information, including research evidence, is communicated and disseminated. Populations of psychiatric clients include growing numbers of mentally ill elders, more people with coexisting substance use disorders, more comorbidities with other chronic illnesses such as HIV/AIDS as well as more people of racial and cultural diversity. The streamlining of psychiatric services has shifted settings in which psychiatric–mental health nurses practice from inpatient units and psychiatric hospitals to services that are community based and rehabilitation oriented including those in jails, homeless shelters, nursing homes, and on the streets. As members of interdisciplinary teams, psychiatric–mental health nurses are challenged to tailor and humanize technologies for traditional as well as new clients within these conditions.

Benner (2000b) reminds us that when a culture places its faith in scientific and technologic cures, chronic illness (e.g., many psychiatric disorders) is often ignored. She advises us that we should be able to respect biomedical cures yet recognize the importance of caring. Benner urges us to integrate the value of clinical wisdom as we respond to contemporary mandates and join the movement toward evidence-based practice.

What Is Evidence-Based Practice?

Evidence-based practice is the integration of individual clinical expertise with the best available external clinical evidence from systematic research. The combined results from clinically relevant research, clinical expertise, and patient preferences produce the best evidence for ensuring effective and yet individualized client care, according to nurse experts Rosswurm & Larrabee (1999) and others who are frequently cited sources on this topic. The outcome of an evidence-based practice system is often found in the form of **practice guidelines**, (practice guidelines for psychiatric–mental health nursing are discussed in Chapter 1) **critical pathways** (also called *clinical pathways*), and **clinical algorithms**. These forms are designed to specify the best procedures or practices for clinical problems and psychiatric diagnoses, in addition to tracking both the process and the outcomes of care.

BEST PRACTICES BASED ON EVIDENCE

Interest in the concept of **best practices** can be traced to concerns about avoiding nursing and medical mistakes and enhancing safety for clients. Best practices are broad consensus statements about values, attitudes, skills, knowledge, and approaches. To avoid mistakes, clinicians need to know the correct course of action. However, until recently, much psychiatric–mental health nursing knowledge was based on:

- Traditions and customs established in specific settings as part of the collective culture or the ideas of psychiatrists or administrators in charge.
- Trial and error if nurses did not necessarily know all the possible approaches and didn't know with certainty what the most effective, safest course of action should be.
- Clinical judgment, the accumulated knowledge that inquiring nurses actively, systematically, and intentionally extract from their practice experience.
- Authority governed by regulations that accrediting agencies or third-party payers required.

The movement toward evidence-based best practices represents an attempt to place the art of caring on a more solid scientific foundation. Consequently, nurse researchers are conducting clinical trials and outcome studies designed to generate a mounting body of evidence on which to base practice decisions. Others are summarizing this accumulating body of evidence in textbooks such as this, in *meta-analyses* (conceptual summaries) that are found in "State of the Science" features in nursing journals, and also in books in which identified experts collect original research evidence, and summarize and evaluate it using identified criteria. The National Institute of Nursing Research (NINR) is also currently funding studies designed to summarize research evidence organized around specific topics. An example of such a synthesis on the subject of sleep appears later in this chapter.

CRITICAL THINKING AND EVIDENCE-BASED PRACTICE

Closing the gap between evidence and practice requires not only the conduct of nursing research and critical syntheses of it, but also competencies among clinical nurses that have at their core the ability to think critically about the evidence. These competencies include the ability to:

- Find meaningful research evidence.
- Conduct an intelligent critique of studies once they are located.
- Summarize studies to accumulate a body of evidence focused on a topic or clinical problem.
- Implement a system for change to evidence-based practice in an organizational setting that includes involving all members of the team to ensure full participation in the design and implementation of new practice guidelines or protocols.
- Follow up and document the impact of changes and adopt, adapt, or discard changes based on additional evidence.

We believe in engaging others in the ongoing discussion about practice and the implications of our science for everyday care. (Study the Using Research Evidence feature that follows to determine how qualitative research evidence can influence the psychiatric–mental health nursing care of Megan, the case example).

PRACTICE GUIDELINES, CRITICAL PATHWAYS, AND CLINICAL ALGORITHMS

As evidence accumulates, psychiatric–mental health nurses have the opportunity to develop strategies for care called practice guidelines, critical pathways, and clinical algorithms. **Clinical algorithms** show a logical progression of decisions and activities that are designed to standardize quality care for a particular clinical problem or condition (see Chapter 15, Figure 15–4 as an example). You can find examples of practice guidelines for psychiatric–mental health nursing in Chapter 1 and practice guidelines and ethical guidelines in Chapter 10. ■ Figure 3–2 (see pages 47–48) offers an example of a critical pathway for a client experiencing panic disorder.

Critical pathways provide a means of accurate documentation and shift the emphasis from depicting nursing as a series of tasks (e.g., monitoring medication side effects, taking vital signs, etc.) to interventions connected to a purpose or client outcome. They offer us an opportunity to best represent our role in treatment. We must be clear and specific about the manner in which we in psychiatric–mental health nursing contribute to client outcomes such as:

- Stabilization of acute psychotic symptoms.
- Restoration of cognitive function.

USING RESEARCH EVIDENCE

Megan is a 26-year-old woman who has recently immigrated to the United States from Ireland. Her background is strongly Roman Catholic, but she has suffered past life events that include pregnancy by her biological father at the age of 15, death of the child a few hours after the baby's birth, and repeated rapes at the hands of boyfriends. Megan is hospitalized because of a current incident of self-harm, which she described as "cutting the bad out of me." She has seriously cut both her arms. She believes literally that the Bible tells her that "if your hand is your undoing, cut it off; it is better for you to enter into life maimed than to keep both hands and go to hell into unquenchable fire" (Mark 9:43). She tells you that after she cuts herself, she feels she has got the bad out and feels absolved and relieved. She needs you to try to understand. Her past experiences with psychiatrists and psychiatric–mental health nurses were ones in which she thought health care providers were hostile and thought she was a waste of their time. She was told repeatedly that she was a "naughty little girl." Your nursing care plan must include all structural supports to ensure Megan's safety, but beyond that goal, you must attempt to understand Megan's cultural framework, her own situated reality, and her logic of self-harm. The study cited below emphasizes that lack of understanding, uncaring attitudes, and ritual humiliation only serve to confirm negative versions of self-harming clients' self-worth. This study doesn't tell us what to do, but rather what to avoid if we are to be helpful to self-harming clients like Megan:

Harris, J. (2001). Self-Harm: Cutting the bad out of me. *Qualitative Health Research, 10*(2), 164–173.

- Establishment of social support for caregivers.
- Management for symptoms of depression.
- Safety from harm.
- Sense of spiritual solace.

It is not possible to remember all the best practice guidelines, clinical pathways, or clinical algorithms, so psychiatric–mental health nurses need to learn to use systems that consistently provide what we want. We have some resistance to this idea because we have always prided ourselves on individualized client care—but we need to recognize that our memories may not be sufficient given the knowledge explosion in nursing science. An example of technologic support for such systems is the personal digital assistant (PDA). A growing number of nurses use these devices (often called palm pilots) to ensure quick, easy access to assessment data, evidence-based clinical guidelines, medication information, and other applications. Drug reference software such as *ePocratesqRx* allows clinicians to dock a PDA to a personal computer with an Internet connection and download the latest information on medications such as when a drug has been recalled or has new indications. This technique is called *HotSynching*.

THE ART OF NURSING EMBEDDED IN THE SCIENCE

Throughout this chapter you will read about a view of the growing science of nursing tempered by a belief in the spiritual and in what has traditionally been called, the art. As Benner (2000) expressed, "the belief that caring practices and astute nursing judgments are called arts is because they are not entirely predictable or perfect" (p. 10). She urges every nurse to tell our stories so that the intangible can become tangible and the artfulness of good nursing practice can be incorporated in a nursing science based on evidence.

THE SARAH COLE HIRSH INSTITUTE FOR BEST PRACTICES BASED ON EVIDENCE

Current authors have identified evidence-based practice as essential for clinical excellence and measurable nursing interventions. One such example is The Sarah Cole Hirsh Institute for Best Practices Based on Evidence at the Frances Payne Bolton School of Nursing, Case Western Reserve University in Cleveland, Ohio. This institution asserts that evidence-based best nursing practices are becoming more important in health care settings. The focus on evidence-based practice is directed by accrediting bodies and payers interested in quality care, reduced costs, and on remaining competitive.

The Hirsh Institute was established in 1998 as a repository of best nursing practices based on research findings. Its purposes are to:

- Improve patient care.
- Guide the national nursing research agenda.
- Provide unique educational experiences.
- Provide the most up-to-date nursing knowledge available.

The Institute achieves its purposes through:

- State of the Evidence Reviews.
- Evidence-based innovation services.
- Certificate programs on implementing best practices including those in psychiatric mental health care.

The following clinical example illustrates the nature of questions addressed to implement evidence-based practice with older adults.

A practice innovation was implemented at Hanna House, Case Western Reserve University, in which older adults administered their own medications. Questions addressed to implement this practice included:

- What criteria should be implemented to select clients suitable for self-medication?
- How does one best educate staff and clients about self-medication?
- What are the best educational materials available for this purpose?
- How can medications be kept at the bedside without violating drug safekeeping laws that protect client safety?

This example resulted in saving time at discharge and enhancement of the dignity and involvement of clients in their own care. Providers concluded that the high level of medication

Critical Pathway for a Client with Panic Disorder: Outpatient Treatment			
Expected length of treatment: 8 weeks			
	Date ______ Weeks 1–2	**Date ______ Weeks 3–6**	**Date ______ Weeks 7–8**
Weekly outcomes	Client will: • Identify initial goals for therapy. • Contract for ongoing treatment. • Participate in treatment plan. • Begin to identify sources of anxiety/ panic.	Client will: • Identify ongoing goals for therapy. • Maintain contract for ongoing therapy. • Participate in treatment plan. • Identify strategies to manage anxiety and panic.	Client will describe ongoing strategies to manage panic disorder. Client will demonstrate ability to cope with ongoing feelings of panic. Client will describe strategies to cope with an inability to cope with stressors.
Assessments, tests, and treatments	Psychosocial assessment to include mental status, mood, affect, behavior, and communication. Assist client to explore factors that precipitate panic attacks.	Psychosocial assessment. Assess recent history of anxiety and panic attacks. Explore contributing factors. Discuss effectiveness of cognitive restructuring strategies.	Psychosocial assessment. Assess recent history of anxiety and panic attacks. Explore contributing factors. Discuss effectiveness of cognitive restructuring strategies.
Knowledge deficit	Orient client to therapy program. Assess learning needs of client. Review initial plan of care. Assess understanding of teaching. Discuss the etiology and management of anxiety and panic disorders. Discuss the physical symptoms of panic and the importance of understanding the meaning of anxiety and panic disorders. Instruct client to maintain journal of anxiety and panic attacks.	Review therapy program and treatment objectives. Review journal of recent panic attacks. Assist client to identify the early signs of anxiety and panic attacks. Discuss strategies to cope with early signs and symptoms of panic attacks, including talking or activity. Discuss additional strategies to cope with panic attacks including expressing anger, positive self-talk, or guided imagery. Teach principles of cognitive restructuring and practice during session. Teach relaxation techniques and practice during session. Discuss use of exercise to alleviate anxiety/panic. Assist client to explore problem-solving strategies. Assess understanding of teaching.	Review plan of care. Review principles of cognitive restructuring. Assess understanding of teaching.
Diet	Nutritional assessment. Encourage well-balanced diet from all food groups. Contract with client to avoid stimulants.	Encourage a well-balanced diet from all food groups. Encourage the avoidance of stimulants.	Encourage a well-balanced diet from all food groups. Encourage the avoidance of stimulants.
Activity	Discuss the importance of regular aerobic exercise. Contract for regular exercise program. Sleep pattern assessment. Discuss strategies to provide sleep-enhancing atmosphere for 45 min prior to sleep.	Review ability to begin and continue exercise program. Maintain contract for regular exercise programs. Encourage client to practice relaxation response. Discuss effectiveness of sleep-enhancing strategies.	Review ability to continue exercise program. Maintain contract for regular exercise programs. Discuss effectiveness of sleep-enhancing strategies.

FIGURE 3–2 ■ *Critical pathway for panic disorder*

Critical Pathway for a Client with Panic Disorder: Outpatient Treatment (continued)

Expected length of treatment: 8 weeks

	Date ____________ Weeks 1–2	Date ____________ Weeks 3–6	Date ____________ Weeks 7–8
Psychosocial	Approach with nonjudgmental and accepting manner. Observe and monitor behavior. Assist client to understand relationship of unexpressed feelings to anxiety and panic experience. Encourage client to express feelings, thoughts, ideas, and beliefs.	Approach with nonjudgmental and accepting manner. Observe and monitor behavior. Encourage client to express feelings, thoughts, ideas, and beliefs. Provide positive feedback for efforts to incorporate coping strategies into daily life. Assist client to understand relationship of feelings to panic. Assist client to realistically identify strengths and limitations. Explore ways of reframing limitations in a positive manner. Assist client to practice and implement effective coping strategies. Assist client to identify potentially stressful situations and role-play coping strategies.	Approach with nonjudgmental and accepting manner. Encourage client to review strategies to manage anxiety and panic.
Medications	Identify target symptoms.	Assess target symptoms. Assess need for medications and refer as indicated. Routine meds as ordered.	Assess target symptoms. Routine meds as ordered.
Consults and discharge plan	Family assessment. Establish objectives of therapy with client.	Review with client progress toward therapy objectives.	Review with client progress toward therapy objectives. Make appropriate referrals to support groups.

FIGURE 3–2 ■ *Critical pathway for panic disorder (continued)*

knowledge at discharge boded well for postdischarge outcomes. Nurse participants commented that working under an evidence-based practice system lifted the curtain that once prevented them from seeing how research can benefit clinical outcomes in the natural setting.

The Hirsh Institute has identified a number of competencies that direct the certificate programs they offer in implementing best nursing practices (see the Nursing Self-Awareness feature).

CHANGE TO EVIDENCE-BASED PRACTICE

Having defined evidence-based practice, identified the contemporary conditions in the mental health/psychiatric care environment that have required it, and examined the competencies to establish it, the section that follows provides a model to guide you in its direction. Evidence-based practice is not a new concept to most nurses; it has been referred to as *using research in nursing*. However, the growth in nursing science and research literature, and our enhanced access to it have intensified the mandate that we use it to discover the most effective approaches to achieve identified client outcomes.

Consensus supports the idea that quality of health care requires delivery based on sound scientific evidence and continuous innovation of new health care practices and approaches. The Surgeon General's *Report on Mental Health* (1999) provided a synthesis of the state of the art of research in the field. This document did not make any evidence-based recommendations for practice, but it did serve to put psychiatric–mental health nurses on alert that we have much to contribute to the growing body of knowledge in mental health care and to influence mental health care policy. It is evident that nurses in the future will be expected to justify their practice with research-based evidence. We must learn to assess client outcomes and clearly link them to nursing interventions.

CONTEXT FOR EVIDENCE-BASED PRACTICE: THE 4 A'S

A review of the contemporary literature identified a number of contextual requirements that should be assessed if evidence-based practice is to flourish. These practice conditions can easily be remembered as the 4 A's:

Nursing SELF-AWARENESS

Am I Ready For Evidence-Based Practice?

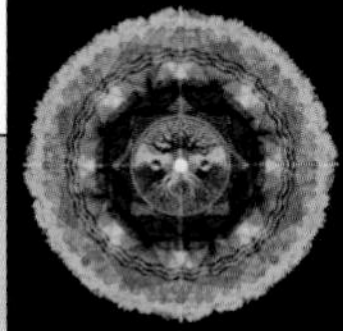

Ask yourself the following questions to determine if you are prepared to implement evidence-based practice in the setting where you care for clients.

1. Do you know how to locate sources of best practices based on evidence?
2. Do you feel confident about your ability to evaluate the usefulness of best practices in the natural setting?
3. Do you have the support and resources necessary to implement best practices in your setting?
4. Can your discoveries about best practices be implemented into organizational protocols and operations?
5. Are you able to muster the expertise and resources necessary to evaluate changes in practice, client outcomes and cost as a result of attempting to introduce best practices?

Source: Adapted from Sarah Cole Hirsch Institute Brochure. (2000). Frances Payne Bolton School of Nursing, Case Western Reserve University, Cleveland, Ohio.

1. Attitudes of open-mindedness to and knowledge of research on the parts of psychiatric–mental health nurses.
2. Access and availability to contemporary and regularly updated research reports or state of the science resources.
3. Administrative support from nurse managers and higher-level executives.
4. Assistance through expert consultants to become critical consumers of research and to use findings in practice.

The increased body of findings from clinical research has brought a variety of choices in nursing interventions to psychiatric–mental health nurses. Standardized language according to the North American Nursing Diagnosis Association (NANDA), the Nursing Outcome Classification (NOC), and Nursing Intervention Classification (NIC) has made such options readily available. Detailed discussion of these standardized nursing languages appears in Chapter 7. The time has come for a shift from what some call "intuition-driven" and "traditional" psychiatric–mental health nursing practice to evidence-based practice. The next section of this chapter provides one model that can be used to guide nurses through this change process.

The Rosswurm and Larrabee Model for Change

Rosswurm and Larrabee (1999) used theoretical and research literature related to evidence-based practice, research utilization, standardized language and change theory to generate a model that guides clinicians through the process of developing and integrating a change to evidence-based practice. Their model endorses qualitative, as well as quantitative research data, clinical expertise, and contextual evidence. It includes the steps summarized in ■ Figure 3–3.

■ Table 3–1 illustrates how Rosswurm and Larrabee applied the six-step model to create an evidence-based protocol for clients with acute confusion.

Rosswurm and Larrabee (1999) developed and tested the usefulness of their model at a regional medical center that provides acute care, but they state it could be used in primary care as well as other settings. A brief overview of the six steps is discussed here.

STEP 1. ASSESSING THE NEED FOR CHANGE

The first step in the process of change to evidence-based practice requires that *stakeholders*, people with a vested interest in the quality of nursing practice, collect internal and external data about current practice to reach consensus that a problem exists. These data may include client satisfaction surveys, risk management data, and other quality assurance data. These data

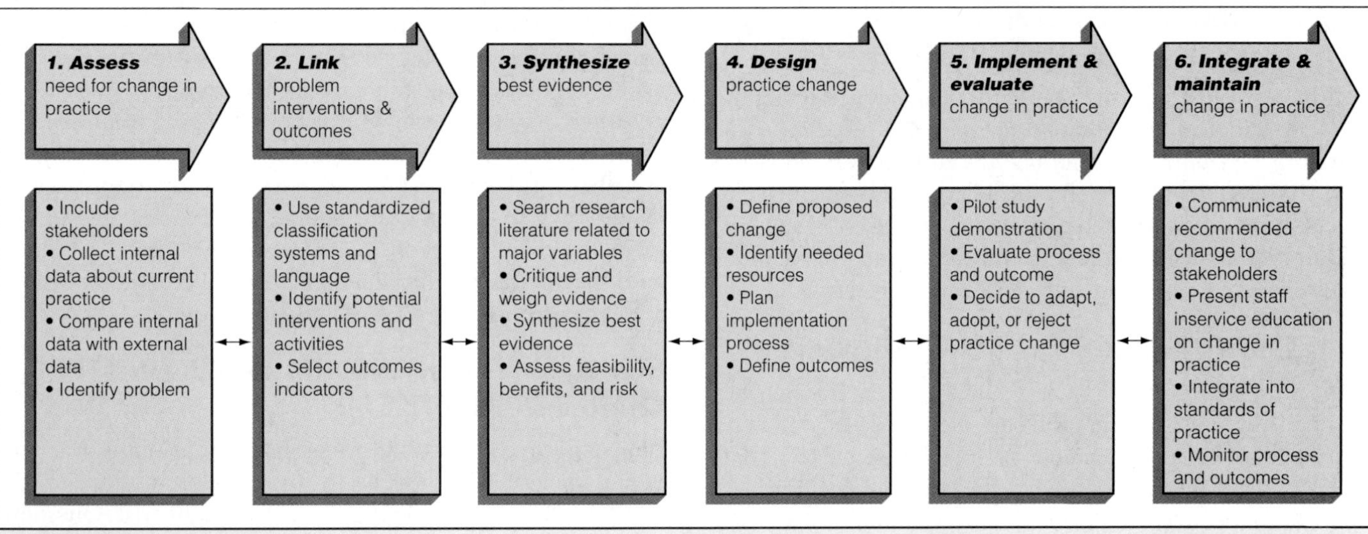

FIGURE 3–3 ■ *Model for evidence-based practice.*

Source: Rosswurm, M. A., & Larrabee, J. H. (1999). A model for change to evidence-based practice. *Image: Journal of Nursing Scholarship, 31*(4), 318. Reprinted with permission from Sigma Theta Tau International.

TABLE 3–1 Application of the Model: Evidence-Based Protocol for Patients with Acute Confusion

Step 1. Assess need for a change
- Discussed clinical problem of acute confusion with nurse managers and nurses
- Reviewed QI & RM data on associated adverse events, i.e., falls, restraints
- Derived from data that patients > 65 years comprised more than 50% of hospital population and were at highest risk for confusion and adverse events
- Assessed nursing knowledge about delirium in elderly patients
- Compared internal data with external data from similar medical centers
- Identified from findings the need to improve nursing staff's knowledge and care of elderly patients at risk for developing confusion during hospitalization

Step 2. Link problem with interventions and outcomes
- Linked acute confusion with the NIC intervention of delirium management
- Included delirium management activities in an acute-confusion protocol
- Identified outcomes of cognitive orientation and safety as measured by a confusion scale, fall rates, and restraints

Step 3. Synthesize best evidence
- Reviewed literature focused on delirium management and safety
- Included nurses in critiquing research literature using worksheets
- Synthesized quantitative research evidence
- Combined quantitative research evidence with qualitative data, clinical judgment, and contextual data
- Assessed system feasibility, patients' benefits, and risks of protocol

Step 4. Design a change in practice
- Included nurses from pilot study units in drafting the evidence-based protocol
- Prepared forms for pilot study and its evaluation with input from unit nurses
- Identified tools for measuring outcomes of cognitive orientation, fall rates, and use of restraints
- Educated all nurses on the pilot study units in use of the evidence-based protocol

Step 5: Implement and evaluate the practice change
- Implemented the pilot study on the two selected hospital units
- Monitored use of the protocol throughout the pilot period
- Collected data and analyzed findings
- Recommended adoption of protocol with minor revisions

Step 6. Integrate and maintain the practice change
- Met with staff nurses on pilot study unit to review revisions
- Presented evidence-based protocol to standards and practice council
- Communicated information to administration and collaborating practitioners
- Conducted inservice education for all nursing staff about the protocol
- Planned ongoing monitoring of outcomes on all units

Source: Rosswurm, M. A., & Larrabee, J. H. (1999). A model for change to evidence-based practice. *Image: Journal of Nursing Scholarship, 31*(4), 319. Reprinted with permission from Sigma Theta Tau International.

are compared to indicators in databases that identify clinical practices that lead to the best outcomes. Such a comparison, called *benchmarking*, either supports current practice or the need for changes.

STEP 2. LINKING THE PROBLEM WITH INTERVENTIONS AND OUTCOMES

In this step, clinicians use standardized language including NANDA and the *Diagnostic and Statistical Manual of the American Psychiatric Association*, 4th edition, Text Revision (DSM-IV-TR) to identify the problem and then link it to selected outcomes and interventions often using NOC and NIC classification systems. Clearly, the outcomes and interventions that are selected rely on the nurse's clinical judgment.

STEP 3. SYNTHESIZING THE BEST EVIDENCE

In the third step, participants search and evaluate research evidence on the topics of the problems, identified outcomes and interventions. Usually, a Medline search is conducted to accomplish the literature search since it is the largest biomedical electronic database, referencing more than 4,000 journals. ■ Figure 3–4 presents a worksheet that Rosswurm and Larrabee have adapted in order to summarize the literature. The purpose of the literature synthesis is to decide whether evidence supports a change in practice. If it does, pilot studies follow to determine the feasibility, risks, and benefits of making the change.

STEP 4. DESIGNING THE CHANGE IN PRACTICE

In the fourth step, a protocol addressing the problem, the outcomes, and the linked interventions is designed. Rosswurm and Larrabee (1999) emphasize that feedback from stakeholders, agency resources, and the practice environment must all be considered when altering a protocol. Keeping it simple and based on the evidence increases the likelihood that it will be accepted. Again, the authors underscore the importance of pilot studies so as to clarify what resources will be needed to implement the change in protocol, what approvals will be needed, and what in-service education of others will be required, as well as what outcomes will serve as evaluation criteria.

STEP 5. IMPLEMENTING AND EVALUATING THE CHANGE IN PRACTICE

This step is most successful when the coordinator, who is providing the leadership, follows the process closely and is consistently available to address questions that might arise. Questions that should be addressed in Step 5 include:

- Are there any differences in outcome indicators before and after the change? For example, is the occurrence of seizures

A Model for Change to Evidence-Based Practice ____________________

Title of Article: ____________________

Purpose/Research Questions/Hypotheses	**Research Variables**	**Design**	**Major Findings and Limitations**
Purpose of Study: **Research Questions/Hypotheses:**	**Independent:** **Dependent:**	**Level I:** Exploratory Descriptive **Level II:** Correlational survey Comparative survey **Level III:** Quasi-experimental Experimental	**Findings:** **Limitations:**
Sample	**Setting**	**Major Tools**	**Quality of Evidence**
Number: **Type:** **Age:** **Gender:** **Health status:** **Diagnosis:** **Other:**	**Type:** Acute care hospital Community Nursing Home Other **Location:** Urban Rural	**Name(s):** #1____ #2____ #3____ **Reliability:** #1____ #2____ #3____ **Validity:** #1____ #2____ #3____	**Evidence Rating:** I. a. Meta-analysis of randomized controlled trials b. One randomized controlled trial II. a. One well-designed controlled study without randomization b. One other type of well-designed quasi-experimental study III. Comparative, correlational, and other descriptive studies IV. Evidence from expert committee reports and expert opinions **Feasibility:** Could this practice change be implemented easily in your organization and with minimal resources? ☐Yes ☐No **Benefit/Risk:** Would the benefits of this practice change outweigh the risks to patients? ☐Yes ☐No **Comments:**

FIGURE 3–4 ■ *Worksheet for critique for research*

Source: Rosswurm, M. A., & Larrabee, J. H. (1999). A model for change to evidence-based practice. *Image: Journal of Nursing Scholarship, 31*(4), 320. Reprinted with permission from Sigma Theta Tau International.

lower among clients detoxifying from alcohol when medicines such as benzodiazapines are prudently administered in addition to provision of psychosocial nursing care?
- Are necessary structural supports (such as technology, equipment, and adequate budget allocations) provided in the setting?
- Was the protocol implemented as it was intended? In other words, was there high compliance among caregivers with the timing and procedure specified in the new protocol?
- What effect did the new protocol have on client outcomes?

Feasibility, risks, and benefits are all assessed by stakeholders when the decision is made to adopt, adapt or reject the change in protocol.

STEP 6. INTEGRATING AND MAINTAINING THE CHANGE IN PRACTICE

In this sixth step, Rosswurm and Larrabee (1999) note that many organizations and people resist change and innovation: They are structured to sustain the status quo. However, they point out that change literature attests to the conclusion that change is more likely to be accepted if stakeholders participate in all steps of the process. Such participation increases their confidence in the feasibility and the potential effectiveness of the change. Clinicians need to know that adequate resources will be available to them, that continuing education will be provided, that the process will be monitored closely by those in leadership positions, and that quality performance will be rewarded. Table 3–1 illustrates the six steps of this model in the case of hospitalized, confused clients.

Obviously, revised protocols must be concisely written and shared widely in order to become integral to any practice environment. Changing to an evidence-based practice system offers a superb opportunity for clinical psychiatric–mental health nurses and nurse researchers to collaborate on their shared concern for clients' well-being.

Building a Knowledge Base for Evidence-Based Psychiatric Nursing Practice

Developing a knowledge base for evidence-based psychiatric nursing practice requires new research, synthesis of research, clinical trials to test the research, and a summary of findings based on the research.

DISCOVERING THE EVIDENCE

MediaLink National Institute of Nursing Research

Research continues to show that new nursing knowledge can improve practice. NINR supports research studies that are creating a cumulative knowledge base that can improve the quality of care for clients. Examples of NINR-funded studies relevant to psychiatric–mental health nursing include research on end-of-life quality issues, easing the transition from hospital to home care for the elderly, and family caregiving for clients with chronic diseases including mental disorders. The overall philosophy of NINR emphasizes that enhancing the scientific basis of nursing is an important strategy not only to improve quality of care but also for the long-term survival of the profession. In the following sections, you will read about two valuable and innovative research initiatives conducted by nurses and funded by NINR. These two studies, in progress at the time of this textbook's publication, illustrate examples of the richness and diversity of efforts to enhance the emerging scientific basis for psychiatric–mental health nursing practice. Such data can also be viewed on the NINR Web site, (www.nih.gov/ninr) which can be accessed through a resource link on the Companion Website for this book. You can also use this Web site to find out what other institutions are organizing knowledge summaries and what other intervention and outcome studies are in progress. However, in keeping with the values of this text, NINR also supports *qualitative studies.* Qualitative studies use interviews, field notes, and observations to generate rather than test hypotheses and/or to interpret meaning under natural conditions. One such study, *An Ethnography of Dying in a Long-Term Care Facility*, is currently being funded not only by NINR, but also by the National Institute on Aging, and the National Cancer Institute. Studies such as this descriptive **ethnography** (the study of human beings and their culture) attest to the recognized contribution of studies that are not designed as **randomized clinical trials,** studies designed to test hypotheses using the traditional experimental approach of randomly assigned subjects to treatment and control groups and then comparing them on identified outcomes that measure outcomes in quantifiable terms. (See our Web site for more information about the differences between qualitative and quantitative/traditional scientific methods.) Psychiatric–mental health nursing stands to benefit most from methodological diversity as we begin to build our knowledge base.

Synthesizing Research Data to Understand Sleep

A disturbance common to many people suffering from psychiatric disorders is disrupted sleep. One nurse investigator has received a $1.2 million grant from NINR to consolidate all the known research into a single reference source. Her team intends to map knowledge of how sleep changes from adulthood to old age with the aim of discovering what variations are normal aspects of aging. Since a significant percentage of our population in the United States is aging, such a consolidating-of-knowledge study is a high priority. Obviously, once normal parameters across the life span are mapped, we have a basis on which to learn about sleep disorders among mentally disordered people. From today and beyond, other nurse scholars will be building a body of research evidence in areas relevant to psychiatric–mental health nursing practice. It is critical that you learn how to access this information as it evolves and refine your own critical thinking skills so that you can evaluate it with confidence.

A Clinical Trial of Wellness Training for Severely Mentally Ill Adults

Severely mentally ill (SMI) adults have many health problems that may not be directly psychiatric in nature because of lifestyles and environmental risk factors, as well as those risks associated with long-term pharmacologic treatment. Chafetz (2001) believes that these general health problems detract from their quality of life and contribute to the use of costly acute health services. Consequently, Chafetz and White (2001) have initiated a randomized clinical trial to study the benefit of adding an active health promotion component to basic primary care services for this population in the city of San Francisco. It is beyond the scope of this chapter to discuss the study's methodology in detail; however, it should be noted that clients will be randomly assigned to usual primary care or to "Wellness Training," and the study will test hypotheses about comparative outcomes between the study groups, including health status, service use, self-efficacy, and overall quality of life. This study's design, a randomized clinical trial, is considered by many to be the *gold standard* or highest level of scientific evidence.

SUMMARIZING THE EVIDENCE

As this chapter emphasized from the outset, psychiatric–mental health nursing research focused on client outcomes must be conducted, located, read, and understood before it can be applied in clinical practice in a systematic manner. Research evidence must also be summarized, critiqued, and synthesized if it is to affect policy development, contribute meaningfully to interdisciplinary knowledge development, and shape standardized practice guidelines. One effort to summarize references divides topics into categories of Health Promotion/Risk Reduction and Pathologic Conditions and Nursing Interventions. In the first category are topics such as biofeedback training, consultation–liaison nursing, grief, and workplace violence, to name a few. Some second category topics include chronic mental illness, correctional mental health, and mentally ill adults with coexisting substance disorders (Fitzpatrick & Wilke, 2001).

The purpose of publications like this one is to make it easier for clinical nurses to locate sources of evidence since the number of journals in which psychiatric–mental health nursing research appears is proliferating. Additional publications that are valuable resources include *Evidence-Based Nursing and Evidence-Based Mental Health* (both published in the United Kingdom) and the Cochrane Collaboration, an electronic library available on the Internet. (See Box 3–1 and our Companion Website for additional resource links.)

EVALUATING THE EVIDENCE

It is essential for all psychiatric–mental health nurses who engage in evidence-based practice to become an intelligent consumer and evaluator of the growing body of science in our field. The amount of what you comprehend in a report of research findings often depends on the amount of active thinking you put into reading research. Box 3–2 on page 54 offers you some helpful tips on techniques for active reading of research.

General criteria useful in evaluating evidence that appear consistently across all research sources include:

1. Is the purpose of the study clear and relevant to a significant nursing problem?
2. Is the study problem stated in such a way as to be researchable (can the investigator collect data about it)?
3. Is the literature adequate and current, and does it reflect a mastery of current knowledge of the topic of inquiry?
4. Is there a match among the study purpose, the study design, and the methods? And are all well detailed and justified?
5. Are the sampling procedures and sample well described and appropriate for the study question and study design?
6. Has the investigator used the correct analytic procedures whether qualitative or quantitative?
7. Are the findings clear and supported by the research data?

The nursing literature abounds with research textbooks that offer guidelines for becoming an intelligent consumer of nursing research evidence. A quick search of *The Cumulative Index to Nursing and Allied Health Literature*, the *International Nursing Index*, and the *Cumulative Medical Index*, as well as a MEDLINE computerized literature search, will reveal many other such books.

USING THE EVIDENCE IN PRACTICE

To date, most psychiatric–mental health nursing practice continues to be based on what has been termed *received wisdom* found in tradition, unsystematic trial and error, and authority rather than being based on evidence. Received wisdom is passive, taken-for-granted knowledge. Studies of research utilization and attitudes toward research reveal that even when psychiatric–mental health nurses report positive attitudes toward research, they rarely state that they use research in daily practice. At present, the goal of evidence-based practice is far from being realized in psychiatric–mental health nursing. In this chapter, you have read that evidence-based practice depends on a number of factors including the nurses' attitudes toward and knowledge of research, the availability and access to relevant research, and an environmental context that provides sufficient resources and managers' support. The Wisconsin Aurora-Metro Health Care Project is one clinical example of integrating research into practice.

The Wisconsin Aurora-Metro Health Care Project

Nurses in eastern Wisconsin have initiated a five-year project to ensure that nursing practice in the five hospitals and numerous other health care agencies was clearly and unequivocally evidence based. A brief overview of the steps of their multisite process is described here.

MediaLink Case Study: Evaluating Evidence

MediaLink International Evidence-Based Resources

BOX 3–1 International Nursing Research Resources

The following are examples of useful resources for evidence-based practice in nursing. (*Note*: This is *not* an all-inclusive list.)

Websites

www.evidencebasednursing.com	An international online journal of nursing research; 24 different summaries in each issue; expert commentators for each	Sponsored by the Royal College of Nursing in the United Kingdom
www.joannabriggs.edu.au	An international research collaboration for evidence based nursing; publish 20 best practice information summary sheets on individual and group therapy, long-term confusion, effectiveness of suicide prevention programs, music as an intervention	Based at the Royal Adelaide Hospital and Adelaide University in Australia with collaborating centers in Australia, New Zealand, and Hong Kong
www.fhs.mcmaster.ca/ceb/acts/ebcp.htm	Extensive resources in teaching with implications for evidence based practice in nursing and other disciplines	McMaster University in Toronto, Canada
www.nih.gov/ninr	The center for nursing research at the National Institutes of Health (see in-text discussion)	United States

BOX 3-2 Techniques for Active Reading

Active reading involves you in a process of actively questioning the material you read. Before you can address the questions of "Is it any good?" and "What does it mean?", you must understand what you are reading. Here are some helpful tips:

1. Quickly read the title page, preface, or abstract to get an idea of the topic of the article or book and categorize it in your mind. Is it really a report of research findings or is it a anecdotal account of somebody's isolated experience? Case studies and case histories count as qualitative research.
2. Study the table of contents or the headings in the article to get a sense of its structure. This alerts you in advance about what to expect.
3. Read any boldface excerpts or boxed summaries (like this one) to ascertain the main points or ideas.
4. Leaf through the whole article, dipping in here and there to follow the logic.
5. Find the important and unfamiliar words and use resources like a glossary or dictionary to determine their meaning.
6. Highlight key points or conclusions by underlining or putting "notes" in the margins.
7. Be able to say with certainty that you understand what you have read before you criticize it.
8. Compare what you have read in one study with what you have read cumulatively on a topic.

Improving Communication. One of the first steps in the process was to build the technology to improve communication. With the assistance of telecommunications staff, nurse researchers obtained state funding to purchase videoconferencing equipment that enabled nurses from the various settings to conduct and share research. They constructed an intranet of Web pages that included requests for proposals, research conferences, and findings from completed research projects. Finally, they upgraded their computer systems, which allowed nurses to search the Internet, the intranet, and the medical library.

Establishing Goals. Discussion groups were conducted with staff nurses, unit managers, clinical nurse specialists, and program directors to:

- Establish review criteria and reward structures that demonstrated that the use of research was expected of all nurses in their daily practice.
- Collect baseline data on the state of research knowledge, attitudes, and practices in the participating agencies.
- Define and implement expectations for research within the five-year time frame.
- Evaluate progress in incorporating research into practice.

Structural Revision. In this step, the project participants redesigned the compensation model, position descriptions, and the performance review criteria, as well as the continuing education curriculum, and decision-making processes to include research use expectations. Of particular value was the development of a Research Resource Manual that describes how research expectations are integrated into Aurora's system structures. For example, the manual:

- Provides instructions for conducting a literature search.
- Provides guidance for evaluating research for use in practice.
- Identifies strategies for finding unit-based research mentors.
- Provides strategies for developing research-based recommendations for changing and sustaining changes in research-based practice.

Conducting Regional Research. A team of researchers conducted a formal study of the Aurora-Metro Research Integration project that included developing, administering, and analyzing results from a survey instrument; implementing an educational intervention (a 16-hour Research Utilization Education Workshop); and comparing before and after scores for participants across multiple settings.

Challenging the Status Quo. Nurses involved in this project have been using research to challenge policies and client care interventions. New research-based guidelines are being implemented. For example, one unit is pilot testing risk management protocols for hospitalized elders; another is reviewing ways of promoting sleep for clients in intensive care. These kinds of research activities contributed toward Aurora-Metro's being honored as the first health care system nationwide to achieve regional magnet status in January 2001.

The story of one regional center's success with integrating research into practice has much to teach us about the complexity and the rewards of taking on such a project. The challenge to psy-

***Nursing* SELF-AWARENESS**

Levels of Research Utilization Competence

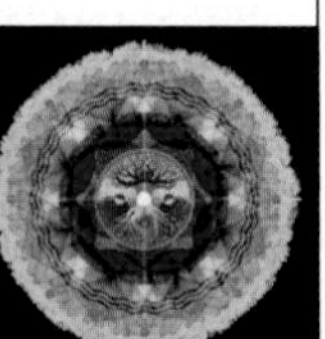

Level 1. Am I aware of the research basis for policies, procedures, and assessment tools that I use in my practice?

Level 2. Do I follow organizational policies and procedures and use valid assessment tools and research-based recommendations to effect positive client and family outcomes?

Level 3. Am I able to apply research-based findings to develop individualized plans of care?

Level 4. Am I able to integrate and translate research-based knowledge into well-designed practice guidelines that help achieve positive client and family outcomes?

Level 5. Do I collaborate with other caregivers to challenge current practices and to synthesize research findings to develop systems for achieving desired client and family outcomes?

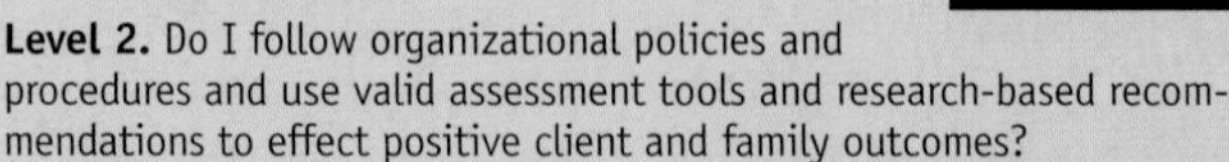

Level 6. (Clinical nurse specialist) Do I participate in expanding the scientific basis of nursing practice by conducting, using and disseminating research?

Level 7. (Manager or director) Do I create an environment for practice that assures research-based nursing (e.g., through budgeting, releasing staff time, and integrating research into organizational goals)?

Source: Adapted from Van Mullem, C., Burke, L. J., Dohmeyer, K., Farrell, M., Harvey, S., John, L., et al. (2001). Integrating research into practice. *American Journal of Nursing, 101*(4), 24E.

chiatric–mental health nurses is to learn from such an example. The Nursing Self-Awareness feature on page 54 challenges you to locate yourself on the ladder of research use expectations for nurses developed by Aurora Health Care, Milwaukee, Wisconsin.

Agenda for the Future

Psychiatric–mental health nurses are on the brink of joining the movement toward evidence-based practice in our field. Yet if we think of research evidence exclusively as evidence that is established in experiments and randomized clinical trials, we may be less likely to become involved in efforts to shift our practice to an evidence-based approach. Psychiatric–mental health nurses deal with less readily apparent client problems and interventions that are more difficult to quantify and measure. Our history, which has valued the intuitive aspects of the interpersonal relationship and caring, also adds to our reluctance to join this movement wholeheartedly. We fear that we may be pushed in a direction that contradicts our philosophical, political, and ethical viewpoints. All human psychosocial experience can't be measured and counted. These ideas have been called "reluctant ideologies" by some, in light of the move in nursing toward evidence-based practice. The authors of this textbook believe that a broad definition of what constitutes legitimate evidence, including clinical wisdom, client preference, and solid qualitative (non-numeric) research findings offers us a meeting ground for the values we attribute to moving toward evidence-based practice.

The future agenda for psychiatric–mental health research will likely follow the target topics for federal funding. Many of the clients with whom we work are among the chronically ill; as our population ages so do those elderly who have been mentally disordered since youth and so do the numbers of older clients who are cognitively impaired due to diseases of the brain; the growing chasm between the rich and the poor in the United States along with increasing populations of ethnically diverse clients put vulnerable populations including adolescents and children at risk for violence and drug abuse. The movement of psychiatric clients away from in-patient care has created a new population in need of our attention—those in jails, in shelters, in group homes, in emergency rooms, in hospice care, and on the streets. Most of the evidence-based practice example stories told in the preceding pages have taken place in well-established agencies and often focused on clients who don't meet diagnostic criteria for mentally disordered. (Refer to our Companion Website for resources and activities designed to keep you informed on the most contemporary advances in evidence-based psychiatric–mental health nursing practice.) The research agenda for psychiatric–mental health nursing is to take this movement not only to our traditional psychiatric clients but also to the jails, shelters, hospice care centers, outreach clinics, drug treatment centers, and the streets. Studies conducted under these natural conditions will help us to learn how what we do makes a difference for client outcomes, to build our body of evidence, and to demonstrate it to others in our clinical practice.

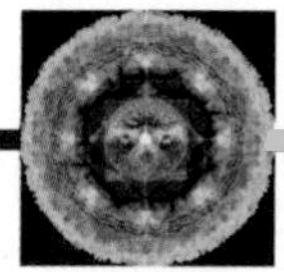

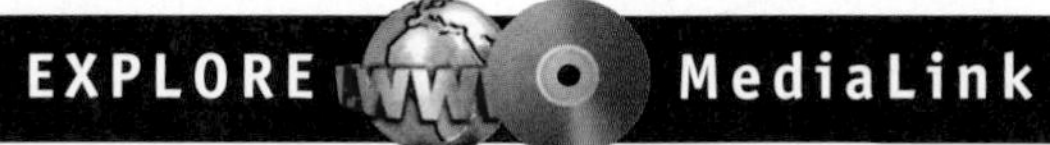

NCLEX review, case studies, and other interactive resources for this chapter can be found on the Companion Website at http://www.prenhall.com/kneisl. Click on Chapter 3 to select the activities for this chapter.

For animations, video tutorials, more NCLEX review questions, and an audio glossary, access the accompanying CD-ROM in this textbook.

BIBLIOGRAPHY

Benner, P. (1999, February). *Keynote address for the center for excellence in chronic illness*. New Haven, CT: Yale University.

Benner, P. (2000a). The language of caring. *Nursing Spectrum, 1*(3), 18W–19W.

Benner, P. (2000b). The wisdom of our practice. *American Journal of Nursing, 100*(10), 99–105.

Chavetz, L. (2001). Personal correspondence.

Chavetz, L., & White, M. (2001). Personal correspondence.

Fitzpatrick, J., & Wilke, P. A. (2001). *Psychiatric mental health research digest.* New York: Springer.

Goode, C. F., & Piedalue, F. (1999). Evidence-based practice. *Journal of Nursing Administration, 29*(6) 15–21.

Grady, P. A. (2000). News from NINR. *Nursing Outlook, 48*, 127.

Harris, J. (2001). Self-harm: Cutting the bad out of me. *Qualitative Health Research, 10*(2), 164–173.

The Hirsh Institute takes research into practice (2000). *Seken Case-Western Reserve University*, 16–18.

President's Advisory Commission on Consumer Protection and Quality in the Health Care Industry (1998). *Fostering evidence-based practice and innovation, quality first. Better health care for all Americans*. Washington, DC: U.S. Government Printing Office.

Rosswurm, M. A., & Larrabee, J. H. (1999). A model for change to evidence-based practice. *Image: Journal of Nursing Scholarship, 31*, 317–322.

U.S. Department of Health and Human Services (1999). *Mental health: A report of the surgeon general*. Rockville, MD: National Institute of Mental Health.

Van Mullem, C., Burke, L. J., Dohmeyer, K., Farrell, M., Harvey, S., John, L., et al. (2001). Integrating research into practice. *American Journal of Nursing, 101*(4), 24A–24H.

Wilson, H. S., & Hutchinson, S. A. (1996). *Consumer's guide to nursing research*. Albany, NY: Delmar.

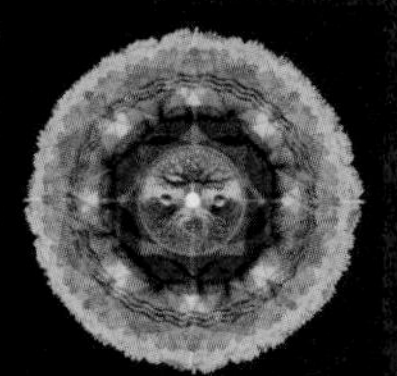

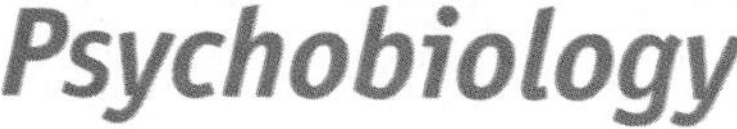

Psychobiology

PAMELA MARCUS
CAROL REN KNEISL
EILEEN TRIGOBOFF

4

Chapter FOUR

FOCUS QUESTIONS

- How do neuroanatomic structures affect thought, behavior, memory, understanding of consequences, and emotions?
- What alterations of the neuromessengers occur in major psychiatric disorders, such as schizophrenia, bipolar disorder, and major depression?
- What are the genetic contributions to mental disorder?
- In which important ways does the communication between the endocrine and immune systems affect mood and behavior?
- How does having the understanding of the biologic contribution to emotional problems contribute to your nursing practice?
- Why is client/family teaching about the biologic implications of psychiatric illnesses important?

KEY TERMS

amygdala
brain stem
cerebellum
cerebrum
DNA
dopamine
hippocampus
hypothalamus
limbic system
neurons
norepinephrine
serotonin

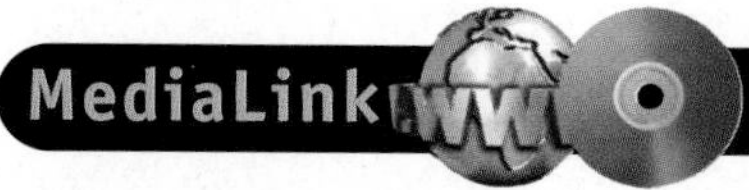

www.prenhall.com/kneisl

Additional resources for this chapter can be found on the Student CD-ROM accompanying this textbook, and on the Companion Website at www.prenhall.com/kneisl. Click on Chapter 4 to select the activities for this chapter.

CD-ROM

- Audio Glossary
- NCLEX Review
- Neurological Synapse Animation
- Serotonin Reuptake Inhibition Animation
- Receptor Sites (Agonists/Antagonists) Animation
- Seizure Videos:
  Seizure
  Complex Seizure
  Grand Mal Seizure

Companion Website

- Additional NCLEX Review
- Case Study: Brain, Mind, and Behavior

CHAPTER OUTLINE

CROSS-REFERENCES

Other topics relevant to this content are: Assessments and brain scans, Chapter 9; Ethics in psychobiology, Chapter 10; History of psychobiology, Chapter 2; Psychobiology of sleep, Chapter 19; Psychopharmacology, Chapter 31; Stress, anxiety, and coping, Chapter 5; Stress management, Chapter 32; For psychobiology specific to each disorder, see Part III, Chapters 12–21.

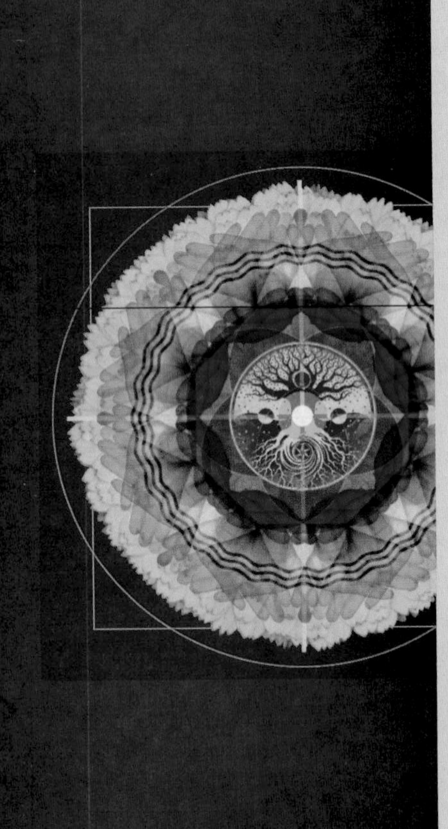

CRITICAL THINKING CHALLENGE

Psychiatric clinicians are expected to provide rapid, in-depth assessment and interventions that move the client quickly through the health care system. Standardized care plans based on a template of outcome criteria have been formulated to support cost-effective care that is based on diagnostic criteria. As developments in neuroscience and psychiatry have emerged, understanding behavior patterns from a biologic perspective is imperative to facilitate the goal of effective care. You would provide the assessment data that can be utilized to determine the most appropriate biologic, as well as interpersonal, interventions.

Imagine you are the nurse at a family care clinic, and Kay, a 30-year-old woman with mood swings, is being assessed. During your clinical interview you discover she is currently a caretaker for several family members: her father who has dementia of the Alzheimer's type, her mother who is depressed and unable to function, and her 38-year-old brother who has severe symptoms of paranoid schizophrenia. Major psychiatric illnesses are now understood as brain diseases that affect behavior, cognition, learning, and emotion. This has ramifications as it relates to your role, since the interventions that are aimed at improving overall functioning must consider Kay's unique biologic, environmental, and psychosocial strengths and weaknesses.

How can you integrate the understanding of the biologic components of Kay's functioning when providing comprehensive care? What is your responsibility to integrate the biologic information with the behavioral and affective components of Kay's life? ■

Psychobiology is neither a new concept nor a recent discovery. It has existed since the birth of humankind and has been a subject of discussion for at least the last 2,000 years. What *is* new in psychobiology is a broader understanding of the biologic basis of the mind and behavior. This understanding lowers the likelihood that people with psychiatric disorders will experience stigma. Current knowledge about the biologic components of behavior is revolutionizing not only psychiatry but also our view of behavior, temperament, and psychiatric disorders and their treatment.

Psychobiology encompasses an enormous amount of information that is growing almost exponentially, based on current research. The study of the brain structures, biochemical foundations, molecular and genetic influences on cognition, mood, emotion, affect, and behavior and the interactions among them make up the realm of psychobiology. This comprehensive view takes into consideration both internal and external influences across a person's life span, including genetics, the effects of other body systems such as the endocrine and immune systems, temperament, and the environment.

A major barrier that inhibits clients and families from seeking care is stigma. Stigma results from the lack of knowledge and misunderstanding of the etiology of severe mental disorder. Parenting styles and lack of character can no longer be blamed as contributors to mental disorders. Understanding the working hypotheses of psychobiology is a social imperative for removing the guilt and stigma associated with psychiatric disorders. Teaching clients and families about the biologic aspects of the disorder increases their understanding of the illness and its treatment, and can increase the client's motivation to continue to seek appropriate treatment.

The *Standards of Psychiatric–Mental Health Nursing Practice* (American Nurses Association [ANA], 2000) urge the inclusion of biologic therapies along with the use of the more traditional psychotherapy, psychosocial therapies, and combination therapies in the ongoing shift to a community-based care system. Excellence-based psychiatric–mental health nursing integrates psychobiologic concepts with our traditional practice to provide holistic caring for both clients and their families. Therefore, understanding the role biologic factors play in the client's illness and recovery can assist the client to increase compliance with medications and other therapeutic interventions through psychoeducation.

In this chapter, we highlight the psychobiologic principles that can be used in the nursing care of a client. It is not possible in one chapter to even touch upon all of the facets of psychobiology in any detail; this chapter will help you to apply psychobiologic principles in your professional work. To help integrate psychobiologic principles into your clinical practice, this chapter will focus on the brain (structure) and the substances and processes (function) that play key roles in behavior and emotional communication.

Brain, Mind, and Behavior

Communication has always been a basis for psychiatric–mental health nursing. Through neurobiologic discoveries, we now know that communication, behaviors, and thought patterns have a molecular, anatomic, and chemical basis. Who we are originates from order or disorder at any of these levels.

The brain encodes or decodes information through complex interactions of neuromessengers, chemical processes, and anatomic systems. When clients say that health care providers told them their symptoms were "a nervous breakdown" or "all in their head," you can reframe those communications and put the message in context with current neurobiologic knowledge. For example, panic attacks are real; they result from the triggering of an overreactive alarm center in the brain, which sends a message of fear via the release of a neurotransmitter, causing a racing heart and shortness of breath.

NEUROANATOMY

Volumes have been written about the anatomy of the brain and the other components of the nervous system. The definition that best suits the perspective of this chapter is that the brain is that part of the central nervous system (brain and spinal cord) encapsulated by the skull. The brain is the core of our humanity. Intercommunication among different parts of the brain yields the experiences of love, hate, joy, fear, and sadness. The brain provides the underlying biology for will, determination, hopes, and dreams, as well as the ability to problem solve, to establish memory, and to learn and use acquired knowledge productively. See ■ Figure 4–1 on page 60 for the major features of brain functioning. www.med.harvard. edu/AANLIB shows an atlas of the brain and can be accessed on the Companion Website of this book.

MediaLink Atlas of the Brain

Cerebrum

The **cerebrum** comprises the largest part of the human brain. It is divided into two components, the *cerebral hemispheres.* The deep furrow that divides the hemispheres is known as the *longitudinal sulcus.* A small but important piece of tissue, the *corpus callosum,* connects the two hemispheres medially and allows communication between them through networks of neurologic fibers. In the past, scientists believed that each hemisphere had separate functions, such as logic or creativity and spatial accommodation. With the advent of new technologies such as positron-emission tomography (PET), it is now possible to assess metabolic activity in the brain as it occurs (see Box 4–1 on page 61). Scientists are able to observe brain activity and have come to realize that creative as well as logical activities require input from both cerebral hemispheres.

The cerebral hemispheres are divided into four lobes, named after the parts of the skull under which they lie: frontal, parietal, temporal, and occipital (see Box 4–2 and ■ Figure 4–2 on page 62). The lobes have pairs on each side of the corpus callosum, which splits the brain in half. These lobes make up the *neocortex.* The neocortex is involved in the subjective experience of emotion, motivation, learning, memory, and gross motor skills. Each lobe has unique functions that contribute to a person's ability to move, process information, and have thoughts and feelings.

The frontal lobe has functional responsibilities for muscular movement and *vegetative effects* (slowing effects) on respiration

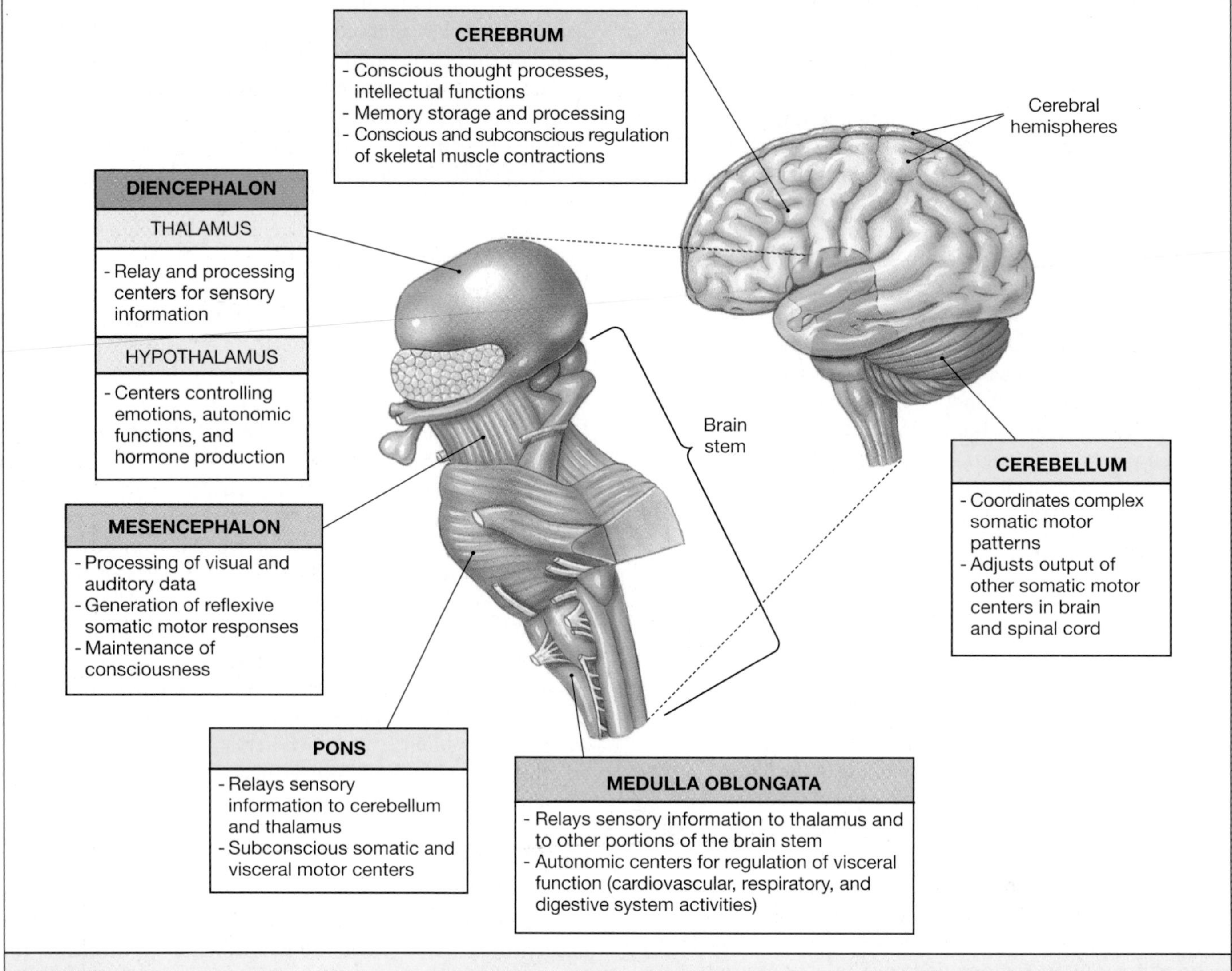

FIGURE 4–1 ■ *Brain functions are listed for the cerebrum, diencephalon, mesencephalon, pons, medulla oblongata, and cerebellum.*

Source: Martini, F. H. (2000). *Fundamentals of anatomy and physiology*. Upper Saddle River, NJ: Prentice Hall.

and circulation. The frontal lobe receives information from the limbic system that results in an effect on thinking, motivation, and understanding consequences to behavior. Lesions in the frontal lobe lead to abnormalities of speech, motor and voluntary movement, a loss of drive, difficulty with thought and planning, and disruption in ability to concentrate and the ability to attend to stimuli in the environment, as well as being able to shift from one mental activity to another. There is a deficit in the motor ability to suck, grasp, and grope. Behavioral changes also occur, such as a dysinhibition of self-control, changes in mood, and apathy.

The temporal lobe is the emotional center and is involved with memory and cognition. This lobe is also important to understanding the acoustic aspects of language as it is the primary auditory cortex. The limbic system, which is involved in emotions, memory, and thought patterns, will be covered in depth later in this chapter.

The parietal lobe facilitates complex motor and cognitive skills, such as a mastery of visual and spatial balance, mathematical ability, and spelling. The parietal lobe is also the primary somatosenory area receiving input from the thalamus. The occipital lobe is involved in visual perception and recognition (Adams, Victor, & Ropper, 1997; Bear, Connors, & Paradiso, 2001; Smock, 1999).

The brain, in general, and the cerebral hemispheres in particular, are well protected not only by the skull but also by a protective fluid, called cerebrospinal fluid (CSF) that circulates around and within the brain. Deep within the brain are three spaces, or *ventricles,* that aid in the circulation of CSF. Normal CSF volume is about 125 mL in an average adult and is replaced approximately four times in 24 hours. The CSF reflects neurochemical activity of the brain and is one method for studying *in vivo* (within the living organism) communications. The purpose of a spinal tap is to measure the volume and pressure of the CSF; to

BOX 4–1 Tools of Psychobiology

Brain Imaging

- *Computed tomography (CT)*. An x-ray beam (radiation exposure) is passed through serial sections of the brain to look at structural images.
- *Magnetic resonance imaging (MRI)*. Reconstructs detailed images of cerebral anatomy from multiple perspectives, including subcortical structures, using radiofrequency signals emitted by relaxing hydrogen atoms. It delineates gray and white matter. New instruments image elements other than hydrogen, allowing MRI to be used for structural, functional, and metabolic imaging. Contraindicated for clients with any metal objects in their bodies such as pacemakers, due to the presence of a magnetic field.
- *Positron emission tomography (PET)*. Imaging of active neurochemical substrates and physiologic processes; regional localization of metabolic functions through the measurement of radioactive labels or tags attached to molecules as glucose; density of neuroreceptors; regional cerebral blood flow (rCBF) of the brain. Operates on the principle that blood rushes to the busiest area of the brain to deliver oxygen and nutrients to the active neurons.
- *Single photon-emission computed tomography (SPECT)*. Measures rCBF; visualizes and measures the density of neuroreceptors, using tracer isotopes such as xenon, a gas; iodine 123; or technetium.

Neurophysiologic Techniques

- *Electroencephalogram (EEG)*. Measures electrical activity patterns of the brain from leads connected to surface electrodes placed on the scalp and nasopharyngeal area.
- *Polysomnography (sleep EEG)*. Measures electrical brain activity data during all-night sleep.
- *Brain electroactivity mapping (BEAM)*. Extends the EEG by generating computerized maps of brain electrical activity to produce images; permits visualization of the brain performing tasks or specific functions. Useful with children.
- *Event-related potential (EPs)*. Repeated auditory or visual stimuli associated with tiny electrical events in the cerebral cortex or subcortical structures, measured by surface electrodes.

Pharmacologic Challenge

The use of a drug (challenge) to provoke a neuronal system for better understanding of its physiologic effects and changes. Examples are the dexamethasone suppression test (DST), thyrotropin-releasing hormone (TRH) challenge, or giving a drug known to have specific receptor affinity such as clonidine to examine the alpha-2-adrenergic system in panic disorder.

Molecular Genetics

- *Linkage map*. A genetic map that represents the relationship between two genes, often revealed by the inheritance of traits in families, to determine the relative position of genes on a given chromosome.
- *Restriction fragment length polymorphisms (RFLPs)*. Method of molecular genetics using restriction enzymes, which cuts a DNA strand at sites where the enzyme recognizes a sequence between coding information. Differences in the lengths of these restriction fragments are believed to be inherited. The transmission can be mapped within families and a genetic pattern of transmission identified.
- *Candidate genes*. Identification of a specific gene thought to have pathophysiologic relevance to the illness being studied.

look for trauma, blood, or infection; and to measure *metabolites*, the products or substances produced from the breakdown of metabolic processes of the brain's neuromessengers.

All of the lobes contain many *gyri* (ridges), fissures, and *sulci* (grooves) that maximize the surface area of the brain. The cerebral hemispheres consist of both white and gray matter. Gray matter consists of fibers that are referred to as *nerves;* bundles of nerves are called *tracts.* The cerebral cortex consists solely of gray matter with underlying white matter. The white matter is an indication of myelination. The white matter increases with age, while gray matter decreases with age. The corpus callosum, a white matter structure, grows in size about 1.8% each year between the ages of 3 and 18 years. This structure integrates the activity between the left and right cerebral hemispheres. The increase in corpus callosum may be a sign of an increased ability for problem-solving abilities (Tamminga, 1999a). The cerebral cortex produces results much like those produced by the central processing unit of a computer. The cortex is the part of the brain that makes sense out of the volumes of input. It processes and synthesizes information, thought, reasoning, will, and choice and is the seat of dreams.

Limbic System

The **limbic system**, often referred to as the "emotional brain," is believed to be responsible for the experience and expression of emotion, as well as memory and some aspects of attention. The limbic system is a functional grouping rather than an anatomic one. The limbic system consists of structures from the cerebral hemispheres and the *diencephalon,* a part of the brain located between the cerebrum and midbrain (Box 4–3 on page 62).

Two limbic structures play an especially important role in the enactment of emotion and memory:

1. Amygdala
2. Hippocampus

Learning and memory are two aspects of the interaction between the amygdala and the hippocampus. The limbic structures also include the olfactory area. Therefore, if the olfactory sensors determine an odor; the memory of the event will include this cue. For example, does the smell of baking cookies trigger a pleasant childhood memory of being in your mother's kitchen when she baked cookies for you? This is the combined effect of amygdala and hippocampal functions using the cue of the smell of the cookies as the stimulus for the memory.

Amygdala. The **amygdala** gauges certain emotional reactions and plays a role in social behavior. It serves as the behavioral awareness center and helps pattern appropriate emotional and behavioral responses such as fear, sexual desire, rage, and appetite. It is hypothesized that the amygdala is also the struc-

BOX 4–2 **Gross Functions of the Cerebral Lobes**

Frontal Lobes

- Responsible for movement; the right frontal lobe controls the left side of the body's movements, and vice versa.
- Contain the premotor cortex, which organizes complicated movement.
- Contain prefrontal fibers with capacities for the ability to plan and problem-solve; also responsible for social judgment, volition, attention, learning, spontaneity, thinking, and affect.

Parietal Lobes

- Contain the sensory cortex, which interprets contact sensations such as touch and pressure.
- Facilitates spatial orientation.

Temporal Lobes

- Involved in hearing, memory, language comprehension, and emotions.
- Connect with the limbic system (the "emotional brain") to allow for the expression of such emotions as rage, fear, sexual and aggressive behavior, and possibly love.

Occipital Lobes

- Facilitate the interpretation of visual images and visual memory.
- Involved in language formation.
- Collaborate with many other brain structures in the formation of memory.

ture that is important in seeking love and sustaining long-term emotional memories.

Hippocampus. The **hippocampus** is also involved in emotional reactions and in learning by helping to process, store, and retrieve information in memory. It provides new information for permanent storage. Hallucinations may, in part, originate from hyperexcitability of psychomotor effects of olfactory, visual, auditory, and tactile stimulation in this region (Smock, 1999). Weak stimuli in the hippocampus can cause epileptic seizures.

The functions of the limbic system are not discrete, and the neuronal connections are so widespread and intricate within the brain that their complex interactions involve many different areas. Other neuronal groups that participate with the limbic system are the thalamus, hypothalamus, and the pituitary gland.

Reticular Activating System. The reticular activating system (RAS) consists of nerve pathways that originate in the spinal cord and connect in the reticular formation, a system of neurons that modulates awareness and states of consciousness. By screening stimulation from the environment, the RAS enables us to concentrate. The RAS also permits routine inattention, allowing for sleep. During sleep, excitatory neurons of the RAS gradually become more and more excitable because of prolonged rest, while inhibitory neurons of sleep centers become less excitable because of their overactivity, leading to a new cycle of wakefulness. This helps explain the rapid transitions between sleep and wakefulness. Arousal, as experienced by

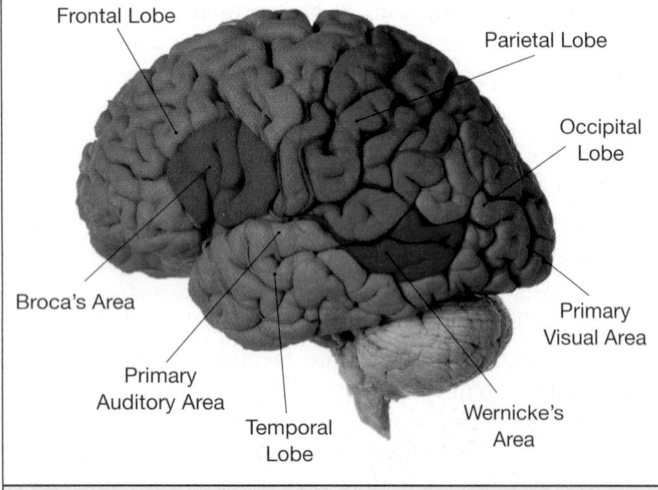

FIGURE 4–2 ■ *There are four major lobes of the brain: frontal, parietal, occipital, and temporal. Broca's area (found on the left frontal lobe) is the area responsible for the ability to speak but not the comprehension of speech. Wernicke's area in the left temporal lobe relays speech comprehension information to the frontal lobe.*

Source: Smock, T. K. (1999). *Physiological psychology: A neuroscience approach*. Upper Saddle River, NJ: Prentice Hall.

BOX 4–3 **The Limbic System**

Functions

Processing of memories; creation of emotional states, drives, and associated behaviors

Cerebral Components

Cortical areas: Limbic lobe (cingulate gyrus, dentate gyrus, and parahippocampal gyrus)
Nuclei: Hippocampus, amygdaloid body
Tracts: Fornix

Diencephalic Components

Thalamus: Anterior nuclear group
Hypothalamus: Centers concerned with emotions, appetites (thirst, hunger), and related behaviors

Other Components

Reticular formation: Network of interconnected nuclei throughout brain stem

Source: Martini, F. H. (2000). *Fundamentals of anatomy and physiology* (p. 454). Upper Saddle River, NJ: Prentice Hall

people with psychiatric conditions, can be the insomnia that occurs when a person's mind becomes preoccupied with a thought. In states of mental disorder, there is obviously some biologic disequilibrium of the RAS because it involves motivation and levels of arousal. However, the details of this imbalance are complex and not well understood at this time.

Extrapyramidal System. The extrapyramidal system consists of tracts of motor neurons from the brain to parts of the spinal cord. This system has complex relays and connections to areas of the cortex, cerebellum, brain stem, and thalamus. These tracts play an important role in gross movements and responses of emotional tone, such as smiling and frowning.

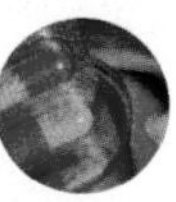

Antipsychotic drugs create side effects that affect the extrapyramidal system; hence the terms *extrapyramidal symptoms (EPS)* and *extrapyramidal side effects (EPSE)*. The four general classes of EPS are:

1. Parkinsonism
2. Dyskinesias and Dystonias
3. Akathisia
4. Tardive Dyskinesia

A complete discussion of extrapyramidal side effects can be found in Chapter 31.

Diencephalon

The diencephalon is composed of the thalamus and the hypothalamus. Both of these structures are illustrated in Figure 4–1 on page 60.

Thalamus. The thalamus functions as a relay station, receiving many impulses from the spinal cord, brain stem, and cerebellum. With the aid of numerous connections in the cerebral hemispheres and cortex, the thalamus regulates activity and movement, sensory experience (except smell), and emotional expression.

Hypothalamus. The **hypothalamus** is a "hub" between the mind and body, giving physical form to thoughts and emotions. It weighs approximately 4 grams and accounts for less than 1% of the total volume of the brain. Its size, however, is not a good indication of importance. The hypothalamus regulates many of the body's critical activities, including hormone levels, appetite (hunger), body temperature (thermoreceptors), sex drive (libido), water balance (thirst), circadian rhythms, pleasure, and pain.

The hypothalamus is the critical link between the cerebral cortex, the limbic system, and the endocrine system. It serves as a pipeline to the brain stem and acts as a conduit for control of the autonomic nervous system. The mammillary bodies, located at the back of the hypothalamus, help transfer information about the activities of the hypothalamus to other parts of the brain. The amygdala controls hypothalamic impulses due to the direct neurologic connection. This is important in the regulation of hunger, thirst, sexual behavior, rage, and/or pleasure. The hypothalamus is involved with the hormonal balance along with the pituitary gland. This is imperative during a time when the individual experiences a stress response (Smock, 1999). The infundibulum, a narrow stalk, connects the hypothalamus to the pituitary gland, a part of the endocrine system. The thalamus and hypothalamus, as well as the pituitary gland, are illustrated in ■ Figure 4–3 on page 64.

Pituitary Gland

The pituitary gland, under the direction of the hypothalamus, secretes hormones. These hormones are carried through the bloodstream and trigger the activities of other glands. The pituitary also receives input from the fornix and includes connections to the thalamus, which, in turn communicates to and from the frontal cortex (see Figure 4–3). The pituitary gland is the primary link between the nervous and endocrine systems.

Basal Ganglia

The basal ganglia are collectively a complex of structures that include the caudate nucleus, putamen, globus pallidus, and substantia nigra. Their functions include initiating and terminating movement, planning motor activities, mediating hallucinations and delusions, and processing emotions and memories. The basal ganglia have a high concentration of dopamine receptors, acetylcholine, gamma-aminobutyric acid, and peptides. A deficit of dopamine from this area is associated with Parkinson's disease. Parkinson's disease is characterized by rhythmic tremors of the extremities, slurred speech, and an unchanging facial expression much like that of former boxer Muhammad Ali, who sustained numerous blows to his head resulting in damage to the basal ganglia.

Cerebellum

The **cerebellum** lies below the posterior section of the cerebrum. It is the second largest structure within the brain. Like the cerebral hemispheres, the cerebellum has an outer layer of gray matter and is mainly composed of underlying white matter. The main function of this highly specialized part of the brain is movement, posture, balance, and sensory–motor coordination. The hand–eye coordination of a diamond cutter, the fluid movements of a ballerina, and the success of a quarterback's moves all depend on cerebellar functions.

Brain Stem

Beneath the limbic system is the **brain stem.** The brain stem consists of three smaller structures: the medulla oblongata, the pons, and the midbrain (as seen in Figure 4–3).

Medulla Oblongata. The medulla oblongata (Latin for "oblong marrow" or the inner portion of the organ shaped as an oblong) is the connecting piece of tissue between the brain stem and the spinal cord. It is less than 5 cm long but is responsible for controlling many vital functions, including respiration, regulation of blood pressure, and partial regulation of heart rate. It also controls the perception of pain, vomiting, swallowing, and some aspects of talking. Incoming fibers from the spinal cord cross over in the medulla, yielding left cerebral hemispheric control of the right side of the body, and vice versa.

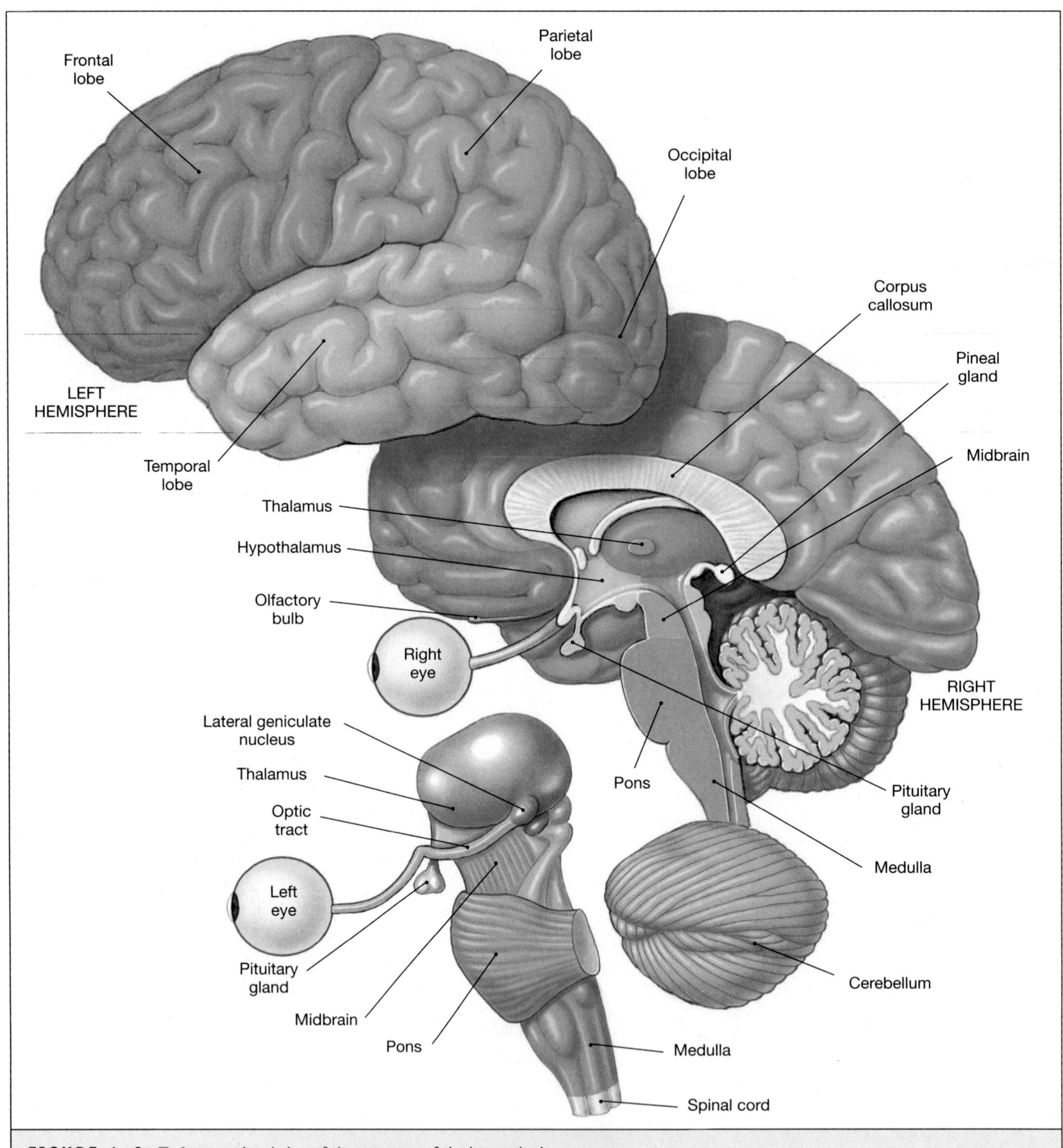

FIGURE 4–3 ■ *Cross-sectional view of the structures of the human brain.*

Source: Smock, T. K. (1999). *Physiological psychology: A neuroscience approach*. Upper Saddle River, NJ: Prentice Hall.

Pons. The pons (Latin for "bridge") contains conduction paths between the spinal cord and the brain, and bridging is its function. It also contains reflex centers that mediate sensations of the face, chewing, abduction of the eyes, facial expressions, balance, and the regulation of respiration. Located within the pons is the locus ceruleus, a tiny oval structure that contains 70% of the neurons (nerve cells) that release norepinephrine, the influence of which extends throughout the brain. One projection is to the amygdala, resulting in emotional and cardiovascular control. Activation of the locus ceruleus is associated with fear, pain, and alarm.

Midbrain. The midbrain is above the pons and below the cerebral hemispheres. The midbrain is a reflex center for the regulation of eye movement, visual accommodation, and regulation of pupil size. The midbrain is also essential for relaying impulses to the cerebral cortex and sending behavior-producing messages back to the rest of the body.

Certain portions of the brain function in concert with other parts to create a system with a given function; the limbic system is a good example. Other systems that are of special interest to psychiatric–mental health nurses include the reticular activating system and the extrapyramidal system, discussed previously in this chapter.

Autonomic Nervous System. Within the brain stem are areas called the autonomic nervous system (ANS). There are two divisions: the sympathetic division and the parasympathetic division. In stressful emotional circumstances, the sympathetic division of the ANS (also called the sympathetic nervous system) prepares for fight or flight; the parasympathetic initiates the relaxation response with the aid of the endocrine system. Researchers have established that prolonged stress can weaken the immune system and may trigger mood disorders (Bailey, 1999; DeVane, 2001). Chapter 5 includes a complete review of stress reactions. The goal of meditation and other forms of stress management is to inhibit the sympathetic response and strengthen the parasympathetic response.

GENETICS

Often, clients may tell you that others in their family experience "moodiness," "crazy thoughts," or that they "worry constantly for no reason." These disclosures are important clues about how major psychiatric disorders tend to run in families. A new area of research is exploring the genetic material to find clues to a possible heritable basis of behavior. What are the molecular consequences of abnormal genes? The application of genetic strategies to clinical practice will bring many new challenges and ethical dilemmas. Alterations in genetic coding, or designer genes, are currently being used with diseases such as cancer and cystic fibrosis to supply healthy genes or block a defective gene. In the future, perhaps the following questions will be answered for practitioners in psychiatry–mental health:

- How can understanding the biological markers determine what medications may help an individual?
- What specific steps can a family take to decrease the incidence of a severe mental disorder if there is a high genetic loading based on history?
- How can nurses help clients understand the role genetics may play in emotional illness?
- Do the same genes, but a different environment, result in depression or an anxiety disorder?
- Does a stressful life event trigger genetically vulnerable neurons to promote rapid-cycling mood disorder or panic disorder?

To begin to answer these questions, a review of the chemical composition of genes and certain aspects of cell structure and function is necessary.

Gene Structure

In 1990, the Human Genome Project was established to discover gene structure, provide a map of how genes work, and locate the chemical base pairs that make up DNA, and the spaces between the chemical pairs, to determine abnormal or disease-linked genes. The gene is the functional unit of information of the chromosome.

The human genome consists of 23 pairs of chromosomes, one from each parent; 22 pairs are the somatic chromosomes, and one pair is the sex chromosome (XX female, XY male). Genes are segments of DNA (deoxyribonucleic acid), the complex molecule that makes up chromosomes, and are found in all of the body's cell nuclei. Each cell uses the complement of genes selectively. The genes make proteins that are necessary for the cell to do its assigned task. For example, a bone cell gene differs from a brain cell gene in structure and function.

RNA (ribonucleic acid) is another complex molecule that plays a role in translating DNA's coding instructions for making protein. Each strand of the complex molecule of DNA is compactly formed into a double helix. The strand of DNA is composed of chemical nucleotides consisting of one sugar molecule (DNA or RNA), one phosphate group, and one of four nitrogen bases. The nucleotides are:

- Adenine (A)
- Thymine (T)
- Guanine (G)
- Cytosine (C)

The nucleotides line up next to each other like two sides of a zipper, with the phosphate and sugar forming the outer strand; the bases (A, T, G, and C) act like interlocking teeth (■ Figure 4–4 on page 66). The sequence of amino acids, which are proteins, is coded by genes. The sequence or code is like a language and is not arbitrary. The nucleotides, or two sides of the zipper, can fit together in only one way: A pairs with T, and G pairs with C. This base pairing allows for the known sequence of one strand to predict the partner strand. Each strand of the double helix thus specifies its complement and allows for the duplication of genetic information in dividing cells.

Gene Function

Variations in the chemical composition of the genes can produce abnormal structural proteins or enzymes, altering the sending or receiving of signals and resulting in dysfunction or disease. The main component of all living matter is protein, which consists of large molecules or long chains of amino acids linked together. The sequence of amino acids along the chain determines each protein's physical and biologic properties, acting as information molecules.

The transfer of DNA from the nucleus requires messenger RNA (mRNA), which serves as the instructor for the making of proteins outside the nucleus. Ribosomes, which float in the cytoplasm or sit on the rough endoplasmic reticulum, translate the mRNA into proteins. Also in the cytoplasm are the mitochondria, which generate energy, via ions and adenosine triphosphate (ATP), from the oxidation of fats and sugars, and

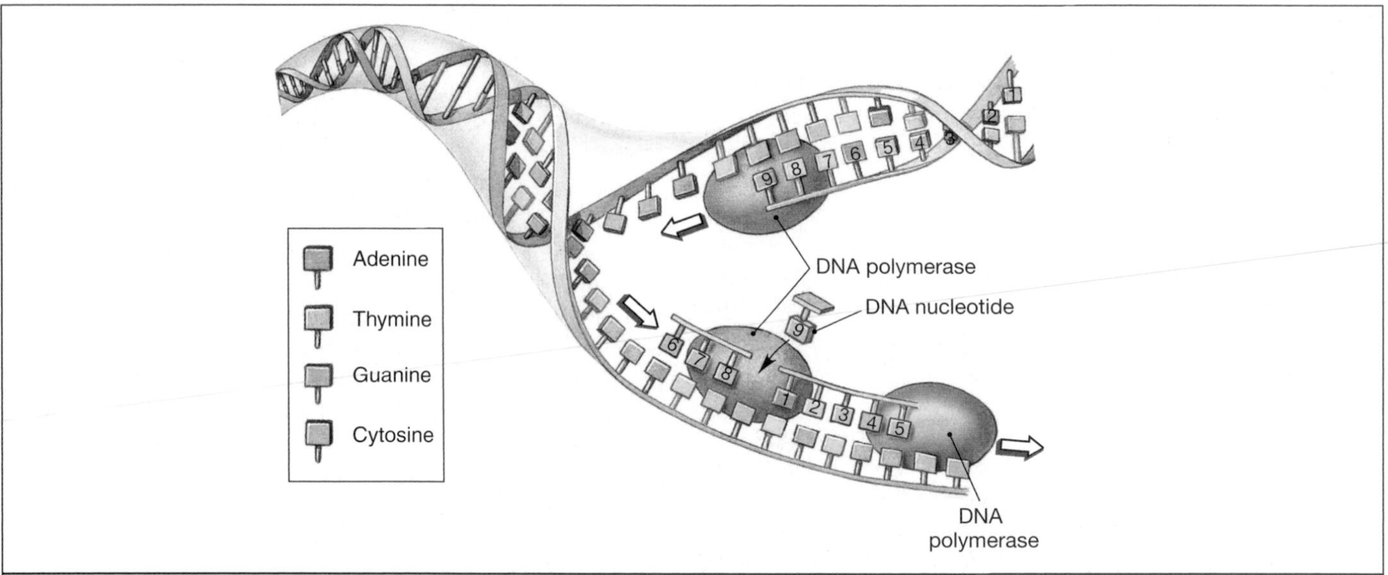

FIGURE 4–4 ■ *The structure of DNA shows how each strand of the complex molecule is compactly formed into a double helix and the strand of DNA is composed of the chemical nucleotides adenine (A), thymine (T), guanine (G), and cytosine (C).*

Source: Martini, F. H. (2001). *Fundamentals of anatomy and physiology*. Upper Saddle River, NJ: Prentice Hall.

also contain RNA and DNA. The process of protein synthesis is diagrammatically illustrated in ■ Figure 4–5.

Instructions for the synthesizing and metabolizing of the molecular messengers of the brain are coded in the DNA. One of the premises of neurobiology is that major mental disorders are brain diseases. A typical protein has a useful life of about two days; thus, new protein molecules are constantly being synthesized. Genes can be mutated by a single mismatch of the wrong base in the DNA, or a piece of the DNA can be mistakenly repeated, deleted, or altered. This could cause the cell to function in a changed manner. This concept may help explain how a client's symptoms or behavioral expression can change over time. New messages among the complex combinations of proteins change the code in the physical environment, resulting in different expressions of temperament, behavior, and individuality.

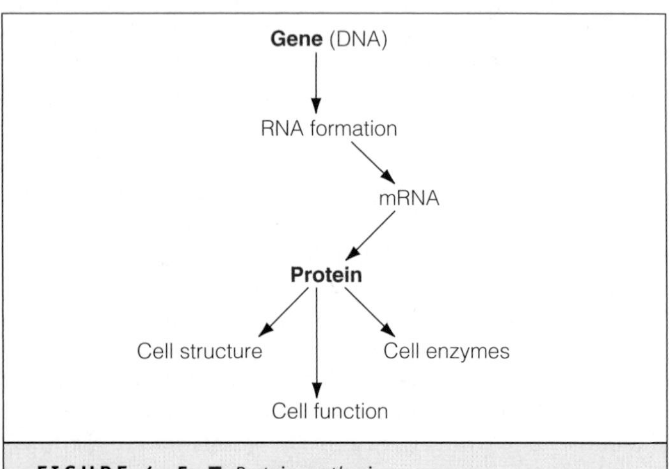

FIGURE 4–5 ■ *Protein synthesis.*

New technologies enable researchers to modify DNA and RNA so that both the messages and the expression of the messages can be manipulated experimentally. DNA markers, from fragments of DNA (restriction fragment length polymorphisms, or RFLPs), are making it possible to identify and localize the genes involved in a disease process. RFLPs represent a direct reflection of the DNA sequence and can be used to determine accuracy on kinship and group relationships. RFLP separation has led to a large library of DNA sequence markers and a human mutation database. This information has assisted researchers in determining the probability that a mutation can take place at any secific area of the genome (Rannala & Reeve, 2001). Those data gathered in the mutation database help us to understand the pathophysiology of a disease and its treatment and possibly, in the future, its prevention.

The polymerase chain reaction (PCR) is another technology used with DNA. Even a single cell would be enough to start the process of analyzing a DNA fragment with PCR as the amounts needed for analysis can be generated from that cell. This process reproduces individual fragments of DNA and is used in genetic engineering efforts and research investigations (Yamaguchi et al., 2002). PCR was used to develop a number of diagnostic tests to detect disease-causing agents, and it is used in determining paternity. Also, forensic medicine finds PCR to be indispensable for criminal investigations.

Genetic Research

Psychiatric-focused genetic studies are conducted by examining the blood of family members who have mental disorder. Linkage studies are a type of genetic blood study used to locate genes that are thought to be involved in susceptibility to emotional illness. These studies examine the inheritance patterns of known DNA markers. This research assists in understanding the possible location of a suspect gene for an identified disorder, although the results thus far have not shown one particular gene as the culprit for any major mental disorder.

In linkage-disequilibrium studies, isolated populations are used to examine suspected genes for an identified disorder that is thought to have come from a few members of the study population (Kendler, Thornton, & Gardner, 2000). The population investigated in a linkage-disequilibrium study may be a geographic or cultural group with possibly fewer variations of the disease gene. Association studies are used to test a hypothesis that a specific gene or group of genes influence a particular disorder.

Ethics in Genetic Research

When a genetic loading component has the potential to create a mental disorder, the ethical implications can be controversial:

- How should a mental health professional proceed in discussions about heritability of the illness?
- What treatments are offered if, in the future, a gene is identified as causing a mental disorder and a child with no symptoms has that gene?

The ethical dilemmas include waiting until the child experiences symptoms and then treating or treating before symptoms appear. These are not clear choices. But overall, action taken by nurses includes the need to be familiar with the biologic mechanism of the illness to help clients make decisions about their care, their choices about childbearing, and to avoid the potential stigma associated with the genetics of mental disorders.

The ethics of genetic research is another area under examination. Consent for study participation includes information about the study, the risks and benefits of the research, what is involved in study participation, and what will be done with this genetic information obtained during the course of the study. Researchers must define how the information that is gathered during the study is secured, how the client's identity will be protected, and what will be reported. Confidentiality in keeping the genetics of the study sample anonymous is an essential consideration for the participants. Study participants have the right in every study to ask questions of the research's principal investigator. Further questions might include, among others:

1. An explanation of individual results.
2. What implications the genetic results may have on children.
3. What implications the genetic results may have on developing physical illnesses.
4. How these results compared to other participants in the research.
5. How these results compared to people in the general population (Beskow & Burke, 2001).

More on this topic is included in Chapter 10, "Ethical Reasoning."

The Genetic Basis of Psychiatric Illness

Research on the genetic basis of inherited psychiatric illnesses has been a focus of the National Institutes for Mental Health's (NIMH) Genetic Workgroup. This group has set goals for genetic research and directions for using the research in the clinical setting. In a report (1997), the Workgroup outlined the current research findings that will set the stage for future understanding of the complexity of the genetic and environmental influences of mental disorder. In all the genetic models, the roles of environmental influences, perinatal events, trauma, infections, and stress have to be considered. When evaluating clients and families for possible genetic links to an emotional disorder, it is important to consider the interaction between the genetic factors and the environment.

Scientists have discovered that:

1. There is no single gene responsible for a mental disorder.
2. There may be several susceptibility genes that interact with one another.
3. Environmental influences interact with genes to increase the risk of developing a mental disorder.

Genetic research is often done with twin studies to predict the impact of heredity. The rate of occurrence of the emotional disorder is compared between *monozygotic* (MZ—identical) twins and *dizygotic* (DZ—fraternal) twins. If the illness occurs more in MZ twins than in DZ twins, then heredity is an important factor to consider in the development of the mental disorder.

NIMH genetic research (1997) shows when evaluating bipolar disorder if one monozygotic twin has the illness, the other twin has a 60 to 80% chance of developing bipolar disorder. The dizygotic twin data shows an 8% chance of having bipolar disorder. When evaluating the statistics for schizophrenia; a monozygotic twin has a 45% chance of developing schizophrenia if they have a twin with this disorder; the dizygotic twin has a 14% chance of being affected. The NIMH data from over 40 family and twin studies demonstrated consistently that the risk of developing schizophrenia is greater in a family that has relatives with this emotional disorder as opposed to the population of normal controls.

Current research is developing in two directions. Due to the Human Genome Project and mapping, researchers are looking for the chromosome that may be implicated in a disease. For example, one group of researchers has identified chromosome 4q35 as an area that is implicated in bipolar disorder in a large linkage study (Adams et al., 1998).

There is no consistently supported single-gene model for the development of schizophrenia. It is hypothesized that there is a polygenetic model (Levinson, et al., 1998) meaning more than one gene may be responsible for this disorder. Recent research has concentrated on determining specific chromosomal locations of those genes. For example, genes 1q22–q24 and 1q42 demonstrate that genetic changes in the brain increase the likelihood of developing schizophrenia or bipolar disorder (Berrettini, 2000; Blackwood, 2000; Brzustowicz, Hodgkinson, Chow, Honer, & Bassett, 2000). Research on genetic location may assist in determining future genetic counseling and treatment.

The second area of current study is to alter the genetic material of a mouse brain to understand the structure and behavior patterns demonstrated in these altered animals. These mice are called "knockout" mice. This body of research is beginning to develop and will be useful in testing hypotheses about the nature of mental disorders as well as testing new medications.

The research on dementia of the Alzheimer's type (DAT) is investigating chromosomal abnormalities. Understanding the causal factors in early-onset DAT has led to assessing mutation in presenilin-1. This research used knockout mice that lacked the gene for presenilin-1. The knockout mice demonstrated that the presenilin-1 did not cleave in the usual way and the beta-amyloid plaques did not occur. The research concluded that when the gene for presenilin-1 is present and overactive there is excessive cleaving of the amyloid precursor protein that forms the plaques (Athan, E. S., Williamson, J., Ciappa, A., Santana, V., Romas, S. N., Lee, J. H., 2001; Dana Alliance for Brain Initiatives, 1999; Naslund, 2000). Further genetic research in DAT is the role amyloid-beta-derived diffusible ligands (ADDLs) have on the nerve cells. ADDLs disrupt the neurons that are responsible for learning and memory and then cause neuronal death (Dana Alliance for Brain Initiatives, 1999). Understanding the changes in the genetic composition of the nerve cells can lead to new medications that can be used to block ADDLs or decrease the excessive cleaving of the amyloid precursor protein. Research will contribute to the information needed to develop effective treatments for this complex disease.

NEURONS, SYNAPSES, AND NEUROTRANSMISSION

The brain's structural complexity increases as one considers the biochemical processes that occur with every thought, emotion, memory, dream, or hope. Thought and feeling are made possible by complex interplay and communication between cells in the central nervous system (CNS) in response to stimuli in the environment. The specialized cells of the nervous system are called **neurons.** Like other cells in the body, each neuron has a cell body that contains the cytoplasm and the nucleus. Unlike other cells, a neuron has at least two other extensions: an axon and one or more dendrites. An axon is the portion of a neuron that conveys electric impulses from the cell body to other neurons. Axons are covered with a white myelin sheath and compose the white matter in the brain and spinal cord. Dendrites are unmyelinated and conduct electrical messages to the cell body. There are approximately 100 billion neurons in the brain and nearly an equal number of supporting (glia) cells.

MediaLink Neurological Synapse Animation

Neurons are classified according to the direction in which they conduct impulses. *Sensory neurons,* also known as afferent neurons, send messages from the periphery to the brain. For example, if you place your foot into a tub of scalding water, the message that the water is too hot is sent to your brain via sensory neuron pathways. *Motor neurons,* or efferent neurons, carry messages that originate in the brain and yield a behavioral change in the periphery. In the example of your foot in the hot water, the message from the brain is to remove the foot (quickly!) from the hot water; this message travels via motor neuron pathways.

Communication among and between neurons is complex and specific. This communication is believed to be the basis of behavior. Each neuron forms anywhere from 1,000 to 10,000 synaptic connections. The synapse is a gap in the synaptic cleft between neurons. See ■ Figure 4–6 for a structural view of how a neuron conveys its messages. These reciprocal synapses form positive and negative feedback loops. Neurons are arranged in networks or pathways whereby neuronal communication is facilitated by repetition. Interneuron communication is electrical and chemical and occurs at synapses, or points of contact between neurons, as well as along the neuron itself.

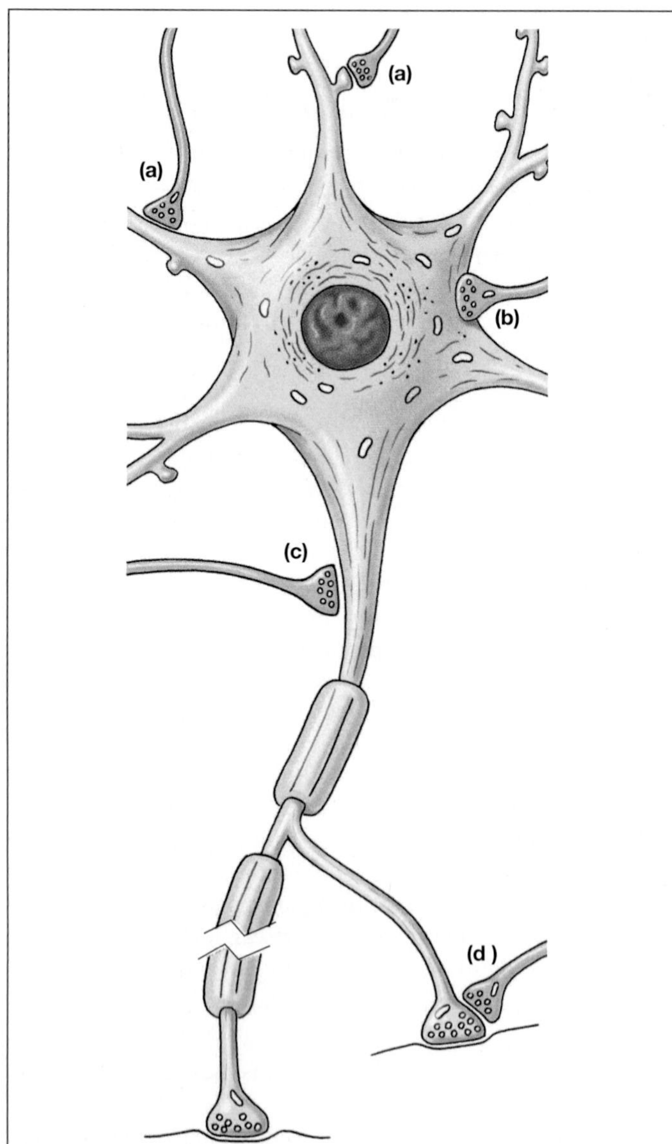

FIGURE 4–6 ■ *There are many different types of synaptic contacts that a neuron is capable of making. Shown here are (a) a synapse onto a dendrite called axodendritic contact, (b) a contact on the soma called axosomatic contact, (c) a synapse onto another axon called axoaxonic contact, and (d) an area where signals are sent and received called axosynaptic contacts.*

Source: Smock, T. K. (1999). *Physiological psychology: A neuroscience approach*, p. 23. Upper Saddle River, NJ: Prentice Hall.

Synaptic Transmission

Neuromessenger is a collective, generic term for neurotransmitters, neuromodulators, and neurohormones. *Neurotransmitters (NTs)* are neuromessengers that are rapidly released at the presynaptic neuron on stimulation, diffuse across the synapse between two neurons, and have either an excitatory or inhibitory effect on the postsynaptic neuron (see ■ Figure 4–7). The membrane of the axon terminal of a neuron contains many saclike projections called synaptic vesicles, which contain the NT molecules that transmit the message across the synapse.

Neurons are encased in cell membranes that function as a complex regulation site. The membranes contain proteins, some of which are phospholipids, enzymes, and ion channels. Ion channels are water-filled molecular tunnels that pass through the cell membrane and allow electrically charged atoms (ions) or small molecules to enter or leave the cell. The neuron exists in a state of tension because of the various ions in its membrane. Changes in ion concentrations cause the nerve impulse, or action potential, which transmits information between neurons. The four major ions are sodium, potassium, calcium, and chloride. Each ion passes in or out of the neuron via its own channel. Nerve impulses involve the opening or closing of the ion channels by gates.

Once the action potential reaches the end of the axon, the electrical transfer of the information ends, and messages are then conveyed by the chemicals, the NT molecules. The signal is mediated by binding to specific receptors on the cell surface (Adams et al., 1997). Depending on the type of channel, the action potential can be:

- Excitatory, influencing the neuron to fire, or
- Inhibitory, preventing it from firing.

Presynaptic axon terminals contain large numbers of calcium channels, which determine the quantity of NT that is released into the synaptic cleft.

At the synapse, the membrane of the postsynaptic neuron contains receptor proteins. Receptors are highly specialized proteins embedded in the membrane of the neuron that are in part exposed to the extracellular fluid and recognize the neuromessenger. Receptors are located on the axon (presynaptic) or on the dendrite (postsynaptic). Neurotransmitters and receptors vary in their affinity for each other, depending on the NT involved. They may bind like a lock and key, or the outcome may depend on what is available. Every neuron is more or less sensitive to a constant amount of neuromessenger, and this is an important principle in pharmacology. The NT that remains in the synapse after the postsynaptic response is either dissolved by synaptic enzymes or reabsorbed for recycling by the presynaptic neuron, a process known as reuptake (Smock, 1999).

MediaLink Serotonin Reuptake Inhibition Animation

Neurotransmitters

Neurotransmitters include these three classes as well as dissolved gases and a number of other compounds:

1. Biogenic amines (monoamines)
2. Amino acids

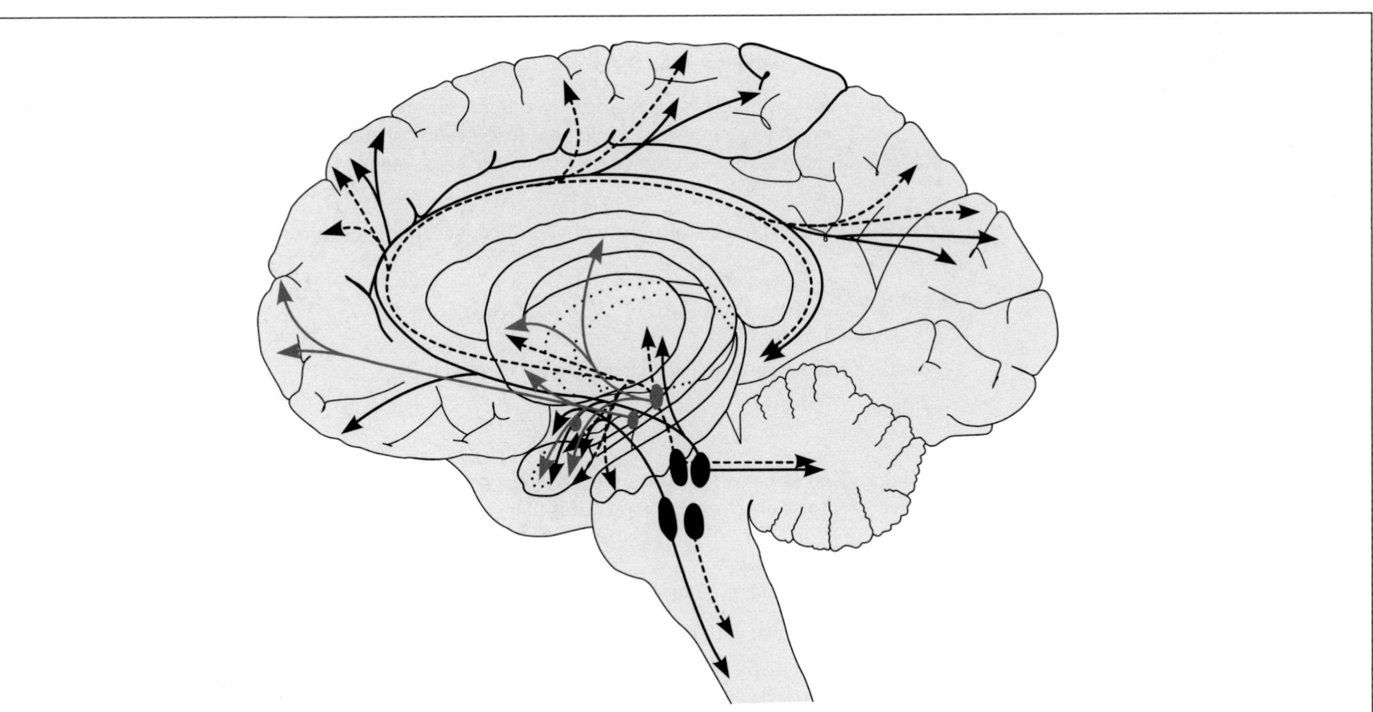

FIGURE 4–7 ■ *Common neurotransmitter pathways. Purple = DA, black = NE, dashed line = 5-HT. Dotted line indicates pons.*

3. Peptides (see ■ Table 4–1)

The biogenic amines include:

- Dopamine (DA)
- Norepinephrine (NE)
- Epinephrine
- Serotonin (5-hydroxytryptamine, or 5-HT)
- Acetylcholine (ACh)
- Histamine (H)

The biogenic amines are synthesized in the axon terminals and released into the synapse. Identification of these neurotransmitters began the era of neuropsychopharmacology.

Functional imaging techniques now enable researchers and clinicians to visualize the pathways of neuron clusters at work, to better understand their functional association with behavior. The original belief that a neuron contained only one NT is no longer valid. Figure 4–7 illustrates the basic pathways of three of the major biogenic amines.

Dopamine. **Dopamine (DA)** is released in a variety of areas in the brain where it influences how we interact in the world. See ■ Table 4–2 for specific DA areas and functions. One example of the excitatory effects of DA is when cocaine inhibits the removal of DA from the neuronal synapse. This causes a rise in the concentration of DA at those synapses, the excitatory impact takes effect, and the "high" associated with cocaine use is created.

Because of the presence of the DA pathways in all of these areas, DA disturbance is involved in psychosis. The efficacy of neuroleptic or antipsychotic drugs used to treat psychoses is correlated with the drug's ability to block DA receptors, although the newer antipsychotics have shown us that DA

TABLE 4–1 The Major Known Neurotransmitters

Neurotransmitter	Function
Biogenic Amines (Monoamines)	
Dopamine (DA) Precursor: tyrosine	Integrates thoughts and emotions; regulates pleasure and reward-seeking stimuli; control of complex movement; motivation; cognition; stimulates hypothalamus to release hormones affecting adrenal, thyroid, and sex hormones.
Norepinephrine (NE) Precursor: tyrosine	Stimulates sympathetic division of the ANS; role in stress response; fluctuates with sleep and wakefulness; role in attention and vigilance, arousal, ability to focus or learn, feeling of reward, regulation of mood and anxiety.
Serotonin (5-HT) Precursor: tryptophan	Inhibits activity and behavior; role in level of arousal; increases sleep time; reduces aggression, play, sexual, and eating activity; temperature regulation; pain control; mood states; role in circadian rhythms; sensory regulation; helps focus the brain; regulates pituitary.
Histamine (H) Precursor: histidine	Mediates allergic and inflammatory responses; smooth muscle constriction; stimulates gastric acid secretion; role in biorhythms and thermoregulation; role in second messenger transmission.
Acetylcholine (Ach) Precursor: choline	Attention; memory; promotes preparation for action; conserves energy; thirst; defense and/or aggression; sexual behavior; mood regulation; REM sleep; stimulates parasympathetic division of the ANS; controls muscle tone in balance with DA in the basal ganglia.
Amino Acids	
Gamma-aminobutyric acid (GABA) Precursor: glutamic acid	Reduces aroused aggression, anxiety, and excitation; sedation; anticonvulsant and muscle-relaxant properties.
Glycine Precursor: serine	Inhibitory.
Glutamate	Excitatory; role in learning and memory; neural degeneration.
Aspartate	Excitatory.
Peptides (Neuromodulators)	
Somatostatin	Mood disorders; Alzheimer's disease; negative feedback control of thyrotropin secretion; role in positive symptoms of schizophrenia. Excites limbic neurons.
Neurotensin	Role in schizophrenia.
Substance P	Excitatory; role in pain syndromes, mood, and movement disorders.
Cholecystokinin (CCK)	Role in schizophrenia; eating and movement disorders; panic disorder.
Vasopressin	Role in mood disorders.
Corticotropin-releasing hormone (CRH)	Stress, mood, memory, and anxiety.
Opioids: endorphins and enkephalins	Alters emotional behavior; pain control; hallucinations; pleasure; motor coordination; water balance.

TABLE 4–2 Dopamine Location and Function

Area/Location	Dopamine Is Associated with:		
Basal ganglia area	The control of complex movement		
Limbic system	Memory Mood	Reward Pleasure	Motivation
Hypothalamic tract	Endocrine functions Circadian rhythms		Food and water intake Temperature
Frontal cortex pathway	Insight Judgment Problem solving		Inhibition Social awareness

receptor blockade is not the only effective treatment for psychosis.

Norepinephrine. Norepinephrine (NE) is also called noradrenalin, and synapses releasing NE are adrenergic synapses. Receptors for the neurotransmitter norepinephrine are widespread in the brain. Locations of the receptors for NE are listed in ■ Table 4–3. NE plays a major role in mediating mood and anxiety. Normally NE is considered to have an excitatory impact. Regulation of norepinephrine has been examined closely in the treatment of mood and anxiety disorders and contributes to current psychopharmacologic interventions.

Serotonin. The serotonin (referred to as 5-HT) neurons arise in the raphe nuclei and project to the same areas as the NE pathways. Serotonin appears to be a modulator. Its effects include and influence the temperature, sensory, sleep, and assertiveness areas of the brain. Serotonin serves as a chemical mediator in pain perception, normal and abnormal behaviors, moods, drives, the regulation of food intake, and in neuroendocrine functions. Receptor subtypes decrease cerebral blood flow during a migraine episode and increase the response to pain.

TABLE 4–3 Norepinephrine Location and Function

Area/Location	Norepinephrine Is Associated with:	
Pons, specifically locus ceruleus	The stress response Arousal	Alertness
Cerebral cortex	Cognitive functioning	
Limbic system	Emotional responses Ability to focus or learn	Reward Regulation of mood Pleasure
Hypothalamus	Endocrine functions Temperature	Appetite Biological rhythms

Acetylcholine. The first chemical to be identified as a true neurotransmitter, acetylcholine (ACh) is the "grandparent" of neurotransmitters. Dopamine and ACh share a concentration of activity within the basal ganglia, and drugs that are used to block EPS are cholinergic stimulants, suggesting a reciprocal relationship between these two neurotransmitters in the modulation of movement and possibly psychosis. ACh plays a major role in the encoding of memory and in cognition. It also plays a mediation role in mood disorders, stress, and sleep regulation. It is considered to be highly significant in neuromuscular transmission.

Histamine. The role of histamine (H) in psychiatric illness is less understood. It is a chemical messenger that mediates a wide range of cellular responses, including allergic and inflammatory reactions, gastric acid secretions, and neurotransmission. Some psychiatric medicines block H receptors, resulting in the side effects of sedation, weight gain, and drowsiness (Barinaga, 2000).

Amino Acids. These neurotransmitters are natural substances found throughout the brain and body and in the proteins of the food we eat. The amino acid gamma-aminobutyric acid (GABA) is the most prevalent inhibitory NT. GABA neurons are widely distributed in the CNS. Glycine, also an inhibitory NT, is primarily in the brain stem, spinal cord, and cerebellum. GABA has a prominent role in arousal; when the neuron is stimulated, GABA acts as a brake, decreasing neuronal excitability. Benzodiazepines act by binding with GABA and benzodiazepine receptors to produce antianxiety, sedative, anticonvulsant, and muscle-relaxant properties.

Glutamate and aspartate are the two primary excitatory amino acid neurotransmitters. Glutamate is primarily located in the cerebral cortex and hippocampus and has a role in long-term memory and learning. Too much glutamate can be a neurotoxin, as seen in Huntington's chorea and phencyclidine (PCP) psychosis.

Psychopharmacologic strategies are becoming more specific with increased understanding of signal transduction. When the NT receptor complex results in a direct change in the membrane potential, it is called first messenger transmission. A rapid, direct membrane change can also initiate a series of intracellular reactions triggering a second messenger transmission. Guanine proteins are large families of receptors that are the links in second messenger cascades. Second messengers are membrane proteins that relay nerve signals from the NT complex through a chain of chemical reactions to the nucleus. Drugs acting at this level allow for greater selectivity in targeting specific enzymes associated with behavior. This cascade of signals is a major mechanism for switching proteins on or off.

PSYCHOENDOCRINOLOGY AND PSYCHONEUROIMMUNOLOGY

This section will examine the interaction of the brain with two subsystems: the body's endocrine system and the immune system. The interaction of the brain with the body's endocrine system is known as *psychoendocrinology*. The interaction of the brain with the body's immune system is known as *psychoneuroimmunology*.

Endocrine System

The endocrine system functions through neurochemical messengers in the bloodstream called hormones. The endocrine system is a communication system. Hormones secreted from the hypothalamus instruct the pituitary to stimulate the target tissues, glands. The major glands of the body are the adrenals, the gonads, and the thyroid; their primary function is releasing hormones. Hormones act as triggers. Each component of the neuroendocrine axis can feed back into any component of the system, including the cortex and limbic system. The amount of hormone produced is partly regulated by a negative feedback mechanism. Feedback regulation exists at all levels of the axis. Thus, the rise or fall in the blood level of one hormone can cause an increase or decrease in the level of another hormone. The immune and endocrine systems are integrated through a shared set of hormone receptors. Hormones have a broader range of responses than nerve impulses and require seconds to days to cause a response that may last from weeks to months.

Irregularities of neuroendocrine function have been linked to depression, postpartum psychosis, schizophrenia, polydipsia in clients with psychosis, panic disorder, obsessive–compulsive disorder (OCD), anorexia nervosa, DAT, and circadian rhythms. Psychopharmacologic challenge tests are described in Box 4–1 earlier in this chapter and enhance our understanding of the pathophysiology of these conditions. One such test is the *dexamethasone suppression test* (DST), which attempts to assess the hypothalamic–pituitary–adrenal (HPA) axis (■ Figure 4–8). Dexamethasone, a synthetic glucocorticoid, is given by mouth at 11:00 PM to "challenge" the axis. By measuring blood samples of the hormone cortisol drawn at 4:00 PM the day before the pill is taken, and at 8:00 AM (highest level of normal rhythm), 4:00 PM (lowest level of rhythm), and 11:00 PM the day after the pill is taken, one can assess a relationship between the pituitary and the hypothalamus.

Dexamethasone "turns off" adrenocorticotropic hormone (ACTH) secretion at the pituitary, which in turn suppresses cortisol secretion from the adrenals. In a normally functioning axis, cortisol is reduced for the next 24 hours. However, nonsuppression, or "escape," is observed by a rise in the 4:00 PM level, when it should be low, in many psychiatric conditions. There are no side effects or long-lasting changes as a result of taking the pill. The results are not diagnostic of the illness, but suggest some pathology in the HPA axis function.

Hormones secreted by the hypothalamus and pituitary are peptides, which are large, complex chains of amino acids linked together and synthesized by ribosomes in the neuronal cell body through the transcription of DNA. Their physiology is complex; they bind to specific receptors, modulating the response of the postsynaptic cell to the NT. These effects are slow, involving such prolonged actions as changes in the number of receptors, synapses, and closures of ion channels. They

MediaLink Receptor Sites (Agonists/Antagonists) Animation

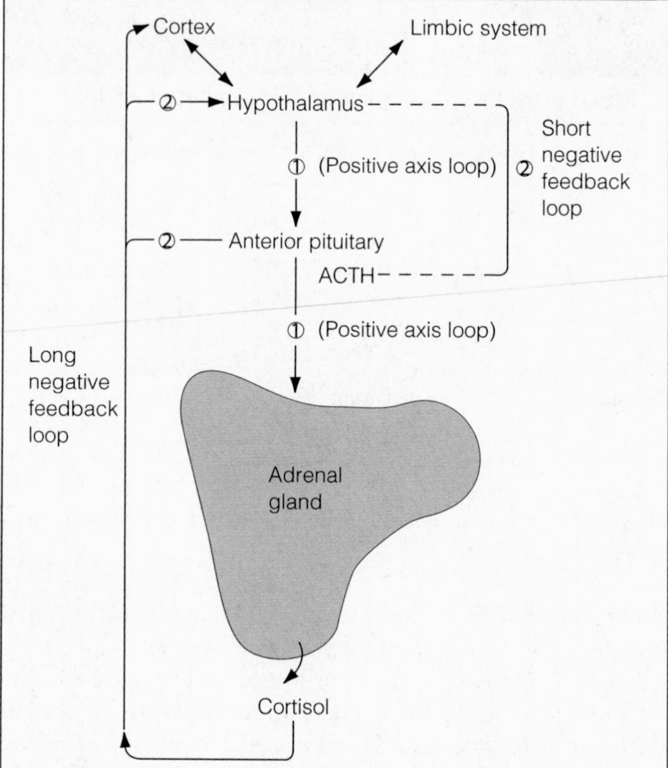

FIGURE 4–8 ■ *Example of neuroendocrine feedback. The positive loop in the axis is depicted by the hypothalamus. Upon stimulation from the cortex or limbic system, the release of trophic peptide CRH (corticotropin-releasing hormone) tells the pituitary gland to signal the adrenal cortex, via ACTH (adrenocorticotropic hormone), to release the glucocorticoid cortisol. Cortisol released into the bloodstream provides negative feedback to the hypothalamus or anterior pituitary. Additionally, ACTH can provide negative feedback to the hypothalamus.*

also have an important role in the memory process (Smock, 1999). The most commonly understood peptides are summarized in Table 4–1.

Researchers have been studying the effect substance P has on human beings. Substance P is a prototype neuropeptide that is thought to co-transmit with serotonin in the neuronal pathways. The role of substance P has been studied in the knockout mice discussed above. The synthesis of substance P along with other neuropeptides is necessary during a neurogenic inflammatory response in mice.

Substance P is released during stress, both physiologic stress, such as pinching the mouse's tail, and environmental stress. In human beings, substance P is thought to contribute to changes in the CNS that predispose the individual to anxiety and depression. As we begin to understand substance P's role in signaling the intensity of pain and aversive stimuli, a new approach to treating pain is evolving. There is also new information about substance P's involvement with depression and psychological stress. The direction of this research will lead to the development of medication compounds that are substance P antagonists that may treat diseases that have an emotional response to aversive stimuli (DeVane, 2001).

Immune System

Psychoneuroimmunology (PNI) is the study of the links between thoughts, emotions, the nervous system, and the immune system. The relationships between these systems have been known by clinicians for a long time. New research is being dedicated to further the *why* of the interactions. The National Institutes of Health (NIH) National Center for Complementary and Alternative Medicine investigates methods and techniques of alternative and complementary treatments. The goal for most practitioners is to combine effective treatments from the alternative options with commonly understood mainstream medicine to provide the best care. This combination is referred to as an integrative approach. An enormous reservoir of choice for promoting health for an individual can be opened up by determining how these, and other, alternative and complementary techniques discussed in Chapter 32 can influence the healing process :

- Ethnic healing practices
- Therapeutic touch
- Massage
- Guided imagery
- Relaxation
- Nutritional counseling

This field holds much potential for nursing and clinicians in all specialties. The area of practice extends to psychiatry as we strive to understand the influence stress has on mental disorders.

The most common psychological problems reported by clients seeking medical consultation are depression and anxiety. These two psychological clusters of symptoms increase the usage of medical diagnostic services. Stress-related symptoms account for 60% of all primary care visits.

Our understanding of chemical communication between the brain and immune system comes from the study of receptors. Cells in the limbic system have many receptors for neuropeptides such as endorphins, and immune system cells contain receptors for endorphins and other peptides such as corticotropin-releasing hormone (CRH).

The brain can directly influence the immune system by sending messages along nerve cells. The series of communication affects the cell nucleus, producing changes in the DNA and RNA that alter the shape of the neuron or even cause cell death. In the fight-or-flight response, immune system function is slowed, and energy is directed toward helping the body meet the immediate challenge.

KINDLING AND BEHAVIORAL SENSITIZATION

Kindling is the repeated administration of a subconvulsant stimulus to the neuron. The stimulus may be a chemical cascade from stress, which results in sensitizing the neuron rather than tolerance of the stimulus. *Behavioral sensitization* is a chemical phenomenon whereby changes occur in behavior as part of short-term and long-term memory. Following a series of these "seizures," the neuron requires less stimulus to produce the seizure-like response. Kindling appears to be a kind of learning, independent of cognition, and it can set off an autonomous process.

Although kindling has not been demonstrated definitively in humans, there is indirect support for these biologic interactions. Alcohol withdrawal, posttraumatic stress disorder (PTSD), panic disorder, and rapid-cycling mood disorders are similar in that stress or a chemical substrate produces kindled seizures in the amygdala region, which over time produce behavior changes (Bailey, 1999; Becker, 1998; Kalynchuk, Treit, & Pinel, 1999; Kendler et al., 2000). Carbamazepine, an anticonvulsant, and the benzodiazepines act on kindled episodes. Future clinical implications of this research require more formal conceptualization. However, it applies as a working hypothesis because bipolar disorder correlates with a stressful life event around the first episode about 60% of the time. Thus, repetitions of illness (episode sensitization) may trigger further psychopathology and also provide some explanation for why people with rapid-cycling mood disorders become refractory to medications over time. The neuron actually goes through changes, so different drugs or combinations are required to stabilize the progressive course (Stahl, 2000).

Circadian Rhythms

Biologic rhythms, or biorhythms, program our 24-hour day–night cycles. Chronobiology is the relationship between time and biologic rhythms and their effect on living systems. There are rhythms in endocrine secretion, NT synthesis, receptor number, enzyme levels and affinities, brain electrical activity, duration of cell cycle times, and the transcription regulation of DNA. Rhythms can have different cycle lengths:

- Ultradian: less than 24 hours
- Circadian: 24 hours
- Infradian: more than 24 hours

Zeitgebers are time cues or synchronizers, and they set the biological rhythms (Smock, 1999). See Box 4–4 for examples of zeitgebers.

One of the major functions of circadian timing is the sequencing and coordination of metabolic/physiologic events. The suprachiasmatic nucleus (SCN), a cluster of neurons in the hypothalamus, is the body's own internal synchronizer for temperature and sleep. External influences include the light–dark cycle, mealtime patterns, and work schedules (Smock, 1999).

One theory of depression is that it represents a phase advance disorder (as evidenced by early morning awakening), decreased onset of rapid eye movement (REM) sleep, and neuroendocrine changes. Mechanisms of sleep, both normal and

BOX 4–4 Zeitgebers

Zeitgebers are the external environmental synchronizers that help us adjust to a 24-hour day and include:

- Light
- Dark
- Feeding schedules
- Social activities
- Work
- Other time-enforced activities

The solar light–dark cycle is considered the most important environmental cue.

pathologic, are covered in Chapter 19. Research into the question of whether estrogen shortens the circadian period, lengthening the sleep phase, advancing sleep onset, and consolidating sleep would help our understanding of the phenomenology of depression and menopause related to changes in the sleep–activity cycle for women. Symptoms of people with seasonal affective disorder (SAD) vary, but the common ones are increased sleep and appetite, decreased energy, weight gain, low self-esteem, and negativism. A common treatment for this desynchronization is exposure to broad-spectrum light. Melatonin, synthesized from tryptophan in the pineal gland, allows the individual to become drowsy and promotes sleep. Light suppresses melatonin production. Therefore, broad-spectrum light can decrease the physiologic source of increased sleep.

Nurses can teach clients who have a recurrent pattern of winter depression to begin preparing for their symptoms by seeking light treatment in the early fall. Usually, exposure to a light of 2,000 lux for two or more hours in the morning (Smock, 1999) is sufficient to promote a change. Additional strategies include:

- Cautioning individuals with bipolar disorder to not stay up all night studying or partying as that disrupts the sleep–wake cycle.
- Helping postpartum mothers with a history of mood disorders to have options prepared for night feedings to avoid becoming sleep deprived.
- Advocating that people with mood disorders not work irregular shift patterns.

The Americans with Disabilities Act (ADA) supports the idea that people with psychiatric disabilities should have a "reasonable" work schedule. This could include a stable shift assignment.

As our understanding of biorhythms increases, we can expect that certain clinical decisions, such as when it is best to perform surgery and the optimal time to administer medications, will change. Knowing a client's circadian patterns will help you administer appropriate medication dosages, resulting in greater efficacy and minimal side effects.

Psychobiology and Mental Disorders

This section examines current hypotheses about the psychobiologic basis of schizophrenia, mood disorders (major depression and bipolar disorder), anxiety disorders (panic disorder and OCD), and DAT. Research is continuing to examine most major psychiatric problems for issues related to biologic changes. The disorders described in this section are examples of how the information that has been gleaned by the biologic research is being understood and utilized in the treatment of these disorders.

SCHIZOPHRENIA

The evolution of the diagnosis of schizophrenia has been dramatic: a shift from a narrowly focused definition of the illness to the requirement of specific criteria of quantifiable symptoms over time. No single neurobiologic hypothesis as the etiologic variable exists. Different domains of psychopathology are directing clinical decisions using multifocal treatments.

Researchers are trying to determine why there is a loss of neurons in the brain tissue of people with schizophrenia (Andreasen, 1999; Woods, 1998). There are fewer nerve cells overall but more pyramidal cells (containing DA, ACh, and glutamate) that are excitatory in nature, bringing sensory inputs (sights, sounds, thoughts) to the cerebral cortex. This suggests that the illness may result from an increased flow of activity up to the cortex, explaining why people with schizophrenia become overwhelmed by stimuli such as hallucinations and misperceptions.

Kwon et al. (1999) found changes in electroencephalograms (EEGs) that may mean a deficit in the processing of data with individuals with schizophrenia. There is an indication of abnormalities in the GABAergic system that can result in cognitive abnormalities, such as hallucinations, and association problems in the thought pattern. Studies of DA receptors, especially DA type II (D_2) receptors, provide clues to the neuropathology of schizophrenia. Most D_2 receptors are in the basal ganglia, as observed with in vivo neuroimaging studies. The presence of D_2 receptors in structures with receptors having connections to the limbic and cortical pathways helps link the functions or behaviors of the cognitive and emotional aspects of schizophrenia. Postmortem studies and PET scans are trying to unravel the issue of whether the postmortem findings are a result of antipsychotic drug treatment or primary to the pathophysiology of the disease syndrome (Glantz & Lewis, 2000).

The conventional and less used antipsychotic drugs, haloperidol and fluphenazine, bind to block D_2 receptors in the basal ganglia and target the symptoms of hallucinations, delusions, and loose associations (also referred to as positive symptoms). From the application of molecular genetics techniques, the cloning of other DA receptors (D_3, D_4, and D_5) has led to more specific psychotropic medications. The newer antipsychotics (sometimes referred to as atypical antipsychotics) clozapine, risperidone, olanzapine, quetiapine, and ziprasidone are targeting such behaviors as restricted emotional expression, attention deficits, poor grooming, lack of motivation, social withdrawal, and poverty of speech (collectively called negative symptoms). They were referred to as atypical because they selected receptor subtypes other than D_2 as the conventional, more typical, antipsychotics did and therefore have less risk in causing EPS.

A second major hypothesis about schizophrenia is that there are structural brain abnormalities associated with the syndrome. Brain computed tomography (CT) scans show enlarged ventricles and widened sulci and fissures that appear to have been present from the onset of symptoms and are thus not a result of treatment. When a twin has schizophrenia, the nonaffected twin's ventricles appear normal in size; the ventricles of the twin with schizophrenia are larger. Postmortem and magnetic resonance imaging (MRI) studies support a left-sided brain abnormality, as seen in a bilateral reduction in the temporal cortex, and reduced hippocampal and amygdala regions (Kleinman & Hyde, 1993). A prenatal injury, postnatal maturational change in brain cells, or delayed myelination of nerve cells may explain the delay of the syndrome until adolescence. Myelin forms the insulating lining of axons and is associated with the maturation of behavior during normal development. Myelination is thought to assist with the emotional component of cognition and behavior. The ability to think abstractly is related to myelination in the limbic system and is thought to be established by mid-adolescence, with full maturity taking place during adulthood. A decrease in myelination would cause an increase in anxiety, difficulty socializing, and difficulty in modulating affect (Tamminga, 1998b, 1999b). See the Using Research Evidence feature regarding brain structures and beliefs.

Neurochemical findings implicated in schizophrenia show increases in glutamate receptors and decreased 5-HT subtype receptors in the cortical and mesolimbic neurons. This may explain the increase in suicide rates among members of this population; further research is currently trying to validate this connection.

Contemporary treatment of schizophrenia is primarily influenced by a stress-diathesis model (a biologic predisposition to a disease). What might be the interactions between the psychobiologic vulnerability and environmental events that stress the person's adaptive abilities and precipitate the onset of the syndrome or the recurrence of symptoms? Nurses should target interventions that alter the neurochemical systems with pharmacotherapy and psychosocial treatments (such as social skills, case management, client and family education) for the external stressors or negative symptoms. Refer to Chapter 14 for further information.

MOOD DISORDERS

Because of the variability in genetics and symptoms of major depression and bipolar disorder, the psychobiologic basis of mood disorders is difficult to determine. Research has focused on 5-HT and NE receptors. Brain stem nuclei that project to the amygdala, hippocampus, mammillary bodies, and cerebral cortex help account for the symptoms of appetite change, insomnia, depressed affect, loss of interest and pleasure (anhedonia), decreased problem-solving skills, and suicide attempts. Postmortem findings show reduced 5-HT reuptake sites in the hypothalamus and hippocampus. Because decreased 5-HT is associated with aggression, it may account for the suicide potential of this population.

Neuroendocrine challenge tests report increased cortisol, blunted ACTH response, hypothalamic–pituitary–thyroid axis alterations, and a higher-than-expected rate of autoimmune thyroiditis. When clients ask you, as their nurse, what these results indicate, you can emphasize they are state-dependent findings, markers that occur while the person is in a depressed mood (state), not diagnostic or a genetic characteristic of the illness.

Recent NT studies suggest that complex interactions among NE, 5-HT, DA, ACh, GABA, peptides, and second messengers contribute to bipolar disorder. There may be as many as six different types of bipolar disorders; further research to distinguish between them will refine our assessments and clinical treatments. Bipolar disorder tends to accelerate over time if left untreated. Early episodes tend to be precipitated by stress, but once recurrent episodes have occurred, the illness accelerates independently of external causes. Even with a genetic predisposition, there can also be changes in gene expression based on life experiences. The genetics, pathophysiology, and neurochemistry studies will yield more effective outcomes (Trippitelli, Jamison, Folstein, Bartko, & DePaulo, 1998).

Somatic therapies other than medications are used in the treatment of mood disorders. Electroconvulsive therapy (ECT) is used for psychotic depression and mania. Exactly how ECT works is not well understood. Evidence suggests that it may resynchronize circadian rhythms, like a "brain defibrillator"; it may act as an anticonvulsant like carbamazepine; or it may restore the equilibrium between cerebral hemispheres. Historically, ECT caused some controversy, probably due to its

MediaLink Case Study: Brain, Mind, and Behavior

USING RESEARCH EVIDENCE

Kenneth is a 28-year-old single male who has been hospitalized three times in the last eight months for paranoid schizophrenia. After each discharge from the hospital he stops taking his medications. Kenneth feels he does not have an illness. He has command auditory hallucinations once he stops taking his medications. His behavior is often bizarre and he is easily frightened. His family is concerned that he will either hurt someone or will be hurt due to his bizarre behavior.

As a nurse, you begin to wonder about Kenneth's denial of his illness. Discussions have always assumed that an actual clinical denial was in operation and that it may have beneficial aspects. Comments such as, "The mind allows you to find out when you can cope with it," have guided demands made on clients. However, your literature review led you to an article by Flashman et al. (2000) that states that several neuropsychological studies indicate that frontal and parietal lobe involvement in schizophrenia can cause an unawareness of the illness. This is thought to be due to having a smaller brain and intracranial volumes of brain tissue and CSF than the normal comparison subjects.

The implications for Kenneth's care may be that while he is symptomatic, he may need to be evaluated for being a danger to self and others, and he may require an emergency hospitalization. Once he is stabilized on medications, an agreement could be made with his parents about how to facilitate his access to care if he stops his medications and becomes symptomatic.

These suggestions stem from the following research:

Flashman, L. A., McAllister, T. W., Andreasen, N. C., & Saykin, A. J. (2000). Smaller brain size associated with schizophrenia. *American Journal of Psychiatry, 157*, 1167–70.

crude beginnings. Current use is not the physiologic event it used to be. Contrary to popular belief, ECT causes no tissue damage or neuronal cell loss (structural brain damage). Most clients report general improvement in cognition, in addition to relief from depression, several weeks following ECT.

Transcranial magnetic stimulation (TMS) uses magnetic fields to stimulate the brain with an indirect electric current (ECT uses a direct electric current). This disrupts neuronal firing and is being examined as an alternative to ECT. TMS is not a precise tool for targeting areas of the brain but may create enough of a disruption to change patterns of thinking. There is no seizure involved and no need for anesthesia (Wright, 2001). Preliminary results from active research indicate that there may even be less memory loss with this treatment. TMS is approved for treating depression in Canada and Europe but is currently only experimental in the United States.

Because of the various clinical symptoms associated with mood disorders, the nurse has an excellent opportunity to assess clients for their unique psychobiologic profile. The outcome of this specific assessment with each client over time will promote improved efficacy of treatment for the target symptoms and potentially prevent disruptive episodes. Promoting client self-care, which involves the client's becoming aware of his or her symptoms in order to report clinical changes early into a reoccurrence of the depression, will assist in the decrease of severity of the mood disorder (see Chapter 15).

ANXIETY DISORDERS

Anxiety disorders have many subtypes, and a complete review will not be undertaken in this chapter. As discussed earlier, the question of whether anxiety disorders are a separate type of disorder or a variant of a depressive spectrum is still unanswered. MRI and PET scans reveal right hippocampal changes, high brain metabolism, and an abnormal sensitivity to hyperventilation in people with panic disorder.

Neurochemical changes are associated with NE, 5-HT, GABA, and peptides in panic disorder. The discharge of NE in the brain stem, chemoreceptors in the medulla, and 5-HT set off a series of communications that extend through the limbic system, rich in benzodiazepine receptors, to the prefrontal cortex. This pathway may explain the rapid pulse from the NE discharge being interpreted by the cortex as a life-threatening heart attack. These neural connections allow for a hypervigilant cognitive appraisal or inability to integrate the sensory information with any biologic sensation. The behavioral outcome is anticipatory anxiety and avoidance of stimuli that might be the associated precipitant of the arousal (an inappropriate behavioral response).

PET scans show higher metabolic rates in the left prefrontal cortex and caudate nuclei in people with OCD. The caudate or "gating station" dysfunction may lead to overactive circuits that fail to properly integrate cognitive, emotional, and motor responses to sensory inputs. The prefrontal hyperactivity may be related to the tendency to ruminate and plan excessively, as well as to think in an abstract way. Increased frontal lobe activity manifests as a heightened sense of judgment (guilt and worry), intense affect (depression), and hyperjudgmental rigidity. See the various brain structures in ■ Figure 4–9.

Abnormal regulation of the 5-HT subsystem has a role in the pathophysiology of OCD. This hypothesis is supported by the improved treatment response to selective serotonin reuptake inhibitors (SSRIs). In addition, increased levels of arginine,

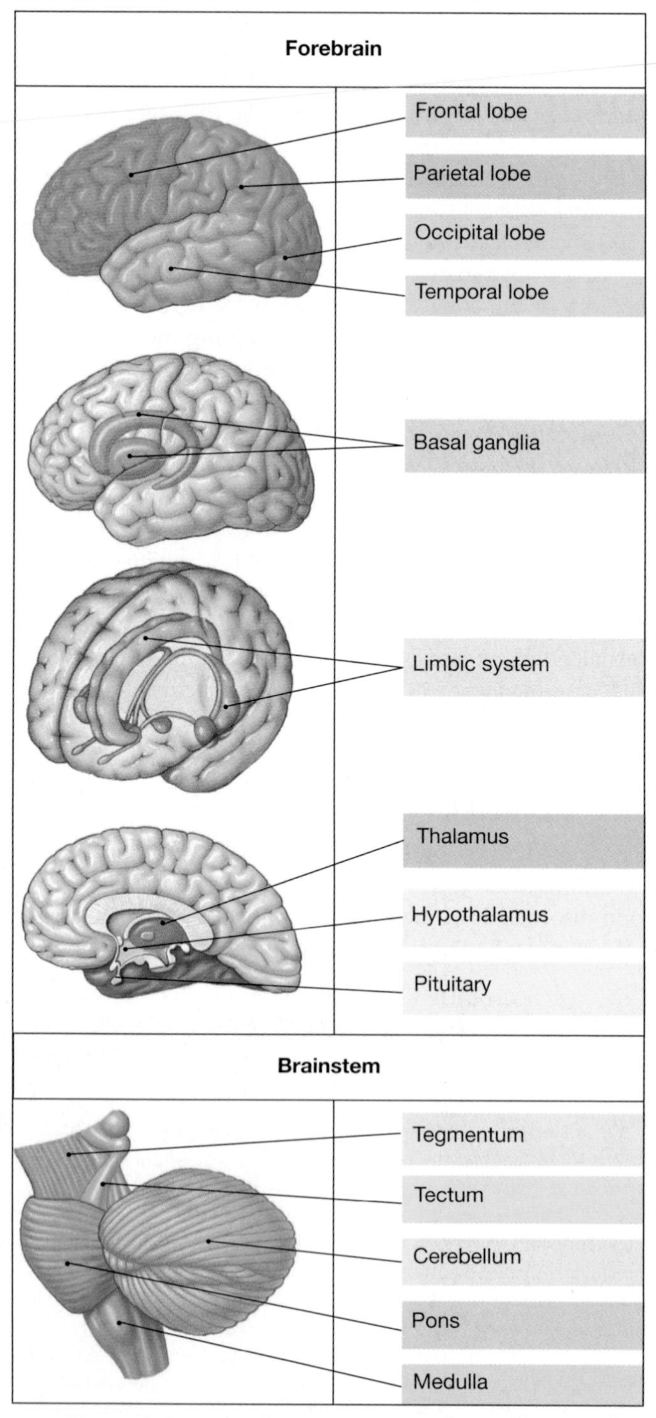

FIGURE 4–9 ■ *Brain structures.*

Source: Smock, T. K. (1999). *Physiological psychology: A neuroscience approach*. Upper Saddle River, NJ: Prentice Hall.

vasopressin, somatostatin, and CRH are found in the CSF of people with OCD. These neuropeptides promote grooming activity and perseverative motor behaviors and increase arousal (anxiety), which are part of the OCD symptomatology.

How do nurses differ in their approaches to mildly anxious clients versus clients with moderate, high, or crisis levels of anxiety? Provided that nurses assess the client's anxiety accurately, how prescriptive are the interventions, and what objective evaluative measures of anxiety control do nurses use?

Anxiety is a psychobiologic condition that responds to both behavioral and pharmacologic interventions and is recognized as amenable to nursing care. Through the use of nursing science, a nurse conducts a thorough assessment of a client's symptoms of anxiety including the use of various assessment tools. Cognitive–behavioral and supportive approaches have been effective interventions for clients with thoughts and verbal expressions of anxiety. Clients with any of the anxiety disorders benefit from assistance with teaching about the use of medications to decrease anxiety symptoms. Refer to Chapter 16 for further information about caring for an individual with an anxiety disorder.

DEMENTIA OF THE ALZHEIMER'S TYPE

People with DAT show a decrease in cerebral blood flow or metabolic function in the posterior temporoparietal regions. It is the only major mental disorder to show this characteristic pattern of hypometabolic function. Thus, PET and SPECT studies may be useful in differentiating DAT from other disorders that include confusion and intellectual deterioration as symptoms. Structural neuronal degeneration occurs, producing neurofibrillary tangles and amyloid deposits, or plaques. The nerve receptor density and the distribution studies offer promise for improved diagnostic accuracy.

Decreases in cholinergic neurons in a region of the basal ganglia that connect to the amygdala, hippocampus, and cortex are seen. Functionally, this results in the short-term memory loss characteristic of the disease. While the deficits are considered central, there are other NT systems involved in the pathology, including NE, 5-HT, DA, peptides, and nerve growth factor. If receptors in the limbic structures are affected, depression or labile mood results; a decrease in social skills, inhibition, and impaired judgment can also be a part of the behavioral pattern.

In assessing and intervening with this client, be aware that disorientation results in fear and agitation. Thus, any change, such as bed reassignment or facility transfer, is a major stressor. For those with parietal involvement, walking down a hall with a patterned carpet, stepping up on a weight scale, or managing steps is difficult because they cannot orient themselves in relation to the space around them.

Working with clients suffering from DAT and their family caregivers calls for your creativity and knowledge of the structure and function of the brain in order to assist with identifying and responding to their needs. Refer to Chapter 12 for further information on the nursing care of an individual with DAT.

Psychobiology and Nursing

Integrating psychobiologic principles into your psychiatric–mental health nursing practice will link body, mind, brain, and behavior. Because nursing examines the person from a psychobiologic perspective, nursing practice is holistic. When performing a comprehensive assessment, it is important to determine the appropriate questions to ask the client in order to obtain information that can lead to the understanding of the client's thoughts, emotional, and behavioral patterns.

The nurse's attitude about the underlying neurobiology of behavior can influence therapeutic outcomes. It is important to consider how treatment outcomes are potently influenced by both the style and the knowledge incorporated into nursing interventions. If the comprehensive nursing assessment, interpretation of the assessment, client teaching, and evaluation of the intervention are done using the knowledge of the role of the biologic, cognitive, and behavioral aspects of the client, the client has a greater opportunity for successful reduction of symptoms. If the nurse views biologic or somatic therapies in an ambivalent manner, he or she will communicate this attitude to the client and the family, and the effectiveness of the interventions may not be as powerful. The nurse integrates his or her viewpoint into client teaching, and its expression can hinder or promote improvement.

The nurse must assess the client with an open mind and interpret and communicate the information to the rest of the multidisciplinary team in a comprehensive manner. To understand client needs necessitates the full synthesis of communication, from molecular to verbal. An understanding of clients' physical and social environment rounds out the mind–body connection. To function as a professional nurse, it is important to be aware of any dualistic issues that may be present, as presented in the Nursing Self-Awareness feature on page 78, and how those attitudes may diminish your nursing ability to be an advocate and support person to clients and their families.

Integrating psychobiology into nursing care exceeds the practice of administering medications. Incorporating psychobiology will enable the nurse to fine-tune assessments, diagnoses, interventions, and evaluations of human response patterns. The synthesis of this critical thinking will provide clients and families with quality care in a cost-effective manner.

Nursing science is still evolving and you are in a position to contribute to our knowledge base by further incorporating this area of science. How would you deduce that psychoeducation assists in client compliance? The following questions will help you:

1. What type of nursing research will provide some solid data that can be used as evidenced-based interventions?
2. How do people with positive symptoms learn?
3. What clinical decision tree do you use to assess whether a client needs a PRN medication for agitation, is having EPS, is anxious, or is trying to communicate?
4. How do you anticipate the client's needs when he or she is having severe negative symptoms and is unable to communicate due to apathy and difficulty with associative thought mechanisms?

Nursing SELF-AWARENESS — Your Attitudes and Feelings About Psychiatric Clients

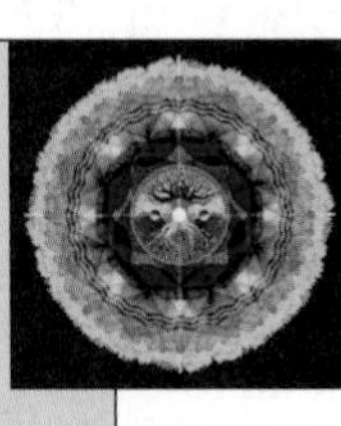

To assist you in examining your view and feelings about psychiatric clients, answer the following:

- How do you describe an individual with a mental disorder? Do you refer to the person by his/her diagnosis?
- How do you describe the person's behavior to another team member when the individual is walking down the street nude, is hostile, or has delusions that other people are trying to "clone" him?
- How would you react if a transitional living facility for people with psychiatric problems bought a house in your neighborhood?
- How do you react when you think an individual is manipulating you? What do you think causes manipulative behavior?
- Are people with psychiatric problems more violent than the general population?
- Do you become angry at clients when they do not take their medications and become symptomatic?
- Do you think that individuals with major emotional disorders can contribute in their families and in society?
- Do you feel hopeless when working with individuals with severe chronic emotional illness?
- Can diet, exercise, and a regular daily pattern of living enhance mental health?
- Do you think that depressed individuals do not try hard enough to "pull themselves up by their bootstraps"?
- Do you think that when people say they are suicidal that they are really attempting to receive attention?
- Do you want to work with people who have psychiatric problems?

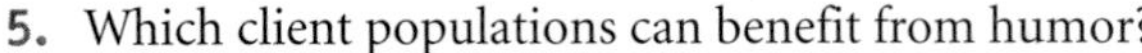

5. Which client populations can benefit from humor?
6. Which stress management interventions are best for someone with panic disorder versus someone in crisis?
7. What early interventions in circadian dysregulation can promote healing for abused individuals?
8. Does a caffeine challenge trigger physiologic arousal in people with PTSD as in people with panic disorder?

Being a nurse is an opportunity for you to be flexible, creative, and a visionary. Keep a diary of how you made a difference for a client. Was a biologic variable involved? Articulate how you made that difference, and link it with cost-effective care. The care of people with psychiatric disorders often incorporates technology to find the neuropathology. However, throughout psychiatric nursing care, nursing practice is the nurse–client relationship and all the communication involved.

The exact biologic determinants for psychiatric disorders and behaviors remain elusive. To date there is no definitive biologic test to identify a psychiatric disorder. However, multifocal and multidisciplinary care incorporating psychobiologic dimensions will advance our ability to offer new, more effective assessments and interventions for our clients.

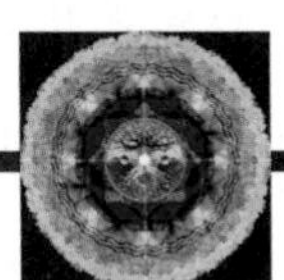

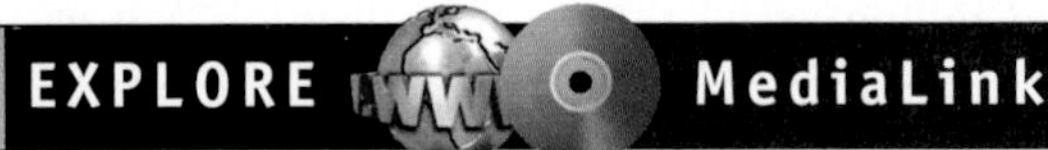

EXPLORE MediaLink

NCLEX review, case studies, and other interactive resources for this chapter can be found on the Companion Website at http://www.prenhall.com/kneisl. Click on Chapter 4 to select the activities for this chapter.

For animations, video tutorials, more NCLEX review questions, and an audio glossary, access the accompanying CD-ROM in this textbook.

BIBLIOGRAPHY

Adams, L. J., Mitchell, P. B., Fielder, S. L., Rosso, A., Donald, J. A., & Schofield, P. R. (1998). A susceptibility locus for bipolar affective disorder on chromosome 4q35. *American Journal of Human Genetics, 62*(5):1084–1091.

Adams, R. D., Victor, M., & Ropper, A. H. (1997). *Principles of neurology* (6th ed.). New York: McGraw-Hill.

American Nurses Association (2000). *Scope and standards of psychiatric–mental health clinical nursing practice*. Washington, DC: Author.

Andreasen, N. (1999). A unitary model of schizophrenia: Bleuler's fragmented phrene as schizencephaly. *Archives of General Psychiatry, 56*, 781–787.

Athan, E. S., Williamson, J., Ciappa, A., Santana, V., Romas, S. N., Lee, J. H., et al. (2001). A founder mutant in presenilin-1 causing early-onset Alzheimer's disease in unrelated Caribbean Hispanic families. *Journal of the American Medical Association, 286*, 2257–2263.

Bailey, K. P. (1999). Electrophysiological kindling and behavioral sensitization as models for bipolar illness: Implications for nursing practice. *Journal of the American Psychiatric Nurses Association, 5*, 62–66.

Barinaga, M. (2000). Synapses call the shots. *Science, 290*, 736–738.

Bear, M. F., Connors, B. W., & Paradiso, M. A. (2001). *Neuroscience: Exploring the brain* (2nd ed.). Baltimore: Lippincott.

Becker, H. C. (1998). Kindling in alcohol withdrawal. *Alcohol Health and Research World, 22,* 25–33.

Berrettini, W. H. (2000). Susceptibility loci for bipolar disorder: Overlap with inherited vulnerability to schizophrenia. *Biological Psychiatry, 47,* 245–251.

Beskow, L. M., Burke, W., Merz, J. F., Barr, P. A., et al. (2001). Informed consent for population based research involving genetics. *Journal of the American Medical Association, 286,* 2315–2321.

Blackwood, D. (2000) P300, a state and a trait marker in schizophrenia. *Lancet, 355,* 771–772.

Brzustowicz, L. M., Hodgkinson, K. A., Chow, E. W., Honer, W. G., & Bassett, A. S. (2000). Location of a major susceptibility locus for familial schizophrenia on chromosome 1q21–q22. *Science, 288,* 678–682.

Dana Alliance for Brain Initiatives. (1999). Update 1999: New connections. Retrieved December, 2002, from the World Wide Web, http://www.dana.org/books/press/progressreport/update99.cfm.

DeVane, C. L. (2001). Substance P: A new era, a new role. *Pharmacotherapy, 21,* 1061–1069.

Flashman, L. A., McAllister, T. W., Andreasen, N. C., & Saykin, A. J. (2000). Smaller brain size associated with schizophrenia. *American Journal of Psychiatry, 157,* 1167–1170.

Glantz, L. A., & Lewis, D. A. (2000). Decreased dendritic spine density on prefrontal cortical pyramidal neurons in schizophrenia. *Archives of General Psychiatry, 57,* 65–73.

Kalynchuk, L. E., Treit, D., & Pinel, J. P. J. (1999). Characterization of the defensive nature of kindling-induced emotionality. *Behavioral Neuroscience, 113,* 766–775.

Kendler, K., Thornton, L. M., & Gardner, C. O. (2000). Stressful life events and previous episodes in the etiology of major depression in women: An evaluation of the "kindling" hypothesis. *American Journal of Psychiatry, 157,* 1243–1251.

Kleinman, J. E., & Hyde, T. M. (1993). Structural foundations of mental illness and treatment: Neuroanatomy. In D. L. Dunner (Ed.), *Current psychiatric therapy.* Philadelphia: Saunders.

Kwon, J. U. S., O'Donnell, B. F., Wallenstein, G. V., Greene, R. W., Hirayasu, Y., Nestor, P. G., et al. (1999). Gamma frequency #150 range abnormalities in auditory stimulation in schizophrenia. *Archives of General Psychiatry, 56,* 1001–1005.

Levinson, D. F., Mahtani, M. M., Nancarrow, D. J., Brown, D. M., Krugylak, L., Kirby, A., et al. (1998). Genome scan of schizophrenia. *American Journal of Psychiatry, 155*(6), 741–750.

Naslund, J. (2000). Amyloid beta-peptide levels associated with early dementia. *Journal of the American Medical Association, 283,* 1571–1577.

NIMH Genetics and Mental Disorders Report of the National Institute of Mental Health's Genetics Workgroup. Retrieved September, 1997, from the World Wide Web, http://www.nimh.nih.gov/research/genetics.htm.

Rannala, B., & Reeve, J. P. (2001). High-resolution multipoint linkage-disequilibrium mapping in the context of a human genome sequence. *American Journal of Human Genetics, 69,* 159.

Smock, T. K. (1999). *Physiological psychology: A neuroscience approach.* Upper Saddle River, NJ: Prentice Hall.

Stahl, S. M. (2000). *Essential psychopharmacology: Neuroscientific basis and clinical applications.* Cambridge, UK: Cambridge University Press.

Tamminga, C. A. (1998a). Images in neuroscience: Brain development III, cerebral cortex. *American Journal of Psychiatry, 155,* 714.

Tamminga, C. A. (1998b). Images in neuroscience: Human brain growth spans decades. *American Journal of Psychiatry, 155,* 1498.

Tamminga, C. A. (1999a). Images in neuroscience, brain development, IX: Human brain growth. *American Journal of Psychiatry, 156,* 4.

Tamminga, C. A. (1999b). Images in neuroscience, brain development X: Pruning during development. *American Journal of Psychiatry, 156,* 168.

Trippitelli, C. L., Jamison, K. R., Folstein, M. F., Bartko, J. J., & DePaulo, J. R. (1998). Pilot study on patients' and spouses' attitudes toward potential genetic testing for bipolar disorder. *American Journal of Psychiatry, 155,* 899–904.

Woods, B. (1998). Is schizophrenia a progressive neurodevelopmental disorder? Toward a unitary pathogenetic mechanism. *American Journal of Psychiatry, 155,* 1661–1670.

Wright, K. (2001). Brain rx: Magnets. *Discover, 11,* 28–29.

Yamaguchi, S., Shinmura, K., Saitoh, T., Takenoshita, S., Kuwano, H., & Yokota, J. (2002). A single nucleotide polymorphism at the splice donor site of the human MYH base excision repair genes results in reduced translation efficiency of its transcripts. *Genes to Cells, 7,* 461–474.

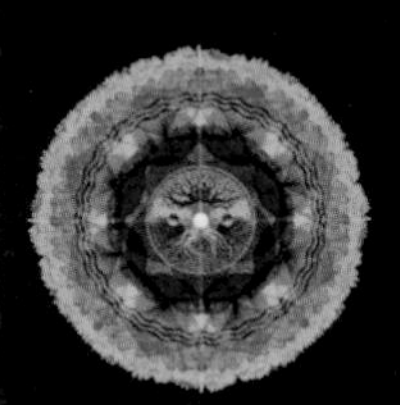

5

Chapter FIVE

Stress, Anxiety, and Coping

CAROL REN KNEISL

KEY TERMS

anxiety
cardiac neurosis
conflict
coping strategies
defense mechanisms
denial
displacement
dissociation
false memory
fantasy
fight-or-flight
general adaptation syndrome (GAS)
identification
intellectualization
introjection
mental disorder due to a general medical condition
projection
psychological factors affecting medical condition
psychoneuroimmunology
rationalization
reaction formation
recovered memory
repression
selective inattention
stress
stressor
suppression
type A personality

FOCUS QUESTIONS

- **How does stress affect an individual?**
- **From where does anxiety stem?**
- **What are the everyday methods people use to cope with stress and anxiety?**
- **What are the common defense-oriented behaviors (defense mechanisms) people use to cope with stress and anxiety?**
- **Which common medical conditions have an onset or a course influenced by psychological and behavioral factors?**

MediaLink 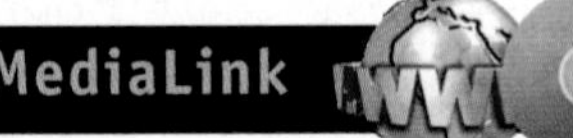 www.prenhall.com/kneisl

Additional resources for this chapter can be found on the Student CD-ROM accompanying this textbook, and on the Companion Website at www.prenhall.com/kneisl. Click on Chapter 5 to select the activities for this chapter.

CD-ROM
- Audio Glossary
- NCLEX Review

Companion Website
- Additional NCLEX Review
- Case Study: Assessing Anxiety

CHAPTER OUTLINE

CROSS REFERENCES

Other topics relevant to this content are: Applying the nursing process to the care of anxious clients, Chapter 16; Assessing the severity of stress according to Axis IV of DSM-IV-TR, Chapter 9 and Appendix A; Behavioral and cognitive interventions, Chapter 30; Crisis intervention, Chapter 33; Posttraumatic stress disorder and acute stress disorder, Chapter 16; Relaxation and stress-management techniques, Chapter 32.

CRITICAL THINKING CHALLENGE

At the scene of an auto accident in which a couple in their eighties lost control of the RV trailer they were towing, the husband remained immobile in the driver's seat, hands firmly fixed to the steering wheel, eyes focused on some distant spot despite the threat of explosion from the smoking car. The wife ran around in circles. She had lost her shoes in the accident, but despite numerous bleeding cuts, she was unaware she was running barefoot through broken glass from the windshield.

The nurses who happened on the scene had differing opinions about which was the healthier response. One said the elderly gentleman's "control" was positive, but the wife's "hysteria" was negative. What do you think? ■

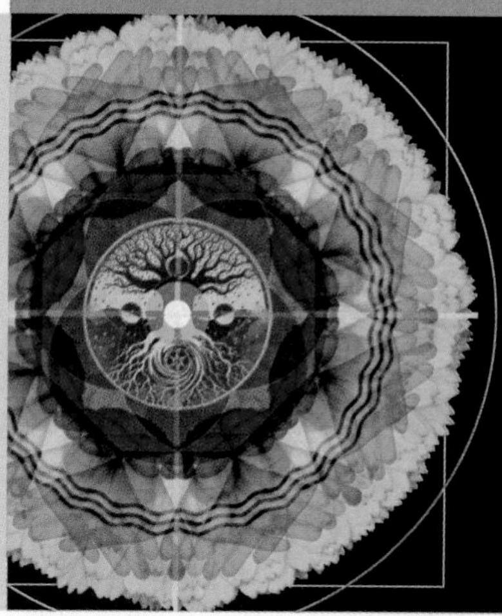

Health care professionals have long been interested in stress and anxiety and in the ways that healthy and dysfunctional people cope or fail to cope with them. Stress and anxiety affect a person's well-being. Various behavioral and physiologic disorders have been linked to stress and anxiety. Some behavioral manifestations are discussed here and elaborated in later chapters (see especially Chapter 16). The cost of stress and anxiety can be quite high: They can cost a woman her job; a man the love and respect of his family. When sufficiently prolonged, stress can kill.

Stress

Stress is part of being alive. Standing erect stresses the muscles and bones that must work together to keep the body erect; eating stresses the digestive system, which must produce enzymes and absorb nutrients; and breathing stresses the respiratory system, which must exchange carbon dioxide and oxygen. More broadly and holistically, **stress** designates a broad class of experiences in which a demanding situation taxes a person's resources or coping capabilities, causing a negative effect. This broader definition approximates the humanistic perspective of this textbook. In this view, stress is a person–environment interaction. The source of the stress, the demanding situation, is known as a **stressor.** The internal state the stress produces is one of tension, anxiety, or strain. See ■ Figure 5–1 for an example of stress as a person–environment situation.

There is no universally accepted definition of stress among stress theorists and researchers. An interactional view of stress, such as the one given above, is consistent with how nurses view human experiences. The theories of stress that follow are the perspectives in common use. Although they do tell us a great deal about responses to stressful situations, it is crucial for nurses to recognize that these explanations are not necessarily consistent with nursing's orientation. Such factors as causes, the situational context in which the stressful event occurs, and the psychologic interpretation of the demanding situation must be considered in a holistic, humanistic approach to the client. These and other important factors related to stress are illustrated in ■ Figure 5–2. Axis IV of DSM-IV-TR offers some general parameters for assessing the severity of stress.

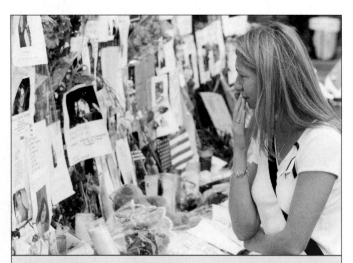

FIGURE 5–1 ■ *A woman looks at the posters listing the missing at a memorial in Union Square in New York, September 18, 2001, one week after the nightmare attacks in New York and Washington. It was one week after the World Trade Center collapsed after hijacked jetliners crashed into each of the two towers on September 11.*

Source: Kai Pfaffenbach/Getty Images Inc.–Hulton Archive Photos.

CONFLICT AS A STRESSOR

The concept of conflict is useful in identifying the stresses that help cause disturbed coping patterns. Conflict often explains such observable behaviors as hesitation, vacillation, blocking, and fatigue. **Conflict**—the coexistence of opposing desires, feelings, or goals—is frequently seen in the behavior of psychotic clients, who may have difficulty making even the simplest decisions.

These conflicts are the most likely to cause stress:

- Conflicts that involve social relations with significant people.
- Conflicts that involve ethical standards.
- Conflicts that involve meeting unconscious needs.
- Conflicts that involve the problems of everyday family living.

A conflict proceeds according to these four steps:

1. The person holds two goals simultaneously.
2. The person moves in relation to both of the goals, using (a) approach–avoidance movements or (b) avoidance–avoidance movements.

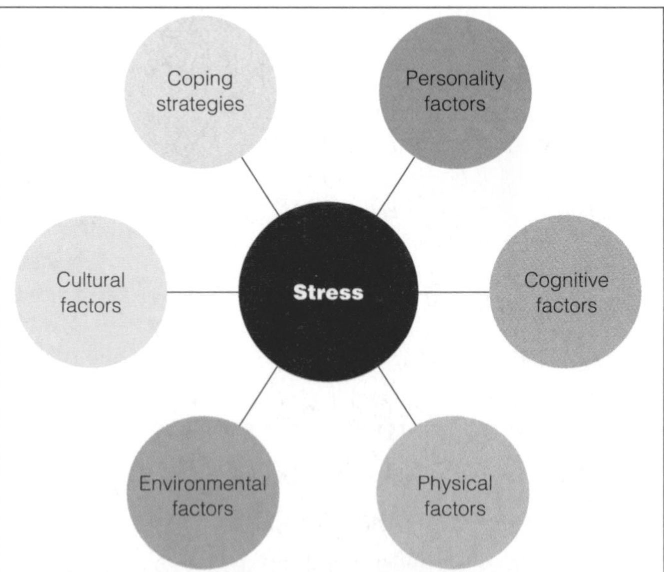

FIGURE 5–2 ■ *Factors involved in stress. Several important factors are involved in understanding stress. They include personality factors (such as how we handle anger), cognitive factors (such as whether we perceive an event as a challenge or threat), physical factors (such as how the body responds to stress), environmental factors (such as fog, fire, or snow), cultural factors (such as our learned beliefs about religion, health, and family), and coping strategies (such as what we do to manage stress).*

3. The person shows hesitation, vacillation, blocking, or fatigue.
4. Resolution occurs either temporarily or permanently.

Conflict with Approach–Avoidance Movements

When a person holds two incompatible goals at the same time, the goals usually constitute an either-or situation. If the person chooses one goal, the other goal is rejected or abolished automatically. Here is an example:

CLINICAL EXAMPLE

Mrs R holds two goals. She wants to talk with the nurse about her fears of going back to work. At the same time, she wants not to be perceived as weak or "a bother." Mrs R makes a movement in relation to her first goal—talking to the nurse—by walking up to her. When the nurse stops and turns toward her, Mrs R asks some superficial question about the time of the next group meeting. In this way she avoids discussing her real concerns. When the nurse offers an opening to talk further, Mrs R avoids the conversation she needs by saying she wants to rest. An hour later, she approaches the nurse with an apologetic but vague question about her medication.

Vacillation describes Mrs R's behavior.

Principles that Explain Vacillation

To understand how vacillation comes about and what is going on during a conflict situation like the one that was described above, we need to understand the following four key principles:

1. As you near a desirable goal, the approach tendency is strengthened.
2. As you near an undesirable goal, the avoidance tendency is strengthened.
3. The strength of the avoidance tendency always increases more rapidly with nearness to the goal than does the strength of the approach tendency.
4. The strength of both tendencies varies with the strength of the need basic to the tendencies. That is, an increased need can strengthen both tendencies and intensify the conflict, whereas a decreased need can weaken both tendencies and lessen the conflict.

Avoidance–Avoidance Conflict

In avoidance–avoidance conflict, a person is faced with two undesirable goals at the same time. The person attempts to avoid the nearer of these two goals, but with the retreat from the nearer goal, the tendency to avoid the second goal increases. Unless the tendency to avoid one of the goals overpowers the tendency to avoid the other goal, or unless there is a third way out of the conflict, the person feels trapped by the conflict.

CLINICAL EXAMPLE

Robert P, the 35-year-old son of well-to-do parents, was strongly attracted to "the good life." He wanted to live in a creative, esthetic environment; read good books; attend the opera; drink quality wine. Simultaneously, he wanted both to avoid working to earn the money for the lifestyle he desired and to not depend on his parents for support. His lifestyle became one of waiting to find a resolution to his conflict. He neither worked nor accepted "handouts" from his family, but his preferred lifestyle became one that he talked about rather than lived.

Biopsychosocial Theories of Stress

Each of the theories discussed in this section contributes to our understanding of stress and coping. However, none is complete in and of itself. Psychoneuroimmunology, the final theory discussed in this section, offers a comprehensive framework for understanding stress–disease relationships by taking the best of what the other theories offer and integrating them with the increasing body of evidence on how stress can alter immunologic functioning and, consequently, disease susceptibility and pathology.

THE FIGHT-OR-FLIGHT RESPONSE TO STRESS

Beyond the routine and essential stress of everyday life, humans risk encountering undesirable or excess stress that threatens well-being and may even be life threatening. They cope with such threats through either a fight (aggression) or flight (withdrawal) response. The **fight-or-flight** response was first discussed by the physician Walter Cannon in 1932, when he identified stress as an actual cause of disease. Consider the following situation of extreme stress: A woman is walking down a dark, deserted street when a man with a knife emerges from the shadows just in front of her. Does she try to defend herself? Does she run away? Whichever action she takes is a result of a variety of physiologic responses to extreme danger. The following are likely to happen when a person faces such a situation:

- The heart beats strong and fast to circulate the blood more quickly.
- Airways in the lung dilate so that the extra blood becomes oxygenated.
- Glucose is released into the blood by the liver.
- The blood vessels dilate to permit the oxygen-rich blood to get to where it is needed most.
- The pupils of the eye dilate to let more light through, making vision more acute.

- Peristalsis in the gastrointestinal system is inhibited so that the energy peristalsis would consume becomes available for other purposes.
- Norepinephrine-containing cells in the central nervous system are active.
- The palms become sweaty; the mouth becomes dry.

Although these physiologic responses seem appropriate for the situation described, imagine the wear and tear on the body if humans responded to all stress in all of these ways. Many specialists in the field of behavioral medicine believe the fight-or-flight response to be maladaptive. For example, some forms of hypertension are caused or made worse by chronic activation of the heart due to either an excessive amount of stress or an excessive response to stress. See the section on Psychological Factors Affecting Medical Conditions later in this chapter for a discussion of the relationship between stress and hypertension, heart disease, and a variety of other medical conditions.

SELYE'S STRESS-ADAPTATION THEORY

Hans Selye, a Canadian endocrinologist and the most well-known and widely recognized stress researcher, developed a response-oriented framework for understanding how people respond to stress. According to Selye, each person has a limited amount of energy to use in dealing with stress. How quickly it is used and, therefore, how quickly one adapts to stress depend on several factors such as heredity, mental attitude, and lifestyle, among others.

Selye defines stress as the rate of wear and tear on the body (1956). He disputes the idea that only serious disease or injury causes stress. Selye thinks that any emotion or activity requires a response or change in the individual. Stressors can be physical, chemical, physiologic, developmental, or emotional. Playing a game of tennis, going out in the rain without an umbrella, having an argument, and getting a promotion are all examples of stressful events. Life itself is basically stressful because it involves a process of adaptation to continual change. Though the experience of adaptation is stressful, it is not necessarily harmful. Indeed, it can be exciting and rewarding under certain circumstances; and although we cannot avoid the stress of living, we can learn to minimize its damaging effects.

Selye observed that, regardless of the diagnosis, most physically ill had certain symptoms in common; they lost their appetite, they lost weight, they felt and looked ill, they were anxious and fatigued, and they had aches and pains in their joints and muscles. A long series of experiments (1956) led to more objective evidence of actual body damage: enlargement of the adrenal glands; shrinkage of the thymus, spleen, and lymph nodes; and the appearance of bleeding gastric ulcers.

Feelings of anxiety, fatigue, or illness are subjective aspects of stress. Though stress itself cannot be perceived, Selye found that it can be objectively measured by the structural and chemical changes that it produces in the body. These changes are called the **general adaptation syndrome (GAS)** because when stress affects the whole person, the whole person must adjust to the changes. The GAS occurs in three stages: alarm, resistance, and exhaustion. The three stages of the GAS are illustrated and summarized in ■ Figure 5–3.

Exhaustion may be reversible if the total body is not affected and if the person can eventually eliminate the source of stress. However, if stress is unrelieved, or if the body's defenses are totally involved, the person may not regain psychologic stability and may become physically ill.

Selye's theory has stimulated extensive research on the neuroendocrine mechanisms underlying stress. The consequent research into psychoendocrinology has brought Selye's model into question (McCain & Smith, 1994). Now classical research has demonstrated that neuroendocrine response differs for different stressors, and that there is individual variance in the sensitivity to psychosocial stimuli (Lazarus & Folkman, 1984; Smith, 1993). The response-based model of stress is not consistent with nursing's view that each individual is unique and people respond differently to similar situations (Fitzpatrick & Wilke, 2001).

LIFE CHANGES AS STRESSFUL EVENTS

Most people are accustomed to thinking of untoward events as stressful, but they do not realize that desirable events such as job promotions, vacations, or outstanding personal achievements may also prove stressful. Holmes and Rahe (1967) studied life changes as stressful events to learn the amount of social readjustment required to cope with them. These authors believe that life events that require coping behavior tend to decrease a person's ability to handle illness or subsequent stress. Since Holmes and Rahe began their research, other investigators have raised cautions about applying this stimulus-based explanation indiscriminately. These cautions are discussed later in this section.

Their research assigned ratings to 43 different life changes, called *life change units (LCUs)*. They asked subjects to indicate what life changes had occurred in the past year and then to add up the points assigned to each one. According to these researchers, a low score indicated that the subject was not likely to have an adverse reaction. A "mild" score meant that there was a 30% chance that the person would manifest the impact of stress through physical symptoms. People in the "moderate" category had a 50% chance of a change in health status, and a "high" score meant an 80% chance of major illness in the next two years. High LCU scores also correlated with an increased probability of accidental injury. This example demonstrates the LCU model:

CLINICAL EXAMPLE

Marcia M, a 22-year-old woman in group therapy, had recently been divorced from her husband (LCU 73) after attempting to achieve a marital reconciliation (LCU 45). Marcia's pregnancy (LCU 40) earlier in the year was uneventful, and the couple's healthy son was born on June 2 (LCU 39). At 6 weeks of age, the child suddenly and unexpectedly died in his crib (LCU 63). The couple began to argue

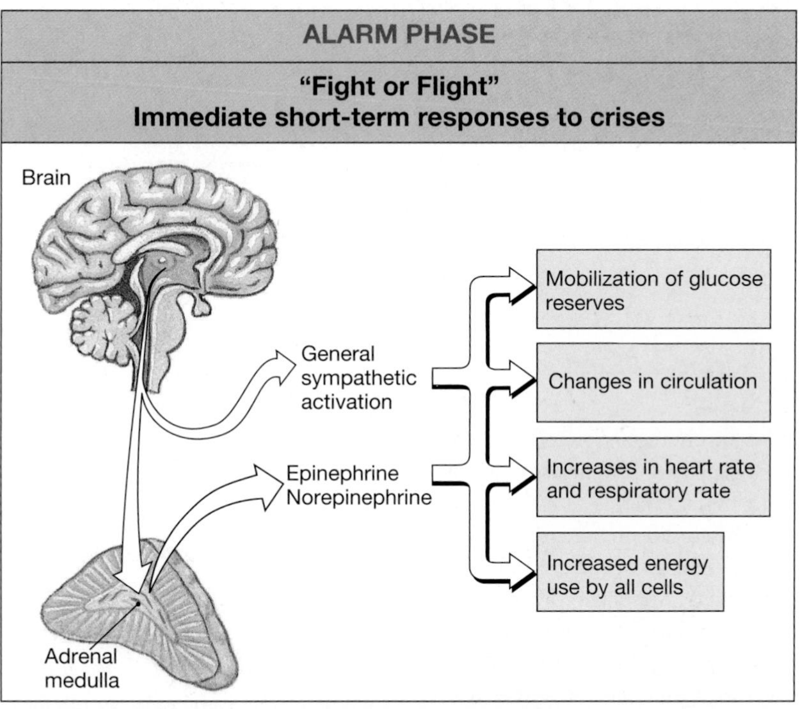

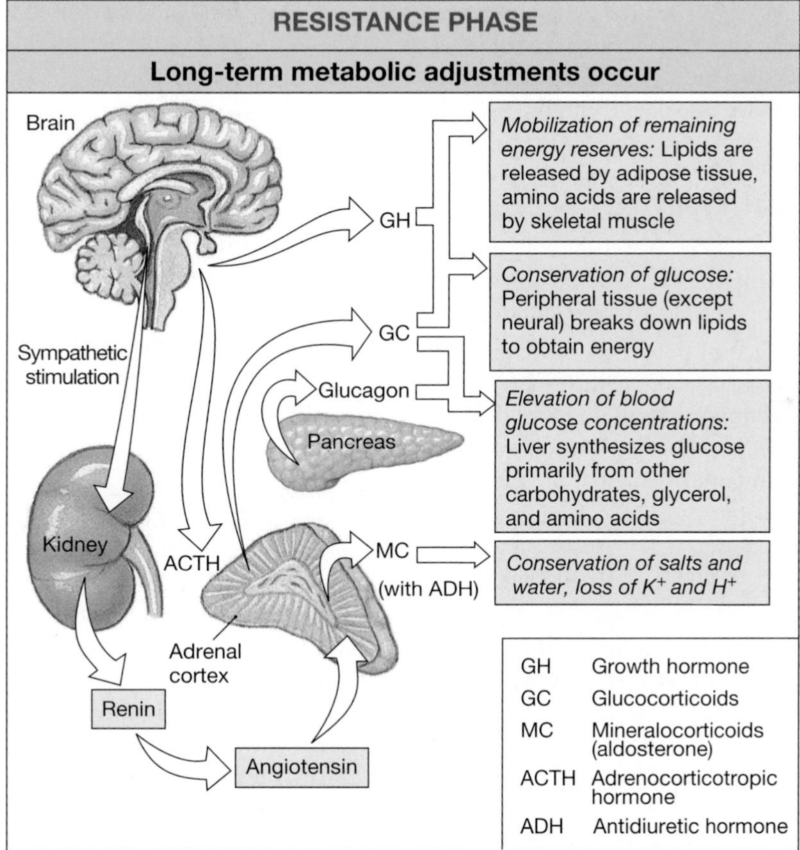

EXHAUSTION PHASE

Collapse of vital systems

Causes may include:
- Exhaustion of lipid reserves
- Inability to produce glucocorticoids
- Failure of electrolyte balance
- Cumulative structural or functional damage to vital organs

FIGURE 5–3 ■ *The general adaptation syndrome.*

Source: Martini, F. H. (2000). *Fundamentals of anatomy and physiology* (5th ed.) (p. 613). Upper Saddle River, NJ: Prentice Hall.

frequently (LCU 35) before they made the decision to divorce. After the divorce, Marcia found herself short of funds (LCU 38) and went to work as a waitress in a pizza restaurant (LCU 36). She found it necessary to move to a less expensive apartment (LCU 20). In the period of one year, Marcia accumulated an LCU score of 390 and was in the high-risk group.

In the early 1970s, other researchers correlated life stress events and mental health. In a study of 720 households in a metropolitan area, Meyers and his associates (1972) found a relationship between a high number of life changes and changes in the mental status of individuals. For example, an increase in the number of life changes preceded worsening of psychiatric symptoms, whereas a decrease in life changes brought improvement. The more stressful the life changes, the greater the likelihood of mental illness. Meyers and his associates also found that entrance-related life events (those involving the addition of a new person into one's social sphere, perhaps through marriage or the birth of a child) produced less symptomatology than did exit-related events (those associated with the loss of a valued individual or status).

Application to Clinical Practice

Nurses applying the Holmes and Rahe model should be aware of the following cautions. This model is based on several assumptions that depict a person as a passive recipient of stress.

- It assumes that events affect all people in the same way, regardless of how the individuals perceive the event.
- It assumes that there is a common threshold beyond which disruption occurs.
- It assumes that the same amount of adaptation is required for each event among all people.
- It equates "change" with "stress."
- It accounts for only 2 to 4% of illness (Fitzpatrick & Wilke, 2001).

To understand the effects of life changes on health, you need to identify what each individual perceives as stressful. Only then can you help people become aware of the stress they face in their lives and plan for the future. To return to the example of Marcia M who had accumulated an LCU score of 390:

CLINICAL EXAMPLE

During the course of group therapy, Marcia shared her desire to return to college and complete the junior and senior years of a medical technology program in which she had been enrolled before her marriage. To do so, she would have to make a number of changes: move to an apartment close to the college because she could not afford to own a car, change her working hours or job so that she could attend day classes, change her sleeping habits, change her recreational and social activities, and reduce her other expenses to pay school costs. The changes required would add almost 200 LCUs to her score.

In group, Marcia was able to consider this information and reevaluate her goals. She decided to delay her return to school until she could get on her feet financially. She chose not to make any other changes in her life for the present time.

Clients can use this information, much as Marcia did, to help decide when it is advantageous or disadvantageous to engage in a life change. This knowledge helps them make responsible decisions about the directions their lives will take. The Client/Family Teaching feature below includes some strategies based on the interrelationship between life changes and stressful events.

STRESS AS A TRANSACTION

Richard Lazarus, a pioneering theorist and researcher in stress, coping, and health, is known for his transaction-based approach to understanding stress. His view is reflected in the definition of stress given at the beginning of this chapter and his transactional model is consistent with nursing's holistic approach. Monat and Lazarus (1991), see perceived threat—what the person appraises as taxing or exceeding his or her resources and endangering his or her well-being—as the central characteristic of stressful situations, and in particular, a threat to a person's most important goals and values. Once a person has perceived a threat, the person evaluates it by thinking about it. This process is termed *cognitive appraisal.* According to Lazarus, the process works like this:

CLIENT / FAMILY TEACHING

Counseling Clients About Life Changes

You can assist clients by incorporating the guidelines below:

- Help clients recognize when a life change occurs.
- Encourage clients to think about the meaning of the change and identify some of the feelings associated with the change.
- Discuss with clients the different ways they might best adjust to the event.
- Encourage clients to take time in arriving at decisions.
- If possible, encourage clients to anticipate life changes and plan for them well in advance.
- Encourage clients to pace themselves. It can be done, even if they are in a hurry.
- Encourage clients to consider the accomplishment of a task as a part of daily living and to avoid looking at such an achievement as a stopping point or a time for letting down.

1. The person assesses the potential for benefit, harm, loss, threat, or challenge in a situation. This is termed *primary appraisal.*
2. The person then evaluates his or her coping resources and options in the situation. This is termed *secondary appraisal.*
3. The person applies the coping resources and options at his or her disposal. This is termed *coping.*
4. The person engages in ongoing reinterpretation of the situation based on new information. This is termed *reappraisal.*

Cognitive appraisal and coping style are influenced by the person's culture. Providing culturally competent care requires understanding the client's perspective and recognizing that a client's cognitive appraisal of a situation may, and probably will, differ from your own.

Lazarus believes that stress depends not only on external conditions but also on the person's physical vulnerability and the adequacy of that person's coping styles.

PSYCHONEUROIMMUNOLOGY FRAMEWORK

Psychoneuroimmunology (PNI) offers a comprehensive framework for understanding the relationship between stress and disease and the biopsychosocial nature and complexity of the stress process. As discussed in Chapter 4, PNI is concerned with interaction among the neurologic, endocrine, and immune systems and takes into account the nature of the influence of psychosocial factors on immune function and health outcomes. Cells in the brain and the endocrine and immune systems produce neuropeptides, the chemical messengers that are links between the mind and the body. The Caring for the Spirit special feature in Chapter 24 is an example of the multifaceted nature of the psychoneuroimmunology framework.

Self-Healing Personalities

Neuropeptide manufacture is activated by positive mental states and suppressed by negative mental states. Several stress and coping-related studies have suggested that some people have *self-healing personalities,* while others have *disease-prone personalities.* Self-healers are emotionally stable people who bounce back from stressful situations (Friedman & VandenBos, 1992). These are people whom others describe as enthusiastic, joyful, secure, energetic, alert, and content. They are likable and have close, warm relationships with others. Borysenko (1993) reports a doubling of N-K cell activity (natural killer lymphocytes that attack virally infected cells and tumor cells in the body) in people with a sense of connectedness as opposed to people who are lonely and isolated.

Hardiness and Health

A now classic study on hardiness and health found that individuals who have strong feelings of confidence in their ability to control circumstances, a willingness to see life events as challenges rather than as obstacles, and a strong commitment to the experiences and demands of daily living have fewer illnesses than those who lack these qualities (Kobasa, 1979).

Disease-Prone Personalities

Disease-prone personalities, on the other hand, tend to display negative emotions. They are suspicious of others and tend to be chronically anxious, angry, or depressed. These chronic negative emotional patterns are linked with various physiologic changes such as activation of the sympathetic nervous system, increase in the level of cortisol, and suppression of the immune system, leading to increased vulnerability to illness.

Anxiety

Anxiety is a state of varying degrees of uneasiness or discomfort. It is frequently coupled with guilt, doubts, fears, and obsessions. Beyond the mild level, anxiety is often described as a feeling of terror or dread; anxiety is believed to be the most uncomfortable feeling a person can experience. In fact, anxiety is so uncomfortable that most people try to get rid of it as soon as possible.

Anxiety is a potent force because the energy it provides can be converted into destructive or constructive action. When used constructively, anxiety can stimulate the action necessary to alter a stressful situation, fill a painful need, or arrange a compromise. A client who understands the source of anxiety is best able to use it constructively.

NEUROBIOLOGIC BASIS OF ANXIETY

Contemporary thinking about anxiety includes a neurobiologic component. Anxiety is now thought to result, at least in part, from dysregulation of one or more neurotransmitters and their receptors. Most research has focused on the BZ–GABA–chloride complex, although several other neurotransmitters and their receptors such as serotonin, norepinephrine, and the neuropeptide cholecystokinin may play a role in the development of anxiety. Other research using MRIs and PET scans focuses on brain structure itself. The neurobiologic component of anxiety is more fully discussed in Chapter 16.

SOURCES OF ANXIETY

Anxiety is an inevitable result of the attempt to maintain equilibrium in a changing world. People experience anxiety in many different situations and interpersonal relationships. However, the general causes of anxiety have been classified into two major kinds of threats:

1. Threats to biologic integrity: actual or impending interference with basic human needs such as the needs for food, drink, or warmth.
2. Threats to the security of the self:
   a. Unmet expectations important to self-integrity.
   b. Unmet needs for status and prestige.
   c. Anticipated disapproval by significant others.
   d. Inability to gain or reinforce self-respect or to gain recognition from others.
   e. Guilt, or discrepancies between self-view and actual behavior.

It is crucial to understand that *either* actual *or* impending interference may cause anxiety; actual interference with a biologic or psychosocial need is not a necessary condition. All that is necessary is the *anticipation* of one of these major threats.

Threats to biologic integrity or to the fulfillment of such basic human needs as food, drink, warmth, and shelter are a general cause of anxiety. Threats to the security of self are not as easily categorized. In some instances, they are obvious; in others, they are more obscure because each person's sense of self is unique. To one person, power and prestige may be essential; to another, independence; to a third, being of service to others.

Consider the last category—being of service to others.

CLINICAL EXAMPLE

Mrs. C, a nurse, is convinced that a client would feel much better if he expressed his fears to her. But no matter how often she provides the opportunity, he insists, "This is not the time to talk about it," and thwarts her attempt. She is not able to help him in a way that is important to her sense of self. In addition, she believes that the unit's nurse manager (whose communication skills she admires) expects her to have been successful in this endeavor.

Mrs. C is worried and anxious. When unmet needs or expectations related to essential values (such as being of service to the client) are coupled with the actual or anticipated disapproval of others who are important (the nurse manager), anxiety is generated.

ANXIETY AS A CONTINUUM

Many theorists conceptualize anxiety as a continuum (■ Figure 5–4). Mild to moderate anxiety can be functionally effective in that it helps us focus our attention and generates energy and motivation. Thus, anxiety is an aspect of problem solving in that it alerts us to the need to concentrate our resources. However, severe anxiety and panic narrow our attention to a crippling degree. Under these conditions alertness is greatly reduced, and learning does not usually take place.

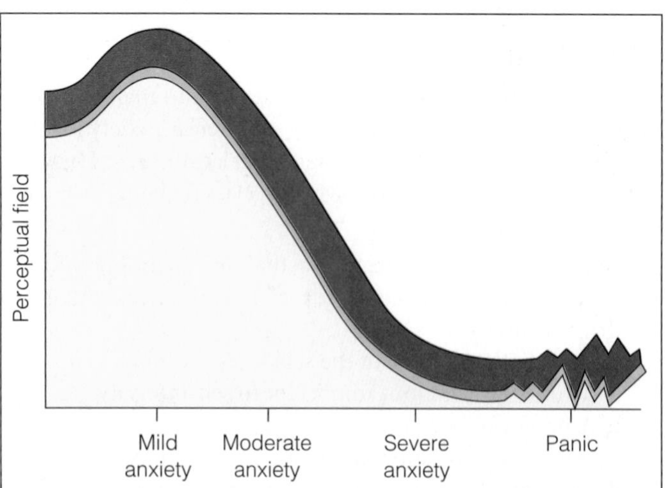

FIGURE 5–4 ■ *The effect of anxiety on the perceptual field. Notice that the perceptual field is increased in mild anxiety, becomes increasingly constricted as anxiety increases, and is completely disrupted at the panic level.*

Mild Anxiety

Mild anxiety helps one deal constructively with stress. A mildly anxious person has a broad perceptual field because mild anxiety heightens the ability to take in sensory stimuli. Such a person is more alert to what is going on and can make better sense of what is happening with others and the environment. The senses take in more; the person hears better, sees better, and makes logical connections between events. The person feels relatively safe and comfortable. Because learning is easier when one is mildly anxious, mild anxiety helps clients learn, for instance, how best to administer their own insulin. Mild anxiety can also help a nursing student review psychiatric–mental health nursing before a final examination.

Moderate Anxiety

In moderate anxiety, a person remains alert, but the perceptual field narrows. The moderately anxious person shuts out the events on the periphery while focusing on central concerns.

CLINICAL EXAMPLE

A nursing student who is moderately anxious about the final examination may be able to focus so intently on studying that she or he is not distracted by an argument between roommates, loud music on the stereo, and a rousing chase scene on television. The student shuts out the chaos in the environment and focuses on what is of central personal importance—preparing for the exam.

This process of taking in some sensory stimuli while excluding others is called **selective inattention.**

People also use selective inattention to cope with anxiety-provoking stimuli. This phenomenon may account for the anxious preoperative client who fails to remember what the nurse said about postoperative pain or the need to cough and deep-breathe after surgery.

Although the perceptual field is narrowed and the person sees, hears, and grasps less, there is an element of voluntary control. Moderately anxious individuals can, with direction, focus on what they have previously shut out.

Severe Anxiety

In severe anxiety, sensory reception is greatly reduced. Severely anxious people focus on small or scattered details of an experience. They have difficulty in problem solving, and their ability to organize is also reduced. They seldom have the complete picture. Selective inattention may be increased and may be less amenable to voluntary control. The person may be unable to focus on events in the environment. New stimuli may be experienced as overwhelming and may cause the anxiety level to rise even higher.

The sympathetic nervous system is activated in severe anxiety, causing an increase in pulse, blood pressure, and respiration and an increase in epinephrine secretion, vasoconstriction, and even body temperature. A multitude of physiologic changes may be observed, which are described in the section that follows.

Panic

The panic level of anxiety is characterized by a completely disrupted perceptual field. Panic has been described as a disintegration of the personality experienced as intense terror. Details may be enlarged, scattered, or distorted. Logical thinking and effective decision making may be impossible. The person in panic is unable to initiate or maintain goal-directed action. Behavior may appear purposeless, and communication may be unintelligible.

ASSESSING ANXIETY

Anxiety can be assessed in the physiologic, cognitive, and emotional/behavioral dimensions. This observation illustrates the relationship between the mind and the body. Anxiety is a multidimensional phenomenon in that the total person is involved in every aspect of it. Objective data, particularly nursing observations, may be critical because of the nature of anxiety. Selective inattention and dissociation interfere with the client's awareness of anxiety and ability to give accurate reports. Families and friends also can contribute data useful to the assessment of anxiety.

Physiologic Dimension

Observations of the client's physiologic state are likely to indicate autonomic nervous system responses, particularly sympathetic effects. Sympathetic nervous system dominance is associated with arousal as occurs during anxiety or as the body's response to a physical emergency. The parasympathetic nervous system maintains normal, smooth functioning. Various organs may be affected, such as the adrenal medulla, heart, blood vessels, lungs, stomach, colon, rectum, salivary glands, liver, pupils of the eyes, and sweat glands. ■ Figure 5–5 on page 90 illustrates the sympathetic and parasympathetic nervous systems in detail. Anxious clients may have an increased heart rate, increased blood pressure, difficulty breathing, sweaty palms, trembling, dry mouth, "butterflies in the stomach" or a "lump in the throat," as well as other symptoms.

Laboratory tests are not routinely done to evaluate anxiety because observation is faster and more accurate. However, anxiety affects the results of laboratory tests done for other purposes. Blood studies may show increased adrenal function, elevated levels of glucose and lactic acid, and decreased parathyroid function and oxygen and calcium levels. Urinary studies may indicate increased levels of epinephrine and norepinephrine.

Cognitive Dimension

Assessment of cognitive function may indicate difficulty in logical thinking, narrowed or distorted perceptual field, selective inattention or dissociation, lack of attention to details, difficulty concentrating, or difficulty focusing. The level of anxiety determines the extent to which cognitive function is affected. Mild, moderate, severe, or panic level of anxiety is assessed according to the descriptions earlier in this chapter.

Emotional/Behavioral Dimension

In the emotional/behavioral dimension, clients may be irritable, angry, withdrawn, and restless, or they may cry. The affective response can often be assessed through the client's subjective description. Clients may describe themselves as "on edge," "uptight," "jittery," "nervous," "worried," or "tense." They may feel dizzy or faint and may experience a feeling of impending doom as if something terrible were about to happen.

Coping with Stress and Anxiety

Nurses can be helpful if they understand the changes their clients are undergoing. Reactions to threatening situations, such as illness and hospitalization, can be divided into two general categories: task-oriented responses and defense-oriented responses. When we feel competent to deal with stress and the situation is not too threatening to our sense of self, our behavior tends to be task-oriented. Task-oriented behavior is geared toward problem solving. Consider the situation of a student who is majoring in mathematics and fails his courses. If he is not too frightened by the possibility that he may not be suited for a career in this field, he can assess the situation and change his major. This is a task-oriented reaction. It is based on a realistic appraisal of the situation and involves a series of carefully thought-out judgments about what course of behavior would be most effective.

MediaLink Case Study: Assessing Anxiety

When we feel inadequate to cope with stress and the situation is extremely threatening to our sense of self, we tend to engage in defense-oriented behavior. The diagnosis of a terminal illness, for instance, may be so overwhelming that a person must temporarily defend against acknowledging this reality. Everyone uses defense-oriented behavior from time to time as a protective measure. Such behavior becomes harmful only when it is the predominant means of coping with stress. In such cases, problem-solving and reality-based behavior are continually avoided. Defense-oriented behavior is discussed later in this chapter.

Coping strategies are a set of behaviors people under stress use in struggling to improve their situations. Once you have finished reading this section, thoughtfully consider how you cope with stress by answering the questions posed in the Nursing Self-Awareness feature on page 91. Coping strategies can be thought of simply as ways of getting along in the world.

EVERYDAY WAYS OF COPING WITH STRESS

Everyday coping strategies offer an immense repertoire of defenses to maintain control and balance in the face of stress. A person can cope on different levels, including physical, social, cognitive, and emotional levels. However, the devices people choose to cope with stress depend on many factors. Among them are the external circumstances, the suddenness and intensity of the stress, the resources available to the person, and the person's predisposition to certain coping patterns, established over the course of one's development. One man who is late for an appointment because he gets caught in a traffic jam may

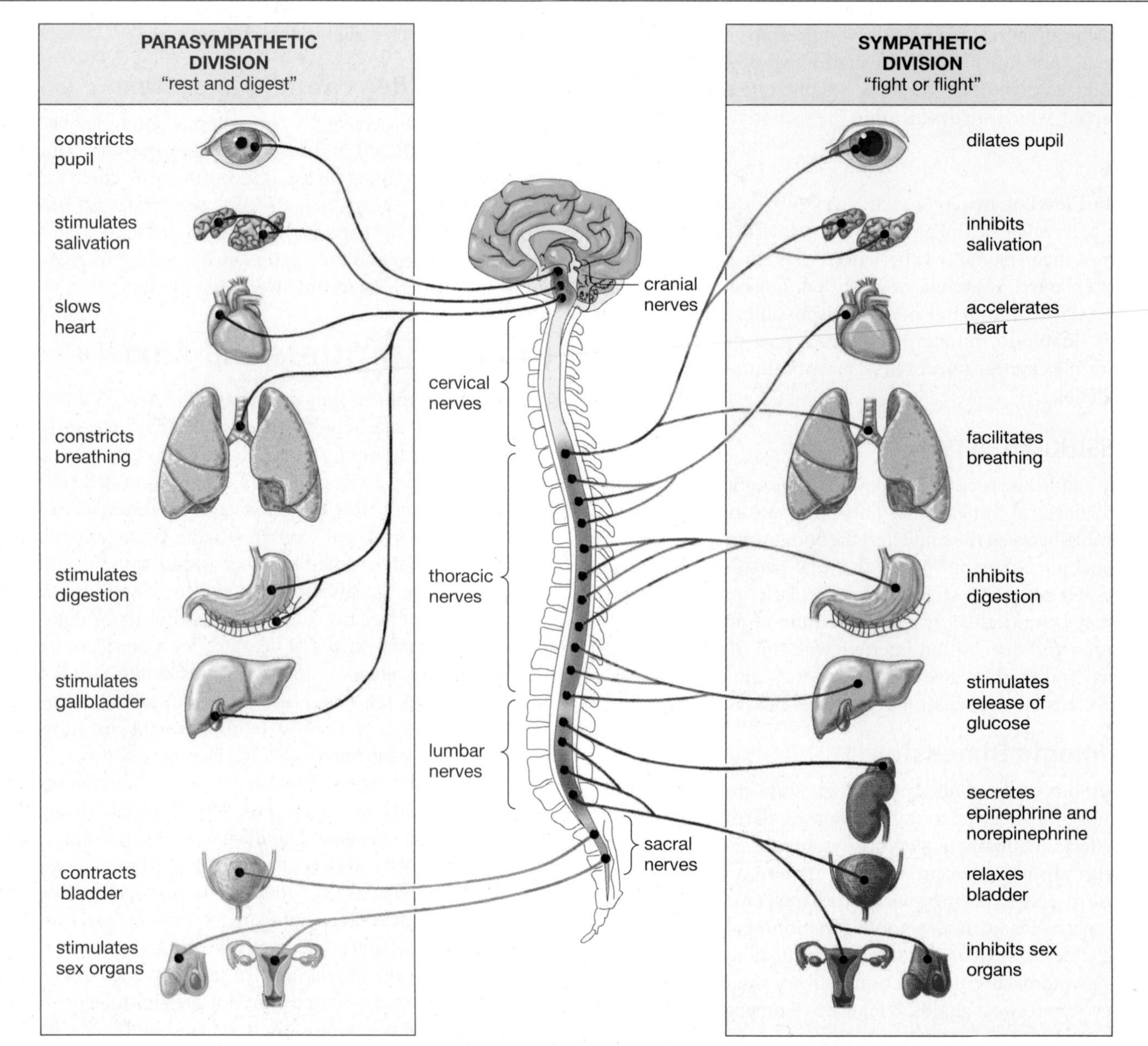

FIGURE 5–5 ■ *Involuntary Control of Bodily Functions. The autonomic nervous system has two divisions, the sympathetic and the parasympathetic, which exercise automatic control over the body's organs, generally in opposing ways. The parasympathetic generally has inhibitory or relaxing effects, while the sympathetic has stimulatory effects. Axons of the parasympathetic division emerge not only from the spinal cord, but from the brain as well.*

Source: Krogh, D. (2000). *Biology: A guide to the natural world,* p. 515. Upper Saddle River, NJ: Prentice Hall.

react with a furious outburst of anger. Another may begin to daydream and forget where he is going. A third may use the time to solve some problem.

Most often, individuals use behaviors that have worked well for them in the past. Sometimes they behave in a certain way because it is the only method they have of coping with stress or because other coping strategies failed to work. Some people learn to turn to others for protection and nurturance; some learn to turn to chemicals or food; some rely on self-discipline and keeping a stiff upper lip; others feel better after the intense expression of feelings; some withdraw physically and/or emotionally; still others exercise or talk the problem out. Common coping methods are discussed below.

Turning to a Comforting Person

The earliest coping strategy is probably the familiar method of turning to a nurturing person for soothing and protecting. Receiving love is being reassured that one is lovable. Love from supportive others may take the form of physical touching, rocking, patting, or verbal reassurances of various kinds ("Don't be afraid, I'll stay with you"). Bible study or listening to religious tapes is comforting to many

Nursing SELF-AWARENESS — What Coping Strategies Do You Use?

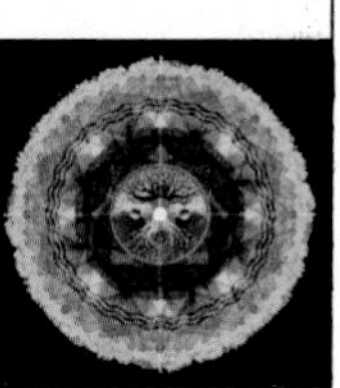

When you are feeling competent to deal with stress and the situation is not too threatening to your sense of self, which task-oriented coping strategies do you use? Review the everyday ways of coping with stress discussed on pages 89–92 and answer the following questions:

- Which everyday ways of coping with stress do you use most often? Be specific.
- Can you identify a pattern or common thread among them?
- What effects do they have on your sense of comfort or well-being?
- What effects do they have on your interpersonal relationships with others (include professional relationships)?

When you are feeling inadequate to cope with stress and the situation is extremely threatening to your sense of self, which defense-oriented behaviors do you use? Review the defense-oriented ways of coping (defense mechanisms) discussed on pages 93–100 and answer the following questions:

- Which defense-oriented ways of coping do you use most often? Be specific.
- Can you identify a pattern or common thread among them?
- What effects do they have on your sense of comfort or well-being?
- What effects do they have on your interpersonal relationships with others (include professional relationships)?

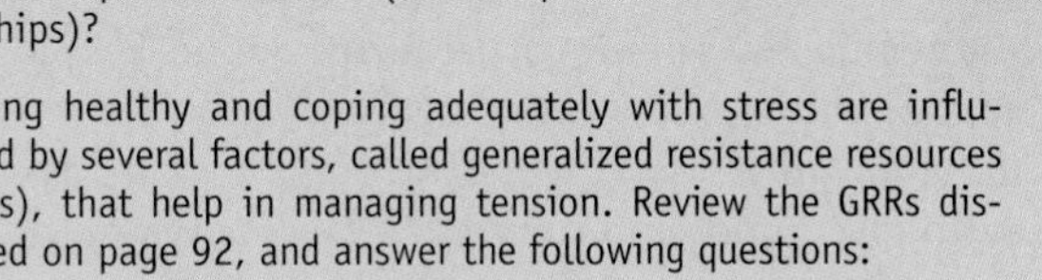

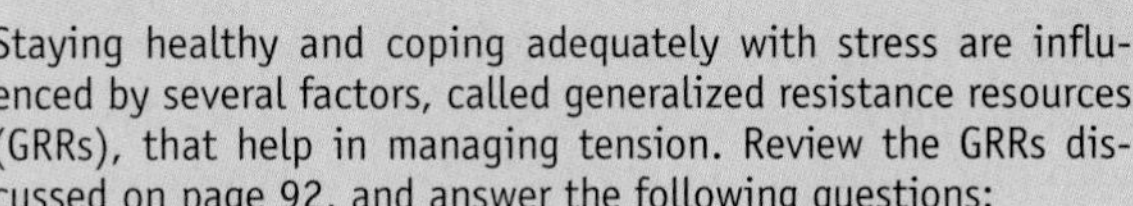

Staying healthy and coping adequately with stress are influenced by several factors, called generalized resistance resources (GRRs), that help in managing tension. Review the GRRs discussed on page 92, and answer the following questions:

- Which GRRs most commonly influence the way in which you manage tension? Be specific.
- In which ways have these GRRs influenced your life course?
- How can you mobilize these personal resources to strengthen control over your life and your sense of personal coherence?
- What effects do they have on your interpersonal relationships with others (include professional relationships)?

people. This category also includes eating in times of stress and for general support. Alcohol, nicotine, and other chemicals are often used to enhance well-being in the face of stress. Many theorists view these alternatives as substitutes for the dependent comfort of being a baby in the care of a nurturing parent.

Relying on Self-Discipline

Whereas some people under stress tend to turn to the comfort of friendly company, food, or alcohol, all of which are reminiscent of childhood dependence, others rely on self-discipline. Self-control ranks high in the value system of many cultures and subcultures. This coping style involves pride in the ability to laugh off problems, endure frustrations, and discount anxiety. Keep a stiff upper lip, bite the bullet, and get over it are all admonitions that people address to themselves when self-discipline is their patterned response to stress. These people are unlikely to want the company of supportive others and may even push them away. They are often unresponsive when others seek comfort from them, for they see such dependent behavior as weak.

Intense Expression of Feeling

Crying, swearing, and laughing all tend to relieve tension. Swearing loses its usefulness as an escape valve if it becomes a habit. This is less true of both crying and laughing. Crying and laughing tend to release energy and exert a soothing effect on a person who is experiencing tension.

Avoidance and Withdrawal

While some people find it hard to sleep when they are under tension, others react to worries, bad news, or an argument with somnolence. Still others respond with a form of waking sleep like apathy or emotional withdrawal, which accomplishes the same thing.

Talking It Out

Many people relieve tension by talking it out. Talking implies establishing and maintaining a contact of sorts with another human being. In addition, it enables new ideas to emerge and new perspectives to be entertained. Obviously, this device is the medium of most therapeutic intervention. This has profound implications for nursing because nurses are the health care providers who spend the most time with clients. It also has profound implications for clients whose communication is dysfunctional or whose ability to communicate freely is restricted. Psychiatric clients generally fall into these categories.

Privately Thinking It Through

Some people believe that the unexamined life is not worth living. When faced with a problem that causes them anxiety, these individuals become introspective about it. The rationalizations that emerge serve as effective tension relievers.

Working It Off

Physical activity to relieve tension may range from simple gestures like finger tapping, floor pacing, and door slamming to activities purposely designed to alter the tension-producing circumstances, such as aerobic exercise. In addition, some tense individuals feel a lot of aggressive energy. Physical exertion in the form of demanding sports, like jogging or racquetball, or manual labor, like scrubbing the floor, is a way to use this energy constructively.

Engaging in Self-Healing Mind/Body Practices

Increasing numbers of people are integrating self-healing practices such as yoga, meditation, massage, visualization, and relaxation exercises into their everyday lives. While Western medicine continues its explosive growth in psychobiologic knowledge and technology, more of us are finding that these ancient principles and practices have significant therapeutic value. A thorough discussion of healing practices is in Chapter 32.

Prayerfulness

Prayer can be individual or communal, private or public. People pray for different reasons—to ask for something for oneself, to ask for something for others, to repent of wrongdoing and ask for forgiveness, to give honor and praise to a Higher Power, to offer thanksgiving. Recent research shows that praying can positively affect high blood pressure, the course and extent of heart attacks, migraine headaches, and anxiety. Further, nursing activities that support prayer as a coping measure may support mental health (Meisenhelder & Chandler, 2000).

Using Symbolic Substitutes

Stress may be relieved by ascribing symbolic values to acts or objects. These acts or objects may or may not have other meanings. There are symbolic devices for the management of tensions in religious practices such as confession, prayer, or sacrifice. For some people, the automobile has a symbolic significance; others ascribe symbolic significance to their annual income or their physical appearance.

The list is almost endless, but the principle is always the same. Some people attach a meaning beyond the obvious one to objects, experiences, and people, through which they find a means to reduce their tensions.

Somatizing

Many organs of the body have an expression and communication function. This is sometimes known as *somatizing* or *organ language*. Some organs communicate their messages only to their owner. For example, the heart may communicate by means of palpitation. Other demonstrations are public, such as blushing or stuttering. Urination and defecation, increased sweating, and altered sexual activity are other familiar examples of organ language.

COPING RESOURCES

Early research on coping was concerned with how people respond to specific stresses in a laboratory setting. More recent studies that consider the whole being in interaction with the environment have led to viewing coping as a dynamic process that involves the demands and restrictions on a person as well as the resources available.

Generalized Resistance

According to Antonovsky (1991), people stay healthy or cope adequately with stress because they possess what he calls *generalized resistance resources (GRRs)*, factors in the person, group, or organization that help in managing tension.

Physical and biochemical GRRs are physiologic characteristics, such as genetic features and levels of immunity. These GRRs also include interaction of the nervous and endocrine systems that help in adaptation; for example, interactions involving ACTH, thyroid-stimulating hormone (TSH), vasopressin, norepinephrine, and insulin and their influence on human behavior. Not only are individuals different in their genetic and biochemical makeup, but the physiologic effects of illness and stress may also alter a person's ability to use physical and biochemical GRRs positively.

Material goods and relative wealth constitute the *artifactual and material GRRs*; having these attributes makes it easier to cope with illness. Money helps to ensure the best health care available. Effective coping is often interrelated with one's socioeconomic status simply because the higher the status, the greater the resources to help the person cope. For example, household help not only relieves an ill person's worries but also reduces the practical burden.

Cognitive GRRs have to do with intelligence and knowledge. When people know about stressors, they can avoid them. They can also predict when periods of stress are imminent and thus reduce their impact. Knowing what community services are available is also a cognitive GRR.

People who are self-aware—who know their own capacities and potentials and have a well-developed sense of themselves—possess *emotional GRRs*. Emotional GRRs determine the extent of psychological hardiness. In general, they have to do with how competent and self-assured one feels.

Valuative and attitudinal GRRs are the products of a person's culture and environment. People are apt to respond in learned ways. The attitudinal aspect also is related to how flexible, rational, and farsighted the person is. The more rational or accurate one's appraisal of a threatening situation and the more flexible one is in approaching the situation and envisioning the consequences, the greater one's resources for coping.

Interpersonal–relational GRRs are available social support systems. The greater a person's social contacts, the greater the social resources available to augment the ability to deal with stress. Love, affection, and nurturance are hallmarks of interpersonal–relational GRRs.

Institutional structures that facilitate coping are called *macrosociocultural GRRs*. These resources include government programs such as Aid to Dependent Children as well as cultural institutions such as death and funeral rites, religious rituals, and ceremonies.

According to this model, the ability to cope is determined by the extent and effectiveness of each person's generalized resistance resources and sense of coherence or the ability to influence one's life course (Landsverk & Kane, 1998). The Using Research Evidence special feature on page 93 illustrates one way in which nurses can help clients influence the course of their lives. Yet the actual process of coping remains unclear. Theorists and researchers still do not fully understand exactly which personal resources should be mobilized and under which conditions.

USING RESEARCH EVIDENCE

As the nurse in a day treatment unit located in a suburb of a large city in the southeastern United States, you are especially aware of the difficulty your clients have in handling stress. Most of your clients are diagnosed with a psychotic disorder and have difficulty in maintaining relationships with friends and family and finding or keeping a job. Thus, most have become marginalized, and the day treatment unit has become the core of their daily activities.

You understand that it is important to strengthen life control among those who have become marginalized. People who are in charge of their lives have a sense of coherence. They are more likely to be able to cope with stressful situations in ways that decrease, or even eliminate, their distress. To help your clients strengthen control over their lives you develop a psychoeducation program for them focusing on the following:

1. Achieving understanding of the internal environment (what thoughts, feelings, and wishes drive the individual).
2. Achieving understanding of the external environment (what forces affect what an individual is able to accomplish).
3. Exploring human relationships to include client-family, client-friend, client-client, client-employer, client-staff, client-landlord, and whatever other dyads are active relationships or potential relationships in the clients' lives.
4. Exploring the meaning of present events, that is, focusing on the here-and-now, rather than the there-and-then, to gain an understanding of what the stressors are in the lives of the clients.

The psychoeducation program you developed is based on the following research citation:

Bengtsson-Tops, A., & Hansson, L. (2001). The validity of Antonovsky's sense of coherence measure in a sample of schizophrenic patients living in the community. *Journal of Advanced Nursing, 33*(4), 432–438.

Landsverk, S. S., & Kane, C. F. (1998). Antonovsky's sense of coherence: Theoretical basis of psychoeducation in schizophrenia. *Issues in Mental Health Nursing, 19*(5), 419–432.

DEFENSE-ORIENTED WAYS OF COPING: DEFENSE MECHANISMS

The coping strategies described above are considered normal. They are simply ways of getting along. In some people, however, what passes for a normal adjustment is actually a very tenuous one with few outlets for controlled aggression, few love objects, few opportunities for satisfaction and growth. These people find it more and more difficult to cope with additional stress. Ultimately, the external stress the person is trying unsuccessfully to ward off is matched by a mounting internal stress. The person suffers both from increased anxiety and from the strain on overworked stabilizers. And what happens to the person who has no one to talk with, who can't jog five miles, or who can't laugh off the problem?

When a person is unable to ward off stress or reduce tension in the usual way, anxiety mounts as the person feels increasingly inadequate to cope with the situation. Under these circumstances, the person is more likely to engage in *defense-oriented behavior*. Defense-oriented behavior is not a specific attempt to solve a problem; it consists of using mental mechanisms to lessen uncomfortable feelings of anxiety and to prevent pain regardless of cost. These characteristic mental mechanisms are commonly called **defense mechanisms.** They are automatic psychological processes that protect the self by allowing the person to deny or distort a stressful event or to restrict awareness and reduce the sense of emotional involvement. But they can also interfere with rational decision making. People who use defense mechanisms are excluding some information about the situation they are in. They are also denying their own feelings about it.

Defense mechanisms are mostly unconscious and often inflexible coping patterns that protect a person through intrapsychic (coming from within) distortions that are really self-deceptions. The person usually has little awareness of what is happening or even less control over events. Although these reactions may help keep the lid on anxiety, they also limit the ability to grow from and savor the experience, they interfere with rational decision making and the ability to work productively, and they impair and erode interpersonal relationships. Even adaptive devices can go wrong.

Because human behavior is so complex and varied, defense mechanisms can be classified in many ways. Often, they are classified according to whether they are simple or complex, whether they are most likely to arise in a specific phase of development, or whether they are commonly associated with a particular form of psychopathology. Definitions of various defense mechanisms overlap, and the same observed behavior may often be explained by more than one type of defense. And people do not use one method of defense at a time; they usually rely on a combination of defenses. For study purposes, the common defense mechanisms discussed here are repression, suppression, dissociation, identification, introjection, projection, denial, fantasy, rationalization, reaction formation, displacement, and intellectualization. They are summarized in ■ Table 5–1 on page 94.

Repression

Repression, the basis of all defense mechanisms, is the dynamic behind much of "forgetting." When people repress, they unconsciously exclude distressing emotions, thoughts, or experiences from awareness. Repression bars access to conscious awareness of feelings and thoughts that would cause anxiety and disrupt the self-concept. It also affords protection from a sudden trauma until the person can deal with the shock. From the individual's point of view, a repressed memory is "forgotten" and cannot be deliberately brought to awareness (see the Caring for the Spirit special feature on page 95). Although the repressed

TABLE 5–1 Defense Mechanisms

Name	Definition	Example
Denial	Blocking out painful or anxiety-inducing events or feelings.	A manager tells an employee he may have to fire him. On the way home, the employee shops for a new car.
Displacement	Discharging pent-up feelings on people less dangerous than those who initially aroused the emotion.	A student who has received a low grade on a term paper blows up at his girlfriend when she asks about his grade.
Dissociation	Handling emotional conflicts, or internal or external stressors, by a temporary alteration of consciousness or identity.	A woman has amnesia for the events surrounding a fatal automobile accident in which she was the speeding driver.
Fantasy	Symbolic satisfaction of wishes through nonrational thought.	A student struggling through graduate school thinks about a prestigious, high-paying job she wants.
Identification	Unconscious assumption of similarity between oneself and another.	After hospitalization for minor surgery, a girl decides to be a nurse.
Intellectualization	Separating an emotion from an idea or thought because the emotional reaction is too painful to be acknowledged.	A man learns from his doctor that he has cancer. He studies the physiology and treatment of cancer without experiencing any emotion.
Introjection	Acceptance of another's values and opinions as one's own.	A woman who prefers a simple lifestyle assumes the materialistic, prestige-oriented values of her husband.
Projection	Attributing one's own unacceptable feelings and thoughts to others.	A man who is quite critical of others thinks that people are joking about his appearance.
Rationalization	Falsification of experience through the construction of logical or socially approved explanations of behavior.	A man cheats on his income tax return and tells himself it's all right because everyone does it.
Reaction formation	Unacceptable feelings disguised by repression of the real feeling and by reinforcement of the opposite feeling.	A woman who dislikes her mother-in-law is always very nice to her.
Repression	Unconsciously keeping unacceptable feelings out of awareness.	A man is jealous of a good friend's success but is unaware of his feelings.
Suppression	Consciously keeping unacceptable feelings and thoughts out of awareness.	A student taking an examination is upset about an argument with her boyfriend but puts it out of her mind so she can finish the test.

feelings remain unconscious, they continue to exert pressure for expression. The self tries to maintain the repression, but in people experiencing extreme stress or anxiety, or in febrile (feverish) or toxic states, repression may begin to fail. Clients who are intoxicated by alcohol or drugs or who are emerging from anesthesia may verbalize feelings that they usually repress.

CLINICAL EXAMPLE

Susan was raped. She was brought to an outpatient clinic by her roommate. Susan said she felt very anxious and could not recall the circumstances surrounding her rape or what the rapist looked like. Her use of repression protected her from facing her fears and humiliation.

Nursing Intervention Strategies. Nursing intervention in such cases should be supportive and protective of the client's defenses. After the initial shock has lessened and the client's anxiety level has been reduced, you can help the client examine the traumatic event.

Suppression

Suppression is an intentional act that helps keep thoughts, feelings, wishes, or actions that cause anxiety out of conscious awareness. Suppression is the conscious form of repression.

CLINICAL EXAMPLE

A woman who is an only child learns that her elderly widowed mother has been diagnosed with cancer. The woman recognizes that she will be the sole support of her mother during this trying time. She also has some professional responsibilities that cannot be put off. The woman decides to put off worrying about what the future may bring or anticipating her mother's death until her mother's diagnostic studies are completed, an accurate staging of the cancer can be performed, the first chemotherapy sequence has

CARING FOR THE SPIRIT

Repressed Memories: Controversial, Unusual, and Sometimes Bizarre Occurrences

Over 100 years ago, Sigmund Freud proposed that we actively and deliberately bury painful or dangerous memories beyond the reach of consciousness. He called this process repression.

According to Freud, repressed memories influence behavior, thinking, and emotions, and produce mental symptoms. Early in his career Freud wrote that sexual abuse in childhood was common and was the cause of repression. This abuse, and the resulting repression, caused the "hysteria" he diagnosed in his patients. After 1897, Freud abruptly abandoned his theory on repression. Instead, he said, children have fantasies of being seduced. These imagined seductions, according to Freud, cause internal conflict, and repression is a way of coping with this internal conflict.

It is unclear why Freud abandoned his theory. Some of his critics believe that Freud bowed to social pressure and the threat of professional ostracism because the notion of rampant childhood sexual abuse was outrageous. Others of his critics believed that Freud himself distorted his patients' stories because of his own psychological problems.

To understand the concept of repression, we need to understand how memory works. Memories are stored in a portion of each of the thousands of neurons in the brain. Each neuron represents a little bit of memory. Because the brain is such a complex organ, it parcels out bits and pieces of an experience to different parts of the brain. For example, memories of sound are parceled out to the auditory cortex, memories of appearance to the visual cortex, memories of sensation to the sensory cortex, memories of smell to the olfactory cortex, and source memory to the frontal cortex. All scattered memory fragments remain physically linked. It is the limbic system that takes on the job of assembling these bits and pieces. The limbic system actually acts as a neural file clerk by pulling memory fragments from various file drawers. Intensely traumatic events produce unusually strong nerve connections.

Memory can go awry if the terror of an experience is so great that the biologic processes underlying information storage are disrupted. However, the right biologic stimulus can set the nerve circuits firing and trigger fear. The source of the fear is *not* remembered. Memory blocks come at great cost. They leave a person without an explanation for bewildering emotional distress that causes turmoil.

Memory can also be confounded; that is, snippets of memory from a real event can be interwoven with snippets of an imagined event. Recent research has demonstrated that the mere suggestion that you could have once been lost in a shopping mall can leave a memory trace in the brain. This memory trace can then become linked to the memory of a friend's or sibling's story of being lost or a fairy tale such as Hansel and Gretel, as well as actual memories of shopping malls. Under stress and over time, the knowledge that being lost in a mall was only a suggestion deteriorates. If you're asked at a later time if you were ever lost in a mall, your brain will activate these assorted images, and eventually you "remember" being lost in a mall as a child.

These findings—that memories are open to faulty recollection or that they can be created through a suggestion from another—have caused great distress for survivors of childhood sexual abuse who experience the phenomenon called **recovered memory.** Recovered memories of childhood sexual abuse are those that emerge into consciousness after being repressed for a period of time, sometimes for years. Imagine what it must be like having recalled long-forgotten memories of painful and humiliating sexual abuse by a trusted or loved adult. Imagine further what it must be like to have your unsettling memories viewed with suspicion. You might feel helpless, hopeless, and lost. Your sense of self would be fragmented, and your self-esteem diminished; your spiritual distress would be heightened.

The recent rise in reported cases of recovered memory has led to a large number of lawsuits against perpetrators accused of having committed acts of abuse years ago. Essentially, people who have recovered repressed memories are pitted against alleged perpetrators who claim these memories are actually manufactured **false memories.** Therapists who work to help people recover repressed memories are pitted against memory researchers who claim that false recovered memories are fabricated in the highly charged atmosphere of mental health therapy.

Psychiatric–mental health nurses need to be aware of both sides of the issue. Remember that many persons who have experienced sexual abuse have a history of not being believed by parents or others they love or trust. Expressing disbelief will only cause the client further pain. Being compassionate will help clients in the struggle to examine their own lives.

been completed, and a realistic prognosis is made of her mother's chances for a remission. As she puts it: "I've got too much to do and can't afford to fall apart right now."

Clients may refuse to consider their difficulties by saying that they "don't want to talk about it" or that they will "think about it some other time." This, too, is suppression.

Nursing Intervention Strategies. Suppression can be dealt with in the same way as repression. Suppression is generally easier to deal with because the material remains conscious. You can be somewhat more directive in assessing why the client avoids talking about a situation. Suggest that the client try to look at the situation because it affects future plans. Offering information about the situation may help clients look at their situations objectively. As they learn more, they may feel less threatened.

Dissociation

In **dissociation,** the individual handles emotional conflicts, or internal or external stressors, by a temporary alteration of consciousness or identity (see Chapter 16 for specific mental dysfunctions in which dissociation is the major mental mechanism). Dissociation resembles repression, but it has a different origin. The self is formed through the process of disapproval and approval from significant other people. Therefore, the self *dissociates*, or refuses awareness of, the expression of personal qualities and experiences of which significant others disapprove. These feelings come to exist separately from the person's self-concept. A little girl with artistic abilities that are not validated by her parents will not think of herself as artistic. She may deny her abilities even when other people point them out.

People who dissociate do not "notice" what they are doing. This limitation of awareness is maintained because the person experiences anxiety whenever permissible levels for the self are trespassed.

CLINICAL EXAMPLE

Ms. T consciously believes that sexual overtures are wrong, yet she behaves seductively toward men. She cannot understand why men see her behavior as a sexual invitation. The use of dissociation complicates Ms. T's problems. She needs to ignore or deny aspects of her situation to feel comfortable in it. Other people notice and point out Ms. T's seductive behavior, but she cannot recognize it because it is not a part of her self-concept. If Ms. T admitted her sexual feelings, she would experience severe anxiety and personality disorganization.

Nursing Intervention Strategies. For a discussion of nursing intervention strategies for dissociation, see Chapter 16.

Identification

Identification is the wish to be like another person and to assume the characteristics of that person's personality. It represents a turning away from our own personality. Identification is unconscious. In this it differs from *imitation*, which is the conscious copying of another person's qualities. Identification with people we admire can serve an important function in maturation by evoking latent qualities. For instance, a little girl who identifies with her mother and sisters learns the behavioral characteristics of womanhood.

The most primitive type of identification is seen in the infant's relationship with the mother. Infants seem to perceive no difference between their mothers and themselves and only gradually become aware that their mothers exist apart from them. Small children deal with people in terms of how these people meet their needs. They do not see them as separate individuals with needs of their own. Such identifications may persist into adult life in people who have not differentiated themselves psychologically from seemingly powerful parents.

One specific manifestation of identification is passiveness in relationships. People who feel they have no resources of their own will overvalue the resources of others and expect to be taken care of. People who are most identified with their parents tend to be people who were not allowed to develop their own individuality. Part of the process of self-realization occurs in adolescence, when we discard, with much anxiety and insecurity, our identification with the parents on whom we have been so dependent. Some clients may not have achieved a degree of self-identity sufficient to do this. Identification can inhibit our usefulness, because it prevents us from focusing on our own capacities.

Identification can be seen in clients who rely heavily on the nurse's advice and support. They expect that all their needs will be met and that nothing will be expected of them.

CLINICAL EXAMPLE

Mr. L has bipolar disorder and is taking lithium. He is not interested in learning about the medication he must take, dietary recommendations, or blood tests he needs. He expects the nurse to take responsibility for seeing that he gets the right medicine and that everything else is in order. Identification prevents him from being self-reliant.

Nursing Intervention Strategies. Nurses who work with clients like Mr. L should clarify what the client's expectations of the nurse are and then correct any misperceptions about the nurse's role. It is important to help Mr. L increase his own skills and take responsibility for his own care. Initially, you can offer the client collaboration and interdependence. The long-term goal in dealing with identification is for the client to formulate a self-care plan independently.

Introjection

Introjection is closely related to identification. It is the process of accepting another's values and opinions as one's own if they contradict the values one had previously held.

CLINICAL EXAMPLE

Joe Kaufmann, a cabinet maker, has worked for his employer who owns a furniture manufacturing company for 10 years. Joe's employer has asked him to cut some corners to help stem the company's financial losses. Afraid of losing his job, Joe compromises his values in providing shoddy workmanship.

Introjection also occurs in severe depression following the death of a loved one. The depressed person may assume many of the deceased person's characteristics, and in so doing lose some self-awareness.

Nursing Intervention Strategies. As a nurse, you can treat introjection like identification, remembering that introjection is more primitive and more intractable. It originates in our experience of being fed as infants. We incorporate people and objects into ourselves in the same way that we swallowed food. We felt a sense of oneness with everything in the external world and could not differentiate ourselves from others. Because thinking processes are not involved in the first experience of introjection, this defense mechanism tends to be difficult to explore on the verbal level.

Projection

Projection is an unconscious means of dealing with personal difficulties or unacceptable wishes by attributing them to others. We blame other people for our shortcomings or see them as harboring our own unacceptable feelings or thoughts. In the course of development, the child, needing parental approval, will identify with the parents and will also deny what they seem to condemn or fail to acknowledge. For instance, if her parents do not openly express and recognize angry feelings, a little girl will tend to regard anger as dangerous. She will then deny awareness of her own anger. Anger in others will disturb her, and she will tend to condemn in others the anger she cannot accept in herself. It is common knowledge that people often tend to criticize others for their own unacknowledged inferiorities. The person who fears being taken advantage of is often an opportunist.

In adult life, projection can be destructive if it interferes with our ability to acknowledge our own feelings. The tendency to attribute our own undesired feelings to others also blurs the boundaries between ourselves and others. This, in turn, makes it difficult to understand other people's feelings. People who make excessive use of projection tend to attribute to others hostile or seductive motives that do not actually exist. This prevents them from forming trusting and reciprocal relationships.

CLINICAL EXAMPLE

Linda G is wary and suspicious of every man she meets. Regardless of how they behave toward her, Linda says: "They only want one thing." She interprets their behavior as sexually suggestive but has no awareness of her own sexual interest in them.

A tendency to projection may also interfere with problem solving. A young woman who believes she is failing a course because of her teacher will not focus her energies on her studies.

Nursing Intervention Strategies. Clients who must deal with the stress of serious illness may shift the blame for their condition onto you, the nurse. They may complain of poor nursing care to a nurse who is actually very skillful. They may believe that they are being "paid back" for wrongdoing in the past. If such a client is accusing you falsely, do not show anger or retaliate but show, through consistency and attention, that you respect the client and are concerned about his or her welfare.

As clients feel more secure in the nurse–client relationship, encourage them to explore the realistic aspects of their situation. For example, you can help a man who blames his family for his alcoholism objectively explore what is known about the etiology of alcoholism. This may help him come to terms with his feelings of guilt and anger. This type of intervention helps the client separate his own feelings from the objective facts of the situation.

Denial

Denial of reality is one of the simplest of the defense mechanisms. In denial, painful or anxiety-producing aspects of awareness are blocked out of consciousness. The reality of a situation is either completely disregarded or transformed so that it is no longer threatening. Denial is one of the most common defenses against the stress of diagnosis and illness and is typically present in the first few minutes of adjustment to the death of a loved one. It may be helpful as a temporary protection against the full impact of a traumatic event.

CLINICAL EXAMPLE

A father reacts with denial when he shouts, "No, it can't be true; there must be a mistake," when told his 8-year-old son has just died in the trauma unit of injuries incurred when his bicycle collided with an automobile.

A young woman admitted to a psychiatric hospital because of acute anxiety and frightening hallucinations says she just "needs a rest."

Nursing Intervention Strategies. Sometimes denial is the best solution for the client. In such situations, support the denial. A terminally ill client who believes she will soon recover and who cannot think about her illness should be allowed the protection of denial. Not all clients need to face up to reality. You should recognize that the use of denial may be preventing serious personality disorganization.

Sometimes, however, denial is directly harmful to the client, as when a man refuses to take medication that is crucial to his survival or to his mental health. In such cases, the motivation for the client's behavior should be assessed. After discovering the protective function the denial is serving, focus on helping the client meet these needs in a way that is not self-destructive. You can also help by not reinforcing patterns of denial but rather focusing on instances when the client seems to be dealing with reality.

Fantasy

Fantasy is a form of nonrational mental activity that enables the individual to temporarily escape the demands of the everyday world. Fantasies are not confined by the reality considerations of cause and effect and time and space. Fantasy normally characterizes the thinking of children before they are able to engage in consensually validated communication. Adults revert to fantasy during times of stress to obtain a symbolic satisfaction of wishes.

CLINICAL EXAMPLE

A businesswoman facing financial difficulties temporarily escapes by daydreaming that she is enjoying a luxurious vacation on a Caribbean island.

Another woman with advanced multiple sclerosis imagines herself a famous ballerina with complete control of her body.

A man whose wife has told him she wants a divorce imagines how much his wife will appreciate him now that he has been diagnosed with cancer.

Fantasy may offer temporary relief from pressures, but people who spend too much time in fantasy may be unable to meet the requirements of reality.

Clients who are very ill may fantasize that when they recover, many good things will happen to them. They may imagine that they will receive special recognition in their work or that they will get along better with their families. These fantasies may help such clients deal with the deprivations caused by illness. However, they may also create unrealistic expectations. The fantasies may make one feel good temporarily but interfere with problem solving.

Nursing Intervention Strategies. Clients who engage in fantasy related to their illness need gradual help in assessing the responses others are likely to make and the achievements they themselves may realistically expect. Clients who fail to adjust to reality will be disappointed when their expectations are not met.

A helpful approach that will not devastate clients who need to hold on to some fantasy is to ask them to discuss their specific future plans. Examining the details of work and interpersonal adjustment may help a person relinquish unrealistic expectations and make more realistic plans. For example, the man who believes that a diagnosis of cancer will improve his marriage because his wife will appreciate him more fully must recognize that this is improbable. He needs to examine the real effects his illness will have on her. He must plan how to make specific improvements in their communication by anticipating problem areas.

Imagination does have a creative aspect, however. Fantasies have a richness and variety that is lacking in the everyday world. Certain artists, such as Dalí and Picasso, enriched their works of art through fantasy. Evidence also exists that insights leading to scientific discovery do not come about as the result of step-by-step logical thinking. Rather, they are created through fantasy.

Rationalization

Rationalization is the attribution of "good" or plausible reasons for questionable behavior to justify it or to deal with disappointment. Rationalizing helps us avoid social disapproval and bolster flagging self-esteem.

CLINICAL EXAMPLE

A nurse fails to return to the bedside of an elderly nursing home client despite a promise to do so before leaving work. She believes her behavior is justified because the client has problems with recent memory and probably wouldn't remember anyway.

Many people use rationalization because they wish to prove to themselves or others that their actions are governed by reason and common sense, even though they may not fully understand the reasons for their own behavior. Such explanations may be essential to maintaining personal integrity. They are not destructive as long as they do not prevent one from solving everyday problems.

Rationalization becomes more of a hindrance when it prevents us from making necessary changes in our behavior by interfering with our ability to examine that behavior. One sign of rationalization is an active search for reasons to justify our behavior or beliefs. Another is an inability to recognize inconsistencies in our beliefs. A third is being upset when our reasons are questioned, since each questioning threatens our defenses.

Clients may use rationalization to soften the blow of losses caused by illness. For instance, a man who is ill may give up work prematurely after rationalizing that he wouldn't have been successful in that field anyway. Such unnecessary restrictions deprive us of possible achievements.

Nursing Intervention Strategies. Nurses must respect the client's need to rationalize fears and insecurities they cannot face. However, hold out to clients the possibility for change. You can help clients face the reality of their situation by encouraging them to explore ways they can deal with it more effectively. One way is to help them explore in detail past instances in which they did change in order to cope with a stressful situation. Believing and recognizing that we have real strengths helps us face our areas of insecurity.

Reaction Formation

Reaction formation is a defense whereby we keep an undesirable impulse out of awareness by emphasizing its opposite. To protect ourselves from recognizing dangerous feelings, we develop conscious attitudes and behavior patterns that are just the opposite of those feelings. For example, the desire to be sexually promiscuous may be concealed behind a moralistic demeanor. Some people who crusade passionately against alcohol or pornography may have an underlying wish to enjoy these things. Hostility may be concealed behind a facade of love and kindness.

CLINICAL EXAMPLE

Sue has been married to Colin for 25 years. Sue's friends and family view Colin as a typical chauvinist. Although both of them are professional people—Colin is a banker and Sue is a freelance writer—Colin seldom lifts a hand around the house or drives the children to any of their lessons or sporting events. He drops his clothing all over the bedroom floor and expects Sue to clean up after him. One day, while Sue and her colleague were polishing an article for a travel magazine, Colin arrived home after lunch in a restaurant and rushed upstairs to the bathroom. In a few minutes, he rushed out the door, saying, "Sorry, Susie, but there's a bit of a mess in the upstairs bathroom." Colin had been nauseated and vomited and did not clean the toilet or the towels he used. Although Sue's colleague's astonishment at Colin's behavior moved to anger, Sue remained unnaturally sweet and loving and unable to consider the possibility of being angry with him. Sue is probably using this excess sweetness and loving kindness to counteract an unacceptable (to her) degree of anger.

People who use this defense are not conscious of their true feelings.

Clues that reaction formation is occurring are an inappropriate intensity of feeling and the inability to consider alternative points of view.

Nursing Intervention Strategies. A client manifesting reaction formation requires essentially the same approach as one manifesting repression. Respect and support the client's defenses while providing a secure relationship in which to explore feelings and new behavioral alternatives. Also be aware that it is easy to be annoyed at clients who cannot face their true feelings. The rigid and excessive display of what seems to be an insincere emotion can be frustrating. Remember that these clients are not "lying" or pretending. They are unconsciously protecting themselves against recognizing threatening feelings.

Displacement

Displacement is the discharging of pent-up feelings, generally hostility, on an object less dangerous than the object that aroused the feelings. This defense is used when emotions are aroused in a situation in which it would be dangerous to express them.

CLINICAL EXAMPLE

John has just failed an important examination. He believes his failure was the instructor's fault. He cannot express the full extent of his anger, because that would get him into worse trouble with the instructor. John goes quietly back to the dormitory. But when his roommate turns the stereo on too loud, John explodes. He doesn't fear retaliation from his roommate—they are peers and friends.

In some cases, we turn our anger toward another person inward on the self. When this happens, we experience exaggerated self-accusations and guilt.

Nursing Intervention Strategies. Clients may express inappropriate anger to the nurse when they are actually angry at someone or something else. The client may feel more secure with the nurse, who offers a safe target for displaced feelings. Displacement differs from projection in that people who use displacement are not distorting their feelings and attributing them to someone else. The feelings are clear, and the person acknowledges them. They are simply being directed at the wrong person. Therefore, it may be easier to help these clients acknowledge the real situation by remaining calm and accepting during an angry outburst. For example, after the outburst is over, say, "You seem so angry; I wonder if you really are angry because your breakfast is cold or if there might be some other reason." Opening up the possibility for a discussion of anger may help these clients to sort out just why and at whom they are angry.

Intellectualization

Intellectualization is the process of separating the emotion aroused by an event from ideas or opinions about the event because the emotion itself is too painful to acknowledge. The painful emotion is avoided by means of a rational explanation that divests the event of any personal significance. Failures are less significant if one believes that the situation could have been worse.

CLINICAL EXAMPLE

A woman whose husband recently died deals with her grief by telling her friends in a rational manner that it was better that he died suddenly by heart attack rather than to have died at the end of a long, chronic illness.

A boy who breaks his pelvis while skiing consoles himself after the accident by saying, "I would rather have a broken hip than a broken neck."

Clients may use intellectualization to blunt the emotional impact of their problems. This may be difficult for the nurse to perceive, because such clients often seem to know a great deal about their condition. They may be able to discuss in great detail the metabolic processes in diabetes or the psychodynamics of anxiety. At the same time, they cannot apply these concepts to their own situation in an emotional sense.

Nursing Intervention Strategies Intellectualization resembles rationalization in that it provides a verbal means of dealing with anxiety. Its use closes off the possibility of accepting and working out problems. Clients often use intellectualization at the onset of a crisis, and the need for this defense may decrease in a supportive nurse–client relationship. You can help the client relate emotionally to a problem by not forcing the expression of feeling. This will only frighten the client further. Asking these clients to explain how their knowledge relates to them personally may encourage them to accept and explore their emotional reactions.

Psychological Factors Affecting Medical Conditions

Physical illnesses with a major emotional component are often referred to as psychophysiologic or psychosomatic disorders. Because these terms are vague and have limited value for diagnosis, treatment, and research, the term **psychological factors affecting medical conditions** (PFAMC) is used in the DSM-IV-TR (American Psychiatric Association [APA], 2000). The essential feature of this category is the presence of one or more specific psychologic or behavioral factors that adversely affect a medical condition. These factors may influence the course of a medical condition, interfere with the condition's treatment, or constitute an additional health risk. They may be any one or a combination of the following:

- A mental disorder affecting the course or treatment of a general medical condition, such as bipolar I disorder (manic episode) complicating hemodialysis.
- A psychological symptom affecting the course or treatment of a general medical condition, such as anxiety complicating the ability to carry out self-care for diabetes mellitus.
- A personality trait or coping style affecting the course or treatment of a general medical condition, such as denial interfering with the timely treatment of cancer.
- A maladaptive health behavior affecting the course or treatment of a general medical condition, such as sedentary lifestyle and overeating affecting treatment for coronary artery disease.
- A stress-related physiologic response affecting the course or treatment of a general medical condition, such as stress-related dysrhythmias in a person recovering from myocardial infarction.

According to the DSM-IV-TR (APA, 2000, p. 732), the PFAMC category should be reserved for situations in which:

1. The psychological factors significantly affect the course or outcome of the medical condition, or
2. The psychological factors place the individual at significantly higher risk for an untoward outcome.

In addition, there should be evidence of a relationship between the psychological factors and the medical condition even though it may not be possible to specifically pin-point the psychological factors as a direct cause or to identify exactly how they operate.

The DSM-IV-TR distinguishes PFAMC from several related disorders. A **mental disorder due to a general medical condition** can be defined as the presence of mental symptoms that are judged to be the direct physiological consequence of a general medical condition. In mental disorder due to a general medical condition, the presumed causality is in the opposite direction. For example, an individual may have catatonic disorder due to a neurologic condition such as a neoplasm, encephalitis, or cerebrovascular disease. Personality change may be due to HIV disease, head trauma, or lupus erythematosus. For situations in which delirium, dementia, amnestic disorder, mood disorder, psychotic disorder, anxiety disorder, sleep disorder, or sexual dysfunction are factors, see the appropriate chapters related to these diagnoses in this text. While somatoform disorders are characterized by both psychological and physical symptoms, no medical condition completely accounts for the physical symptoms seen in people with this disorder. Other psychiatric disorders excluded from PFAMC include conversion disorder, hypochondriasis, physical complaints associated with a mental disorder, and substance-related physical complaints.

The psychiatric diagnostic criteria for PFAMC are discussed in the DSM-IV-TR box below.

DSM-IV-TR

Diagnostic Criteria for Psychological Factors Affecting Medical Condition

A. A general medical condition (coded on Axis III) is present.

B. Psychological factors adversely affect the general medical condition in one of the following ways:

1. The factors have influenced the course of the general medical condition as shown by a close temporal association between the psychological factors and the development or exacerbation of, or delayed recovery from, the general medical condition.
2. The factors interfere with the treatment of the general medical condition.
3. The factors constitute additional health risks for the individual.
4. Stress-related physiologic responses precipitate or exacerbate symptoms of the general medical condition.

Source: Reprinted with permission from American Psychiatric Association (2000). *Diagnostic and statistical manual of mental disorders*. (4th ed., Text Revision) (DSM-IV-TR). Washington, DC: Author.

HOLISTIC THEORY OF ILLNESS

Because all illnesses may ultimately stem from multiple factors, a holistic theory of illness serves as a basis for understanding all human disorders. By appreciating the complex, interwoven pattern of emotional and physical elements, the nurse can more fully comprehend the essential unity of the body and the mind. For a partial list of physical conditions having psychological components, see ■ Table 5–2.

Clients who come to the attention of health care professionals because of physical complaints frequently have their psychological needs neglected. Those unmet needs may be contributing to the complaint, may be the primary cause of symptom development, or may be the reason for the client's decision to seek help. Even if the most technologically advanced diagnostic and treatment approaches are applied, ignoring the psychological components of illness can be as disastrous as ignoring the biological components. Such psychological components can undermine medically appropriate treatment.

■ Figure 5–6 and the following clinical example illustrate these ideas.

CLINICAL EXAMPLE

Peter G, 5 years old, was admitted for the fourth time in 6 months because of an acute asthma attack. While Peter was being treated medically, his parents waited in the family room. Mrs. G sat crying and wringing her hands while Mr. G paced the floor with a strained expression on his face. A staff nurse was able to talk to them and trace the sequence of events leading up to Peter's admission to the hospital.

It was a Saturday afternoon, and Mr. and Mrs. G had been arguing about whether to send Peter to kindergarten in the fall. Two points of view had emerged. Mr. G was all for it. He wanted Peter to grow up quickly and leave his "babyish ways" behind. Mrs. G was against it. Peter was the baby of the family, and Mrs. G felt that her husband was always pushing him to do things too advanced for a 5-year-old. Peter had awakened from his nap to hear his parents shouting at each other. The quarrel ended abruptly when Peter started to wheeze, and both parents rushed to his bedside, united in their concern for him.

What factors brought on Peter's asthma attack at that particular time?

1. The biologic factors include Peter's physiologic makeup. His mother had been asthmatic as a child. She and Peter are both allergic to chocolate, eggs, feathers, and dust. Peter inherited certain genetic features that make him susceptible to certain environmental stressors—in this case, the specific allergens.
2. Sociologic components of Peter's illness revolve around his family's functioning. Mr. and Mrs. G have different viewpoints on what Peter's role in the family should be. Their conflicts create a second source of stress for Peter.
3. A third component is Peter's psychological state. A 5-year-old boy views the integrity of his family as extremely important, and parental conflicts may threaten his sense of security. Peter had discovered that his parents rallied together when he was ill.

In view of these contributing factors, the treatment plan for Peter should not end when Peter stops wheezing. To reduce the number of such emergencies, caregivers need to devise a long-range treatment plan. This plan should encompass the physiologic, psychological, and sociologic components of Peter's

TABLE 5–2 Examples of Physical Conditions Having Psychological Components

System	Condition
Cardiovascular	Essential hypertension, angina pectoris, tachycardia, arrhythmia, cardiospasm, coronary artery disease, mitral valve prolapse, myocardial infarction, migraine headache.
Gastrointestinal	Irritable bowel syndrome, gastric ulcer, duodenal ulcer, pylorospasm, regional enteritis (Crohn's disease), ulcerative colitis, nausea and vomiting, gastritis, chronic diarrhea.
Hormonal	Hypoglycemia, diabetes mellitus, hyperthyroidism, hypothyroidism, hyperparathyroidism, hypoparathyroidism, premenstrual syndrome, obesity.
Immune	Allergic disorders, cancer, autoimmune disorders (systemic lupus erythematosus, rheumatoid arthritis, Hashimoto's thyroiditis, myasthenia gravis, psoriasis), AIDS.
Integumentary	Neurodermatitis (atopic dermatitis), pruritus, psoriasis, hyperhidrosis, urticaria, alopecia, acne, herpes, genital warts.
Neuromuscular/skeletal	Chronic pain, headache, sacroiliac pain, temporomandibular joint (TMJ) pain, rheumatoid arthritis, Raynaud's disease.
Respiratory	Asthma, hyperventilation syndrome, tuberculosis.

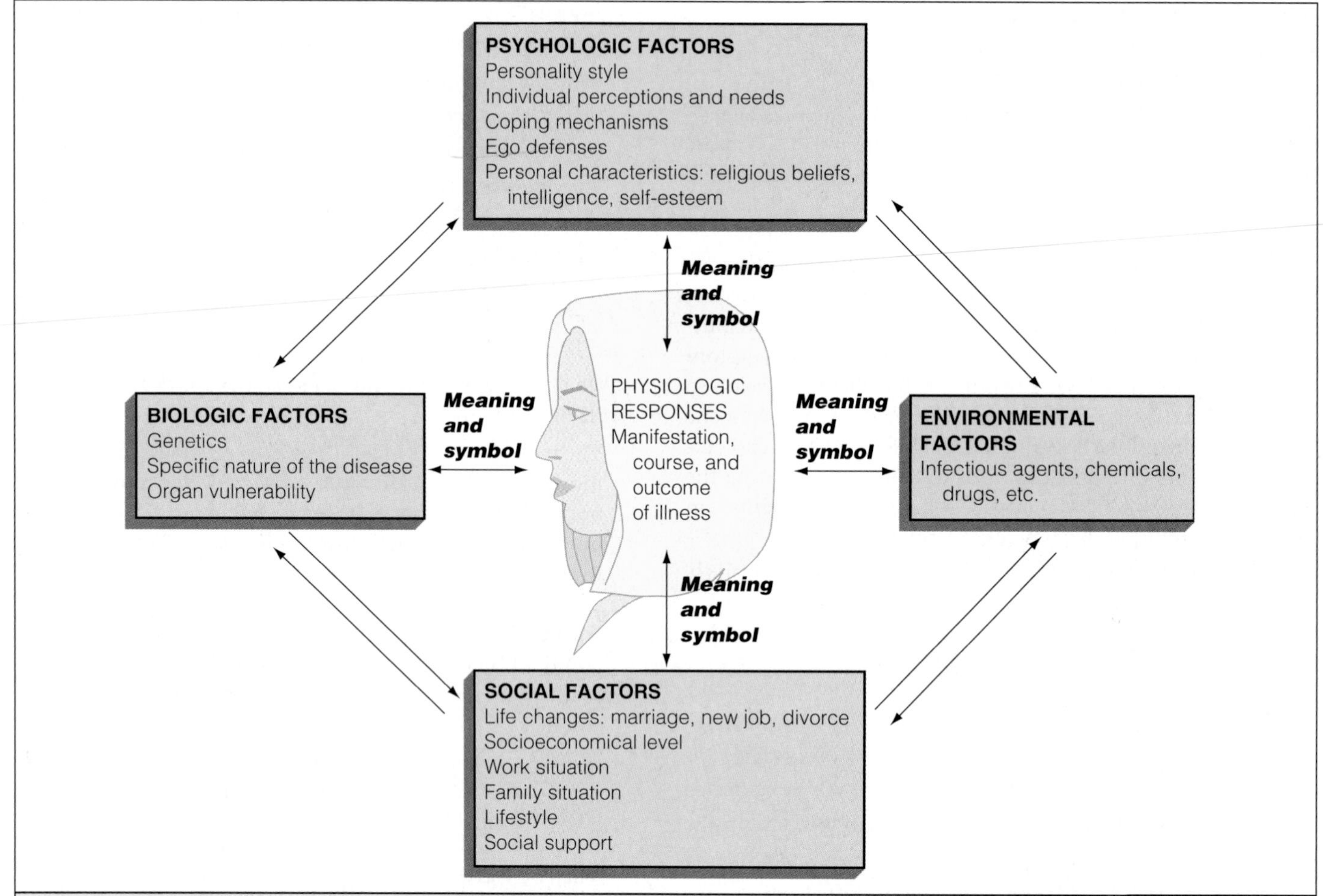

FIGURE 5–6 ■ *The multicausational concept of the illness process. The phrase meaning and symbol refers to the fact that clients interpret all experiences in a highly individual manner according to their specific meaning and the broader meaning in the client's culture.*

asthma attacks. Peter's condition further illustrates the importance of examining cultural, environmental, developmental, genetic, constitutional, and historical factors in all disease processes.

Therefore, in all illness, a holistic approach is necessary if each facet of the client's overall problem is to be addressed. For each of the disorders, we suggest nonmedical interventions that reduce stress while increasing the client's understanding and control over trouble-some symptoms. Promoting a healthy lifestyle and advocating lifestyle modifications are important nursing responsibilities regardless of the clinical area in which you practice.

SELECTED CONDITIONS AFFECTED BY PSYCHOLOGICAL FACTORS

The following sections review the characteristics of several conditions often considered to be affected by psychological factors. For most of these conditions, an exact etiology is unknown. Current research focuses on the complicated interrelationships among such factors as stress, personality, environment, hormones, and genetic susceptibility.

Gastrointestinal Disorders

Gastrointestinal (GI) functional disorders are chronic or recurrent GI symptoms with no identifiable physiological basis. GI symptoms are widespread throughout the population and vary according to such factors as gender and socioeconomic status. Women, for example, tend to more frequently report irritable bowel syndrome or functional constipation, while men more frequently report bloating symptoms. Social, economic, and lifestyle factors all appear to affect susceptibility to GI disorders to varying degrees, although whether such increased susceptibility results from differences in social stress, dietary factors, or other socioeconomic factors is unclear. The medical literature is replete with studies demonstrating a relationship between psychological factors and the GI system, particularly such conditions as irritable bowel syndrome, regional enteritis, ulcerative colitis, dyspepsia, and peptic ulcer.

Peptic Ulcer Disease. Peptic ulcer disease (PUD) has been one of the most thoroughly studied illnesses thought to be influenced by psychological factors. (It is noteworthy that some individuals' peptic ulcer disease has been attributed to the bacterium *Heliobacter pylori,* which can be treated with antimicrobial medication.) PUD is prevalent among people with stressful lifestyles and is associated with "getting ahead" in Western cultures. PUD appears to run in families and may be brought on or exacerbated by diet, stress, and certain infections. Duodenal ulcers, seen more frequently in men, are associated with hypersecretion of hydrochloric acid, probably stimulated by stress and anxiety.

Emotions such as anxiety and anger are also associated with the secretion of acid and pepsin, predisposing susceptible individuals to duodenal ulcer formation. Personality features of hostility, irritability, hypersensitivity, and impaired coping ability may also contribute to ulcer formation.

While studies of the relationship between psychological factors and ulcer formation and chronicity are somewhat controversial, psychological intervention is often recommended for PUD clients. Such intervention is often directed toward resolving dependence conflicts and may include biofeedback and relaxation therapy, individual and group educational approaches, and pharmacologic and dietary management.

Inflammatory Bowel Disorders. The role of psychological factors in inflammatory bowel disorders is unclear. Autoimmune factors and infections, coupled with psychological factors, may contribute to these disorders (Ringel & Drossman, 2001). Clients with ulcerative colitis tend to have a compulsive personality style with the following features: neatness, orderliness, punctuality, indecisiveness, emotional guardedness, humorlessness, conscientiousness, obstinacy, conformity, moral rigidity, and worry. Recent research, however, raises many questions about the validity of these personality features. Contemporary researchers say that the psychological traits these clients display are similar to those of clients with other chronic illnesses, with dependence being the most common trait. In many cases, onset and flare-ups seem linked to stressful life events, such as separations, failures, and disappointments.

Regardless of the source of the client's illness, treatment should focus on present troublesome areas, particularly concerns about the uncertain nature of the disease. Because of inherent differences between Crohn's disease and ulcerative colitis, the clinician must consider different approaches in planning treatment. The plan may include individual psychotherapy, family therapy, and environmental manipulation along with the medical regimen. These clients do best when they are involved in solid and long-term supportive relationships with their nurses and physicians who help them develop coping and self-care skills.

Cardiovascular Disorders

The cardiovascular system is a sensitive indicator of emotional arousal, whether it be fear, anger, or pleasurable excitement. High levels of stress are suspected to have harmful effects on the heart and vascular system, especially if stress is chronic or repeated. Experience, learning, and symbolic meaning, along with their emotional content, can influence heart rate, heart rhythm, and blood pressure. These cardiovascular changes can in turn create emotions, mostly unpleasant, that affect perception and ideation. A number of indicators have been identified as high-risk factors for heart disease. They include genetic, physiologic, social, and psychological influences.

A variety of psychosocial factors are believed to contribute to coronary artery disease (CAD). Many of these have been studied extensively, including affective states, personality or coping style, psychological reaction to environmental stimuli, sociocultural factors, and interpersonal factors. Psychological factors that have been linked to CAD, sudden death, and ventricular arrhythmias include anxiety and depression, a behavior pattern involving feelings of hostility and anger, work overload, life stress, and a lack of social support.

The highly competitive, driving **type A personality** displays the classic constellation of personality characteristics associated with CAD, angina pectoris, and myocardial infarction. Adverse conditions in the client's environment, either social or economic, can also create the stress that leads to cardiac dysfunction.

Essential hypertension, cardiac dysrhythmias, and so-called cardiac neurosis are three syndromes of cardiovascular functioning with major psychological inputs. The classical hypothesis in hypertension has been that people have conflict between their dependent and aggressive inclinations. This causes chronic repression of all displays of anger or resentment. The repressed emotions are eventually transformed into disorders of blood pressure regulation. Although this specific hypothesis has been difficult to prove, experiments have shown that fear, anger, frustration, and guilt (along with several medical conditions) all cause rises in diastolic blood pressure in vulnerable individuals. Likewise, anxiety, hostility, depression, interpersonal conflict, and disruptive life events have all been shown to potentially precipitate dysrhythmias, such as sinus tachycardia, paroxysmal atrial tachycardia, and both atrial and ventricular ectopic beats.

Cardiac neurosis is a syndrome consisting of cardiac distress, exercise intolerance, easy fatigability, respiratory discomfort, and dizziness. These features are similar to those found in panic disorder and mitral valve prolapse.

The treatment of cardiac disease must be multifaceted. In addition to medical or surgical treatment, other approaches involve stress management, relaxation training, biofeedback, weight control through diet and exercise, and behavioral interventions to help people give up smoking. More efforts are being geared toward prevention, including programs by industry and corporations to promote healthy lifestyles among employees.

Asthma

Asthma is among the most widely studied illnesses of the respiratory system. Because breathing is essential to life, there has been much speculation about the emotional and symbolic significance that can become attached to the processes of air exchange.

There are allergic, immunologic, and emotional inputs to asthmatic attacks. The emotional components may lead directly to alterations in bronchus size. Contemporary researchers examine the interplay of both psychological and physiologic aspects of asthma, particularly the neurologic and humoral bases of asthma pathogenesis. However, certain personality types are linked by some researchers and clinicians to asthma susceptibility: those with extreme inhibition, covert aggression, marked dependence needs, a high need for affection, and those prone to depression, anxiety, and disturbances of self-esteem.

Asthmatic people may be extremely frightened by asthmatic attacks, particularly in childhood. This fear may make them feel helpless and vulnerable. In response, they often adopt a clinging style of relating. The emotional and physical aspects of the illness seem to interrelate in a complex system of feedback loops. See the clinical profile of Peter G (p. 100–101) for an example.

Each person with asthma must be assessed individually to determine what factors are contributing to the disease process. A treatment plan may include, along with medication, family therapy, relaxation training, behavior modification, and hypnosis.

Arthritis

Rheumatoid arthritis (RA) has long been identified as an illness that is strongly influenced by emotional life. Its etiology remains uncertain. Psychological stresses are thought to precipitate attacks and flare-ups. The mechanism of transformation from idea or affect into tissue alteration appears to be via hormonal and autonomic nervous system pathways. Specifically, levels of growth hormone, sex hormones, thyroid hormone, and adrenal corticosteroids all change in stages of emotional arousal, and all are involved in the production of connective tissue, especially collagen. The hypothalamus and the limbic system also mediate.

Early psychological studies of individuals with RA attempted to define the "rheumatic personality." These people were described as self-sacrificing, masochistic, inhibited, perfectionistic, and retiring. While a high percentage of people with RA are depressed, they do not differ from others with chronic illness in this respect; that is, chronic illness increases the risk of depression. Thus, in RA, depression may stem from actual and perceived functional and other losses (such as mobility). The diagnosis cannot be based on personality type, however, because there are many exceptions to the rule. Physical findings, deformities, subcutaneous nodules, and blood studies remain the criteria for identification.

A treatment plan for clients with arthritis may include pain control, surgery, drugs, vocational counseling, occupational therapy, and interventions to alleviate or prevent depression and to deal with depression and anger more directly.

Headache

The experience of headache resulting from emotional tension is common. Headaches account for many physician visits and for job absenteeism. Headaches are also highly associated with depressive and anxiety disorders. Headaches may be divided into the five following types:

1. Vascular headache of migraine type.
2. Muscle contraction headache (tension headache).
3. Combined vascular–muscle contraction headache.
4. Delusional, depressive, conversion, or hypochondriacal headache.
5. Structural or disease-related headache.

The mechanism of vascular headache seems to involve the release of various vasoactive substances in the brain, such as serotonin, catecholamines, histamine, bradykinin, and prostaglandins. This release frequently occurs with stress. In genetically susceptible individuals, the substances cause vasodilation and inflammation of the arterial walls. There are generally early warning symptoms of migraine attacks. These range from mood changes and GI upset to gross neurologic findings in the visual and contralateral sensorimotor systems. A number of upsets in physiologic functioning can actually be migraine equivalents. These include nausea and vomiting, diarrhea, tachycardia, cyclical edema, vertigo, periodic fever, pain, depression, confusion, and insomnia.

A tension headache results from muscular contraction in the neck, shoulders, face, or scalp. These are steady, persistent headaches with no warning signs that commonly feel like a "band wrapped around the head." Some theorists support the notion that headache sufferers are likely to maintain rigid control over emotions, feel hostility toward others, use introjection as a defense, and be perfectionists.

Structural or disease-related headache arises from systemic infections, primary or metastatic tumors, hematomas, abscesses, cranial infections, cranial nerve inflammations, and eye, ear, nose, sinus, or tooth diseases.

Interventions are based on the diagnosis and the contributing factors that have been identified. Possible treatments and approaches include measures that increase circulation, such as massage or heat application; use of medications; alterations in diet, rest, and exercise patterns; psychotherapy; and biofeedback, meditation, hypnosis, relaxation, and other stress-management approaches.

Endocrine Disorders

A large number of disorders of endocrine functioning are associated with psychologic factors. The endocrine system has particular significance for psychiatry, because there is a close relationship between the emotions and a variety of active chemical substances released in tissues by nerve impulses (Hellhammer & Wade, 1993). In physical medicine, the feedback loop has long been accepted as the model for the functioning of the endocrine organs.

Extensive research on the endocrine feedback system has led to a sophisticated model that includes several kinds of feedback loops. The levels of circulating hormones released by endocrine glands, such as the thyroid and gonads (the sex glands), are controlled by long feedback loops that send information to the cerebral cortex and limbic system. Short feedback loops of pituitary hormones affect the hypothalamus. Very short loops of releasing hormones from the hypothalamus determine their own production and control. Studies on the relationship between emotions and endocrine function have shown that:

- Various neurotransmitters affect hormone-releasing factors.

- Psychoactive drugs whose action is mediated by neurotransmitters also affect the release of releasing factors.
- Stress stimulates the autonomic nervous system, which can stimulate the adrenal medulla to produce epinephrine or the pancreas to secrete insulin.
- Corticosteroid production of the adrenal cortex increases greatly during some psychotic episodes of schizophrenic clients.
- Steroid levels also increase in agitated or anxious depressive people.

It seems fair to conclude that the emotional centers of the brain—the cerebral cortex and limbic system—are intimately tied to the endocrine organs, through the axis of the hypothalamus and the anterior pituitary. Their secretions act as communication messengers. It is not surprising, then, to find expressions of emotional arousal through endocrine changes and major effects on emotional states from endocrine diseases. These are both, in fact, common. Endocrine disorders and their physical and mental symptoms are listed in the Assessment box below.

Adrenal dysfunction characteristically produces prominent mental as well as distinctive physical symptoms. Thyroid disorders are commonly accompanied by cognitive or emotional changes. Stress has been implicated, though inconclusively, in the precipitation of thyrotoxic crises. Stress may influence the course of diabetes, either directly by promoting a flare-up or indirectly by causing the client to neglect a usually rigid medical regimen. So many mental symptoms are associated with hypoglycemia that many clients are classified and treated as "classic neurotics."

It is evident that numerous problems can be caused by endocrine dysfunction. The treatment approach must be individualized to meet the client's physical and psychological needs. An important role for the nurse is primary prevention. Adequately preparing a person for developmental changes by offering accurate information about likely physical and emotional alterations can help prevent severe psychiatric disturbances during these periods. Reliable support and open channels of communication are necessary. New coping strategies can be successful if their design, timing, and presentation are appropriate.

Skin Disorders

Allergic illnesses, particularly those involving the skin, have been shown to have psychological elements in etiology or course (Buske-Kirschbaum, Geiben, & Hellhammer, 2001). The skin, with its critical sensory functions, mediates between the outside world and internal states. Itching (pruritus), excessive sweating (hidrosis), urticaria, and atopic dermatitis are all commonly classified as psychophysiologic conditions.

A variety of stressful or emotional states are associated with flare-ups of allergic skin disorders. Attempts have been made to correlate the following specific emotional states or stresses with individual disorders:

- Generalized pruritus: aggression.
- Genital and anal pruritus: sexuality (heterosexual and homosexual).
- Hyperhidrosis: anxiety.
- Urticaria: anger.
- Atopic dermatitis: longing for love.

In truth, these feelings and conflicts are seen in normal, disordered, and other psychophysiologic states. Nurses should therefore be cautious about accepting pathogenic mechanisms and explanations.

ASSESSMENT — Common Features of Endocrine Disorders

Disease	Physical Symptoms	Mental Symptoms
Addison's disease (adrenal insufficiency)	Weakness, fatigue, anorexia, weight loss, nausea and vomiting, pigmentation of skin, hypotension.	Depression, irritability, psychomotor retardation, apathy, memory defect, hallucinations.
Cushing's syndrome (adrenal cortex hyperfunction)	Truncal obesity, moon facies, abdominal striae, hirsutism, amenorrhea, hypertension, osteoporosis, weakness.	Impotence, decreased libido, anxiety, increased emotional lability, apathy, insomnia, memory deficits, confusion, disorientation.
Diabetes mellitus	Polydipsia, polyuria, polyphagia, weight loss, blurred vision, fatigue, impotence, fainting, paresthesia.	Stupor, coma, fatigue, impotence.
Hyperthyroidism	Staring, exophthalmos, goiter, moist warm skin, weight loss, increased appetite, weakness, tremor, tachycardia, heat intolerance.	Anxiety, tension, irritability, hyperexcitability, emotional lability, depression, psychosis, or delirium.
Hypoglycemia	Tremor, light-headedness, sweating, hunger, nausea, pallor, tachycardia, hypertension.	Anxiety, fugue, unusual behavior, confusion, apathy, psychomotor agitation or retardation, depression, delusions, hallucinations, convulsions, coma.
Hypothyroidism	Dull expression, puffy eyelids, swollen tongue, hoarse voice, rough dry skin, cold intolerance.	Psychomotor retardation, decreased initiative, slow comprehension, drowsiness, decreased recent memory, delirium, stupor, depression or psychosis.
Premenstrual syndrome	Headache, breast engorgement, lower abdominal bloating, GI complaints, increased sweating, craving for sweets, other appetite changes.	Irritability, depression, anxiety, emotional lability, fatigue, crying spells.

The location of the lesions has, historically, had symbolic significance. Thus, conflict over an extramarital affair has been associated with dermatitis in the wedding ring area. Head and face locations have been classically associated with conflict over affective display. Affliction of the hands is associated with practical or professional conflicts. A genital distribution of lesions may be associated with sexual concerns.

RESISTANCE TO PSYCHOSOCIAL INTERVENTION

Behavioral therapy, cognitive therapy, biofeedback, hypnotherapy, and psychotherapy have all been used successfully with appropriate clients. However, despite the wealth of psychosocial interventions available to people with psychophysiologic disorders, many are resistant to approaches that are not strictly medical. Reasons for this include:

- These clients are believed to lack insight because they express conflict through somatic complaints rather than verbalization.
- Conflicts over unresolved dependence and aggressive wishes may make it difficult to relate to these clients interpersonally.
- These clients focus steadfastly on their somatic complaints, apparently indicating that alternative defense mechanisms are unavailable or inadequate.
- They are rarely highly motivated to heighten their self-awareness, which is the goal of many forms of psychotherapy.
- Even when they are somewhat motivated, they may be unable or unwilling to delay gratification and thus are impatient with the slow process of growth usually required in psychotherapeutic work.

For these reasons, traditional psychotherapy is not the most useful intervention. Approaches that enhance medical and surgical intervention and allow the client's primary bond to remain with nonpsychiatric health care providers are more successful. Programs geared toward stress management (such as those discussed in Chapter 32) are very useful because they present stress as part of the human condition and the participants do not feel labeled as having psychiatric problems. Behavioral and cognitive approaches have also gained favor because they may alleviate symptoms over a short period of time and thus prove effective in terms of outcome and cost. Behavioral and cognitive approaches are discussed in Chapter 30.

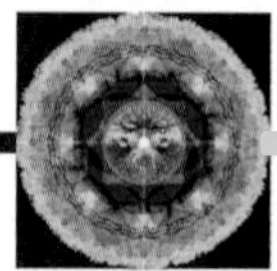

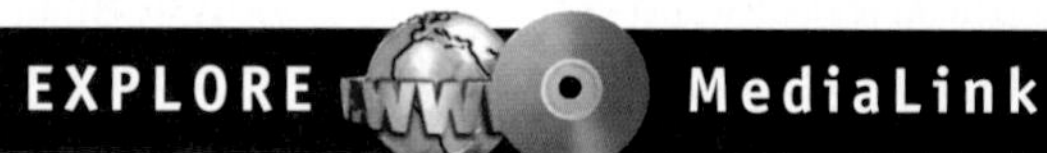

NCLEX review, case studies, and other interactive resources for this chapter can be found on the Companion Website at http://www.prenhall.com/kneisl. Click on Chapter 5 to select the activities for this chapter.

For animations, video tutorials, more NCLEX review questions, and an audio glossary, access the accompanying CD-ROM in this textbook.

BIBLIOGRAPHY

American Psychiatric Association (2000). *Diagnostic and statistical manual of mental disorders* (4th ed., Text Revision) (DSM-IV-TR). Washington, DC: Author.

Antonovsky, A. (1991). *Unraveling the mystery of health: How people manage stress.* Boston: Jossey-Bass.

Baum, A., & Posluszny, D. M. (1999). Health psychology: Mapping biobehavioral contributions to health and illness. *Annual Review of Psychology, 50,* 137–163.

Bengtssen-Tops, A., & Hansson, L. (2001). The validity of Antonovsky's sense of coherence measure in a sample of schizophrenic patients living in the community. *Journal of Advanced Nursing, 33*(4), 432–438.

Benner, P., & Wrubel, J. (1986). *The primacy of caring: Stress and coping in health and illness.* Menlo Park, CA: Addison-Wesley.

Borysenko, J. (1993). *Fire in the soul: A new psychology of spiritual optimism.* New York: Warner Books.

Buske-Kirschbaum, A., Geiben, A., & Hellhammer, D. (2001). Psychobiological aspects of atopic dermatitis: An overview. *Psychotherapy and Psychosomatics, 70*(1), 6–16.

Dossey, L. (1997). *Healing words.* New York: HarperCollins.

Faun, G. A., & Sonino, N. (2000). Psychosomatic medicine: Emerging trends and perspectives. *Psychotherapy and Psychosomatics, 69*(4), 184–197.

Fitzpatrick, J. J., & Wilke, P. A. (2001). *Psychiatric–mental health nursing digest.* New York: Springer.

Fontaine, K. L. (2000). *Healing practices: Alternative therapies for nursing.* Upper Saddle River, NJ: Prentice Hall.

Friedman, H., & VandenBos, G. (1992). Disease-prone and self-healing personalities. *Hospital and Community Psychiatry, 43*(12), 1177–1179.

Hellhammer, D., & Wade, S. (1993). Endocrine correlates of stress vulnerability. *Psychotherapy and Psychosomatics, 60,* 8–17.

Holmes, T. H., & Rahe, R. H. (1967). The social readjustment rating scale. *Journal of Psychosomatic Research, 11,* 213–218.

Kaye, J., Morton, J., Bowcutt, M., & Maupin, D. (2001). Stress, depression, and psychoneuroimmunology. *Journal of Neuroscience Nursing, 32*(2), 93–100.

Kobasa, S. C. (1979). Stressful life events, personality, and health: An inquiry into hardiness. *Journal of Personality and Social Psychology, 37,* 1–11.

Landsverk, S. S., & Kane, C. F. (1998). Antonovsky's sense of coherence: Theoretical basis of psychoeducation in schizophrenia. *Issues in Mental Health Nursing, 19*(5), 419–431.

Lazarus, R. S., & Folkman, S. (1984). *Stress, appraisal, and coping*. New York: Springer.

Meisenhelder, J. B., & Chandler, E. N. (2000). Prayer and health outcomes in church members. *Alternative Therapies in Health and Medicine, 6*(4), 56–60.

Meyers, J. (1972). Life events and mental status. *Journal of Health and Human Behavior, 1*, 398–406.

Monat, A., & Lazarus, R. S. (1991). *Stress and coping* (3rd ed.). New York: Columbia University Press.

Rahe, R. H. (1979). Life change events and mental illness: An overview. *Journal of Human Stress, 5*, 2–10.

Ringel, Y., & Drossman, D. A. (2001). Psychosocial aspects of Crohn's disease. *Surgical Clinics of North America, 81*(1), 231–252.

Selye, H. (1956). *The stress of life*. New York: McGraw-Hill.

Smith, J. C. (1993). *Understanding stress and coping*. New York: Macmillan.

Smock, T. K. (1999). *Physiological psychology: A neuroscience approach*. Upper Saddle River, NJ: Prentice Hall.

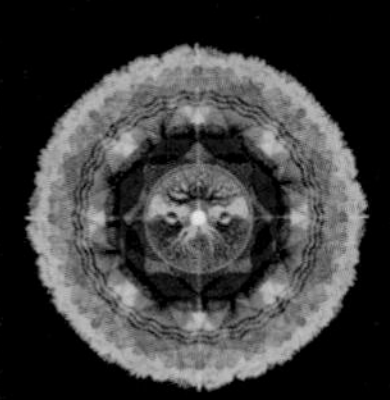

Cultural Competence and Psychiatric Epidemiology

BETH MOSCATO

Chapter SIX

KEY TERMS

acculturation
comorbidity
cultural competence
cultural sensitivity
ethnicity
ethnocentrism
global burden of disease
primary prevention
psychiatric epidemiology
risk factor
secondary prevention
tertiary prevention

FOCUS QUESTIONS

- What does cultural competence mean?
- Which personal strategies can you use to develop cultural competence in your work with specific cultural groups?
- What risk factors associated with mental disorders affect the experience, expression, reporting, and evaluation of mental disorders among culturally diverse groups?
- How would you explain the natural history of disorder, including its four stages?
- How do psychiatric–mental health nurses incorporate the three levels of prevention in their practice?
- When and how would you apply epidemiologic principles in your psychiatric–mental health nursing practice?

MediaLink 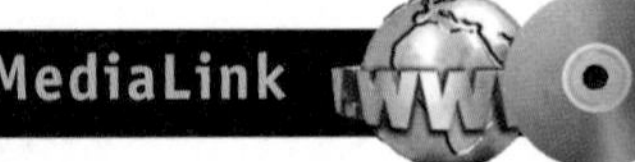 www.prenhall.com/kneisl

Additional resources for this chapter can be found on the Student CD-ROM accompanying this textbook, and on the Companion Website at www.prenhall.com/kneisl. Click on Chapter 6 to select the activities for this chapter.

CD-ROM
- Audio Glossary
- NCLEX Review

Companion Website
- Additional NCLEX Review
- Case Study: Developing Cultural Competence

CHAPTER OUTLINE

CROSS REFERENCES

Other topics relevant to this content are: Assessment, Chapter 9; Clients with a dual diagnosis, Chapter 21; Communication skills, Chapter 8; Ethics, Chapter 10; Non-Western therapies, Chapter 32; Nurse's values, Chapter 1; Psychiatric theories, Chapter 2; Psychobiology, Chapter 4.

CRITICAL THINKING CHALLENGE

Psychiatric–mental health nurses often focus on a particular client in a clinical setting. How might the client's cultural beliefs, values, practices, and healing traditions influence this process? Does such a client represent "what kind" and "how much" mental disorder is "out there" in the community? Are you willing to expand your nursing skills by considering the community itself as a potential "client" for mental health assessment and services? How can you apply principles of cultural competence and psychiatric epidemiology to your psychiatric nursing experiences with culturally diverse groups as well as clients? ■

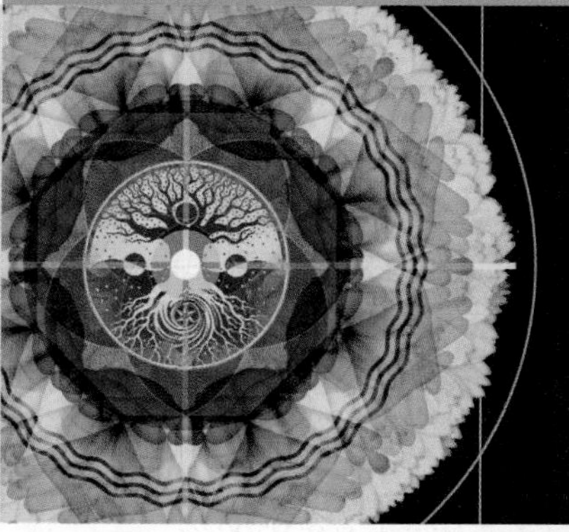

To meet global needs and opportunities in the twenty-first century, nursing is addressing cultural diversity in a health care system in which multicultural individuals are both recipients of care as well as care providers. America is undergoing demographic shifts that include increasing numbers of diverse cultural groups. The population of the United States will continue to grow but at a slower rate. Fifty-year projections (2000 to 2050) from the U.S. Bureau of the Census highlight increases in each of the major cultural groups (African-Americans, Native American, Eskimo, and Aleut, Asian and Pacific Islander, and those with Hispanic origins) other than Caucasian. It is estimated that these diverse cultural groups will represent almost half (47%) of the population by 2050. Population trends reveal that Hispanics will represent the largest minority group by 2005 and comprise 25% of the population by 2050.

MediaLink U.S. Census Bureau

Culture shapes human behavior and assigns unique meanings to the world around us. Nurses need to be aware that these cultural forces are powerful determinants of health-related behaviors in any population. Census information can be found on the U.S. Census Bureau Web site (www. census. gov) and accessed through the Companion Website for this book.

Thus, culture can influence the experience, expression, reporting, and evaluation of mental disorders. Symptoms related to major depression, as highlighted by the DSM-IV-TR, may illustrate this point. Depression may be experienced in somatic terms, rather than with sadness or guilt, in some cultures. People of Latino and Mediterranean cultures may complain of headaches and "nerves." People of Chinese and Asian cultures may emphasize weakness and tiredness. Middle Easterners may refer to problems of the "heart." The Hopi may express the depressive experience by being "heartbroken." Cultures may differ regarding the seriousness placed on symptoms and share distinctive culture-specific experiences (such as the feeling of being hexed). It is essential to identify those cultural factors that may facilitate, or deter, desired health-related behaviors.

As a nurse, you are called upon to participate in a health care system comprising individuals from different national, regional, ethnic, generational, socioeconomic, religious, and health status backgrounds. The range and variety of health care beliefs, rituals, traditions, and healing practices across cultures are staggering (see ■ Figure 6–1). It is the nurse's professional responsibility to understand, respect, and work with these cultural differences. Professional effectiveness in this multicultural health care environment requires the development of essential skills related to an understanding and integration of cultural phenomena in all aspects of your professional nursing care. Thus, this chapter has two sections. The first section will emphasize developing an understanding of cultural competence, especially in relation to nursing practice. The subsequent section will highlight psychiatric epidemiology in our culturally diverse society.

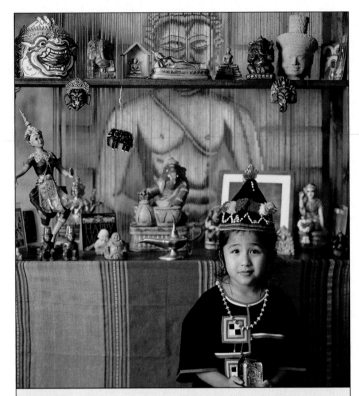

FIGURE 6–1 ■ *This young American girl's parents were born in Thailand. Their home contains many cultural artifacts that help their daughter to understand and appreciate the rituals and traditions associated with her cultural heritage.*

Source: Duane Rieder/Getty Images Inc.—Image Bank

Developing an Understanding of Cultural Competence

In the Western biomedical model, illness is often reduced to a particular disease, pathophysiology is emphasized, and the focus is on the client's body rather than on the whole individual. (See Chapter 32 for a discussion of non-Western traditions.) To understand the client's experience of illness, you must attempt to enter the client's world, understand the client's beliefs about "what is wrong, what happened, and what should be done" to achieve well-being. Thus, the client's perceptions, understandings, and approaches to health and disease are an integral part of any nursing care plan activities.

CULTURAL COMPETENCE

Cultural competence refers to the capacity of nurses or health service delivery systems to effectively understand and plan for the needs of a culturally diverse client or group. Spector (2000a) views cultural competence as a complex combination of knowledge, attitudes, and skills used by the health care provider to deliver services that attend to the total context of the client's situation across cultural boundaries. With cultural competence, you are able to move beyond a superficial analysis of cultural differences, having the capacity to understand and work with cultural nuances.

The concept of cultural competence may be applied to health service delivery systems as well. It embraces the notion that health care systems should be able to understand and plan for the health needs of a specific cultural group. Thus, agencies that acknowledge, accept, and work with cultural differences may be viewed as "culturally competent," whereas those agencies that ignore culture when delivering services are viewed as "culturally blind." The National Center for Cultural Competence assists health care and mental health organizations in promoting culturally competent values, policy, structures, and practices (National Center for Cultural Competence, 2002). Their Web site (www.gucdc.georgetown.edu/nccc/cultural.html) can be accessed through the Companion Website for this book.

Worldview

Simply put, cultural competence incorporates the client's worldview. A *worldview* is the way a group of people (culture or subculture) see their social world, symbolic system, and physical environment and their own place in each. Worldview is revealed in people's religion, art, language, values, and health care beliefs and practices. A people's worldview provides a sense of identity as a Native American, a Puerto Rican, or a Masai tribesman. It promotes a group's survival and gives members a generally useful picture of the universe.

Ethnicity and Ethnocentrism

Ethnicity refers to one's sense of identity, providing social belonging and loyalty to a particular reference group within society. This sense of identity may be based on common ancestry, and religious, national, language, tribal, or cultural origins. The terms *culturally diverse, multicultural,* and *ethnic* are used throughout this chapter. In contrast, **ethnocentrism** is the belief that one's own cultural values and behaviors are superior and preferable to any other cultural group. The nurse may be unaware of personal ethnocentric behavior that can undermine establishment of a balanced and respectful partnership with a multicultural client or group.

CULTURAL SENSITIVITY

Related to cultural competence is the concept of **cultural sensitivity,** the process of increasing professional effectiveness through understanding, respecting, and appreciating the importance of cultural factors in the delivery of health services. These cultural factors may include health beliefs, values, practices, and healing traditions of a culturally diverse client or group. *Cultural openness* may be a synonym for cultural sensitivity.

It is also important to appreciate the subculture, or culture within a culture. Recently researchers have referred to the "culture" of the hospital, the operating room, or the nursing school and the "subculture" of the mentally ill, the physically handicapped, or the elderly. Anthropologists point out that simply sharing some common characteristics does not make people members of a culture or subculture. There must be considerably more homogeneity in the group for it to be considered a culture or a subculture. For example, the Choctaw Indians living on a reservation in Philadelphia, Mississippi, are a subculture because they share a language, values and beliefs, and behavioral patterns. They are part of the larger Native American culture. In contrast, the physically handicapped are not a subculture because they have various disabilities, come from different socioeconomic levels, and may only rarely come into contact with other physically handicapped people.

A case can be made for viewing a hospital or part of it as a culture or subculture. The transient inhabitants of the hospital share a language, standards of acceptable behavior, and a similar worldview. This can be seen even more clearly in specialty units, such as intensive care or psychiatric units. People can be viewed as working within a hospital culture while living within the American culture. Applying the term *culture* or *subculture* to these environments may help us understand a hospital, an emergency room, a school, or a church. Some nurse anthropologists view nursing as a subculture (the health care providers subculture) and document its definite set of beliefs, practices, habits, rituals, and values, often stemming from dominant American cultural values.

MediaLink National Center for Cultural Competence

GLOBAL BURDEN OF DISEASE

Cultural competence and sensitivity are increasingly essential skills as we address mental health in the global community. The **global burden of disease** (Murray & Lopez, 1996) represents comprehensive estimates of patterns of mortality and disability from diseases and injuries. Traditionally, a population's health status has been measured by number of deaths (i.e., "who's dying from what"). The goal of this study was to measure health status by measuring disease burden in years of life lost to premature death (i.e. "who dies sooner") and disability (i.e., "who's living with a disability of known severity and duration"). Here, disability plays a central, rather than invisible, role in determining the overall health status of a population. This extensive five-year study provides information on disease burden by age, gender, cause, and region, including estimates for developing countries.

When looking at number of deaths alone, self-inflicted injuries rank among the top 10 leading causes of death in developed countries. However, this study shows that the burden of psychiatric disorders has been heavily underestimated by traditional approaches that account for death but not disability. Psychiatric disorders emerge as a highly significant component of global disease burden. Of the 10 leading causes of disability in the world in 1990, five were mental health conditions. These conditions, outlined in ■ Table 6–1 on page 112, included unipolar depression, alcohol use, manic depression, schizophrenia, and obsessive–compulsive disorder. In fact, unipolar depression was responsible for more than 1 in every 10 years of life lived with a disability globally. Depression was women's leading cause of disease burden worldwide.

This study also provides projections of disease burden to 2020. Unipolar depression, plus several types of injuries (including war, violence, and suicide) are likely to increase (see ■ Figure 6–2) on page 112. Tobacco is expected to cause more premature death and disability than any single disease by 2020. These projections help to anticipate future mental health needs globally.

TABLE 6–1 Leading Causes of Disability in the World: Documenting the Global Burden of Disease

All Causes	Percent of Total Disability
1. Unipolar major depression	10.7
2. Iron-deficiency anemia	4.7
3. Falls	4.6
4. Alcohol use	3.3
5. Chronic obstructive pulmonary disease	3.1
6. Bipolar disorder	3.0
7. Congenital anomalies	2.9
8. Osteoarthritis	2.8
9. Schizophrenia	2.6
10. Obsessive–compulsive disorders	2.2

Source: Adapted from Murray, C. J. L., & Lopez A. D. (1996). *The global burden of disease: A comprehensive assessment of mortality and disability from diseases, injuries, and risk factors in 1990 and projected to 2020.* Cambridge, MA: Harvard University Press.

CULTURAL VALUES

Be aware that perceptions of health, disease, prevention, and treatment may differ among multicultural groups and that many interpretations of reality exist in the world (see Chapter 32). Acknowledging divergent values can be a significant first step toward improving one's cultural competence and sensitivity to differences, especially when the nurse is from the dominant culture (i.e., of white Anglo-American origin). ■ Table 6–2 highlights common values that may differ between dominant Anglo-American and other nondominant cultural groups.

TABLE 6–2 Common Values That May Differ Between Dominant and Nondominant Cultural Groups

Anglo-American (Dominant)	Other Cultural Groups (Nondominant)
Competition	Cooperation
Control over environment	Fate
Directness/Honesty	Indirectness/"Saving face"
Doing	Being
Efficiency	Idealism
Future orientation	Past or present orientation
Human equality	Hierarchy/Ranking
Individualism	Group welfare
Informality	Formality
Mastery over nature	Harmony with nature
Materialism	Spiritualism
Self-help	Birthright inheritance
Time dominates	Personal interaction dominates
Youth	Elders

Source: Adapted from Huff, R. M., & Kline, M. V. (1999). *Promoting health in multicultural populations: A handbook for practitioners*. New York: Sage.

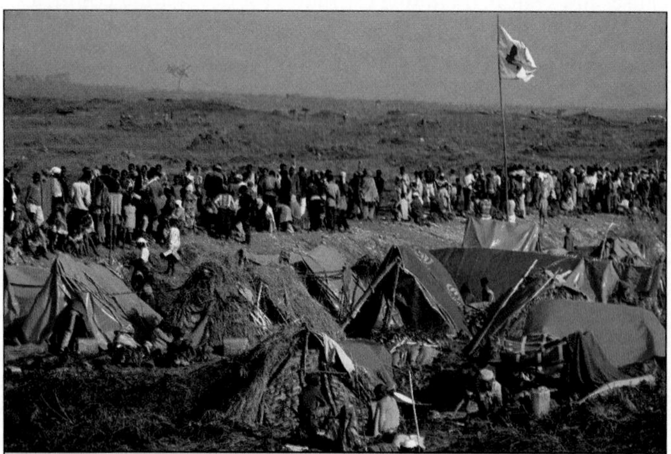

FIGURE 6–2 ■ *Addressing the global burden of disease includes concern for the 35 million refugees and internally displaced persons around the world. Fleeing one's home to avoid war and massacres presents many complex problems—psychological, physiologic, political, and environmental.*

Source: Wesley Bocxe/Photo Researchers, Inc.

CROSS-CULTURAL COMMUNICATION

Consider the challenge of learning to communicate across cultures. The need to increase awareness of your own communication style is important in becoming competent and sensitive to cultural differences. For example, you may carefully choose a rate of speaking that promotes understanding and respect of the client. Other helpful techniques may be to speak in simple sentences and avoid use of slang, jargon, or technical words. Practical suggestions to improve cross-cultural communication skills may include:

- Attending multicultural events.
- Reading about different cultural groups.
- Talking to members of the cultural group.
- Spending time in a particular ethnic community.
- Learning another language.

Language and Dialect

You may need to determine the client's level of fluency in English and assess the degree to which another language is used as the primary language. Such language use may vary by age, gender, or generational level. In a given setting, language differences represent a serious barrier to all aspects of health care delivery. When you are unfamiliar with the client's language, great care must be taken to pay attention to nonverbal communication. The linguistically isolated client may look to your nonverbal behavior in an attempt to understand what is expected in an unfamiliar situation. The use of a well-trained, effective interpreter is essential if the client does not speak the language or dialect of the dominant culture. In this instance, allow extra time for careful translation and back-translation. It is useful to expect some discomfort and uncertainty when working in a cross-cultural health care setting. Specific information on medical interpretation and resources for promoting language and cultural competence to improve the care for minority, immigrant, and ethnically diverse communities can be found at www.diveristyrx.org and accessed through the Companion Website for this book.

Degree of Literacy

Determine the client's reading ability in English or other languages before using written materials related to health care. If the client cannot read English, then determine how best to provide appropriate translated materials that are culturally relevant in the particular setting.

OTHER CULTURAL PHENOMENA AFFECTING HEALTH

In addition to cross-cultural communication, Giger and Davidhizar (1999) call attention to the following five cultural phenomena that also affect health and health care among diverse cultural groups: environmental control, biological variations, social organization, space, and time orientation. Attend to each phenomenon summarized below during any cultural assessment, since each may influence health perceptions, beliefs, practices, and healing traditions.

Environmental Control

Environmental control refers to the ability to organize activities that attempt to control nature or environmental factors. Thus, a multicultural group may embrace specific health and illness beliefs, practices, use of folk healers, and healing traditions in attempts to intervene with the complex environment.

Biologic Variations

There may be distinct genetic and physical differences from one multicultural group to another. Examples of such differences include: nutritional habits and preferences, skin color, body build and structure, and selective susceptibility to certain diseases.

Social Organization

Social organization describes the type of family unit (e.g., extended, nuclear, or single-parent family) and type of social organizations (e.g., religious or multicultural) that shape the identity of a culturally diverse client or group. Socialization from one's early family life strongly contributes to cultural identification and development.

Space

Use of space may be defined and have different meanings based on one's particular culture. There may be different norms for intimacy as well as personal, social, and public distances among various cultural groups.

Time Orientation

Emphasis on the past, present, or future varies among culturally diverse groups. As noted in Table 6–2, nondominant cultural groups may value the past and present, whereas the dominant Anglo-American culture may emphasize the future.

CULTURAL ASSESSMENT

An appropriate cultural assessment is essential to culturally competent nursing care. This cultural assessment may be incorporated into routine assessment procedures as the first step of the nursing process when working with any client or group.

Degree of Acculturation

The degree of acculturation should be assessed for any client or group in a multicultural setting. **Acculturation** may be defined as the degree to which a particular culturally diverse client or group has adopted the values, attitudes, and behaviors of mainstream U.S. culture. Acculturation may be one of the most important factors that explain health status and risk behaviors. One cannot assume that because a culturally diverse client or group is in the United States, there is acculturation into the mainstream culture. There is likely to be a range of acculturation levels from the very traditional to the very acculturated. The more traditional the client or group, the less likely for the client or group to be familiar with, understand, or practice Western approaches. It is important to assess the degree of acculturation in a multicultural setting because there may be a natural tendency on the part of many culturally diverse clients to resist acculturation. The measurement of acculturation is an important assessment activity and a variety of scales can be used, such as the following assessment tool.

Heritage Assessment

The term *cultural care*, incorporates professional health care that is culturally sensitive, culturally competent, and culturally appropriate. Within this framework, the Heritage Assessment Tool for the multicultural client in Box 6–1 on page 114 represents a practical, useful way for you to investigate a client's (or your own) ethnic, cultural, and religious heritage. Such assessment may be used to understand a client's health traditions and reveal how deeply a client may identify with any particular tradition. It is important to emphasize that multicultural clients may embrace health beliefs and traditions from more than one culture, based on their unique heritage (Spector, 2000b).

A heritage assessment will help you to identify positive elements that can be reinforced to facilitate health promotion and disease prevention and anticipate rigid adherence to health beliefs and traditions that may conflict with effective Western practices.

Cultural assessment applies to agencies and health service delivery systems as well as to individuals or groups. Thus, you may have an opportunity to assess where a particular agency stands in terms of cultural competency and sensitivity.

MediaLink Language Interpretation

BOX 6–1 **Heritage Assessment Tool**

Note: The greater the number of positive responses, the greater the person's identification with a traditional heritage. The one exception to positive answers is the question about family name change. This question may be answered negatively.

1. Where was your mother born? ______
2. Where was your father born? ______
3. Where were your grandparents born?
   (1) Your mother's mother? ______
   (2) Your mother's father? ______
   (3) Your father's mother? ______
   (4) Your father's father? ______
4. How many brothers _____ and sisters _____ do you have?
5. What setting did you grow up in? Urban _____ Rural _____ Suburban _____
6. What country did your parents grow up in?
   Father _____
   Mother _____
7. How old were you when you came to the United States? _____
8. How old were your parents when they came to the United States? Mother _____ Father _____
9. When you were growing up, who lived with you? _____
10. Have you maintained contact with
    a. Aunts, uncles, cousins? (1) Yes _____ (2) No _____
    b. Brothers and sisters? (1) Yes _____ (2) No _____
    c. Parents? (1) Yes _____ (2) No _____
    d. Your own children? (1) Yes _____ (2) No _____
11. Did most of your aunts, uncles, cousins live near your home?
    (1) Yes _____ (2) No _____
12. Approximately how often did you visit your family members who lived outside your home?
    (1) Daily _____ (2) Weekly _____ (3) Monthly _____ (4) Once a year or less _____ (5) Never _____
13. Was your original family name changed?
    (1) Yes _____ (2) No _____
14. What is your religious preference?
    (1) Catholic _____ (2) Jewish _____ (3) Protestant _____
    (4) Denomination (5) Other _____ (6) None _____
15. Is your spouse the same religion as you?
    (1) Yes _____ (2) No _____
16. Is your spouse the same ethnic background as you?
    (1) Yes _____ (2) No _____
17. What kind of school did you go to?
    (1) Public _____ (2) Private _____ (3) Parochial _____
18. As an adult, do you live in a neighborhood where the neighbors are the same religion and ethnic background as yourself?
    (1) Yes _____ (2) No _____
19. Do you belong to a religious institution?
    (1) Yes _____ (2) No _____
20. Would you describe yourself as an active member?
    (1) Yes _____ (2) No _____
21. How often do you attend your religious institution?
    (1) More than once a week _____ (2) Weekly _____
    (3) Monthly _____ (4) Special holidays only _____
    (5) Never _____
22. Do you practice your religion at home?
    (1) Yes _____ (2) No _____
    (If yes, please specify)
    (3) Praying _____ (4) Bible reading _____
    (5) Diet _____ (6) Celebrating religious holidays _____
23. Do you prepare foods of your ethnic background?
    (1) Yes _____ (2) No _____
24. Do you participate in ethnic activities?
    (1) Yes _____ (2) No _____
    (If yes, please verify)
    (3) Singing _____ (4) Holiday celebrations _____
    (5) Dancing _____ (6) Festivals _____
    (7) Costumes _____ (8) Other _____
25. Are your friends from the same religious background as you?
    (1) Yes _____ (2) No _____
26. Are your friends from the same ethnic background as you?
    (1) Yes _____ (2) No _____
27. What is your native language? _____
28. Do you speak this language?
    (1) Prefer _____ (2) Occasionally _____ (3) Rarely _____
29. Do you read your native language?
    (1) Yes _____ (2) No _____

Source: Spector, R. E. (2000). *CulturalCare: Guide to heritage assessment and health traditions* (5th ed.). Pearson Education/PH College.

Developing Cultural Competence in Nursing Practice

Developing an understanding of cultural competence requires paying attention to considerations of global health, cultural values, cultural phenomena affecting health, and the importance of cultural assessment as part of the nursing process. Cultural competence in nursing practice requires practical strategies (in general as well as specific to a particular cultural group), considerations of community-based health care promotion and disease prevention programs, and the need to advocate for cultural diversity in nursing practice, research, and education. At the same time, it is important to be aware that there are varying degrees of acculturation and individual differences—assessment of one Chinese person may be dramatically different than another and from one generation to another.

The Transcultural Nursing Society (TCNS) promotes knowledgable culturally based care. You can obtain information on this organization through their Web site (www.tcns.org), which can be accessed through the Companion Website for this book. Certification as a transcultural nurse can also be obtained through TCNS.

GENERAL STRATEGIES FOR DEVELOPING CULTURAL COMPETENCE

An essential step toward developing cultural competence is to examine your own perceptions, prejudices, and stereotypes regarding the particular cultural group of interest. It is helpful to suspend personal judgments in favor of learning more regarding "who these people really are." Become informed regarding the culture's history, migration, and immigration patterns. Learn about specific cultural beliefs, values, practices, and healing traditions as these may relate to particular lifestyle habits (e.g., religion, gender, dietary patterns, use of alcohol and drugs, use of touch, use of time, etc.). Be careful of your own ethnocentrism because culturally diverse groups may initially view you as foreign and uneducated regarding their proper forms of address, social customs, and appropriate ways for dealing with their concerns and health problems. If possible, attempt to identify issues related to access to health care for this cultural group as well. Such issues may include usual patterns of care, barriers to care (including accessibility, availability, and acceptability), and use of social assistance services.

The Nursing Self-Awareness feature below outlines several helpful suggestions for working with culturally diverse clients and groups. Such strategies will help you to apply principles of cultural competence and sensitivity to a particular health care setting.

DEVELOPING CULTURAL COMPETENCE WITH SPECIFIC CULTURAL GROUPS

Summaries of cultural health beliefs and practices for five major cultural groups (Hispanic, African-American, Native American and Alaska Native, Asian-American, and Pacific Islander populations) are in ■ Table 6–3 on page 116. Helpful suggestions to consider when working toward cultural competence are provided for each of the above groups. It is advantageous to consult with a nurse anthropologist, whenever possible. (Spector, 2000b; Huff & Klein, 1999).

MediaLink Transcultural Nursing Society

COMMUNITY-BASED HEALTH CARE PROMOTION AND DISEASE PREVENTION PROGRAMS

Often, the nurse may be able to plan, implement, and/or evaluate a program designed to meet the complex nursing needs of a specific cultural group. Examples of such community-based programs may include:

- A community-level anger-management program in an urban barrio to reach Mexican-Americans using the media as part of a mental health campaign.
- An HIV sexual risk reduction intervention among young adult African-American women.
- Working with Native Americans to develop a "talking circle" program to reduce alcohol-related injuries and alcoholism.

A useful planning framework for health promotion and disease prevention programs in multicultural populations is provided in ■ Table 6–4 on page 118. The first formal step of any program planning process is to involve those individuals affected by the problem. This principle of participation appears to be the most important component of any program development. Collaboration between planner and participants can be achieved only if there is respect for each other's values and for the agenda to be accomplished. As you become involved in any community-based program, remember to utilize the group's cultural unique-

Nursing SELF-AWARENESS — Applying Principles of Cultural Competence and Sensitivity

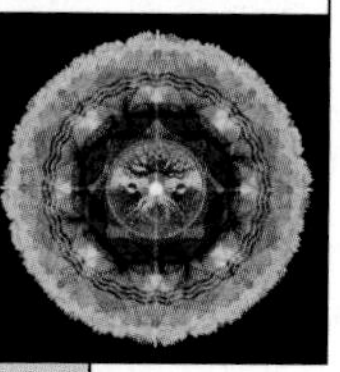

Assess your ability to carry out these suggestions when working with a culturally diverse client or group. Which of these suggestions are most useful to you as you develop cultural competence and sensitivity in your particular setting?

- Learn about the culture of interest by making multiple visits to the community to become familiar with the community's way of life. Activities may include talking to community leaders and residents, eating at local restaurants, visiting cultural sites, and attending local events.
- Learn specifically about the culture's orientation to health, disease, health traditions, and traditional healing practices.
- Identify and learn about the traditional healers within the community. Note the healers' ease of access, medicines used, cultural acceptability, and cost of care.
- Be open and nonjudgmental regarding specific cultural practices that are not part of your cultural heritage.
- Add questions to your assessment tools that reflect these cultural values, beliefs, rituals, and practices.
- Practice cross-cultural communication skills.
- Learn how to work with a competent interpreter as necessary.
- Take time to explain Western concepts of health, disease, treatment, and prevention that are relevant and understandable to the culture of interest.
- Use educational materials that are culturally appropriate and relevant to this culture.
- Work with, and learn from, indigenous health care providers when addressing the needs of this culture.
- Learn how to work with peer educators from the community.
- Seek ways to improve access to services for multicultural groups with emphasis on availability, accessibility, and acceptability.

TABLE 6–3 Developing Cultural Competence with Specific Cultural Groups

Cultural Groups/ Nations of Origin	Health Beliefs and Practices	Suggestions to Consider
Hispanic (including Spain, Cuba, Puerto Rico, Mexico, Central and South America)	Belief in folk illnesses may characterize many traditional Hispanic groups. *Curanderismo* is the traditional health care system that may be used first, but not discussed, with a Western health care provider. Traditional folk healers may be the first health practitioners consulted. They are culturally acceptable, much less expensive than Western health care, and are willing to make house calls. *Fatalism*, i.e., the belief that an individual cannot control one's health, may be a common attitude among traditional groups. Health care decisions may involve the head of the household who decides what is best for the family.	Be aware that family and family support are very important core values. Respect is an extremely important factor in all relationships. Avoiding conflict and achieving harmony are strong cultural values.
African-American (including West Indian Islands, Haiti, Dominican Republic, Brazil, England, many West African countries)	Traditional explanations for disease and illness may involve natural causes (e.g., stress, poor eating habits) and unnatural causes from witchcraft practices (e.g., voodoo, bad spirits, other works of the devil). The Western health care system is generally well respected and used for serious illness, although folk healing traditions may also be utilized. Traditional folk healers may be the only health practitioners used by African-Americans of low income.	Be aware that there may be caution to use programs from inside and outside of some black communities. Prior programs and services may have lost funding and personnel. African-Americans who have been trained "outside" the community may need to earn trust by demonstrating sincere interest in the community's particular needs and concerns. Churches often have been used as sites for health education and intervention.
Native American and Alaskan Native (including First Nation and indigenous American Indian Nations, Alaskan Aleuts and Eskimos)	Traditional ceremonies may be practiced among tribal groups to promote wellbeing and balance. Many tribal groups feel distrustful and exploited by Westerners. Medicine men, traditional healers, and herbal treatments are very important to some groups. Taboos and modesty are important in tribal life.	Be aware that every tribal group has its own unique history, traditions, and values. Become familiar with acceptable verbal and nonverbal communications of the group. Respect tribal sovereignty and work within the tribal group. Be aware that use of "talking circles" together with tribal stories have been useful for culturally appropriate educational interventions.
Asian American (including Asian Indians, Chinese, Cambodians, Thais, Vietnamese, Laotians, Filipinos, Hmong, Koreans, Japanese)	A central concept of the traditional health care system is the need to attain a harmonious relationship with nature. This traditional health care system may be the first one used for any illness. There may be a tendency not to discuss this with a Western health care practitioner. Teachings of Buddhism, Confusianism, and Taoism may emphasize upholding a public presentation that avoids admission of physical or mental illness. Many Asians may prefer traditional forms of native medicine, seeking help from Chinatown "masters" who treat with traditional herbs and other methods. Asians may not use the Western health care system because of painful diagnostic tests and lack of information.	Be aware that balance or equilibrium and kinship solidarity are two beliefs that may be prominent in Asians. Kinship solidarity refers to the belief that an individual is subservient to the family or kinship-based group. Thus, separation from family members may be stressful. Respect for elders and male authority may determine decision-making practices regarding health care for recent immigrants. Use "active listening" and watch for nonverbal cues since some Asian groups may not disagree openly with health care providers. Likewise, conflicts are generally handled within the family and may not be shared with a health care provider unless a trust is established. It is helpful if outreach workers are perceived as nonthreatening and nonintrusive.

(continued)

TABLE 6–3 Developing Cultural Competence with Specific Cultural Groups *(continued)*

Cultural Groups/ Nations of Origin	Health Beliefs and Practices	Suggestions to Consider
Pacific Islander (including Guamanian, Samoan, Hawaiian, Pacific Islander American)	Health beliefs and practices among these cultural groups may vary greatly. Thus, knowledge of the geographic location and particular ethnic group is essential. In general, indigenous illnesses may be treated with traditional healing practices, whereas Western illnesses may be treated with Western medical approaches. Taboos, modesty, and traditional healing practices are very important to these cultural groups.	Be aware that there may be a lack of health data available for the particular Pacific Islander group of interest. It may be helpful to involve women in all aspects of health care since many island cultures are matriarchal. Emphasize concepts of wholeness and interconnectedness which are central features of several Pacific Islander groups. Culturally acceptable and appropriate strategies for health promotion may include use of "talk stories," role playing, pictures, and folk media (e.g., song, dance, music).
Anglo-American/European American (including Germany, Ireland, England, Italy, the former Soviet Union, and all other European countries)	Often the dominant cultural group which influences the determination of health care needs, beliefs, practices, and programs in communities. Primary reliance on a "modern" or "Western" health care system, emphasizing use of technology and diagnostic tests. There may be reliance on traditional health beliefs and practices that may vary greatly, depending upon the country of ancestry. There is a recent increased interest in complementary and alternative (CAM) practices which emphasize holistic, naturalistic healing. Judeo-Christian beliefs may influence health practices.	Individualism, materialism, and emphases on time and youth may be strong cultural values. Directness and efficiency may be factors in relationships with health care providers. Assess the utility of self-help literature and groups when planning health care interventions.

Sources: Adapted from Huff, R. M., & Kline, M. V. (1999). *Promoting health in multicultural populations: A handbook for practitioners*. New York: Sage; and Spector, R. E. (2000). *Cultural diversity in health & illness* (5th ed.). Upper Saddle River, NJ: Prentice Hall.

ness by incorporating how group members define health problems, identify proposed solutions, and select types of activities to be emphasized. Group members are invaluable participants in identifying how health-promoting behavioral changes, once achieved, can be sustained in that community.

ADVOCATING ISSUES OF CULTURAL DIVERSITY IN NURSING

Nurses need to make a conscious decision to acknowledge and value the diversity in others. Developing cultural competence and sensitivity needed for comprehensive care is based on new knowledge, personal self-assessment, supervised practice, mentoring experiences, experience in culturally diverse clinical practice settings, participation in discussions, and diversity training. The starting point to advocate for cultural diversity in nursing is right now.

Nursing Practice

Nursing competencies must include the ability to actively and effectively work with culturally diverse clients. Look for opportunities for meaningful dialogue and relationship building across cultures. You may seek out practicing nurses of a particular cultural background to serve as resource consultants. You may mentor nurse colleagues from other cultures who work in your setting. You may seek information from transcultural health care nurses with experiences in third world countries, such as the nurses who sponsor www.culturediversity.org, which can be accessed through the Companion Website for this book.

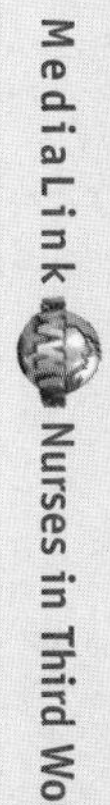

You may read transcultural journals (e.g., *Journal of Transcultural Nursing, Journal of the Black Nurses Association,* etc.) to familiarize yourself with critical culture-based issues and opportunities. You may become a member of an organization such as TCNS or a certified transcultural nurse. Make every attempt to openly discuss cultural conflicts in order to actively address suspicions and distortions. Avoiding conflict may result in chronic strained communication, insensitivity, and exclusion that thwarts culturally competent care.

Nursing Research

Gary, Sigsby, and Campbell (1998) assert that nurses can use research training and development to seek collaboration, coali-

TABLE 6–4 A Planning Framework for Health Promotion and Disease Prevention Programs Involving a Specific Cultural Group

Therapeutic Task	Nursing Interventions
1. Planning the Program	Involve those affected by the problem.
	Assess the needs of the cultural community.
	Diagnose health-related concerns (problems and needs) in the community.
	Prioritize and select the target cultural group, problem, and setting.
	Assess the specific needs of your target cultural group.
	Develop appropriate target group goals and objectives.
	Select health promotion program intervention activities that consider the unique characteristics of the target group, health problem, and setting.
2. Implementing the Program	Preimplementation preparation.
	Program implementation.
	Implementation administration and monitoring.
3. Evaluating the Program	Assess the immediate impact of the program (impact evaluation).
	Assess the long-term target group health and social outcomes (outcome evaluation).
	Assess the quality of the program inputs during the development and implementation phases (process evaluation).

Source: Adapted from Huff, R. M., & Kline, M. V. (1999). *Promoting health in multicultural populations: A handbook for practitioners*. New York: Sage.

tion, and compassion across cultures. Nursing research may define what knowledge is meaningful for a particular multicultural group. Through research, nurses can become informed regarding which interventions might be useful in specific community-based programs. Research may contribute to the development of more inclusive theories to account for behaviors observed in multicultural groups. Finally, research may better identify important health-related distinctions among numerous cultural groups that are currently classified into one category (e.g., various values and traditions of specific Native American Indian Nations such as the Cherokee, Navajo, and Sioux).

MediaLink Case Study: Developing Cultural Competence

Nursing Education

Vinson (2000) advocates development of an appreciation of how cultural identity influences health and illness as a professional education competency. Although the nursing profession remains a field dominated by white females, accrediting agencies are now encouraging nursing faculty to integrate content that emphasizes cultural diversity. Educators need to work within multicultural and multidisciplinary frameworks to tackle issues in the "real world." Yet, recruitment and retention of culturally diverse students continue to be problems in schools of nursing. Educational institutions need to recruit and mentor culturally diverse students to serve as clinicians, managers, faculty, and leaders who can then serve as role models for other students. One way to attract and educate a diverse student group is to practice diversity in faculty recruitment. When considering nursing curricula, it is important to note that knowledge of a foreign language will be essential as we strive to meet global needs in the twenty-first century. Refer to the Using Research Evidence feature on page 119 for practical strategies when addressing cultural diversity in the classroom.

Finally, while it may be easy to discuss strategies, make recommendations, and pay "lip service" to the value of developing cultural competence and sensitivity, nurses need to step out of their personal frames of reference, confront their own stereotypes and biases, and be open to different worldviews. Nurses also need to accept the challenge to incorporate cultural competence and sensitivity into all aspects of professional nursing care.

Psychiatric Epidemiology in a Culturally Diverse Society

The practice of psychiatric–mental health nursing traditionally focuses on the individual, group, family, and therapeutic use of the surrounding environment (milieu). Various disciplines, such as psychiatric nursing, can be grouped according to their underlying principles and methods. Epidemiology represents an emerging specialty that focuses on human populations rather than on individual clients per se. "Epidemiology" consists of these three Greek word roots: *epi*, meaning "among"; *demos*, meaning "people"; and *logos*, meaning "doctrine"—the doctrine of what is among or happening to people.

Epidemiologists often study the biopsychosocial factors that influence health status in populations. Epidemiologic information for the United States is available through the Centers for Disease Control and Prevention (www.cdc.gov) and for Canada

USING RESEARCH EVIDENCE

Juireith is a 24-year-old African-American female beginning the baccalaureate nursing program at your local university. She was born in Jamaica and then moved to Bronx, New York, to live with extended family. She now lives alone in your town, determined to earn a university degree in nursing. She sits with the few other African-American nursing students in class. As a student interested in the development of cultural sensitivity in professional nursing education and practice, you practice the following strategies as a way of demonstrating the personal value you place upon diversity:

- Eliminate stereotyping by understanding your attitudes, evaluating your assumptions, and learning about differences in others.
- Listen to the concerns and issues of culturally diverse students.
- Establish collaborative efforts by offering opportunities for participation in scholarly efforts to culturally diverse students.
- Confront feelings of racism since most individuals in mainstream U.S. culture may not be aware of passive racism. Words or actions can be discussed and explained if misinterpreted.
- Acknowledge and appreciate cultural differences. Welcome and value change and a new approach.
- Contribute toward building a student learning environment that accommodates cultural differences.

These strategies are drawn from historic and current perspectives addressing a growing consciousness of cultural diversity in nursing as reported in the following research:

Hagey, R., Choudhry, U., Guruge, S., Turrittin, J., Collins, E., & Lee, R. (2001). Immigrant nurses' experiences of racism. *Journal of Nursing Scholarship*, 33(4), 384–394.

through Health Canada (www.hcsc.gc.ca) and can be accessed through the Companion Web site for this book. The CDC also partners with other nations around the world. Epidemiologic principles and methods may be applied to determine the cause of a disorder (such as HIV), to assess risks associated with a harmful exposure (such as rape), to determine whether a particular treatment (such as behavior therapy) is effective, and to identify health service utilization needs and trends. Psychiatric epidemiology is particularly useful to the psychiatric nurse as the basic discipline for preventive and community psychiatry. Information on psychiatric epidemiologic studies is available through the National Institute of Mental Health (www.nimh.gov) and can be accessed through the Companion Website for this book.

Hundreds of millions of people worldwide in both developing and developed countries suffer from psychiatric disorders causing personal suffering, social disruption, and economic losses. The worldwide occurrence of psychiatric disorders prompts nurses to address multicultural diversity as principles of psychiatric epidemiology are applied to various human populations. The United States represents a multicultural country consisting of numerous subgroups who have brought unique cultural traits with them from waves of immigration over years.

An important premise of psychiatric epidemiology is that mental illness is not randomly distributed across populations. Not all people are at equal risk for developing mental disorders. One client may be depressed, another may be psychotic, while a third may suffer from debilitating physical illness. Such differences in the occurrence of mental disorders are of prime interest in epidemiology.

DEFINITION OF PSYCHIATRIC EPIDEMIOLOGY

Psychiatric epidemiology is the study of the distribution and determinants of mental disorders (or other health-related conditions or events) in human populations. Purposes include prevention, surveillance (monitoring), and the control of mental disorders. Epidemiology traditionally investigated the cause of disease. More recently, "disease" has been generalized to include a wide variety of mental disorders and health-related problems. Health-related conditions or events may include injuries; exposure to environmental pollutants, natural and manmade disasters, and traumatic or violent events; behavioral problems; and the nonuse or misuse of mental health services. This chapter uses the word *disorder* rather than *disease* to reflect current perspectives in the field of psychiatric epidemiology.

A psychiatric epidemiologist is an investigator who studies mental disorders or other health-related conditions or events in defined populations to develop a comprehensive picture of mental health problems and to evaluate interventions. An advanced professional degree (master's or Ph.D.) from a school of public health or similar institution is required. Epidemiologists ask, "Which characteristics among individuals (such as genetic) or their environment (such as exposure to stressful life events) explain differences in morbidity from specific mental disorders?" Nursing provides an excellent background for investigating disease occurrence and its relation to various characteristics of individuals or their environment.

MediaLink Psychiatric Epidemiological Studies

Within the context of psychiatric epidemiology, cultural diversity refers to varied cultural and ethnic backgrounds that may influence the experience, expression, reporting, and evaluation of mental disorders. Considerations of cultural diversity related to mental disorders will be interwoven throughout this section. Examples of important concepts frequently emphasize depression because it is among the most common disorders in the United States today.

USES OF PSYCHIATRIC EPIDEMIOLOGY

Psychiatric epidemiology is used to do the following:

- Determine causative factors for specific disorders.
- Identify groups of people (populations) at high risk of developing specific disorders.
- Recognize changes in health problems, especially the emergence of new problems.

- Plan for current health needs and predict future needs.
- Evaluate preventive and therapeutic measures.

It is important to note that both the patterns of occurrence of mental disorders in a community and the patterns of delivery of psychiatric care are studied. The services offered influence, and are influenced by, the amount and nature of the disorders and by changes in modes of therapy.

Key Epidemiologic Concepts

Several key concepts commonly used in epidemiology may serve as a foundation for applying epidemiologic principles to your work in psychiatric nursing. Knowledge of these terms is also useful when reviewing current medical literature. (You may wish to use an epidemiology resource such as Bernier, Watson, Nowell, Emery, and St. Pierre [1998] to further your understanding of epidemiologic concepts and their applications.)

PREVALENCE

Here is a formula for determining prevalence rate:

$$\text{Prevalence rate} = \frac{\text{Number of existing cases of disorder at a point in time}}{\text{Total population}}$$

Prevalence rates may be used for the following purposes:

- To express the burden of a disorder in the population.
- To identify population subgroups (by age, sex, etc.) for prevention strategies.
- For the planning and evaluation of mental health services.
- To track changes in patterns of a disorder over time.

INCIDENCE

An incidence rate measures the number of *new* cases of a disease or disorder in a population over a period of time. Here is a formula for determining incidence rate:

$$\text{Incidence rate} = \frac{\text{Number of new cases of disorder over a period of time}}{\text{Population at risk}}$$

Incidence is a direct measure of the rate at which individuals in a given population develop a disease or disorder. Thus, incidence is a direct measure of risk. Clues to the causes of a disorder may be obtained as new "incident" cases are studied.

Studies of chronic diseases, such as schizophrenia, generally use prevalence measures; studies of acute disorders or events, such as rape, generally use incidence measures. One can examine prevalence or incidence rates by age, sex, race/ethnicity, and other biopsychosocial factors to determine which subgroups are at greatest risk for specific diseases. The identification of vulnerable subgroups may be the first step in the development of intervention strategies that target resources for people at greatest risk.

RISK FACTORS

A critical issue related to cultural diversity in psychiatric epidemiology is that important factors reflecting varying cultures need to be assessed in clinical practice and research. Ethnicity, race, dietary patterns, the use of alcohol and drugs, health and healing practices, other lifestyle habits, religious or spiritual beliefs, the use of time, and migration patterns may differentially affect the experience, expression, reporting, and evaluation of mental disorders among culturally diverse groups. The field of research has been criticized in retrospect for studying white males and, to a lesser extent, white females, and then generalizing the results to all other groups.

The notion of biopsychosocial risk factors is common in psychiatric literature. A **risk factor** is a factor whose presence is associated with an increased chance or probability of mental disorder. Some risk factors cannot be modified, such as age. Other risk factors are susceptible to change, such as personal lifestyle habits regarding the use of alcohol and tobacco. A limited review of numerous risk factors associated with the occurrence of many psychiatric disorders is outlined by Bromet (1998).

Gender

Differences in rates between males and females are found for substance abuse, anxiety disorders, and depression. The male-to-female ratios are estimated at 6:1 for alcoholism, 1:2 for depression, and 1:2 for phobias.

Age

Age is associated with the occurrence of mental disorders. An important finding from the ECA studies (Bruce, Leaf, Rozal, Floris, & Huff, 1994) was that young adults (age 25–44) had the highest prevalence estimates for most disorders. Alcoholism is known to peak in the early forties. Heavy drinking associated with driving or fighting while intoxicated appears to peak in the early twenties.

Social Class

Lower social class status is associated with increased rates of depression, alcohol and other substance abuse, and antisocial personality disorder. Although risk factors vary among mental disorders, studies indicate that adults in poverty are at higher risk for an episode of at least one mental disorder compared with those not in poverty.

Ethnicity

Ethnicity appears to be indirectly associated with mental disorders because different ethnic groups share different social and physical environments. The Epidemiologic Catchment Area (ECA) studies (Bruce, Leaf, Rozal, Florio, & Hoff, 1994) found similar prevalence rates for most mental disorders between African-Americans and Caucasians. For major depression, Caucasian men tended to have higher rates than African-American men, while African-American women had higher prevalence rates than Caucasian women. Caucasians of all ages have higher suicide rates than African-Americans, with Native American youth at increased risk for suicide.

Marital Status

Marital status, especially being single, may be associated with psychiatric disorders such as schizophrenia. The highest rates of depression occur among those recently divorced or separated. Married women are more depressed than nonmarried women. In contrast, married men are less depressed than unmarried men.

Physical Health Status

The link between physical and mental health is noteworthy. Studies provide evidence that psychiatric clients may have an increased mortality rate. Medically hospitalized clients have increased rates of mental disorder as well. Major depression is associated with many chronic medical conditions and is predictive of shortened life expectancy.

Positive Family History

Depression and schizophrenia appear related to a history of such disorders in the family. Evidence points to a genetic vulnerability for developing alcoholism. There is some evidence that dementia of the Alzheimer's type may show a familial pattern. Findings regarding bipolar disorder (manic depression) and anxiety disorders are currently controversial with regard to family history. Recent developments in genetics may contribute to further understanding regarding the contribution of family history to the development of mental disorders.

Season of Birth

Seasonal variation is well studied in relation to stillbirths and neonatal deaths. Studies in some countries, including the United States, reveal that individuals with schizophrenia are more likely to be born during winter or spring.

Social Environment

Higher levels of stress associated with particular events in one's social environment may be associated with increased rates of mental disorder. Loss of life or property is a risk factor related to *natural disasters,* such as earthquakes, floods, and tornadoes. *Single traumatic events,* such as bereavement or unemployment, may produce adverse mental health consequences. The diagnosis of posttraumatic stress disorder (PTSD) represents a response to an unusual, intense stressor. *Adverse life events* are known to contribute to some forms of depression. A stressful family environment is an established risk factor for behavioral problems in children.

Physical Environment

High-level *chemical exposures* to mercury, carbon monoxide, carbon disulfide, and lead are related to serious central nervous system disturbances. Environmental exposure to lead is related to deleterious effects on children. When considering *homelessness,* rates of mental disorder among homeless adults and children are remarkably high.

It is important to note that the presence of one particular risk factor does not inevitably lead to the development of a mental disorder. Rather, a number of factors occurring in a defined time period may cause a disorder. Multifactorial causation is the term used to describe the requirement that a combination of causes or factors may be needed to produce the disorder.

Lifestyle Habits

It is important to reemphasize that culturally diverse lifestyle habits should be incorporated in any nursing assessment. Such habits may influence the experience, expression, reporting, and evaluation of mental disorders. Lifestyle habits may include dietary patterns, use of alcohol and drugs, health and healing practices, religious and spiritual beliefs, use of time, and migration patterns.

THE NATURAL HISTORY OF DISORDER

Many disorders, especially chronic disorders, have a natural life history. The natural history of disorder refers to the course of disorder over time in the absence of intervention. Chronic disorder may be viewed in a sequence of stages. Risk factors favoring the development of a disorder may be present early in life, preceding the appearance of symptoms by many years. It is important to note that we do not have a complete understanding of the natural history of many psychiatric disorders. Every disorder has its own life history, but in general, disorders have these four basic stages: 1. stage of susceptibility, 2. stage of presymptomatic disorder, 3. stage of clinical disorder, and 4. stage of disability (■ Figure 6–3) on page 122.

1. *Stage of Susceptibility.* During this stage, the groundwork has been laid by the presence of risk factors that favor the occurrence of disorder. The individual is susceptible to the disorder, but the disorder has not yet developed. Identification of those at high risk for developing a disorder is a major mental health care challenge. For example, the following risk factors may "set the stage," placing a woman at increased risk for depression: lack of a primary relationship, not employed outside the home, having three or more children under the age of 6, and having endured the loss of a parent in childhood.
2. *Stage of Presymptomatic Disorder.* During this stage, there is no apparent disorder, but pathological changes have started to occur. The disorder has begun but remains unrecognized because it may be asymptomatic. If signs of the disorder are present, they may be considered to be the ordinary discomforts of daily living. Mild depression serves as an example of this presymptomatic stage.
3. *Stage of Clinical Disorder.* This stage is characterized by recognizable signs and symptoms of disorder. For some disorders, people regularly come under nursing or medical care at some point over the course of an illness. These disorders are "high-profile" because they cause such symptoms as peculiar behavior, failure to thrive, severe or chronic distress, or pain. Classification may be based on laboratory findings or on functional or therapeutic considerations. Cancer is usually classified by the location, extent,

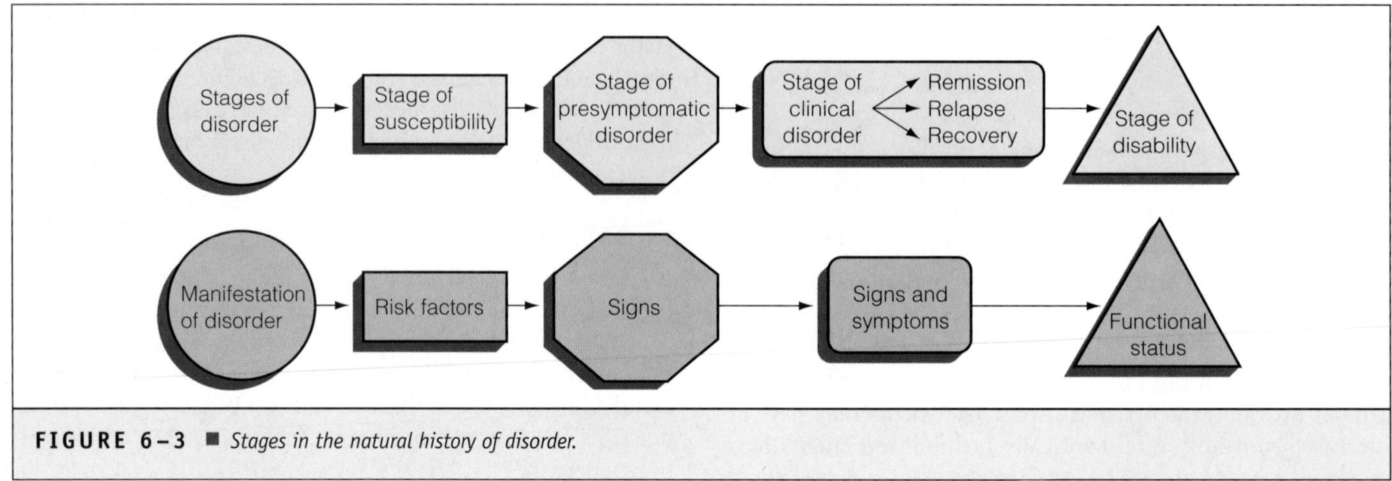

FIGURE 6–3 ■ *Stages in the natural history of disorder.*

and type of tumor. The most current source of classification of psychiatric disorders is the American Psychiatric Association's *Diagnostic and Statistical Manual of Mental Disorders*, 4th edition, Text Revision, or DSM-IV-TR (American Psychiatric Association, 2000). DSM-IV-TR criteria for psychiatric disorders rely on a descriptive diagnostic classification scheme. It is important to note that "clinical disorder" describes a disorder that has come under nursing or medical care and is then treated in a variety of ways that may alter the subsequent course of events.

4. *Stage of Disability.* Some disorders run their course and resolve completely, either spontaneously or in response to therapy. However, some disorders leave residual impairment or disability of short or long duration. While there is a substantial amount of disability associated with acute disorders, the extended disability resulting from chronic disorders is of greater significance to society.

LEVELS OF PREVENTION

Understanding the stages of the natural history of disorder can serve as a basis for applying prevention strategies. Emphasis here is on preventive, rather than curative, nursing interventions. Prevention simply means keeping the disorder from occurring. The meaning of the word has been extended to include measures that interrupt or slow the progression of disorder. Three levels of prevention are usually possible, depending on when clinical efforts are made. Although these concepts apply to mental disorders in this chapter, they may be effectively applied to any medical disease or condition.

Primary Prevention

Primary prevention involves avoiding the occurrence of disorder by removing the risk factors. The goals of primary prevention are mental health promotion and the prevention of disorder. Mental health promotion addresses conditions at home, work, and school that favor healthy living. Emotional support, adequate shelter, a safe environment, and good nutrition are examples. Mental health education programs, including counseling in preparation for major life events (such as independent living programs and parent training in child development) are an integral aspect of mental health promotion. The prevention of disorder is usually carried out through specific protective measures. These may involve training in specific skills and competence building for high-risk individuals (stress management seminars, Big Brother/Big Sister programs) or may emphasize healthy behaviors (lifestyle counseling, Students Against Drunken Driving programs, and "Say No to Drugs" programs).

It is important to note that primary prevention is often accomplished outside the mental health care system. Nurses may be directly involved in many primary prevention activities, including client referral to specific appropriate community resources to reduce the risk of mental disorder.

Secondary Prevention

Secondary prevention involves the early detection and prompt treatment of disorder. An important caution is that *prognosis is affected by the duration of any mental disorder.* Thus, secondary prevention strategies are crucial in mental health care. Because of a current inability to prevent certain disorders, efforts to control many of these disorders focus on secondary prevention. In the presymptomatic stage, screening surveys by health departments and other community agencies may target individuals in order to alter the natural history of the condition detected. At the stage of clinical disorder, prompt, thorough diagnosis and treatment are essential. A large number of secondary prevention services include inpatient units, emergency services, outpatient clinics, and day treatment programs. Psychiatric case-finding efforts in walk-in clinics, primary practice, and hospital settings are further examples of secondary prevention strategies that can be employed.

In general, there are three clinical outcomes regarding mental disorders: remission, relapse, or permanent recovery. Much of your effort as a psychiatric–mental health nurse will focus on achieving the overall goal of secondary prevention, that is, termination or limitation of the course of a mental disorder.

Tertiary Prevention

Tertiary prevention involves the limiting of disability and rehabilitation when a disorder has occurred. Ideally, this level of prevention is restorative in nature; in reality, the emphasis may be on sustaining basic functions. Goals of tertiary prevention include restoring functional status, limiting progression, and preventing complications. An interdisciplinary team addressing nursing care, medical care, rehabilitation (physical, vocational), occupational therapy, and other support services may be involved. Two specific examples of tertiary prevention are suicide prevention associated with an inpatient's severe major depressive episode, and independent living programs for the frequently admitted chronic psychiatric patient. The interrelationships between the stages of the natural history of disorder and the levels of prevention are illustrated in ■ Figure 6–4.

EPIDEMIOLOGIC/CULTURAL STUDIES

Two common types of studies that examine the distribution and determinants of mental disorders are descriptive studies and cross-sectional studies.

Descriptive Studies

Knowing about patterns of occurrence is a useful first step in identifying factors that may play a causative role or otherwise contribute to the development of a disorder. A descriptive study identifies the amount and distribution of a disorder within a population by answering the following questions related to person, place, and time:

- *Who* is affected? (person)
- *Where* do the cases occur? (place)
- *When* do cases occur? (time)

"*Who*" addresses important personal characteristics (such as age, gender, and ethnicity/race) to determine which of these characteristics differ in comparisons of disorder frequency across populations. Age is generally the most important personal characteristic associated with disorders. Gender is also a factor among disorders; depression, for example, shows male–female differences in patterns of disorder and death. Rates of depression are almost twice as high in women com-

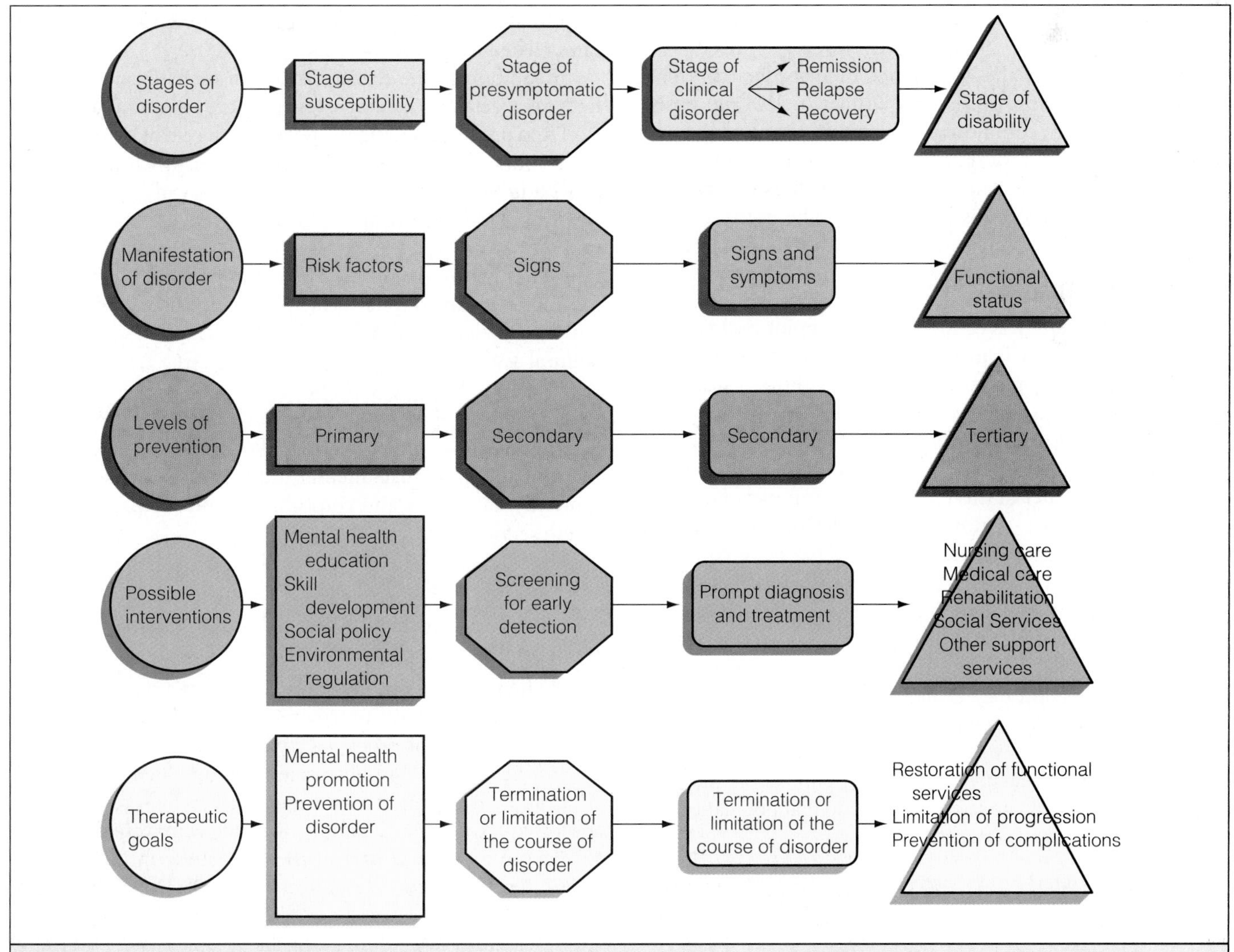

FIGURE 6–4 ■ *Stages in the natural history of disorder, with corresponding levels of prevention, possible interventions, and therapeutic goals.*

pared to men. Women also have a higher rate of attempted suicide, but completed suicides are more common in men.

Many disorders differ markedly in frequency and severity by racial group. Like race, ethnicity may influence the development of disorder. For example, cultural differences are believed to influence use of alcohol among different groups, which may explain why alcoholism is less common among Jews compared to many other ethnic groups. Psychological stress among Hispanics may be related to mal de ojo, thought to be the result of a witch purposefully casting a spell by looking admiringly at a child. Native Americans may suffer such culture-bound syndromes as pibloqtok (active, convulsive hysterical seizures) or ghost sickness (confusion, dizziness, and fear). Some Asians express psychological disharmony through somatic complaints (headaches, stomachaches, and palpitations).

"*Where*" addresses the geographic location where disorders are clustered. Variations in location can provide clues to factors associated with the occurrence of disorders. International comparisons are widely used to assess relative progress in the control of disorders. "Where" also may address political subdivisions, such as entire nations, states, counties, and towns. Location, such as a remote rural setting, may influence access to mental health services.

"*When*" addresses the occurrence of disorders by time, which is usually expressed on an annual or lifetime basis. Prevalence rates are commonly presented in terms of lifetime and one-year periods for various disorders. Incidence rates may be reported in terms of a one-year time span. Seasonal fluctuations in the frequency of disorders may also be noted, such as the seasonal patterns associated with some mood disorders.

Cross-Sectional Studies

A cross-sectional study is conducted at one point in time. The prevalence of disorder is measured by surveying a group that consists of some people with and some without a disorder. These studies, often called prevalence studies, are relatively inexpensive, simple to carry out, and may provide clues to factors associated with disorder. The National Comorbidity Survey (NCS), discussed later in this chapter, is an example of a cross-sectional (prevalence) study (Kessler, McGonagle, & Zhao, 1994). Cross-sectional studies are among the most common types of research designs reported in the psychiatric literature.

Often, the ideal population to be studied is either too large or too spread out over time, and there is a need to select a smaller group of individuals for study. A sample or representative portion of the population may actually participate in the study. A representative sample resembles the population in relation to important characteristics such as age and gender. If the study sample is truly representative of the larger population, then the results of the study can be safely extended to that population.

Recent Developments Incorporating Cultural Diversity

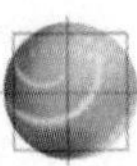

Several recent developments in psychiatric epidemiology are assessment and diagnostic advances in relation to cultural diversity, key findings from major recent studies, and patterns in the use of mental health services.

USING DSM-IV-TR FOR CULTURAL ASSESSMENT

In psychiatric epidemiology, a "case" is a person in the population or study group identified as having a particular mental disorder. The definition of a case in epidemiology is not necessarily the same as the ordinary clinical definition. Cases may be identified by clinical nursing diagnoses, by psychiatrists' clinical diagnoses, by clinical records, by surveys of the general population, and by population screening (Last, 2000).

Although discussions regarding the DSM-IV-TR are incorporated throughout this textbook, DSM-IV-TR features relating to cultural diversity deserve emphasis. DSM-IV-TR field trials were carried out in more than 70 diverse sites. Representative groups of subjects were selected from a range of sociocultural and ethnic backgrounds to test diagnostic categories as a whole, as well as specific items within each category. A DSM-IV-TR section for each disorder entitled "Specific Culture, Age, and Gender Features" systematically offers guidance concerning variations that may be attributable to one's cultural setting. The section also provides information on differential prevalence rates related to culture.

In addition to the earlier discussion on assessment, guidelines for a detailed cultural assessment are offered in the DSM-IV-TR to provide a systematic review of the client's cultural and ethnic background and to identify ways in which the cultural context influences nursing care. The glossary of culture-bound syndromes to help identify any local patterns of experience that may or may not be linked to a specific DSM-IV-TR category are reproduced in Appendix A. The accompanying Nursing Self-Awareness feature applies principles of psychiatric epidemiology to a particular clinical setting and client with emphasis on cultural assessment.

KEY FINDINGS FROM RECENT MAJOR STUDIES

Key findings from recent major studies on mental disorders are relevant to psychiatric–mental health nurses in these areas: mortality, morbidity and comorbidity, and the use of mental health services.

Mortality

Information on mortality associated with psychiatric diagnoses is important for two reasons.

1. An increased risk of mortality represents a serious negative outcome that may contribute information about the natural history of disorder.
2. Information on mortality may be used to identify high-risk groups in community settings. Researchers recently followed a community sample of adults who were first interviewed in 1980 as part of the ECA study in New Haven, Connecticut (Bruce, Leaf, Rozal, Florio, & Hoff, 1994). Nine years later, the researchers determined who was living or deceased. A key finding was the greater risk of mortality among adults with the following disorders: major depression, alcohol abuse or dependence, and schizophrenia. The

Nursing SELF-AWARENESS | **Applying Principles of Psychiatric Epidemiology**

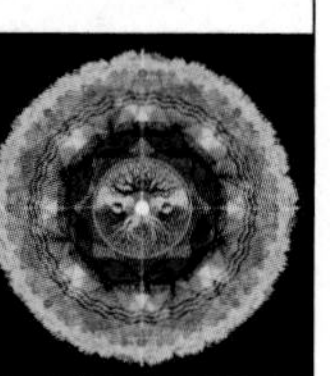

Attempt to identify the following concerns regarding a particular population that is served:

- Am I able to identify groups of people (such as children, elderly, or homeless) at high risk for the development of specific psychiatric disorders?
- Have I obtained information on any changes in health problems at this setting, especially the emergence of new problems?
- In what ways might I be involved in the identification of current health needs of this population, and the prediction of future needs of this population?
- Are there particular care-seeking patterns related to the utilization of mental health services (including nonuse or misuse of services) that I need to be aware of?
- How might I be involved in the evaluation of preventive and therapeutic measures aimed at this population?

Attempt to answer the following questions regarding a particular client that is served:

- Have I assessed which risk factors associated with psychiatric disorders may relate to this client?
- Have I obtained information about this client's cultural identity as part of my psychiatric nursing assessment?
- Do I have an understanding of this client's lifestyle habits which may impact on mental health care (such as health and healing practices, religious and spiritual beliefs, and use of alcohol and drugs)?
- Can I identify cultural resources that might be useful in the planning and provision of mental health services for this client?
- Am I able to formulate goals targeting one or more of the three levels of prevention (primary, secondary, tertiary)?

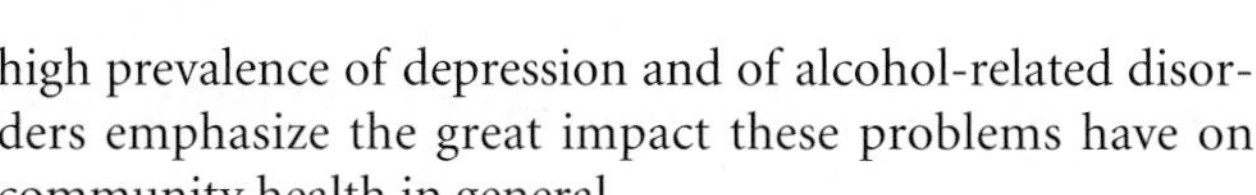

high prevalence of depression and of alcohol-related disorders emphasize the great impact these problems have on community health in general.

Morbidity and Comorbidity

There is increasing awareness of the issue of comorbidity among people with mental disorders, particularly depression, anxiety, and alcohol and other substance abuse. **Comorbidity** is defined as the occurrence of two or more psychiatric disorders over an individual's life span.

The National Comorbidity Survey (NCS). The landmark National Comorbidity Survey, a congressionally mandated survey conducted with a representative national sample, is the most extensive and current research regarding psychiatric disorders to date (Kessler, McGonagle, & Zhao, 1994). The goals of the NCS included:

- Carrying out a national survey to estimate the prevalence of psychiatric morbidity and comorbidity in the United States.
- Investigating the implications of comorbidity for mental health service utilization and course of illness.
- Investigating the risk factors for comorbidity.

More specifically, this survey of the noninstitutionalized U.S. household population (age 15–54) reported on about 10,000 subjects using a study design that enabled investigation of seasonal variation in the prevalence of mental disorders. A structured psychiatric interview was used to generate DSM-III-R psychiatric diagnoses (the version in use at that time).

The prevalence of psychiatric disorders was greater than previously thought. Nearly half the subjects reported at least one mental disorder in their lifetime. The most common disorders were major depression and alcohol dependence. The following findings were consistent with previous research:

- Women had higher rates of affective and anxiety disorders.
- Men had higher rates of substance abuse disorders and antisocial personality disorder.
- Most disorders declined with age and with higher socioeconomic status.
- Fewer than 40% of those with a lifetime disorder had ever received professional treatment.

A most striking finding is that mental disorders are more highly concentrated than previously recognized in approximately one-sixth (14%) of the population who have had a history of three or more comorbid disorders. When severity is considered, this group also includes the great majority of those with severe disorders. Less than 50% of this highly comorbid group ever obtained specialty mental health treatment, despite the number and severity of their disorders. Findings point to the need for community-based preventive programs aimed at more outreach. There is also a need for more research on barriers to mental health services.

The Epidemiologic Catchment Area (ECA) Studies. Additional findings from the ECA studies provide information from community and institutional samples regarding the comorbidity of mental disorders related to alcohol and other drug abuse. Regier et al. (1990) reported that, in general, 37% of those with a mental disorder also had an alcohol abuse disorder. Among mental disorders associated with alcoholism, anxiety disorders were most prevalent (19%), followed by antisocial personality disorder (14%), and depressive disorder (13%). The relationship between mental disorder and drug abuse (other than alcohol) is also noteworthy: A comorbid mental disorder was found among more than half of those with drug (other than alcohol) abuse disorders.

Expressed in terms of risk, those having a mental disorder in their lifetime had more than twice the risk of having an alcohol abuse disorder and over four times the risk of having another drug abuse disorder. Individuals treated in specialty mental health and addictive disorder clinics were at significantly higher risk for having comorbid disorders. Helzer and Pryzbeck (1988) found that comorbidity of alcoholism with other disorders was more common for women compared to men. Issues related to comorbidity will receive significant attention in future psychiatric research.

The Use of Mental Health Services. Care-seeking patterns need to be especially addressed in the conduct of epidemiologic studies. Patterns may be summarized as follows:

- Most people with mental disorders do not seek professional treatment.
- Comorbidity increases the likelihood that a person will seek treatment. Still less than half of the highly comorbid group identified in the National Comorbidity Study ever obtained specialty mental health treatment, despite the number and severity of their disorders.
- When seeking treatment, most people with mental disorders seek treatment from primary care physicians, who prescribe the majority of psychotropic medications. Yet there is a current decrease in primary care physicians, especially in impoverished and rural areas.
- Individuals with chronic mental disorders comprise the majority of those who seek treatment.
- Psychiatrists tend to treat individuals with severe disorders, yet there is a current undersupply of psychiatrists in the United States.

Awareness of these care-seeking patterns is essential in order to address the nonuse or misuse of mental health services. Knowledge of such patterns is also useful for selection of the most appropriate subjects for a given epidemiologic study. Pivotal issues are the availability, accessibility, cost, and quality of mental health services, especially since prognosis is affected by the duration of any mental disorder.

Cost is the most frequently addressed mental health topic in current literature on medical care organization. Financial incentives appear to drive the services provided to those with mental disorders, and funding sources appear to drive the entire health care industry. Insurance coverage for mental health care appears to lag behind that for other medical care. Severely underserved groups in relation to mental health services include:

- Substance abusers.
- Older adults (especially if minority).
- Uninsured persons.
- Homeless persons.

Current mental health policy appears reactive rather than proactive, situational rather than long term and strategic, and rehabilitative rather than preventive.

IMPLICATIONS FOR PSYCHIATRIC–MENTAL HEALTH NURSING PRACTICE

In general, epidemiologic principles extend nursing skills by considering the community itself as a potential "client" for mental health assessment and services. More specifically, epidemiologic principles may be applied to each step of the nursing process. Assessment may include collecting information on the natural history of disorder, potential risk factors, and the client's cultural and ethnic background. Nursing diagnoses may involve the use of one or more psychiatric instruments as part of diagnostic procedures. The levels of prevention may serve as a comprehensive framework for planning and implementing nursing interventions, as well as for evaluation and outcome criteria.

Because most people with mental disorders never seek professional treatment, there is a need for more outreach to ensure availability, accessibility, reasonable cost, and quality of mental health services for all subgroups of the population. Psychiatric nurses may advocate for more outreach aimed at high-risk groups, such as the impoverished, the homeless, and those with comorbid conditions.

IMPLICATIONS FOR PSYCHIATRIC–MENTAL HEALTH NURSING RESEARCH

The results from studies suggest that the causes and consequences of high comorbidity should be the focus of continued research. More research on potential barriers to professional care seeking is needed, including care-seeking patterns that consider ethnic and cultural differences.

The research contains gaps. There appears to be a lack of systematic, evaluative study aimed at determining which treatments are most effective for which disorders in which groups at any given time. Research into productivity and efficiency is important: Most clients, especially those with severe or persistent mental disorders, have found a fragmented, underfinanced, uncoordinated, and frequently inaccessible system of care.

Potential areas for future psychiatric–mental health nursing research include:

- Expanded cross-national comparisons.
- Genetics and neurobiology.
- Environmental factors (e.g., physical illness, traumatic life events, lack of support).
- The development of preventive programs.
- Advances in psychopharmacology.
- Child and adolescent studies.
- Use of various study designs.
- Development of brief interview instruments for use in screening programs.

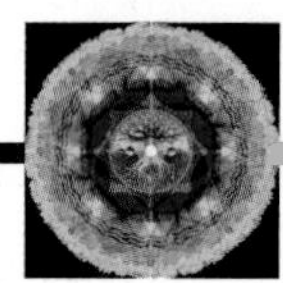

EXPLORE MediaLink

NCLEX review, case studies, and other interactive resources for this chapter can be found on the Companion Website at http://www.prenhall.com/kneisl. Click on Chapter 6 to select the activities for this chapter.

For animations, video tutorials, more NCLEX review questions, and an audio glossary, access the accompanying CD-ROM in this textbook.

BIBLIOGRAPHY

American Psychiatric Association (2000). *Diagnostic and statistical manual of mental disorders* (4th ed., Text Revision) (DSM-IV-TR). Washington, DC: Author.

Bechtel, G. A., Davidhizar, R., Tiller, C. M., & Quinn, M. E. (1999). Future realities in nursing: Partnerships, practice, and economics. *Nursingconnections. 12*(1), 19–26.

Bernier, R. H., Watson, V., Nowell, A., Emery, B., & St. Pierre, J. (1998). *Episource: A guide to resources in epidemiology* (2nd ed.). Roswell, GA: Epidemiology Monitor.

Bromet, E. J. (1998). Psychiatric disorders. In R. B. Wallace (Ed.). *Maxcy–Rosenau–Last Public Health and Preventive Medicine* (14th ed.). Stamford, CT: Appleton & Lange.

Bruce, M., Leaf, P., Rozal, G., Florio, L., & Hoff, R. (1994). Psychiatric status and 9-year mortality data in the New Haven Epidemiologic Catchment Area Study. *American Journal of Psychiatry, 151*(5), 716–721.

Gary, F. A., Sigsby, L. M., & Campbell, D. (1998). Preparing for the 21st century: Diversity in nursing education, research, and practice. *Journal of Professional Nursing 14*(5), 272–279.

Giger, J. N., & Davidhizar, R. E. (1999). *Transcultural nursing: Assessment and intervention* (3rd ed.). St. Louis: Mosby.

Hagey, R., Choudhry, U., Guruge, S., Turrittin, J., Collins, E., & Lee, R. (2001). Immigrant nurses' experiences of racism. *Journal of nursing scholarship, 33*(4), 384–394.

Helzer, J. E., & Pryzbeck, T. R. (1988). The co-occurrence of alcoholism with other psychiatric disorders in the general population and its impact on treatment. *Journal of Studies on Alcohol, 49*(1), 219–224.

Huff, R. M., & Kline, M. V. (1999). *Promoting health in multicultural populations: A handbook for practitioners.* Thousand Oaks, CA: Sage Publications, Inc.

Kessler, R., McGonagle, K., & Zhao, S. (1994). Lifetime and 12-month prevalence of DSM-III-R psychiatric disorders in the United States: Results from the National Comorbidity Survey. *Archives of General Psychiatry 51*, 8–18.

Last, J. M. (2000). *A dictionary of epidemiology* (4th ed.). New York: Oxford University Press.

Murray, C. J. L., & Lopez, A. D. (1996). *The global burden of disease: A comprehensive assessment of mortality and disability from diseases, injuries, and risk factors in 1990 and projected to 2020.* Cambridge, MA: Harvard University Press.

National Center for Cultural Competence (2002). Developing cultural competence in health care settings. *Pediatric Nursing*, 28(2), 133–137.

Regier, D., Farmer, M. E., Rae, D. S., Locke, B. Z., Keith, S. J., Judd, L. L., & Goodwin, F. K., et al. (1990). Comorbidity of mental health disorders with alcohol and other drug abuse. *Journal of the American Medical Association, 264*, 2511–2518.

Rothman, K. J., & Greenland, S. (1998). *Modern epidemiology* (2nd ed.). Philadelphia: Lippincott-Raven.

Spector, R. E. (2000a). *Cultural diversity in health & illness* (5th ed.). Upper Saddle River, NJ: Prentice Hall.

Spector, R. E. (2000b). *CulturalCare: Guide to heritage assessment and health traditions* (5th ed.). Upper Saddle River, NJ: Prentice Hall.

Valanis, B. (1999). *Epidemiology in nursing and health care* (3rd ed.). Stamford, CT: Appleton & Lange.

Vaughan, J. (1997). Is there really racism in nursing? *Journal of Nursing Education, 36*(3), 135–139.

Vinson, J. A. (2000). Nursing's epistemology revisited in relation to professional education competencies. *Journal of Professional Nursing, 16*(1), 39–46.

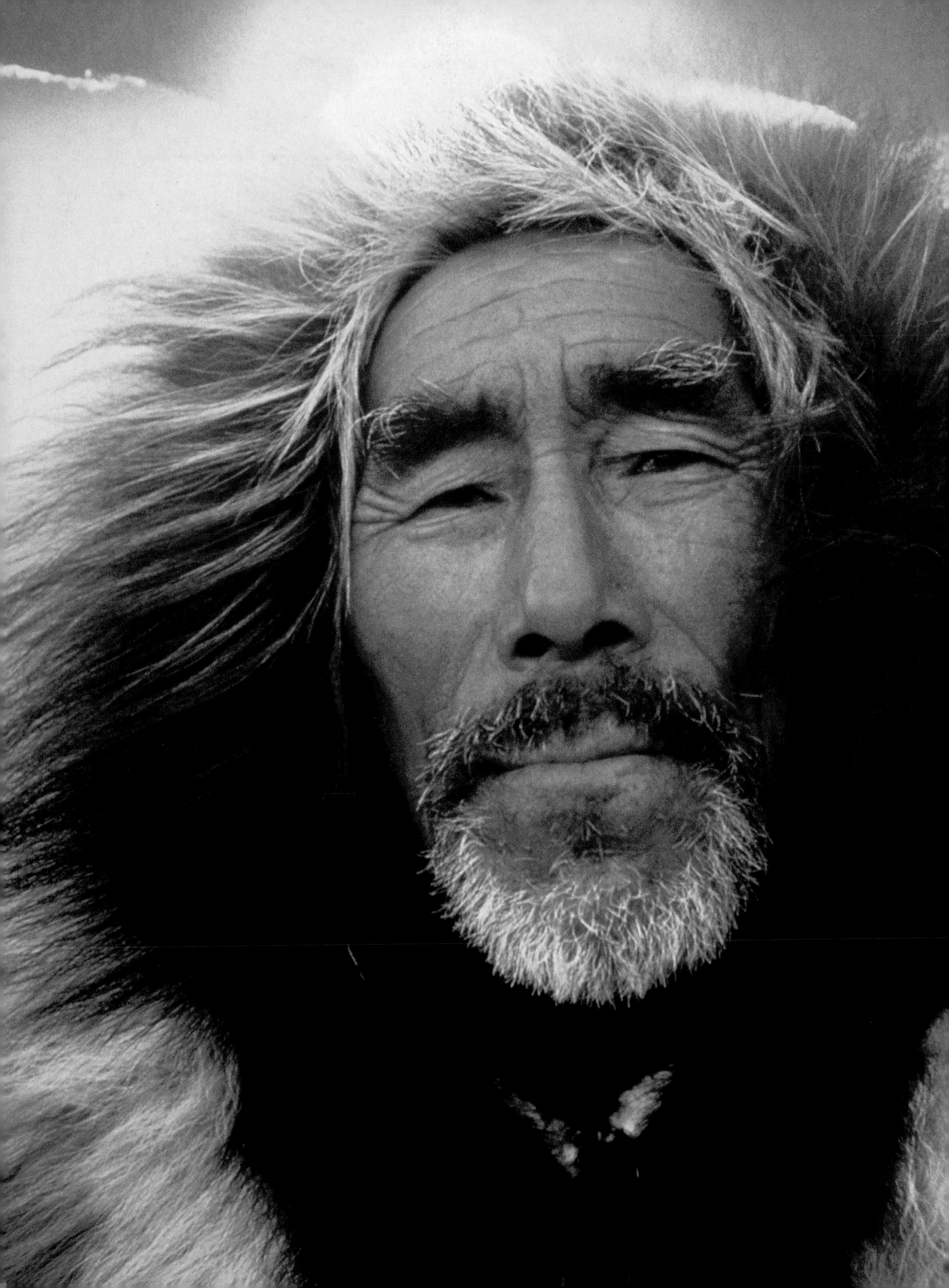

CHAPTER 7 *The Nursing Process with Psychiatric–Mental Health Clients*
CHAPTER 8 *Therapeutic Communication*
CHAPTER 9 *Assessment*
CHAPTER 10 *Clients' Rights, Ethics, and Advocacy*
CHAPTER 11 *Creating a Therapeutic Environment*

UNIT *Two*

Applying Psychiatric–Mental Health Nursing Processes and Competencies

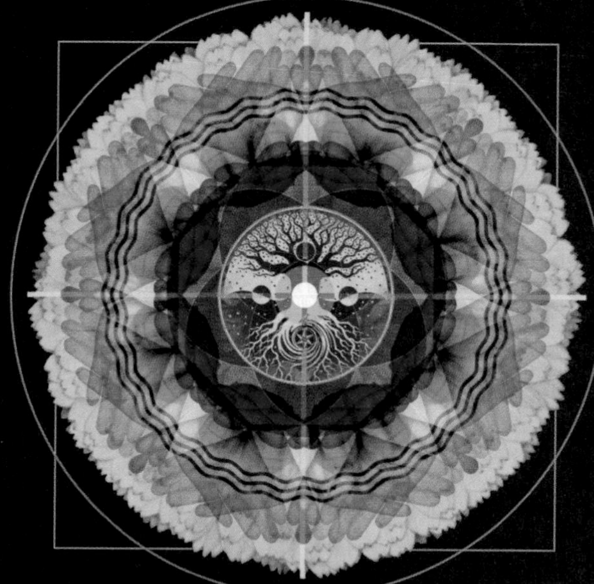

Vlad is an Eskimo man who lives and works under the midnight sun in the harsh conditions of northern Alaska. His family tells us that he suffers from periods of brooding that are often followed by violent aggressive outbursts. As psychiatric–mental health nurses we have the power to project shadow or light onto some part of the world and into the lives of the people who dwell there. Our challenge is to bridge the boundaries and borders of meaning that surround others. Great value can be gleaned from poets and storytellers in various wisdom traditions as well as from the stories of people like Vlad and his family. Crossing boundaries can mean venturing beyond conventional views or it can mean pursuing different boundary-crossing strategies. Culturally competent communication incorporates the client's worldview. In Unit Two, you will learn about assessing, communicating, advocating, and creating a therapeutic environment that reflects sensitivity to the ways in which culture affects our ability to see how other people are doing and how our actions can affect their hearts, minds, and health.

←

Source: Harald Sund/Getty Images, Inc.—Image Bank

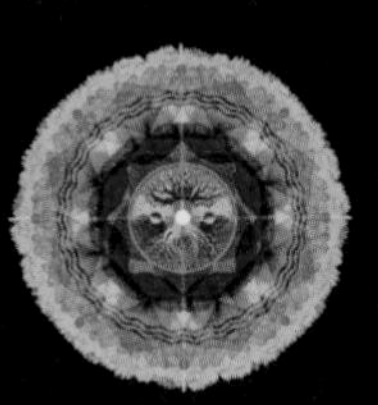

7

The Nursing Process with Psychiatric–Mental Health Clients

HOLLY SKODOL WILSON

Chapter SEVEN

KEY TERMS

chief complaint
nursing process
objective data
primary data source
secondary data source
Standards of Psychiatric–Mental Health Nursing Practice
subjective data

FOCUS QUESTIONS

- **How are the American Nurses Association Standards of Psychiatric–Mental Health Nursing Practice related to the nursing process?**
- **Are you able to use the standardized language of NANDA, NOC, and NIC linkages to provide and document care for clients with psychiatric diagnoses?**
- **What measurement criteria would you use to determine that the care you provide to psychiatric clients meets each of the standards?**
- **Why is a common vocabulary to describe psychiatric–mental health nursing care important?**

MediaLink 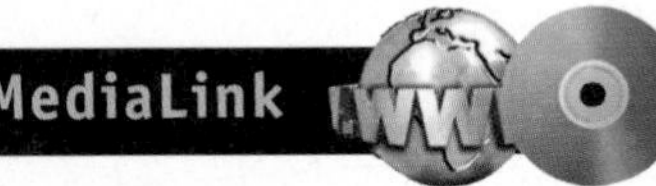 www.prenhall.com/kneisl

Additional resources for this chapter can be found on the Student CD-ROM accompanying this textbook, and on the Companion Website at www.prenhall.com/kneisl. Click on Chapter 7 to select the activities for this chapter.

CD-ROM
- Audio Glossary
- NCLEX Review

Companion Website
- Additional NCLEX Review
- Case Study: Obtaining a Client History

CHAPTER OUTLINE

CROSS REFERENCES

Other topics relevant to this content are: Assessment, Chapter 9; Evidence-based practice, Chapter 3; Scope and Standards of Psychiatric–Mental Health Nursing Practice, Chapter 1; Theories, Chapter 2.

CRITICAL THINKING CHALLENGE

Imagine yourself as nurse manager on an unlocked psychiatric inpatient unit committed to maintaining high standards of care. A 55-year-old man with a 30-year history of alcohol abuse and cigarette smoking is admitted for alcohol detoxification. Because he had pulled out his IV fluids on the preceding shift, managed to get hold of a cigarette lighter in order to smoke, and fallen out of bed, he is now in a posey vest (soft restraints). Your assessment of his current mental status, and his background history and mental status examination results, convince you that he is at risk for harming himself. Your hospital policies justify one-to-one supervision because he meets the criteria. Yet the staff situation is such that you are unable to assign a member of your nursing team to be with him constantly. What are your options? What would you do to provide an acceptable standard of care for this client? ■

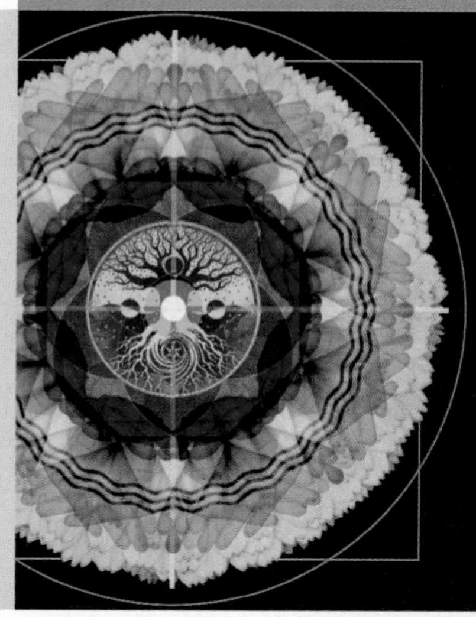

How does a nurse approach the following clinical problems? Obviously, there are no quick and easy formulas for responding to situations that involve genuine human complexities. The 2000 American Nurses Association (ANA) **Standards of Psychiatric–Mental Health Nursing Practice** reflect the current state of knowledge in the field and offer some guidance in providing nursing care to clients like those described below.

CLINICAL EXAMPLE

Diane S., a 23-year-old woman, is admitted to a medical unit with severe anorexia nervosa and thoughts of suicide. She is agitated and tearful and says life looks so bad that she just wants to get out of it.

J. is a 27-year-old man who walked into the hospital emergency room because he sees the walls sparkling and weaving around, he feels like people are laughing at him, and he tastes petroleum in his mouth, which he describes as the "taste of afterbirth." He was on his way to jump off the George Washington Bridge when he saw the hospital and decided to come in for help.

The client is a 52-year-old, disheveled woman dressed in ragged street clothes and wearing a turban on her head. She believes that there are radio waves in her teeth reporting of a plot to have her committed to mental hospitals. She has lived on the streets for the past two years with all her possessions and clothing in four large brown paper bags. She speaks in an uninterrupted monotone and is hostile toward the nurse.

The word *process* suggests movement toward a goal in phases or stages. The **nursing process** is the "foundation of clinical decision making and encompasses all significant action taken by nurses in providing developmentally and culturally relevant psychiatric–mental health care to all patients" (American Nurses Association [ANA], 2000). It is adapted from the scientific approach to problem solving. The steps are depicted in ■ Figure 7–1.

This chapter describes the ways that the nursing process approach is applied in psychiatric–mental health nursing practice. We urge that the nursing process become the way in which you think about clients, with the human responses discussed in other chapters of this text. Nursing process is currently used in most nursing curricula and included in most nurse practice acts. The nursing process is flexible and adaptable. It can be applied in a variety of settings with individual clients, families, groups, and aggregates. It requires you to use judgment and creativity in caring for clients in an organized and systematic way.

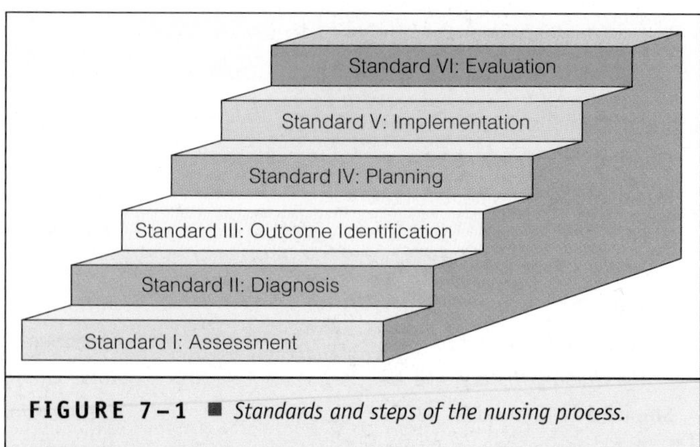

FIGURE 7–1 ■ *Standards and steps of the nursing process.*

Standards of Psychiatric–Mental Health Nursing Practice

The six standards of psychiatric and mental health nursing practice (ANA, 2000) are the focus of this chapter. Together they guide the nurse in the use of the nursing process to make clinical decisions in the practice of psychiatric–mental health nursing.

STANDARD I: ASSESSMENT

The psychiatric–mental health nurse collects patient health care data.

Rationale

The assessment interview, which requires linguistically and culturally effective communication skills, interviewing, behavioral observation, record review, and comprehensive assessment of the patient and relevant systems, enables the psychiatric–mental health nurse to make sound clinical judgments and plan appropriate interventions with the patient.

Measurement Criteria

Criteria you can use to judge that Standard I have been met are:

1. The priority of data collection is determined by the patient's immediate condition or need.
2. The data may include but are not limited to the patient's:
   a. ability to remain safe and not be a danger to oneself and others.
   b. central complaint, symptoms, or focus or concern.
   c. physical, developmental, cognitive, mental, and emotional health status.
   d. demographic profile and history of health patterns, illnesses, and past treatments.
   e. family, social, cultural, race, ethnicity, and community systems.
   f. daily activities, functional health status, substance use, health habits, and social roles, including work and sexual functioning.
   g. interpersonal relationships, communication skills, and coping patterns.

h. spiritual, religious, or philosophical beliefs and values.
i. economic, political, legal, and environmental factors affecting health.
j. significant support systems and community resources, both available and underutilized.
k. health beliefs and practices.
l. knowledge, satisfaction, and motivation to change, related to health.
m. strengths and competencies that can be used to promote health.
n. current and past medications, including prescribed and over-the-counter.
o. medication interactions and history of side effects.
p. complementary therapies used to treat health and mental illness.
q. other contributing factors that influence health and mental health.

3. Pertinent data are collected from multiple sources using various developmentally and culturally appropriate assessment techniques, standardized instruments, and diagnostic and laboratory tests. Multiple sources of assessment data can include not only the patient, but also family, social network, other health care clinicians, past and current medical records, and community agencies and systems (with consideration of the patient's confidentiality).
4. The patient, significant others, and interdisciplinary team members are involved in the assessment process and data analysis.
5. The patient and significant others are informed of their respective roles and responsibilities in the assessment process and data analysis.
6. The assessment process is systematic and ongoing.
7. The data collection is based on clinical judgment to ensure that relevant and necessary data are collected.
8. The database is synthesized, prioritized, and documented in a retrievable form.

Data collection requires astute observation, purposeful listening, a broad knowledge of human behavior, and an understanding of what needs to be known and where to obtain the information. The tools used in psychiatric assessment of individual clients include the following:

- Psychiatric history
- Mental status examination
- Psychosocial assessment, including culture
- Neurologic assessment
- Psychologic testing

These assessment tools, among others, are discussed in Chapter 9.

Subjective Data

Subjective data are reported by the client and significant others in their own words. An example is the **chief complaint** expressed by clients in the course of an intake interview or psychiatric history. Here are some examples of chief complaints:

CLINICAL EXAMPLE

I was in "warp 5" and pretending to be an undercover cop.

My brother doesn't think I take good enough care of myself.

My husband has been beating me and I think I am losing my mind.

Objective Data

Objective data are collected and verified by people other than the client and family. Here are some examples:

- Physical examination findings, such as hearing loss.
- Neurologic examination findings, such as those observed when testing for reflexes or observing for tremors.
- Results of psychometric tests, such as the Temporal and Personal Orientation Test or the Global Cognitive Function and Language Comprehension Tests used to assess functional status among the elderly.
- Scores on rating scales developed to quantify the severity of disabilities among the chronically mentally ill.
- Laboratory test results, including complete blood count, sedimentation rate, blood chemistry, thyroid function studies, serum vitamin B_{12}, folate levels, computed tomography (CT) brain scan, chest x-ray films, and electrocardiograms.

The Nursing History

The nursing history is the foremost method of collecting data from the primary source (the client). Nursing histories summarize client information that the nurse can use to individualize care. They differ from medical or psychiatric histories, which are records of previous illness and hospitalizations, in that they focus on *client perceptions and expectations* related to their illness, hospitalization, and care.

The **primary data source** is the client. **Secondary data sources** include laboratory and psychologic test results, family members, and other members of the mental health team. Together, these data sources provide a rationale for determining the client's nursing diagnosis direction for identifying outcomes, and a basis for planning, implementing, and evaluating nursing care. The assessment phase of the nursing process culminates in the formulation of a nursing diagnosis.

STANDARD II: DIAGNOSIS

The psychiatric–mental health nurse analyzes the assessment data in determining diagnoses.

Rationale

The basis for providing psychiatric–mental health nursing care is the recognition and identification of patterns of response to actual or potential psychiatric illnesses, mental health problems, and potential comorbid physical illnesses.

MediaLink 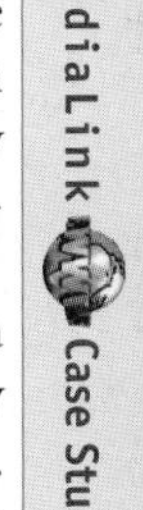 Case Study: Obtaining a Client History

Measurement Criteria

Criteria you can use to judge that Standard II have been met are:

1. Diagnoses and potential problem statements are derived from assessment data.
2. Interpersonal, systematic, or environmental circumstances that affect the mental well-being of the individual, family, or community are identified.
3. The diagnosis is based on an accepted framework that supports the psychiatric–mental health nursing knowledge and judgment used in analyzing the data.
4. Diagnoses conform to accepted classifications systems, such as NANDA or other nursing classifications, *International Classification of Diseases and Statistical Manual of Mental Diseases* (WHO 1993), and *The Diagnostic and Statistical Manual of Mental Disorders, IV Edition* (APA 1994) used in the practice setting.
5. Diagnoses and risk factors are discussed and verified with the patient, significant others, and other health care clinicians when appropriate and possible.
6. Diagnoses identify actual or potential psychiatric illness and mental health problems of patients.
7. Diagnoses and clinical impressions are documented in a manner that facilitates the identification of patient outcomes and their use in the plan of care and research.

Note, however that the World Health Organization and the American Psychiatric Association updated both the *International Classification of Disease* and the *Diagnostic and Statistical Manual* in the year 2000.

NANDA Diagnoses in Psychiatric Nursing

Since 1973 NANDA has been the formal organization that reviews and endorses regularly updated lists of accepted diagnoses used to describe client problems using a standardized language. The 2003–2004 list of nursing diagnoses appears in Box 7–1. Asterisks indicate those most commonly identified among psychiatric clients according to the authors of this text. Wilkinson (2000) states that:

> Nursing diagnosis highlights critical thinking and decision-making and provides a consistent and universally understood terminology among nurses working in various settings. . . . (p. ix)

The increasing use of computerized client records requires a concise, standardized language for labeling client problems. Nursing diagnoses, according to the most recent NANDA taxonomy, may be actual or potential problems that are called "Risk for." The following clinical example illustrates the components of a NANDA nursing diagnosis made with a psychiatric client.

CLINICAL EXAMPLE

Scott is a student of economics preparing to apply to law school. He appears at the campus mental health clinic complaining of difficulty sleeping; a vague, uneasy feeling of dread and apprehension; difficulty working on his final course papers; irritability; and hypervigilance. From time to time, he is sweaty and feels his heart pounding. He spends a lot of time ruminating about the wrongs done to him and tends to blame his parents and teachers for his distress. He describes himself as "stressed out" and smokes pot to calm down almost every day.

Scott clearly meets the definition for anxiety defined by NANDA as "a vague, uneasy feeling of discomfort or dread accompanied by an autonomic response; the source is often nonspecific or unknown to the individual; a feeling of apprehension caused by anticipation of danger."

Scott's diminished productivity, insomnia, and vigilance are *behavioral* defining characteristics; his distress and irritability are *affective* defining characteristics. His insomnia and sense of his heart pounding can be viewed as *physiologic* defining characteristics. Focus on the self, rumination, and his tendency to blame others all exemplify *cognitive* defining characteristics. It is important that the nurse assess related factors such as stress due to law school applications and the college senior projects, unconscious conflict about his goals in life, unmet needs, and the impact of substance abuse on his anxiety level.

Chapters throughout this text illustrate NANDA diagnoses common to clients with major DSM-IV-TR mental disorders, vulnerable populations, and developmental age groups.

Relationship of NANDA Diagnoses to DSM-IV-TR Diagnoses

The standard interdisciplinary psychiatric diagnosis manual text revision or DSM-IV-TR (APA, 2000) is used by the whole mental health team. DSM-IV-TR provides a label for a client's psychiatric disorder and thus facilitates communication among team members. The NANDA diagnosis for a psychiatric client is the conceptualization of a client's human response from the unique nursing perspective. Psychiatric–mental health nurses must be knowledgeable about both psychiatric diagnostic nomenclature and the expanding efforts of nurses to develop our own diagnostic nomenclature. Both are essential for communication with colleagues and for developing an individualized nursing care plan. The Nursing Self-Awareness feature on page 136 raises some issues on the trend toward standardized nomenclatures that you may want to think about and discuss with your peers. ■ Table 7–1 on page 137 compares a DSM-IV-TR diagnosis with related psychiatric nursing diagnoses according to NANDA.

STANDARD III: OUTCOME IDENTIFICATION

The psychiatric–mental health nurse identifies expected outcomes individualized to the patient.

Rationale

Within the context of providing nursing care, the ultimate goal is to influence mental health outcomes and improve the patient's health status.

BOX 7–1 2003–2004 NANDA-Approved Nursing Diagnoses

Activity Intolerance
Activity Intolerance, Risk for
Adaptive Capacity: Intracranial, Decreased
*Adjustment, Impaired
Airway Clearance, Ineffective
Anxiety
Anxiety, Death
Aspiration, Risk for
Attachment, Parent/Infant/Child, Risk for Impaired
*Body Image, Disturbed
Body Temperature: Imbalanced, Risk for
Bowel Incontinence
Breastfeeding, Effective
Breastfeeding, Ineffective
Breastfeeding, Interrupted
Breathing Pattern, Ineffective
Cardiac Output, Decreased
*Caregiver Role Strain
*Caregiver Role Strain, Risk for
Communication, Readiness for Enhanced
*Communication: Verbal, Impaired
*Confusion, Acute
*Confusion, Chronic
Constipation
Constipation, Perceived
Constipation, Risk for
*Coping: Community, Ineffective
*Coping: Community, Readiness for Enhanced
*Coping, Defensive
*Coping: Family, Compromised
*Coping: Family, Disabled
Coping: Family, Readiness for Enhanced
Coping (Individual), Readiness for Enhanced
Coping, Ineffective
Decisional Conflict (Specify)
*Denial, Ineffective
Dentition, Impaired
*Development: Delayed, Risk for
Diarrhea
Disuse Syndrome, Risk for
Diversional Activity, Deficient
Dysreflexia, Autonomic
Dysreflexia, Autonomic, Risk for
Energy Field, Disturbed
Environmental Interpretation Syndrome, Impaired
Failure to Thrive, Adult
Falls, Risk for
*Family Processes, Dysfunctional: Alcoholism
*Family Processes, Interrupted
Family Processes, Readiness for Enhanced
*Fatigue
*Fear
Fluid Balance, Readiness for Enhanced
Fluid Volume, Deficient
Fluid Volume, Deficient, Risk for
Fluid Volume, Excess
Fluid Volume, Imbalanced, Risk for
Gas Exchange, Impaired
*Grieving, Anticipatory
*Grieving, Dysfunctional
Growth, Disproportionate, Risk for
Growth and Development, Delayed
Health Maintenance, Ineffective
Health Seeking Behaviors (Specify)
*Home Maintenance, Impaired
*Hopelessness
Hyperthermia
Hypothermia
Identity: Personal, Disturbed
Infant Behavior, Disorganized
Infant Behavior: Disorganized, Risk for
Infant Behavior: Organized, Readiness for Enhanced
Infant Feeding Pattern, Ineffective
Infection, Risk for
*Injury, Risk for
*Knowledge, Deficient (Specify)
Knowledge (specify), Readiness for Enhanced
Latex Allergy Response
Latex Allergy Response, Risk for
*Loneliness, Risk for
*Memory, Impaired
Mobility: Bed, Impaired
Mobility: Physical, Impaired
Mobility: Wheelchair, Impaired
Nausea
Neurovascular Dysfunction: Peripheral, Risk for
*Noncompliance (Specify)
*Nutrition, Imbalanced: Less than Body Requirements
Nutrition, Imbalanced: More than Body Requirements
Nutrition, Imbalanced: More than Body Requirements, Risk for
Nutrition, Readiness for Enhanced
Oral Mucous Membrane, Impaired
Pain, Acute
Pain, Chronic
Parenting, Impaired
Parenting, Readiness for Enhanced
Parenting, Risk for Impaired
Perioperative Positioning Injury, Risk for
Poisoning, Risk for
*Post-Trauma Syndrome
*Post-Trauma Syndrome, Risk for
Powerlessness
*Powerlessness, Risk for
Protection, Ineffective
*Rape-Trauma Syndrome
*Rape-Trauma Syndrome: Compound Reaction
*Rape-Trauma Syndrome: Silent Reaction
Relocation Stress Syndrome
*Relocation Stress Syndrome, Risk for
Role Conflict, Parental
*Role Performance, Ineffective
*Self-Care Deficit: Bathing/Hygiene
*Self-Care Deficit: Dressing/Grooming
Self-Care Deficit: Feeding
Self-Care Deficit: Toileting
Self-Concept, Readiness for Enhanced
*Self-Esteem, Chronic Low
*Self-Esteem, Situational Low
*Self-Esteem, Risk for Situational Low
Self-Mutilation
Self-Mutilation, Risk for
*Sensory Perception, Disturbed (Specify: Visual, Auditory, Kinesthetic, Gustatory, Tactile, Olfactory)
*Sexual Dysfunction
*Sexuality Patterns, Ineffective
Skin Integrity, Impaired
Skin Integrity, Risk for Impaired
*Sleep Deprivation
*Sleep Pattern Disturbed
Sleep, Readiness for Enhanced
*Social Interaction, Impaired
*Social Isolation
*Sorrow, Chronic
*Spiritual Distress
*Spiritual Distress, Risk for
*Spiritual Well-Being, Readiness for Enhanced
Spontaneous Ventilation, Impaired
Sudden Infant Death Syndrome, Risk for
Suffocation, Risk for
Suicide, Risk for
Surgical Recovery, Delayed
Swallowing, Impaired
Therapeutic Regimen Management: Community, Ineffective
Therapeutic Regimen Management, Effective
Therapeutic Regimen Management: Family, Ineffective
Therapeutic Regimen Management, Ineffective
Therapeutic Regimen Management, Readiness for Enhanced
Thermoregulation, Ineffective

(continued)

BOX 7-1 **2003–2004 NANDA-Approved Nursing Diagnoses *(continued)***

*Thought Processes, Disturbed
Tissue Integrity, Impaired
Tissue Perfusion, Ineffective (Specify type: renal, cerebral, cardiopulmonary, gastrointestinal, peripheral)
Tissue Perfusion, Ineffective (Peripheral)
Transfer Ability, Impaired
*Trauma, Risk for
*Unilateral Neglect
Urinary Elimination, Impaired
Urinary Elimination, Readiness for Enhanced
Urinary Incontinence, Functional
Urinary Incontinence, Reflex
Urinary Incontinence, Stress
Urinary Incontinence, Total
Urinary Incontinence, Urge
Urinary Incontinence, Risk for Urge
Urinary Retention
Ventilatory Weaning Response, Dysfunctional
*Violence: Other-Directed, risk for
*Violence: Self-Directed, risk for
Walking, Impaired
Wandering

*Asterisks indicate those most commonly identified among psychiatric clients.

Source: NANDA Nursing Diagnoses: Definitions and Classification, 2003-2004. Philadelphia: North American Nursing Diagnosis Association. Used with permission.

Measurement Criteria

Criteria you can use to judge that Standard III has been met are:

1. Expected outcomes are derived from the diagnoses.
2. Expected outcomes are patient-oriented, evidence-based therapeutically sound, realistic, attainable, and cost-effective.
3. Expected outcomes are documented as measurable goals using standard classifications when available.
4. Expected outcomes are formulated by the nurse and the patient, significant others, and interdisciplinary team members when possible.
5. Expected outcomes are realistic in relation to the patient's present and potential capabilities and quality of life.
6. Expected outcomes are identified with consideration of the associated benefits and costs.
7. Expected outcomes estimate a time for attainment.
8. Expected outcomes provide direction for continuity of care.
9. Expected outcomes reflect current scientific knowledge in mental health care.
10. Expected outcomes serve as a record of change in the patient's health status.

Iowa Project Nursing Outcomes Classification

The responsibility for total quality management (TQM) and an increasing emphasis on cost containment along with requirements established by the Joint Commission on the Accreditation of Healthcare Organizations (JCAHO) have resulted in a number of outcome classifications for use in clinical and practical evaluation research. The most well known of the Nursing-Sensitive Outcomes Classification (NOC) systems is the one developed under the leadership of a research team at the University of Iowa. NOC as used in this text is a comprehensive list of standardized concepts, definitions, and measures that describe patient/client outcomes influenced by nursing interventions. The most recent classification of 260 NOC outcomes have been linked to NANDA diagnoses. Such linkages assist nurses in identifying possible outcomes when a diagnosis is made. Field testing of the current outcomes classification emphasizing reliability, validity, sensitivity, specificity, and usefulness is ongoing. Work continues on the NOC system so that nursing's contribution to health care, including mental health care will be documented and visible. Box 7–2 illustrates NOC outcomes for the NANDA diagnosis of anxiety as it relates to Scott, the subject of the clinical example presented

***Nursing* SELF-AWARENESS** **Does Standardized Terminology Conflict with Individualized Client Care?**

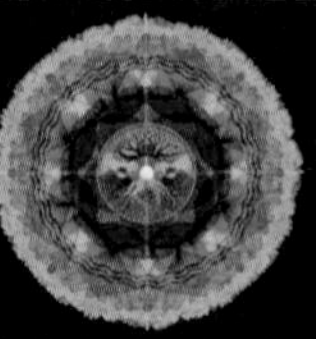

This textbook challenges psychiatric–mental health nurses to engage in reflective and creative responses to complex mind–body–spirit problems. We are challenged to face issues of global mental health with intelligence, stamina, creativity, and moral courage. The word *courage* is rooted in a French word meaning "heart." In this chapter and in this book, you are presented with a vocabulary of standardized language including NANDA, NIC, NOC, and DSM-IV-TR. As you know, language and symbols are critical in creating the assumptions, emotional climate, and behavioral norms that define people and their environments and what is possible within them. Reflect on your own ideas about the following questions:

- Do you believe that any standardized vocabulary dismisses the unique stories of clients and their families?
- What do you think are the advantages and disadvantages of using an accepted language or vocabulary when working as a mental health team member?
- When evaluating the categories and language in NANDA, NIC, NOC, and DSM-IV-TR, do you think they adequately portray the diversity of people's lived experience and contribute to nurses' ability to plan effective care?
- Do you think that standardized language systems are compatible with bringing "heart" to psychiatric–mental health nursing?

TABLE 7–1 Comparison of DSM-IV-TR and NANDA Diagnoses

DSM-IV-TR Diagnosis	NANDA Diagnoses
300.02 Generalized Anxiety Disorder	Anxiety
	Coping: Individual, Ineffective
	Fatigue
	Fear
	Role Performance, Altered
	Sleep Pattern Disturbance

previously in this chapter. Other NOC outcomes appear throughout this text.

STANDARD IV: PLANNING

Standard IV states that the psychiatric–mental health nurse develops a plan of care that is negotiated among clients, nurses, family, and health care team and prescribes evidence-based interventions to attain expected outcomes.

Rationale

A plan of care is used to guide therapeutic intervention systematically, document progress, and achieve the expected client outcomes.

Measurement Criteria

Criteria that you can use to judge that Standard IV have been met are:

1. The plan is individualized according to the patient's characteristics, needs, health problems and condition, and
    a. Identifies priorities of care in relation to expected outcomes.
    b. Identifies effective interventions to achieve outcomes.
    c. Specifies evidence-based interventions that reflect current best practices and research.
    d. Reflects the patient's motivation, health beliefs, and functional capabilities.
    e. Includes an educational program related to the patient's health problems, stress management, treatment regimen, relapse prevention, self-care activities, and quality of life.
    f. Indicates responsibilities of the nurse, the patient, the family and other significant persons, and the interdisciplinary team members in implementing the plan.
    g. Gives direction to patient care activities designated by the nurse to the family, significant others, and other care clinicians.
    h. Provides the appropriate referral and case management to ensure continuity of care.
    i. Considers the benefits and costs of interventions in relation to outcomes.
2. The plan is developed in collaboration with the patient, significant others, and the interdisciplinary team members when appropriate.
3. The plan is documented in a format that allows modification, as necessary, interdisciplinary access to its information, and retrieval of data for analysis and research.

BOX 7–2 NOC Suggested Outcomes

Aggression Control: Ability to restrain assaultive, combative, or destructive behavior toward others

Anxiety Control: Ability to eliminate or reduce feelings of apprehension and tension from an unidentifiable source

Coping: Actions to manage stressors that tax an individual's resources

Impulse Control: Ability to self-restrain compulsive or impulsive behaviors

Self-Mutilation Restraint: Ability to refrain from intentional self-inflicted injury (nonlethal)

Social Interaction Skills: An individual's use of effective interaction behaviors

Source: Wilkinson, J. M. (2000). *Nursing diagnosis handbook* (p. 23). Pearson Education/PH College.

Hints for Negotiating a Plan of Care

The first step is to determine whether to try to convince the client that your plan is the right plan or to alter your goals and plan. One way to do so is to ask clients what their goals are and how you can help them achieve their goals. Some clients respond that they just came along to appease a significant other who is the one with the real problem. Others believe they are there for a "rest" or a "checkup." Some want to be taken care of and protected, and some believe they have been tricked or betrayed and locked up against their will. Having asked, you must *listen*. Sometimes the simple experience of being heard and understood without being invalidated and dismissed out of hand becomes the basis for subsequent negotiations and eventual agreement about mutually determined goals and a plan to achieve them. One such plan appears in the Using Research Evidence feature on page 138.

STANDARD V: IMPLEMENTATION

Standard V states that the psychiatric–mental health nurse implements the interventions identified in the plan of care.

Rationale

In implementing the plan of care, psychiatric–mental health nurses use a wide range of interventions designed to prevent mental and physical illness, and promote, maintain, and restore mental and physical health. Psychiatric–mental health nurses select interventions according to their level of practice. At the basic level, the nurse may select counseling, milieu therapy, promotion of self-care activities, intake screening, and evaluation of psychobiologic interventions, health teaching, case management, health promotion and health maintenance crisis-

USING RESEARCH EVIDENCE

Ruby Ann is a 19-year-old African-American mother of three small children. She lives with her 30-year-old boyfriend in a one-room apartment located in a rough area of a major southern city. Ruby Ann has been treated on numerous occasions in the city hospital's emergency room for bruises, lacerations, and broken bones, which she attributed to falling down the steps of her building. She has called 911 four times in the past year because her boyfriend was threatening to kill her and her babies. Ruby Ann appears at the battered women's shelter where you are the psychiatric–mental health nurse responsible for providing her care. Your assessment interview reveals that Ruby Ann has experienced severe and frequent verbal and physical abuse including rape. She reports that she is unable to sleep, has no appetite, has lost 20 pounds over the past 9 months, and suffers from anxiety and depression. Ruby Ann also confides that her spiritual beliefs had sustained her despite her suffering and distress. She says, "If God wasn't with me, I wouldn't have got outta there, but I'm startin to doubt Him cause how could He let all this happen to me and my babies!"

Based on these data and research on the relationship between spiritual beliefs and distressing symptoms among battered women, your care plan for Ruby Ann includes the following:

Nursing Diagnosis: **Spiritual Distress, Risk for**
Outcome: **Hope, Spiritual Well-Being**
Interventions: **Support Group** (to prevent isolation), **Presence** (to offer comfort and compassion), **Resiliency Promotion, Identification of Resources that have been a Source of Spiritual Support in the Past** (prayer, church attendance, choir)

Addressing Ruby Ann's need for spiritual support holds the potential for reducing her feelings of shame, fear, and helplessness according to research cited below:

Humphreys, J. (2000). Spirituality and distress in sheltered battered women. *Journal of Nursing Scholarship, 23*(3), 2000, 273–278.

management, and a variety of other approaches to meet the mental health needs of clients (See Chapter 1). In addition to the intervention options available to the basic-level psychiatric–mental health nurse, at the advanced level the certified specialist may provide consultation, engage in psychotherapy, and prescribe pharmacologic agents where permitted by state statutes or regulations.

Measurement Criteria

Criteria that you can use to judge that Standard V have been met are:

1. A therapeutic nurse–patient relationship is established and maintained throughout treatment.
2. Interventions are based on research when available.
3. Interventions are implemented according to the established plan of care.
4. Interventions are performed according to the psychiatric–mental health nurse's level of education and practice.
5. Interventions are performed in a safe, timely, ethical, and appropriate manner.
6. Interventions are modified based on continued assessment of the patient's response to treatment and other clinical indicators of effectiveness.
7. Interventions are documented in a format that is related to patient outcomes, accessible to the interdisciplinary team, and retrievable for future data analysis and research.

Iowa Classification of Nursing Interventions

Iowa Classification of Nursing Interventions (NIC) is a standardized vocabulary and classification of nursing interventions. The NIC language includes all interventions performed by nurses, both independent and collaborate and through direct and indirect care. Each NIC intervention consists of a label name, a definition, and a set of actions that go into the delivery of the intervention and a short list of background literature. There are a total of 486 interventions grouped into 7 domains. The domains (see ■ Figure 7–2) are:

1. Physiologic: Basic
2. Physiologic: Complex
3. Behavioral
4. Safety
5. Family
6. Health System
7. Community

An example of NIC for NANDA anxiety diagnosis appears in Box 7–3.

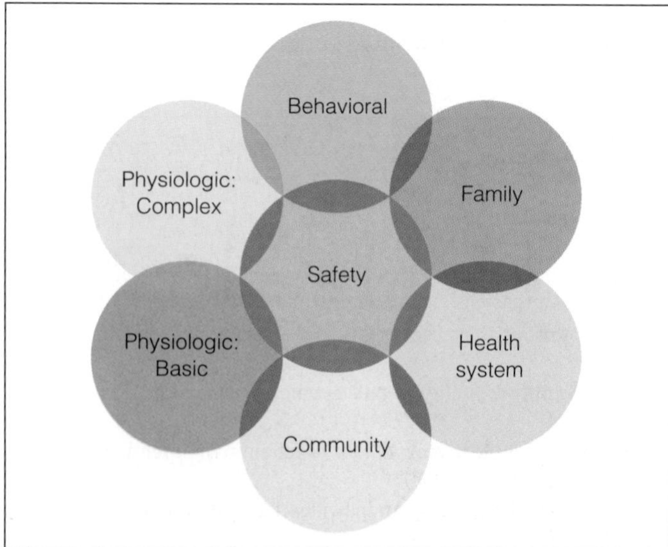

FIGURE 7–2 ■ *Domains of Nursing Intervention Classification (NIC).*

BOX 7-3 One Example of an NIC Intervention

Anxiety Reduction

Definition: Minimizing apprehension, dread, foreboding, or uneasiness related to an identified source of anticipated danger

Activities

Use a calm, reassuring approach
Clearly state expectations for patient's behavior
Explain all procedures, including sensations likely to be experienced during the procedure
Seek to understand the patient's perspective of a stressful situation
Provide factual information concerning diagnosis, treatment, and prognosis
Stay with patient to promote safety and reduce fear
Encourage patients to stay with child, as appropriate
Provide objects that symbolize safeness
Administer back rub/neck rub, as appropriate
Encourage noncompetitive activities, as appropriate
Keep treatment equipment out of sight
Listen attentively
Reinforce behavior, as appropriate
Create an atmosphere to facilitate trust
Encourage verbalization of feelings, perceptions, and fears
Identify when level of anxiety changes
Provide diversional activities geared toward the reduction of tension
Help patient identify situations that precipitate anxiety
Control stimuli, as appropriate, for patient needs
Support the use of appropriate defense mechanisms
Assist patient to articulate a realistic description of an upcoming event
Determine patient's decision-making ability
Instruct patient on the use of relaxation techniques
Administer medications to reduce anxiety, as appropriate

Source: Reprinted from *Nursing interventions classifications,* 3rd ed., McCloskey, J. C. & Bulechek, G. M. Copyright 2000, with permission from Elsevier Science.

Measurement Criteria

Criteria that you can use to judge whether Standard VI have been met are:

STANDARD VI: EVALUATION

The psychiatric–mental health nurse evaluates the patient's progress in attaining expected outcomes.

Rationale

Nursing care is a dynamic process involving change in the patient's health status over time, giving rise to the need for data, different diagnoses, and modifications in the plan of care. Therefore, evaluation is a continuous process of appraising the effect of nursing and the treatment regimen on the patient's health status and expected outcomes.

Measurement Criteria

1. Evaluation is systematic, ongoing, and criterion-based.
2. The patient, family or significant others, and other health care clinicians are involved in the evaluation process, as possible, to ascertain the patient's level of satisfaction with care and evaluate the benefits and costs associated with the treatment process.
3. The effectiveness of interventions in relation to outcomes is evaluated, using standardized methods as appropriate.
4. The patient's responses to treatment are documented in a format that is related to expected outcomes, accessible to the interdisciplinary team, and retrievable for data analysis and future research.
5. Ongoing assessment data are used to revise diagnoses, outcomes, and the plan of care as needed.
6. Revisions in the diagnoses, outcomes, and plan of care are documented.
7. The revised plan provides for the continuity of care.

Example of Using NOC Language to Evaluate

In the clinical example of Scott, discussed earlier in this chapter, a nursing care plan would include the following evaluation criteria using NOC language.

- *Anxiety* relieved, as evidenced by consistently demonstrating Aggression Control, Anxiety Control, Coping, Impulse Control, Self-Mutilation Restraint, and substantially effective Social Interaction Skills
- Demonstrates Anxiety Control, as evidenced by the following indicators (specify 1–5: never, rarely, sometimes, often, or consistently demonstrated):

  Plans coping strategies for stressful situations
  Maintains role performance
  Reports absence of sensory perceptual disorders
  Reports absence of physical manifestations of anxiety
  Behavioral manifestations of anxiety absent

Other Examples. Patient will:

- Continue necessary activities even though anxiety persists
- Demonstrate ability to focus on new knowledge and skills
- Identify symptoms that are indicators of own anxiety
- Not demonstrate aggressive behaviors
- Communicate needs and negative feelings appropriately

Such standardized language enhances the clarity of communication among nurses caring for a client like Scott.

Putting Psychiatric–Mental Health Nursing Standards into Practice by Using the Nursing Process

The contemporary climate for psychiatric–mental health care is one that demands accountability in terms of client outcomes and cost containment. While the therapeutic use of self and the art of caring remain the cornerstones of practice. They are based on an informed decision-making process that has a theoretical and research base. Applying the nursing process, according to the ANA standards, is a critical competency basic to quality professional practice in psychiatric–mental health nursing.

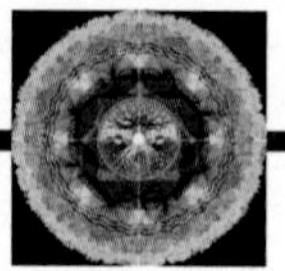

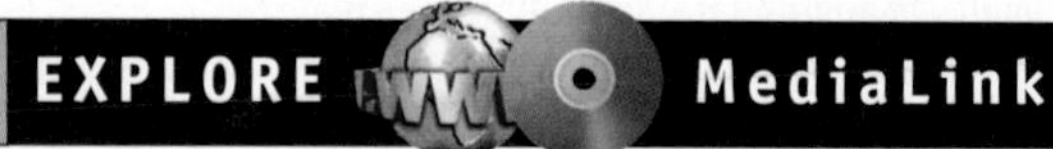

NCLEX review, case studies, and other interactive resources for this chapter can be found on the Companion Website at http://www.prenhall.com/kneisl. Click on Chapter 7 to select the activities for this chapter.

For animations, video tutorials, more NCLEX review questions, and an audio glossary, access the accompanying CD-ROM in this textbook.

BIBLIOGRAPHY

American Nurses Association (2000). *Scope and standards of psychiatric–mental health nursing practice*. Washington, DC: Author.

American Psychiatric Association (2000). *Diagnostic and statistical manual of mental disorders* (4th ed., Text Revision) (DSM-IV-TR). Washington, DC: Author.

American Psychiatric Association. (1994). *Diagnostic and statistical manual of mental disorders* (4th ed.) (DSM-IV). Washington, DC: Author.

Humphreys, J. (2000). Spirituality and distress in sheltered battered women. *Journal of Nursing Scholarship, 32*(3), 273–278.

Johnson, M., Maas, M., & Moorhead, S. (2001). *Nursing diagnoses, outcomes and interventions (NANDA, NOC and NIC linkages)*. St. Louis: Mosby.

Johnson, M., Maas, M., & Moorhead, S. (2001). *Nursing outcomes classification (NOC)*. St. Louis: Mosby.

McCloskey, J. C., & Bulechek, G. M. (2000). *Nursing interventions classification (NIC)* (3rd ed.). St. Louis: Mosby.

North American Nursing Diagnosis Association. (1999). *Nursing diagnoses: Definitions and classifications*. Philadelphia: Author.

Wilkinson, J. M. (2000). *Nursing diagnosis handbook*. Upper Saddle River, NJ: Prentice Hall.

World Health Organization (1993). *International classification of diseases and statistical manual of mental diseases*. Washington, DC: Author.

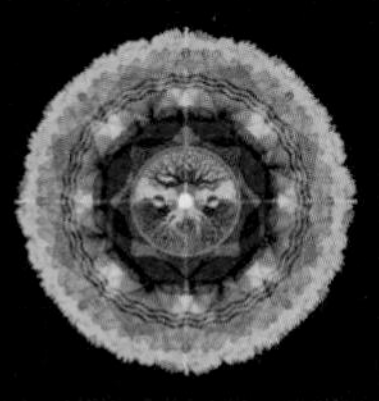

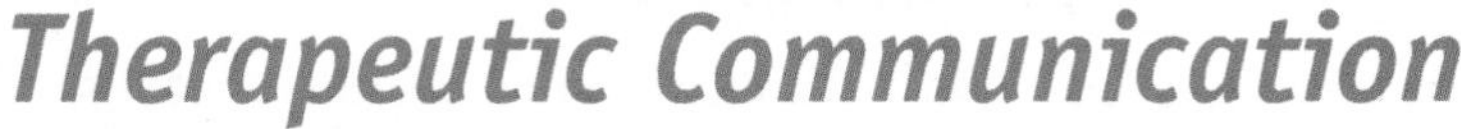

Therapeutic Communication

CAROL REN KNEISL

8

Chapter EIGHT

FOCUS QUESTIONS

- What factors influence the process of human communication?
- Why is nonverbal communication as important as verbal communication?
- How do the theories of human communication discussed here relate to humanistic psychiatric–mental health nursing?
- Why are the concepts of facilitative communication essential ingredients of interpersonal relationships?
- How do the skills discussed here foster effective communication throughout the nursing process?

KEY TERMS

feedback
illusion
interpersonal communication
intrapersonal communication
mixed message
neologism
nonverbal communication
overload
perception
subculture
tangential reply
underload

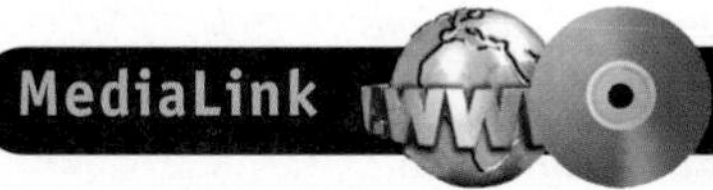

Additional resources for this chapter can be found on the Student CD-ROM accompanying this textbook, and on the Companion Website at www.prenhall.com/kneisl. Click on Chapter 8 to select the activities for this chapter.

CD-ROM
- Audio Glossary
- NCLEX Review

Companion Website
- Additional NCLEX Review
- Case Study: Communication Skills

CHAPTER OUTLINE

CROSS REFERENCES

Other topics related to this content are: Assessment, Chapter 9; Confidentiality of communication, Chapter 10; Qualities of effective psychiatric–mental health nursing, Chapter 1; Role of human values in the communication of the nurse, Chapter 1; Therapeutic nurse–client relationship, Chapter 28.

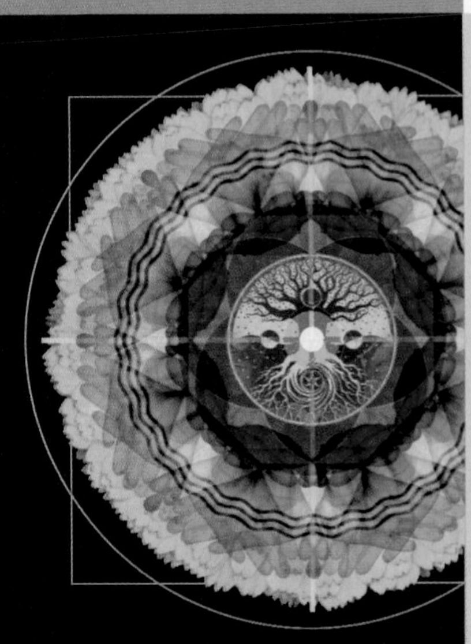

CRITICAL THINKING CHALLENGE

You are about to embark on your first inpatient psychiatric nursing experience. You feel anxious because although you've read the facilitative communication techniques described in this chapter, you feel uncomfortable about using them. They seem artificial, stilted, and "not you." What can you do to help make your psychiatric–mental health nursing experience a positive learning experience for you as well as for your clients? ■

When John Bowlby discovered in the 1950s that infants in foundling homes were literally dying for lack of contact and affection, the scientific community began to attach new importance to the old saying that *people need people.* We recognize today that the mechanism for establishing, maintaining, and improving human contacts is interpersonal communication. Communication is a very special process and the most significant of human behaviors. Moreover, it is the main method for implementing the nursing process.

When they tell "their story," clients explain themselves, the events of their lives, and the circumstances they face. Psychiatric nurses help clients tell their stories, help them explore the circumstances of their lives, and help them resolve the things that have gone wrong.

Psychiatric–mental health nurses are instructed to engage in "therapeutic use of self." They are told that their "relationship" with a client is the primary therapeutic tool, that they should demonstrate qualities of sensitivity and caring. For many students, like the student in the clinical example below, these instructions are mysterious jargon quite unlike the clear-cut step-by-step procedures they learn for some physical treatments.

CLINICAL EXAMPLE

I found myself watching the nurses on the unit and my instructors closely when they talked with the clients. Somehow I thought maybe by imitating things that they did or said I'd figure out what "being therapeutic" was supposed to mean. I knew it had something to do with things the nurse said or didn't say when she talked with the clients. But it all got very fuzzy to me beyond that very elementary grasp of it. I used to latch onto ideas like "Agreeing is untherapeutic. So is giving advice or opinions." The only entries I felt safe in putting down in my process recording were stiff-sounding reflections, like "You sound angry."

The process of communication is complex and has many dimensions. It cannot be reduced to a few simple steps that nurses can memorize and perform.

The Process of Human Communication

Communication is an ongoing, dynamic, and everchanging series of events, each of which affects and is affected by all the others. Communication is not simply the transfer of information or meaning from one human being to another. Meaning cannot be transferred; it must be mutually negotiated, because meaning is influenced by a number of significant factors.

ROLE OF PERCEPTION

A person's image or perception of the world is an essential element in communicating. The term **perception** refers to the experience of sensing, interpreting, and comprehending the world in which one lives. This makes perception a highly personal and internal act.

People process through their senses all the information they have about the world around them. However, seeing is not always believing. Communication specialists have discovered that because of human physiologic limitations, the eye and brain are constantly being tricked into seeing things that are not really what they seem; these are called **illusions.** ■ Figure 8–1 shows an illusion that reflects physiologic constraints. Before continuing to read, stare at Figure 8–1 for 20 seconds. The illustration will appear to swing back and forth. You can verify that the movement is an illusion by checking your visual perception against your tactile sensations.

What people "see" or sense is strongly influenced by many factors. For example, past experiences have prepared us to see things, people, and events in particular ways.

Also, people tend to observe more carefully when a purpose guides the observation. The purposes or reasons for engaging in an observation also determine what we observe. The nurse in an intensive care unit observes a cardiac surgery client differently than a family member does.

Finally, when understandings differ, you and I can look at the same object and see different things. Mental set helps determine how and what a person perceives. Before you read any further, look at the picture of the young woman in ■ Figure 8–2 on page 144. Do you see the silhouette of a young woman? Do you also see the face of an elderly woman? Using the phrase "the picture of the young woman in Figure 8–2" encouraged you to perceive the illustration in a particular way. Now you should also be able to see the elderly woman in the illustration.

As the illustrations demonstrate, the old axiom might be better stated: "Believing is seeing." Because we tend to perceive in

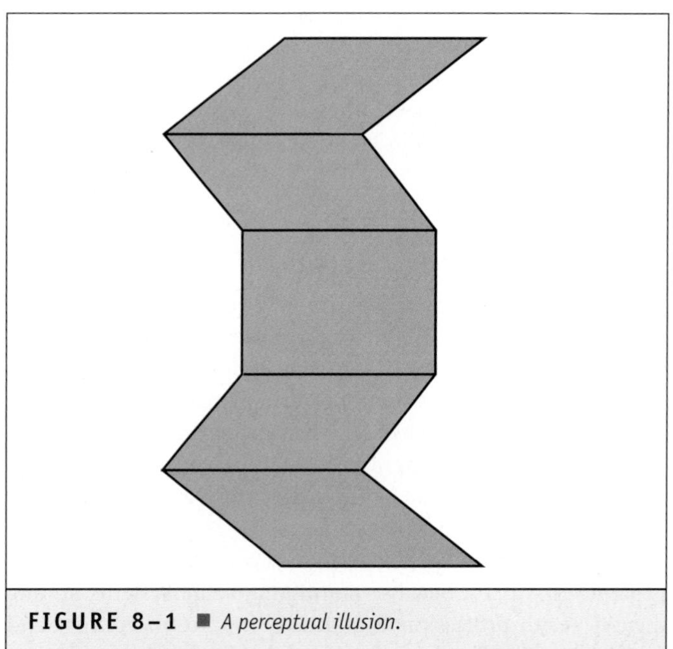

FIGURE 8–1 ■ *A perceptual illusion.*

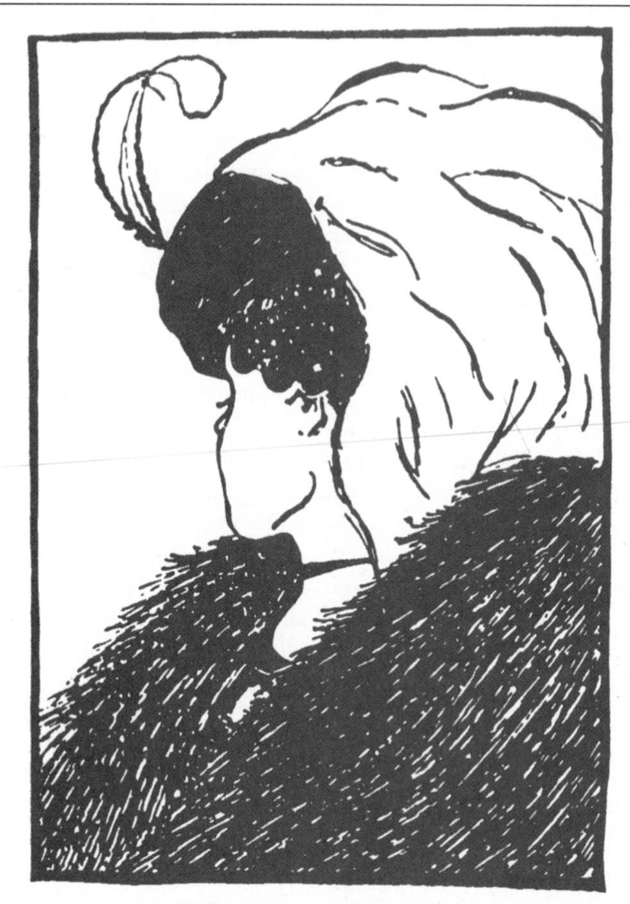

FIGURE 8–2 ■ *The influence of mental set on perception.*

terms of past experiences, expectations, and goals, perceptions may be a prime obstacle to communication. No two individuals perceive the world in exactly the same way, and the meanings of events differ because people's perceptions of them differ. Perceptions of other human beings are of particular importance because human communication is inevitably affected by how we perceive one another. To see others at all as they are, people need to know themselves and to know how the self affects their perceptions of others.

ROLE OF VALUES

Values are concepts of the desirable. People value what is of worth to them. Values influence the process of communication because people's values, like their perceptions, differ.

Value systems differ for a number of reasons. Age is one. Children's values shift when they become teenagers. The college or work experience generally influences values in yet other directions. Marrying or being a parent or grandparent may cause other value changes or shifts.

Psychiatric nurses must ultimately come to terms with the problem of values, because conflicting value systems among mental health professionals expose clients to uncertainty and confusion. Consider the following examples:

CLINICAL EXAMPLE

The parents of a 15-year-old girl were upset to find a small plastic bag of marijuana in her dresser drawer. She had been playing hooky from school and wore jeans that her parents considered sloppy. After a series of lengthy, angry discussions with her parents, she was confined to her room. During this period she refused to eat or drink.

When the teenager was seen by a mental health treatment team, the members' opinions were divided. Some said that her behavior signaled an emotional disturbance. They labeled her antisocial, depressed, and anxious. Others believed the parents were too rigid in attempting to force her to accept their values.

In another instance, a 35-year-old man was firmly committed to prayer. Most of his spare time involved church-related activities. Staff members at a mental health clinic where he sought counseling told him that he was resorting to an early infantile attitude about God as the magic worker.

Clearly, these staff members were influenced by their own values.

The daily roles people take also influence their values. In any one day a man may be a student, husband, father, nurse, citizen, speaker, artist, son, and teacher.

ROLE OF CULTURE

Each culture provides its members with notions about how the world is structured and what it means. These preconceptions, learned at an early age, are so subtle that they often go unrecognized. They nonetheless set limits on communication and interaction with others. Relying on culturally determined generalizations or stereotypes can have profound effects on one's relationships with others.

Communication is culture-bound in a wide variety of ways. The culture and the **subculture** (the culture within the culture) teach people how to communicate through language, hand gestures, clothing, and even in the ways they use the space around them. The nurse who does not know that "run it by me" means to explain something, that a "close-knuckle drill" is a fistfight, or that "he's really phat" means that the person is Pretty Hot And Tempting may be confused by conversations with members of certain subcultures—adolescents and street people, for example. The nurse who overhears two clients talking about "angel dust" is likely to come to erroneous conclusions if unaware that the term refers not to something religious, but to PCP—an animal tranquilizer. In some cultures, belching after dinner is a compliment to the host. In other cultures, belching may be considered uncouth or an insult. When Americans make a circle with thumb and forefinger and extend the other fingers, they mean "OK." To Brazilians, the same gesture is an obscene sign of contempt.

These examples make it obvious that communicating with meaning requires that the participants take culture well into account. How people communicate with others who do not share similar histories, heritages, or cultures is of critical importance in humanistic psychiatric nursing practice.

THE SPOKEN WORD

Verbal language, the ability to utter the spoken word, makes people human and distinguishes them from other animals. Yet problems arise when we discover that words mean different things to different people. That is, *words* do not "mean" something; *people* do.

If communication between nurse and client is to be mutually negotiated, the nurse must understand the four concepts discussed next.

Denotation and Connotation

A *denotative meaning* is one that is in general use by most people who share a common language. A *connotative meaning* usually arises from a person's personal experience. While all Americans are likely to share the same general denotative meaning of the word *pig*, the word may have completely different connotation for a farmer, a consumer of meat, a person of the Moslem faith, an orthodox Jew, a prisoner, and a police officer. These positive and negative connotative meanings can evoke powerful emotions.

Private and Shared Meanings

For communication to take place, meaning must be shared. People can use private meanings to communicate with others only when the parties agree about what the word means. The private meaning then becomes a shared meaning. It is common for families, two friends, or members of larger social groups (military personnel, drug users, adolescents) to use language in highly personal and private ways. Problems arise when the assumption is made that people who are outside the group share these meanings.

People who are schizophrenic may use language in an idiosyncratic way or may use a private, unshared language referred to as **neologisms**. Such people are unaware that others don't share this use of language. People who use neologisms expect to be understood and may become upset when they are not.

CLINICAL EXAMPLE

A young man who was hospitalized on a psychiatric unit complained to other clients and staff members that he had been odenated, *and he became increasingly frustrated and anxious when it became apparent that he wasn't being understood. With some help he was able to explain that he was upset about having been moved to a private room. The room was, he said, so dark and dingy that it looked like a cave. Animals live in caves that are called* dens. *In his view he had been* o-den-ated—*put into a cave.*

In trying to make private meanings shared, make an effort to reach mutual understanding of the client's message. It is insufficient, and quite possibly inaccurate, to attach meaning based solely on the nurse's (or the client's) interpretation of an event, a word or phrase, or a gesture.

NONVERBAL MESSAGES

Most researchers agree that **nonverbal communication** channels carry more social meaning than verbal channels. Nonverbal cues help us judge the reliability of verbal messages more readily, especially in the presence of a **mixed message** (inconsistency between the verbal and nonverbal components).

There is a wide variety in nonverbal channels: body movements, including facial expressions and hand gestures; pitch, rate, and volume of the voice; the use of personal and social space; touch; and the use of cultural artifacts (such as clothing and cosmetics).

Body Movement

The study of body movement as a form of nonverbal communication is called *kinesics*. Facial expressions, gestures, and eye movements are the most common categories.

Facial expressions are the single most important source of nonverbal communication. They generally communicate emotions. The silent film comedians—blank-faced Buster Keaton and comic, endearing Charlie Chaplin—and the great mime Marcel Marceau communicate not only isolated acts but complete sequences of behavior with kinesics alone.

Body movements and gestures provide clues about people and about how they feel toward others. Hand gestures can communicate anxiety, indifference, and impatience, among other things. Foot shuffling and fidgetting may express the desire to escape. Body position gives cues about how open a person is to another person, or how interesting and attractive one person is to another. People tend to position their bodies according to their feelings about the person with whom they are communicating.

Eye contact is another very important cue in communicating. For example, proper sidewalk behavior among Americans is for passers-by to look at each other until they are about eight feet apart. At this distance, both parties look downward or away so they will not appear to be staring. Several common but unstated rules about eye contact are:

- Interaction is invited by staring at another person on the other side of the room. If the other person returns the gaze, the invitation to interact has been accepted. Averting the eyes signals a rejection of the looker's request.
- A person's frank gaze is widely interpreted as positive regard.
- Greater mutual eye contact occurs among friends.
- People who seek eye contact while speaking are usually perceived as believable and earnest.

- If the usual short, intermittent gazes during a conversation are replaced by gazes of longer duration, the person looked at is likely to believe that the person gazing considers the relationship between the two people to be more important than the content of the conversation.

Voice Quality and Nonlanguage Sounds

Voice quality, such as pitch and range, and nonlanguage vocalizations, such as sobbing, laughing, or grunting—noises without linguistic structure—are components in addition to language itself.

Vocal cues can differentiate emotions. Who hasn't heard the injunction, "Don't speak to me in that tone of voice!" Sometimes people use vocal cues to make inferences about personality traits. For example, people who increase the loudness, pitch, timbre (overtones), and rate of their speech are often thought to be active and dynamic. Those who use greater intonation and volume and are fluent are thought to be persuasive. Status cues in speech are based on a combination of word choice, pronunciation, grammar, speech fluency, and articulation, among other factors.

Personal and Social Space

Proxemics is the study of space relationships maintained by people in social interaction. It includes the dimensions of *territoriality* (fixed and permanent territory that is somehow marked off and defended from intrusion) and *personal space* (a portable territory surrounding the self that others are expected not to invade). ■ Figure 8–3 illustrates the various relationships between intimacy and personal space.

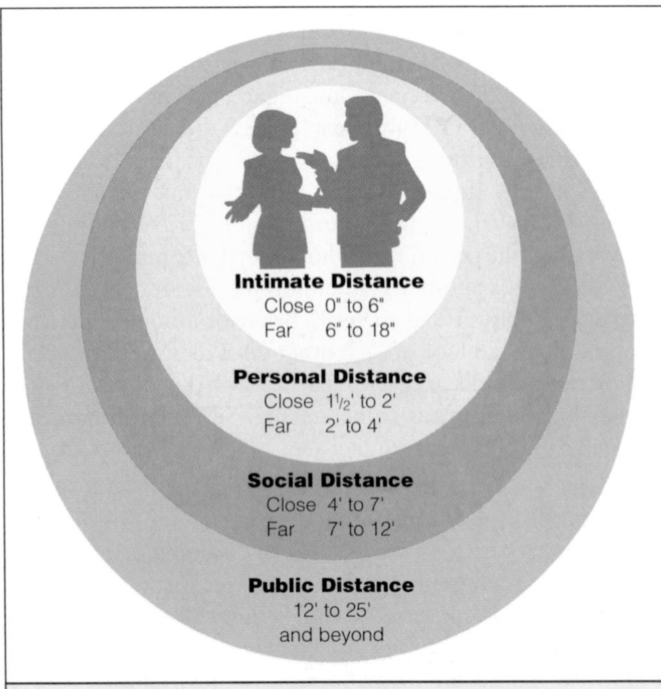

FIGURE 8–3 ■ *Intimacy and personal space.*

Knowing something about proxemics is useful, for example, in planning the physical space in which communication is to occur. Nurses can arrange furniture to increase or decrease interpersonal distance. A cozy, open seating arrangement encourages interaction; chairs in a row that face the front of a room discourage interaction. Nurses should be especially sensitive to the constraints imposed on communication by physical objects. Nurses can use proxemics to decipher verbal communication by paying attention to how others use interpersonal space.

Touch

Touching behaviors, because they tend to personalize communication, are extremely important in emotional situations. In North American society, the use of touch is governed by strong social norms. Unwritten guidelines control who, when, why, and where people touch.

Most of the taboos against touching seem to stem from the sexual implications of touching behavior. However, although touching is a physical act, it may or may not be sexual in nature. A realization of the importance of touch and an understanding that touching is not necessarily a sexual behavior may make this channel of communication available to more people. It is equally important to be sensitive to the other person's disposition toward touching, so as not to alienate another by infringing on the person's right not to be touched. The use of touch in therapeutic work is discussed in Chapters 28 and 32.

Cultural Artifacts

Artifacts are items in contact with interacting people that may function as nonverbal stimuli: clothes, cosmetics, perfume, deodorants, jewelry, eyeglasses, wigs and hairpieces, beards and mustaches, and so on.

Think about what information is communicated through artifacts such as a full-length mink coat, hair that is dyed purple, a gold band on the third finger of the left hand, a military uniform, or a Phi Beta Kappa key.

VERBAL AND NONVERBAL LINKS

The verbal and nonverbal elements of human communication are inextricably linked. Six different ways in which verbal and nonverbal systems interrelate are discussed below.

1. A nonverbal cue may *repeat* a verbal cue but in a different way. The deep-sea fisherman who verbally describes the size of the sailfish he caught may also extend both hands to indicate its length. The gesture repeats the idea.
2. Nonverbal behavior may also *contradict* verbal behavior. Consider the woman who meets a college roommate she hasn't seen for quite some time. She says, "You haven't changed a bit," but her tone of voice and facial expression convey sarcasm. When verbal and nonverbal cues contradict one another, it is usually safer to put more faith in the nonverbal cues.
3. Nonverbal messages may *add to or modify* verbal messages. When a man says he is a "little" irritated about being kept waiting, his tone of voice and body actions may indicate a more profound anger.

4. Certain nonverbal cues *accent or emphasize* verbal cues. A woman shrugs her shoulders when she says she doesn't really care which movie she and her companion see. A master of ceremonies holds up his hand when he asks for quiet. These gestures and body movements emphasize the words.
5. Cues that *regulate*, such as those that tell people when to start talking or when to stop talking, are usually nonverbal. A woman who keeps opening and closing her mouth briefly while others are talking is indicating that she wants a turn too.
6. Sometimes nonverbal cues are used to *substitute* for words. A wave from a friend at a distance replaces "hello." Applause at the end of a play tells the actors that they have pleased the audience.

Biopsychosocial Theories and Models of Human Communication

Communication takes place on at least three different levels: intrapersonal, interpersonal, and public (such as communication through the mass media or giving a public speech). Psychiatric–mental health nurses are more concerned with intrapersonal and interpersonal communication. **Intrapersonal communication** occurs when people communicate within themselves. A nurse who walks into a client's room and thinks, "The first pint of blood is almost finished. I'd better get the next one ready for infusion," is communicating intrapersonally.

Interpersonal communication, which this chapter discusses in depth, takes place in dyads (groups of two people) and small groups. This level of person-to-person communication is at the heart of psychiatric nursing.

One of the easiest ways to illustrate the nature of human communication and the elements of the process is through a model, or visual representation. People use models frequently for many purposes. They might use a map, which is a visual representation of a geographic location, to find their way to the community mental health center they plan to visit. Health professionals use electroencephalagrams (EEGs) to see a visual representation of the electrical activity in the brain. However, models provide incomplete views—a map does not show all the trees, buildings, or park statues in the territory; and an EEG tracing does not show the color, size, or blood supply of the brain. It is important to keep this in mind when looking at models. They sometimes make a process look simpler than it is.

SYMBOLIC INTERACTIONIST MODEL

A symbolic interactionist model is based on a transactional perspective. It views human communication on the social–interpersonal level and accounts for the whole persons involved in the process. Communication is viewed as a process of simultaneous mutual influence, rather than as a turn-taking event. The participants are products of their social system and integral parts of it. In the communication, some events take place *within* the participants (they are intrapersonal), and some take place *between* the participants (they are interpersonal).

Participants are who they are in relationship to the other person with whom they are communicating. For example, in each dyadic (two-person) communication event there are at least *six* perceptions involved:

1. Jeff's perception of himself
2. Jeff's perception of Sarah
3. Jeff's impression of the way Sarah sees him
4. Sarah's perception of herself
5. Sarah's perception of Jeff
6. Sarah's impression of the way Jeff sees her

Therefore, in addition to the content message, a relationship message also exists. Suppose Jeff passes Sarah in the corridor and Jeff says, "Hi, how are you?" Sarah answers, "Just fine, thanks," but moves down the corridor and away from Jeff as quickly as possible. Their subsequent communication will be affected by whether Jeff perceives Sarah as walking away because she wanted to get home before a rainstorm, or because he believes that Sarah is angry with him and her behavior is a comment on their relationship. The symbolic interactionist model helps explain what takes place between Jeff and Sarah.

A model constructed by Hulett (1966) according to symbolic interactionist principles, and adapted for this text, is shown in ■ Figure 8–4 on page 148. It shows five phases in each person's communication sequence: input, covert rehearsal, message generation, environmental event, and goal response.

During the phase of *input*, the person is motivated through some stimulus, either external or internal, toward some goal that requires engaging in a social interaction with another. Let's say that Jeff is attracted to Sarah and would like to get to know her better.

In the *covert rehearsal* phase, the person moves to make sense of the input received and develops and organizes a message *before* generating it. ■ Figure 8–5 on page 149 represents the covert rehearsal phase of the symbolic interactionist model. The individual first scans the information about self and others (Jeff enjoys movies and remembers hearing Sarah tell a friend that she'd really like to see the new Steven Spielberg movie in town) and then mentally rehearses possible actions to take (role playing) and possible reactions of the other (role taking). This gives Jeff the chance to think of four or five different ways to approach Sarah. This process is represented by the intrapersonal feedback loop.

The covert rehearsal phase is really the core of the communication process. In it, Jeff decides what to say, how to say it, and even whether to send the message to Sarah at all.

During *message generation*, the third phase, the instrumental act of giving a message is performed. (Jeff asks Sarah to the movie.) A message generated by one person serves as the input or the stimulus for another person. (Sarah thinks about Jeff's invitation, decides whether she wants to go to the movie with him, and considers what response to make to Jeff.) Once the second person completes the covert rehearsal and generates a message, this message becomes an *environmental event* for the first person. In our example, the environmental event is the fourth stage in the sequence for Jeff, whose *goal response* serves as an environmental event for Sarah, and so on.

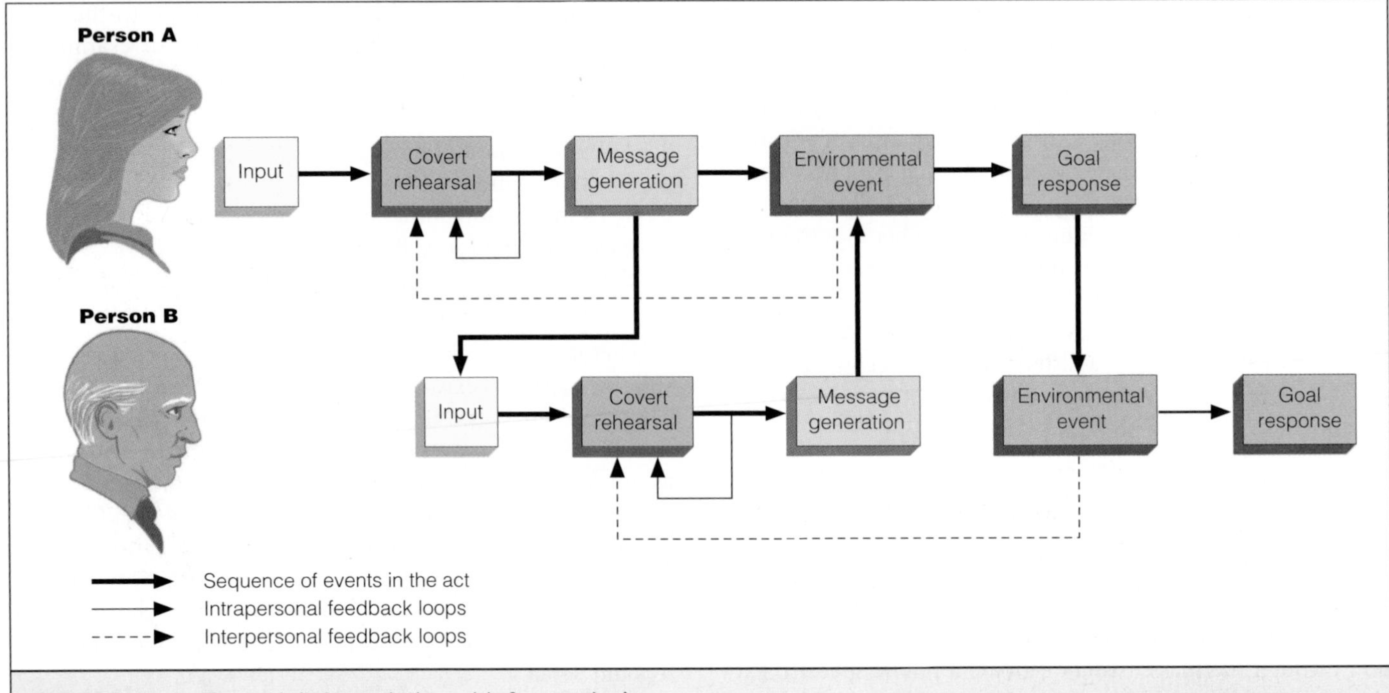

FIGURE 8–4 ■ *A symbolic interactionist model of communication.*

Source: Adapted from Hulett, J. E., Jr. (1966). A symbolic interactionist model of human communication. *AV Communication Review, 14,* 5–33. The Association for Educational Communications and Technology.

A second, or interpersonal, feedback loop connects the person's environmental event phase to the covert rehearsal stage. It allows the person an opportunity to determine whether he or she has made an error in the approach to the other and to make appropriate corrections by repeating the covert rehearsal and devising an altered message. (Jeff carefully considers Sarah's response. He listens to what she says and watches her behavior toward him. If her response is less than enthusiastic, he will try to determine what went wrong and how to correct it.)

In summary, the symbolic interactionist view of communication includes the following concepts:

- People run through a series of internal trials in the process of organizing a message.
- People select and transmit the message that will, in their view, have the highest probability of success.
- Success depends on the accuracy and completeness of the cognitive map and the accuracy and efficiency of the intrapersonal and interpersonal feedback loops.
- Communication is a dynamic (ever-changing) process that is unrepeatable and irreversible.
- Communication is complex.
- The meaning of messages is not transferred; it is mutually negotiated.

Communication is, at the very least, a very complicated process.

NEUROBIOLOGIC FACTORS

Looking at communication in its broadest sense requires us to go beyond the spoken word, the written word, and motor activity to the molecular level. In this broad view, communication can also be thought of as the movement of neurotransmitters within a synapse between neurons (Restak, 2000). Neurobiology researchers believe that communication at the molecular level may be the root of all brain functioning, including communication.

The neuron, the functional unit of the brain, differs from other cells in the body in that it is specialized for the function of information processing. The flow of information from one nerve cell to another involves the passage of electrically charged chemical particles—sodium, potassium, calcium, and chloride—across the cell membrane of the neuron. Neurotransmitters released by the presynaptic membrane of the axon cross the synaptic cleft and bind to their receptors on the postsynaptic membrane of the dendrite of the target cell. This process is more fully described in Chapter 4.

Therefore, brain activity can also be thought of in terms of messages and receptors or communicators and receivers. It makes sense to acknowledge that when communication is disrupted at one level—for example, when a crucial chemical in the brain undergoes an alteration—the end result can be felt at other more obvious communication levels of the individual (such as verbal and nonverbal communication and intrapersonal and interpersonal communication). To put this into perspective, your understanding of the words on this page is related not only to your understanding of written English, but also to the chloride ion channel activity on the membranes of millions of your brain cells.

The neurobiology of human communication is very complex and not yet fully understood. For example, we know that there is a speech circuit in the brain between the auditory cortex on the left, which passes to Wernicke's area in the temporal cortex, and from

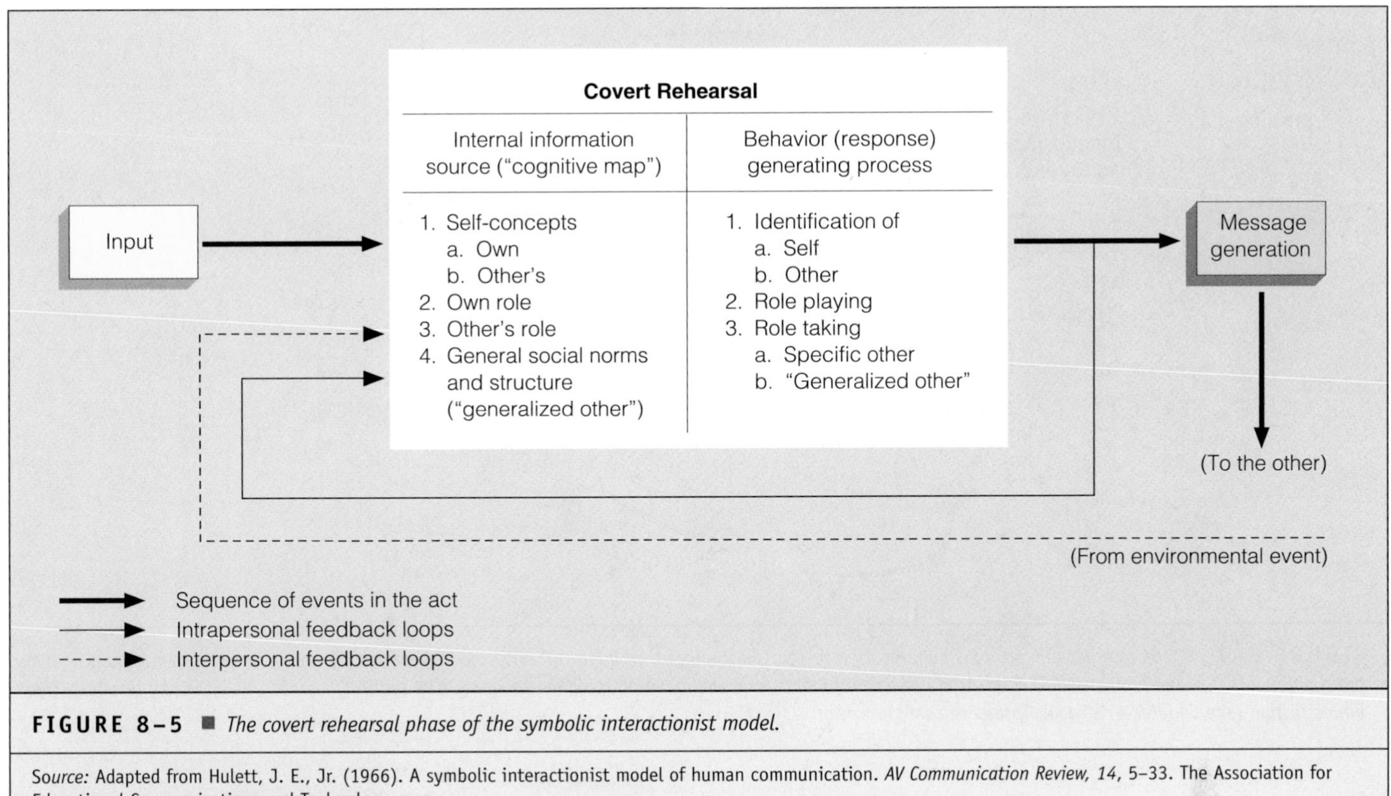

FIGURE 8–5 ■ *The covert rehearsal phase of the symbolic interactionist model.*

Source: Adapted from Hulett, J. E., Jr. (1966). A symbolic interactionist model of human communication. *AV Communication Review, 14*, 5–33. The Association for Educational Communications and Technology.

there to Broca's area in the left frontal lobe via the arcuate fasciculus (a pathway composed mainly of axons that synapse with other neurons). This speech circuit is detailed in ■ Figure 8–6.

However, knowing about the speech circuit does not go far enough in explaining the complexities of the neurobiologic basic of human communication. Communication is distributed much more than was previously believed. To add to the complexity, these areas are not the same in all of us. Therefore, there is no specific map of the brain that can locate specific communication functions with absolute certainty. Nor does it mean that damage in a specific region will necessarily cause a deficiency in a function thought to be contained in that region. ■ Figure 8–7 elaborates the interdependence of various regions of the brain thought to influence communication.

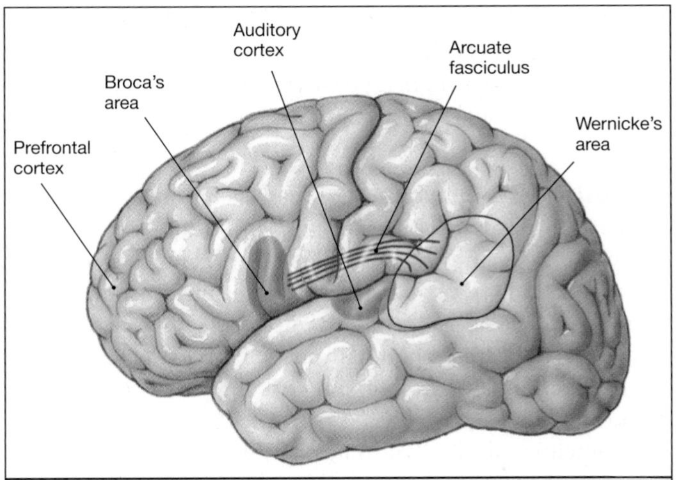

FIGURE 8–6 ■ *The speech circuit.*

Source: Smock, T. K. (1999). *Physiological psychology: A neuroscience approach*. Upper Saddle River, NJ: Prentice Hall.

RUESCH'S THERAPEUTIC COMMUNICATION THEORY

In the view of psychiatrist Jurgen Ruesch (1961), communication includes all the processes by which one human being influences another. Ruesch's theory takes into account the perceptions and interpretations that influence one person's view of the other. Further, Ruesch assumes that, to survive, the individual must communicate successfully.

According to Ruesch, communication is one of the most difficult human skills to master. It takes a long time to learn because it occurs in a series of steps, each building on the previous one. To communicate effectively requires decades of continuous practice. It is believed that interference hampers development and leaves an indelible mark.

Basic Concepts

The basic concepts of Ruesch's theory are as follows:

- Communication occurs in four different settings: intrapersonal, interpersonal, group, and societal.
- The ability to receive, evaluate, and transmit messages is influenced by perception, evaluation (which involves memory, past experiences, and value systems), and the transmission quality of messages (amount, speed, efficacy, and distinctiveness).

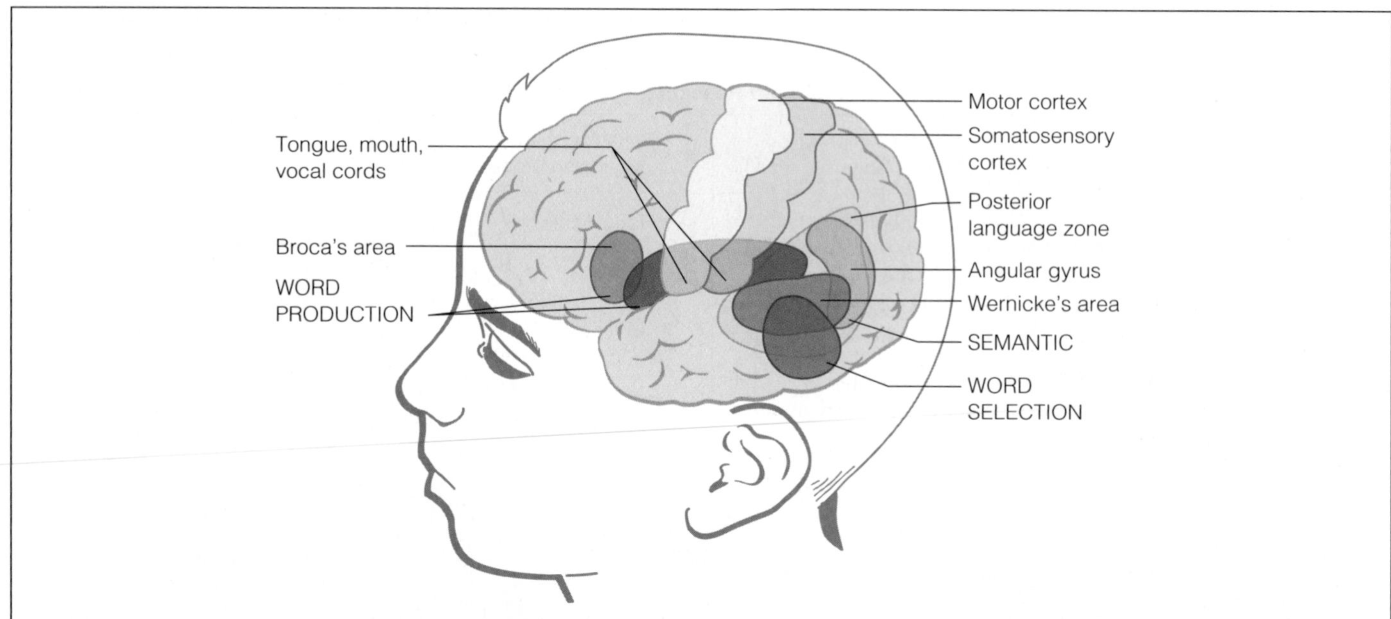

FIGURE 8–7 ■ *The interdependency of communication systems in the brain. In addition to Wernicke's and Broca's areas, several other regions of the brain are involved in the production of words, the selection of words, and the meaning assigned to words. The brain's emotion circuits in, for example, the limbic system (see Chapter 4) strongly influence communication.*

- Messages achieve meaning when they are mutually validated or verified between the two parties.
- Correction through feedback is basic to adaptive, healthy behavior and successful communication.

Successful Versus Disturbed Communication

The four formal criteria for successful communication are efficiency, appropriateness, flexibility, and feedback. When these criteria are not met, communication is disturbed.

Efficiency. Simplicity, clarity, and correct timing are all components of efficient messages. Psychiatric–mental health nurses and other mental health professionals may find themselves using complex and scientific words or professional mental health jargon to convey messages. Obscure or clumsy language and irrelevant or useless information may also prevent others from understanding a message.

Clear messages give a sense of order or structure and reduce ambiguity by narrowing the number of possible interpretations of meanings. Emphasizing the important ideas helps.

Proper timing is also important. It is best to give messages when the other person is able to "hear" them, when there are no intervening noises or inputs, and when the other person can interpret them without undue haste. Problems occur if the interval between the messages is either too short or too long.

Appropriateness. Messages are appropriate when they are relevant to the situation at hand and when there is mutual fit of overall patterns and constituent parts. Communication is inappropriate when it does not fit the circumstance, is irrelevant, or is misconstrued.

Communication can also be inappropriate in amount. Since every individual has both high and low tolerance levels for stimulation, a person's ability to cope with ideas, make decisions, and act is affected by the amount and rate of sensory input received. Exceeding a tolerance level is called **overload.** A person who is overloaded by too many messages or by messages too closely spaced cannot handle incoming messages. **Underload** occurs when delay or lack of information interferes with a person's ability to comprehend the message of another.

The **tangential reply** is another example of inappropriateness. A tangential reply to a statement disregards the content of the message and is directed toward either an incidental aspect of the initial statement, the type of language used, the emotions of the sender, or another facet of the same topic.

Flexibility. People cannot always be sure how a message will be received, because each person with whom they communicate is unique and changing. Since they cannot expect constancy from others, people need to be flexible. In communication, lack of flexibility manifests itself as either exaggerated control or exaggerated permissiveness. Both extremes increase the likelihood of frustrating, ungratifying, or disturbed communication.

Maintaining flexibility can be difficult if doing so requires a person to abandon or temporarily lay aside a carefully planned goal. To be flexible, a person must have the ability to set new priorities and to move to meet immediate goals. People who practice humanistic psychiatric nursing work to achieve flexibility in their relationships with clients and colleagues.

Feedback. Feedback is the process by which performance is checked and malfunctions corrected. It performs a regulatory function in the communication process. One example of how feedback can help to correct a system malfunction is illustrated in the Using Research Evidence special feature below. Feedback allows people to decide which messages have been understood as intended. It requires the cooperation of two people—one to give it and one to receive it.

Under certain circumstances of disturbed communication, feedback either fails or functions poorly. When messages do not get through or are distorted, appropriate replies cannot be obtained, and corrective feedback does not occur. Content that elicits anxiety, fear, shame, or any of several other strong emotions is likely to hamper feedback.

PRAGMATICS OF HUMAN COMMUNICATION THEORY

Watzlawick, Beavin, and Jackson (1967) base their theory of human communication on the assumption that communication is synonymous with interaction. These authors maintain that, in the presence of another, all behavior is communicative. This theory is concerned with the pragmatics, or the behavioral effects, of human interaction. What makes this theory particularly useful for this book is its conception of human communication as a reciprocal process.

Communication Levels

According to this theory, one cannot *not* communicate. Both activity and inactivity, verbalizations and silences, convey messages. This communication occurs on two levels. The *content level* of a communication is the report aspect, in which information is conveyed. The *relationship level* is communication about a communication.

All interchanges can be viewed as either *symmetric* (based on equality) or *complementary* (based on difference). In symmetric relationships, the partners usually mirror each other's behavior, thus minimizing difference. Complementary relationships, in contrast, maximize difference.

Communication Disturbances

Communication can be disturbed when a person attempts *not* to communicate. In this framework, the basic dilemma in schizophrenia is the schizophrenic person's attempt not to communicate. However, because it is impossible not to communicate, schizophrenics are faced with the need to deny that they are communicating while denying that this denial is a communication.

Another disturbance occurs when a person communicates in a way that invalidates the messages sent to or received from the other person. Such communications, called *disqualifications,* include a wide range of behavior such as self-contradictions, inconsistencies, subject switches, incomplete sentences, and misunderstandings.

A person may communicate in a way that confirms, rejects, or disconfirms the other person's view of self. Confirmation of one person's self-view by another is thought to be the greatest single factor in ensuring mental development and stability. Rejection of the other's definition of self essentially conveys this message: "You're wrong." Disconfirmation, by contrast, conveys this message: "You don't exist." Disconfirmation questions the other's authenticity. Disconfirmation leads to alienation and has been found to occur with some regularity in the experiences of schizophrenic persons.

Although all relationships are necessarily either symmetric or complementary, *runaways* (exaggerations to the point of disturbance) may occur in either of the patterns. For example, the

USING RESEARCH EVIDENCE

Julie Rodriguez, a staff nurse in the psychiatric emergency department of a large metropolitan hospital, has been concerned because of the unfavorable evaluations left in the comment box by visitors to the emergency department. Although the waiting room has been newly remodeled and has comfortable seating, visitors to the department view themselves as ignored for long periods of time while waiting to be seen. Their view of the staff is that staff members are very busy and seem to be working very hard. This doesn't seem to make up for the visitors' feelings that nurses and other staff are emotionally distant or "just there to do a job." The majority of visitors believe that they have waited longer to be seen than what the documented records show; for them time seems to pass very slowly.

Julie believes that the emergency department staff should be rated as highly as the physical environment. To achieve this goal, Julie has come up with the following plan, which she presented to her colleagues in their weekly meeting:

1. Provide a staff member presence at intermittent intervals—a nurse attuned to client needs and concerns related to their condition or to their care, and a volunteer to assist visitors with other questions or concerns such as those related to insurance, transportation, hospital admission, and so on.
2. Provide relaxing music, educational videos, books and puzzles, magazines and newspapers, and games for visitors' use. The volunteer would be responsible for maintaining these activities.

Julie's rationale for her proposal contains the following elements: providing more than a physical presence in the waiting room avoids the perception that staff members are emotionally distant or just there to do a job and, in conjunction with the additional activities transforms a technical, potentially impersonal setting into a more human place. Her rationale is based on knowledge she gained from several recent research articles, including:

Roper, J. M., & Manela, J. (2000). Psychiatric patients' perceptions of waiting time in the psychiatric emergency service. *Journal of Psychosocial Nursing and Mental Health Services, 38*(5), 18–27.

Snyder, M., Brandt, C. L., & Tseng, Y. (2000). Use of presence in the critical care unit. *AACN Clinical Issues, 11*(1), 27–33.

danger of competitiveness is ever-present in symmetric relationships. Symmetric interactions that lose their stability may enter a spiral in which each individual attempts to be just a little bit "more equal" than the other. Runaways are seen in quarrels between people or wars between nations, behaviors that are relatively open. Rejection of the other's self generally occurs when a symmetric relationship breaks down.

Breakdowns in complementary relationships, however, are generally characterized by disconfirmation of the other. For this reason, they are usually viewed as more serious.

NEUROLINGUISTIC PROGRAMMING THEORY

Neurolinguistic programming (NLP) is a communication model developed in the early 1970s by Richard Bandler and John Grinder. The model is derived from theory in linguistics, neurophysiology, psychology, cybernetics, and psychiatry.

Bandler and Grinder first observed psychotherapists who were known as expert communicators to discover what made them so effective as therapists. They concluded that people take in, or *access*, information in three sensory modalities:

1. auditory
2. visual
3. kinesthetic.

Further, each person prefers one mode over the others. Sounds may facilitate communication with one person, while touch or sight may be more effective with another person. In addition, people process information, or make sense out of it, according to the representational system (the NLP phrase for sensory modality) through which they receive it.

They also found that the expert communicators they observed were able to adapt themselves to match the client's representational system and to imitate the client in a natural and respectful way. Bandler and Grinder theorized that by tuning in to and then using the other person's preferred sensory mode, one could greatly enhance the ability to establish rapport. The most effective communicators, according to NLP theory, are those who can use all three modalities and easily move from one representational system to another.

Determining the Representational System

To determine whether a client's representational system is auditory, visual, or kinesthetic, one identifies the client's:

- Preferred predicates (verbs, adjectives, adverbs that tell something about the subject).
- Eye-accessing cues.
- Gross hand movements.
- Breathing pattern.
- Speech pattern and voice tones.

Preferred Predicates. The Assessment box categorizes predicates according to the auditory, visual, and kinesthetic modes. A necessary first step before attempting to link words with nonverbal behavior is observing the client to see which set of predicates is preferred.

ASSESSMENT

Preferred Predicates

Auditory	Visual	Kinesthetic
Argue	Appear	Attach
Chant	Bright	Breathless
Debate	Colorful	Calm
Eavesdrop	Glimpse	Excite
Hassle	Image	Fondle
Hear	Observe	Hurt
Listen	Pretty	Rough
Overhear	Scan	Sharp
Praise	Sight	Soft
Quiet	Spy	Sore
Scream	Stare	Support
Silent	Ugly	Tension
Tell	View	Throw
Whine	Watch	Touch
Whisper	Wink	Warm

Eye-Accessing Cues. Eye-accessing cues correlate with an individual's thinking process. People who are visualizing generally turn their eyes upward or look straight ahead, focusing on nothing. Someone processing auditory information usually moves the eyes from side to side. A person engaging in intrapersonal communication usually focuses the eyes down in the direction of the nondominant hand. A person in the kinesthetic mode looks down toward the dominant hand when experiencing sensations or emotions.

Gross Hand Movements. Gross hand movements also give clues to the client's sensory mode. People have a tendency to point toward or touch the sense organ that matches their current sensory mode. The person in a visual mode often points toward the eye, and the person in an auditory mode often points toward or touches the ear.

Breathing Pattern. Assessing the breathing patterns helps the observer understand the client's representational model. Shallow, thoracic breathing is often associated with visual accessing. Even breathing or prolonged expiration is associated with auditory accessing, and deep abdominal breathing is associated with kinesthetic accessing.

Speech Pattern and Voice Tones. Visual accessing often correlates with quick bursts of words that are high pitched, strained, or nasal. Auditory accessing is often associated with a clear, midrange voice tone or with a rhythmic tempo and clearly enunciated words. Kinesthetic accessing is associated with a slow voice and a low volume or deep tone, or with a breathy tone and long pauses.

Therapeutic Use of NLP

Using NLP theory in psychiatric–mental health nursing practice gives us yet another way to empathize with clients by "trying on" their style. People tend to be less anxious with the familiar. Nurses who mirror the client's sensory mode are likely to be experienced as more comfortable and safer to be with, conditions that facilitate rapport.

Nurses can use mirroring to help the client follow the nurse's lead. For example, with an anxious client, the nurse might begin by mirroring the behaviors that indicate the client's anxiety and then shift into a more relaxed posture and less anxious behaviors. The nurse can lead the client from a more anxious state to a less anxious state by employing the NLP principles discussed here.

An important benefit of the NLP approach is that it allows nurses to assess the client's style and preferred sensory mode and to communicate more effectively with clients by using both verbal and nonverbal communication in the client's preferred mode. The following examples express the same nursing intervention with different predicates, depending on the client's preferred mode:

Visual—"Yes, I can *see* that you are much better. You *look* good, your eyes are *clear*, your *appearance* has certainly changed."

Auditory—"Yes, I can *hear* from the *sound* of your voice that you are better. *Talking* with you today is quite different from yesterday."

Kinesthetic—"Yes, you do seem to be *feeling* much better today, you're *holding* your head up, and your *grasp* is certainly *firmer* than yesterday."

By expanding their abilities to communicate with clients in all three modes, nurses can become more effective communicators.

Facilitative Communication

Facilitative communication aims at initiating, building, and maintaining fulfilling and trusting relationships with other people. Communicating ideas and feelings with clarity, efficiency, and appropriateness helps a person be interpersonally effective. In reading the rest of this chapter, try to relate the therapeutic communication principles and practices discussed earlier to these ideas about facilitative communication.

Don't forget about using appropriate nonverbal skills. Your verbal and nonverbal messages should be consistent with one another. Nonverbal messages should enhance, not detract from, verbal messages. The Nursing Self-Awareness special feature presents some guidelines for you in achieving this goal.

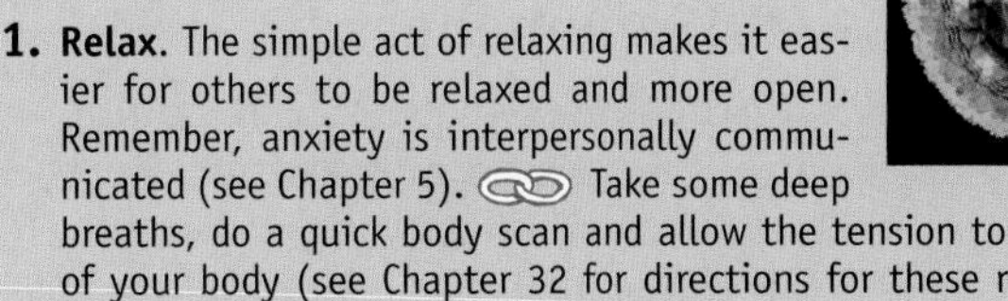

Nursing SELF-AWARENESS

Guidelines for Improving Nonverbal Communication

1. **Relax.** The simple act of relaxing makes it easier for others to be relaxed and more open. Remember, anxiety is interpersonally communicated (see Chapter 5). Take some deep breaths, do a quick body scan and allow the tension to flow out of your body (see Chapter 32 for directions for these relaxation techniques).
2. **Use facial, hand, and body gestures judiciously.** Nonverbal gestures that are used indiscriminately lose their effectiveness. Overdoing a gesture—constantly smiling, constantly nodding your head—may become annoying to the other person and make it more difficult for them to talk with you.
3. **Get feedback on your nonverbal communication.** Your classmates and instructors are sources of feedback. Ask them to comment on the facial expressions and body gestures that you use when you converse with them. Consider being videotaped so that you can see for yourself any mannerisms or gestures that intrude on your ability to be an effective communicator.
4. **Practice.** Once you've identified any intrusive facial expressions or body gestures, practice blending your verbal message with appropriate nonverbal cues such as hand gestures, body posture, facial expression, and tone of voice. Then, role play with your classmates and ask them to comment on your effectiveness.

SUPERFICIALITY VERSUS INTIMACY

Most relationships between people begin at the level of social superficiality. In a nurse–client relationship, we try to develop facilitative intimacy, which differs from social intimacy. For example, the interdependence that characterizes the social relationship is greatly reduced. In social relationships, participants may "tell their stories" to one another. In facilitative relationships that have therapeutic goals, only the client is engaged in storytelling with the nurse. The progress is specifically focused. Clients not only explain themselves, the events of their lives, and the circumstances they face, they do so with a purpose in mind—understanding the circumstances through exploring them and moving to improve the circumstances of their lives.

Movement toward therapeutic intimacy may be difficult at first. For one thing, such intimacy violates certain social taboos. For example, at a party it may be socially incorrect to comment on a person's anxiety, stuttering, or facial tic. During facilitative and therapeutic communication, all messages, including these nonverbal ones, are heeded and may be discussed.

Therapeutic intimacy also requires that the participants move beyond social "chitchat" into meaningful areas of concern for the client. Therapeutic intimacy requires high involvement and commitment.

FACILITATING INTIMACY

Several interpersonal principles and practices are essential to the achievement of facilitative intimacy.

Responding with Empathy

Most theorists believe that empathy is the most important dimension in the helping process. Without a high level of empathic understanding, nurses have no real basis for helping. Empathy facilitates interpersonal exploration.

Responding with Respect

Responding with respect demonstrates that you value the integrity of the client and have faith in the client's ability to solve problems, given appropriate help. By encouraging clients to put forward possible plans of action, you convey respect for their ability to take charge of their own destiny. Giving advice, by contrast, conveys a directly opposite message.

Responding with Genuineness

Genuineness refers to the ability to be real or honest with another. To be effective, genuineness must be timed properly and based on a solid relationship. Honesty is not always the best policy, especially if it is brutal or if the client is not capable of dealing with it.

Clients who can experience your authenticity can risk greater genuineness and authenticity themselves. The nurse who is genuine is more likely to deal with and eventually help the client resolve real problems, rather than just those that are safe or socially acceptable.

Responding with Immediacy

Responding with immediacy means responding to what is happening between the client and yourself in the here-and-now. Because this dimension may involve the feelings of the client toward you, it can be one of the most difficult to achieve. For example, the client may confront you with overt or implied criticism of your role or competence. If you respond in a defensive or evasive way, the relationship may be threatened. If you are open, reasonable, and concerned, the relationship may be strengthened. However, focusing attention on the relationship too early can hinder the formation of an adequate base.

Responding with Warmth

Warmth is so closely linked with empathy and respect that it is seldom communicated as an independent dimension. It is important, however, to note some additional points about the expression of warmth. Effusive, chatty, "buddy-buddy" behavior should not be confused with warmth. Warmth is most often conveyed in communications of respect and empathy.

Be aware of and accept the client's right to maintain distance (refer to Figure 8–4). Warmth and intimacy cannot be forced. Initially high levels of warmth can be counter-productive for clients who have received little warmth from others in their lives or have been taken advantage of by others. Warmth alone is insufficient for building a relationship and solving problems.

FACILITATIVE COMMUNICATION SKILLS

Presenting a how-to manual or a "cookbook" of communication skills goes against the thrust of this book. Using a set of communication skills as a sort of relationship "magic" will probably doom you to failure. Relationships, and the people in them, are unique and much too complex to rely on a formula for facilitative communication. The following skills are therefore presented with many misgivings. It is important to remember that a holistic approach is inconsistent with the rigid, inflexible application of communication techniques. The communication techniques presented here should be viewed as having the potential to foster effective communication. They must be adapted individually for each human encounter. Blend them with the understandings you have gained from the interpersonal communication principles and practices discussed earlier in this chapter.

Empathizing

Nurses are taught skills of active listening. But listening without *empathy* is not enough. Empathic understanding not only increases the nurse's grasp of the client's difficulties but also helps the nurse offer feedback on how the client affects others. Empathy can best be understood as *role taking*, a process through which people feel with one another. They are able to sense the feelings of another because they have evoked in themselves the attitude of the person to whom they are relating.

The term *empathy* is often mistakenly used synonymously with *sympathy*. Empathy contains no elements of condolence, agreement, or pity. When nurses sympathize, they assume that there is a parallel between their feelings and those of the client. The perceived similarity makes good judgment and objectivity difficult.

A nurse's empathic involvement with troubled clients can have a number of stressful consequences. Problems can arise at any phase in the empathy process. Each of the common obstacles to achieving an empathic concern for clients can be understood as a failure to cope with one of the four phases of achieving empathy. The four phases of therapeutic empathizing are discussed in Box 8–1. The nurse may overidentify and lapse into sympathy for the client. The nurse may fail to incorporate the client's feelings and instead project personal ones. The nurse may bypass the reverberation phase and substitute gut-level intuitions for rational problem solving. At the detachment phase, the nurse may experience overdistancing or burnout.

Actively Listening

Actively listening is paying undivided attention to what the client says and does. Paying undivided attention is the major goal of active listening. A common error made by inexperienced psychiatric–mental health nurses is being too busy planning what they are going to say next. Focusing on yourself prevents you from hearing what the other person is saying and gives the client the nonverbal message that what he or she is say-

BOX 8–1 Phases of Therapeutic Empathizing

The process of empathic understanding has four phases:

1. *Identification.* Through the relaxation of conscious controls, we allow ourselves to become absorbed in contemplating the client and the client's experiences.
2. *Incorporation.* We take in the experiences of the client rather than attribute our own experiences and feelings to the client.
3. *Reverberation.* We interplay the internalized feelings of the client and our own experiences or fantasies. While fully absorbed in the identity of the client, we still experience ourselves as separate personalities.
4. *Detachment.* We withdraw from subjective involvement and totally resume our own identity. We use the insight gained from the reverberation phase as well as reason and objectivity to offer responses that are useful to the client.

ing is not very important. In fact, what the client is saying is very important. If you don't listen, you won't be able to comprehend the message. If you don't comprehend the message, you will not be able to effectively use the facilitative communication techniques that follow.

Active listening is best accomplished when environmental distractions are minimized. Consider finding a quiet place, turning off the television, or closing the door. Avoid taking extensive notes; they take your attention away from the client, and you will miss some of what is being said on the verbal level and done on the nonverbal level. Face the client, use eye contact, show interest, and listen objectively while minimizing your own personal responses.

Using Silence

Do not feel obligated to respond after every statement a client makes. *Using silence* goes beyond active listening and can be a very effective facilitative technique when it encourages the client to communicate, when it allows the client time to ponder what has been said or a connection the client has made, when it allows the client time to collect his or her thoughts, or when it allows the client time to consider alternatives. Looking interested while maintaining an open posture or a questioning look will encourage the client to use the time effectively.

Uncomfortable silences should be broken and analyzed. You would not want a client to become increasingly anxious or resistive. (See Chapters 5 and 16 for suggestions on handling anxiety and Chapter 28 for suggestions on handling resistance.)

Remember, silence is an effective communication technique only when it is used as an appropriate and purposeful therapeutic intervention. Nurses who are silent because they are uncomfortable or because they lack the knowledge or the skill to communicate effectively must seek an experienced clinical supervisor to help them analyze their own personal and professional growth needs.

Reflecting

Reflecting is repeating the client's verbal or nonverbal message for the client's benefit. It encourages the client to become more actively involved.

Reflecting Content. Reflecting the *content* of the message basically repeats the client's statement. This gives clients the opportunity to hear and mull over what they have told you.

- "You believe things will be better soon."
- "You think it would be better to take a part-time job."

Content reflection is perhaps one of the most misused and overused methods in mental health counseling. It loses its effectiveness when used for lack of other choices.

Reflecting Feelings. Reflecting *feelings* is verbalizing the implied feelings in the client's comment.

- "Sounds like you're really angry at your brother."
- "You're feeling uncomfortable about being discharged from the hospital."

In reflecting feelings, you attempt to identify latent and connotative meanings that may either clarify or distort the content. Reflection is useful because it encourages the client to make additional clarifying comments.

Imparting Information

Imparting information is helping the client by supplying additional data. This therefore encourages further clarification based on new or additional input.

- "Group therapy will be held on Tuesday evening from 6:30 until 8:00."
- "I am a psychiatric nurse."

It is not constructive to withhold useful information from the client or to reply "What do you think?" to a straight-forward, information-seeking question. However, be careful not to cross the line between giving information and giving advice, or give information as a way of avoiding an area of interpersonal difficulty. Also, the nurse who gives personal, social information may move out of the realm of therapeutic intervention. Information that is important to disclose to the client to protect the client's rights includes your title and position. Denying you are new to the field may only cause mistrust.

Remember that clients' participation in decision making begins when they take in and understand information about their own condition. The goal of imparting information should be to provide effective education that empowers clients and their families. Studies have shown that an educated, empowered client is more likely to achieve positive mental health outcomes and less likely to need admission or readmission to an acute care facility. You can help clients by utilizing each teachable moment.

MediaLink Case Study: Communication Skills

Clarifying

Clarifying is an attempt to understand the basic nature of a client's statement.

- "I'm confused about. . . . Could you go over that again, please?"
- "You say you're feeling anxious now. What's that like for you?"

Asking the client to give an example to clarify a meaning helps you understand the client's intended message better. A person who describes a concrete incident is more likely to see the connections between it and similar occurrences. Illustrations are also very useful qualifiers.

Paraphrasing

In *paraphrasing*, you assimilate and restate what the client has said.

- "In other words, you're fed up with being treated like a child."
- "I hear you saying that when people compliment you, you feel embarrassed. If they knew the real you, they'd stay away."

Paraphrasing gives you the opportunity to test your understanding of what a client is attempting to communicate. It is reflective in nature, in that it lets the client know how another person is understanding the message.

Checking Perceptions

Checking perceptions means sharing how one person perceives and hears another. After sharing perceptions of the client's behaviors, thoughts, and feelings, ask the client to verify the perception.

- "Let me know if this is how you see it too."
- "I get the feeling that you're uncomfortable when we're silent. Does that seem to fit?"

Nurses use perception checks to make sure that they understand a client. An effective perception check conveys the message, "I want to understand. . . ." It gives the other person the opportunity to correct inaccurate perceptions. It also allows you to avoid actions based on false assumptions about the client.

Questioning

Questioning is a very direct way of speaking with clients. But when used to excess, questioning controls the nature and range of the client's responses. Questions can be useful when you are seeking specific information. When your intent is to engage the client in meaningful dialogue, however, questions should be limited.

When using questions, it is best to make them open-ended rather than closed. An *open-ended question* focuses the topic but allows freedom of response.

- "How were you feeling when your mother said that to you?"
- "What's your opinion about . . . ?"

The *closed-ended question* limits the client's choice of responses, generally to "yes" or "no" ("Were you feeling angry when your mother said that?"). Closed-ended questions limit therapeutic exploration. Clients whose thinking is disorganized may need to be guided by closed-ended questions, e.g., questions on suicidal thoughts (see Chapter 22).

"Why" questions usually have the same effect. They are often impossible to answer and rarely lead to a clearer understanding of the situation. However, "who," "what," "when," and "how" questions may be helpful when used judiciously.

Be careful when questioning clients not to steer the client to answer in a certain way. For example, "You don't drink alcohol to excess, do you?" suggests that the client should answer "no."

Structuring

Structuring is an attempt to create order or evolve guidelines. It helps the client become aware of problems and the order in which the client might deal with them.

- "You've mentioned that you want to improve your relationships with your wife, your sister, and your boss. Let's put them in order of priority."
- "No, I won't be giving you advice, but we can discuss the possible solutions together."

Structuring is particularly useful when clients introduce a number of concerns in a brief period and have little idea of which to begin work on. Nurses use structuring not only to explore content but also to delimit the parameters of the nurse-client relationship and to identify how the nurse will participate with the client in the problem-solving process.

Pinpointing

Pinpointing calls attention to certain kinds of statements and relationships. For example, you may point to inconsistencies among statements, to similarities and differences in the points of view, feelings, or actions of two or more people, or to differences between what one says and what one does.

- "So, you and your wife don't agree about how many children you want."
- "You say you're sad, but you're smiling."

Linking

In *linking*, you respond to the client in a way that ties together two events, experiences, feelings, or people. You can use linking to connect past experiences with current behaviors. Another example is linking the tension between two people with current life stress.

- "You felt depressed after the birth of both your children."
- "So, the arguments didn't really begin until after you got your promotion."

Giving Feedback

Feedback helps others become aware of how their behavior affects us and how we perceive their actions. Responding with feedback can be therapeutic self-disclosure. It allows you to offer clients constructive information that makes them aware of their effect on others. Total self-disclosure by the nurse is inappropriate in the nurse-client relationship. It places a burden of interdependence on the client and limits the time and energy available to work on the client's concerns. Reciprocal self-disclosure is more appropriate in friend and colleague relationships.

- "When you wring your hands, I feel anxious."
- "Sometimes when you turn your head away from me, I think you're angry."

It is important to give feedback in a way that does not threaten the client, resulting in increased defensiveness. The more defensive the client, the less likely the client will hear and understand the feedback. The Intervention box on page 157 lists some characteristics of helpful, nonthreatening feedback.

Confronting

Constructive confrontations often lead to productive change. *Confronting* is a deliberate invitation to examine some aspect of personal behavior that indicates a discrepancy between what the person says and what the person does. Confrontation requires careful attention to nonverbal communication and the discrepancies between nonverbal and verbal messages.

Confrontations may be informational or interpretive, and they may be directed toward both the resources and the limitations of the client. An *informational confrontation* describes the visible behavior of another person. An *interpretive confrontation* expresses thoughts and feelings about the other's behavior and draws inferences about the meaning of the behavior.

INTERVENTION

Characteristics of Helpful, Nonthreatening Feedback

Strategy	Rationale
Focus feedback on behavior rather than on client.	Refer to what client actually does rather than how you imagine client to be.
Focus feedback on observations rather than inferences.	Refer to what you actually see or hear client do; inferences refer to conclusions or assumptions you make about client.
Focus feedback on description rather than judgment.	Report what occurred rather than evaluating it in terms of good or bad, right or wrong.
Focus feedback on "more or less" rather than "either/or" descriptions of behavior.	"More or less" descriptions stress quantity rather than quality (which may be value-laden).
Focus feedback on here-and-now behavior rather than there-and-then behavior.	The most meaningful feedback is given as soon as it is appropriate to do so.
Focus feedback on sharing of information and ideas rather than advice.	Sharing ideas and information helps client make decisions about own well-being; giving advice takes away client's freedom to be self-determining.
Focus feedback on exploration of alternatives rather than answers or solutions.	Focusing on a variety of alternatives for accomplishing a particular goal prevents premature acceptance of answers or solutions that may not be appropriate.
Focus feedback on its value to the client rather than on catharsis it provides you.	Feedback should serve needs of client, not your needs.
Limit feedback to amount of information client is able to use rather than amount you have available to give.	Overloading will decrease effectiveness of feedback.
Limit feedback to appropriate time and place.	Excellent feedback presented at an inappropriate time may be ineffective or harmful.
Focus feedback on what is said rather than why it is said.	Focusing on why things are said or done moves away from observations and toward motive or intent (which can only be assumed, unless verified).

- "You say you're 'the dummy in the family,' yet none of your brothers or sisters made the honor roll like you did."
- "Ever since Sally and Joe criticized the way you conducted the meeting, you haven't spoken to them. It looks like you're feeling angry."

Six skills to be incorporated in constructive confrontations are:

1. Use of personal statements with the words *I*, *my*, and *me*.
2. Use of relationship statements expressing what you think or feel about the client in the here and now.
3. Use of behavior descriptions (statements describing the visible behavior of the client).
4. Use of description of personal feelings, specifying the feeling by name.
5. Use of responses aimed at understanding, such as paraphrasing and perception checking.
6. Use of constructive feedback skills (see the Intervention box).

Summarizing

Summarizing is the highlighting of the main ideas expressed in an interaction. It shows the client that you understand. Both the client and the nurse benefit from this review of the main themes of the conversation. Summarizing is also useful in focusing the client's thinking and aiding conscious learning.

- "The last time we were together you were concerned about. . . ."
- "You had three main concerns today."

You can use this technique appropriately at different times during an interaction. For example, it is useful to summarize the previous interaction in the first few minutes you and the client spend together. Early summarizing helps the client recall the areas discussed and gives the client the opportunity to see how you have synthesized the content of a previous session. Summarizing is useful because it keeps the participants directed toward a goal.

Injudicious use of summarizing is a common pitfall. You may rush to summarize despite other, more pressing and immediate client concerns. In this instance, summarizing is likely to meet your needs for structure but does nothing to address the client's here-and-now concerns.

Processing

Processing is a complex and sophisticated technique. Process comments direct attention to the interpersonal dynamics of the nurse-client experience. These dynamics are illustrated in the content, feelings, and behavior expressed.

- "It seems that important things that need to be taken care of come up in the last five minutes we have together in our session."
- "Today is the first day our session has started out with silence. Last week it seemed there wouldn't be enough time."

Processing is most useful when therapeutic intimacy has been achieved.

CULTURALLY COMPETENT COMMUNICATION STRATEGIES

Cultural and social class differences between client and nurse may impede a nurse's best intentions. Quality nursing care is culturally sensitive; that is, aware of cultural issues that are important to the client and may affect the client's response to treatment. In planning nursing interventions do not follow a predetermined plan but plan care that is culturally competent for each person. For example, if a Hispanic teenage girl is obese and wants to lose weight, you would not hand her a printed 500-calorie diet plan but would work with her and a nutritionist to plan a diet based on the foods she prefers. You would also discuss the care plan with the girl's father (because of the patriarchal dominance in the Hispanic culture) and would expect many family members at visiting time. If an Asian client who is a Buddhist wants time each day to meditate, you would allow for that time in the care plan rather than filling every hour with "constructive," "growth-producing" activity.

Taking a client's culture into consideration when planning care is not an easy task. It is time-consuming and requires patience, insight, and creativity.

Understanding One's Own Sociocultural Heritage

Gaining awareness of sociocultural differences requires that you first come to understand your own background and the influence of that background on your practice. Nurses are better able to meet the sociocultural needs of a client when they acknowledge that a culture and a society influence their beliefs, values, attitudes, and behavior. The questions in the Nursing Self-Awareness special feature are designed to facilitate acknowledgment of the your own sociocultural heritage (see also the Nursing Self-Awareness special feature on page 115 in Chapter 6). Answering these questions honestly and completely is the important first step in self-awareness. The second step involves exploring beliefs and attitudes that may be different from or the same as those held by the client.

Nursing SELF-AWARENESS

Questions That Acknowledge Sociocultural Heritage

- What ethnic group, socioeconomic class, religions, age groups, and community do you belong to?
- What experiences have you had with people from ethnic groups, socioeconomic classes, religions, age groups, or communities different from your own?
- What were those experiences like? How did you feel about them?
- When you were growing up, what did your parents and significant others say about people who were different from your family?
- What about your ethnic group, socioeconomic class, religion, age, or community do you find embarrassing or wish you could change? Why?
- What sociocultural factors in your background might contribute to being rejected by members of other cultures?
- What personal qualities do you have that will help you establish interpersonal relationships with persons from other cultural groups?
- What personal qualities may be detrimental?
- What assumptions do you hold about the people who populate our world?

Avoiding Misdiagnosis

Clients from different cultures may be misdiagnosed by Western health care providers. Culturally competent nurses can play a role in assessing clients' social, psychologic, and behavioral symptoms in the light of clients' own cultural norms. For example, a psychiatrist may diagnose a man who talks to the dead as schizophrenic, but for a Puerto Rican who believes in espiritismo, talking to the dead is a common practice. A client who is a charismatic Christian may lapse into an altered state of consciousness and speak in tongues. To interpret these behaviors as evidence of schizophrenia is inappropriate. Obtaining a cultural profile helps to prevent misdiagnosis.

Circumventing Potential Cultural Barriers to Communication

The guidelines in Box 8–2 will help you determine and remove potential barriers to communication. Emphasizing similarities can help to form a therapeutic relationship. Differences may serve as topics for discussion. An open, ongoing dialogue is beneficial for both parties because it promotes understanding.

When English is not the client's primary language and you are a monolingual provider, it will help if you select the words you use carefully, avoiding buzz words and jargon. Speak clearly, pacing yourself to be neither too fast nor too slow. Words that are slurred, have many syllables in them, or are too technical make communication more difficult. Speaking too fast may overload the client and make it difficult for the client to follow. Speaking too slowly may lose the client's attention.

Select the gestures you use with care, using your non-verbal behavior to underscore your words and your actions. The proper use of gestures can clarify a message, and drawings can sometimes be helpful. Be careful however; as discussed earlier in this chapter, not all gestures mean the same thing in all cultures.

Listen to your client's words and watch your client's gestures carefully. Do your best to understand and validate the meaning they have for you. Listening carefully to the client helps you avoid focusing on what you will say or do next and demonstrates your genuine concern for the client's distress.

If the client attempts to speak English, his or her thoughts may appear distorted when language is the real problem. There have been a number of documented instances in which people have been diagnosed as mentally disordered and confined to a mental hospital because mental health professionals erroneously diagnosed a language problem or value difference as disordered thinking or psychosis.

An interpreter may be necessary if language is a barrier. If the client does not have his or her own interpreter, you may be able to enlist the aid of a bilingual staff member. For the sake of confidentiality and the client's privacy and reputation, avoid using family members as interpreters. Clients may not want family members privy to personal information, for example, sexual preference, drug or alcohol use, content of hallucinations (what the voices say). Health and social services departments, international institutes, college language departments, neighborhood houses, or cultural centers will often know of people who are willing to volunteer as interpreters.

BOX 8-2 Strategies for Assessing and Removing Potential Cultural Barriers to Communication

- Determine the client's level of fluency in English.
- Arrange for an interpreter, if needed.
- Allow the client to choose seating for comfortable personal space and eye contact.
- Avoid using body language that may be offensive or misunderstood.
- Speak directly to the client, whether or not an interpreter is present.
- Choose a speech rate and style that promotes understanding and demonstrates respect for the client.
- Avoid slang, technical jargon, and complex sentences.
- Use open-ended questions or questions phrased in several ways to obtain information.
- Determine the client's reading ability before using written materials. If the client cannot read English, translate the materials.
- Check for client understanding.
- Be aware of cultural phenomena that affect etiquette:
  1. Know the proper forms of address for people from a given culture and the ways by which people welcome one another.
  2. Know when touch, such as an embrace or handshake, is expected and when physical contact is prohibited.
  3. Remember that gestures do not have universal meaning—what is acceptable to one cultural group may be unacceptable to another.
  4. Smiling may indicate friendliness to some; to others it may be taboo.
  5. Know in which cultures avoiding eye contact is a sign of respect.

Source: Adapted from Spector, R. E. (2000). *CulturalCare: Guide to heritage assessment and health traditions* (5th ed.) (pp. 15, 41–42). Pearson Education/PH College.

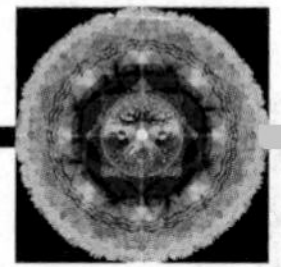

EXPLORE MediaLink

NCLEX review, case studies, and other interactive resources for this chapter can be found on the Companion Website at http://www.prenhall.com/kneisl. Click on Chapter 8 to select the activities for this chapter.

For animations, video tutorials, more NCLEX review questions, and an audio glossary, access the accompanying CD-ROM in this textbook.

BIBLIOGRAPHY

Bandler, R. (1993). *Time for a change*. Denver: Meta Publications.

Dilts, R., Bandler, R., & Bandler, L. C. (1990). *Neurolinguistic programming*. Denver: Meta Publications.

Gregory, R. (2001). Listening. *Journal of Psychosocial Nursing and Mental Health Services, 39*(2), 48–51.

Hulett, J. E., Jr. (1966). A symbolic interactionist model of human communication. *AV Communication Review, 14*, 5–33.

Klagsbrun, J. (2001). Listening and focusing: Holistic health care tools for nurses. *Nursing Clinics of North America, 36*(1), 115–130.

Northouse, P. G., & Northouse, L. L. (1998). *Health communication: Strategies for health professionals* (3rd ed.). Stamford CT: Appleton & Lange.

Poss, J. E., & Beeman, T. (2000). Effective use of interpreters in health care: Guidelines for nurse managers and clinicians. *Seminar for Nurse Managers, 7*(4), 166–171.

Ratey, J. J. (2001). *A user's guide to the brain*. New York: Pantheon Books.

Restak, R. M. (2000). *Mysteries of the mind*. New York: National Geographic Society.

Reynolds, W. J., & Scott, B. (2000). Do nurses and other professional helpers normally display much empathy? *Journal of Advances in Nursing, 31*(1), 226–234.

Reynolds, W., Scott, P. A., & Austin, W. (2000). Nursing, empathy, and perception of the moral. *Journal of Advances in Nursing, 32*(1), 235–242.

Roper, J. M., & Manela, J. (2000). Psychiatric patient's perceptions of waiting time in the psychiatric emergency service. *Journal of Psychosocial Nursing and Mental Health Services, 38*(5), 18–27.

Ruesch, J. (1961). *Therapeutic communication*. New York: Norton.

Ruesch, J., & Bateson, G. (1968). *Communication: The social matrix of psychiatry*. New York: Norton.

Ryan, M., Twibell, R., Brigham, C., & Bennett P. (2000). Learning to care for clients in their world, not mine. *Journal of Nursing Education, 39*(9), 401–408.

Schuster, P. M. (2000). *Communication: The key to the therapeutic relationship*. Philadelphia: Davis.

Snyder, M., Brandt, C. L., & Tseng, Y. (2000). Use of presence in the critical care unit. *AACN Clinical Issues, 11*(1), 27–33.

Spector, R. E. (2000a). *CulturalCare: Guide to heritage assessment and health traditions* (5th ed). Upper Saddle River, NJ: Prentice Hall.

Spector, R. E. (2000b). *Cultural diversity in health & illness* (5th ed.). Upper Saddle River, NJ: Prentice Hall.

Stone, D. F., Patton, B., & Heen, S. (2000). *Difficult conversations: How to discuss what matters most*. New York: Viking Penguin.

Tamparo, C. D., & Lindh, W. Q. (2000). *Therapeutic communications for health professionals*. Albany, NY: Delmar.

Wachtel, P. L. (1998). Therapeutic communication: Knowing what to say when. Philadelphia: Guilford.

Watzlawick, P. (1993). *The language of change: Elements of therapeutic communication*. New York: Norton.

Watzlawick, P., Beavin, J., & Jackson, D. (1967). *The pragmatics of human communication*. New York: Norton.

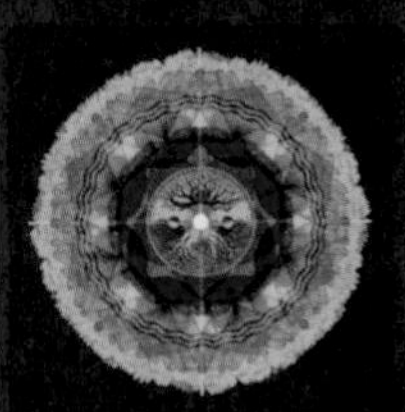

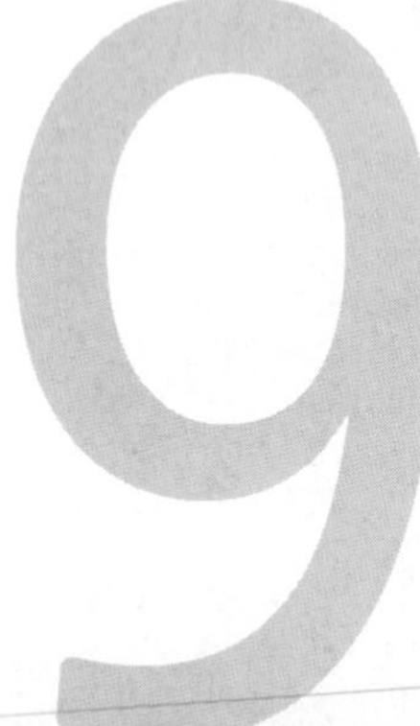

Chapter NINE

Assessment

EILEEN TRIGOBOFF
CAROL REN KNEISL
HOLLY SKODOL WILSON

KEY TERMS

Beck Depression Inventory
Benton Visual Retention Test
blocking
circumstantiality
compulsions
confabulations
daydreams
delusions
fantasy
flat affect
flight of ideas
Global Assessment of Functioning (GAF) Scale
hallucinations
intelligence tests
Mental Status Examination (MSE)
Millon Clinical Multiaxial Inventory–II (MCMI-II)
Mini-Mental State Exam (MMSE)
Minnesota Multiphasic Personality Inventory–2 (MMPI-2)
mutism
Nurses' Observation Scale for Inpatient Evaluation (NOSIE)
objective personality tests
obsessions
perseveration
projective personality tests

continued on next page

FOCUS QUESTIONS

- **When does assessment take place?**
- **What steps would you take to conduct a psychiatric history and a mental status examination on a client?**
- **Under which circumstances would you use the Mental State Examination or the Mini-Mental State Exam?**
- **Where would a psychosocial stressor be placed on the DSM-IV-TR multiaxial system for making a psychiatric diagnosis?**
- **How would you apply the principles of quality assurance to your assessments and interventions?**

MediaLink 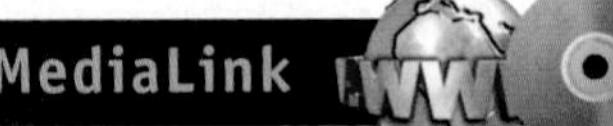 www.prenhall.com/kneisl

Additional resources for this chapter can be found on the Student CD-ROM accompanying this textbook, and on the Companion Website at www.prenhall.com/kneisl. Click on Chapter 9 to select the activities for this chapter.

CD-ROM
- Audio Glossary
- NCLEX Review
- Extrapyramidal Side Effects:
  Hands & Arms Tremor Video
  Grasping Tremor Video
  Lateral Tremor Video

Companion Website
- Additional NCLEX Review
- Case Study: Preparing an Assessment

CHAPTER OUTLINE

Key Terms continued

psychiatric history
Raven's Progressive Matrices Test
Rorschach Test
Sentence Completion Test
State–Trait Anxiety Inventory
Thematic Apperception Test (TAT)
Weschler Adult Intelligence Scale–III (WAIS-III)

CROSS REFERENCES

Other topics relevant to this content are: Assessing clients with delirium or dementia, Chapter 12; Assessing clients with mood disorders, Chapter 15; Assessing clients with schizophrenic disorders, Chapter 14; Assessing clients with substance-related disorders, Chapter 13; Brain imaging; Chapter, 4; Counseling the individual, Chapter 28; Cultural competence, Chapter 6; Family characteristics and dynamics, Chapter 29; Group process, Chapter 29; Nursing process, Chapter 7; Suicide assessment, Chapter 22; Therapeutic communication, Chapter 8.

CRITICAL THINKING CHALLENGE

You are responsible for an intake assessment with Jared, a 35-year-old male client. He is being admitted to inpatient care because he has been transferred from an emergency room after driving his car off a freeway ramp into a building. His psychiatric diagnosis is major depression with psychotic features and he has had prior hospitalizations for what in his chart are termed "suicidal gestures." Most guidelines for conducting a mental status intake examination emphasize the importance of conducting a suicide assessment. This assessment includes questions like, "Have you ever thought of ending it all?", "Have you ever considered suicide?", or "Do you plan to hurt yourself?"

Jared is single, unemployed, and has a problem with alcohol abuse. In your interview you ask if he is considering hurting himself again, and he says "no." He seems anxious and does express feelings of hopelessness. He also hopes to find a new life as a result of his hospitalization. What recommendations do you make for his first few days on the psychiatric inpatient unit, and why? ■

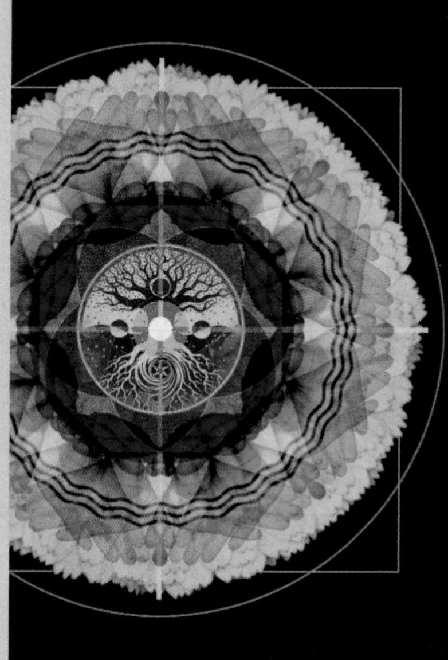

The systematic scientific approach known among nurses as the *nursing process* has evolved as the cornerstone of clinical practice. The nursing process begins with assessment for the purpose of collecting and analyzing objective and subjective data about the clients with whom nurses work. One of the chief rationales for nursing assessment is described in our Scope and Standards of Practice (American Nurses Association [ANA], 2000). A comprehensive assessment enables the nurse to make sound clinical judgments and plan appropriate interventions. The primary sources of client data in most instances are the clients themselves. Nurses' documentation, psychological evaluations and tests, physicians' orders, social workers' information, and other secondary data sources can enlarge, clarify, and substantiate data obtained directly from the client. A nurse's assessment skills are utilized throughout an individual client's care. They are used constantly and are essential to the success of a treatment regimen.

Psychiatric Examination

MediaLink Psychiatric Assessment Skills (UK)

Systems of data collection and assessment vary among mental health agencies. The psychiatric examination consists of two parts: the psychiatric history and the mental status exam. It is most often done during initial or early interactions with a client. The traditional psychiatric examination is discussed in this chapter because it is still used in settings where psychiatric nurses work and is considered the counterpart of the physical examination and history. An introduction to the basics of psychiatric assessment skills can be found at www. psychiatry.ox.ac. uk/medicalstudents/learning/psychassessment.pdf and can be accessed on the Companion Website of this book.

PSYCHIATRIC HISTORY

The psychiatric history gathers information about the client's current condition and previous diagnoses, interventions, and treatment along with a family history.

Data Sources

Not all data gathered during psychiatric history taking are obtained from the client. There are several other sources. Family, friends, police, mental health personnel, and others may contribute data to the psychiatric history. When the sources are varied, the psychiatric history focuses on the perceptions of others: how they see the client and the circumstances of the client's life. The sources of the information to be included in the psychiatric history and their relationship to the client should always be clearly indicated. Information given by these collateral sources should be reviewed and understood in terms of that relationship.

The **psychiatric history** generally includes the following categories of data:

- *Complaint*—the main reason the client is having a psychiatric examination. The client may have personally initiated the psychiatric examination, or others (such as courts, hospital staff, family, referral from school or industry) may have initiated it. The "chief complaint" should be recorded verbatim and indicated as such with quotation marks in the write-up ("I just don't want to live any longer" or "My drug use has become unmanageable").
- *Present symptoms*—the nature of the onset and the development of symptoms. These data are usually traced from the present to the last period of adaptive functioning.
- *Previous hospitalizations and mental health treatment.*
- *Family history*—generally, whether any family members have ever sought or received mental health treatment.
- *Personal history*—the person's birth and development; past and recent illnesses; schooling and educational problems; occupation; sexual development, interests, and practices; marital history; the use of alcohol, drugs, caffeine, and tobacco; and religious or spiritual practices.
- *Personality*—the client's relationships with others, moods, feelings, interests, and leisure activities.

Input from family and friends can give a better perspective of the client you are interviewing and can give you some insight into the psychosocial aspects of the circumstances with which the client lives. The value of this input includes perceptions of the client by others (how they see the client), how symptoms are expressed in that environment, and patterns of interactions. Keep in mind that family and friends have their own perspectives through which they filter events. All information from family and friends is treated as important data to be contributed to the whole assessment and not necessarily a total picture of the client.

The main purpose of history taking is to gather information, although it is often effective in establishing rapport with a client. The information offered by the client will not likely emerge in the exact order of the forms to be completed. You can shape and guide the interview while allowing the client to provide information at a comfortable pace. You can also promote rapport by avoiding an interrogative approach and allowing the client's story to unfold naturally. For the most part, the assessment process involves inserting all collected data for documentation without maintaining a rigid structure.

MENTAL STATUS EXAMINATION

The **Mental Status Examination (MSE)** is usually a standardized procedure in agencies that use it. The primary purpose of the MSE is to help the examiner gather more objective data to be used in determining etiology, diagnosis, prognosis, and treatment, and to deal immediately with any risk of violence or harm. The sections of the MSE that deal with sensorium and intellect are particularly important in establishing the existence of delirium, dementia, amnestic, and other cognitive disorders. The purpose of this examination differs from that of the psychiatric history in that it identifies the person's present mental status.

The mental status examiner generally seeks the following categories of information (not necessarily in the sequence presented here):

1. *General behavior, appearance, and attitude*—a complete and accurate description of the client's physical characteristics, apparent age, manner of dress, use of cosmetics, personal hygiene, and responses to the examiner. Postures, gait, ges-

tures, facial expression, and mannerisms are included in the description. The examiner also notes the client's general activity level.

CLINICAL EXAMPLE

A 35-year-old white male, dressed in torn, disheveled jeans. Presented a blank facial expression, slouched posture, shuffling gait, generally low activity level, and sullen behavior.

Other descriptors that may be used include *frank, friendly, irritable, dramatic, evasive, indifferent,* and so forth. Details should be sufficient to identify and characterize the client.

2. *Characteristics of talk*—the form, rather than the content, of the client's speech. The speech is described in terms of loudness, flow, speed, quantity, level of coherence, and logic. A sample of the client's conversation with the examiner may be included in quotation marks. The goal is to describe the quantity and quality of speech to discern difficulties in thought processes. The following patterns, if present, should be particularly noted.
   a. **Mutism**—no verbal response despite indications that the client is aware of the examiner's questions.
   b. **Circumstantiality**—cumbersome, convoluted, and unnecessary detail in response to the interviewer's questions.
   c. **Perseveration**—a pattern of repeating the same words or movements despite apparent efforts to make a new response.
   d. **Flight of ideas**—rapid, overly productive responses to questions that seem related only by chance associations between one sentence fragment and another. Associated with flight of ideas might be rhyming, clang associations, punning, and evidence of distractibility.
   e. **Blocking**—a pattern of sudden silence in the stream of conversation for no obvious reason but often thought to be associated with intrusion of delusional thoughts or hallucinations.
3. *Emotional state*—the person's pervasive or dominant mood or affective reaction. Both subjective and objective data are included. Subjective data are obtained through the use of nonleading questions, for instance, "How are you feeling?" If the client replies with general terms, such as *nervous*, the interviewer should ask the client to describe how the nervousness shows itself and its effect, since such words may mean different things to different individuals. The examiner should observe objective signs, such as facial expression, motor behavior, the presence of tears, flushing, sweating, tachycardia, tremors, respiratory irregularities, states of excitement, fear, and depression. The attitude of the client toward the examiner sometimes offers valuable clues. Attitudes of hostility, suspiciousness, or flirtatiousness, a desire for bodily contact, or outspoken criticisms should be noted.

   The psychiatric client is apt to have a persistent emotional trend reflective of a particular emotional disorder, such as depression. If this is true, the examiner should probe further to discover the intensity and persistence of this reaction, in keeping with *Diagnostic and Statistical Manual of Mental Disorders*, 4th edition, Text Revision (DSM-IV-TR) criteria.

   It is desirable to record verbatim the replies to questions concerning the client's mood. The relationship between mood and the content of thought is particularly significant. There may be a wide divergence between what clients say or do and their emotional state as expressed by attitudes or facial expressions.

   Note whether intense emotional responses accompany discussion of specific topics. Shallowness or **flat affect** is indicated by an insufficiently intense emotional display in association with ideas or situations that ordinarily would call for a stronger response. *Dissociation* or *disharmony* is often indicated by an inappropriate emotional response, such as smiling or silly behavior, when the attitude should be one of concern, anxiety, or sadness. It is difficult to evaluate emotional reactions in clients who use *simulation* or play-acting. Clients who are trying to cover up a deep depression may feign cheerfulness and good spirits. The reverse may also be true.

   The client's emotional reactions may be constant or may fluctuate during the examination. Try to specify the ease or readiness with which such changes occur in response to pleasant or unpleasant stimuli. The following terms can be used to describe intensity of response:

   - Composed, complacent, frank, friendly, playful, teasing, silly, cheerful, boastful, elated, grandiose, ecstatic
   - Tense, worried, anxious, pessimistic, sad, perplexed, bewildered, gloomy, depressed, frightened
   - Aloof, superior, disdainful, distant, defensive, suspicious
   - Irritable, resentful, hostile, sarcastic, angry, furious
   - Indifferent, resigned, apathetic, dull, affectless

   Pay attention to the influence of content on affect, and note especially disharmony between affect and content or thought. Also important is constancy or change in the emotional state.
4. *Content of thought: special preoccupations and experiences*—delusions, illusions, or hallucinations, depersonalizations, obsessions or compulsions, phobias, fantasies, and daydreams. You can elicit these data by asking such questions as, "Do you have any difficulties?" or "Have you been troubled or ill in any way?"

   Delusions are false beliefs. If the client has delusions of being the object of environmental attention, some of the following questions might reveal them: "Do people like you?" "Have you ever been watched or spied on or singled out for special attention?" "Do others have it in for you?" Delusions of *alien control* (passivity) are feelings of being controlled or guided by external forces. If you suspect these delusions, ask the client such questions as "Do you ever feel your thoughts or actions are under any outside influences or control?" or "Are you able to influence others, to read their minds, or to put thoughts in their minds?" See the Rx Communication feature below for examples and rationales for these interactions.

A client with *nihilistic delusions* more or less completely denies reality and existence. The client states that nothing exists, or that everything is lost. Statements such as "I have no head, no stomach," "I cannot die," or "I will live to eternity" suggest nihilistic delusions.

Delusions of *self-deprecation* are often seen in connection with severe depressions. The client describes feeling unworthy, sinful, ugly, or foul smelling. *Delusions of grandeur* are associated with elated states such as great wealth, strength, power, sexual potency, or identification with a famous person or a god. *Somatic delusions* are focused on having cancer, obstructed bowels, leprosy, or some horrible disease. These are to be distinguished from a preoccupation with normal, visceral, or peripheral sensations.

Hallucinations are false sensory impressions with no external basis in fact. Try to elicit the clearness of the projection to the outside world—for example, the source of the voices (from outside or inside the head), the clarity and distinctness of the perception, and the intensity. Be subtle in approaching the client for evidence of hallucinatory phenomena, unless the client is obviously hallucinating. In the case of obvious hallucinations, it's appropriate to ask about them directly.

Obsessions are insistent thoughts recognized as arising from the self. The client usually regards them as absurd and relatively meaningless, yet they persist despite endeavors to get rid of them. **Compulsions** are repetitive acts performed through some inner need or drive and supposedly against the client's wishes, yet not performing them results in tension and anxiety.

Fantasies and **daydreams** are preoccupations that are often difficult to elicit from the client. The difficulty may be that the client misunderstands what the examiner wants, but often people are ashamed to talk about their fantasies and daydreams because of their content.

5. *Orientation*—orientation in terms of time, place, person, and self or purpose to determine the presence of confusion or clouding of consciousness. You may introduce such questions by asking, "Have you kept track of the time?" If so, "What is today's date?" Clients who say they don't know should be asked to estimate approximately or to guess at an answer. Many clinicians begin the MSE with these questions because disorientation should cause the examiner to question the validity and reliability of data obtained subsequently.
6. *Memory*—the person's attention span and ability to retain or recall past experiences in both the recent and the remote past. If memory loss exists, determine whether it is constant or variable and whether the loss is limited to a certain time period. The examiner should be alert to **confabulations**—invented memories to take the place of those the client cannot recall. It is useful to introduce questions relating to memory by some general statement, such as "Has your memory been good?" or "Have you had difficulty remembering telephone numbers or appointments?"
   a. *Recall of remote past experiences.* Ask for a review of the important events in the client's life. Then compare the response with information obtained from other sources during the history taking.
   b. *Recall of recent past experiences.* These are events leading to the present seeking of treatment.
   c. *Retention and recall of immediate impressions.* The examiner might ask the client to repeat a name, an address, or a set of objects—for example, rose, teacup, and battleship—immediately and again after 3 to 5 minutes. Another test is to have the client repeat three-digit num-

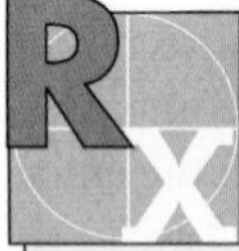

COMMUNICATION

Assessing Your Client

CLIENT: "I don't trust you."

NURSE RESPONSE #1: "You're very uncomfortable, so let's get this done efficiently."

RATIONALE: Empathic reflection, redirection, guidance, and limit setting.

NURSE RESPONSE #2: "That tells me how hard this is for you, but let's put it into your words."

RATIONALE: Accurate empathy, therapeutic reframe.

CLIENT: "They're all out to get me."

NURSE RESPONSE #1: "How does that make you feel?"

RATIONALE: Focus on process, ventilation/catharsis of feelings, induction of positive transference.

NURSE RESPONSE #2: "Tell me the ways you've been coping so we can figure out what would be best for you."

RATIONALE: Focus on emotional process, seeking details of client's behaviors and planned actions.

bers at a rate of one per second, or to repeat a complicated sentence.

d. *General grasp and recall.* You might ask the client to read a story and then repeat the gist with as many details as possible.

In a classic, concise guide for conducting a psychiatric examination, S. M. Small (1980) includes the following story as an example:

CLINICAL EXAMPLE

A cowboy from Arizona went to San Francisco with his dog, which he left at a friend's while he purchased a new suit of clothes. Dressed in the new suit, he went back to the dog, whistled to him, called him by name, and patted him. The dog would have nothing to do with him in his new hat and coat, but gave a mournful howl. Coaxing had no effect, so the cowboy went away and donned his old garments. Then the dog immediately showed his wild joy on seeing his master as he thought he ought to be.

7. *General intellectual level*—a nonstandardized evaluation of intelligence. The examiner looks for the person's ability to use factual knowledge in a comprehensive way.
   a. *General grasp of information.* You may ask the client to name the five largest cities of the United States, the last four presidents, or the governor of the state.
   b. *Ability to calculate.* Tests of simple multiplication and addition are useful for this purpose. Another test consists of subtracting from one hundred by sevens until the person can go no further (serial sevens test).
   c. *Reasoning and judgment.* A common test of reasoning is to ask clients what they might do with a gift of $10,000. Examiners must be particularly careful to correct for their own biases and values in assessing each client's answer.
8. *Abstract thinking*—the distinctions between such abstractions as poverty and misery or idleness and laziness. It is common to ask the client to interpret simple fables or proverbs, like "Don't cry over spilled milk."
9. *Insight evaluation*—whether clients recognize the significance of the present situation, whether they feel the need for treatment, and how they explain the symptoms. Often, it is helpful to ask clients for suggestions for their own treatment.
10. *Summary*—the important psychopathologic findings and a tentative diagnosis. Any pertinent facts from the medical history and/or physical examination should be added to the summary.

MINI-MENTAL STATE EXAM

If there is not enough time to complete a full MSE, it is possible to fairly accurately assess and evaluate a client's functioning in a streamlined manner. The **Mini-Mental State Exam (MMSE)** (Folstein, Folstein, & McHugh, 1975) provides a framework for such an assessment. Box 9–1 shows four sections of the MMSE with the general area of information the questions are explaining. A total of 11 questions cover the scope of the way a client thinks and reacts. There are scores assigned to each question and the total score indicates the likelihood and level of cognitive decline.

For the test to be efficient and valid you must ask the questions in the order they are listed. The main focus of the exam is cognitive functioning, although the client's mood can be ascertained in the process. The maximum score is 30 points, and the score is represented as a fraction with the actual points scored as the numerator and 30 points as the denominator (i.e., 28/30, 20/30, 17/30, etc.). It is important to note that there are limitations to using the MMSE with people who have certain disabilities with sight or motor movement allowing writing. If a client is not able to perform one of the activities, it may be necessary to conduct a full MSE or to document the results of the relevant aspects of the MMSE without a score.

NURSES' OBSERVATION SCALE FOR INPATIENT EVALUATIONS

An assessment tool designed specifically for use by inpatient nurses is the **Nurses' Observation Scale for Inpatient Evaluations (NOSIE)**. Developed and determined to be a valid and reliable tool in 1966 (Honigfeld, Gillis, & Klett, 1996), it has been useful in quickly assessing client functioning in six areas, three on positive features, three on negative features. The NOSIE has two forms, a longer and a shorter version. This assessment takes place within proscribed time periods, typically within three days of admission.

BOX 9–1 MMSE Sample Items

Orientation to Time
"What is the date?"

Registration
"Listen carefully, I am going to say three words. You say them back after I stop.
Ready? Here they are . . .
HOUSE (pause), CAR (pause), LAKE (pause). Now repeat those words back to me."
[Repeat up to 5 times, but score only the first trial.]

Naming
"What is this?" [Point to a pencil or pen.]

Reading
"Please read this and do what it says." [Show examinee the words on the stimulus form.]
CLOSE YOUR EYES

Scoring the NOSIE, after interrater reliability has been established, is convenient and can give valuable information regarding likelihood for behaviors and interactions while in inpatient settings. Interrater reliability is the process of making sure that all of the raters have similar scoring measures and techniques. These measures and techniques are usually established when all raters score the same client at the same time, or score a videotape of the same client and compare scores for consistency. If the NOSIE is incorporated into an inpatient setting as a regular feature of assessing client assets, routine interrater reliability checks need to take place. This assessment tool has remained useful across the decades. It reinforces the value of nursing determinations made when assessing behavior.

Physiologic Assessment

As the summary of the MSE suggests, nurses must carefully consider the possibility that a client's symptoms may have a physiologic, a biologic, and, in particular, a neurologic basis. In some reported instances, clients with brain tumors or bromide intoxication have been hospitalized on psychiatric units and treated exclusively for their seemingly psychiatric symptoms. Such a critical oversight obviously delays and seriously hampers appropriate treatment of the correct biologic or neurologic problem. The value of careful assessment regarding general health issues and screening for biologic disorders cannot be overemphasized. In many community settings, psychiatric–mental health nurses are the only mental health care providers prepared to undertake a biologic and neurologic assessment and interpret the results.

MediaLink Case Study: Preparing an Assessment

The objectives of a biologic and neurologic assessment are:

1. Detection of underlying and perhaps unsuspected organic disease that may be responsible for psychiatric symptoms.
2. Understanding of disease as a factor in the overall psychiatric disability.
3. Appreciation of somatic symptoms that reflect primarily psychological rather than physiologic problems.

www.priory.com/psycont discusses psychiatric assessments and can be accessed on the Companion Website of this book.

BIOLOGIC HISTORY TAKING

Of several procedures that enlighten the nurse who is attempting to account for biologic aspects of psychiatric symptoms, the client's history is certainly a major one. The nurse should inquire into three primary areas of biologic history:

MediaLink Tremor Videos

1. Facts about known physical diseases and dysfunction
2. Information about specific physical complaints
3. General health history

Information about previous illnesses may provide essential clues. Clients with comorbidities of substance abuse and mental disorder are particularly challenging. For example, suppose the presenting symptoms include paranoid delusions and the client has a history of similar episodes. During each previous episode, the client responded to diverse forms of treatment and demonstrated no residual symptoms. This history suggests a strong possibility of amphetamine- or other drug-related psychosis, and a drug screen laboratory test may be indicated. An occupational history may provide information about exposure to inorganic mercury, leading to symptoms of psychosis, or exposure to lead, resulting in mental disorder.

The second area of emphasis in biologic history taking is eliciting information from the client about specific physical complaints. Again, it is crucial for the nurse to consider symptoms in terms of both psychiatric conditions and physical diseases. Symptoms that are atypical of psychiatric disorders are particularly revealing clues. For example, suppose a client with hallucinations and delusions also complains of a severe headache at the onset of the symptoms. The symptoms together suggest possible brain disease and call for careful and repeated neurologic assessment and use of brain imaging techniques.

History taking should also include information about the medications the client is currently taking. Digitalis intoxication may result in impairment. Reserpine may produce symptoms generally considered psychiatric in nature.

The third area is that of the general health history. As mentioned above, psychiatric nurses need to be able to assess for a variety of general health problems and therefore need to have medical–surgical nursing skills. During your assessment of any client, assess for medical problems as well as the psychiatric symptomatology. Keep in mind that some medical problems are masked by psychiatric symptoms and psychiatric symptomatology can be the result of a medical disorder.

OBSERVATION

Observation also yields important data bearing on the possible presence of organic disorders.

- An unsteady gait may suggest diffuse brain disease or alcohol or drug intoxication.
- Asymmetry—dragging a leg or not swinging one arm—might be a sign of a focal brain lesion.
- Although inattention to proper hygiene and dress, particularly mismatched socks or shoes, is common in people with emotional disorders, it is also a hallmark of dementias.
- Frequent, quick, purposeless movements are characteristic of anxiety, but they are equally characteristic of chorea and hyperthyroidism.
- Tremors accompanied by anxiety may point to Parkinson's disease.
- Recent weight loss, although often encountered in depression and schizophrenia, may be due to gastrointestinal disease, carcinoma, Addison's disease, and many other physical disorders.

Observe skin color, pupillary changes, alertness and responsiveness, and quality of speech and word production, keeping in mind the possibility of delirium, dementia, substance intoxication, or other medical conditions.

Neurologic Assessment

A careful neurologic assessment is mandatory for each client suspected of having brain dysfunction. Its goal is to discover signs pointing to circumscribed, focal cerebral dysfunction or diffuse, bilateral cerebral disease.

BRAIN IMAGING TECHNIQUES

As previously introduced in Chapter 4, a range of brain imaging techniques are now available for viewing the living brain to detect seizure activity; evaluate sleep disorders; detect disorders such as multiple sclerosis; detect tumors, trauma, and strokes; examine the blood flowing to the brain; and identify cerebral atrophy, cerebral hemorrhage, cerebral infarct, hematomas, and abscesses. All of these conditions may present as psychiatric or behavioral symptoms. The most frequently used brain imaging techniques are described in the Tools of Psychobiology Box (see page 61) in Chapter 4. The positron-emission tomography (PET) scan brain image (see ■ Figure 9–1A, ■ B) shows two scans of the same brain tumor (glioma) at different areas (levels) of the brain.

Authorities in mental health practice consistently remind clinicians of the need for thorough biologic and neurologic assessment of clients seen in psychiatric settings. The psychiatric literature abounds with accounts of clients whose symptoms were initially considered exclusively psychiatric but ultimately proved medical, especially neurologic. Assessment errors occurred not because the features did not suggest medical disease but because such features were given too little weight or were misinterpreted. Changes in the American Psychiatric Association's (APA's) DSM-IV-TR (2000) require that both medical condition and substance abuse be ruled out as conditions resulting in psychiatric symptoms.

Psychological Testing

Clinical psychologists administer and interpret a wide variety of psychological tests. There are two types of psychological tests: those concerned with intelligence and those concerned with personality. Both intelligence and personality tests are typically included in a comprehensive psychological evaluation. Both types of tests are summarized in ■ Table 9–1 on page 168.

INTELLIGENCE TESTS

Intelligence tests may be useful particularly in evaluating the presence and degree of mental retardation and to assess cognitive functioning. Commonly used intelligence tests are the Wechsler Adult Intelligence Scale–III, Stanford–Binet Test–IV, the Wechsler Intelligence Scale for Children–III, Raven's Progressive Matrices Test, and the Wide Range Achievement Test–Revised (WRAT-R).

PERSONALITY TESTS

There are objective and projective personality tests. **Objective personality tests** provide data on various aspects of the client's personality, which is scored or analyzed using empirically derived criteria; an example is the Minnesota Multiphasic Personality Inventory–2 (MMPI-2). **Projective personality tests** involve presenting the client with a somewhat ambiguous stimulus, often a visual one, to which the client responds with an idiosyncratic perception. For example, the client states what the stimulus looks like or makes up a story about it. It is thought that in this process the client projects something of herself or himself into the response. An example is the Rorschach Test.

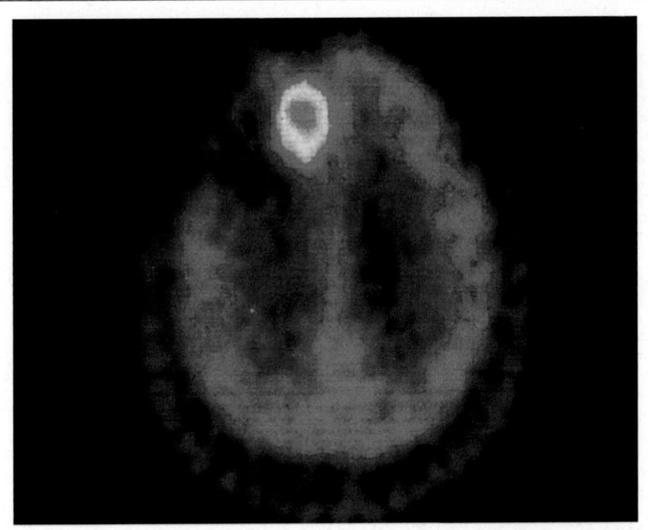

A

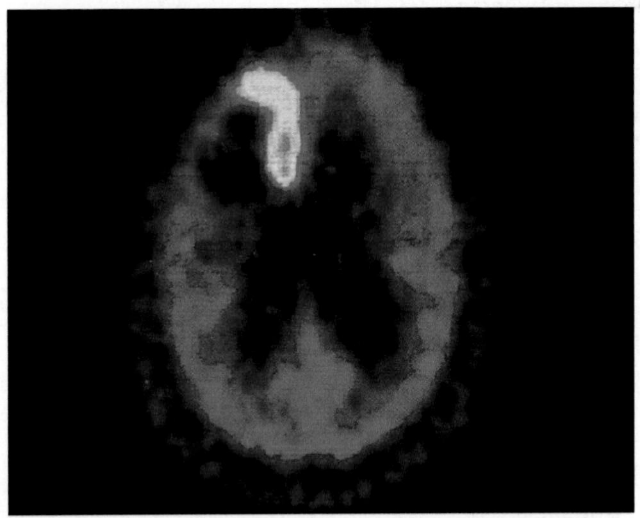

B

FIGURE 9–1 ■ *This frontal lobe glioblastoma multiforme, a primary tumor, is metabolically very hot. (A) Note the large red area of the tumor. (B) The same tumor at a different level in the brain.*

Source: Courtesy of Dr. Giovanni DiChiro and Dr. Ramesh Raman of the Neuroimaging Branch, National Institute of Neurological Disorders and Stroke, National Institute of Health.

TABLE 9–1 Common Psychological Tests in Clinical Use

Name of Test	Description	Method
Stanford-Binet Intelligence Test	A general intelligence test based on an age-level concept from 2 years to about 15 years. It is particularly useful to test children and to evaluate mental retardation.	The client is asked to do a graded series of tasks designed to correlate with the abilities of children of a particular age group. Each set is more difficult than the one before it.
Wechsler Adult Intelligence Scale-III (WAIS-III)	A general intelligence test for people 16 and older. It is the most widely used and best standardized intelligence test.	The client completes 11 subtests, which yield both verbal and performance scores as well as full-scale IQs. Subtest raw scores may also be compared to reveal variability in functioning. The subtests are: information, comprehension, arithmetic, similarities, memory for digits, vocabulary, digit symbol, picture completion, block design, picture arrangement, and object assembly.
Wechsler Intelligence Scale for Children–III(WIS3-III)	A general intelligence test for children.	Similar to the WAIS-III for adults, this test asks the client to complete subtests, which yield separate verbal, performance, and full-scale IQ scores.
Rorschach Test	A projective test that is thought to reveal aspects of inner psychodynamic functioning. It reveals personality features and symptoms and is commonly used as a diagnostic tool.	The client responds to 10 cards, one at a time, consisting of black-and-white or colored standardized inkblots. Responses include the impressions, thoughts, and associations that come to mind while the client looks at the inkblot.
Thematic Apperception Test (TAT)	A projective test offering a standardized set of stimuli for exploring the client's emotional life. Themes and interpersonal problems emerge in the client's responses.	The client is shown a series of ambiguous pictures of people in various significant situations and is asked to respond by describing what is happening in the picture and telling a story about it. Adaptations have been designed for use with children. In these, the central figure is a child or the pictures are cartoons of animals.
Minnesota Multiphasic Personality Inventory–2 (MMPI-2)	A self-administered objective (as opposed to projective) personality test designed to yield a broad examination of personality functioning that is amenable to statistical interpretation, such as profiles of symptoms or psychopathology.	The client responds to 567 statements by indicating either "true" or "false." The client's personality profile is formulated using 10 major clinical scales and dozens of subscales.
Sentence Completion Test	A projective test designed to elicit conscious associations to specific areas of functioning, thus illustrating the fears, preoccupations, ambitions, and idiosyncrasies of the client.	The client is asked to spontaneously complete sentences such as "I feel guilty about . . .," "Sex is . . .," "My mother . . .," "Sometimes I wish . . .," Both mood and content are noted.
The State–Trait Anxiety Inventory	Measures state and trait anxiety. State anxiety is conceptualized as a transitory emotional state or condition, trait anxiety refers to relatively stable individual differences in vulnerability to anxiety.	This is a paper-and-pencil, self-report instrument.
Millon Clinical Multiaxial Inventory–II (MCMI-II)	Profiles the presence and intensity of personality traits consistent with the DSM-IV-TR Axis II personality types.	Like the MMPI-2, this test consists of true-false questions.
The Beck Depression Inventory	This test is a quick, reliable, and valid measure of the extent to which depression may be present.	Questions ask the client to rate the presence and intensity of various symptoms of depression.
Raven's Progressive Matrices Test	This test is designed to provide data on intellectual ability in a relatively culturally unbiased manner.	Test asks the client to solve two-dimensional visual-spatial items of increasing difficulty.

Examples of Objective Personality Tests

Common objective personality tests are discussed below.

Minnesota Multiphasic Personality Inventory–2. The Minnesota Multiphasic Personality Inventory–2 (MMPI-2) is a psychological test that consists of 567 items to which the test-taker responds with "true" or "false." It is an actuarial test, which means that the test taker's patterns of responses to groups of items are compared to the response patterns generated by standardization samples of psychiatric clients with different diagnoses. A rigorous effort was made to incorporate cross-cultural considerations in the test's construction, including the use of ethnically and culturally diverse standardization samples. The test includes 10 major clinical scales, which measure aspects of different psychopathologies. See ■ Table 9–2 for the 10 major clinical scales.

The test taker's item responses are scored according to complex formulas that permit the construction of a profile of scores on the 10 major clinical scales. This profile can then be interpreted, with the help of several different profile code books, and individual features of the profile can be closely examined to permit a comprehensive interpretation. This interpretation can include the following:

- A behavioral description of probable courses of action in which the test taker may engage
- Information about psychodynamics and internal motivating factors
- Information concerning relationships with friends and with significant others
- Diagnostic formulation
- Treatment recommendations as needed

The MMPI-2 has a very large number of empirical studies supporting its use in clinical settings and may, in fact, be the most researched psychological test in existence today. Some other uses suggested for the MMPI-2 include personnel screening, employment screening, and prediction of response to medical and surgical treatment, as well as a screening measure for colleges and universities, industry and business, and government agencies; however its use in these contexts is not as well researched.

TABLE 9–2 The 10 Major Clinical Scales Measured by the MMPI-2

The MMPI-2 measures aspects of different psychopathologies:

1. Hypochondriasis
2. Depression
3. Hysteria
4. Antisocial personality features
5. Comfort with sexual orientation
6. Paranoia
7. Anxiety
8. Schizophrenia
9. Mania
10. Social introversion

State–Trait Anxiety Inventory. The State–Trait Anxiety Inventory is a paper-and-pencil self-report instrument that measures state and trait anxiety. State anxiety is conceptualized as a transitory emotional state or condition characterized by subjective and consciously perceived feelings of tension and apprehension, and heightened autonomic nervous system activity. Trait anxiety refers to relatively stable individual differences in vulnerability to anxiety (Spielberger, 1976).

Millon Clinical Multiaxial Inventory–II. Like the MMPI-2, the Millon Clinical Multiaxial Inventory–II (MCMI-II) test consists of true–false questions. The responses of the client permit the deriving of a profile referencing the presence and intensity of personality traits consistent with the DSM-IV-TR Axis II personality types. This test can provide valuable assistance in clarifying underlying stable personality features that can strongly influence the way clients interact with, and present symptoms to, health care providers.

Beck Depression Inventory. The Beck Depression Inventory consists of questions that ask the client to rate the presence and intensity of various symptoms of depression. A score is calculated, which can then be compared against empirically derived cutoff scores. The comparison can then permit a classification of the extent to which the client may be depressed. This test is a quick but reliable and valid measure of the extent to which depression may be present.

Examples of Projective Personality Tests

Note how the following selected projective personality tests differ from the objective personality tests above.

The Rorschach Test. The Rorschach Test consists of 10 standardized inkblots in black and white or color on separate cards, displayed one by one. Clients are asked to respond in terms of their associations, thoughts, and impressions. Because each card contains only inkblots, clients' responses are thought to be *projections* of important aspects of their inner psychodynamic functioning. The examiner scores the responses according to:

- *Location.* Where on the blot area was the response seen?
- *Content.* What did the client see?
- *Determinant.* What characteristic of the blot prompted the response?
- *Form level.* How closely did the response correspond to the contour of the blot area used?
- *Originality.* How common a response is it?

Interpretation is based on a complicated system of scoring responses and analyzing content. In recent years, there have been efforts to develop empirically based systems of content analysis to enable greater standardization of Rorschach scoring and interpretation.

Thematic Apperception Test. The Thematic Apperception Test (TAT) also consists of a series of cards shown one by one. However, TAT cards are pictures of people in various situations as illustrated in ■ Figure 9–2. Clients are asked to describe what seems to be happening in the picture, what the people are feeling and thinking, and how the situation that is seen will be resolved. Because the pictures are ambiguous, the responses are thought to reveal aspects of the clients' own emotional lives. The psychologist who interprets and scores the TAT looks for themes, threads, and patterns in the responses. Some adaptations of the TAT for use with children are available.

Sentence Completion Test. The Sentence Completion Test asks clients to complete an extensive series of incomplete sentences with the first thoughts that come to mind. The sentences are designed to elicit responses concerning fantasies, fears, daydreams, and aspirations, among other things.

COGNITIVE FUNCTION TESTS

Cognitive function tests generally assign a level of how well, or poorly, a person is able to think and process information.

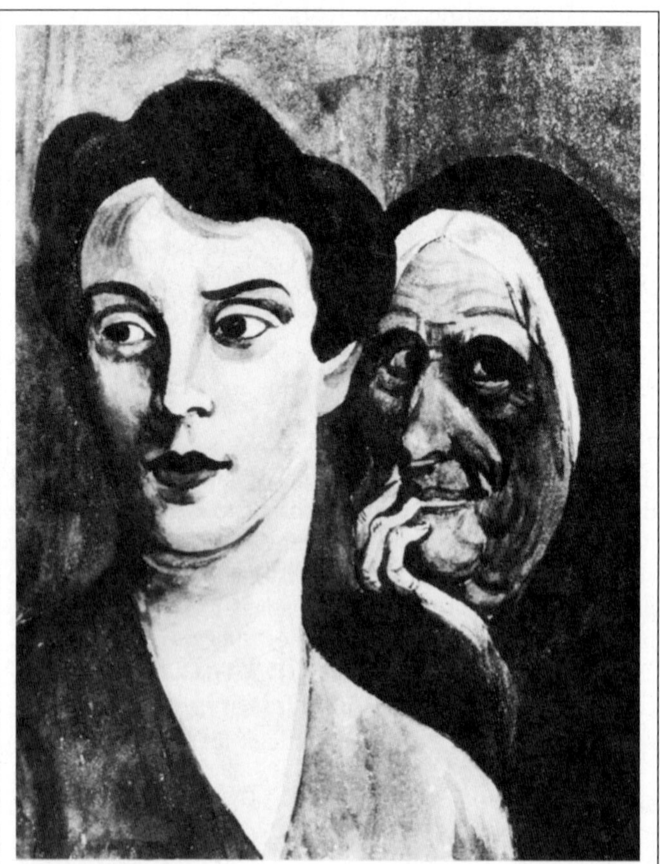

FIGURE 9–2 ■ *Card 12 GF of the Thematic Apperception Test.*

Source: Reprinted by permission of the publishers from Henry A. Murray, *Thematic Apperception Test,* Cambridge, MA: Harvard University Press. Copyright © 1943 by the President and Fellows of Harvard College, © 1971 by Henry A. Murray.

Examples of Cognitive Function Tests

Common cognitive function tests are discussed below.

Wechsler Adult Intelligence Scale–III. The Wechsler Adult Intelligence Scale–III (WAIS-III) consists of 14 subtests. Most frequently, only the 11 subtests that are necessary and sufficient for the derivation of the IQ scores are administered. The 11 subtests are picture completion, vocabulary, digit symbol, similarities, block design, arithmetic, matrix reasoning, digit span, information, picture arrangement, and comprehension. In addition to providing information on the verbal and nonverbal (performance) abilities of the client, comparisons between individual subtest scores can be evaluated to yield data on relative specific cognitive strengths and weaknesses of the client.

Raven's Progressive Matrices Test. The Raven's Progressive Matrices Test is designed to provide data on intellectual ability in a relatively culturally unbiased manner. Many other intelligence tests depend on knowledge and skills that are somewhat culturally bound. The Raven's Progressive Matrices Test asks the client to solve two-dimensional visual–spatial items of increasing difficulty, items that are relatively culturally unbiased. Scores on this test can be translated into empirically derived categories of intellectual ability.

Benton Visual Retention Test. The Benton Visual Retention Test is an example of a neuropsychological assessment instrument that can yield valuable data on aspects of a person's cognitive functioning. It is sometimes used as a quick screening device to see if the test taker may be manifesting signs of cognitive dysfunction. It is more often used to provide details on the nature of cognitive dysfunction being manifested by someone who has already been determined to have a cognitive problem or difficulty. The test taker is asked to reproduce various geometric designs after examining the designs for a few seconds. The type and frequency of different kinds of errors, as well as the number of designs reproduced correctly, are compared with empirically based frequency tables to determine the extent to which cognitive dysfunction may be possible, probable, or strongly indicated. The test performance is strongly influenced by any difficulties in the test taker's visual processing, organization, memory, and visual–motor skills.

Psychiatric Diagnostic Practice According to the DSM-IV-TR

The American Psychiatric Association (APA) in 1952 published the first edition of the *Diagnostic and Statistical Manual.* The second edition, published in 1968, attempted compatibility with the *International Classification of Diseases, Injuries, and Causes of Death* (ICD-9) published by the World Health Organization. DSM-II was criticized for its low reliability and tendency to reflect an individual psychiatrist's philosophy. The APA published a third edition entitled the *Diagnostic and Statistical Manual of Mental Disorders III* in 1980 and a revised edition in 1987. Important features distinguished the DSM-III-R from its predecessors. It used specified diagnostic criteria to improve the reliability of diagnostic judgments and offered a multiaxial or multidimensional approach to clinical assessment of psychiatric clients in which five different classes of data are collected and assessed. The DSM-IV was published in 1994 and further clarified and codified psychiatric diagnostics.

The DSM-IV-TR (the "TR" stands for Text Revision), published in 2000, represents the current state of knowledge about diagnosing mental disorders. The continual evolution of this specialty area is represented in the changes made from DSM-IV. DSM-IV-TR is composed of a list of all the official numeric codes and terms for all recognized mental disorders, along with a comprehensive description of each and specified diagnostic criteria that must be present in order to make each diagnosis. Box 9–2 provides an example of a change from DSM-IV to DSM-IV-TR. Highlights of the changes made in the DSM-IV-TR are listed and discussed in the manual's Appendix D. Updated information regarding numerous clinical issues such as prevalence and comorbidity, among others, have been incorporated in this latest edition. (For a complete list of codes and diagnoses according to the DSM-IV-TR, see this text's Appendix A.)

BASIC PRINCIPLES OF THE MULTIAXIAL SYSTEM

DSM-IV-TR's multiaxial assessment is congruent with holistic views of people, recognizes the role of environmental stress in influencing behavior, and requires that the clinician collect data about client adaptive strengths as well as about symptoms or problems. One of the most important features of the DSM-IV-TR is increased interclinician reliability resulting from the use of specified observable criteria that have been field tested for interrater reliability. Its multiaxial approach is of significance to psychiatric nursing because it expresses the multidimensionality of human responses to environment, one of the hallmarks of nursing process.

The following example illustrates the principle behind a multiaxial system:

CLINICAL EXAMPLE

A 35-year-old man came to an outpatient mental health clinic for evaluation. He came in for treatment for severe fear and avoidance of flying that amounted to a phobia. However, he also had a long-term personality disturbance and had noticeable eczema.

Suppose three different clinicians were asked to evaluate this man. A biologically oriented clinician would certainly diagnose the eczema but might fail to notice the personality disturbance and make little of the phobia. A psychodynamically oriented clinician would be sure to diagnose the personality disorder but might overlook the eczema and the phobia, considering them to be merely manifestations of the underlying personality disturbance. Finally, a clinician who was behaviorally oriented would notice the phobia but might not diagnose the personality disturbance and the eczema. It is clear, then, that because of their differing theoretic orientations, these clinicians have a rather high likelihood of diagnostic disagreement.

Now suppose this same man were presented to the same three colleagues, but this time the clinicians were required to evaluate him in each of three different areas of functioning: behavioral or psychological, personality, and physical functioning. In this case, all three clinicians would be much more likely to diagnose all three conditions and thus agree on the total evaluation of the individual.

In the DSM-IV-TR multiaxial system, every person is evaluated on five axes, each dealing with a different class of information about the client (see Box 9–3 on page 172). A multiaxial evaluation system provides a much more comprehensive evaluation of an individual and increases the likelihood that clinicians will agree among themselves about the condition of the person being evaluated.

BOX 9–2 DSM-IV to DSM-IV-TR Crosswalk

This box demonstrates examples of the changes made in a diagnostic category from the DSM-IV to the DSM-IV-TR.

DSM-IV	DSM-IV-TR
Multiaxial Assessment	• Instructions for making a Global Assessment of Functioning (GAF) rating have been greatly expanded • Discussion about applying the GAF to the current time frame and about the underlying structure of the scale has been added. • A four-step method ensuring that no elements of the GAF have been overlooked has been added.
Mental Disorders Due to a General Medical Condition	• Error corrected in the exclusion criterion which does not allow a diagnosis of Personality Change Due to a General Medical Condition to be given comorbidly with a diagnosis of dementia
Adjustment Disorders	• Associated Features and Disorders section has been updated to clarify comorbidity with other disorders • Prevalence section is expanded to include rates in children and in particular settings • Course section now includes text about risk of progression to other disorders

BOX 9–3 DSM-IV-TR Axes

Axis I:	Adult and Child Clinical Disorders Conditions not attributable to a mental disorder that are a focus of clinical attention Additional codes
Axis II:	Personality Disorders Mental Retardation No diagnosis on Axis II (V codes)
Axis III:	General Medical Conditions
Axis IV:	Psychosocial and Environmental Problems
Axis V:	Global Assessment of Functioning (GAF)

Source: Reprinted with permission from the Diagnostic and Statistical Manual of Mental Disorders, Fourth Edition, Text Revision. Copyright 2000 American Psychiatric Association.

The DSM-IV-TR multiaxial system includes the five axes listed in the accompanying box. Axes I and II include all the mental disorders in the DSM-IV-TR and therefore might be said to represent the intrapersonal or *psychological* area of functioning. Axis III is for recording general medical conditions related to understanding the cause of psychiatric symptoms or managing the individual and thus represents the area of *physical* functioning. Axes IV and V, for identifying psychosocial and environmental problems and the Global Assessment of Functioning (GAF) scale, include an assessment of the person's social functioning. In this sense, the multiaxial system provides a comprehensive biopsychosocial approach to assessment.

Description of the Axes

To use the multiaxial system effectively, nurses must understand its components.

Axis I: Clinical Disorders. Axis I includes all of the Adult and Child Clinical Disorders. Axis I also contains other conditions that may be a focus of clinical attention, but there is not universal agreement that these conditions actually constitute clinical syndromes. Nevertheless, the symptoms elucidated in these conditions are observed often enough to warrant their inclusion in the diagnostic array available to the clinician. These include psychological factors that would affect a physical condition, medication-induced movement disorders, relational problems, and others. More specific examples include such conditions as marital problems, occupational problems, and parent–child problems, in which the problem being evaluated or for which clinical care is sought is not due to a mental disorder.

A mental disorder is differentiated from other problems as a clinically significant behavioral or psychological syndrome or pattern that occurs in an individual. A mental disorder is associated with either a painful symptom (distress) or impairment in functioning (disability), or with an increased risk of suffering, death, pain, disability, or loss of freedom. Further, the distress or disability does not primarily reflect a sanctioned response to an event, deviant behavior, or conflict between an individual and society.

CLINICAL EXAMPLE

A man with bipolar disorder that has been in remission for many years develops marital difficulties for reasons unrelated to his psychiatric history or condition. He and his wife have been arguing about her intent to resume a career.

Both "Marital problem" and "Bipolar disorder in remission" could be recorded on Axis I. If, however, the bipolar disorder is not in complete remission, and marital conflict develops as a result of his changeable moods and other symptoms associated with the mental disorder, the marital problem would not be recorded in addition to the bipolar disorder, since the marital problem in this case is due to the person's mental disorder.

Axis II: Personality Disorders. Axis II contains the personality disorders, usually diagnosed in adults, and developmental disorders including mental retardation, diagnosed in children and adolescents. Axis II is also used to report maladaptive personality traits. All the remaining mental disorders of adults and children and associated conditions are recorded on Axis I.

The classes of disorders on Axis II were given their own axis because their usually mild and chronic symptomatology is often overshadowed by a more florid Axis I condition. DSM-IV-TR clarifies the conceptual distinction between Axis I and Axis II by noting that Axis II conditions have an early onset and have a stable, not episodic, course. Axis II also has options for describing the lack of a diagnosis or condition on the axis. Examples of evaluations using only Axes I and II are presented in Box 9–4.

Axis III: General Medical Conditions. Clinicians use Axis III to record physical disorders and medical conditions

BOX 9–4 Examples of DSM-IV-TR Multiaxial Evaluation on Axes I and II

Example 1

Axis I:	303.90	Alcohol dependence, in remission in a controlled environment
Axis II:	301.7	Antisocial personality disorder

Example 2

Axis I:	V71.09	No diagnosis
Axis II:	301.22	Schizotypal personality disorder

that must be taken into account in planning treatment, or that are relevant to understanding the etiology or worsening of the mental disorder. A clinician might also want to record other significant physical findings, such as "soft" neurologic signs or even a single symptom (such as vomiting).

If there is a lack of information on Axis III, that fact should be stated: "No information," or "Diagnosis deferred—not evaluated," or "Referred to Dr. Smith for evaluation." In any event, *something* should be noted on this axis; omitting it for lack of information undermines the purpose of a holistic, multiaxial system. Of course, recent advances in psychobiologic knowledge make Axis III findings particularly important for psychiatric mental health nursing. Box 9–5 provides an example of multiaxial evaluation on Axes I, II, and III.

Axis IV: Psychosocial and Environmental Problems. Axis IV provides the categories of psychosocial problems that may affect the diagnosis and treatment of mental disorders as discussed in Box 9–6.

In addition to identifying the type of problem(s), evaluators should also note in their own words the specific problems they consider pertinent. Thus, a multiaxial evaluation, up through Axis IV, might look like the example in Box 9–7.

Axis V: Global Assessment of Functioning. Axis V, The Global Assessment of Functioning (GAF) is for reporting the client's overall level of functioning. This information is useful in planning treatment and measuring its impact, and in predicting outcome. The reporting of overall functioning on Axis V can be performed using the **Global Assessment of Functioning (GAF) Scale** as shown in Box 9–8 on page 174. This GAF Scale gives the clinician an opportunity to examine the overall impact of the client's circumstances on psychological, social, and occupational performance. The ratings on this scale fall within decile ranges and track both symptom severity and the functional level of an individual. When symptoms and functioning are at different levels, the worse of the two is shown through the score. For example, if a client had moderate symptoms and severe problems functioning, your rating would demarcate the severe problems in functioning. If a client's functioning was basically unimpaired but the symptoms experienced were significant, the symptom level would be represented in your GAF rating. Generally, ratings on the GAF reflect the client's current level of functioning, meaning the lowest level of functioning within the last seven days.

One of the most accurate indicators of clinical outcome is the level of premorbid functioning that an individual sustained. For this reason, the GAF Scale can be used to rate the highest level of psychological, social, and occupational functioning that an individual was able to sustain for at least a few months during the past year as well as at the time of evaluation.

BOX 9–5 Example of DSM-IV-TR Multiaxial Evaluation on Axes I, II, and III

Axis I:	312.8	Conduct disorder, moderate childhood-onset type
Axis II:	V71.09	No diagnosis
Axis III:		Diabetes

In this example, the client, a child in this case, will probably not be very compliant with the diabetes treatment regimen because of psychologic problems (conduct disorder, noted on Axis I).

BOX 9–6 Axis IV: Psychosocial and Environmental Problems

Problems with primary support group
Problems related to the social environment
Educational problems
Occupational problems
Housing problems
Economic problems
Problems with access to health care services
Problems related to interaction with the legal system/crime
Other psychosocial and environmental problems

Source: Reprinted with permission from the Diagnostic and Statistical Manual of Mental Disorders, Fourth Edition, Text Revision (p. 32). Copyright 2000 American Psychiatric Association.

PSYCHIATRIC–MENTAL HEALTH NURSING AND DSM

From the perspective of psychiatric–mental health nursing, the DSM-IV-TR represents some progress toward values that psychiatric–mental health nurses have espoused for decades. It

- Provides a framework for interdisciplinary communication.
- Represents progress toward a more holistic view of mind–body relations.
- Bases revisions on a series of formative evaluations.
- Represents a collaborative achievement.
- Provides for diagnostic uncertainty.
- Incorporates biologic, psychologic, and social variables.
- Achieves positive results in extensive field testing for validity and reliability.
- Considers adaptive strength as well as problems.
- Reflects a descriptive, phenomenologic perspective rather than any psychiatric theory.

The Using Research Evidence feature (see page 175) provides an example of the rigorous scientific work on which DSM-IV-TR decisions were made.

BOX 9–7 Example of a DSM-IV-TR Multiaxial Evaluation on Axes I, II, III, and IV

Axis I:	300.01	Panic disorder without agoraphobia
Axis II:	301.83	Borderline personality disorder
Axis III:		No diagnosis
Axis IV:		Unemployment

BOX 9–8 **Global Assessment of Functioning (GAF) Scale**

Consider psychological, social, and occupational functioning on a hypothetical continuum of mental health–illness. Do not include impairment in functioning due to physical (or environmental) limitations.

Code	(Note: Use intermediate codes when appropriate, e.g., 45, 68, 72.)
100–91	Superior functioning in a wide range of activities, life's problems never seem to get out of hand, is sought out by others because of his or her many positive qualities. No symptoms.
90–81	Absent or minimal symptoms (e.g., mild anxiety before an exam), good functioning in all areas, interested and involved in a wide range of activities, socially effective, generally satisfied with life, no more than everyday problems or concerns (e.g., an occasional argument with family members).
80–71	If symptoms are present, they are transient and expectable reactions to psychosocial stressors (e.g., difficulty concentrating after family argument); no more than slight impairment in social, occupational, or school functioning (e.g., temporarily falling behind in schoolwork).
70–61	Some mild symptoms (e.g., depressed mood and mild insomnia) OR some difficulty in social, occupational, or school functioning (e.g., occasional truancy, or theft within the household), but generally functioning pretty well, has some meaningful interpersonal relationships.
60–51	Moderate symptoms (e.g., flat affect and circumstantial speech, occasional panic attacks) OR moderate difficulty in social, occupational, or school functioning (e.g., few friends, conflicts with peers or coworkers).
50–41	Serious symptoms (e.g., suicidal ideation, severe obsessional rituals, frequent shoplifting) OR any serious impairment in social, occupational, or school functioning (e.g., no friends, unable to keep a job).
40–31	Some impairment in reality testing or communication (e.g., speech is at times illogical, obscure, or irrelevant) OR major impairment in several areas, such as work or school, family relations, judgment, thinking, or mood (e.g., depressed man avoids friends, neglects family, and is unable to work; child frequently beats up younger children, is defiant at home, and is failing at school).
30–21	Behavior is considerably influenced by delusions or hallucinations OR serious impairment in communication or judgment (e.g., sometimes incoherent, acts grossly inappropriately, suicidal preoccupation) OR inability to function in almost all areas (e.g., stays in bed all day; no job, home, or friends).
20–11	Some danger of hurting self or others (e.g., suicide attempts without clear expectation of death; frequently violent; manic excitement) OR occasionally fails to maintain minimal personal hygiene (e.g., smears feces) OR gross impairment in communication (e.g., largely incoherent or mute).
10–1	Persistent danger of severely hurting self or others (e.g., recurrent violence) OR persistent inability to maintain minimal personal hygiene OR serious suicidal act with clear expectation of death.
0	Inadequate information

The rating of overall psychological functioning on a scale of 0–100 was operationalized by Luborsky in the Health-Sickness Rating Scale (Luborsky, L.: Clinicians' judgments of mental health. Archives of General Psychiatry *7:407–417, 1962). Spitzer and colleagues developed a revision of the Health-Sickness Rating Scale called the Global Assessment Scale (GAS) (Endicott, J., Spitzer, R. L., Fleiss, I. L., and Cohen, J.: The Global Assessment Scale: A procedure for measuring overall severity of psychiatric disturbance.* Archives of General Psychiatry *33:766–771, 1976). A modified version of the GAS was included in* DSM-III-R *as the Global Assessment of Functioning (GAF) Scale.*

Source: Reprinted with permission from the Diagnostic and Statistical Manual of Mental Disorders, Fourth Edition, Text Revision. Copyright 2000 American Psychiatric Association.

Psychosocial Assessment

Psychosocial assessment is a dynamic process. It begins during the initial contact with the client, and it continues throughout the nurse–client experience. Psychosocial assessments may be made of an individual, or may be completed on a family or a group. In any case, they begin with the identifying characteristics, such as name, sex, age, marital status, and ethnic and cultural origins. Problem identification and definition are also necessary phases in the assessment process. The method for assessment described below has been adapted from the classic problem-solving model of Compton and Galaway (1998).

INDIVIDUAL ASSESSMENT

During the individual assessment, consider the following factors:

1. *Physical and intellectual.*
   a. Presence of physical illness and/or disability.
   b. Appearance and energy level.
   c. Current and potential levels of intellectual functioning.
   d. How the client sees his or her personal world and translates events around self; client's perceptual abilities.
   e. Cause-and-effect reasoning, ability to focus.
2. *Socioeconomic factors.*
   a. Economic factors—level of income, adequacy of subsis-

USING RESEARCH EVIDENCE

You are doing the initial assessment with a 45-year-old client who is having difficulties with depression and his primary personal relationship. These problems are more clearly delineated through your interview and during the MSE. You also notice a number of telling signs of alcohol use such as having no recollection of certain events (blackouts), sexual dysfunction unrelated to the depression or previous treatment, and input from his wife that "he enjoys a drink now and then" and that he might be trying "on his own" to treat the depression.

Your information gathering must be efficient and effective in determining the nature and extent of this client's problems. If this client is indeed using alcohol to self-medicate, your assessment must register that complicating feature of this man's psychiatric problem. You know from your journal reading that research has shown an abbreviated form of the Alcohol Use Disorders Identification test (AUDIT) and the CAGE questionnaire in combination form a useful alcohol screening and history tool set. The four CAGE questions (when one or more are answered "yes," indicates a problem with alcohol) and the multiple-choice questions of the abbreviated AUDIT, are recommended by experts for routine screening. This assessment effort on your part is succinct and effective for early detection of alcohol consumption behaviors and identifies an alcoholic history.

Once identified in your assessment as a feature of his current condition, treatment can be crafted to provide assistance, support abstinence, and individualize interventions. The antidepressant protocol used will take this client's difficulties with addicting substances into account. Appropriate family therapy can be instituted as well as recreating recreational and social habits to maximize an optimal outcome.

These suggestions stem from the following research:

Henderson-Martin, B. (2000). No more surprises: Screening patients for alcohol abuse. *American Journal of Nursing, 100*, 26–33.

tence: their effect on lifestyle, sense of adequacy, and self-worth.

b. Employment and attitudes about it.

c. Racial, cultural, and ethnic identification; sense of identity and belonging.

d. Religious identification can be linked to significant value systems, norms, and spiritual practices. Spirituality and its meaning for the client are a part of the Psychosocial Assessment. Attachment to a system of meaning, whatever that system may be, can be an asset and a strength. See the Caring for the Spirit feature for sample questions that can used during a spiritual health assessment.

3. *Personal values and goals.*
   a. Presence or absence of congruence between values and their expression in action; meaning of values to individual.
   b. Congruence between the individual's values and goals and the immediate systems with which the client interacts.
   c. Congruence between the individual's values and the assessor's values; the meaning of this for the intervention process.
4. *Adaptive functioning and response to present involvement.*
   a. Manner in which the individual presents self to others—grooming, appearance, posture.
   b. Emotional tone and change or constancy of levels.
   c. Style of communication—verbal and nonverbal; ability to express appropriate emotion, follow train of thought; factors of dissonance, confusion, uncertainty.
   d. Symptoms or symptomatic behavior.
   e. Quality of relationships the individual seeks to establish—direction, purposes, and uses of such relationships for the individual.
   f. Perception of self.
   g. Social roles that are assumed or ascribed; competence in fulfilling these roles.

CARING FOR THE SPIRIT

Spiritual Health Assessment

For these first five statements, indicate whether you *never, sometimes, often*, or *nearly always* agree.

1. I trust myself.

2. I feel my life has meaning and purpose.

3. Other people give meaning to my life.

4. I trust other people.

5. I have close friends.

6. I have experienced the following in my life:

Loss _____ Separation _____ Divorce _____
Geographic moves _____ Rejection _____ Death _____

7. Do *religion* and *spirituality* mean the same thing to you? If not, what are the differences to you?

8. With 1 being the lowest and 10 the highest, place an X on the scale below to indicate your relationship with your higher power, and circle the place on the scale that you feel would be ideal for your relationship with your higher power. Explain why you chose each of these points.

1 2 3 4 5 6 7 8 9 10

(no relationship) (turn only problems over) (turn total self over)

9. My religious upbringing and background can be described as (check as many as apply):

Nurturing _____ Helpful _____ Strict _____
Conservative _____ Liberal _____ Punishing _____
Negative _____ Had very little _____ Had none _____

h. Relational behavior:
   - ► Capacity for intimacy
   - ► Dependence/independence balance
   - ► Power and control conflicts
   - ► Exploitiveness
   - ► Openness

5. *Developmental factors.*
   a. How role performance is equated with life stage.
   b. How developmental experiences have been interpreted and used.
   c. How the individual has dealt with past conflicts, tasks, and problems.
   d. Whether the present problem is unique in the person's life experience.

THE PLACE OF ASSESSMENT IN PRACTICE

Assessment is essential in clinical practice and serves several purposes:

- Identifying problems.
- Identifying client motivations, strengths, and resources.
- Identifying forces (both internal and external to the client) that may hinder the therapeutic plan.
- Setting reasonable goals given who the client is at this time.
- Determining appropriate intervention strategies.
- Providing continuous evaluation of the process and indicating when the therapeutic plan should be changed.

MediaLink Navigating Health Care

Assessment is an ongoing, dynamic process that utilizes all your senses and all your skills. When your observations are combined with all the information you receive from the client and other collateral sources, it provides an opportunity for nurse and client to engage in a partnership based on mutual definition of problems and goals. Information and services that help nurses, physicians, consumers, other providers, and health plans navigate the complexity of the health care system can be found at www.webmd.com and can be accessed on the Companion Website of this book.

Documentation

When recording client data, the nurse has the responsibility to protect the client from identification and unwarranted exposure. The client's name should not be discussed out of the treatment area unless it is a secure environment and the discussion is among treatment providers for that client. Documentation is a legal and clinically relevant expression of care given to the client and how the client responds to that care. The use of any of this information in other arenas must be in the context of delivering that care. The nurse's respect for the client's self-disclosures is one way for the client to gauge the nurse's trustworthiness. See specific information on this in Chapter 10.

NURSING CARE PLANS

Nursing care plans are a means of providing nursing personnel with information about the needs and therapeutic plans for each client. They are of major importance when an agency uses source-oriented documentation, because they provide an ongoing, up-to-date record of goal-directed, individualized nursing care. When problem-oriented documentation is used, nursing care plans may be an outgrowth of that documentation. Facilities may also choose to have interdisciplinary treatment planning where nursing care is specifically delineated, as are certain other professions' (i.e., medicine, social work).

CRITICAL PATHWAYS

Critical pathways are an innovation on the more familiar and traditional nursing care plan. They are usually formatted in columns and emphasize patient outcomes tied to target dates. See Figure 3–2 on pages 47–48. Critical pathways in general specify the following categories of information:

1. Daily client outcomes (short-term goals).
2. Assessments, tests, and treatments.
3. Knowledge deficit (daily prescriptions for nursing interventions focused on client teaching).
4. Diet (daily prescriptions).
5. Activity (daily prescriptions for nursing interventions).
6. Psychosocial considerations (daily prescriptions for nursing interventions).

The precise format for critical pathways may vary from setting to setting or may be based on the client's condition. As is the case with nursing care plans, critical pathways are not set in stone and must be modified based on changes in client assessment data. Furthermore, standardized critical pathways should always be individualized for individual clients.

ALGORITHMS

Algorithms are behavioral steps, or step-by-step procedures, for the management of common problems. Algorithms have proved to be useful protocols, particularly in settings that employ large numbers of paraprofessionals. At intake points in community mental health settings, such as walk-in neighborhood clinics, mental health workers often make the initial psychosocial assessment and may plan and implement treatment strategies.

Clinical algorithms for common mental health problems provide the nonprofessional with structured, standardized guidelines for decision making. Professional nurses in nonpsychiatric settings find clinical algorithms particularly useful. Algorithms for depression and suicidal lethality have been found to be reliable and valid in these circumstances.

Quality Assurance

Quality Assurance can be known by many names. Some of these names include Performance Improvement (PI), Total Quality Management (TQM), Continuous Improvement (CI), and Continuous Quality Improvement (CQI). (For our purposes we will use the term Quality Assurance [QA] in this text.) No matter what name is used, the basis of QA is to assure that quality is maintained through an ongoing effort to find new and better ways of doing things and achieving better results.

Whenever QA is properly conducted, it involves the entire organization, whether it is a large bureaucratic hospital setting or a small private practice. All members of the workforce are involved in evaluating procedures, looking for ways to improve the process, and then improving them. As a matter of fact, QA is best conducted by the people doing the work rather than by supervisors and administrators.

You will hear QA referred to as a process. This is because QA is evolving as it improves clinical practice. It does not have a fixed or rigid plan. QA involves four basic steps—Plan, Do, Check, and Act—that are continuously in progress (see ■ Figure 9–3). (This explains why "continuous" is sometimes in the title: Continuous Improvement or Continuous Quality Improvement.)

Quality assurance is about asking questions, using perception surveys and questionnaires, and listening carefully to both compliments and complaints of the people involved in the process. The recipient of your clinical services can be imagined as your customer; someone who can make choices to a certain extent about from whom they receive services. And customers are the best judges of quality. They know best whether their needs and expectations are being met.

When you assess a client, are your procedures the best they can be? Have you utilized all possible and available resources to form the most comprehensive impression of this individual and how to approach treatment? One useful strategy for applying QA to assessment procedures is to compare the outcome of a clinical case with the assessment. Were the recommendations for treatment from the assessment helpful in treating the individual? The involvement of several clinicians in this effort can shape more and more advantageous procedures. If you have a QA format when examining your practices, then you are more likely to be able to create a truly quality assessment.

The *psychiatric audit* is one way to evaluate the quality of mental health services consumers receive. An audit consists of a review of the client's chart to compare criteria for quality care with actual practice. Problem-oriented documentation provides the descriptive documentation necessary for such QA programs. Although documentation may not always accurately indicate the quality of the care given, it is an important part of the process as it keeps the mental health care workers accountable to consumers of their services.

When QA is utilized in this way, it benefits everyone. Recipients and their families have an opportunity to receive a higher quality of care, which means better health and greater satisfaction with treatment. You and your coworkers find better ways to do things, which can lead to greater job satisfaction. The facility where care is given benefits from QA as an ongoing focus on improving quality which helps the facility fulfill its mission and do its job.

Correct problem identification and intervention strategies often depend on the quality of the assessment. Psychiatric client information is gathered, assessed, and communicated through the various interdisciplinary assessments. Your assessment's primary purpose is to gather data to formulate a psychiatric diagnosis, prognosis, and treatment plan. All of the information gathered on your client can be incomplete or even incorrect if misinterpreted. Read the Nursing Self-Awareness feature to determine your abilities to assess clients with minimal interference from your own cultural background and views.

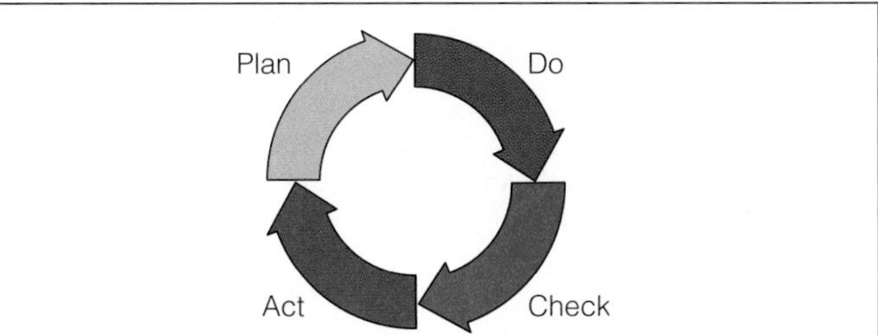

FIGURE 9–3 ■ *The Quality Assurance Cycle of Activities. The four steps of Quality Assurance are labeled Plan, Do, Check, and Act and are performed in a cyclic fashion.*

Nursing SELF-AWARENESS

Evaluating Your Own Assessment Skills

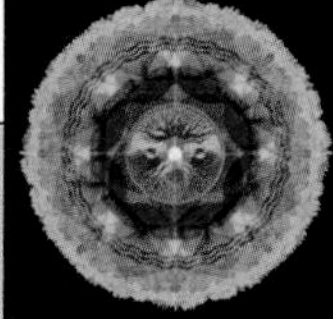

Evaluate your assessment skills by responding to the following:

1. Can you ask an open-ended question and not anticipate the answer?
2. Are you able to remain silent during an interview without being uncomfortable?
3. Do you accept information given to you without criticism or judgment?
4. Can you show empathy, not sympathy, for others' problems?
5. Gauge your tolerance for unusual or abnormal behavior.
6. Evaluate how aware you are of other cultures and their expressions of distress.
7. What is your skill level for understanding the content of what is said to you along with the process of how things are said, not said, done, and not done?
8. Do you have success getting your message across to others?
9. Have you been able to make necessary changes when you received feedback on your interactions?
10. Rate your skills for assessing someone accurately on a scale of 0 to 10, with 0 being the lowest level and 10 being the highest level. (For example, use a brief interaction with a new colleague and then discuss your assessment with the colleague). Discover your weak assessment areas and work on improving them (and raising your score). Repeat regularly.

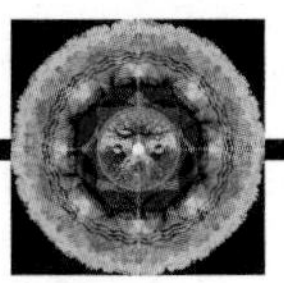

EXPLORE MediaLink

NCLEX review, case studies, and other interactive resources for this chapter can be found on the Companion Website at http://www.prenhall.com/kneisl. Click on Chapter 9 to select the activities for this chapter.

For animations, video tutorials, more NCLEX review questions, and an audio glossary, access the accompanying CD-ROM in this textbook.

BIBLIOGRAPHY

American Nurses Association (2000). *Scope and standards of psychiatric–mental health nursing practice*. Washington, DC: Author.

American Psychiatric Association (2000). *Diagnostic and statistical manual of mental disorders* (4th ed., Text Revision) (DSM-IV-TR). Washington DC: Author.

Bender, L. (1938). *A visual–motor gestalt test and its clinical use*. Research monograph 3. American Orthopsychiatric Association.

Compton, B. R., & Galaway, B. (1998). *Social work processes* (6th ed.). Belmont, CA: Wadsworth.

Cowman, S., Farrelly, M., & Gilheany, P. (2001). An examination of the role and function of psychiatric nurses in clinical practice in Ireland. *Journal of Advanced Nursing, 34*, 745–753.

Draper, B., Brodaty, H., Low, L. F., Saab, D., Lie, D., Richards, V., & Paton, H. (2001). Use of psychotropics in Sydney nursing homes: Associations with depression, psychosis, and behavioral disturbances. *International Psychogeriatrics, 13*, 107–120.

Drew, B. L. (2001). Self-harm behavior and no-suicide contracting in psychiatric inpatient settings. *Archives of Psychiatric Nursing, 15*, 99–106.

Ehmann, T. S., Holliday, S. G., MacEwan, G. W., & Smith, G. N. (2001). Multidimensional assessment of psychosis: A factor-analytic validation study of the Routine Assessment of Patient Progress. *Comprehensive Psychiatry, 42*, 32–38.

Folstein, M., Folstein, S, & McHugh, P. (1975). Mini-mental state: A practical method for grading the cognitive state of patients for the clinician. *Journal of Psychiatric Residents, 12*, 189.

Henderson-Martin, B. (2000). No more surprises: Screening patients for alcohol abuse. *American Journal of Nursing, 100*, 26–33.

Honigfeld, G., Gillis, R. D., & Klett, C. J. (1966). NOSIE-30: A treatment-sensitive ward behavior scale. *Psychological Reports, 19*, 180–182.

Lemmer, B. (2000). A review of violence and personal injury legal cases in psychiatric and mental health nursing to identify a practical framework for risk assessment. *Journal of Psychiatric & Mental Health Nursing, 7*, 43–49.

Murray, H. A. (1943). *Thematic apperception test*. Cambridge, MA: Harvard University Press.

Raichle, M. E. (1994, April). Visualizing the mind. *Scientific American*, 58–64.

Small, S. M. (1980). *Outline for psychiatric evaluation*. New York: Sandoz/Novartis.

Spielberger, C. D. (1976). The nature and measurement of anxiety. In C. D. Spielberger & R. Diaz-Guerrero (Eds.), *Cross cultural anxiety* (pp. 3–12). Washington, DC: Hemisphere/Wiley.

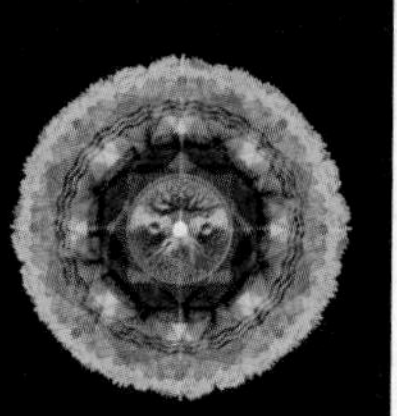

Clients' Rights, Ethics, and Advocacy

CAROL REN KNEISL

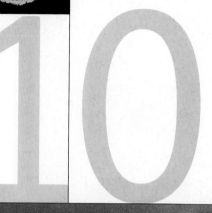

Chapter TEN

FOCUS QUESTIONS

- How do the five principles of bioethics relate to the practice of psychiatric–mental health nursing?
- What ethical guidelines should be applied in reconciling crucial ethical dilemmas?
- Why do psychiatric–mental health nurses need to be knowledgeable about the mental health statutes and regulations in the state in which they practice?
- What responsibilities do psychiatric–mental health nurses have in protecting the rights of mental health consumers?
- For what acts can psychiatric–mental health nurses be held legally liable?
- In which circumstances should psychiatric–mental health nurses act as advocates for mental health consumers?

MediaLink 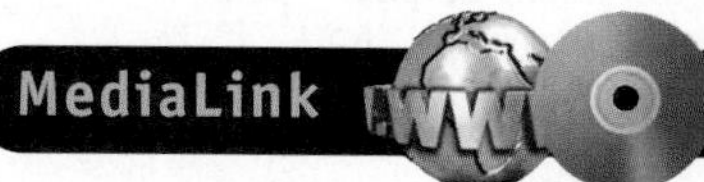 www.prenhall.com/kneisl

Additional resources for this chapter can be found on the Student CD-ROM accompanying this textbook, and on the Companion Website at www.prenhall.com/kneisl. Click on Chapter 10 to select the activities for this chapter.

CD-ROM
- Audio Glossary
- NCLEX Review

Companion Website
- Additional NCLEX Review
- Case Study: Involuntary Commitment

KEY TERMS

competency
habeas corpus
informed consent
involuntary commitment
least restrictive setting
malpractice
negligence
privileged communication
psychiatric advance directives (PADs)
voluntary admission

CROSS REFERENCES

Child abuse, elder abuse, and domestic abuse, Chapter 23; Cultural considerations, Chapter 6; Dilemmas in using physical and chemical restraints, Chapter 34; Ethics in managed care and milieu therapy, Chapter 11; Forensic psychiatric nursing, Chapter 35; History of moral treatment, Chapter 2; Legal insanity, diminished capacity, and competence to stand trial, Chapter 35.

CHAPTER OUTLINE

CRITICAL THINKING CHALLENGE

Sue Aberdeen is a client of a mental health outreach clinic. She was diagnosed with bipolar disorder more than 20 years ago. At one time or another during this period, various mental health care providers have prescribed several different medications for Sue. Most have been only slightly helpful or ineffective. Most recently, Sue has been taking lithium, which seems to be the most helpful. Her long-time friend brought Sue to the clinic because Sue has not been taking her medication. She has been unable to sleep and is distracted and agitated. Sue has been to a different bar every night this week, and has gone home with and had sex with a different man each night. The nurse assigned to her case has been attempting to persuade Sue to take her lithium. Sue has continued to refuse, and the nurse has continued to explain and cajole. Finally, Sue shouted: "You just don't get it, do you? Buzz off, you bitch!" and stomped out of the clinic. How can you reconcile the desire and duty to help with a client's refusal for treatment? When do you think it is acceptable for a client to refuse to be treated? How do you think refusal to cooperate with treatment should be handled? ■

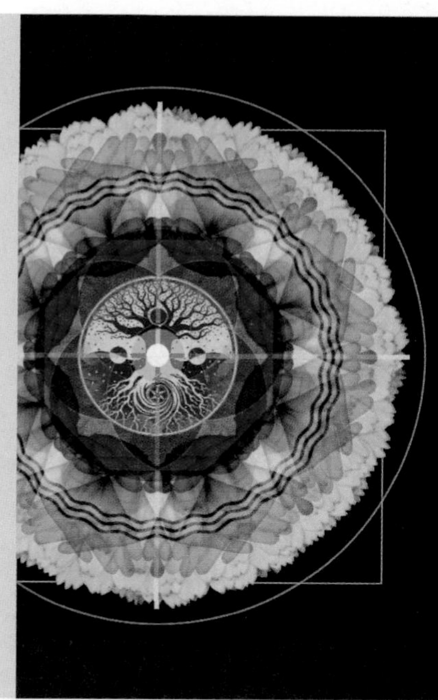

Ethical, judicial, legislative, political, and economic decisions profoundly influence mental health practice. Many factors bring about changes in the understanding and practice of mental health intervention. These changes challenge the psychiatric–mental health nurse to examine central issues, such as how does one balance the common and the individual "good" in health care, how does one define mental health, and what are nurses', mental health consumers', and society's rights, liability, and accountability?

An examination of these issues generally improves care, but it often confuses the boundaries of ethical behavior, mental health practice, and the law. This confusion entraps mental health care professionals, mental health consumers, families, lawyers, and the public in a muddle of conflicting policies and procedures. In addition, a client's right to privacy, to receive and refuse treatment, and to define happiness and growth pivot on society's values.

This chapter will bring some clarity to the ever-changing relationship between the law and mental health services so that psychiatric–mental health nurses can not only practice ethically and with confidence, but also exercise their power as citizens, professionals, and advocates to influence the direction of mental health care.

Ethics

Psychiatric–mental health nurses must often identify alternative courses of action and decide what to do when there is a conflict of rights and obligations between clients and families, between themselves and other mental health care workers, or between the client's good and the community or social good. *Ethics* is a branch of philosophy that deals with the values that are related to human conduct, the rightness or wrongness of actions, the goodness and badness of one's motives, and the goodness and badness of the results of one's actions. *Bioethics* is a field that applies ethical reasoning to issues and dilemmas in the area of health care.

The predominant character of ethical conflicts is, according to Redman and Fry (2000), disagreement with the quality of care given to clients:

- Differences in the definition of adequacy of care among professionals, the institution, and society
- Differences in the philosophical orientations of nurses, physicians, and other health care professionals involved in the care of clients
- A lack of respect for the knowledge and expertise of nurses
- Difficulty in carrying out the nurse's advocacy role for clients

These conflicts involve complex ethical issues and dilemmas that are tempered by the need to provide culturally congruent care (Zoucha & Husted, 2000).

ETHICAL ANALYSIS

One of the major difficulties in ethical analysis is that there are no definite, clear-cut solutions to ethical dilemmas. For centuries moral philosophers—beginning with Socrates, Plato, and Aristotle—have struggled with two main ethical questions: What is the meaning of right or good? and What should I do? To identify, clarify, define, and defend a stand on an ethical issue, we must engage in a process of ethical reasoning about data that can be gathered by using the framework of six critical questions set out in Box 10–1 on page 182.

Taking a stand on an ethical issue involves much more than merely accepting the moral position or personal values of another. It requires an understanding of the principles of bioethics.

BOX 10–1 Framework of Questions for Analyzing an Ethical Issue

1. Who are the relevant actors in the situation?
2. What is the required action?
3. What are the probable and possible consequences of the action?
4. What is the range of alternative actions or choices?
5. What is the intent or purpose of the action?
6. What is the context of the action?

PRINCIPLES OF BIOETHICS

The five principles of bioethics discussed here are autonomy, beneficence, fidelity or nonmaleficence, justice, and veracity.

Autonomy

Autonomy is the freedom to choose a course of action, to act on that choice, and to live with the consequences of that choice. Helping clients, their families, and their significant others make choices, fosters autonomy. You help clients by providing them with the information they need in order to choose, helping them to understand and sort through the information, and by supporting their choice, even when that choice is one that you may not have made. Professional autonomy for you, as a psychiatric–mental health nurse, means having to account for and accept the consequence of professional decisions and actions. Professionals must balance the goal of more autonomy in nursing with efforts to achieve what providers and consumers determine is the common and the individual good in health care.

Beneficence

Beneficence is the principle of attempting to do things that benefit others or that promote the good of others. You operate under the principle of beneficence whenever you help people who cannot decide for themselves or are incapacitated or incompetent. Protecting people from harming themselves because of thoughts, feelings, or behaviors that lead to self-harm is done in a spirit of beneficence.

MediaLink American Nurses Association

Fidelity

Fidelity means that you maintain loyalty and commitment to your clients and are faithful to your promises, duties, and obligations. Fidelity is crucial to establishing trusting relationships with clients, their families, and other mental health workers.

Justice

Justice is the principle of treating others fairly and equally. It is the fair and equitable distribution of burdens and benefits. The principle of justice has always been a cornerstone of bioethics (Botes, 2000a) and has become even more important when considered in issues related to health care reform and managed care. The principle of justice raises questions such as: Should indigent persons receive electroconvulsive therapy (ECT) to treat depression, but those who can afford it be treated with newer and costly psychotropic drugs? Is insurance coverage for psychiatric–mental health services a basic service or a luxury? Should mental health care be given to those who need it or only to those who can pay for it?

Nonmaleficence

Nonmaleficence is the intention to do no wrong. Your motives for actions should be in the direction of helpfulness based on sound knowledge of psychiatric–mental health theory. Nonmaleficence requires you to be self-aware and is the principle behind the Nursing Self-Awareness features throughout this text.

Veracity

Veracity is the intention to tell the truth. Veracity is critical to establishing trust with clients, their families, and other mental health care workers. If you cannot be trusted to tell the truth, you cannot be depended on; what you say and what you do will be open to suspicion. Veracity means that you do not lie to clients to "humor" them.

ETHICAL GUIDELINES FOR PSYCHIATRIC–MENTAL HEALTH NURSES

Most professions develop guidelines for the behavior of their members. Ethical guidelines for psychiatric–mental health nurses stem from two sources. The first source is the *Scope and Standards for Psychiatric–Mental Health Nursing Practice* published by the American Nurses Association (ANA) (2000). (These standards are reproduced and discussed in detail in Chapters 1 and 7.) The standard of professional performance that deals specifically with ethics for psychiatric–mental health nurses, Standard V, is reproduced in Box 10–2. The second source is the code of ethics for nurses also developed by ANA (2001). The ANA Code of Ethics is reproduced in Box 10–3. Use these two sources to make clinical judgments and to engage in ethical reasoning.

You may also find ANA's ethics and human rights issues online journal helpful in your practice. The journal is available at www.nursingworld.org/ethics/update, which can be accessed through the Companion Website for this book.

CLINICAL JUDGMENT AND ETHICAL REASONING

The judgments that lead people to label someone's experience as paranoid rather than simply unpopular are based on shifting criteria. Behavior that is considered bizarre or unreasonable in one cultural context may be considered desirable in another. The definitions of those who need psychiatric help are constantly changing. Nurses are necessarily guided in therapeutic work by a belief system—some vision of what kinds of changes would improve a client's life. Nurses are further guided by some moral principles that limit the extent to which they will help a client obtain happiness at the expense of others, and the extent to which they will participate in the oppression of an individual in the interests of societal control. Laws represent yet another source of limits. They are discussed later in this chapter in the section on clients' rights.

BOX 10-2 ANA Standard of Professional Performance: Standard V. Ethics

The psychiatric-mental health nurse's assessments, actions, and recommendations on behalf of patients are determined and implemented in an ethical manner.

Rationale

The public's trust and its right to humane psychiatric-mental health care are upheld by professional nursing practice. Ethical Standards describe a code of behaviors to guide professional practice. People with psychiatric-mental health needs are a vulnerable population. The foundation of psychiatric-mental health nursing practice is the development of a therapeutic relationship with the patient. Boundaries need to be established to safeguard the patient's well-being.

Measurement Criteria

1. The psychiatric-mental health nurse's practice is guided by the ANA *Code for Nurses*.
2. The psychiatric-mental health nurse establishes appropriate boundaries and maintains a therapeutic and professional relationship with patients at all times.
3. The psychiatric-mental health nurse maintains patient confidentiality within ethical, legal, and regulatory parameters.
4. The psychiatric-mental health nurse functions as a patient advocate.
5. The psychiatric-mental health nurse monitors any personal biases and seeks consultation or supervision as needed in order to deliver care in a nonjudgmental and nondiscriminatory manner sensitive to patient diversity.
6. The psychiatric-mental health nurse seeks to prevent ethical problems, identifies ethical dilemmas that occur within the practice environment, and seeks available resources to help resolve ethical dilemmas.
7. The psychiatric-mental health nurse reports abuse of patients' rights, and incompetent, unethical, and illegal practices.
8. The psychiatric-mental health nurse participates in the informed consent process (including the right to refuse) for patients' procedures, tests, treatments, and research participation, as appropriate.
9. The psychiatric-mental health nurse carefully monitors and manages self-disclosure in a therapeutic manner.
10. The psychiatric-mental health nurse does not promote or engage in intimate, sexual, or business relationships with current or former patients, and recognizes that to engage in such a relationship is unusual and an exception.
11. The psychiatric-mental health nurse guards against the exploitation of information furnished by the patient.
12. The psychiatric-mental health nurse is aware of and avoids the dangers of using the power inherent in the therapeutic relationship to influence the patient in ways not related to the treatment goals.

Source: Reprinted with permission from American Nurses Association, American Psychiatric Nurses Association, International Society of Psychiatric-Mental Health Nurses, Scope and Standards of Psychiatric-Mental Health Nursing Practice, © 2000. American Nurses Publishing, American Nurses Foundation/American Nurses Association, Washington, DC.

Nursing is frequently faced with two goals:

1. Responding to the therapeutic needs of individuals.
2. Serving society by preserving social order.

Often these two goals are in conflict, and nurses must face the dilemma of placing one above the other. The only way to resolve the conflict is for us to clarify our own values through a process of ethical reasoning.

Situations that involve ethical dilemmas require you to understand the concept of *moral claims*. Ethical reasoning is the process you can use when there is a conflict of claims and you have to make a choice favoring one claim over another. Anyone who is responsible for moral choices is obliged to recognize the reason, virtue, ideal, rule, or principle on which he or she makes a decision.

BOX 10-3 ANA Code of Ethics for Nurses

1. The nurse, in all professional relationships, practices with compassion and respect for the inherent dignity, worth, and uniqueness of every individual, unrestricted by considerations of social or economic status, personal attributes, or the nature of health problems.
2. The nurse's primary commitment is to the patient, whether an individual, family, group, or community.
3. The nurse promotes, advocates for, and strives to protect the health, safety, and rights of the patient.
4. The nurse is responsible and accountable for individual nursing practice and determines the appropriate delegation of tasks consistent with the nurse's obligation to provide optimum patient care.
5. The nurse owes the same duties to self as to others, including the responsibility to preserve integrity and safety, to maintain competence, and to continue personal and professional growth.
6. The nurse participates in establishing, maintaining, and improving health care environments and conditions of employment conducive to the provision of quality health care and consistent with the values of the profession through individual and collective action.
7. The nurse participates in the advancement of the profession through contributions to practice, education, administration, and knowledge development.
8. The nurse collaborates with other health professionals and the public in promoting community, national, and international efforts to meet health needs.
9. The profession of nursing, as represented by associations and their members, is responsible for articulating nursing values, for maintaining the integrity of the profession and its practice, and for shaping social policy.

Source: Reprinted with permission from American Nurses Association, *Code of Ethics for Nurses with Interpretive Statements,* © 2001 American Nurses Publishing, American Nurses Foundation/American Nurses Association, Washington, DC.

ETHICAL DILEMMAS IN PSYCHIATRIC–MENTAL HEALTH NURSING

Ultimately, nurses must reconcile a number of crucial ethical dilemmas with their personal and professional values. Among these issues are:

- The potential stigma of psychiatric diagnostic labels.
- Psychiatry's right to control individual freedom.
- The justification for involuntary treatment.
- The use of restrictive treatment interventions.
- The client's right to suicide.
- The client's right to privacy.

Practicing psychiatric–mental health nursing requires ethical responsibility. The quality of a nurse's moral commitment is a measure of professional excellence. However, problems arise when there is conflict about the ground rules for behavior, whether the conflict is between client and social group, nurse and profession, or nurse and agency. These problems are phrased in the ethical language of right and wrong. Circumstances likely to give rise to such problems include the following:

- The professional and the client are from different social classes and may have different cultural values.

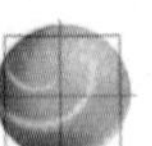

- The voluntary nature of the client's participation is compromised.
- The client's competence to enter into an agreement about intervention is questionable, or the client does not realize that certain interventions are being implemented.

Every nursing relationship begins with an unusual burden of ethical responsibility. The following pages explore some of these moral issues.

Stigma of Psychiatric Diagnoses

The list of stereotypes associated with diagnostic categories is well known to most nurses. Equally familiar are the consequences to people with these diagnoses. People labeled as drug addicts, alcoholics, convicts, paranoids, and so on acquire a discredited social identity because of the character flaws often associated with the labels. To much of society, the labels used in psychiatry suggest decadence, immorality, and wanton disregard for society's values. It is important to consider how and when psychiatric–mental health nurses, while advocating humane treatment for clients, indirectly contribute to discrediting a client's social identity by participating in the arbitrary use of oppressive labels.

Need for Diagnostic Labels. Diagnosis has considerable value in psychiatric practice. Putting clients into diagnostic categories makes it easy for health care professionals to communicate with each other about the client. The diagnosis often dictates a particular course of treatment and enables the mental health team to prognosticate about a client's recovery. Diagnostic categories enable nurses to plan comprehensively for client care and to conduct research.

Nurse's Moral Stance on Diagnoses. Does labeling with psychiatric diagnoses merely provide psychiatric professionals with some additional sense of control in their dealings with clients? Is it true that a diagnosis gives staff members an increased sense of being able to predict client behavior and a way of calmly viewing what might otherwise be upsetting behavior: "That's just her hysterical personality coming out," or "Those complaints are just paranoid delusions." The consequences of psychiatric labels for clients and their families, however, raise moral questions about their legitimacy when they are used arbitrarily or without current knowledge of diagnostic criteria.

Nurses have a moral responsibility to question practices that exact a price from clients far in excess of the benefits. Every moment of moral injustice takes its toll on nurses as well as clients. Every moment of moral responsibility strengthens their sense of personal integrity.

Controlling Individual Freedom

Involuntary hospitalization and treatment of psychiatric clients are usually considered humanitarian efforts to help "the mentally ill." Yet any practice that directly and coercively deprives a person of freedom has political implications. In some states clients have no guarantee that they will ever be released from the hospital. This ethical issue is further complicated by the fact that psychiatric professionals can no longer argue that involuntary hospitalization is necessary to restore mental health. Instead, the confinement must be justified as necessary to protect the client or others from harm.

Violence Against Others. Psychiatric–mental health nurses are faced with the dilemma of trying to be both healer-helpers and agents of social control. In dealing with violently destructive clients, they must balance the value of life against the value of liberty. A thorough discussion of violence in the psychiatric setting is in Chapter 34.

Suicide. Traditionally, nurses have felt that they should do everything possible to preserve life. We have relied on this imperative to justify intervention in suicide attempts as well as heroic technical measures to avert impending deaths. The treatment given to dying clients is often in conflict with the treatment they desire. For example, a physician may disregard a client's protests against treatment. The physician may assert that the client's medical condition is causing the client to behave irrationally. There is not necessarily an ethical difference between clients dying of physical deterioration and clients dying of emotional or mental deterioration. Many of the same ethical questions emerge about the suicidal client:

- How is *quality of life* defined?
- Is the definition limited to physical factors?
- Who should have the right to make the definition?
- How is rationality to be measured?
- Are people always in conscious control of their choices?

A thorough discussion of suicide is in Chapter 22.

An individual's right to choose when and how to die is a complex biomedical issue. The thoughtful professional nurse needs to clarify the issues, give them careful consideration, and search for a personal position. There are many ways in which people can deliberately shorten or end their own lives. They can destroy themselves quickly with a gun, or slowly through the chronic use of drugs such as tobacco or alcohol. When is coercive intervention by psychiatric practitioners justified?

Psychosurgery. The most dramatic of restrictive measures is *psychosurgery*, the surgical removal or destruction of brain tissue with the intent of altering behavior even though there may be no direct evidence of structural disease or damage in the brain. Psychosurgery has become the subject of marked controversy on ethical grounds. Advocates claim that it is done to restore rather than destroy individual freedom. They argue that before psychosurgery, the client is crippled by mental illness. Individual autonomy is compromised by the client's bizarre behavior or internal psychologic state. After the surgery, clients supposedly are more autonomous than before, by their own and others' criteria. Advocates of the selective use of psychosurgery, even against the client's will, outline three conditions that must be met to justify it:

1. The illness being treated is seriously disabling and untreatable by nonsurgical means such as medication or psychotherapy.
2. The treatment is undertaken with some sort of systematic investigative protocol; it is accompanied by evaluation research.
3. The treatment occurs in settings with as many safeguards as possible to arrive at informed consent, if possible, perhaps using a client advocate during the procedure.

The most common psychosurgery in the mid-1900s was prefrontal lobotomy (severing of the prefrontal tracts in the cortex) to treat schizophrenia. Although this form of surgery is now obsolete after having been found to be ineffective in treating schizophrenia, there are older mental health clients who still must contend with the untoward aftereffects—memory loss, personality changes—of this treatment. Today, the case for psychosurgery is most likely to be made in instances of severe and resistant depression (Malhi & Bartlett, 2000), or when obsessive–compulsive disorder is not helped by behavior therapy or psychotropic medications and is severely disabling (Jenike, 2001).

Psychotropic Drugs. The discovery that certain drugs can radically alter the expression of human emotions has had an enormous impact on psychiatry. The mental hospital is no longer seen as a "warehouse" for storing society's deviants; it is now a "clearinghouse" where clients are sorted, renovated, and dispatched back into their communities with symptomatic behavior under control through one or another of the current psychiatric medications.

Psychiatric professionals have associated the advent of psychotropic medications with a new optimism and less fear about working with people labeled mentally ill. Conceivably, the impact of the drugs on the attitudes of nurses may increase the amount of humane contact clients are given while in the hospital. Furthermore, it might be argued that the drugs have helped keep people out of the hospital and have decreased the need for other more dramatic measures, such as electroshock treatment.

Drugs that make people feel better, however, can lessen their motivation to confront an oppressive situation. This can have serious implications for the political and moral climate of society. It is conceivable that pills could be developed to keep a person quietly enslaved. Suppose drugs were coercively given to anyone whose unhappiness was rooted in social oppression?

The cautious and judicious use of drugs with the client's consent can be helpful. Used irresponsibly, they can close off moral and political confrontations. Decisions about the use of drugs must be made in the context of the social situation and environment.

In hospital settings, medications are regularly used to reduce symptoms and make client behavior more manageable. Most staff members justify their use of chemical controls by defining violent or bizarre behavior as an indirect request for limits. By assigning this meaning to the use of drugs, practitioners can feel that their actions to suppress symptoms are based on the needs of the client rather than on the staff's management motives.

CLINICAL EXAMPLE

After pacing angrily up and down the hall in front of the nurses' station for 20 minutes or so, Carlotta kicks over some mops in a bucket. A male staff member shouts to the nurse to get her PRN medication ready and strides into the hall telling the client to stop it. Carlotta cries and shouts, and they begin struggling. Several other staff members rush over to assist. They drag and carry Carlotta into her room, where she is given Haldol (10 mg). She continues fighting and screaming. Staff members continue to wrestle with her in her room. Finally they decide to transfer her to the unit downstairs, where she can be put into a seclusion room. In a report, a staff member describes the incident as: "Carlotta blew up and needed controls."

It is possible that all these controls would not have been necessary had a nurse behind the glass windows of the nurses' station responded to the nonverbal cues of mounting tension that the client communicated before kicking over the mops (see Chapter 34).

Restraints. Even the physical characteristics of psychiatric inpatient settings convey the notion that clients are not expected to be capable of self-control and that staff members have the responsibility for providing it. Many clients view these interventions as forms of abuse, while the staff sees them as "helping people who can't take care of themselves."

All the judgments that must be made about restraints involve moral decisions. What other techniques have been tried? Is the client obviously out of control? How does the nurse decide? Is the client cognitively compromised? What will be the effects on the client of such a dramatic intervention? What are the effects on others in the milieu? Legal factors that influence judgments about restraints are discussed later in this chapter.

Client Privacy and Confidentiality

When people seek psychiatric help, they must usually reveal highly personal, possibly embarrassing, and potentially damaging information about themselves. Almost all modes of therapeutic intervention rely on the client's willingness to talk openly and honestly about personal concerns, feelings, or problems. The solo therapist in private practice with voluntary clients is usually able to avoid compromising the client's right to confidentiality. In fact, many private therapists view themselves as vigilant protectors of their clients' privacy. You, however, may encounter a serious ethical conflict in being both the confidant of the client and the employee of the organization. Nurses have dual allegiances—to the client and to the agency.

Clients usually assume that health care professionals have no other purpose than to help them. They lose sight of the fact that nurses are often asked to collect data about them that might be highly influential in determining their medications, their disposition, and even their civil rights. While it is often the psychiatrist who makes final pronouncements about a client's mental health status, diagnosis, prognosis, and the like, such pronouncements rest on information collected and communicated to the physician by nurses. This information-gathering process merits serious scrutiny.

Information gathering and sharing are part of the psychiatric–mental health nurse's role. Thoughtful handling of patient confidentiality is facilitated by three safeguards:

1. Nurses must convey to clients the limit of confidentiality in their exchanges—that is, what the nurses do with the information a client shares.
2. Nurses must attempt to portray accurately to others the reliability, validity, and representativeness of the data they communicate about a client.
3. Strict confidentiality may have to be violated when an innocent third party is endangered.

Confidentiality is discussed further in this chapter in the section on client rights.

Legislation, Commitment, and Hospitalization Issues

In the last 30 years, the courts have had an impact on the direction of mental health legislation and state statutes. As a review of history tells us, the courts have traditionally been concerned with the possibility of wrongful commitment. Little attention was paid to the restrictions placed on the legal and civil rights of an individual once hospitalized. In recent years, however, the courts have become more concerned with the substantive rights of psychiatric clients whether hospitalized or not, including the right to treatment, the right not to perform institutional labor, and retention of civil rights such as the rights to communication, visitation, religious activities, and medical self-determination. This is reflected in many state statutes, along with an emphasis on procedural safeguards focused on involuntary commitment.

A review of mental health laws and judicial decisions underscores the fact that there is *great variability from state to state.* Because of this variability, it is critical to safe practice that nurses be knowledgeable about the mental health statutes and regulations in the state in which they practice. Most mental health agencies and psychiatric facilities maintain copies of these statutes, as do local law libraries. Nurses may also refer to the agency in their state that oversees mental health care.

ADMISSION AND COMMITMENT CATEGORIES

The two major categories of hospitalization are **voluntary admission** and **involuntary commitment.** Admission and release procedures differ accordingly. They are described below and compared in ■ Table 10–1.

Voluntary Admission to a Mental Hospital

Voluntary admission comes about by written application for admission by prospective clients, or someone acting in their behalf, such as a parent or guardian, a partner, or a mental health agent appointed through a psychiatric advance directive. As the word *voluntary* implies, the client has a right to demand and obtain release. Depending on the state, the client agrees to give notice, usually in writing, of the intention to leave during a grace

TABLE 10–1 Voluntary Admission and Involuntary Commitment Compared

	Voluntary Admission		*Involuntary Commitment*			
	Informal	**Voluntary**	**Emergency**	**Temporary**	**Extended**	**Outpatient**
Released	Anytime	Usually conditional	Average after 3–5 days	48 hours to 6 months	After 60–180 days or an indeterminate time	Can be indeterminate
Use	Limited	Increasing	Increasing	Increasing	Decreasing	Increasing
Criteria for admission	Client request	Client request	Usually client dangerousness	Client dangerousness or need of care and treatment	Client dangerousness or need of care and treatment	Client condition deteriorating or client in need of treatment

period from 24 hours to 15 days. It is justified on the grounds that the hospital staff needs time to examine the client to determine whether a change to involuntary status is indicated. The extra time also gives family and staff the opportunity to persuade the client to remain voluntarily. This "conditional provision" is seen by some as a covert form of involuntary hospitalization. There are now statutory assurances in most states, that voluntary clients must be adequately informed of their rights and status.

Informal voluntary admission, an alternative to the structure and personal concessions required in voluntary admission, is an option in several states. This procedure is similar to that required in a medical admission. The prospective inpatient verbally requests admission and is free to leave the institution at any time. Informal voluntary admission procedures are more likely to be an option in general hospital psychiatric units and private facilities than in state institutions, and they account for a small percentage of all admissions in states that have this provision.

Involuntary Commitment to a Mental Hospital

The state's ability to hospitalize or *commit* an individual involuntarily is sanctioned by one of two state powers:

1. Police power enables the state to hospitalize people who are considered dangerous to others because of their illness.
2. Parens patriae power enables the state to take on the role of protector and assume reponsibility for people considered dangerous to themselves or unable to care for themselves in a potentially dangerous situation because of a mental disability.

Most states provide for more than one involuntary hospitalization procedure. Involuntary hospitalization can come about if the designated body, such as a court, an administrative tribunal, or the required number of physicians find that the prospective client's mental state meets the statutory criteria for involuntary commitment. The criteria vary from state to state according to the type of involuntary hospitalization. However, all state involuntary commitment statutes can be expected to include one or more of the following criteria:

- Dangerous to self or others.
- Unable to provide for basic needs.
- Mentally ill.

In an increasing number of states, involuntary commitment is justified only if the individual is dangerous to self or others because of a mental disorder. The remaining states augment this by stating that the client's need for care and treatment may also justify commitment.

Involuntary commitment can be divided into four categories:

1. Emergency.
2. Temporary or observational.
3. Extended or indeterminate.
4. Outpatient commitment.

Emergency. Emergency involuntary hospitalization is available in almost all states. It is a temporary measure with limited, short-range goals, and it deals largely with the prevention of behavior likely to create a "clear and present" danger to the client or others. Under common law, any official or private person has the right to detain a dangerous mentally disordered person.

Some formal application is required to initiate emergency detention. In some states, any citizen may make the application. In others, it is limited to police officers, health officers, and physicians. Because this type of involuntary admission is an emergency measure and is warranted only until the appropriate legal steps can be taken, the statutes limit the amount of time an individual can be detained. The usual practice is to allow detention for 3 to 5 days, although some states set a limit of 24 hours.

Temporary or Observational. Temporary or observational involuntary hospitalization is the involuntary commitment of an allegedly mentally deranged individual for a specified period of time to allow for adequate observation so that a diagnosis can be made and treatment instituted. The actual time period can vary from 48 hours to as long as 6 months.

In some states, any citizen can make an application for the temporary hospitalization of a person in need of aid. Others require a family member or guardian, a health or welfare officer, or a physician to apply. Temporary hospitalization may be brought about by the medical certification of one or two physicians, or it may require further approval by a judge, justice, or district attorney in some jurisdictions.

At the end of the observation period, several options are available. The treating physician may (a) discharge the client, (b) have the client stay voluntarily, or (c) file an application for extended hospitalization. In some states, observational hospitalization is mandatory before a court ruling may be made in favor of extended hospitalization.

Extended or Indeterminate. Extended or indeterminate involuntary hospitalization can come about through either judicial or nonjudicial procedures. *Judicial hospitalization procedures* require that a judge or jury determine whether the person is mentally ill to a degree that requires extended hospitalization. If so, the court orders the client hospitalized for an extended period (60 to 180 days) or an indeterminate time.

Proceedings are usually initiated by an application for hospitalization of an allegedly mentally ill person. About half the states permit any responsible person or citizen to make or swear to the application. Others allow only one or more of the following groups: relatives, public officers, physicians, and hospital superintendents. Supporting medical evidence may or may not be required at the time of application.

Most states having judicial hospitalization procedures make some provision for a prehearing medical examination in addition to the medical certification required to support the application. In all jurisdictions having judicial hospitalization procedures, it is mandatory to notify the person proposed to be hospitalized of the hearing. Most states also require notice to the client's attorney, family, or guardian.

A hearing is mandatory in most states, although a few states leave it to the client to request it. While the client's presence is required at the hearing in a few states, most states merely permit attendance if it is not thought to be harmful to the client's

MediaLink Case Study: Involuntary Commitment

condition or if the client in fact demands it. Few states require the hearing to be held in a courtroom. Most say the place is entirely discretionary. Jury trials are no longer mandatory in any state, but 15 states still have provisions for the use of a jury to decide the question of hospitalization.

Nonjudicial hospitalization procedures for extended or indeterminate involuntary hospitalization include both administrative and medical certification, but such procedures are now much less prominent on the statute books. Extended hospitalization brought about by an administrative board follows the same procedure used in judicial hospitalization.

Involuntary hospitalization by *medical certification*, an alternative to the more traditional judicial commitment, is usually advocated for clients who are incapable of consenting to voluntary treatment, although they do not protest hospitalization. The need for hospitalization is usually determined by an examination by one or more physicians and documented by a medical certificate. All states having medical certification provide either for judicial proceedings, if the client contests the hospitalization at any time after certification, or for expanded habeas corpus proceedings described later in this chapter in the section on client rights.

Involuntary Outpatient Commitment

A growing number of states (now at 37), in response to several highly publicized and dramatic instances of violent acts by mentally disordered persons, have modified their statutes and regulations to allow for court-ordered outpatient treatment (Appelbaum, 2001). In most states allowing for involuntary outpatient commitment (IOC), the criteria are similar to that necessary for inpatient commitment: proof of mental illness and dangerousness. A few states have passed statutes permitting preventive commitment. In these instances, IOC is used to avert a further deterioration of the person's mental health that would require inpatient hospitalization. IOC has also been used to ensure that mentally ill offenders follow through with outpatient treatment once they are released from prison. Conditional release, a concept related to IOC, is discussed later in this chapter.

The effectiveness of IOC has been questioned on the basis that it may actually drive people away from treatment (Allen & Smith, 2001). IOC may also be vulnerable to legal challenge on the basis of constitutional standards.

Dilemmas Associated with Involuntary Commitment

Involuntary hospitalization is an exercise of power, and like all forms of power, it can be abused. Because of this potential for abuse, commitment criteria are important. In this country, a person's loss of liberty can be justified only under certain circumstances.

As the review of mental health statutes shows, a degree of "dangerousness" is the favored justification for loss of liberty by involuntary hospitalization. The "dangerousness" criterion is not without its inherent problems. Some of these are considered to be the following:

- Definitions of "dangerousness" vary from state to state.
- It is impossible to predict dangerous behavior reliably.
- In the absence of other criteria, "dangerousness" will be overused to justify admission.
- The stigma of *dangerous* will be added to that of *mentally ill*.
- The stereotype of *mentally disabled* will be reinforced and thus will work against the development of community programs.
- The media will be encouraged to continue selective reporting of instances in which mental illness and criminal behavior appear to be linked.
- Clinical practice shows that "dangerous" individuals are often not treatable, while the most treatable individuals are not dangerous.

In at least one state, a National Alliance for the Mentally Ill (NAMI) board of directors has come out against IOC. Their concern is that an emphasis on IOC will detract from the necessity of funding assertive outreach programs, housing, and other basic community services.

DISCHARGE OR SEPARATION CATEGORIES

A client can separate from a mental institution in one of three ways: discharge, transfer, and escape.

Discharge

Like admission, discharge from a mental hospital can have various layers of complexity. Discharges occur in one of two ways—conditionally or absolutely.

Conditional. As implied by the word *conditional*, complete discharge in this situation depends on whether the person fulfills certain conditions over a specified period of time, usually 6 months to 1 year. Compliance with outpatient care, demonstrated ability and willingness to take medications, and the ability to meet the needs of daily living are a few of the many possible prerequisites.

A person who is unable to meet the specified conditions can be reinstitutionalized without going through any legal admission procedure. An individual committed for an extended or indeterminate time is more likely to be a candidate for conditional than absolute discharge.

Absolute. The legal relationship between the institution and the client is terminated by an absolute discharge. If the client should require readmission to the hospital at any time, even a few hours after discharge, a new hospitalization proceeding would be required.

An absolute discharge can be achieved in three ways:

1. An administrative discharge is issued by the hospital officials.
2. A judicial discharge is ordered by the courts.
3. A writ of habeas corpus is ordered by the courts on the client's application.

As a rule, the authority for discharging involuntary clients rests in the hands of the hospital director, and these clients are given administrative discharges. However, a few statutes extend this power to the central agency responsible for supervising mental institutions in the state, such as the Department of Mental

Health. The client has no formal method of initiating an administrative discharge.

The majority of states have provisions for judicial discharge, which is initiated by an application to the court by the client, the client's family, or any citizen who is in disagreement with hospital authorities over the client's need to be hospitalized. A few states require the application to be accompanied by a medical certificate supporting the idea that the client is ready for discharge. In many states, judicial discharge does not depend on complete recovery. A degree of improvement may be sufficient. Some states guard against frequent applications for discharge by the same clients by imposing a 3-month to 1-year waiting period between requests.

Transfer

Transfers account for a small number of separations from a mental health care facility. Most are transfers within the state and county mental health system. A smaller number are transfers from state to federal facilities or from one state to another.

Escape

A client may take the initiative and decide to terminate the relationship with the institution by informally leaving the hospital grounds. This is commonly referred to as escape, elopement, or being AWOL (absent without leave). Voluntary clients cannot generally be returned to the hospital against their will. However, involuntarily committed clients may be brought back to the hospital against their will with the assistance of the police, if necessary.

Client Rights

The current concern for client rights has not developed overnight. It actually has been evolving since the 1960s, when there was an increased interest in underrepresented minority groups, the poor, women, and the mentally disabled. This section focuses on client rights. Specific information on the legal definition of sanity, diminished capacity, and competence to stand trial can be found in Chapter 35.

LEGISLATION AND CLIENT RIGHTS

In 1980, the United States Congress passed the Mental Health Systems Act, which included a model mental health client's bill of rights. This piece of legislation can be thought of as a set of recommendations; it is not a requirement that individual states follow its recommendations. In 1990, the American Hospital Association published a Patient's Bill of Rights that many health care settings throughout the United States have adopted. Consumer groups and professional organizations have, at various times, published their own versions of a bill of rights. A mental health consumer's bill of rights has been developed and supported by 15 professional organizations, including nursing, for those seeking mental health and substance abuse treatment. This particular bill of rights can be found on www.apa.org/pubinfo/rights/rights. html and accessed through the Companion Website for this book. However, there is no one standard mental health client bill of rights at the national level, and the variability among states is great. Some states guarantee several important rights while some states guarantee only a few rights. In other words, there is no consistency among states. The rights that mental health consumers should have in practice are outlined in Box 10–4. A discussion of several of these important rights follows later in this chapter. One means of helping clients protect some of their rights is through the execution of a psychiatric advance directive.

PSYCHIATRIC ADVANCE DIRECTIVES

Psychiatric advance directives (PADs) are modeled after advance directives for end-of-life care. Any person can prepare a PAD as a contingency plan to put in place should the person be incapacitated, found to be incompetent, or unable to make decisions about psychiatric care. Some people *expect to become incapacitated* in the future, for example, a person with symptoms of early Alzheimer's or Pick's disease (see Chapter 12). Others may simply *anticipate the possibility of becoming incapacitated* in the future, for example, a person with a family history of Alzheimer's or Pick's disease. Still others have experienced an episode of mental disorder—perhaps depression requiring a period of hospitalization during which the person received ECT—and wish to register their preferences for any future psychiatric intervention. See Box 10–5 on page 190 for the elements that comprise a PAD.

A written PAD allows a person to:

1. Register refusal of certain psychiatric interventions such as ECT, psychotropic medications, psychosurgery, and the like.
2. Register consent and desire for certain psychiatric interventions.
3. Specify the conditions under which these interventions are acceptable.
4. Appoint a trusted surrogate decision maker, a person(s) authorized to give consent on the person's behalf.

BOX 10–4 The Rights of Mental Health Consumers

- Right to informed consent
- Right to treatment
- Right to refuse treatment
- Right to treatment in the least restrictive setting
- Right to communicate with others
- Right not to be subjected to unnecessary mechanical restraints
- Right to privacy
- Right to periodic review of status
- Right to independent psychiatric examination
- Right to participate in legal matters including making a valid contract, executing a will, marrying or divorcing, voting, driving a motor vehicle, practicing a profession, suing or being sued, managing or disposing of property
- Right to habeas corpus
- Right to legal representation
- Right to keep clothing and personal effects
- Right to religious freedom
- Right to education
- Right to civil service status

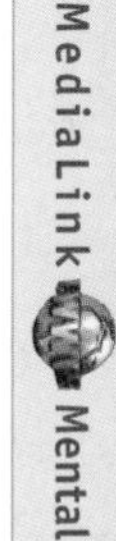

BOX 10–5 Components of a Psychiatric Advance Directive (PAD)

The following PAD components are recommended by the Bazelon Center for Mental Health Law.

Part I: Statement of Intent
Part II: Appointment of an Agent for Mental Health Care
Part III: Statement of My Desires, Instructions, Special Provisions, and Limitations Regarding My Mental Health Treatment and Care
Part IV: Statement of My Preferences Regarding Notification of Others, Visitors, and Custody of My Child(ren)
Part V: Statement of My Preferences Regarding Revocation or Termination of This Advance Directive
Part VI: Signature Page

5. Register whether the person is willing or unwilling to participate in psychiatric research studies.
6. Improve communication between the person and the mental health care provider.
7. Possibly shorten a hospital stay (Bazelon Center for Mental Health Law, 2001; Swanson, Tepper, Backlar, & Swartz, 2000).

Increasing numbers of mental health professionals favor PADs because in addition to guiding family members, significant others, and professionals, they respect the client's autonomy. Advance directives become even more important when the surrogate decision maker is other than the client's next of kin (see the accompanying Using Research Evidence feature). In this instance, a PAD can also reduce the use of court proceedings.

While PADs are becoming more popular (they first came into existence in the 1990s), they are legally recognized in only a few states. However, many mental health consumers who are now using these documents find that a PAD increases the likelihood that mental health care providers, hospitals, and judges honor their choices. All states have a provision for a durable power of attorney for health care to which a PAD can be attached. An advance directive such as a PAD provides written direction for ethically sensitive judgment on the part of professionals and surrogates even in states in which they are not legally recognized. ■ Figure 10–1 illustrates a step-by-step process that you can use to help a client develop and implement a PAD.

RIGHT TO INFORMED CONSENT

A client has the right to understand and participate in the treatment process prior to consenting to treatment. **Informed consent** is required by all states. The main purpose of the doctrine of informed consent is to encourage individual autonomy and sound decision making. Client self-determination is the basic principle of informed consent.

Key elements of informed consent are **competency**, information, and voluntariness. A client must be cognitively able to understand the situation and the implications of treatment. If a client's competency is in question, a mental status examination may be necessary. The medication record may need to be reviewed to determine if the client received medication that might interfere with cognitive ability. Any deficits in the client's reception and processing of information need to be taken into account. The client must be competent to understand the problem, along with the negative and positive effects from the proposed treatment, and the likely outcome with and without treatment.

Many illnesses impair the ability to acquire new information. At times, this is a response to the biologic components of the illness or the effects of medication. Other times, there may be an educational deficit. For some long-term clients, the presence of a mental illness may have affected the educational experience. This does not mean that intelligence is affected, but that reading and writing skills may not be consistent with chronological age. Developing plans for offering information that would be needed in the decision-making process helps to ensure a client's right to informed consent. It may be necessary to present information in small pieces using simple language and pictures. Several short presentations may be required with some mechanism to assess learning to determine whether the client understands the proposed treatment.

USING RESEARCH EVIDENCE

Heather Adams is a neighbor in your apartment building. On weekends, the two of you sometimes get together for morning coffee. Last weekend, Heather shared with you a concern that has been troubling her for a few weeks. She is 31 years old, unmarried, and lives alone. Her father died three years ago in a construction accident. Since that time, Heather's mother has become increasingly incapacitated with Alzheimer's disease and is now a resident in a long-term care facility for the cognitively impaired. When she was in her early 20s, Heather was hospitalized and treated for depression. Heather's next of kin is her brother, Ed, from whom she has been estranged for five years. Her fear is that should she become incapacitated again with depression, the brother whom she actively dislikes, and with whom she does not get along, will make treatment decisions as next-of-kin.

As her neighbor, a citizen, an advocate, and an ethical psychiatric–mental health nurse you have decided to invite Heather for coffee on Saturday. Because Heather seems to be a person who would benefit from a formal PAD, you intend to educate her about her choices. You've located a sample PAD from the Bazelon Center for Mental Health Law (see the bibliography at the end of this chapter) to form the basis of a discussion with Heather and to help her to formalize her wishes concerning any possible future psychiatric treatment such as medication and ECT, treatment setting, the selection of a trusted surrogate, and whether or not she is willing to participate in psychiatric research studies. This way, as suggested in the study below, you can serve as an active resource for Heather:

Swanson, J. W., Tepper, M. C., Backlar, P., & Swartz, M. S. (2000). Psychiatric advance directives: An alternative to coercive treatment. *Psychiatry, 63*(2), 160–172.

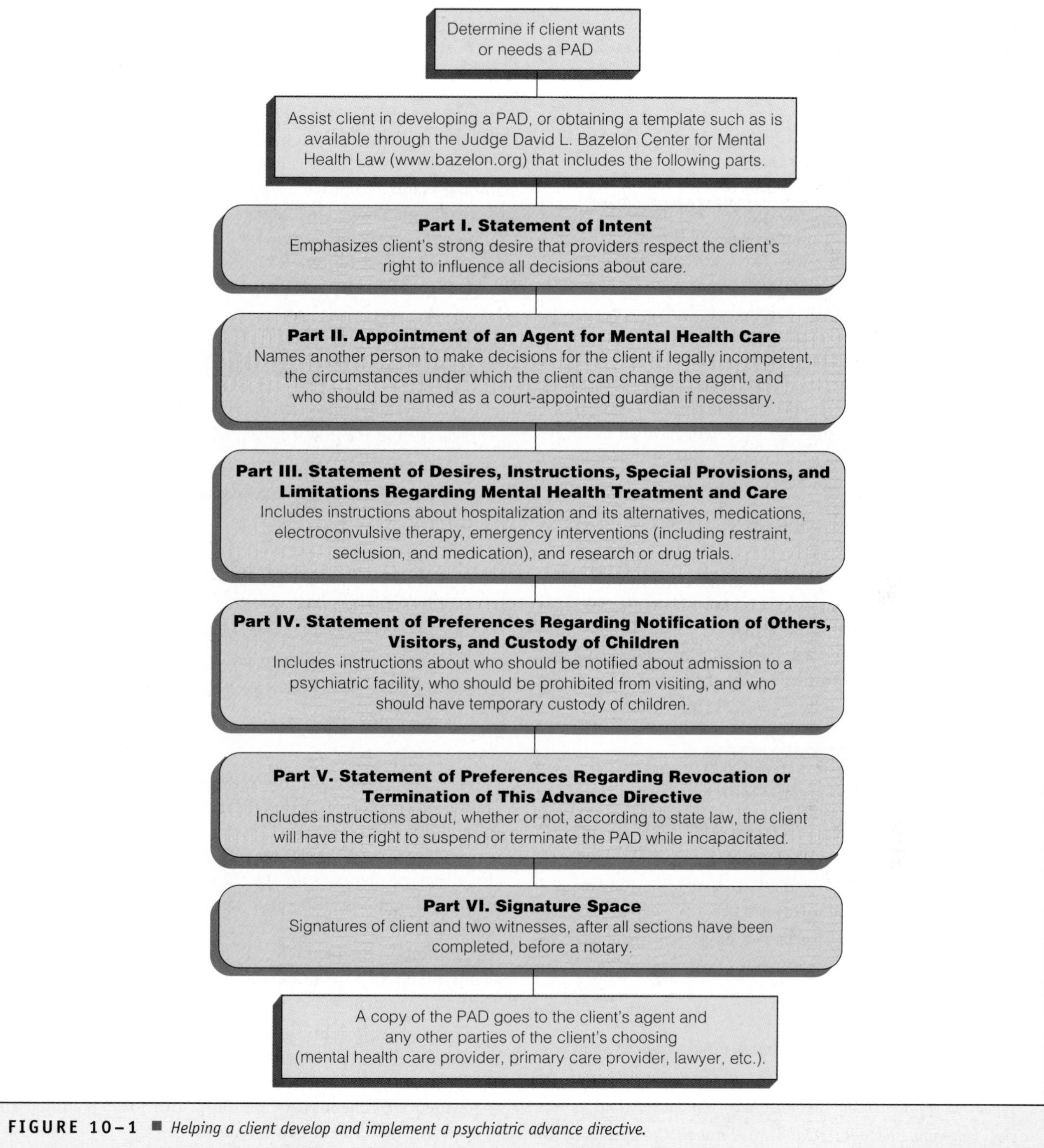

FIGURE 10–1 ■ *Helping a client develop and implement a psychiatric advance directive.*

All clients must be offered choices and given the advantages and disadvantages of each. While members of the mental health team can offer suggestions, it must be clear to the client that there is no self-serving bias on the part of the treatment team for one choice or another. The client must have the opportunity to ask questions or gain a second opinion. The client should not be rushed or coerced into giving consent.

Informed consent must be documented in writing through the use of a specific form signed by the client, or by an entry into the client's medical record. While written documentation of informed consent will likely fulfill the legal obligation, it is helpful to think of informed consent as more of a reoccurring process. While hospitalized, clients should be offered many chances to participate in their own care.

BOX 10–6 Informed Consent Requirements

Informed consent requires that the client:

- Is of the age of consent.
- Is deemed mentally competent.
- Can state that he or she is acting voluntarily.
- Can repeat the elements of the condition.
- Can repeat the treatment options.
- Can repeat the benefits and consequences of each treatment.
- Can repeat the consequences of inaction.
- Is not impaired by alcohol or other drugs.
- Can complete the specific written forms such as consent forms, treatment plans, and discharge plans.

At times, it may become clear that the client lacks the ability to offer consent. In this case, it is important to interact with legal counsel to determine what should be done. Some states will allow legal relatives to participate for a client who cannot consent. Other states demand that the client have an advocate appointed to serve as decision maker. For a summary of informed consent requirements, see Box 10–6.

RIGHT TO TREATMENT

The first argument for a right to treatment for involuntarily committed individuals came from Morton Birnbaum, a lawyer and a physician, in an article published in 1960. However, the ground-breaking cases did not come from the familiar circles of civil commitment but from people who had been sidetracked from the prison system into hospitals.

CLINICAL EXAMPLE

Instead of being convicted for carrying a dangerous weapon and receiving a maximum sentence of one year, a man in Washington, D.C., who pleaded "not guilty by reason of insanity" was sent to a maximum security unit of a federal psychiatric hospital for treatment on an involuntary commitment basis. Four years later, he questioned his detention on the basis of not having received any psychiatric treatment.

A man, indicted for murder, was sent to a Massachusetts state hospital after having been found incompetent to stand trial. He requested transfer to another facility on the grounds that he was not receiving adequate treatment. Through the testimony of experts, his attorneys were able to show that he was simply receiving custodial care.

An involuntary client in a Florida mental hospital for over 14 years brought suit against the hospital director, claiming that he had been deprived of his constitutional right to liberty. At trial, the jury found that (a) he had received not merely inadequate treatment, but no treatment at all; (b) he was not dangerous; (c) acceptable community alternatives were available; and (d) the hospital director, knowing all this, had "maliciously" deprived him of liberty.

In these instances, the courts found a constitutional rationale for treatment. Depriving a citizen of liberty on the attruistic theory that the loss of liberty is for the purpose of therapy, and then failing to provide adequate therapy, violates the rights of citizens guaranteed by the constitution.

Right to treatment issues also have to do with inappropriate releases, or passes to leave a hospital when prudent care would indicate that freedom was inappropriate.

CLINICAL EXAMPLE

Eight days after admission to a New Orleans hospital for severe depression, a client was given a weekend pass, during which she attempted suicide. She sued the hospital and psychotherapists for allowing her to leave the hospital when she was not in a fit mental condition.

In Washington, D.C., a client, who had been committed to a hospital after being acquitted of murder by reason of insanity, left the hospital grounds and stabbed his wife. The hospital was found liable based on its failure to take reasonable measures to ensure that the client did not leave the hospital grounds.

The concept of right to treatment is an outgrowth of the philosophic point of view that the deprivation of liberty, whether voluntarily or involuntarily, must have an overriding purpose. A review of court cases indicates that the right to treatment came about because there was no overriding purpose: Because of overcrowded conditions, inadequate staffing, financial and programmatic deficiencies, there were not enough resources to deliver the bare minimum of treatment. "Right to treatment" ensures that clients are not in a treatment setting for custodial purposes only. The necessary elements in a treatment-oriented program are:

- Physical examination and psychosocial assessment on admission and then as indicated.
- Treatment plans with clear objectives and interventions.
- Evidence of client participation in treatment planning and consent for all treatment methods.
- Up-to-date medical records.
- Treatment in as normal an environment as possible.
- Staff in adequate numbers and with sufficient training to provide quality care.
- Availability of treatment that meets client needs as identified in the treatment plan.
- Necessary support services such as dental, speech, physical, and rehabilitation therapy.
- Ongoing treatment plan evaluations.

- Programs to help clients develop skills needed for independent versus institutional living.
- Adequate planning for discharge to a less restrictive setting, according to client needs.

RIGHT TO REFUSE TREATMENT

At some time in their lives, all people experience the kind of excessive stress that makes them feel miserable or even desperate. But some people communicate these feelings in ways that are inappropriate, troublesome, unreasonable, or frightening to others. A young woman who in times of stress mutilates her body by burning it repeatedly with cigarettes; a teenager who breaks everything in sight during violent, destructive outbursts; and a belligerent male who initiates physical fights with anyone and everyone without provocation—all usually become candidates for *symptomatic treatments,* behavioral control measures often used against a person's will.

CLINICAL EXAMPLE

One of the first cases against restrictive treatment was brought in Minnesota in 1976. In this case, ECT was felt to be an "intrusive" treatment and was not allowed to be given against a competent client's wishes.

An involuntarily committed client at a New Jersey state hospital claimed that his constitutional rights were violated by forcibly administering medication. He objected to the side effects produced by chlorpromazine (Thorazine) and lithium carbonate. The judge ruled in the client's favor, noting that a person subjected to the harsh side effects of psychotropic drugs should have control over their administration.

Clients at a Massachusetts state hospital initiated a class action suit, contending that their constitutional rights were being violated by the hospital's practice of using forced seclusion and medication in nonemergency situations. The court granted competent clients and guardians of incompetent clients an absolute right to refuse medication in nonemergency situations.

An issue that captured public attention was the notorious case of a homeless New York woman forcibly removed from the streets because of her self-neglect and provocative behavior. She was judged competent, however, to refuse medication despite her status as an involuntary patient.

In another case, the court found that a nurse who forcibly administered medication to a competent adult client had committed an intentional tort. The client was involuntarily committed to a mental hospital. She was a practicing Christian Scientist and refused medication. The court held that medication could be given over the client's religious objections only if she were harmful to herself or others. The court allowed her damages for assault and battery.

In almost all states, ECT is closely regulated by statute. Most state statutes specify that ECT can be administered only if informed consent is obtained from the client. In the case of an incompetent client, consent must be obtained from the guardian or next of kin. The client's right to refuse ECT is specifically mentioned in many state statutes.

Psychosurgery, referred to in various state statutes as "brain surgery," "lobotomy," or "experimental" or "hazardous" procedures, is also closely regulated by state statute. Most state statutes specify that psychosurgery can be performed only if informed consent is obtained from the client. In several states, psychosurgery can be performed only upon a court order if the client is incompetent. The client's right to refuse psychosurgery is also specifically mentioned in many state statutes.

If written consent is withheld by a client already declared "legally incompetent" by the court or certified "functionally incompetent" by a treating psychiatrist, the decision to medicate forcibly would be referred to a client advocate. It would be up to the client advocate's discretion to request a hearing before an independent psychiatrist. In the case of a competent though involuntarily hospitalized person, a hearing before an independent psychiatrist would be required at which the client would have the right to legal counsel. It is vital to remember that overriding a client's right to refuse treatment is legally complicated and related to safeguards that are in place to manage such situations. These legal safeguards serve to protect the rights of all people.

Dilemmas Associated with the Right to Refuse Treatment

There are a number of areas of judicial disagreement in the right to refuse treatment that will create dilemmas for the mental health care professional. Consider the other dilemmas outlined in the Nursing Self-Awareness feature on page 194. For example, there is no common definition of the term *psychiatric emergency.* The traditional definition of *emergency* refers to an overt and immediate threat to a person's life. The contemporary definition focuses on the immediate, impending, and significant deterioration of the client's condition.

Another area of controversy is: At what point can the state override an involuntarily committed client's right to refuse psychotropic medication in a nonemergency? Is it only when a person has been judged incompetent, or does danger to self or others provide a legitimate reason under the state's police power to administer treatment?

In the case of an incompetent individual, there is disagreement over who should decide for the person and what standard should be used. Is it to be a guardian, the hospital staff, or the judiciary? Is the standard to be what the best interests of the client seem to be as judged by an informed outsider, or is it what the client would want if competent to make the choice?

Here are some criteria a court is likely to use in ruling on a case involving the right to refuse treatment:

- *Client competency.* If the client is competent, informed consent is possible.
- *Intrusiveness of treatment.* As the intrusiveness increases, so does the court's scrutiny.
- *Permanence of treatment effect.* If side effects are adverse and permanent, the court is less likely to override refusal.
- *Experimental nature of treatment.* The treatment must have scientific merit, and the client must give informed consent.
- *Risk–benefit ratio.* The benefits of treatment must outweigh the risk.
- *Motivation for treatment.* The treatment cannot be used to punish or "quiet" the client for the staff's benefit.
- *Motivation for refusal.* Religious objections are usually upheld.

Despite the difficulties and issues raised by the client's right to refuse treatment, some very real positive outcomes are these:

- Clients must be involved in treatment choices, process, and outcome.
- Clients must be informed of choices and offered alternatives.
- Staff members must acquire a second opinion on potentially harmful procedures.

RIGHT TO TREATMENT IN THE LEAST RESTRICTIVE SETTING

The idea of least restrictive setting or alternative has become an important component of both the deinstitutionalization and client rights movements. The term **least restrictive setting** generally refers to the placement of clients in the therapeutic setting that will provide care while allowing maximum freedom. By extension, it also means providing for the least amount of limitation or interference in an individual's thought and decision making, physical activity, and sense of self as necessary to provide for safety.

CLINICAL EXAMPLE

A 61-year-old District of Columbia woman had difficulty caring for herself because of confusion secondary to arteriosclerotic brain disease. While not considered a danger to others, she did wander when confused and was subsequently admitted to the federal psychiatric hospital. The court ruled that she did not need 24-hour psychiatric supervision and that a less restrictive form of treatment should be found. Today, such clients can be supervised in assisted living facilities for the cognitively impaired.

The American Nurses Association's Standards of Psychiatric–Mental Health Nursing Practice (2000) expect that the nurse will choose the least restrictive limit and use it only for as long as it is necessary for the safety of the client and others.

Treatment Setting

Treatment setting is evaluated on such criteria as the limitations it places on physical freedom (locked or unlocked), choice of activities, and the presence of "adult status" as shown by locked bedrooms and the unsupervised use of private bathroom facilities. In this scheme, total institutions would be considered the most restrictive, halfway houses less so, and family or independent living the least.

Institutional Policy

Institutional policy is the degree of restriction imposed by the rules and regulations necessary to run the institution. Criteria to evaluate a setting would include such items as the amount of supervision in daily living tasks, the amount of client involvement in treatment planning, and the priority of activities that increase the client's autonomy.

Enforcement

The enforcement dimension includes the methods sanctioned to enforce the institution's rules. Is coercion or threat of punishment used? Is the standard for socially acceptable behavior higher in the institution than it would be in the client's own environment? For example, a nurse says to a client, "We don't use that foul language here . . . I don't think you're ready for that pass." How readily and to what extent is the client's autonomy compromised to meet organizational needs?

Nursing SELF-AWARENESS

Right to Refuse Treatment

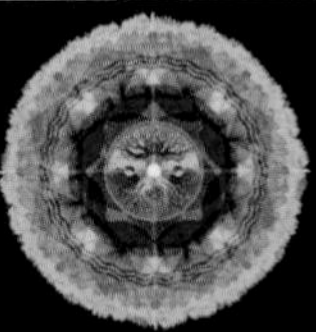

To increase self-awareness of your own opinions about a client's right to refuse treatment, think about the following questions:

- How do I feel when a client's legal right to leave a treatment setting is deemed more important than the client's need for treatment?
- Should clients whose behavior disrupts and frightens other clients be allowed to refuse treatment even when interventions like medication would definitely reduce their symptoms?
- In the case of a client judged to be mentally incompetent, what standard should be used to make decisions about treatment? Should it be the hospital staff? A guardian? According to the best interests of the client? What the client would want if competent to make the choice?
- Does society have an obligation to care for a seriously mentally ill person even if this requires limiting that person's freedom to refuse treatment?
- Should a person on the street who is gesturing and talking to himself or herself and who is carrying a few belongings in a plastic bag be allowed to continue living on the street or be mandated into outpatient commitment?

Treatment

The treatment dimension has to do with the intrusiveness of the treatment used. Psychosurgery and ECT would be considered more intrusive than medication. Long-acting medication such as fluphenazine decanoate would be considered more intrusive than oral medication. The clarity of treatment goals is also a consideration. Nebulous or nonexistent goals increase restrictiveness.

Client Characteristics

The client's illness characteristics are seen by some as restricting behavior to a much greater degree than any locked door. Some believe it is simplistic to think that moving a client from an institutional setting to the community will automatically result in less restriction. Without effective community-based treatment, including safe housing, many chronically ill clients frequently end up on the streets (see Chapter 11).

RIGHT TO COMMUNICATE WITH OTHERS

The basis for laws granting communication rights is that such communication can expose cases of wrongful hospitalization. Generally, communication is unrestricted or guaranteed to named public officials or the central hospital agency for the state. Most states extend this guarantee to include correspondence with attorneys. Most states also require that any correspondence limitation be part of the client's clinical record. Approximately half the states require the client to have reasonable access to writing materials and postage.

Most states have some statutory provisions concerning visitation. However, hospital authorities are generally given broad discretionary powers to curtail this right. Before implementing any restriction in communication or visitation, the nurse should ask: Is it fair and reasonable? Could I defend it to a noninvolved professional?

RIGHT NOT TO BE SUBJECTED TO UNNECESSARY MECHANICAL RESTRAINTS

Though improvements in treatment have decreased the use of mechanical or physical restraints, such restraints still play a role in some treatment programs. Most states have attempted to regulate their use by statute through specifying that restraints can be used when the client presents a risk of harm to self or others. Some states specifically say restraints are not to be used for punishment or staff convenience. In those states not having statutory provisions regarding restraints, the procedures to be followed are usually found in the administrative regulations.

Half the states have laws relating to seclusion. Prevention of harm to self or others is the most common criterion, followed by treatment or therapeutic reasons. The use of either restraints or seclusion must be documented in the client's medical record. Nursing organizations such as the American Nurses Association (ANA) (2001) and the American Psychiatric Nurses Association (APNA) (2000) have developed position statements on the use of seclusion and restraint. The position statements are available at www.nursingworld.org/readroom/position/ethics/restrnt.htm, the Web site for ANA, and at www.apna.org/papers/position_paper7.htm, the Web site for APNA, which can be accessed through the Companion Website for this book. See also Chapter 34.

RIGHT TO PRIVACY

Almost all states have a specific statute regarding the mental health consumer's right to keep personal information secret, and the specific steps to be taken for release of that information. The confidential nature of the client information is also cited in the American Nurses Association Code of Ethics—maintaining client confidentiality within ethical legal, and regulatory parameters—as it is in most professional codes (refer to Box 10–2).

The goal of confidentiality is to ensure the client's privacy. There is a significant amount of stigma attached to being the recipient of psychiatric treatment. Though professionals may argue that this is unfair, it is a fact. Because of this, it is important that clients be the ones to give out this information about themselves. Instructors, students, supervisors, or team members who receive information about a client in the course of supervision or in providing treatment for the client are also obligated to treat this material as confidential.

In order for the disclosure of information to occur, a client must sign a release form. To be a valid release, the client must be told as specifically as possible what information is to be released. The client should know the following prior to signing.

- What information is going to be released?
- Who needs it?
- Why do they need it?
- When will they need it?
- How will it be used?

■ Figure 10–2 illustrates situations in which signed consents are necessary.

Emergency situations may arise. For example, a client may be in a car accident or take an overdose while out on pass and

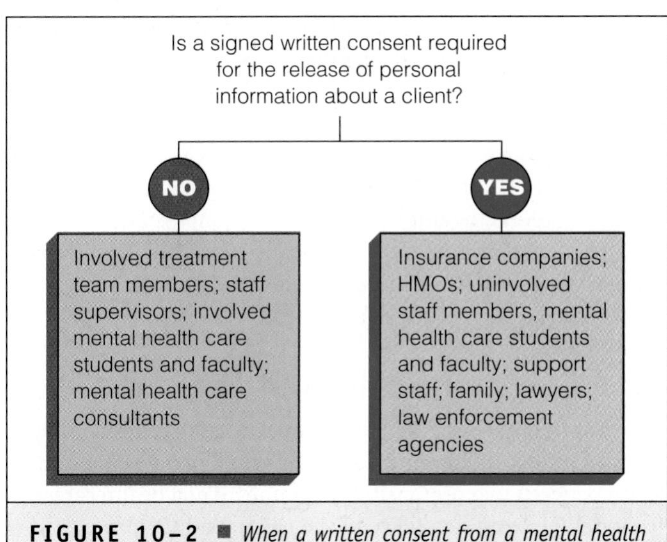

FIGURE 10–2 ■ *When a written consent from a mental health consumer is required for release of personal information.*

end up being treated in another hospital's emergency room. In these situations, the release of information can occur without the client's approval. It is important to document such a breach of confidentiality.

Confidentiality of information is not easy to maintain. Medical records are generally kept, not in locked files, but at an easy access point in the nurses' station. Medical files usually travel all over the hospital with the client and are often available for the perusal of others not directly involved in the client's treatment. The increased use of computers for communication and data storage, along with the information requested by the government, third-party payers, and employers, often poses a threat to a client's privacy. More mundane, but equally serious, incidences of breaches of confidentiality occur when staff members talk about clients in the halls, elevator, and cafeteria.

Privileged Communication

Privileged communication is a narrower concept than confidentiality. It is established by state statute to protect possibly incriminating disclosures made by the client to specified professionals.

CLINICAL EXAMPLE

A minister brought suit because his former psychiatrist disclosed confidential information about him to his clerical superiors. The court held that unless a client poses a serious threat to himself or to others, the psychiatrist owes a duty of confidentiality. The client was able to recover damages for lost earnings, harm to his reputation, and emotional distress.

Privileged communication has traditionally existed between husband and wife, attorney and client, clergy and church member, and physician and client. In some states, communication between psychologist and client is also accorded privileged status. Only a few states recognize privileged communication between nurse and client. Be sure that you are informed about the law in your state. The privilege is the client's and can be claimed only if a therapeutic relationship exists. The professional can reveal the information at the client's request.

Each state that grants a privilege also specifies exceptions to that privilege. Box 10–7 discusses when the right to privacy can be breached.

Disclosure to Safeguard Others

An exception to confidentiality and privilege that has developed from a California Supreme Court decision illustrates the competition between two responsibilities of the mental health care professional: (1) confidentiality to the client, and (2) protection of the public from the "violent" client. The court's ruling underlines the mental health care professional's responsibility to balance confidentiality with the "duty to warn" and the "duty to protect."

CLINICAL EXAMPLE

The classic case involves the parents of a young woman who successfully sued the University of California, claiming that a psychotherapist from the student counseling center had a responsibility to warn their daughter that his client had threatened to kill her. At the time, the psychologist did notify campus security officers that he believed his client was dangerous and should be involuntarily committed for observation and treatment. However, the man appeared rational to the police and promised them he would stay away from the young woman. He then terminated treatment, and two months later killed her. The California Supreme Court said that, despite the unsuccessful attempt to confine the client, the therapist knew that he was at large and dangerous and had a duty to warn the young woman of the danger. The court recognized the client's right to confidentiality but said this must be weighed against the public's need for safety against violent assault, especially when an individual in danger can be identified.

In a number of cases, therapists were held liable for not taking some action to protect potential unidentified victims. The Intervention box on page 197 shows a model to help mental health caregivers decide on a course of action in implementing the duty to warn or protect.

The duty to warn has stirred up controversy in the mental health community. There is a concern about the fact that clients with aggression problems will drop out of therapy, not use it effectively, or be less likely to seek treatment for fear of being betrayed. Remember also that no mental health care professional can reliably predict the future violence of a mentally disordered person.

BOX 10–7 When the Right to Privacy Can Be Breached

The release of information without the client's consent can be made under the following conditions:

- When acting in the client's best interests in an emergency situation
- When acting to protect third parties
- During commitment proceedings
- When making a court-ordered evaluation or report
- When a client is incompetent and consent is given by a guardian, or when the guardian is not available
- When reporting child abuse, gunshot wounds, or contagious diseases, as required by state law
- During criminal proceedings
- In child custody disputes
- During child abuse proceedings
- When a client introduced a defense of mental illness into litigation proceedings

INTERVENTION

A Model for Implementing the Duty to Warn or Protect

Action	Implementation
Assess dangerousness	Compare data to factors believed to correlate with dangerous behavior, such as increasing use of drugs and/or alcohol, current and past threats of violence and/or assaultive behavior, presence of command hallucinations.
	Be sure to review past and current treatment records. Interview client, family, and significant others.
	Ask: Is the threat serious? Are the threats repeated? Are the means to carry out the threat available? Can the victim be identified? Is the victim accessible?
Select a course of action to protect the victim	Consider either voluntary hospitalization, or, if necessary, initiate involuntary commitment.
	If the client is already hospitalized, is a more secure unit needed to prevent escape?
	If the client is an outpatient, is medication needed? Are more frequent visits needed? Is a more intensive outpatient care needed, such as a day program?
	Because threats often involve family members, is intensive, systems-oriented therapy indicated to include the intended victim?
	If containment or control is not possible, contact the identified victim. Consider also alerting the police.
Implement decision	Continue to monitor: If initial course of action fails, take other measures. Be sure to document this decision-making process in the client's record.

RIGHT TO PERIODIC REVIEW

Most states have some provision for periodic review of involuntary clients. Periodic review provides some protection for the individual against spending more time than necessary in the hospital. Review is required every 30 days in some states, every year in others. A few states require review "as frequently as necessary," or "from time to time." The actual scope of the review is usually not governed by statute. The trend in recent years has been away from hospitalization for indeterminate periods of time. In New York and California, short-term commitment is the rule, and court review is necessary to extend commitment for another short period.

RIGHT TO INDEPENDENT PSYCHIATRIC EXAMINATION

Mental health consumers have the right to an independent psychiatric assessment by a physician of their own choosing. The client must be released if the physician determines the client is not mentally ill.

RIGHT TO PARTICIPATE IN LEGAL MATTERS

Mental health consumers have rights to participate as citizens in legal matters.

Contracts

Clients committed to a mental hospital generally maintain their right to make a valid contract, unless they have also been judged incompetent. In most states, commitment proceedings are separate from those for competence. Therefore, an individual who is "legally incompetent" is not necessarily subject to commitment, and an individual committed to an institution is not automatically legally incompetent. Even though the issue of contracts may seem clear-cut, in reality a client's right to contract may be restricted by the administrative regulations of hospitals and state mental health agencies. A contested contract would most likely be a matter for the court to decide.

Wills

To make a valid will, a person must:

- Be aware of making a will.
- Be familiar with the property being disposed of.
- Know the names, identities, and relationships of the people named in the will.

A person with a psychiatric diagnosis, whether in or out of the hospital, can make a valid will as long as these requirements are met. Psychosis with accompanying delusions does not by itself negate a valid will. The delusions have to produce a significant distortion of the person's perception of the property, family, or personal relationships to invalidate the will.

Marriage and Divorce

According to statute and common law, a valid marriage contract hinges on the individual's possession of sufficient mental capacity to give consent. Sufficient mental capacity implies that the person:

- Understands the nature of the marriage relationship.
- Knows the duties and obligations involved.

The statutes of a small number of states prohibit marriage by mentally disordered people because they are believed to be incapable of making a contract. More states, however, prohibit marriage by the mentally disordered on the grounds that they are "insane" or "of unsound mind," without specifically defining these terms. Despite these prohibiting statutes, few states even try to enforce the prohibition outside mental institutions.

Most states have provisions for annulment or divorce on the grounds of prenuptial mental disability. Within the last 25 years, divorce on the grounds of postnuptial mental disability has been incorporated in the statutes of most states.

Voting

Most states do not actually prohibit hospitalized people from voting. In fact, some specifically preserve this right by legislation. The hospitalized client's right to vote is probably more restricted by caretaker and community apathy than it is by statute.

RIGHT TO DRIVE

Statutes on driving privileges are difficult to interpret. Most states will not issue a driver's license to mentally disturbed people. In some states this restriction also applies to epileptics, drug addicts, and alcoholics. Several states suspend a driver's license as soon as the individual enters a mental institution. Other jurisdictions limit the restriction to those admitted involuntarily, while still others base suspension on legal competency.

RIGHT TO PRACTICE A PROFESSION

The ability of a hospitalized client to practice a profession is usually impaired simply by the physical confinement. However, most states have some statutes prohibiting the practice of a profession by a mentally disturbed person. The vagueness of the statutes often makes it difficult to know when they are applicable. As a rule, it is up to the professional licensing board to suspend or revoke the license of a member who is believed to be too mentally incapacitated to practice a profession safely, even though not hospitalized.

RIGHT TO HABEAS CORPUS

Mental health consumers in all states have the protection of the constitutional right of **habeas corpus.** Habeas corpus requires the speedy release of any person who has been illegally detained. Any client can petition for release on the grounds of being sane. If found sane in a hearing, the client must be discharged.

RIGHTS OF CHILDREN OR MINORS

The rights of children have been the subject of judicial and legislative action over the last twenty years. In most states, an individual is considered a minor or juvenile if younger than 18 years of age. As a minor the person is considered legally incompetent. Legal consent for medical treatment must come from parents or a guardian. There are, however, a number of exceptions to this general rule of presumed legal incompetency in some state statutes. These include the rights to:

- Seek treatment for drug abuse.
- Consent to contraception.
- Seek psychiatric treatment.

Other factors, such as military service, marriage, emancipation, pregnancy, and parenthood, may also affect the age at which a minor may be considered competent.

The most controversial issue of a minor's role in the mental health system involves involuntary commitment. Like adults, minors can be committed to a mental hospital against their will. But, unlike adult admissions, the admission of a minor who objects is considered "voluntary" if the parents have authorized it. Because of the realization that parents may not always be acting in the best interests of the child, a number of lawsuits challenging this practice were filed. It was argued that the "voluntary" admission of minors without procedural safeguards was unconstitutional, and that a court hearing should always be held to determine if commitment is warranted. The United States Supreme Court upheld the rights of parents to admit their children to psychiatric facilities as long as a "neutral factfinder" (physician) believes medical standards for admission have been met.

The trend for inclusion of procedural safeguards continues as an increasing number of states have modified their "voluntary" parental commitment statute by one or more of the following factors:

- Lowering the age of required consent. The majority of states specify age 16 to 18.
- Requiring the consent of the child.
- Providing for a court hearing if the child protests.
- Providing for self-initiated institutionalization for minors.

Liability and the Psychiatric–Mental Health Nurse

Criminal and civil are the two main classes of law. *Criminal law* pertains to behavior considered to be a threat to the order of society as a whole, such as murder, assault, and robbery. *Civil law* is concerned with the legal rights and duties of private parties. Most legal actions against nurses are civil actions.

An important division of civil law is known as *tort law*. The term *tort* comes from the Latin word for "twisted." A tort is a wrongful act resulting in injury for which the injured party files a civil suit requesting legal redress, usually in the form of monetary damages. Torts may be intentional, as in assault, battery, defamation of character, invasion of privacy, false imprisonment, fraud, and misrepresentation; or unintentional, as in negligence. Under tort law, nurses can be held responsible for their own actions. Therefore, all nurses should carry their own malpractice insurance.

NEGLIGENCE

The concepts of duty and responsibility permeate human relationships. In healthy relationships, expectations are negotiated between individuals that delineate the responsibilities of each person. People who experience times of stress and illness may have difficulty forming realistic expectations, accepting responsibility for actions, and understanding the roles and limits of those who would like to help.

There are times when two people may experience problems understanding and meeting the duties and responsibilities of the relationship. The resolution of such problems is often a therapeutic issue. At times, however, the legal system may become involved. This is particularly true if the client, or the client's family, perceives that the nurse failed to provide the quality of care expected.

All nurses are responsible for determining the quality of care as experienced by their clients. If lapses in the quality of care occur, they should be addressed. The term negligence is used whenever a nurse fails to act in a manner in which most reasonable and prudent people would act or when a nurse acts in a way that a reasonably prudent person would not have done under similar circumstances. How does one determine what is reasonable and prudent? First, the nurse is accountable to external legal authorities such as the nurse practice acts of the state in which she or he practices, and civil and criminal codes. The nurse is also accountable to the Standards of Psychiatric–Mental Health Nursing Practice (2000) published by the American Nurses Association, and to the employing agency or hospital. Nurses are also accountable for familiarizing themselves with current journal and textbook information related to the care of mental health clients.

Conditions for Establishing Negligence

A simple breach in the quality of care does not necessarily mean that a nurse was negligent (Lee, 2000). Certain conditions must be met to determine negligence and hold the nurse accountable. These conditions are discussed below and summarized in Box 10–8.

Contract for Care. A contract for care must have been established between the nurse and the client. A nurse may also begin this contract by accepting a client assignment, having a discussion with the client, offering information or education, providing treatment, serving as a group leader, accepting a client into an activity, or supervising the activities of a mental health worker. It is important to note that entering into a therapeutic relationship creates a legally binding contract between the nurse and the client.

Duty of Care. There must be identifiable, explicit, and manifest duty of care in which the intentions of the nurse are to help the client. This intention to help is termed *good faith*. One example is the "good faith" use of the nursing process, including pertinent and timely assessment, planning, outcome identification, intervention, and evaluation of the client. Another example is a nursing care policy that indicates a course of action. A policy of a given mental health agency might state that each nurse must perform an assessment that includes information related to the emotional, physical, and social health of each client. Failure to use the nursing process and to follow the procedure to provide such an assessment (and take actions based upon this assessment) might be grounds for a charge of negligence.

Ignorance of a policy or procedure is not an acceptable rationale for not following a policy or procedure. For example, all nurses are expected to assess clients for the potential to commit suicide. All reasonable, prudent nurses perform an assessment for suicide potential. The nurse must act to safeguard the life of the client within the limits of the law. Failure to perform such an assessment or take actions to protect the client might be deemed negligent, if harm is present.

Presence of Harm. The client must suffer harm that can be directly linked to the failure of the nurse to act in a reasonable and prudent manner. A nurse who fails to assess for suicide potential, thus failing to protect the client, can be held negligent only if the client suffers harm in a suicide attempt or dies as a result of self-inflicted action.

Common Practice. There may be no written policy or procedure, nor a law to guide a practitioner in acting, but there is strong indication for action based on what is generally considered *common practice*. Consider a client who lacks any contact with reality. The client cannot perform activities of daily living such as eating, bathing, toileting, or making decisions about safety. It is common practice to provide care in which the nurse will perform the activities of daily living for the client. Conversely, it is common practice to encourage clients to do as much for themselves as possible. Psychiatric–mental health nurses generally do not bathe clients who can bathe alone.

Boundary Violation. Another example concerns the boundaries of personal relationships between clients and mental health care professionals. Some states fail to define the boundaries of personal relationships between clients and mental health care professionals. In these cases, each nurse must define the nature of the nurse–client relationship. Nurses do not form social relationships with mental health clients with whom there is or has been a professional relationship. This implies that nurses do not date nor engage in sexual activity with a client. Any suggestion or promise that the relationship might be personal can be considered negligence—the failure to explain the limits of the relationship to the client and to act within the boundaries of that relationship.

Acting Against the Nurse's Advice. There are times when clients contribute to the harm they suffer. A client may be informed of the dangers of certain actions and yet may decide to act against the advice of the nurse. Each client maintains the civil rights of freedom of speech, movement, and action unless there are grounds to curtail these rights, as in the case of harm to self and others. Consider the following Clinical Example.

BOX 10–8 Determining Negligence

- Did a contract for care exist?
- Was the care reasonable and prudent?
- Did the care follow guidelines suggested by external sources such as nurse practice acts, the ANA Code of Ethics, the ANA Standards for Psychiatric–Mental Health Nursing, the state Mental Health Act?
- Was the care consistent with internal sources such as policies and procedures of the agency or physician orders?
- Was there evidence of thorough assessment of the client, including old records and interviews with family members?
- Did the action taken reveal appropriate ongoing monitoring of the client's condition?
- Did harm result to the client?
- Was the harm due to violation of the duty to care?

CLINICAL EXAMPLE

A client had been beaten by her boyfriend and was informed about the pattern of escalating abuse, given the phone numbers of agencies that were available on a 24-hour basis, encouraged to form a safe plan, and offered alternative living arrangements. She decided to return to her boyfriend and suffered paralysis from another beating. She claimed the staff did not act to protect her.

Use Box 10–8 on page 199 to help you determine if the staff was negligent.

MALPRACTICE

Malpractice refers to the negligent acts of health care professionals when they fail to act in a responsible and prudent manner in carrying out their professional duties. The most common sources of liability in psychiatric–mental health services are identified in Box 10–9.

Need to Document

The following cases illustrate a breach of the ANA's Standards of Psychiatric–Mental Health Nursing Practice and emphasize the importance of written communication between nurse and physician.

CLINICAL EXAMPLE

A man was admitted to a hospital after becoming increasingly depressed and suicidal secondary to the medication used to treat his hypertension. As a new client, he was not allowed to leave the unit. Four days later the nursing staff assumed without a verifying written medical order (later a verbal order would be claimed) that he was allowed to leave the unit, unescorted, to attend Mass with permission of the nurse on duty. The following morning he was allowed to go to breakfast unescorted. This time, however, he committed suicide by jumping from a seventh floor window. The court ruled that the nurse involved with his care breached the standard of care due under Alaska law. The nurse failed to exercise reasonable care to protect a suicidal client against foreseeable harm to himself.

Another case shows the importance of nursing observation and documentation, even though in this case it did not prevent a tragedy.

CLINICAL EXAMPLE

Distraught with problems and a pending divorce, a 35-year-old man was voluntarily admitted to a psychiatric hospital. During this admission he expressed thoughts of suicide and also thoughts of killing his wife and her mother. Three weeks after his discharge, he was readmitted voluntarily after a suicide attempt. Nurses' notes revealed his repeated homicidal threats. Three weeks after his second admission, he was given a pass. He subsequently secured a gun and shot and killed his wife and her friend. He was tried and convicted on two counts of murder. The children brought a wrongful death action against the hospital, seeking damages for the murder of their mother by their father. The court granted substantial damages to the children. No liability was attributed to the nurses involved, but the physician was judged negligent.

It is important to remember the nature and purpose of hospital records and to follow prudent, appropriate, and ethical procedures in record maintenance. Records that have been changed for whatever reason need to include the date, the reason for the change, and the signature of the person making the change. A dishonest change could result in the charge of fraud or misrepresentation as occurred in the next Clinical Example.

CLINICAL EXAMPLE

A 23-year-old woman was admitted with a diagnosis of schizophrenia. She spent three days in a bare, quiet room for safety reasons. On the fourth day the bed was returned to the room, but no rationale was noted in the chart. A few days later, an order on the client's chart for an antipsychotic medication was not noted, and the client was without medication for three days. The client was later found in a semicomatose condition with her head lodged between the side rails and mattress. Subsequently, the nursing director ordered the nursing staff to "rewrite" the nursing notes. The substituted record clearly conflicted with other records and staff testimony. A $3.6 million verdict against the hospital was upheld.

Many factors contribute to the initiation of a malpractice suit by a client. As long as you are involved in practice, lawsuits are a possibility. You may be sued without necessarily being singled out. A number of ways to protect against a successful lawsuit are discussed in Box 10–10.

Client Advocacy

The rights clients have in theory and those in actual practice are often quite different. The gap between the rights clients have in theory and in practice may be the result of a knowledge deficit on the part of treatment providers. The remedy is simple: Educate the treatment providers so that they in turn can edu-

BOX 10-9 Common Sources of Liability in Psychiatric–Mental Health Services

1. Client suicide
2. Improper treatment
3. Misuse of psychotropic medications
4. Breach of confidentiality
5. False imprisonment
6. Injuries or problems related to ECT
7. Sexual contact with a client
8. Failure to obtain informed consent
9. Failure to report abuse
10. Failure to warn potential victims

cate their clients. Another possibility that may not be so amenable to an easy solution is that direct care treatment providers are threatened by the expansion of client rights. Mental health staff have been heard to say that new regulations not only hampered treatment but made their job both more difficult and more dangerous.

The federal government has encouraged states to develop ombudsmen (a person who speaks for or champions the cause of another) or advocacy programs. These state advocacy programs have the authority to investigate reported incidents of neglect and abuse to the mentally ill in public or private hospitals, research facilities, and nursing homes. Private advocacy organizations such as the Bazelon Center for Mental Health Law (www.bazelon.org) can be accessed through the Companion Website for this book.

Two recent pieces of federal legislation have implications for the rights of clients. In 1990, the Americans with Disabilities Act (ADA) extended federal protection to individuals with physical and/or mental health disabilities for access to public services, employment, and benefits. In an effort to increase the involvement of individuals in directing their own medical care, the Patient Self-Determination Act (PSDA) of 1991 was ratified by Congress as part of the Omnibus Budget Reconciliation Act. The PSDA was designed to inform competent patients at the time of their admission to a hospital of their rights to accept or reject aspects of their medical care.

Although laws can protect certain aspects of human rights, there is a far greater area that laws cannot protect. Laws rarely have a direct effect on a person's beliefs, values, and attitudes, which to a great extent determine whether the letter or the spirit of the law will be carried out. Remember that while the letter of the law may require reading clients their rights on admission it doesn't necessarily mean they understand or remember the information. Psychiatric–mental health nurses practicing from a humanistic perspective are often in a position to advocate both the letter and the spirit of clients' rights.

BOX 10-10 How to Protect Yourself Legally

- Be aware of provisions in your state nurse practice act.
- Follow standards of care.
- Know the relevant law.
- Review agency procedures and policies with both the ANA standards of care and relevant law in mind, clarify any conflict with legal counsel if necessary, and then follow procedures.
- Practice protective documentation:
  1. Document the nursing process, chart accurately and precisely, and chart any significant change as soon as possible. Remember that any omission is presumed not to have occurred.
  2. Chart objectively and be specific, avoiding phrases such as "doing well" or "having a good day."
  3. Be sure to adequately describe methods used in client education and evaluation of client comprehension.
  4. Make sure your nursing documentation reflects the precautions taken during intensive nursing actions, such as the use of seclusion and restraints or the administration of psychoactive agents.
  5. Never alter a client's record after the fact.
- Question the physician about any ambiguous orders before carrying them out.
- Be sure to carry your own malpractice insurance.

PHYSICAL AND PSYCHOLOGICAL ABUSE OF CLIENTS

Clients are particularly vulnerable to both physical and psychological abuse and often do not have the ability or power to defend themselves. There is little actual information on how much client abuse exists in treatment settings. One advocate group ranked client abuse to be the most frequent rights violation complaint. Another ranked it third. These are the types of abuse reported to occur with some frequency:

- Supplying clients with drugs or alcohol in return for favors.
- Making privileges contingent on favors from clients.
- Slapping and kicking clients when staff members felt frustrated.
- Using restraints when other less intrusive alternatives were available.
- Verbal harassment, including threats, sarcasm, and other "put-downs."
- General threats of harm if clients do not behave "appropriately" or as they are told.
- Inhumane physical facilities.

Sexual misconduct with clients is also a form of abuse.

MediaLink Client Advocacy Program

ADVOCACY STRATEGIES

Psychiatric–mental health nursing intervention would be directed at some of the identifying causes that may lead to client abuse, including:

- Unsuitability of certain staff members who do not have the patience or understanding to work with clients having trouble with control.
- A buildup of stresses that have reduced both the staff's patience and ability to problem-solve (burnout).
- An actual lack of knowledge of other means of interacting with clients in a high-stress situation.

Other areas of advocacy include:

- Educating clients and their families about their legal rights.

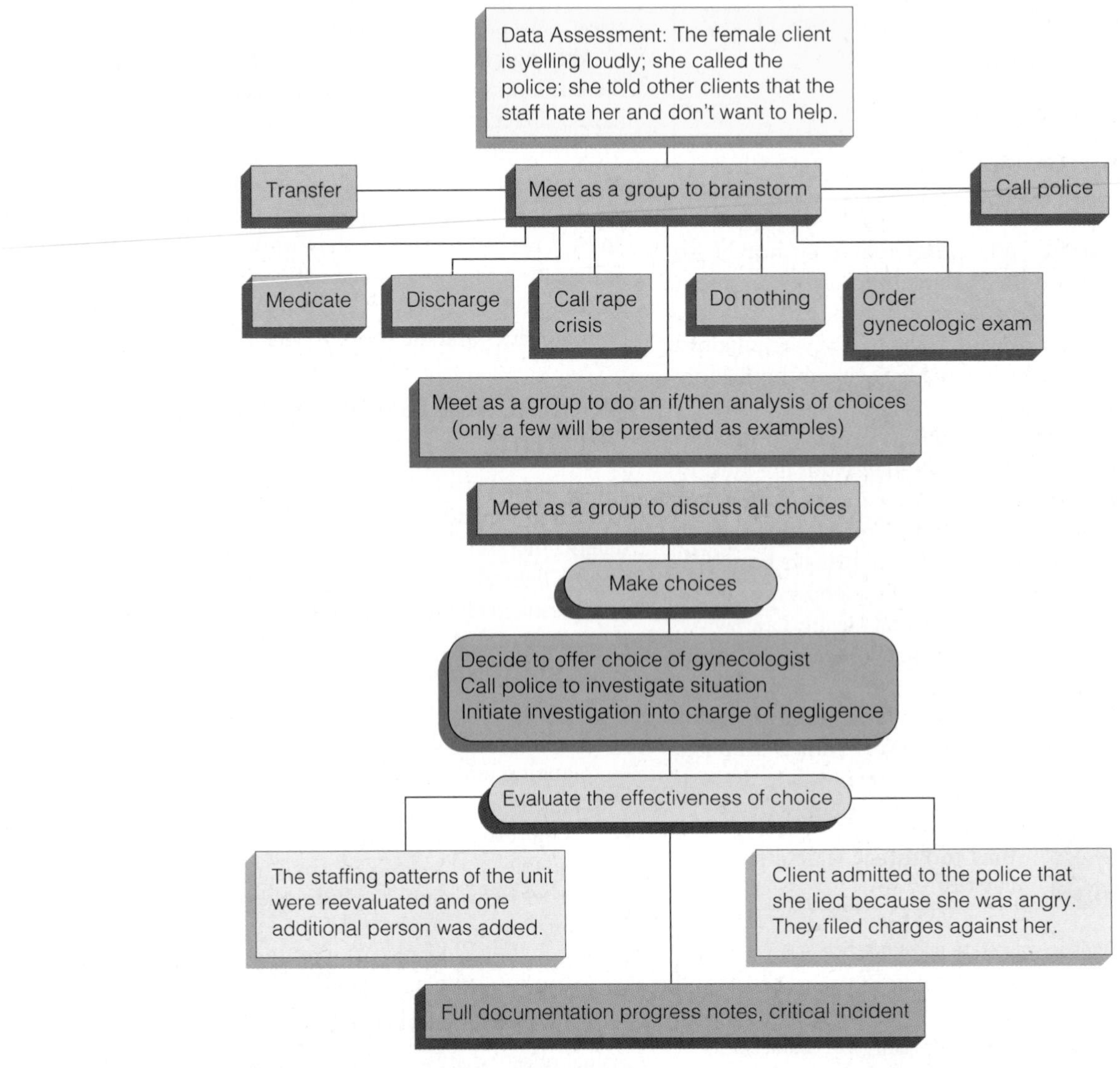

FIGURE 10–3 ■ *"If/then" analysis as a model in decision making.*

- Monitoring treatment planning and delivery of service for the abuse of client rights.
- Evaluating policies and procedures regarding client rights infringement.
- Making sure clients have the necessary information to make an informed decision or give informed consent.
- Questioning other health care professionals when their care is based more on stereotypic ideas than an assessment of the client's needs.
- Speaking out for safe practice conditions when threatened by budget cutbacks.
- Supporting an organization such as the Bazelon Center for Mental Health Law that defends the rights of children and adults with mental disabilities through policy advocacy.

DUTY TO INTERVENE

In medical–surgical nursing, it is often very easy to determine when and how to help clients. If a client has low blood sugar, you offer food to increase the blood sugar level. In psychiatric–mental health nursing, it is often difficult to determine when and how to intervene in particular situations. What is my

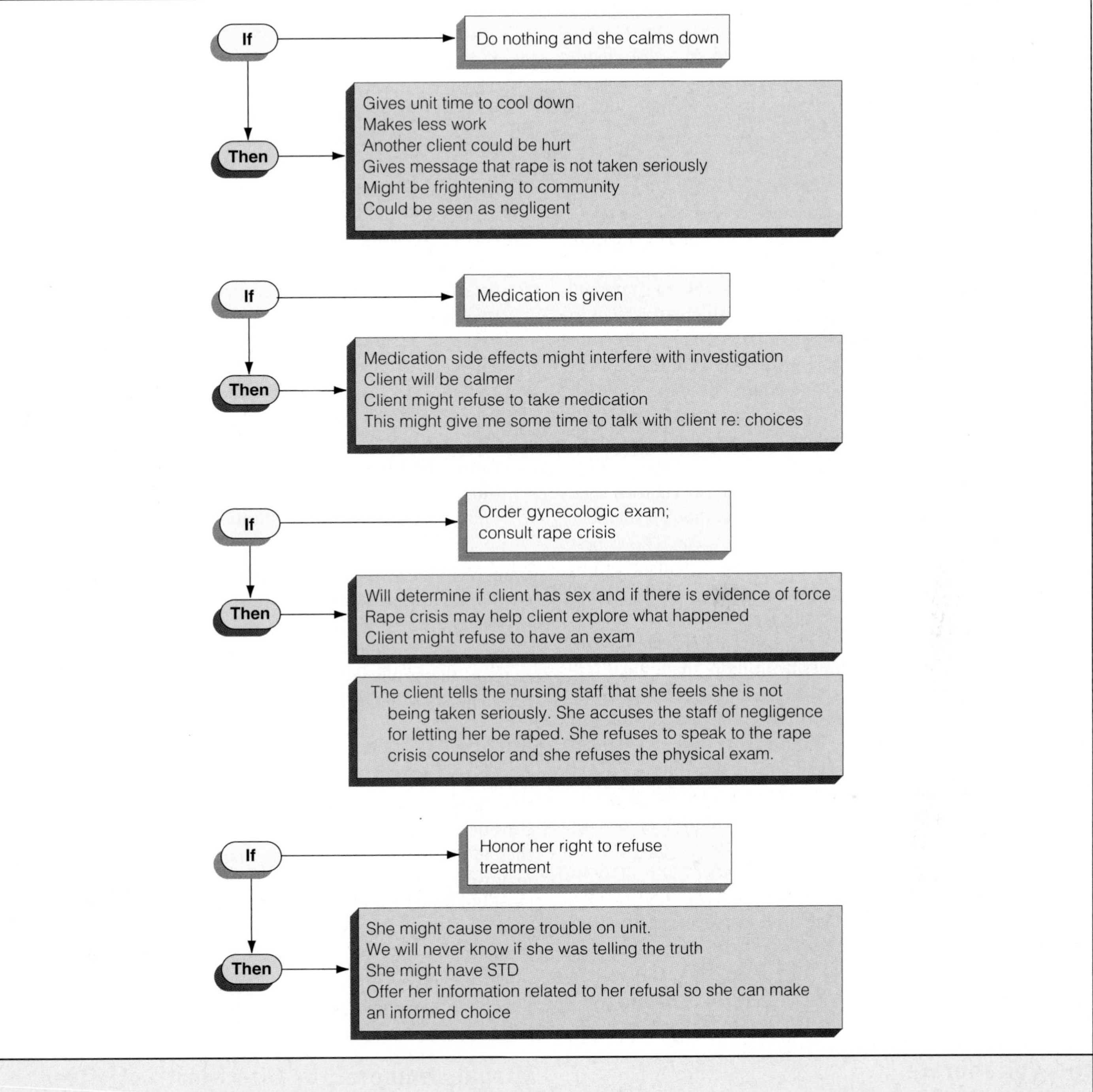

responsibility? What should be done? Who should do it? What are the appropriate legal choices? What is an appropriate ethical response? Am I going to get sued for doing this? Am I going to get sued if I don't?

If
Do nothing and she calms down
Then
Gives unit time to cool down
Makes less work
Another client could be hurt
Gives message that rape is not taken seriously
Might be frightening to community
Could be seen as negligent
If
Medication is given
Then
Medication side effects might interfere with investigation
Client will be calmer
Client might refuse to take medication
This might give me some time to talk with client re: choices
If
Order gynecologic exam; consult rape crisis
Then
Will determine if client has sex and if there is evidence of force
Rape crisis may help client explore what happened
Client might refuse to have an exam
The client tells the nursing staff that she feels she is not being taken seriously. She accuses the staff of negligence for letting her be raped. She refuses to speak to the rape crisis counselor and she refuses the physical exam.
If
Honor her right to refuse treatment
Then
She might cause more trouble on unit.
We will never know if she was telling the truth
She might have STD
Offer her information related to her refusal so she can make an informed choice

Contract for Care

A contract for care implies that the client has a need for help and that the nurse has agreed to act in good faith for the interest of the client. Nurses form this contract when they accept the duty to care for a client during the process of working on a mental health unit. This contract focuses on the nurse's professional perception that there is an issue that requires management.

Notice that the client may not have asked for help. There are many times when the client is so ill that asking for help is not a reasonable expectation. When working with mental health clients, one general rule applies: Once a situation has come to your awareness, it is important that you take all reasonable and prudent actions to intervene to be helpful to the client.

The process of admission should prepare a client for the actions that the nurse will take given certain situations such as suicidal threats or acts of violence. Most mental health units have a list of client rights and administrative policies and procedures. For example, material that is confidential is explained and material that must be shared is discussed. At times, clients may attempt to use the mental health unit as a shield against facing legal charges, and the nurse must make relevant policies explicit to the client.

Assessment

All interventions must follow a thorough assessment. The client must be informed that staff members will perform ongoing assessments to facilitate care, and if this is not clear, the client may become suspicious. When clients are not able to cooperate with assessments because of cognitive impairment, it is vital to obtain information from other sources including records from previous hospitalizations, family members, or community therapists (with client permission). The staff may need to review lab work to explore the level of reliability in the information presented by clients with respect to drug or alcohol use, for example.

Lying on the part of the client has several aspects with legal implications. Clients may deliberately mislead the staff member by telling stories that the client knows are not true. This is best dealt with through respectful confrontation. Clients may not actually lie but may frame a situation so that the client is viewed as a victim, without including details pertinent to a full understanding of the situation. In this case, it may be helpful to walk through the situation several times, with more than one interviewer, and ask for further details.

Some mental disorders affect the perception and memory of events so profoundly that only a third party such as a family member can offer an accurate view. Nurses must make a good faith effort to perform a full assessment of a client before intervening. This information must be recorded in the chart with statements not only related to information the nurse was able to obtain but also actions the nurse took to obtain information. Failure to assess the client and the situation may result in errors in judgment. It is essential to take time to collect information essential for decision making. This process requires expert communication skills not only with the client but with others involved in the client's care.

Responsibility to Communicate and Collaborate

The duty to intervene requires that information be communicated clearly to others, particularly those who participate in the decision-making process. The nurse is responsible for informing all individuals involved in the care of a client of the results of the assessment and of the considerations for the intervention phase.

Providing optimal care to clients requires cooperation and collaboration with others. No one professional can make decisions without consultation with others. Each psychiatric–mental health nurse must be able to communicate effectively within the established protocols of the agency of employment. These policies and procedures are often called the chain of command. The chain of command is the expected pattern of communication surrounding the care of clients. Several aspects of the chain of command are important to remember.

1. Nurses are often responsible for the care provided by others. The nurse may work with several nursing assistants or mental health technicians. The nurse must make clear to nonprofessionals the situations that demand immediate attention. The paraprofessionals working on a psychiatric–mental health nursing unit must be able to recognize situations that should be immediately reported.
2. The nurse often serves as a liaison to other departments. The nurse practice act in the state of employment will determine the dependent, independent, and interdependent roles of the nurse. Often these roles need to be explained to other professionals.
3. The ANA's Standards for Psychiatric–Mental Health Nursing Practice (2000) provide standards of care. Many professionals do not know that the psychiatric nurse must judge her practice based on these guidelines. The hospital or mental health agency will provide guidelines for notification and decision making that must be followed. It is vital to know the policies of the institution.

In an untoward situation, these three elements form a framework for actions that need to be taken. Once an event has occurred, you must notify team members who may not be present on the unit. Usually, the nurse manager or supervisor, physician, psychologist, social worker, security department, and at times the family, a person who has been threatened, or the police must all be notified.

Formulating a Plan to Intervene

It is vital to formulate a plan before making a decision to intervene. Nurses often complain of not having "think time," time to consider all options before acting. Many nurses indicate that they respond based on past experience or intuition. While this may work for many expert nurses, beginning nurses need to carefully think through options and learn to assess the clinical and legal implications of actions in a methodical fashion. ■ Figure 10–3a (see pages 202–203) illustrates a model that might be helpful in decision making. Figure 10–3b illustrates possible options and potential results of individual interventions.

Illegal, Immoral, or Unethical Activities of Professionals

At times, the nurse may notice that peers are engaging in illegal activities. While these unfortunate situations may occur, it is vital for each nurse to understand the legal mandate that requires a response from any professional who has knowledge of illegal, immoral, or unethical activities. Normally, this response will be to report the events to others in the agency using the chain of command. At other times, the nurse may need to seek the guidance of the State Board of Nursing or the American Nurses Association.

Nurse impairment is perhaps the most common situation encountered by professional staff. A nurse may be impaired through addiction to alcohol or narcotics, or through an event of personal experience with emotional illness. This impairment may be linked with other illegal acts such as theft of drugs or a client's personal property. Each nurse is first responsible to the client and must report such impairment in a reasonable, prudent, and timely manner. Although some nurses erroneously view this intervention as an invasion of privacy or "tattling," prompt efficient action may safeguard the client from harm while offering the impaired nurse a chance at recovery. Most hospitals have programs to assist impaired nurses to recover. Many state nursing boards or state professional associations have programs to assist the nurse addict or emotionally impaired nurse.

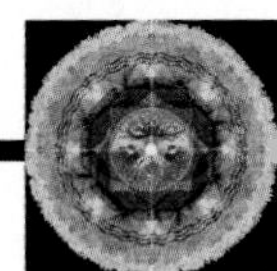

EXPLORE MediaLink

NCLEX review, case studies, and other interactive resources for this chapter can be found on the Companion Website at http://www.prenhall.com/kneisl. Click on Chapter 10 to select the activities for this chapter.

For animations, video tutorials, more NCLEX review questions, and an audio glossary, access the accompanying CD-ROM in this textbook.

BIBLIOGRAPHY

Allen, M., & Smith, V. F. (2001). Opening Pandora's box: The practical and legal dangers of involuntary outpatient commitment. *Psychiatric Services, 52*(3), 342–346.

American Nurses Association (2001). *Code for nurses with interpretive statements.* Washington, DC: Author.

American Nurses Association (2000). *Scope and standards of psychiatric–mental health nursing practice.* Washington, DC: Author.

Appelbaum, P. S. (2001). Thinking carefully about outpatient commitment. *Psychiatric Services, 52*(3), 347–350.

Bazelon Center for Mental Health Law (2001). *Psychiatric advance directive.* Washington, DC: Bazelon Center.

Beauchamp, T. L., & Walter, L. (1999). *Contemporary issues in bioethics* (5th ed.). Boston: Wadsworth.

Edge, R., & Groves, T. (1999). *Ethics of healthcare: A guide for clinical practice* (2nd ed.). Albany, NY: Delmar.

Fry, S. T. (2002). Defining nurses' ethical practices in the 21st century. *International Nursing Review, 49*(1), 1–3.

Giordano, S. (2000). For the protection of others. The value of individual autonomy and the safety of others. *Health Care Analysis, 8*(3), 309–319.

Hamric, A. B. (2000). Moral distress in everyday ethics. *Nursing Outlook, 48*(5), 199–202.

Hamric, A. B. (2000). What is happening to advocacy? *Nursing Outlook, 48*(3), 103–104.

Jenike, M. A. (2001). An update on obsessive-compulsive disorder. *Bulletin of the Menninger Clinic, 65*(1), 4–25.

Lee, N. G. (2000). Proving nursing negligence. *American Journal of Nursing, 100*(11), 55–56.

Malhi, G. S., Bartlett, J. R. (2000). Depression: A role for neurosurgery? *British Journal of Neurosurgery, 14*(5), 415–422.

Marty, D. A., & Chapin, R. (2000). The legislative tenets of the client's right to treatment in the LRE and freedom from harm: Implications for community providers. *Community Mental Health Journal, 36*(6), 545–556.

Redman, B. K., & Fry, S. T. (2000). Nurses' ethical conflicts: What is really known about them? *Nursing Ethics, 7*(4), 360–366.

Segal, S. P., Laurie, J, A., & Segal, M. J. (2001). Factors in the use of coercive retention in civil commitment evaluations in psychiatric services. *Psychiatric Services, 52*(4), 514–520.

Swanson, J. W., Tepper, M. C., Backlar, P., & Swartz, M. S. (2000). Psychiatric advance directives: An alternative to coercive treatment. *Psychiatry, 63*(2), 160–172.

Torrey, E. F., & Zdanowicz, M. (2001). Outpatient commitment: What, why, and for whom? *Psychiatric Services, 52*(3), 337–341.

Watson, A., Hanrahan, P., Luchino, D., & Lurigio, A. (2000). Mental health courts and the complex issue of mentally ill offenders. *Psychiatric Services, 52*(4), 477–481.

Whitmore, R. (2000). Consequences of not "knowing the patient." *Clinical Nurse Specialist, 14*, 75–81.

Zoucha, R., & Husted, G. L. (2000). The ethical dimensions of delivering culturally congruent nursing and health care. *Issues in Mental Health Nursing, 21*(3), 325–340.

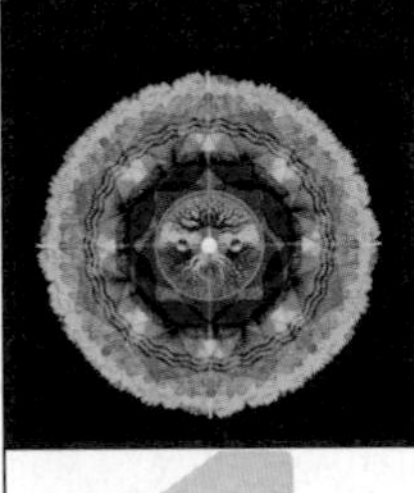

11

Chapter ELEVEN

Creating a Therapeutic Environment

CAROL REN KNEISL

KEY TERMS

case management
client government
critical pathways
deinstitutionalization
National Alliance for the Mentally Ill (NAMI)
psychiatric rehabilitation
severely and persistently mentally ill (SPMI)
therapeutic environment (therapeutic milieu)

FOCUS QUESTIONS

- **In what types of hospital-based and community-based settings do psychiatric–mental health nurses practice?**
- **What specific challenges do psychiatric home care nurses face?**
- **How do managed mental health care organizations influence psychiatric care?**
- **What differentiates case management from other types of care?**
- **How do psychiatric nurses create and manage a therapeutic environment?**
- **Who are the severely and persistently mentally ill and what adaptations in programming are necessary to meet their needs?**

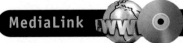

MediaLink 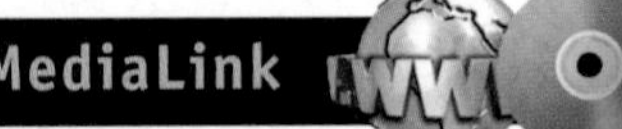 www.prenhall.com/kneisl

Additional resources for this chapter can be found on the Student CD-ROM accompanying this textbook, and on the Companion Website at www.prenhall.com/kneisl. Click on Chapter 11 to select the activities for this chapter.

CD-ROM
- Audio Glossary
- NCLEX Review

Companion Website
- Additional NCLEX Review
- Case Study: Community-Based Treatment

CHAPTER OUTLINE

CROSS REFERENCES

Other topics relevant to this content are: Crisis intervention, Chapter 33; Ethics, Chapter 10; Family burden, Chapter 29; Mood disorders, Chapter 15; Restrictive environments for care, Chapter 10; Schizophrenia, Chapter 14; Substance-related disorders, Chapter 13; Substance-related disorder in combination with mental disorder, Chapter 21; Violence in the psychiatric setting, Chapter 34.

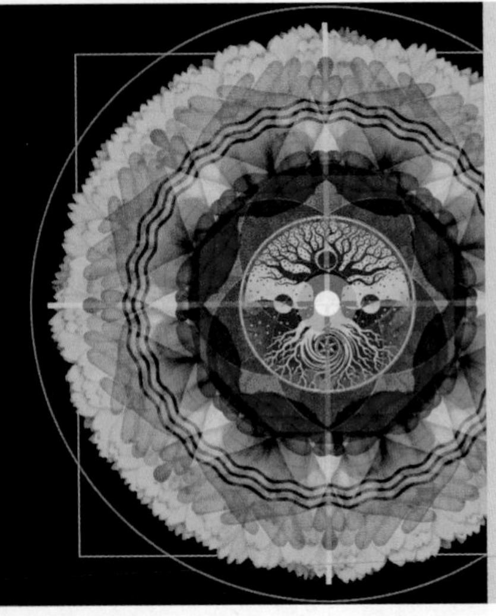

CRITICAL THINKING CHALLENGE

At a nursing care conference, you and your nurse colleague, Sylvia, disagree about the direction of future mental health care for Tommy, a client at the outpatient clinic of the community mental health center where you both work. Tommy, now 53 years old, has been in and out of psychiatric hospitals since he was 18. Tommy now lives in an adult foster care home and visits the clinic monthly for follow-up purposes. Sylvia believes that the number one nursing goal should be to provide support to Tommy so that he can maintain his current level of functioning. You believe that the number one nursing goal should be to make Tommy as independent as possible. Can these two different stands be reconciled? How? Do you see this as a matter of psychiatric nursing practice or as a question of moral beliefs? Why? ■

Economic, political, technologic, legal, and demographic forces are propelling reform and change in the provision of mental health care. Great strides continue to be made in the treatment of mental illness along with a commitment to comprehensive service delivery and innovations in multidisciplinary approaches to care. Our clients and their care are increasingly located in the larger community of which they are a part. In fact, pockets of mentally ill in the community will not seek care within the confines of the four walls of a psychiatric hospital, a comprehensive community mental health center, or even a walk-in clinic in a storefront. Intensive outreach programs currently lead community mental health efforts. The shift away from institutional-based care began with what is known as the community mental health movement.

This chapter discusses the wide variety of hospital- and community-based mental health treatment services and programs in use today and the high-risk populations most likely to use these services. Managed care and case management, psychiatric rehabilitation, and establishing therapeutic environments are discussed as processes by which the goals of services and programs are met. In addition to this chapter, each disorder chapter in Unit II of this text discusses home care, community-based care, and case management.

Deinstitutionalization and the Community Mental Health Movement

From the early nineteenth century until the 1950s, state and county mental hospitals constituted the major treatment resource for the mentally ill (see ■ Figures 11–1 and ■ 11–2). As it often turned out, these hospitals served as the mentally ill client's long-term, and sometimes permanent, residence. **Deinstitutionalization**, bringing mental health clients out of the hospital and into the community, began in the post–World War II period, when large public mental hospitals were overcrowded, had fallen into disrepair, and were widely criticized among humanitarians for "warehousing" their residents.

With the development of psychotropic drugs in 1954, and the enactment of state statutes that restricted involuntary detainment in psychiatric facilities, the resident population of state and county mental hospitals declined. By the late 1970s, only one-third as many people were hospitalized in psychiatric hospitals. This phase-down of large bureaucratic institutions occurred within the context of a much broader movement for community mental health that reached its apex in the 1960s. Box 11–1 is a timeline that summarizes the landmarks in community mental health.

When federal funds became available for the construction of community mental health centers and the provision of acute care and ambulatory services in the community, it was assumed

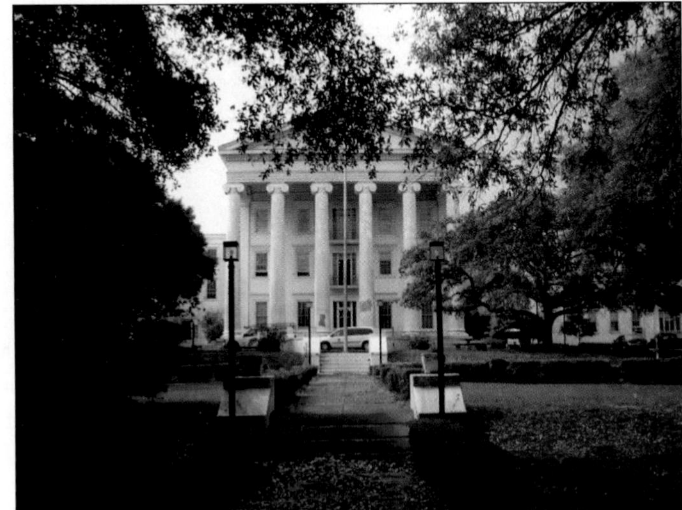

FIGURE 11–1 ■ *One of the first 10 mental hospitals in the country, the Insane Asylum of the State of Louisiana (now East Louisiana State Hospital) was built in the 1840s. Once housing over 5,000 people before deinstitutionalization, this example of Greek Revival architecture and national historic landmark has a current hospital population of 260.*

Source: Photo courtesy of Kay R. Hanks, RN, East Louisiana State Hospital, Jackson, Louisiana.

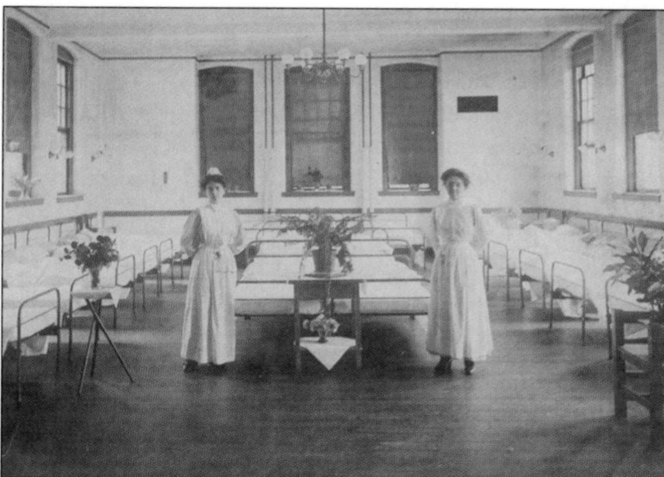

FIGURE 11–2 ■ *Psychiatric nurses in 1901 in a typical ward at the Buffalo State Hospital (now the Buffalo Psychiatric Center). At this time, architecture was believed to be able to influence the course of mental illness. For example, depressed persons were housed in wards with high ceilings such as this one in order to elevate the spirits.*

Source: Photo courtesy of Buffalo Psychiatric Center, Buffalo, New York.

that equal access to all levels of mental health prevention and treatment would exist. However, several disturbing trends cast this assumption into doubt. First of all, hospital care remained the main treatment modality for the severely mentally ill: Repeated readmissions replaced long-term institutional residence. New populations of the mentally ill in the community—the homeless, crack cocaine addicts, mentally ill criminal offenders—were unable or unwilling to use the provided services. It became apparent that aggressive outreach services were needed in order to make both hospital-based and community-based treatments and programs accessible to those individuals who needed them. The greatest problems have been in creating adequate and accessible community resources (Lamb & Bachrach, 2001).

Types of Treatment Services and Programs

Hospital-based inpatient treatment and community-based outpatient treatment constitute the two major umbrellas under which care is provided.

HOSPITAL-BASED TREATMENT

Clients admitted to inpatient settings, such as the one in ■ Figure 11–3 on page 211, must meet admission criteria. The admitting diagnosis is often one that is life threatening. Overall effectiveness of functioning using the DSM Axis V global assessment of functioning scale (GAF; see Chapter 9) determines the acuity of the illness. Impairment in functioning must be in the 10 to 50 range to qualify for admission, in most instances. Clients experiencing this degree of discomfort require intense, skilled nursing care to provide for safety needs. For example, a GAF score of 30 indicates that behavior is strongly influenced by delusions or hallucinations, serious impairment in communication or judgment, or an inability to function in almost all areas. Some managed care organizations (MCOs) have designed their own criteria that require ratings of functioning, physical impairments, family support, and other elements as part of a preadmission assessment.

You can easily see how your role as a nurse in the inpatient psychiatric setting is similar to the role of the critical care nurse in the general hospital. Clients who are admitted to the psychiatric unit with active suicidal ideation, who are psychotic, or who are experiencing withdrawal symptoms require intensive nursing care and case management.

BOX 11–1 Landmarks in Community Mental Health

The 1950s

- The National Mental Health Study Act established the Joint Commission on Mental Illness and Health.
- Psychotropic drugs were introduced to control psychotic symptoms, facilitating a transition to community care and a new emphasis on access to all levels of mental health treatment and prevention in the community.

The 1960s

- The Joint Commission presented its report, *Action for Mental Health,* to Congress, recommending a shift to community-based care.
- The Community Mental Health Centers Act authorized $150 million in federal matching funds to states to develop comprehensive community mental health centers and community services including acute and ambulatory care.

The 1970s

- President Carter established a President's Commission on Mental Health.
- The National Institute of Mental Health (NIMH) began the Community Support Program.
- Congress passed the Omnibus Budget Reconciliation Act, placing services formerly directed by the NIMH in federal block grants to states.
- The NIMH established an Office of Programs for the Homeless Mentally Ill.

The 1990s

- The NIMH funded research demonstration programs authorized by the Stewart B. McKinney Homeless Assistance Act.
- The Federal Task Force on Homelessness and Severe Mental Illness made recommendations for the expansion of housing and service options to the homeless mentally ill.
- The Americans with Disabilities Act affirmed the rights of those with psychiatric disabilities.

COMMUNITY-BASED TREATMENT

There are a wide variety of community-based treatment settings. Box 11–2 gives you several examples of settings in which psychiatric–mental health nurses practice, some of which are discussed next. Several others are discussed in other sections of this chapter.

Community Mental Health Centers

Community mental health centers (CMHCs) vary considerably in their appearance (see ■ Figure 11–3a, b, and c) and in the services they offer. Services offered in CMHCs include:

- Emergency services.
- Medication management clinics.
- Psychoeducation groups.
- Vocational rehabilitation.
- Consultation services to hospitals, nursing homes, primary care centers.
- Other specialty services as determined by the population they serve (programs for the severely and persistently mentally ill, mental health clinics for the homeless, dual diagnosis services for chemically dependent mentally ill clients, elder services, etc.).

A study in Australia (McCann, 2002) indicated that an important function of community mental health nurses is to uncover their clients' hope for the future. These community mental health nurses used two main strategies to enable the process of hopefulness:

1. Enhancing motivation
2. Developing pathways to wellness.

These activities enhance the quality of the nurse–client relationship, and advance client self-determination, education, and planning for the future.

In large metropolitan areas, CMHCs often include:

- Inpatient hospital-based care, and
- Partial hospitalization programs:
    1. Day care services for those who need supervision and assistance during daytime hours.
    2. Night treatment services for those who are able to maintain employment during the day but need supervision and assistance during nighttime hours.

Mobile Outreach Units

Mobile treatment teams go out into the community by car or on foot to deliver services in whatever setting makes the client comfortable—a public place, a jail, a home, a shopping mall, a fast-food restaurant, under a bridge, or in an alley. Common treatment goals of mobile outreach units are:

- Bringing community-based treatment programs to homeless clients and to those who would not otherwise seek mental health services or have little or no access to mental health care.
- Providing medication management prescribed by another mental health professional to clients who have problems in complying with treatment by psychotropic medications.
- Preventing relapse and hospitalization.
- Identifying and assessing persons in the community in need of mental health care and facilitating their entry into a mental health service program.
- Providing emergency intervention or crisis prevention services to mental health consumers, police, employers, landlords, business owners, and so on.
- Satisfying the requirements of court-ordered treatment.

Mobile treatment teams have also been able to reduce the need for hospitalization in many instances. Major mental health consumer characteristics that relate to the likelihood of hospitalization are:

1. Being young and homeless and experiencing acute problems.
2. Having been referred by psychiatric hospitals, the legal system, or other treatment facilities.

BOX 11–2 Community Treatment Settings

- Adult day care settings
- AIDS support programs
- Assisted living facilities
- Child day care centers
- Client's own home
- Community mental health centers
- Correctional facilities (jails, prisons, detention centers)
- Courts (mental health evaluation, mentally ill offenders, victims of violence)
- Crisis services
- Day treatment centers
- Emergency departments of hospitals
- Ethnic cultural centers
- Foster care homes for adults and youths
- Group homes
- Halfway houses
- Hospices
- Houses of worship (churches, synagogues, mosques, temples)
- Immigrant centers
- Industry and business centers
- Mobile outreach teams
- Nursing homes
- Rural mental health clinics
- Partial hospitalization programs
- Primary care centers
- Private practice offices (psychiatric–mental health nurses, psychiatrists, psychologists, social workers)
- Residential facilities for cognitively impaired
- Schools
- Sheltered workshops
- Shelters and residential services (battered women, homeless, youths, people in crisis)
- Substance abuse programs
- Youth centers
- YMCAs/YWCAs

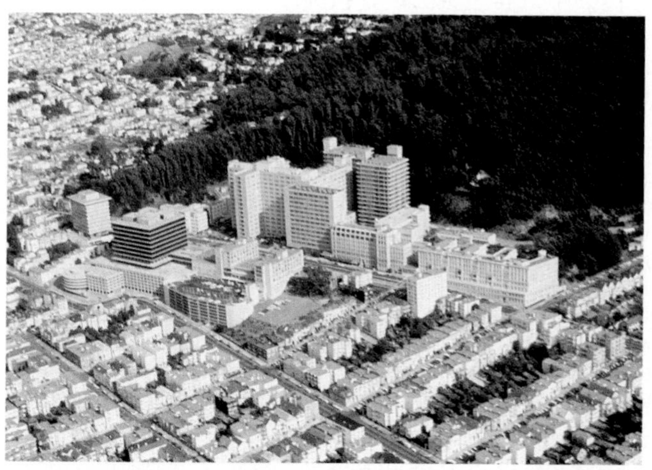

A

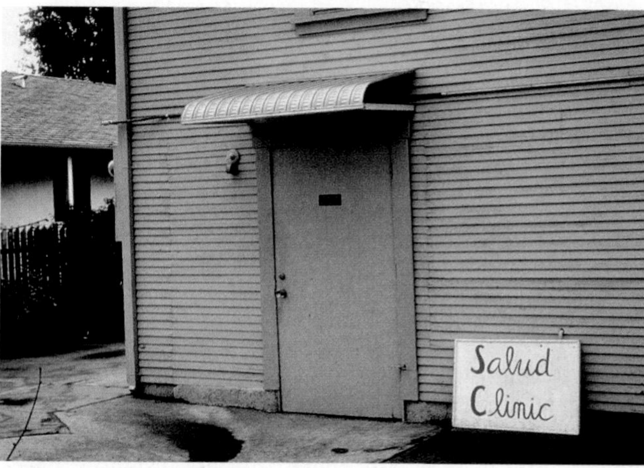

B

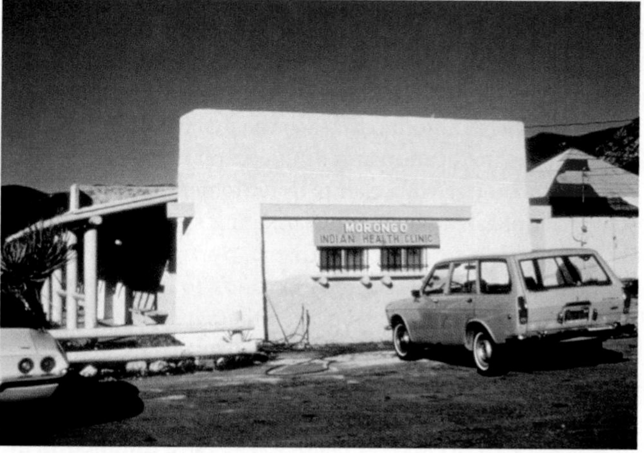

C

FIGURE 11–3 ■ *A community mental health center is more a concept than a place. Community mental health centers cannot be recognized by appearance alone.*
(A) A university-based medical center with a community mental health center and a neuropsychiatric inpatient unit.
(B) An inner-city mental health outreach clinic.
(C) A rural mental health outreach clinic and day treatment program

3. Showing signs of substance abuse, having no income, and being severely mentally disabled (Guo, Biegel, Johnsen, & Dyches, 2001).

Assertive Community Treatment (ACT)

Assertive programs have shown much promise in terms of service delivery to high-risk groups and are believed to prevent psychotic relapse and rehospitalizations (Bustillo, Lauriello, Horan, & Keith, 2001) and reduce arrests, emergency room visits, and homelessness of clients with severe and persistent mental illness (Clarke et al., 2000). These are expensive, sophisticated programs that are believed to be cost-effective because they offset still more expensive hospital episodes. Assertive programs are known by names other than ACT—Continuous Treatment Teams (CTTs), Intensive Case Management (ICM), and Programs for Assertive Community Treatment (PACT) are some of them.

These teams may include interdisciplinary groups of 7 to 12 staff members—nurses, psychiatrists, social workers, peer specialists who are mental health consumers, and mental health paraprofessionals—who deliver service in the client's own environment. Treatment teams not only provide a mobile outreach capacity, they also provide consumers with access to multidisciplinary providers and comprehensive services.

The team structure is believed to reduce stress and burnout of individual case managers by sharing the load of difficult clients. The client benefits from both reduced dependence on an individual clinician and the support of a large multidisciplinary group for backup during crisis. In addition, clients benefit because staff members in these teams must be clinically sophisticated and capable of managing acute care in the community.

Concerns about coercion have arisen with ACT treatment programs. A major concern has been that ACT teams often become actively and directly involved in many areas of the client's life and may control access to resources such as housing and money in return for compliance with medication and treatment programs through outpatient commitment (Torrey & Zdanowicz, 2001). This paternalism interferes with the client's personal autonomy. Members of ACT teams must be sure to look for opportunities to enhance clients' quality of life through personal goal setting and decision making to the extent possible for each individual client. See the Using Research Evidence feature on page 212. Guidelines and standards recommended for assertive community treatment teams, and developed by the National Alliance for the Mentally Ill (NAMI) are available at www.nami.org/about/pactstd.html and can be accessed through the Companion Website for this book.

MediaLink Assertive Community Treatment

Psychiatric Home Care

Psychiatric home care nursing has a long history in community mental health (Fagin, 2001). Some of the most successful programs for the severely mentally ill in the early years of community mental health employed visiting nurses to deliver home-based services. Today, there is growing demand for psychiatric home care nursing as a cost-effective alternative to hospitalization. Medicare, Medicaid, managed care organizations, and pri-

USING RESEARCH EVIDENCE

Angie is a 42-year-old woman who has been hospitalized several times for acute schizophrenic episodes. Each episode has been preceded by a period in which Angie stopped taking her medication. Angie usually becomes argumentative, begins to hallucinate, fails to pay attention to her personal care, does not show up for her job, and withdraws from others, staying in her apartment in the dark. This time, Angie, who has a key to her boyfriend's apartment, entered his apartment when he wasn't there and locked herself in. She played a CD over and over at such a high volume that the neighbors next door and in the apartment below complained to the building superintendent.

When the building superintendent knocked on the door, Angie refused to let him in. His pleas with her to keep the noise down were met with increasing rage. Angie began throwing things in the apartment, broke a window, and damaged the walls. Fortunately, Angie's boyfriend arrived on the scene and called the mental health clinic where Angie was registered as a client. Soon after, the police arrived in response to calls from neighbors. Angie refused to open the door for them.

The mobile mental health team that arrived on the scene was able to persuade Angie to let them in the apartment. They negotiated an agreement among Angie, her boyfriend, the building superintendent, and the police that charges would not be filed against Angie providing that she agreed to assertive community treatment that would involve involuntary outpatient commitment including medication management. Angie's boyfriend agreed to repair the window and any damaged walls. The goals were to avoid hospitalization for Angie, to avoid criminal charges, to help her comply with a medication regimen, and to keep close contact with her and preempt future violent behavior. The mobile mental health team considered the following research study in developing a plan of action for Angie:

Guo, S., Biegel, D. E., Johnsen, A. & Dyches, H. (2001). Assessing the impact of community-based mobile crisis services on previous hospitalization. *Psychiatric Services, 52*(2), 223–228.

vate health insurance all fund psychiatric home care at different levels and with different requirements for reimbursement.

Clients with a primary psychiatric diagnosis should be cared for in the home by an experienced psychiatric–mental health nurse. In fact, Medicare (which funds most psychiatric home care) requires this experience. Basic-level and advanced-level psychiatric–mental health nurses provide direct psychiatric care to mental health consumers through home care agencies. Advanced-level nurses may also provide direct psychiatric care or function as intensive case managers and consultants to staff as well as mental health consumers.

Other requirements for Medicare reimbursement are homebound status and the presence of a diagnosed psychiatric disorder. Homebound status for psychiatric home care would include clients who are immobilized by depression or anxiety attacks, clients who are disoriented or confused, clients with hallucinations or delusions that compromise their safety, or mental health clients whose physical health prevents them from going to other locations where mental health services are offered.

Psychiatric home care is more likely to be used for clients recently discharged from a psychiatric hospital, the homebound elderly, persons with dementia, young adults with severe and persistent mental illness, or clients who have an associated medical condition such as neuropsychiatric problems as a result of infection with HIV (human immunodeficiency virus; see also Chapter 24).

As clients are discharged from hospitals more quickly, the nurse who is providing home care may be providing services that traditionally would have been delivered in a hospital setting. For example, the drug clozapine (Clozaril), used to alleviate symptoms of schizophrenia, requires frequent blood tests to monitor for side effects. The home care nurse draws the blood and monitors the drug protocol in the home setting. Alcohol-related complications such as diabetes may require extensive family teaching to enable family members to successfully manage a chronic alcoholic family member who is also diabetic.

You might encounter your clients in personal care homes or hospices. Clients with AIDS-related dementia often require extensive counseling and supportive services as they struggle with their illness. These types of clients are often quite medically ill, and you may collaborate with another nurse provider in meeting their needs.

In some personal care homes, you may be the only professional who visits an elderly client. In these instances, part of your teaching plan is to work with ancillary staff members who are responsible for running the personal care home. The importance of medication compliance for a severely, persistently mentally ill person cannot be overemphasized. Your method of ensuring that clients in personal care homes receive their medication as ordered is often to teach the managers of these facilities about the medication and its effects on behavior.

If you encounter your clients in retirement complexes, your teaching emphasis may be with an aging spouse. This person may not be able to carry out instructions and may require repetitive teaching plans and other aids to ensure that your client follows treatment protocols. In these instances, your skills in family systems will be useful aids in planning appropriate interventions.

Providing direct psychiatric home care services requires that you are sensitive to several factors. They are outlined in Box 11–3.

Managed Mental Health Care

Managed mental health care, a method for capping the rate of increase in the cost of mental health care, while ensuring access to quality mental health care services, has become an increasingly important force in psychiatric–mental health nursing. As a service delivery system, managed mental health care creates a

BOX 11-3 Challenges for the Psychiatric Home Care Nurse

- Remember that you are a guest in the client's home and that the client has the right to refuse your admittance to that home.
- As a guest in the client's home, be aware of the client's cultural background and strive to be culturally sensitive. Incorporating the client's cultural beliefs into the care you give will not only enhance your relationship with the client and family, but will also positively influence the client's participation in the treatment process.

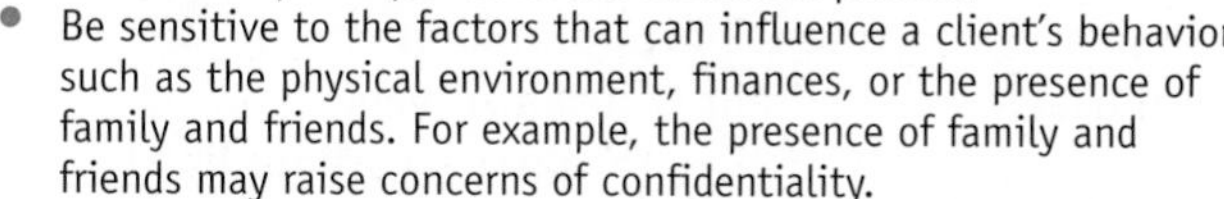

- Be sensitive to the factors that can influence a client's behavior such as the physical environment, finances, or the presence of family and friends. For example, the presence of family and friends may raise concerns of confidentiality.
- Work collaboratively with the psychiatrist, other mental health professional, or the client's primary medical care provider to provide in-depth psychiatric home care.
- Be sensitive to changes in the client's behavior that may indicate relapse or a worsening of symptoms.
- Don't forget to assess for medical problems that may compound or be compounded by the mental disorder.
- Provide psychoeducation, especially in terms of psychotropic medications even for clients who have been on the same medication for years (medication noncompliance accounts for the majority of psychiatric hospital readmissions). Do not assume that clients received adequate instruction, or that they remember the instruction.
- Empower your clients and encourage increasing independence by involving them in the treatment plan.
- Be aware of any factors in the environment that threaten either the client's or your safety. Leave the client's home if your safety seems to be in question (see also Chapter 34) and inform family, caregivers, or other involved mental health professionals or community resources.

rich climate for nurses to become actively involved in primary prevention and education.

MANAGED CARE SETTINGS

The shift in practice settings from inpatient to community settings presents new challenges to you as a psychiatric–mental health nurse. Nursing is responding to pressures to use health care resources more efficiently. Clients are admitted to hospitals in later stages of disease or illness, or perhaps not admitted at all. Criteria for hospitalization are based on medical necessity. For instance, the once standard 28-day program for substance abuse treatment has given way to innovative and shorter models for detoxification services and outpatient treatment that meet the lifestyle needs of clients and their employers. Employer demands, coupled with cost containment, have created an entire range of ambulatory care services that at one time would have been considered ineffective. Substance-abusing clients may have options of day; evening, or weekend partial hospitalization programs. Some programs adhere to a Monday through Friday schedule of 4 to 6 hours per day or evening. Weekend programs are usually 8 hours on Saturday and 8 hours on Sunday.

Inpatient Settings

The admission criteria for inpatient care have been discussed earlier in this chapter. These goals are achieved through shorter, more intense hospital stays, and the use of critical pathways and case management.

Shorter, More Intense Stays. A focus on shorter, more intense stays came about through the emphasis in MCOs on the need to maximize value for the mental health consumer and to keep costs down through the judicious use of available resources. These goals are achieved through the use of critical pathways and case management. Case management is discussed in detail later in this chapter in the section on creating a therapeutic environment.

Critical Pathways. Critical pathways, or road maps of expected outcomes described in Chapter 7, are valuable tools for helping nurses in delivering care within managed-care frameworks. When a client "falls off the map" or falls to meet the desired outcomes, this information can be fed to a quality-improvement program to avoid such deviations in the future. However, since critical pathways are the tools by which MCOs achieve their goals, they have become increasingly important.

Primary Care Centers

Alternatives to hospitalization and accelerated discharge to ambulatory care settings create a demand for sophisticated, comprehensive, and well-coordinated services in the primary care setting. Managed care sites can offer rich concentrations of primary care resources to meet client needs. Such a setting is conducive to delegating responsibility to the most cost-effective, medically appropriate provider. The ambulatory care facilities of MCOs are ideal settings for psychiatric–mental health nurses to function in the role of primary mental health care provider.

Generally, psychiatric–mental health nurses in MCOs perform mental health assessments, monitor chronic illness, provide direct care for acute problems, and facilitate health-promotion groups. Examples of some of the health-promotion activities nurses can initiate in primary care settings are stress management, parenting education, violence prevention, bereavement counseling, suicide prevention, and teen pregnancy prevention.

Triage Services. Psychiatric–mental health nurses provide effective *triage* services in the ambulatory care setting. Triage involves determining the severity of the illness and the need for immediate care in order to direct care and ensure the efficient use of medical and nursing staff and facilities. In the triage role, you often act as the *gatekeeper* of the system. You essentially decide who will use the system and at what level of care. The gatekeeping function is discussed in the case management section of this chapter.

Many factors need to be considered in the role of triage nurse. The common denominator in all instances is allocation of resources for ensuring quality and cost-effectiveness. You may be performing face-to-face assessments or telephone triage. One of the most important required skills is good listening ability, coupled with an ability to collect information for making a decision about appropriate intervention. Information may be fragmented, and interviews with several people may be required to provide a comprehensive view of the client's presenting problem.

Triage clinicians in mental health care settings provide short-term, episodic intervention to members enrolled in the plan and simplify access to appropriate points of service in the system. ■ Figure 11–4 depicts the triage process and the complexity of options available to clinicians in managed care. Collaboration and consultation are important processes nurses use when performing this first-point-of-contact service.

When triaging, you use a variety of nursing skills to evaluate the client's presenting problem. Using listening skills, you combine verbal and nonverbal data with information available in the client's medical record.

CLINICAL EXAMPLE

Margaret, a 35-year-old woman, is referred after several visits for minor medical problems. You note from the record a pattern of medication refills for antianxiety medication from the primary care provider. You also notice she has been referred for mental health care on two other occasions but has failed to keep these appointments. This information is valuable as you begin your assessment.

After completing the assessment, your next step is to decide a course of action. Using the nursing process, you begin to plan appropriate interventions. Choices include no intervention, immediate intervention, intervention within 24 hours, or routine appointment. Your further options include a private office, a public clinic, or a hospital emergency room.

Employer-Based Clinics

As managed health care continues to develop new models, employers are becoming increasingly sophisticated in developing systems to meet the needs of their employees. Employers may establish on-site clinics with an MCO. The office is staffed with MCO employees. Here the psychiatric–mental health nurse might be asked to serve as a consultant, counseling at the site a day or two per week, seeing clients referred through the primary care providers in the employer-based clinic.

MCOs AS A PRACTICE ENVIRONMENT

There are several other aspects of practicing in managed care settings in mental health that are unique to this delivery system. These include boundaries, legal issues, treatment and medication compliance, unrealistic member expectations, and continuity of care.

Boundaries

Boundaries are personal limits we use to differentiate between one event and another. Working as a clinician in the managed-care arena exposes one to demands, crises, time pressures, schedules, and other stressful events inherent in any health care delivery system. It is crucial for you to maintain adequate boundaries to prevent burnout, maintain objectivity, and be comfortable setting limits with consumers.

Psychiatric–mental health nurses working in MCOs need orientation to the structure, goals, and operating philosophy to become part of the culture of the practice setting. Nurses whose own values are congruent with the MCO will be less susceptible to burnout and able to feel satisfied in practice. Burnout prevention is discussed in Chapter 1.

Legal Issues

In traditional fee-for-service practice when a judge mandates treatment, there is usually acceptance of the client into the system for service. Service is delivered on demand, and then a charge is issued to the client. In MCOs, court-ordered treatment is negotiated on a case-by-case basis. What this means is that not every person who presents with a request for court-ordered treatment will automatically receive this service.

CLINICAL EXAMPLE

A transportation worker who has received his third DUI (driving under the influence) citation requests service. The member has already received two previous episodes of treatment and is not covered for services in the current calendar year.

A decision must then be made about how to respond to this request. These sometimes thorny and difficult legal cases are often referred for individual case review to the medical director.

A decision may be made to allow for a "flexing" of benefits or authorization of out-of-plan services. In flexing, an outpatient mental health care benefit may be converted to an inpatient benefit to allow for the needed hospitalization. The psychiatric–mental health nurse is sometimes in the role of client advocate, helping negotiate uncharted territory in these unusual circumstances.

Treatment Adherence

Compliance or adherence issues are more readily observed in MCOs, particularly in closed panel systems where appointment clerks, clinicians, and pharmacists may work side by side. Perhaps because services are prepaid, MCO consumers find it easier not to keep scheduled appointments. This is sometimes referred to as DNKA (did not keep appointment). In mental

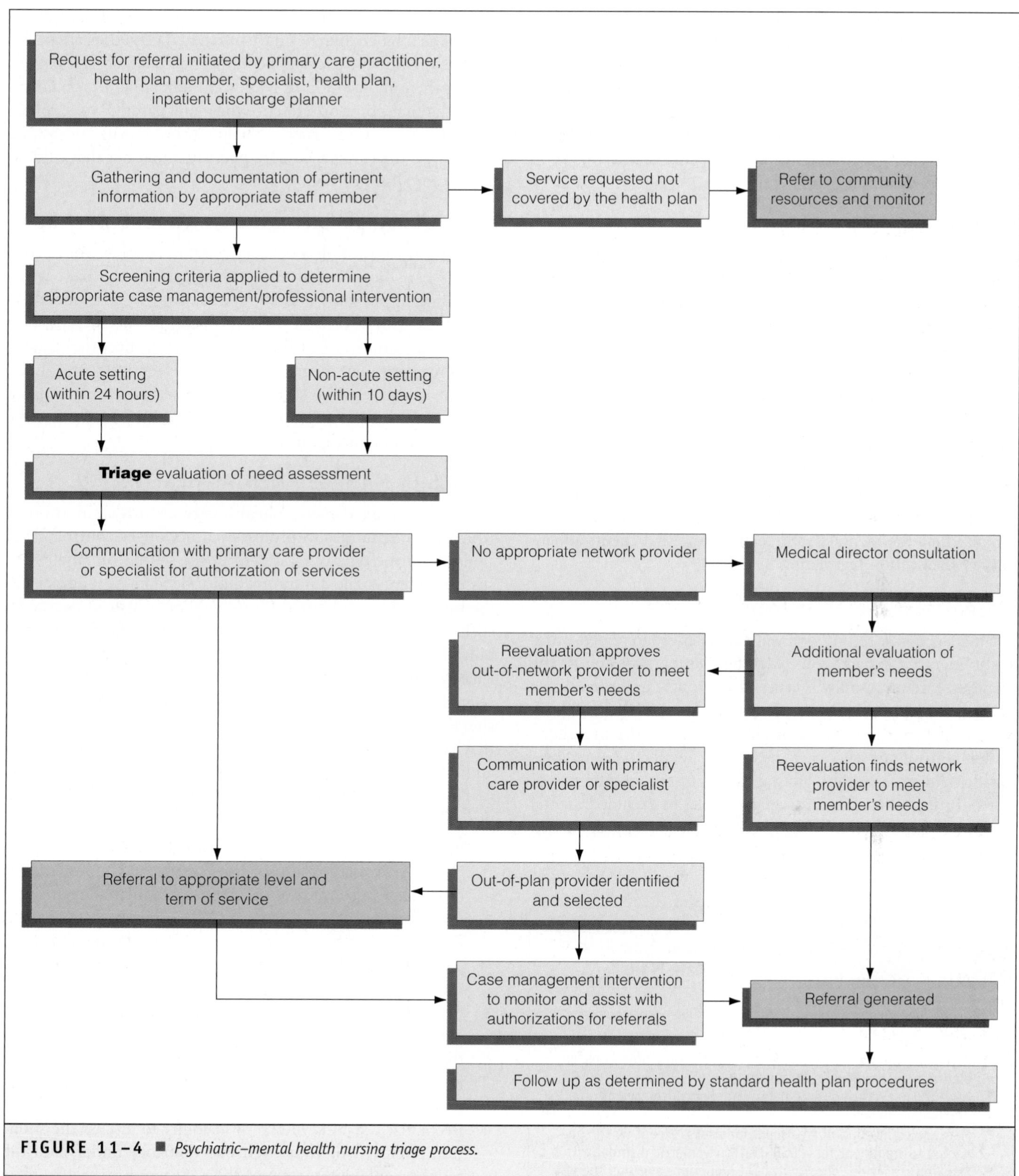

FIGURE 11–4 ■ *Psychiatric–mental health nursing triage process.*

health care, this behavior has clinical and administrative significance. It is important to note that different MCOs deal with this problem in various ways. One alternative is to set strict limits and not allow future appointments to be scheduled until the client makes copayment for all missed appointments. Another is to require clients to wait their turn in line for the next available appointment. Finally, the DNKA must be handled as a therapeutic issue in the therapy.

Some MCOs "double-book" appointments, relying on no-shows to balance out the schedule. When these missed appointments occur following hospitalization for a major psychiatric episode of illness, the clinician must aggressively maintain contact with the client. The importance of adhering to an after-care plan to avoid relapse is crucial. Phone calls, letters, or catching clients while they are visiting another department in the facility are all useful interventions. Some MCOs have developed transportation systems such as a free bus to ensure that clients keep appointments and follow after-care plans.

Medication Adherence

Medication adherence or compliance follows many principles used in other settings. Nurses in MCOs often work in collaborative relationships with other providers to ensure adherence. When medication copayments are low, appointments are available, and transportation is accessible, the likelihood of adherence is increased. In the MCO setting, the primary care provider is an ally of the mental health care team. Primary care providers who see clients for routine medical problems are in a position to reinforce the importance of staying on psychotropic drugs. Often a discussion of side effects eliminates confusion and increases understanding of the medicine's effect. Managed-care pharmacists can also help the mental health team ensure that clients adhere to their medication regimens.

Unrealistic Member Expectations

In a managed-care setting, you will be challenged to resolve unrealistic member expectations. Members' understanding of the managed care philosophy is crucial for effective and responsible health behaviors, including expectations of available services.

The member's entitlement expectations is the member's understanding of the care he or she expects to receive. Entitlement expectations often differ from the specific provisions of the health plan contract. Examples of excluded mental health services of several large MCO contracts appear in Box 11–4.

BOX 11–4 Mental Health Services Often Excluded from Typical Managed Care Plans

Following are some examples of mental health services that are not included in typical MCO plans:

- Psychiatric or substance abuse therapy on court order, unless plan-approved as medically necessary.
- Psychological testing, except for diagnosis or treatment of a psychiatric disorder.
- Marriage counseling or treatment for stress, except when connected to treatment for a DSM-IV-TR psychiatric disorder.
- Smoking cessation, obesity, weight reduction, aversion therapy, custodial care, V code conditions (non–DSM-IV-TR conditions that may be a focus of clinical attention such as noncompliance with treatment, malingering, age-related cognitive decline, etc. discussed in Appendix A), autism, learning disabilities, mental retardation, congenital disorders.
- Experimental treatment (psychosurgery, megavitamin therapy, codependence therapy, or treatment for sexual addiction).

Health plan members often do not consider what type of mental health benefits they have purchased until they are in crisis. The memory of television commercials suggesting inpatient care as the only solution to adolescent adjustment problems is often the first point of reference for many parents. Your role as consumer educator is crucial to helping your clients understand how to use their managed-care plans in a manner that is satisfactory for all concerned.

Continuity of Care and Treatment Breaks

Some MCOs are seamless delivery systems. In other words, consumers can move from one level of care to the next while remaining in the same delivery system. In this sense, members of an MCO can be considered to be in continuous therapy. This has clinical implications that require new conceptual frameworks for treatment. Primary care services tend to focus on the present impasse, while secondary care services are geared to examine the underlying obstacle. It is essential to the healing process that both are coordinated.

ETHICS IN MANAGED MENTAL HEALTH CARE

In effect, managed mental health care creates a situation in which the mental health professional no longer controls decisions about the type of treatment or the setting (inpatient versus outpatient). The autonomy and independent judgment of the nurse are being limited (Smoyak, 2000). Instead decisions, such as two therapy sessions each week or outpatient drug rehabilitation, are monitored by an agent employed by insurers. Clearly, managed psychiatric care raises serious ethical issues related to client autonomy of choice regarding therapist and site, the integrity of the nurse–client relationship, and the risk that noncompliant psychiatric clients may be denied access to additional treatment.

Four principles to guide you through the ethical dilemmas posed by managed mental health care systems are:

1. Recognize that as a clinician, you are dedicated to caring for clients in a relationship of fidelity and, at the same time, must act as a steward of society's scarce mental health care resources.
2. Recognize that it is ethically correct to recommend the least costly treatment unless you have evidence that a more costly intervention will yield a superior outcome.
3. Recognize that you need to advocate for the ethical principle of justice in managed mental health care situations so that cost savings with one client are used to meet the mental health care needs of another, not pay off an insurance company's debts.
4. Recognize that it is your responsibility to discuss the situation openly with your clients so that they understand the reimbursable parameters of their care and can act in their own interests.

A mental health consumer's bill of rights that also examines insurance coverage and managed care plans in light of the principles identified in the bill is located at www.apa.org/pubinfo/rights/rights.html and can be accessed through the Companion Website for this book.

A moral debate about the ethics of applying managed care to psychiatric clients is active. Be prepared to sharpen your ethical reasoning skills and tools.

Case Management

Rapid changes in the health care system have contributed to client feelings of being overwhelmed and confused about how to use services effectively. In many systems, clients no longer rely on a single provider or institution to shepherd them through an episode of illness. **Case management** is one strategy that has evolved to meet the needs of clients, families, employers, and providers. The fundamental focus of case management is to integrate, coordinate, and advocate for individuals, families, and groups requiring extensive services through:

- Assessment and problem identification.
- Planning.
- Procurement, delivery, and coordination of service.
- Monitoring to ensure that the multiple service needs of the client are met.

The central element that differentiates case management from other types of care is the coordination of one episode of care across the multiple settings of the care continuum.

CASE MANAGER ROLE

Nurses who perform this role must be vested with the authority and accountability necessary to negotiate with complex systems and a wide diversity of providers and populations. Nurses are particularly prepared to function in this role by the very nature of the profession.

This is especially evident in the managed care setting where clients from diverse backgrounds sometimes struggle to negotiate a new system of health care delivery. We know that race and poverty are factors that impede a client's access to mental health services and that race and ethnicity affect how clients use mental health services. Our racial diversity as a nation is increasing, and case management can help individuals and families who bring unique needs and cultural experiences to the managed case setting.

As case managers, nurses can provide physical assessment or illness-detection skills. An additional factor contributing to the natural fit between nurses and consumers is the increased emphasis on psychobiology and pharmacology in helping clients cope with alterations in their mental health.

PROCESS OF CASE MANAGEMENT

Like the nursing process, case management focuses on the following elements:

- Assessment
- Outcome development
- Planning
- Intervention
- Monitoring
- Evaluation

The process of case management enhances quality by preventing unnecessary hospitalization, focusing treatment goals in least-restrictive settings, and preventing the duplication and fragmentation of services.

Gatekeeping and Facilitating

The service you provide as a case manager is one of gatekeeping and facilitating. As gatekeeper, you serve as the client's initial contact for care and referrals. For example, the case manager for a client with bipolar disorder may be contacted as that client presents in the emergency department in a manic state. Because of knowledge of prior history and treatment, you are able to determine if inpatient care is required. You would have access to recent laboratory studies regarding lithium carbonate levels and also have an established relationship with family members. In other words, case management helps clients and their caregivers make informed decisions, such as whether the client needs hospitalization, based on client needs, abilities, resources, and personal preferences.

In a case of recurring substance abuse, the nurse case manager can help a family make informed decisions, taking into consideration the client's health status and diagnosis, treatment plan, payment resources, and health care options. This facilitation aspect of case management assures that clients receive care that is appropriate, individualized, cost-effective, and has optimal outcomes.

Client Advocacy

Agencies that provide client services must have clear statements regarding client rights and responsibilities. The case manager often refers to these in negotiating with both client and system regarding appropriate referrals and authorizations for treatment.

A statement of rights helps focus our awareness on the most fundamental aspect of the case manager role, that of being a client advocate. While there are many and varied models of case management, the nurse who defines this role as client advocate will have the greatest chance of success. When you carry out your role in this framework, you bring to the multidisciplinary team skills and knowledge that extend beyond biologic or pathologic aspects of care. You view the client through a holistic perspective. You piece together the fragmented pieces of the client's care. This cannot be done in the isolation of an office or simply by telephone. It requires active, on-site presence, interviews, meetings, attendance at treatment planning conferences, and appropriate documentation.

In the role of case manager the nurse may be caught in the middle of conflicting value systems. For example, clients with alcoholism or bulimia have been treated traditionally with intensive, extended inpatient treatment programs. Managed care plans may authorize this treatment only in an outpatient setting. The nurse must respond to clients' need for autonomy in making decisions regarding treatment as well as negotiate within the limitations of the managed care plan. Case managers must use creativity and flexibility in negotiating among the conflicting needs of several parties. Clients and families who are accustomed to specific treatment models for illnesses with relapse potential often feel confused and misunderstood when new treatment approaches are suggested that appear economically motivated.

Assessment Phase Challenges

Nurses who function as case managers must interact with all members of the health care team. Trust, mutual support, and clear communication among team members is necessary before case management services can be implemented. Meetings with administrative personnel and tactful systems entry strategies must be employed while laying the groundwork for a case management program. Careful introduction of the role, which differentiates it from medical care management, is necessary in clarifying role responsibilities. Other members of the team may feel threatened by the addition of a case manager and view it as an indictment of their own role performance. When system administration can orient its members to the case manager's role, there is a higher level of acceptance of the service as augmenting client care rather than interfering with it.

Planning Phase Challenges

In this phase of care, the nurse can bring valuable information concerning benefits, limits, family resources, expectations, and other pertinent data to the treatment planning table. Using the formal and informal support systems, the treatment team is able to set mutually agreed-upon goals with desired outcomes and can begin to plan action steps using intended time frames or critical pathways as a guide.

Implementation Phase Challenges

The next phase of the case management process is to ensure that the client gets needed care. In some systems the case manager may be asked to deliver care. However, this approach is not in the best interest of the client because the case manager's role is to remain the objective, internal consultant, looking at the whole picture. When pulled into delivering the care, the case manager loses perspective and may find important issues clouded. For example, a case management nurse who is asked to function as the client's primary therapist because the primary nurse is overloaded will sacrifice time and resources needed to monitor the quality of care delivered and perhaps lose objectivity.

Keep in mind during the implementation phase that your role involves conflict resolution. To set limits tactfully, arbitrate differences, and maintain successful outcomes for all, you need patience, maturity, and experience. The case manager is also called on to provide additional data or client/family education where a denial or extension of service is in question. As client advocate, you may identify gaps in care that require action in community, facilities, or nursing systems. Nurse case managers are among the best consultants to nursing departments for improving quality because they view problems in the system from the client's perspective.

Evaluation Phase Challenges

The case manager's role in evaluation consists of continuous monitoring of intervention responses and progress toward desired outcomes. This may include medication monitoring for dosage and adherence, as well as monitoring client response to other therapies. You may interview the client directly to gather this information, and then compare it with what is recorded in the medical record. Inconsistent data are always a red flag for intervention by the case manager. Perhaps the process is moving too slowly or the client is not an active participant in the care plan. Once outcomes are achieved and the client is discharged, there must be a mechanism for ongoing quality improvement based on recommended standards of nursing practice. Critical incidents and inconsistencies in the care must be communicated in an ongoing, systematic program of continuous quality improvement. This information is ultimately used to measure provider and facility performance for contract renewal decisions.

The Therapeutic Environment in Hospital-Based Care

The **therapeutic environment** is the purposeful use of people, resources, and events in the client's immediate environment to:

- Ensure safety.
- Promote optimal functioning in the activities of daily living.
- Develop or improve interpersonal skills.
- Enhance the capacity to live independently outside the institutional setting.

Various terms such as *therapeutic milieu, therapeutic community*, and *milieu therapy* have been used to identify treatment environment philosophies. The terms are often used interchangeably and refer to the impact of the authority structure and the roles and relationships that affect decision making and client interactions.

In milieu therapy models, organizational hierarchy is flattened, therapeutic potential is seen in multiple relationships, and the client assumes personal responsibility for behavior. Originally, therapeutic milieu programs were at least several months long and had homogenous client populations.

A UNIQUE ROLE FOR NURSES

A nurse's 24-hour daily contact with clients provides a unique opportunity for creating and managing the therapeutic environment as a special domain. No other discipline literally shares with clients the living space of the treatment unit. Nurses individually influence the environment through their presence. Nurses provide human contact, support, and direction; they share philosophy and values; and they establish collaborative work relationships. Nurses can indirectly influence client behavior by the assessment and manipulation of both the physical and social environments. These responsibilities make it increasingly important that you review and explore your attitudes about organizational rules (see the Nursing Self-Awareness feature).

While many milieu principles remain relevant in current treatment environments, trends such as short lengths of stay,

Nursing SELF-AWARENESS

Your Attitudes About Organizational Rules

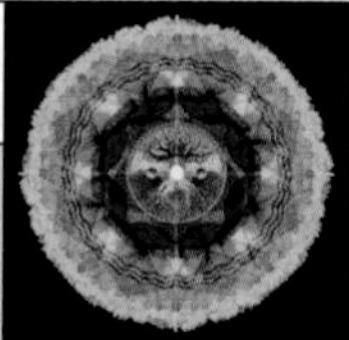

To increase self-awareness about your own attitudes about organizational rules in a treatment setting think about the following questions:

- What kinds of client behaviors make me uncomfortable or angry?
- What unit rules are most important?
- How do I feel when a client breaks a unit rule?
- What do I do in response to a client who breaks a unit rule?

To increase self-awareness about your own attitudes about client autonomy and self-determination, think about the following questions:

- Am I comfortable with clients deciding what the program's schedule, activities, or rules will be?
- Am I comfortable with clients deciding their own treatment goals?
- How do I feel when a client chooses a treatment goal that is not the same as the one I would have selected or that I do not think is in the client's "best interest"?

Should clients be allowed to comment on each other's behavior or treatment goals?

high client acuity, and resurgence of the biomedical model require reexamination of the relevance of the assumptions of the therapeutic community in acute inpatient care. The emergence of subacute treatment settings and community-based rehabilitation programs also offers new arenas to implement therapeutic environment principles. A continuing challenge of psychiatric–mental health nursing is to synthesize a new model that includes the best aspects of both the psychobiologic and the therapeutic milieu models.

EXTERNAL FACTORS AFFECTING THERAPEUTIC ENVIRONMENTS

A variety of external factors have affected the therapeutic environment since the days of its precursor, milieu therapy (see Box 11–5). These issues have an impact on the treatment environment in several ways. It is more difficult to develop group cohesiveness and involvement with other clients' progress when group membership changes frequently. Symptom acuity may also limit a client's ability to be actively involved with the treatment issues of others. Staff roles may be more traditional and typical of medical care settings, and this may create more hierarchical relationships. In actual practice, these factors will be influenced by the program's attitude toward privacy, autonomy, safety, and group well-being.

Privacy

Individuals routinely vary their patterns of contact with and withdrawal from others, as well as the information they share about themselves. The very nature of psychiatric hospitalization conflicts with the need for privacy. Intimate personal details are examined and discussed, and there may be no opportunity to escape staff surveillance or social contact. Nurses must respect a client's privacy by keeping surveillance and monitoring to the minimum necessary for client safety, honoring the confidentiality of personal information, and maintaining routine social practices such as knocking on the door and waiting for an answer before entering a bedroom or bathroom.

Autonomy

The rules and schedules that characterize psychiatric treatment settings usually promote the management of groups of people and may interfere with the personal decision making and autonomy of the individual client. Although the ability of mentally ill clients to carry out age-appropriate roles may be significantly impaired, the therapeutic environment provides opportunities for normal functioning according to each client's abilities.

Safety

Mentally ill clients may pose significant safety hazards to themselves or others because of suicidal or assaultive behaviors, poor judgment, or confusion. Efforts to maintain client safety may deprive clients of privacy and autonomy. For example, clients requiring close surveillance have little or no privacy; nurses may intervene to override decisions made by clients whose judgment is impaired.

BOX 11–5 External Factors That Affect the Therapeutic Environment

- Client groups are not homogenous.
- Clients frequently have dual diagnoses, such as psychiatric and substance abuse problems or psychiatric and medical problems.
- Managed mental health care organizations increasingly limit access to inpatient care to those who are a danger to themselves or others.
- Lengths of inpatient stay have decreased to an average of about seven days.
- Treatment is closely monitored to determine the need for medication, seclusion, restraint, or other intensive supervision.
- Case managers quickly assess discharge planning needs and obstacles and coordinate access to other levels of services.
- There has been a resurgence of the biologic model of care as psychopharmacology (see Chapter 31) and other somatic treatments such as ECT (see Chapter 15) and transcranial magnetic stimulation (see Chapter 32) offer specialized treatment approaches to symptom reduction.
- Clients with multiple medical problems and dementias may also require more traditional medical interventions.
- Staff members now have diverse and specialized training and are expected to work as multidisciplinary teams to address individualized treatment goals.
- Regulatory agencies, client rights groups, and professional practice standards establish criteria for the therapeutic environment.

Group Well-Being

A client's behavior may be disruptive or detrimental to the overall well-being of other clients. Nurses may need to monitor or manage certain clients to maximize the common good. As with the concept of safety, the individual's privacy and autonomy may be violated when group well-being is considered primary. (Some philosophers, however, consider that the group's well-being enhances the individual's autonomy.) Individual autonomy, individual well-being, and group well-being are often conflicting issues. Nurses must be sensitive to situations in which clashes occur.

APPLYING THERAPEUTIC ENVIRONMENT PRINCIPLES

Some of the current ideas about the therapeutic environment, particularly the philosophic values, do not easily lend themselves to quick evaluation or manipulation. Staff must consider the clients' levels of functioning as well as the discrete features of the structural environment. What is suitable for one group of clients may be too strict or too lenient for another. Some general guidelines for incorporating therapeutic environment principles in your work with clients are in the Intervention Box on page 221. Selected guidelines are discussed later in this chapter.

Restrictiveness

The restrictiveness of the treatment environment is characterized according to physical, psychologic, and social dimensions. The physical environment includes the nature of the setting, such as location in the community, security, and options for behavior control (e.g., seclusion). The psychological environment is composed of staff and client backgrounds, behavior, attitudes, and values. The social environment consists of the rules and regulations that govern the operation of the setting as well as the treatment standards for managing client behavior.

The importance of evaluating a program's restrictiveness stems from mental health legislation mandating care according to the least restrictive alternative. This concept is heavily influenced by ethical and legal theories that hold individual autonomy paramount. Thus, program rules or staff attitudes that interfere with a client's autonomy would be considered more restrictive than a program that supported autonomy and self-determination. (See Chapter 10.)

A facility's physical structure is a major focus of attention in pursuing the least restrictive alternatives for treatment. Physical restrictiveness is ranked according to the degree of interference with client independence.

The physical structure of many institutions—such as locked doors, communal living arrangements, and limited access to community resources—interferes with client freedom of movement and individuality. Thus, facilities located in huge hospital complexes, which do not interface with the community's shopping, religious, or entertainment activities or provide for client privacy, have a more restrictive environment than community-based settings.

Orienting Client and Family

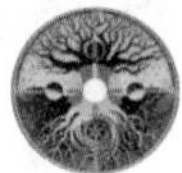

Clients and their family or significant others need to be informed about all aspects of the therapeutic environment. Be sure to accomplish the following:

- Orient and educate client, family, and significant others about hospitalization and treatment by reviewing the clinical problems, treatments, and behavioral outcomes that are the focus of hospitalization or treatment in a community facility.
- Engage clients, family, and significant others in the treatment process by encouraging them to identify personal goals and participate in evaluating the course of treatment.

Encourage them to relate their concerns and questions about what to expect during the treatment experience. The Client/Family Teaching feature on page 222 lists questions they may ask. Be sure to include information on all unasked questions in your health teaching orientation activities.

Safety and the Structural Environment

Although building features are beyond your ability to influence, other aspects of the physical structure are open to your interventions. As the nurse, you should:

1. Evaluate whether security is sufficient.
2. Assess the advantages and necessity of the security.
3. Assess whether the security has any detrimental impact.
4. Consider whether the security advantages could be accomplished through some other intervention that does not have a detrimental impact.
5. Reevaluate structural controls implemented for specific reasons to determine whether they are no longer relevant and should be discontinued.

The following clinical example illustrates a structural control based on an unclear rationale.

CLINICAL EXAMPLE

A 15-bed unit in an inpatient setting had laundry facilities for clients to care for their own clothes. A psychotic and confused client put a potted plant through a wash cycle, causing major damage to the washing machine. Staff members locked the laundry facilities to prevent future damage to the machines. The doors remained locked even after the client was discharged, preventing any independent client access to the facilities. Preventing possible future damage to machines became a predominant staff concern.

While locking laundry room doors was intended to be a short-term structural solution to avoid further environmental damage, the solution itself created a new problem of interference with self-care performance by more independent clients.

INTERVENTION

Guidelines for Working with Clients in the Therapeutic Environment

Strategy	Rationale
Safety and the Structural Environment	
• Appropriate structural security, including locked doors, nonbreakable glass, seclusion room, silent alarms, devices such as concave nonbreakable mirrors to view blind spots.	• Security must be appropriate to client acuity and type of treatment program.
• Unit rules and staff policy related to acceptable conduct.	• Rules should be clearly stated.
• Procedures and training for use of time-outs, seclusion, restraint, special precautions, search and management of client personal belongings such as razors.	• Staff training promotes consistency and safe implementation of security and client management techniques.
Structure	
• Client orientation to behavior expectations through multiple sources, including handbook, bulletin boards, community meeting, identification of a primary nurse.	• Clients are unfamiliar with expectations; new information may need to be repeated.
• Delineation of program schedule and expectations for client participation.	• Clear expectations and written schedule promote client independence.
Support	
• Staff visibility and availability to guide and monitor client activities.	• Demonstrates role-modeling skills and provides an opportunity for informal assessment and interaction.
• Implementation of least restrictive interventions such as confirming messages, calming, personal control, setting limits, and medication to minimize the need for more restrictive behavior management.	• Least restrictive interventions promote client autonomy and demonstrate respect.
• Enhance normality of the environment through use of clocks, calendars, furniture.	• Reduces the institutional qualities of environment.
• Promote opportunities for self-care decision making, and activities that prepare for return to community.	• Reduces dependence on hospital; promotes positive transition to community.
• Integrate client's existing social supports, including family and spiritual support system to reinforce goals and interventions.	• Promotes family involvement and empowerment; extends opportunities for positive outcome by involving social supports.
• Monitor and discuss staff concerns to promote communication, identify parallel issues, ensure a positive social climate.	• Staff interactions affect the general atmosphere and capacity for therapeutic interventions.
• Support cultural diversity and staff self-awareness related to issues of client rights and social control.	• Demonstrates respect and supports client autonomy and independence.
Socialization	
• Orient client and family to the steps and process of inpatient psychiatric treatment.	• Clients and family may be unfamiliar with psychiatric treatment; may have misinformation.
• Identify fears and stereotypes client/family may have about "brain surgery, shock treatment, or padded cells," as well as concerns about how psychotherapy works.	• Reduces fear and encourages engaging in treatment.
• Educate client/family about legal rights of psychiatric clients and confidentiality of information.	• Engages client and family in treatment process.
• Encourage client participation in determining and evaluating treatment goals.	• Promotes involvement and empowerment.
Self-Understanding	
• Encourage formal and informal group participation.	• Provides opportunities to gain social skills.
• Emphasize commonalities of experience.	• Reduces sense of isolation and hopelessness.
• Identify skills gained through hospital experience.	• Offers hope and focuses on the future.
• Instill hope and social connectedness.	• Reduces isolation.
• Encourage client feedback about satisfaction with treatment and hospital experience.	• Promotes empowerment.

CLIENT / FAMILY TEACHING

Orientation to the Therapeutic Environment

Answers to these questions should be individualized to reflect each unit's treatment philosophy and the specific legal rights of the client according to the state.

1. What psychiatric treatment can I expect to receive?
2. Will I receive medications? Do I have to take the medications?
3. Do I have to share a room with someone else?
4. Will I have to tell other clients about my problems?
5. Will you write down information that I tell you about myself or my family?
6. Is this unit a safe place for me?
7. Can I leave the unit on passes?
8. What happens if I no longer want to be a client in this hospital?
9. What happens if I have a disagreement with someone?
10. Who are the staff here? Who can I talk to if I have questions?
11. Can I smoke?
12. When is bedtime?
13. What time are the meals? Can I keep my own snacks?
14. Is there a way for me to wash my own clothes?
15. Is there a telephone I can use?
16. When are the visiting hours?
17. Can I write letters and get mail?
18. Can I keep my money with me? Is my personal property safe?
19. Are religious services available?

Seclusion and restraint are interventions that use structure to control client behavior in order to implement safety measures. Because seclusion and restraint are highly restrictive interventions that interfere with client autonomy and freedom of movement, it is important to implement alternative steps whenever possible. Chapter 34 includes a complete discussion of seclusion and restraint.

The structural environment should not dehumanize its inhabitants; moreover, it should actively contribute to their improved functioning and comfort. Reality-oriented resources such as the following contribute to a sense of normality:

- Clocks and calendars to promote time orientation.
- Newspapers to encourage an awareness of social events.
- Ramps and rails to facilitate mobility and movement.
- Furniture arranged to promote interpersonal interaction.

Healthy people may take these for granted, but they are critical resources to the impaired client.

Program Structure

Program structure, another aspect of the therapeutic environment, is composed of the schedule and expectations for client treatment and participation. Nurses have a number of opportunities to communicate expectations and to address issues that arise. How expectations are communicated and issues assessed and addressed are strongly influenced by the individual nurse's attitudes toward organization rules in a treatment setting (see the Nursing Self-Awareness feature on page 219).

Program Rules. All clients should be given the regulations of the setting either before or as soon after admission as possible. Although written expectations do not automatically ensure acceptable behavior or prevent harmful behavior, they provide a clear baseline, serve as reminders, and provide structure for clients. These rules reinforce the staff's commitment to basic safety and specify obligations for all members of the setting. Written expectations may be presented to clients at the time of admission, discussed in community meetings, and used as a reference if a client violates a rule. Individualized behavioral contracts with clients are discussed in Chapter 30.

While all programs have a set of rules and regulations, not all use community meetings or client government as an integral part of the program. They are more likely to be seen in settings that subscribe to the therapeutic milieu philosophy.

Community Meetings. Groups provide an opportunity for clients to solve problems of conflicting interests, experience cooperation with others, share responsibility, and experience leadership in the group. The most common milieu-oriented group is the community meeting. Its functions include:

- Welcoming new members.
- Identifying and discussing unit rules (expectations).
- Discussing aspects of the unit environment such as cleanliness, privacy, radio and television use, or other interpersonal problems that may interfere with the quality of life for the group.
- Planning activities.

Clients usually chair the community meeting and report on assignments, such as checking for cleanliness of areas of responsibility (e.g., the kitchen or bedrooms).

The community meeting is also used to solve problems related to living with a large group of people or living in the hospital unit.

CLINICAL EXAMPLE

Clients on a 25-bed unlocked unit had access to two pay telephones. Both telephones, however, were near the nurses' station, and conversations could be overheard easily. Clients complained in community meeting of the lack of privacy, and a nurse intervened to help them write a letter to the hospital administration. The administration purchased a new cordless telephone, which allowed clients to make and receive calls in any area of the unit.

Client Government. Some client community groups also grant clients privileges for completing ward jobs or for demonstrating certain behaviors in the community living groups. Clients are expected to take responsibility for themselves and each other and to learn the consequences of their actions. Involving clients in the management of the unit and receiving therapy with other clients provide opportunities for participation, corrective learning experiences, and the development of new behavior patterns. Feedback is an essential technique for increasing insight and promoting learning. This type of community group, known as **client government,** may be most suitable to intermediate and long-term care settings, where the client group is stable and a group culture evolves over time.

CLINICAL EXAMPLE

The community meeting group of a 20-bed adolescent program bases recommendations for weekend passes on members' requests and the individual's functioning in the client community. Lisa, 14 years old, has a history of running away from home, lying, drug and alcohol abuse, prostitution, and suicide threats. She requested a Saturday day pass, although she did not have specific plans for how she would spend the time. Other clients commented that Lisa had not completed her ward job of checking the cleanliness of the kitchen, and the staff noted that she continued to withdraw from social contacts. The group agreed that Lisa should not receive a pass until she could demonstrate some improved ability to structure her time and interact with others.

Supportive Social Climate

The multiple influences on individual and group behavior may come from external sources such as professional practice standards, regulatory agencies, and laws. The client's attitudes, beliefs, and behaviors, as well as styles of interaction between people, also have an impact on the therapeutic environment.

Nursing routines that limit client self-care can be detrimental to the unit atmosphere signaling overinvolvement and loss of client autonomy.

CLINICAL EXAMPLE

Acutely psychotic and chronically mentally ill men and women are admitted to a 20-bed locked unit in a large county hospital. Nurses on this unit seem rushed and complain of having no time to discuss nursing care issues or write nursing care plans. A nurse consultant observed work patterns for several days and noted that the staff were involved (frequently unnecessarily) in intimate details of the clients' daily activities. This involvement extended to lighting matches for cigarettes and squeezing toothpaste onto toothbrushes. Simple routines that interfered with client autonomy also controlled the staff by preventing professional performance and relationships.

The nurse consultant assessed that the staff's complaint of excessive workload while they helped with daily details of client activities actually created self-care deficits for clients. The consultant recommended that the staff promote client self-care skills to be in accordance with their actual ability. This resulted in improvement of client independence and staff performance.

Spirituality

Nurses can use the spiritual beliefs of clients to enhance the therapeutic environment.

Specific assessment of a client's spiritual beliefs and practices provides the nurse an opportunity to understand their clinical impact and to use spiritual resources available to the client to enhance wellness and coping (see the Caring for the Spirit fea-

CARING FOR THE SPIRIT

Incorporating Spirituality into the Therapeutic Environment

Incorporate spirituality into the therapeutic environment by:

- Providing opportunities for ceremonies, such as weekly services or holiday celebrations.
- Facilitating group discussions based on sharing religious or spiritual beliefs.
- Demonstrating tolerance and acceptance of differing beliefs and rituals.
- Encouraging the social support that can be provided by acceptance in a community that shares similar beliefs.
- Being aware of how one's own beliefs may influence client interactions.
- Defining a negative life event in terms of an opportunity for spiritual growth or a divine plan.
- Using spiritual music or ceremonies to promote relaxation and reduce anxiety.
- Collaborating with clergy or a representative of the client's faith who is accepted by the client to (a) correct misinterpretations of spiritual information that the client may be using maladaptively; (b) translate to clinicians spiritual aspects of a client's decision making; or (c) identify options and alternatives consistent with the faith that support adaptive resolution.

ture on page 223). Discussion of beliefs enables the nurse to reassure clients who fear that their beliefs will be challenged or minimized in a psychiatric environment. Finally, acknowledgment of the significant influence of spirituality in American life encourages nurses to recognize and explore their own beliefs in order to minimize the impact of bias in their client interactions.

Remember also that clients come from various cultural backgrounds and their beliefs about spirituality or religion may vary from culture to culture and will be influenced by the degree of cultural assimilation. Strive to provide spiritual resources that are both culturally congruent and culturally competent.

Client and Family Education

It is important to recognize that, in addition to educating the client and family about the client's illness and treatment, you also have a responsibility to teach them how to implement the principles of the therapeutic environment outside the treatment setting. The goal is to help the client and family reach a mutually agreeable plan for a safe, secure, and supportive living arrangement that meets their needs.

Establishing a Healthy Lifestyle and Habits. Requirements for a healthy lifestyle include the following:

- Eat a balanced diet.
- Avoid caffeine, alcohol, cigarettes, and illegal drugs.
- Get adequate rest and sleep.
- Exercise at least three times a week.

Establishing a Daily Schedule. A routine helps clients to keep on track and helps them to organize their thinking as well as their activities. Suggest that clients:

- Have a routine for waking up, eating, accomplishing daily activities, and resting.
- Identify specific tasks that need to be accomplished that day, or skills that need to be performed.
- Complete tasks in small, manageable increments.
- Take medications as prescribed.

Using Positive Communication Skills. Misunderstandings and resentments often result from inadequate, incomplete, or negative communication. They can be eliminated or reduced by following these guidelines as well as those presented in Chapter 8:

- Give instructions or directions at the level of the client's ability. This may include verbal prompting along with physical assistance, verbal prompting alone, and especially, praise for independent performance.
- Avoid criticism, argument, and negative reinforcement (see Chapter 30).
- Be empathic by putting yourself in the client's shoes.
- Help the client to identify feelings by reflecting and making observations.

Identifying and Participating in Support Groups. Support groups help both clients and family to cope (see also Chapter 29). Families need to recognize signs of family stress and have a plan for respite, perhaps by trading off responsibilities with other family members or significant others. Families need to take the following steps:

1. Gather information about resources for the client and the family, including social, health care, and long-term financial resources.
2. Choose mental health care workers on the basis of the degree of comfort in relating to them.
3. Evaluate the client's options for living arrangements and rehabilitation.

Recognizing Relapse or Exacerbation of the Client's Illness. Clients' symptoms can return or worsen. Clients and their families should have:

- A plan for managing symptoms. This might include reducing schedule demands and/or contacting the mental health team or case manager for assistance.
- A plan for emergency behavior management for possible instances of violence or suicide (see Chapters 22 and 34).

Treatment Settings and Programs for Severe and Persistent Mental Illness

The term **severe and persistent mental illness** (SPMI) or serious mental illness (SMI), came into use because it avoids some of the more undesirable features of its predecessor term used to describe clients, the *chronically mentally ill*. Severely and persistently mentally ill individuals have psychiatric disorders that disrupt major role functioning over time, involving some level of disability.

CLINICAL DIVERSITY

There is no common course for SPMI. This is a clinically diverse population, with different diagnoses and varied patterns of illness. Schizophrenic disorders provide the prototype for SPMI; they are typically disabling, on an intermittent or ongoing basis (see Chapter 14). However, even schizophrenic disorders vary considerably in terms of symptom profile, pattern of relapse or acute exacerbations, and quality of long-term functioning. Bipolar disorders, recurrent depressions, and severe personality disorders can be just as disabling as some forms of schizophrenia.

The core feature of a severe and persistent disorder is not diagnosis or prognosis, but the experience of *psychiatric disability*. Whether mild or severe, whether ongoing, recurring, or remitting, these disorders require services that go beyond the limits of an acute disease model.

DEFINING PSYCHIATRIC DISABILITY

In 1980, the World Health Organization (WHO) developed and published a classification system for the phases of a long-term illness. As ■ Figure 11–5 shows, the etiology of the disorder, known or unknown, gives rise to changes in structure or functioning, manifested as signs and symptoms, and collectively

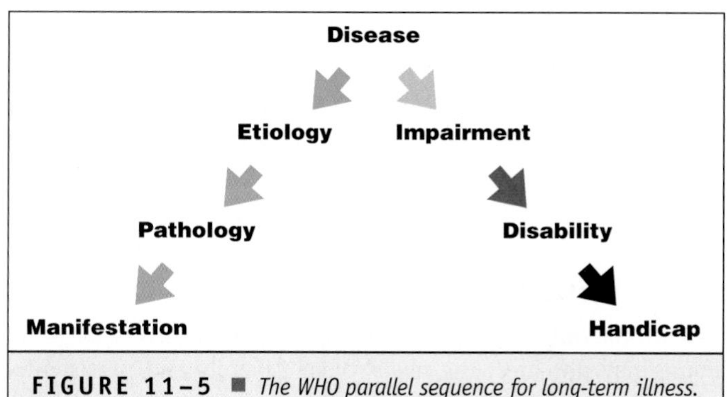

FIGURE 11–5 ■ *The WHO parallel sequence for long-term illness.*

known as *impairment.* If the impairment alters functional performance or behavior, it produces *disability*. When the impairment or disability places the person at a disadvantage within the community, a *handicap* occurs.

The profile that emerges of people with SPMI is that of a highly vulnerable subgroup in our mental health care system, and one of the groups least likely to access social resources to protect that vulnerability. This subgroup of our population accounts for the majority of persons being treated in hospital-based systems and in many community programs. They are at risk for developing secondary or concurrent psychiatric problems and for problems associated with socioeconomic status. They account for 25% of homeless persons in our communities (Dickey, 2000). These multiple, interacting problems require complex approaches to services.

COMMUNITY SUPPORT PROGRAMS FOR SPMI

Community support programs offer a range of treatment and rehabilitation services, with a case management component to assess needs, coordinate care, and monitor outcomes.

Case Management

Case management is the linchpin for community support programs. The case manager remains a consistent figure in the treatment plan. This avoids duplication and overlap of services. It also avoids shunting vulnerable clients between services because of fluctuations in their clinical status.

Case managers often find that they are fulfilling many roles for their clients that have not been satisfied by other clinical resources, including a sense of social support. High-risk groups such as the dually diagnosed, the homeless mentally ill, and frequently hospitalized patients may receive more intensive and clinically sophisticated forms of case management to address their unique service requirements. The case management philosophy has generated enthusiasm in systems for the psychiatrically disabled, because it acknowledges the pervasive nature of their problems, their need for multiple services, and the oscillating or unpredictable course of illness.

Support for Basic Needs

Community mental health programs generally emphasize the importance of self-support and gainful employment whenever possible. However, surveys of the severely mentally ill indicate generally low rates of competitive employment. This situation reflects general economic conditions as well as work disability. In times of high unemployment, people with psychiatric disabilities may be pushed out of jobs that can be performed by competing groups in the labor force. Certainly many mentally ill individuals without "gainful" employment are meaningfully occupied in supported employment and/or volunteer work. However, low rates of competitive employment among members of this population underscore their dependence on income assistance programs such as Supplemental Security Income (SSI).

A community support system helps assure the severely mentally ill both access to and linkage with appropriate services to secure income and obtain other entitlements (such as health benefits) and basic resources such as food, clothing, and transportation. This may be a more complex task than it appears to be because accessing financial resources may mean helping the client through difficult applications procedures and even appeals. It may also involve providing money management services to help the severely mentally ill individuals who cannot budget their monthly income independently.

Residential Services

Recent reports continue to document the lack of affordable and decent housing options for many of the severely mentally ill and their consequent concentration in what may be marginal or unsafe areas. Many of the severely and persistently mentally ill live with families, but those who live alone frequently depend on residential hotels and boarding homes. It is difficult to generalize about the quality of these housing options because they vary a great deal. For example, some boarding arrangements encourage autonomy and provide a warm, stable environment for residents. Other arrangements, however, fall far below standards that should be applied to living environments for the chronically disabled.

The question of housing satisfaction can also be highly subjective. Some people prefer the privacy of a hotel, despite what may be other negative features, such as location or small living space. Other people prefer a more cozy, homelike environment such as the one in ■ Figure 11–6 on page 226. Programs with an active treatment component may be attractive to some people, but others appreciate a fairly calm and nondemanding environment despite its monotony. For this reason, a community support system focuses not only on accessing some form of acceptable housing but on evaluating the quality of that housing for the individual, working with the client to find "a good fit".

Medication Management

Medication regimens are the mainstay of treatment programs for the severely and persistently mentally ill. Research on the efficacy of medication, particularly neuroleptic regimens for schizophrenia, demonstrates that these agents reduce rates of relapse and hospital readmission. However, they have not been problem-free. Drug regimens demand adherence, tolerance of temporary side effects, and

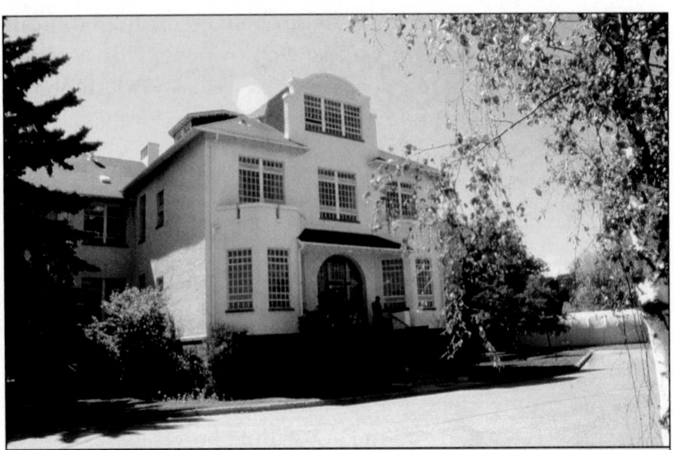

FIGURE 11–6 ■ *A halfway house for transitional care after discharge from a hospital-based unit.*

acceptance of the risk of long-term problems such as tardive dyskinesia. Secondary effects of medications can be uncomfortable and embarrassingly visible (e.g., tongue thrusting).

Medication services for the severely and persistently mentally ill should address the impact of medications on quality of life and should promote collaboration with clients to develop a regimen that is tolerable and beneficial. *Depot medication therapy*, usually consisting of an injection every 2 to 4 weeks, does not require the client to take medications several times a day and is a valuable strategy for some people. Current advances in psychopharmacology have produced new classes of medications that may prove less uncomfortable and socially limiting than standard treatments, and that may help people who have been resistant to medication, or nonadherent, in the past. The introduction of newer therapies makes the medication component of community care all the more important, particularly for advanced practice nurses with prescriptive authority for the severely mentally ill.

CLINICAL EXAMPLE

Ms. Linnea is a 57-year-old widow who came into the medication clinic for her monthly injection, accompanied by her case manager. Ms. Linnea has carried a diagnosis of schizophrenia, paranoid type, for many years but she was maintained well with outpatient care and medications, requiring only brief crisis intervention and two short hospital stays by the time she was 50.

After her husband died, Ms. Linnea had a severe decompensation, experiencing frightening hallucinations and delusions, and was threatening her neighbors. Police were called and she was hospitalized. Ms. Linnea was stabilized on depot medications and was referred to a community-support program for assistance with both housing and rehabilitation. A case manager helped Ms. Linnea apply for SSI, arranged for a shared apartment, facilitated medication and clinic appointments, visited her weekly, and encouraged regular participation in a social rehabilitation program. Ms. Linnea has not required hospitalization in six years. Although she still "hears voices," she is able to monitor her symptoms and advises her son or her case manager when her symptoms increase.

Outpatient Treatment

Traditional outpatient psychotherapies that address *problems in living* may not meet the needs of all severely and persistently mentally ill persons because disabled people often require a broader range of support services to function well in the community. Many of the severely mentally ill also require rehabilitation interventions that address their specific functional deficits and treatment goals, rather than insight-oriented therapies. Nevertheless, these clients need individual, family, and group treatments that are sensitive to their particular problems and needs.

Crisis Stabilization; Emergency and Acute Inpatient Care

The severely and persistently mentally ill are at risk for acute exacerbations of an illness. This may be particularly true during times of stress or transition. But in some cases, acute exacerbations are entirely unpredictable and are probably less indicative of the effects of environmental stressors than of the fluctuations of a disease process. In any case, this population requires access to acute assessment and treatment services as part of a package of community support including twenty-four-hour emergency and crisis units and outreach programs. Nursing expertise is extremely important in these emergency settings because of the need for skilled and comprehensive assessment of acute problems.

General Health Care

The severely mentally ill are a medically underserved group in the community, with needs in the areas of primary health care, dental care, and vision care. Health needs are most pronounced in such subgroups as substance-abusing clients and the elderly mentally ill, who have concurrent physical disorders. However, many of the severely mentally ill are to some extent at risk from lifestyle factors (problematic housing or nutrition) or from the consequences of psychiatric treatment (problematic medication side effects or drug interactions). Any person with a serious psychiatric diagnosis risks underdiagnosis of medical illness by both primary care and psychiatric providers. Wellness centers are a relatively new phenomenon.

In psychiatric services, many clinicians focus on mental disorders with inadequate attention to the total person. Only a small proportion of medical problems are diagnosed in physical assessments. Those most likely to be underdiagnosed were substance abusers, elderly clients, and women. Community support and case management interventions can help the severely mentally ill obtain services despite these problems of "falling between the cracks" in systems that are poorly organized to meet the needs of clients with multiple diagnoses.

Vocational Programs

When the severely mentally ill are surveyed about their preferences, they usually indicate a strong desire to work. Work not only provides income, it also helps create a sense of self-worth and social belonging. However, psychiatric disability limits access to employment by its impact on healthy functioning and because of the stigma attached to mental disorders. Vocational services address this problem by providing training and protected alternatives to the competitive workplace.

Vocational training may occur in specialized programs, or it may be integrated into other mental health modalities such as day treatment. It provides assessment of work capacities and preferences, technical preparation, and social skills training to prepare people for the workplace. However, not all people with psychiatric disabilities enter the competitive workplace. Many, by desire or by necessity, work within protected environments. Sheltered workshop programs have a long history of offering work in a low-stress, low-demand environment. Transitional vocational programs also provide a low-stress environment but emphasize the development of skills for movement to the competitive workplace.

Much recent attention has focused on supported employment, an approach that provides training and support in the place of employment. For example, a job coach might accompany a group of psychiatrically disabled workers to a place of employment where the coach learns the same job as the team, provides on-the-job training, and provides daily backup and support. This approach is based on the principle that the mentally ill learn skills best in the environment where they will be practiced. Supported employment models may become increasingly prominent because the Americans with Disabilities Act (ADA) guarantees people with psychiatric disabilities the right to reasonable accommodation in the workplace. To learn how the ADA applies to people with psychiatric disabilities, use the Companion Website for this book to access the policy guidelines of the Equal Employment Opportunity Commission at www.eeoc.gov.

Day Programs

A complete system of community-based services for the severely mentally ill offers some forms of day programs. Day treatment and partial hospitalization programs provide continuity of care between the hospital and the outpatient sector in a less restrictive setting. These programs can also provide an alternative to hospital care for individuals who need complex treatment monitoring.

Day treatment programs offer groups and activities that provide for recreation and socialization and that help people function in the community. They may be used on a short-term basis for specific goals or on a long-term basis for relapse prevention. Day programs are increasingly incorporating a rehabilitation philosophy that maximizes opportunities for meaningful activities in environments that are as "normal" as possible, focusing on strengths rather than on pathology.

Family and Network Support

Family support interventions are directed at reducing stress in the client's interpersonal environment and minimizing the burden of care for family members. If clients have little contact with families, interventions may target the people in their networks that provide them with support: friends, landlords, service providers.

With this emphasis on support to the supporters, interventions include:

- Psychoeducational activities that increase knowledge about the disorder and reduce family stress.
- Practical assistance with information about homemaking or legal services.
- Respite services (short-term placements to relieve the family of the burden of care).

Such services have been widely recommended as a way to reduce the family's burden and enhance the quality of life of both the client and relatives for the long term.

Nurses working with families of the severely and persistently mentally ill need to become attuned to their concerns. Families may express ambivalence about care giving. For example, they may want to promote the client's autonomy yet feel discomfort or guilt about the type of living situation the client is able to maintain independently. Clear information and nonjudgmental attitudes from nurses and other providers can do much to alleviate a family's distress and assure them that there may not be a single ideal solution to their problems.

MediaLink Americans with Disabilities Act

Advocacy

Many of the difficulties the severely mentally ill experience in the community reflect a poor understanding of psychiatric illness among the general population and inadequate resources for their needs. For example, access to housing is a function of resources and community acceptance. Attention to housing is futile if no residential resources exist; vocational programs require access to employers. For this reason, one component of community support for the severely mentally ill is advocacy, or activities increasing access to resources. Advocacy can occur on an individual basis; for example, a case manager might intervene with a landlord to help a client obtain housing. Advocacy activities also occur at the level of the community, such as in programs for community education or outreach to employers.

Families of the severely and persistently mentally ill have also assumed a much greater advocacy role than in the past. Family advocacy arose in response to problems accompanying the deinstitutionalization process that placed an enormous burden of care on families. It also developed in reaction to the stigmatization of parents by people who attributed serious mental disorders to child-rearing practices. The major family organization for people with severe and persistent mental disorders is the **National Alliance for the Mentally Ill (NAMI)**. The national and local chapters of NAMI have grown tremendously over the past 20 years and have become a recognized force in mental health policy development. Chapter 29 discusses NAMI in greater detail.

REHABILITATION APPROACHES

Although the components of community support models provide the structure for services to the severely and persistently mentally ill, their effectiveness depends on the content of these component services. **Psychiatric rehabilitation,** an emphasis on the prevention or reduction of impairment or handicap as opposed to the treatment of disease serves as a guide for the content of practice at many levels of care, and it includes an overall treatment philosophy as well as specific interventions and programs.

Rehabilitation Philosophy

Psychiatric rehabilitation has its roots in theory about physical disabilities (Anthony, Cohen, Farkas, & Gagne, 2002). Considering WHO's phases of a long-term illness, psychiatric rehabilitation separates the treatment of disease from the prevention or reduction of impairment and handicap. Treatment addresses the disease process and its consequent symptoms. Rehabilitation approaches emphasize specific interventions to address targeted areas of functioning. Rehabilitation approaches are also strongly grounded in beliefs about empowerment of the mentally ill, emphasizing client feelings of control and worth.

Rehabilitation-oriented services begin with functional assessment and identification of highly individualized goals. A plan is developed to meet objectives by behavioral interventions that target specific functional deficits, or by environmental interventions that enable functioning with an existing deficit. From a rehabilitation perspective, it is important to extend support as long as possible. Support is not necessarily withdrawn because a client improves. For example, clients doing well in supported employment programs would not be expected to necessarily "graduate" to independent employment and thereby forfeit the support.

Rehabilitation philosophy is entirely consistent with self-care and symptom management interventions for the mentally ill developed by psychiatric–mental health nurses. In fact rehabilitation theory and conceptual models in nursing share a common focus on functional adaptation in supportive environments.

The Clubhouse Model

Although a rehabilitation philosophy can inform and enhance many treatment modalities, some specific rehabilitation programs make a unique contribution to service systems. One of the most important types of psychiatric rehabilitation programs are psychosocial rehabilitation centers, modeled after clubhouse programs. Under a community support system structure, these would fall at the level of day programming, but may be very different than the program contents of "maintenance" day treatment centers, which do not apply a rehabilitation perspective.

As Anthony, Cohen, Farkas, & Gagne (2002) explain, psychosocial rehabilitation centers grew out of clubs formed by former psychiatric hospital patients in order to provide mutual support and assistance. These evolved into service centers providing multiple services such as group activities, assistance with employment, and housing. Psychosocial centers emphasize a collaborative relationship between staff and members, and provide experiences in a supportive but realistic milieu, for the development of abilities for functioning in the real world.

Vocational Rehabilitation

While all mental health programs have some emphasis on vocational rehabilitation, not all vocational programs conform to a psychiatric rehabilitation model. Supported employment models reflect a rehabilitation perspective because of their emphasis on adding support to the normal environment. This model delineates basic competencies that are necessary for employment and offers classes that prepare the client to set goals and choose a job focus. Once clients are placed, they are supported by job coaches, who act as role models, provide feedback, and act as liaisons to employers.

Social Skills Training

Social skills training methods are based on principles of social learning and use behavioral techniques such as role playing, practicing, and reinforcement to promote the learning of instrumental role behavior as well as problem-solving abilities and interpersonal skills. Social skills training techniques may be incorporated into individual, group, and family treatment modalities, where they may add measurable benefits.

High-Risk SPMI Clients

Subgroups of the severely and persistently mentally ill are at particularly high risk for poor outcomes and are also extraordinarily difficult to serve in conventional programs. These include those with:

- Substance-related problems
- Homelessness
- Frequent readmissions to acute care
- Frequent criminal justice system involvement

The interrelationships among these problems are complex, making it difficult to separate them, or to distinguish root problems from their consequences. For example, substance use may exacerbate symptoms and lead to rehospitalization. This in turn may disrupt stability of residence, increasing the possibility of arrest and reducing the likelihood of medication adherence. In other words, if individuals belong to one subgroup at risk, it is likely that they belong to several, thus increasing their overall vulnerability.

CONCURRENT SUBSTANCE-RELATED DISORDERS

Psychiatric illness greatly increases the odds of having a substance-related disorder. Alcohol has typically been the drug of choice with the severely mentally ill, perhaps because of its relative cheapness and accessibility. Psychostimulant use has also increased among this population, a phenomenon partially attributed to the emergence of crack cocaine as a major drug of abuse. Concurrent substance-related disorders are probably the most consistent predictor of readmission to psychiatric hospitals.

Substance use contributes to a host of undesirable outcomes. It is highly correlated with homelessness and criminal justice system involvement (Zweben, 2000).] It is also a cause of concurrent medical morbidity, including exposure to HIV. Several hospital surveys indicate a high rate of seropositivity among severely mentally ill adults. Triple diagnosis clients—those with HIV disorders, substance-related disorders, and psychiatric disorders—require a complex and demanding range of services.

For a variety of reasons involving different funding streams and different treatment philosophies, substance abuse services and psychiatric care are often poorly integrated (see Chapter 21). In mental health care systems, the dually diagnosed client encounters little specific expertise related to drug or alcohol use. The severely mentally ill sometimes do poorly in substance abuse programs stressing confrontation or demanding sobriety as a precondition to treatment. Integrated programs for the dually diagnosed mentally ill include inpatient programs and some of the assertive treatment models discussed below. Adjusting the psychotropic medications for these clients may help them deal with problems such as dysphoria and anxiety that lead to self-medication with drugs and alcohol.

HOMELESS AND MENTALLY ILL

The mentally ill constitute a prominent subgroup (25%) among the urban homeless (Dickey, 2000). The goal of providing acceptable and long-term housing for the mentally ill remains elusive, particularly in urban centers. The proportion of the mentally ill in the community who are permanently homeless is relatively small. However, a large and heterogeneous group experiences spells of residential instability.

CLINICAL EXAMPLE

Rob is a 29-year-old man who was referred to an intensive case management team after his third hospital admission within one year. Rob has a diagnosis of schizoaffective disorder, but it is unclear whether his diagnosis accounts for his frequent acute episodes or whether the episodes are precipitated by his use of stimulants and alcohol. Rob has no stable place of residence and has used shelters over the past few years. He describes himself as too preoccupied with his survival needs to seek treatment between emergency episodes. He claims that alcohol helps him to manage his anxiety and his "voices" when he is on the streets. The case management team will first address Rob's need for safe housing. The team will then work with Rob to help him acknowledge that alcohol and drugs can increase his discomfort, and to support his use of psychotropic medication. When Rob is stabilized, he will work with the team and consider other treatment goals.

Whether these periods of homelessness involve movement between transient accommodations or actual street dwelling, they impose very harsh living conditions on people who are highly vulnerable. Homelessness interferes with the ability to use services, including the use of psychotropic medications. It increases the risk of trauma, substance abuse, infectious disease exposure, and victimization. Homelessness also makes conventional services unworkable, since the undomiciled can rarely store medication and use regular outpatient services.

Services to the homeless include supported housing models with case management components, shelter-based rehabilitation and substance abuse services, and mobile outreach teams to identify cases and to link them with services. Case management services are particularly important. Clients who formed a positive alliance with their case manager had significantly fewer days of homelessness (Chinman, Rosenheck, & Lam, 2000). While shelters and emergency programs serve a critical short-term need, they also contribute to instability. It is preferable, by far, to develop permanent housing for people with psychiatric disabilities. The National Center on Homelessness and Mental Illness specifically focuses on the delivery of services to people who are homeless and have serious mental illnesses. Their Website, www.nrchmi.com, can be accessed through the Companion Website for this book.

MediaLink Homelessness and Mental Illness

FREQUENT READMISSIONS AND RELAPSE

Recidivism, or frequent readmission, in acute psychiatric settings is a problem for several reasons:

1. It represents a considerable expense.
2. It is a signal of relapse, indicating severe difficulties for the individual.
3. It suggests a failure of the community system to link the client between acute episodes and to institute the type of treatment and monitoring that might manage symptomatic shifts without hospitalization.

Virtually all severe and persistent disorders will involve some kind of relapse at some time; more than one or two admissions in 12 months exceeds norms.

Client-based factors that contribute to recidivism include substance abuse, which may be the best predictor of readmission (see Chapter 13). Cycling through emergency and acute care has been attributed to a "chronic crisis" style among some diagnostic groups, particularly those with severe *DSM* Axis II disorders. However, many younger clients with schizophrenia and bipolar disorder use alcohol and drugs to combat boredom and medication side effects, and to self-medicate or treat symptoms in what they consider to be a "normal" way.

On a systems level, readmission may reflect a failure to link the client with services that he or she considers meaningful and accessible. The system as a whole may respond best to clients who "fit" into programs and benefit from treatment alone. Those with more social needs or less acceptance of their illness may not consider current ambulatory services relevant to their needs and may require more assertive outreach to link with outpatient providers.

FREQUENT CRIMINAL JUSTICE SYSTEM INVOLVEMENT

Prevalence rates of major psychiatric disorders in the jails have increased gradually but continuously, at least in part because of deinstitutionalization policies. Society has a low tolerance for disordered behavior, and the lack of services for the severely and persistently mentally ill in the mental health care system may lead to a funneling into the criminal justice system. According to the Bazelon Center for Mental Health Law (2001), mentally ill persons have a 64% greater chance of being arrested than those who are not mentally ill but have committed the same crime. Four fact sheets offering specific information for advocates on combating the criminalization of people with mental illness can be found at www.bazelon.org/decrim.html and accessed through the Companion Website for this book.

Unemployment, homelessness, and substance abuse contribute to the profile of the severely mentally ill forensic client. Many forensic inpatient services are filled to capacity. Most mentally ill offenders end up in county jails rather than forensic mental hospitals; they rarely become connected with local mental health networks and are frequently counted among the homeless because they have no fixed address.

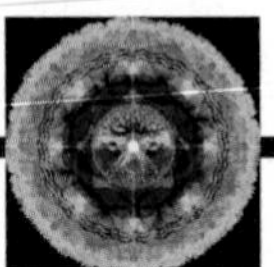

EXPLORE MediaLink

NCLEX review, case studies, and other interactive resources for this chapter can be found on the Companion Website at http://www.prenhall.com/kneisl. Click on Chapter 11 to select the activities for this chapter.

For animations, video tutorials, more NCLEX review questions, and an audio glossary, access the accompanying CD-ROM in this textbook.

BIBLIOGRAPHY

Anderson, C. E. (2000). An insider's perspective of managed mental health care. *Care Management Journal, 2*(2), 93–100.

Anthony, W. A., Cohen, M., Farkas, M., & Gagne, C. (2002). *Psychiatric rehabilitation* (2nd ed.) Boston: Boston University Center for Psychiatric Rehabilitation.

Bazelon Center for Mental Health Law. (2001). Ending the criminalization of people with mental illness. Retrieved July 12, 2000, from www.bazelon.org/decrim.html.

Brimblecombe, N. (2001). *Acute mental health care in the community: Intensive home therapy*. London: Whurr Publishers.

Bustillo, J., Lauriello, J., Horan, W., & Keith, S. (2001). The psychosocial treatment of schizophrenia: An update. *American Journal of Psychiatry, 158*(2), 163–175.

Chinman, M. J., Rosenheck, R., & Lam, J. A. (2000). The case management relationship and outcomes of homeless persons with serious mental illness. *Psychiatric Services, 51*(9), 1142–1147.

Herinckx, H. A., Kinney, R. F., Paulson, R. I., Cutler, D. L., Lewis, K., Clarke, G. N., et al. (2000). Psychiatric hospitalizations, arrests, emergency room visits, and homelessness of clients with severe and persistent mental illness: Findings from a randomized trial of two ACT programs vs. usual care. *Mental Health Services Research, 2*(3), 165–174.

Croze, C. (2000). Managed behavioral healthcare in the public sector. *Administrative Policy in Mental Health, 28*(1), 37–50.

DeLeon, G., Sacks, S., Staines, G., & McKendrick, K. (2000). Modified therapeutic communities for homeless mentally ill chemical abusers: Treatment outcomes. *American Journal of Drug and Alcohol Abuse, 26*(3), 461–480.

Dickey, B. (2000). Review of programs for persons who are homeless and mentally ill. *Harvard Review of Psychiatry, 8*(5), 242–250.

Donegan, K. R., & Palmer-Erbs, V. K. (1998). Promoting the importance of work for persons with psychiatric disabilities—the role of the psychiatric nurse. *Journal of Psychosocial Nursing and Mental Health Services, 36*(4), 13–23.

Fagin, C. M. (2001). Revisiting treatment in the home. *Archives of Psychiatric Nursing, 15*(1), 3–9.

Farrell, S. P., & Deeds, E. S. (1997). The clubhouse model as exemplar. Merging psychiatric nursing and psychosocial rehabilitation. *Journal of Psychosocial Nursing and Mental Health Services, 35*(1), 27–34.

Guo, S., Biegel, D. E., Johnsen, A., & Dyches, H. (2001). Assessing the impact of community-based mobile crisis services on previous hospitalizations. *Psychiatric Services, 52*(2), 223–228.

Jeffrey, M., & Riley, J. (2000). Managed behavioral healthcare in the private sector. *Administrative Policy in Mental Health, 28*(1), 37–50.

Kirsch, D. (2000). Developing outpatient mental health services for managed care. *Psychiatric Clinics of North America, 23*(2), 403–413.

Knowles, C. (2000). Burger King, Dunkin Donuts and community mental health care. *Health Place, 6*(3), 213–224.

Krauss, J. B. (1993). *Health care reform: Essential mental health services*. Washington, DC: American Nurses Publishing.

Lamb, H. R., & Bachrach, L. (2001). Some perspectives on deinstitutionalization. *Psychiatric Services, 52*(8), 1039–1045.

McCann, T. V. (2002). Uncovering hope with clients who have psychotic illness. *Journal of Holistic Nursing, 20*(1), 81–99.

Morrell-Bellai, T., Goering, P. A., & Boydell, K. M. (2000). Becoming and remaining homeless: A qualitative investigation. *Issues in Mental Health Nursing, 21*(6), 581–604.

Odell, S. M., & Commander, M. J. (2000). Risk factors for homelessness among people with psychotic disorders. *Social Psychiatry and Psychiatric Epidemiology, 35*(9), 396–401.

Shern, D. L., Shern, D. L., Tsemberis, S., Anthony, W., Lovell, A. M., Richmond, L., & Felton, C. J., et. al. (2000). Serving street-dwelling individuals with psychiatric disabilities: Outcomes of a psychiatric rehabilitation clinical trial. *American Journal of Public Health, 90*(12), 1873–1878.

Schreter, R. K. (2000). Alternative treatment programs. The psychiatric continuum of care. *Psychiatric Clinics of North America, 23*(2), 335–346.

Smith, N. (2000). Behavioral health home care 2000: Integration and collaboration. *Home Healthcare Nurse, 18*(1), 24–25.

Smoyak, S. (2000). The history, economics, and financing of mental health care. Part 3: The present. *Journal of Psychosocial Nursing and Mental Health Services, 38*(11), 32–38.

Torrey, E. F., & Zdanowicz, M. (2001). Outpatient commitment: What, why, and for whom. *Psychiatric Services, 52*(3), 337–341.

Zweben, J. E. (2000). Severely and persistently mentally ill substance abusers: Clinical and policy issues. *Journal of Psychoactive Drugs, 32*(4), 383–389.

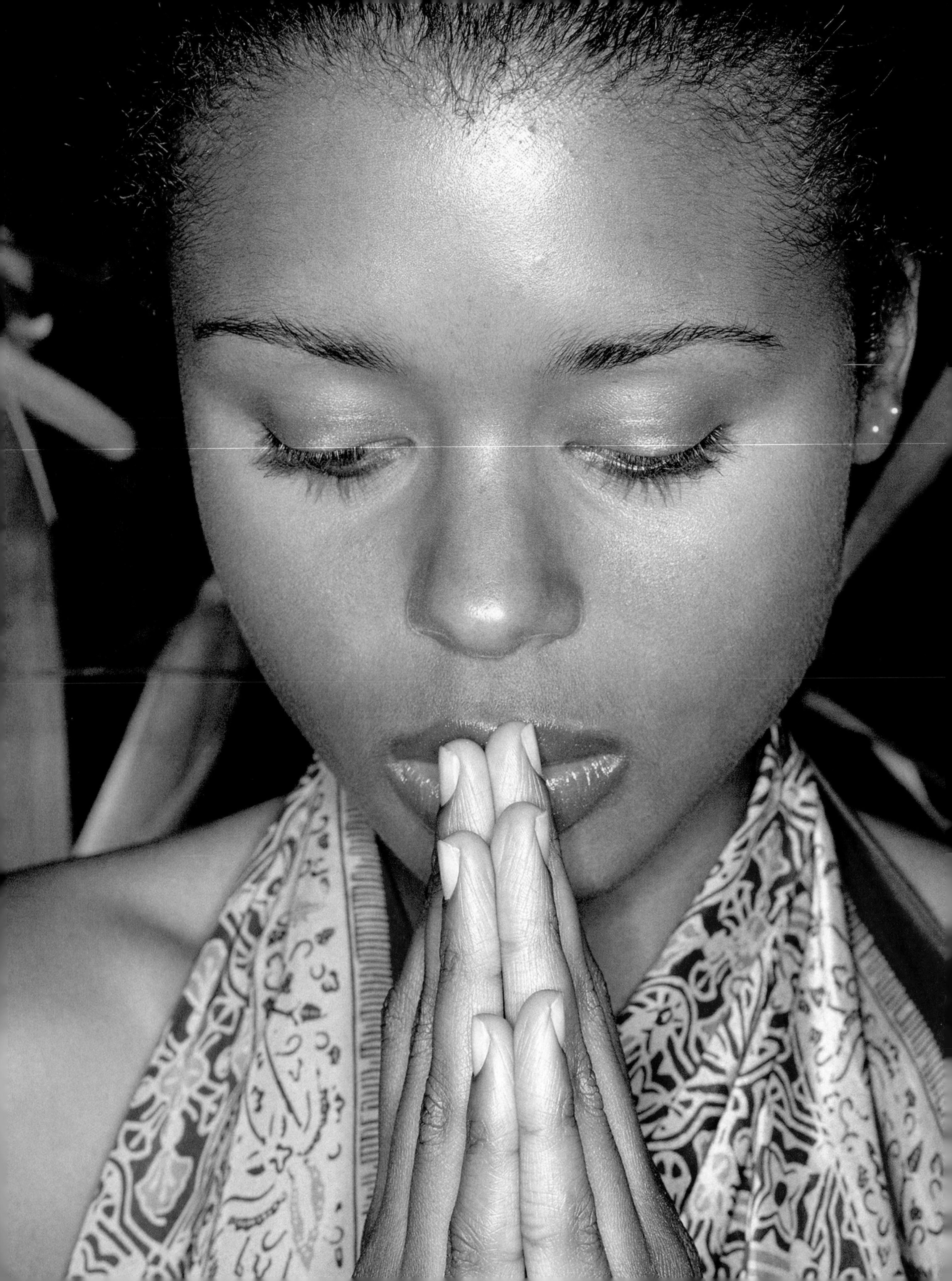

UNIT *Three*

Clients with Mental Disorders

Fatima, the young woman portrayed in this image, lives under difficult and stressful personal circumstances. In her story we learn that she suffers from sleep difficulties, trembling, and tearfulness, as well as headaches and stomach upsets. Her faith offers her solace and reminds us that a commitment to care for the spirit of our clients represents a way of looking at life and connecting with people by being mindful and compassionately present in our transactions with them. This commitment weaves us all together in a shared tapestry. Constructive encounters with others who are different from ourselves are keys to developing the capacity for trustworthy belonging and confident agency in a diverse and complex world. When we encounter differences, we learn to practice what has been called evolved, compassionate empathy. Recognizing resemblance in difference can be a spiritual fact that adds to our sense of responsibility, our willingness to make commitments, and a pattern of engagement with others that supports the transcendent, spiritual domain including, but also going beyond, the logical, rational, and cognitive domains. In Unit Three, you will learn how to understand and be compassionately present with clients who suffer from the recognized major mental disorders.

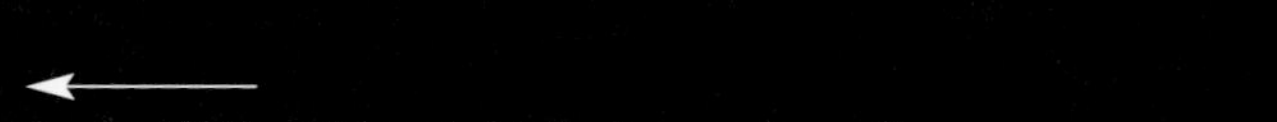

Source: Willie Maldonado/Getty Images, Inc.—Stone

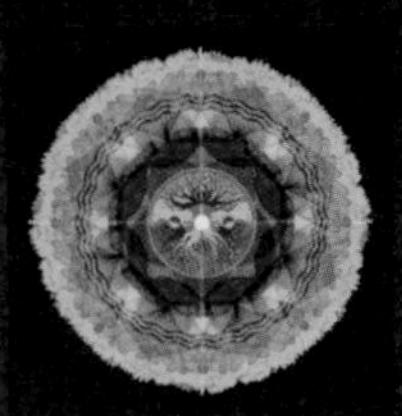

12

Chapter TWELVE

Cognitive Disorders

EILEEN TRIGOBOFF
HOLLY SKODOL WILSON

KEY TERMS

amnestic disorder
aphasia, expressive
aphasia, receptive
Creutzfeldt–Jakob disease
delirium
dementia
dementia of the Alzheimer's type (DAT) or Alzheimer's dementia (AD)
Huntington's disease
new variant Creutzfeldt–Jakob disease (nvCJD)
parkinsonism
Parkinson's disease
Pick's disease
pseudodementia
sundowning
vascular dementia

FOCUS QUESTIONS

- What are the biopsychosocial theories that explain delirium, dementia, amnestic disorders, and other cognitive disorders?
- How would one go about differentiating among the various types of cognitive disorders?
- What are the specific DSM-IV-TR diagnostic criteria for cognitive disorders?
- What would be examples of relevant subjective and objective data for clients with cognitive disorders?
- What causes you the most difficulty when caring for clients with cognitive disorders?

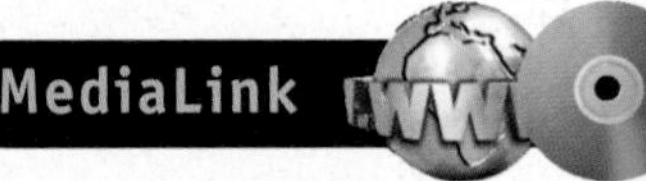

Additional resources for this chapter can be found on the Student CD-ROM accompanying this textbook, and on the Companion Website at www.prenhall.com/kneisl. Click on Chapter 12 to select the activities for this chapter.

CD-ROM
- Audio Glossary
- NCLEX Review
- EPSE: Parkinsonism Video
- PET/SPECT Dementia Animation
- Extrapyramidal Side Effects:
  Hands & Arms Tremor Video
  Grasping Tremor Video
  Lateral Tremor Video
  Akinesia & Pill Rolling Video

Companion Website
- Additional NCLEX Review
- Care Plan: Delirium
- Case Study: Treating Clients with Alzheimer's Disease

CHAPTER OUTLINE

CROSS REFERENCES

Other topics relevant to this content are: Acetylcholinesterase inhibitors, Chapter 31; AIDS-related dementia, Chapter 24; Elders, Chapter 27; Families, Chapter 29; Guidelines in the use of restraining techniques, Chapter 34; Therapeutic environments, Chapter 11; Wernicke–Korsakoff syndrome, Chapter 13.

CRITICAL THINKING CHALLENGE

You are the community mental health nurse for Mrs. Downston, an elderly widow with dementia of the Alzheimer's type (DAT). This client has lived with her daughter Dolores, her son-in-law Don, and their two teenage daughters in their suburban home for the past three years. Throughout this set of circumstances you have been involved with this case. It is notable how the stress of Mrs. Downston's deterioration is affecting the entire family. Dolores and Don have been rearranging and strictly limiting their social activities to make sure Mrs. Downston is supervised. The load of physical care is increasing, and they both have physical problems that will soon make this care impossible. The teenagers have not been able to have friends to the house, as Mrs. Downston is frightened by newcomers and screams in horror.

Psychiatric practitioners frequently advocate institutionalizing clients with DAT. Family caregivers, however, often have difficulty with this decision and may even take offense at this suggestion in spite of the fact that they are mentally and physically exhausted. How would you handle this issue with Mrs. Downston's family? What suggestions or alternatives would you propose? At what point, if ever, should a professional exert pressure on family caregivers to institutionalize their loved one? ■

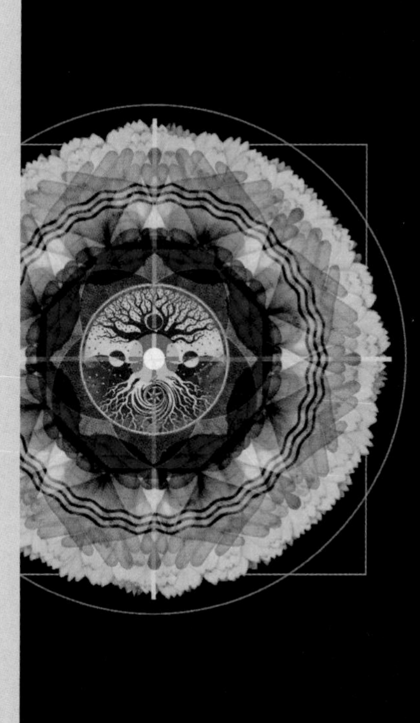

The specialty area of psychiatry has been actively embracing psychobiologic causes and psychobiologic treatments for psychiatric disorders. As a result of this and the aging of our population, psychiatric–mental health nurses are becoming increasingly interested in clients with delirium, dementia, amnestic disorder, and other cognitive disorders. Clients with these disorders provide a special challenge because they frequently cannot speak our language. And as similar challenges have faced psychiatric nurses communicating with a client who has florid psychosis, discovering how to reach these people, how to assess how they feel, and how to care for them are critical nursing skills.

Besides family caregivers, nurses are the most logical advocates for these clients. Frequently, we are in charge of day treatment centers or nursing homes, or we facilitate support groups. Families look to us for suggestions to ease their burdens, for strategies to cope with difficult behavioral symptoms, for education to explain unpredictable behavior, and for resources that might alleviate their situation.

Your knowledge of psychobiology and your holistic approach to client care are unique assets essential to providing quality care for clients with cognitive disorders. Today, because of the recent reconceptualization of the *Diagnostic and Statistical Manual of Mental Disorders*, 4th edition (Text Revision) (DSM-IV-TR), the diagnostic nomenclature includes delirium, dementia, amnestic disorder, and other cognitive disorders.

Before the twentieth century, all organic brain disorders of the aged were categorized as senile dementia. Beginning at the turn of the twentieth century, neuropathologists doing autopsy work distinguished senile dementia from arteriosclerotic conditions and neurosyphilis. Arteriosclerotic brain disease was then considered the primary cause of confusional states in older adults. It was believed to be the result of diseased cerebral vessels.

By the middle of the twentieth century, a new category, organic brain disease (OBD), was added. This category was broader, allowing for a defect both in the vessels and in the brain itself. The category organic brain syndrome (OBS) then followed, which recognized the need for a diagnosis that included symptoms without a known cause. A few years ago, the term *organic mental syndrome* (OMS) referred to a group of psychological or behavioral signs of unknown or unclear etiology, while *organic mental disorder* (OMD) referred to a particular syndrome whose etiology was known or presumed.

Delirium

The elderly, especially those with dementia, are prone to transient cognitive disorders usually referred to as either **delirium** or acute confusional state. It is estimated that 15% to 50% of elderly general medical clients will experience a life-threatening acute confusional state (Hall & Leipzig, 2000; Lawlor, Fainsinger, & Bruera, 2000). More than 2 million elderly people are affected each year. If hospitalized, they remain in the hospital twice as long as elderly clients without delirium, and one-fourth of these older adults with delirium die within one month of admission. Up to 60% of residents over 75 years of age in long-term care facilities may be delirious at any time.

Delirium can be defined as a type of confusional state that is marked by:

1. Prominent disorientation.
2. Disorders of perception.
3. Terrifying hallucinations and vivid dreams.
4. A kaleidoscopic array of strange and absurd fantasies and delusions.
5. Agitated behavior.
6. Inability to sleep.
7. Tendency to convulse.
8. Intense emotional disturbances (Lyketsos et al., 2000).

Additional elements include disorientation, impaired attention and concentration, and diminution of all mental activity. Rage, depression, fear, apathy, and incontinence are common.

Differentiating delirium from dementia can be a difficult process for nurses and physicians; however, failure to recognize delirium in clients can delay appropriate treatment to a dangerous degree. See the DSM-IV-TR Diagnostic Criteria box on page 237 for the taxonomy of delirium.

Because delirium is usually caused by an underlying systemic illness, a prompt search is essential for treatable conditions like pain, dehydration, advanced cancer, diabetes, hyponatremia, hypercalcemia, thyroid crisis, infection, silent myocardial infarction, drug intoxication, or liver or renal failure. If the cause is removed, complete recovery can be achieved (Guttman, 1999).

SIGNS OF DELIRIUM

Detecting delirium requires an examination of cognition, attention and wakefulness, and psychomotor behavior.

Cognition

The three components of cognition—perception, thinking, and memory—are all disrupted in delirium:

1. *Perception*. The person shows reduced ability to distinguish and integrate sensory information and to differentiate it from hallucinations, dreams, illusions, and imagery.
2. *Thinking*. The thinking process is fragmented and disorganized to the extent that the person is unable to reason, judge, abstract, or solve problems.
3. *Memory*. Memory is impaired in all three spheres; the person is unable to register, retain, or recall information.

Attention and Wakefulness

Attention is impaired in all three spheres. The person has difficulty with:

- Alertness or maintaining vigilance.
- Selectiveness, or the ability to focus on and selectively attend to stimuli at will.

DSM-IV-TR Diagnostic Criteria for Cognitive Disorders

DIAGNOSTIC CRITERIA FOR DELIRIUM DUE TO . . . [INDICATE THE GENERAL MEDICAL CONDITION]

A. Disturbance of consciousness (i.e., reduced clarity of awareness of the environment) with reduced ability to focus, sustain, or shift attention.

B. A change in cognition (such as memory deficit, disorientation, language disturbance) or the development of a perceptual disturbance that is not better accounted for by a preexisting, established, or evolving dementia.

C. The disturbance develops over a short period of time (usually hours to days) and tends to fluctuate during the course of the day.

D. There is evidence from the history, physical examination, or laboratory findings that the disturbance is caused by the direct physiological consequences of a general medical condition.

DIAGNOSTIC CRITERIA FOR DEMENTIA OF THE ALZHEIMER'S TYPE (DAT)

A. The development of multiple cognitive deficits manifested by both

1. memory impairment (impaired ability to learn new information or to recall previously learned information)

2. one (or more) of the following cognitive disturbances:

a. Aphasia (language disturbance)

b. Apraxia (impaired ability to carry out motor activities despite intact motor function)

c. Agnosia (failure to recognize or identify objects despite intact sensory function)

d. Disturbance in executive functioning (i.e., planning, organizing, sequencing, abstracting)

B. The cognitive deficits in Criteria A1 and A2 each cause significant impairment in social or occupational functioning and represent a significant decline from a previous level of functioning.

C. The course is characterized by gradual onset and continuing cognitive decline.

D. The cognitive deficits in Criteria A1 and A2 are not due to any of the following:

1. Other central nervous system conditions that cause progressive deficits in memory and cognition (e.g., cerebrovascular disease, Parkinson's disease, Huntington's disease, subdural hematoma, normal-pressure hydrocephalus, brain tumor)

2. Systemic conditions that are known to cause dementia (e.g., hypothyroidism, vitamin B_{12} or folic acid deficiency, niacin deficiency, hypercalcemia, neurosyphilis, HIV infection)

3. Substance-induced conditions

E. The deficits do not occur exclusively during the course of a delirium.

F. The disturbance is not better accounted for by another Axis I disorder (e.g., major depressive disorder, schizophrenia).

Source: Reprinted with permission from the Diagnostic and Statistical Manual of Mental Disorders, 4th edition, Text Revision. Copyright 2000 American Psychiatric Association.

- Directiveness, or the ability to direct and focus one's mental processes.

Wakefulness is usually reduced during the day, and the person experiences sleeplessness, restlessness, and agitation at night. There is a disturbed sleep–wake cycle, with an hour-to-hour variation. Interestingly, delirium and dreaming are characterized by the same electroencephalographic (EEG) changes. The person is then caught between dreaming and hallucinating, sleep and wakefulness.

Psychomotor Behavior

The delirious client is either hyperactive or hypoactive, often alternating between them. Speech may be slurred and disjointed, with aimless vocalizations and repetitions. Tremors and irregular spasmodic (choreiform) movements may be present. See the following clinical examples of delirium.

CLINICAL EXAMPLE

Mr. Robio, an 80-year-old bachelor with bilateral cataracts, lived alone in a small midwestern town with his pet cat Suzy. Mr. Robio was admitted to the community hospital for a hernia repair that he had been putting off for several months. Never hospitalized before, he was extremely anxious on admission and became more so with each preoperative procedure that day. By 10:00 that evening, Mr. Robio was found wandering in the hallway, looking and calling for Suzy. The nurse gave him a barbiturate sleeping preparation and returned him to his room. Three hours later he was again found wandering, this time nude and more disoriented than before. He was again sedated and confined to bed with a vest and soft wrist restraints. By morning, Mr. Robio was so disoriented and agitated that the surgery was canceled. Mr. Robio's physician then ordered diazepam (Valium) for sedation, and the client remained confined to bed. Within one week, Mr. Robio's behavior had deteriorated to the extent that he required institutionalization. He was transferred to a local nursing home for permanent care.

A 55-year-old man, Mr. Bruener, was involved with a difficult divorce and went drinking with his friends. He drank numerous "straight" drinks and shortly thereafter began screaming, crying, and acting aggressively toward others in the bar. At one point he tried to choke a man, and later picked up a chair and threw it. The police took him to jail and, when he began to convulse, to the hospital.

Mrs. Weinstein, a 65-year-old woman, was in the hospital with renal problems. Although previously alert, she rapidly became agitated and confused about where she was. She was unresponsive to the nurse's efforts to orient her and refused to cooperate during her morning care. Within hours after this extreme agitation, she lapsed into a stupor and then a coma.

Differentiating Delirium from Dementia

Several criteria distinguish delirium from dementia (Tschanz et al., 2000):

- *State of consciousness.* People with delirium have fluctuating consciousness, whereas individuals with dementia are as attentive as they can be and do not have clouded consciousness until terminal stages.
- *Stability.* In clients with delirium, the ability to pay attention and respond varies, whereas in clients with dementia, these abilities are relatively stable.
- *Duration.* Delirium is short lived; dementia is prolonged.
- *Rate of onset.* Delirium develops rapidly, whereas dementia is typically an insidious process.
- *Cause.* Delirium may be traced to a recent source, whereas dementia cannot be linked to another cause.

For a summary of the characteristics of delirium and dementia, and the differentiation between them and depression, see ■ Table 12–1. Depression is discussed in Chapter 15.

PSEUDODELIRIUM

In 5% to 20% of the cases of delirium, no organic cause can be identified. As in pseudodementia, the presence of inconsistencies in cognitive functioning (e.g., the client does not know where he or she is but can find the bathroom, bed, etc.) should raise the suspicion of a pseudodelirium. If the client also has a history of psychiatric illness, is grossly and consistently delusional, has marked manic or depressive features, or is unmotivated during cognitive testing, the diagnosis of this cognitive disorder may be appropriate.

Dementia

The prevalence of dementia is 1% starting at 65 years of age and doubles every 5 years. Dementia of the Alzheimer's type (DAT) alone affects as many as 4 million people in the United States. This number is 10 times greater than at the turn of the last century, and it is likely to double by 2030 (Grob, Lorreck, Binder, & Haller, 2000). Over 60% of people in nursing homes have been diagnosed with dementia. A now common clinical syndrome, dementia is marked by the following:

- Global cognitive impairment extending to the areas of abstract thinking, judgment, insight, complex capabilities (language, tasks, recognition), and personality change
- Memory impairment
- Decline in intellectual function
- Altered judgment, in awake and alert states
- Altered affect
- Spatial disorientation

Dementia is a mental disorder involving functional declines in multiple cognitive areas, including memory, along with behavioral and psychological symptoms (Finkel & Burns, 2000). Symptoms related to specific areas of brain damage are shown in ■ Figure 12–1 (page 240). The DSM-IV-TR further differentiates dementia as "sufficiently severe to cause impairment in occupational or social functioning" (American Psychiatric Association [APA], 2000, p. 148).

Dementias are classified according to causal agent or area of neurologic damage. The latter schema distinguishes between cortical and subcortical dementias. Alzheimer's disease is the classic cortical dementia, whereas Huntington's disease and Parkinson's disease are common subcortical types. These categories are quite similar. People with subcortical dementias, however, have a higher order of functioning.

DEMENTIA OF THE ALZHEIMER'S TYPE

Dementia of the Alzheimer's type (DAT), also known as *Alzheimer's disease* or *Alzheimer's dementia (AD)*, a chronic progressive disorder, is the most common form of dementia seen in older adults. See Box 12–1 (page 241) for DSM-IV-TR diagnostic criteria for dementia of the Alzheimer's type (DAT). Reference to this disease with either abbreviation—DAT or AD—is accepted; however, to keep the distinction clear that this is one type of dementia, it will be referred to as DAT throughout this chapter.

One in 10 persons over 65 and nearly half of those over 85 have Alzheimer's disease. Today, 4 million Americans have Alzheimer's disease. Unless a cure or prevention is found, that number will jump to 14 million by the year 2050. Worldwide, it is estimated that 22 million individuals will develop Alzheimer's disease by the year 2025. Caregivers are affected by this disease, too. In a national survey, 19 million Americans said that they have a family member with Alzheimer's disease, and 37 million said they knew someone with the disease (Alzheimer's Association, 2002).

TABLE 12–1 Comparing Delirium, Dementia, and Depression

	Delirium	Dementia	Depression
Diagnostic Features	Disturbance of consciousness accompanied by a change in cognition unaccounted for by a preexisting or evolving dementia. Reduced clarity of awareness of the environment. Impaired ability to focus, sustain, or shift attention. Change in cognition may include memory impairment, disorientation to time and/or place, or language disturbance such as rambling, irrelevant or pressured and incoherent speech. Simple or complex perceptual disturbances may include misinterpretations, illusions, or hallucinations.	Multiple cognitive deficits including memory impairment and either aphasia, apraxia, or agnosia; or a disturbance in executive functioning (the ability to think abstractly, to plan, initiate, sequence, monitor, and stop complex behavior). Impairment in occupational or social functioning that represents a decline from earlier level of functioning.	Dysphoric mood, loss of interest or pleasure in usual activities and pastimes, appetite disturbance, change in weight, sleep disturbance, psychomotor agitation or retardation, decreased energy, feelings of worthlessness or guilt, difficulty concentrating or thinking, thoughts of death or suicide or suicide attempts.
Associated Features	Emotional disturbance: fear, anxiety, irritability, anger, euphoria, apathy. Disturbance in sleep-wake cycle with daytime sleepiness or nighttime agitation and difficulty falling asleep. Disturbed psychomotor behavior including groping or picking at bedclothes, sudden movements, or sluggishness and lethargy. Possible extremes of psychomotor activity during the day.	Spatial disorientation, poor judgment, poor insight, violence, suicidal behavior, disinhibited behavior, slurred speech, anxiety, mood and sleep disturbances, delusions, hallucinations, vulnerability to physical and psychosocial stressors.	Depressed appearance, tearfulness, feelings of anxiety, irritability, fear, brooding, excessive concern with physical health, panic attacks, phobias. Delusion or hallucinations may be present. In elderly, see symptoms suggesting dementia (e.g., disorientation, memory loss, distractibility, apathy, difficulty in concentration, inattentiveness).
Onset	May begin abruptly. Relatively rapid: over hours. Short period of time: a few days. Especially common in children and after the age of 60.	Depends on underlying etiology. May be rather sudden (e.g., head trauma) or insidious in onset and slow, but progress is relentless over several years (e.g., primary degenerative dementia).	Usually able to date onset with some precision. Onset is variable; symptoms usually developing over a period of days to weeks but may be sudden. In some instances, prodromal symptoms may occur over several months.
Course	Fluctuates; symptoms usually worse at night; lucid intervals usually in the morning.	Depends on underlying etiology. May be progressive, static, or remitting.	Often not recognized or misdiagnosed in the elderly. Need to differentiate from dementia.
Duration	May resolve in a few hours, or a few weeks.	May progress to death over several years. May be slowed.	Self-limiting. Median time period is 8 months; may last up to 2 years.
Outcome	Recovery if underlying disease is corrected or self-limiting. If disorder persists, shift to another more stable organic brain syndrome. May cause death.	Generally irreversible. Slowing of deterioration depends on underlying pathology, timely diagnosis, and treatment. The more widespread the structural damage to the brain, the less likely the clinical improvement.	Can be successfully treated. Spontaneous recovery is expected. Severe depression may end in suicide.
Etiologic Factors	Systemic infections. Metabolic disorders (hepatic or renal disease, hypoxia, hypercapnia, hypoglycemia, ionic imbalances, thiamine deficiency). Postoperative states. Substance intoxication and withdrawal. Head trauma. Lesions of the right parietal lobe and occipital lobe. Toxin exposure. Anticholinergic effects of medication.	Primary degenerative dementia, Alzheimer type. Infections of central nervous system. Brain trauma. Virus (e.g., AIDS, Creutzfeldt–Jakob disease). Toxic metabolic disturbance. Vascular disease (e.g., vascular dementia). Normal pressure hydrocephalus. Neurologic conditions such as Huntington's disease, multiple sclerosis, Parkinson's disease. Postanoxic or posthypoglycemic states.	Situational: bereavement, loss of health, major catastrophic event in person's life, trauma.

Source: Blazer, D., Hughes, D. C., George, L. K. (1987). The epidemiology of depression in an elderly community population. *The Gerontologist, 27,* 281–287.

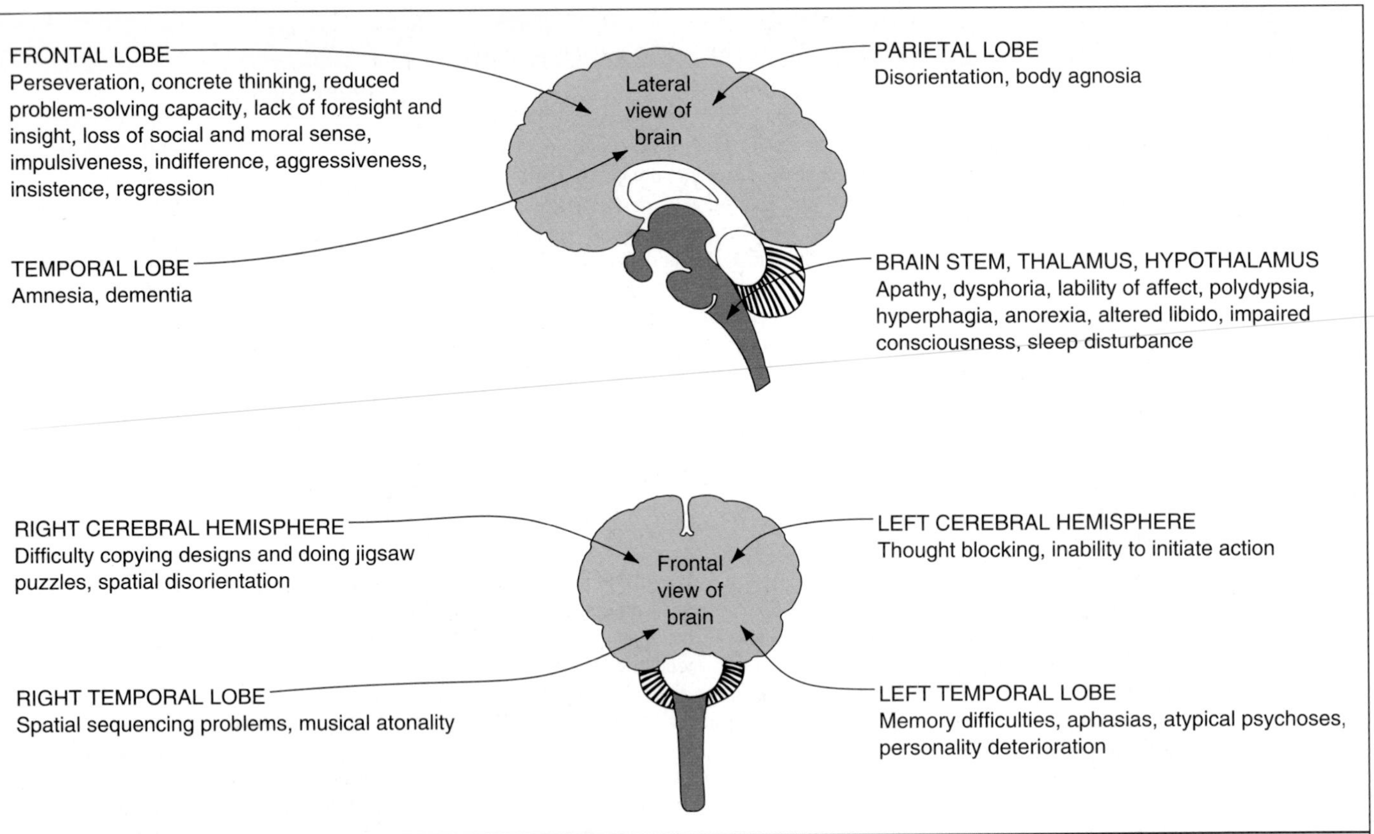

FRONTAL LOBE
Perseveration, concrete thinking, reduced problem-solving capacity, lack of foresight and insight, loss of social and moral sense, impulsiveness, indifference, aggressiveness, insistence, regression

TEMPORAL LOBE
Amnesia, dementia

Lateral view of brain

PARIETAL LOBE
Disorientation, body agnosia

BRAIN STEM, THALAMUS, HYPOTHALAMUS
Apathy, dysphoria, lability of affect, polydypsia, hyperphagia, anorexia, altered libido, impaired consciousness, sleep disturbance

RIGHT CEREBRAL HEMISPHERE
Difficulty copying designs and doing jigsaw puzzles, spatial disorientation

RIGHT TEMPORAL LOBE
Spatial sequencing problems, musical atonality

Frontal view of brain

LEFT CEREBRAL HEMISPHERE
Thought blocking, inability to initiate action

LEFT TEMPORAL LOBE
Memory difficulties, aphasias, atypical psychoses, personality deterioration

FIGURE 12–1 ■ *Behavioral changes related to specific areas of brain damage. Damage to each part of the brain results in specific alterations and deficits in client behaviors and skills.*

MediaLink Alzheimer's Association

Additional data such as these can be accessed through a direct link to the Alzheimer's Association Web site (www.alz.org) through the Companion Website for this book.

In addition to the quality-of-life issues for the clients involved, there are financial realities that affect the individual, the family, the community, and our health care system in general. DAT costs the U.S. economy over $100 billion a year for long-term care.

Alois Alzheimer first recognized the features of what would come to be called dementia of the Alzheimer's Type in 1907 while conducting an autopsy on a 51-year-old woman with a 4½-year history of dementia. He discovered senile plaques in the brain and other pathologic lesions that he called neurofibrillary tangles. Neurofibrillary tangles are illustrated in ■ Figure 12–2. These are now referred to as Alzheimer-type changes. This disease may also destroy those neurons that secrete the neurotransmitter acetylcholine, which plays a role in memory and learning.

Signs of Dementia of the Alzheimer's Type

Signs of this disease include the following:

- *Aphasia:* The loss of language ability.
- *Anomia:* Over time, the person experiences difficulty remembering words.
- *Agraphia:* An inability to express thoughts in writing.
- *Alexia:* An inability to understand written language (eventually, the condition progresses to a loss of all verbal ability).
- *Apraxia:* The loss of purposeful movement without loss of muscle power or coordination in general. The ability to conceptualize or perform motor tasks deteriorates. People with apraxia may have difficulty carrying out complex tasks.

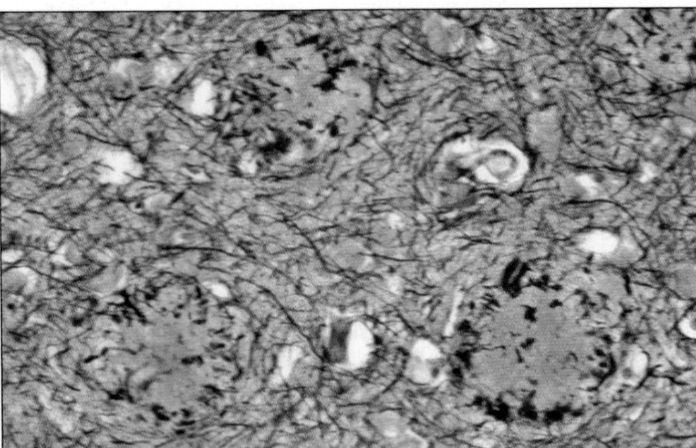

FIGURE 12–2 ■ *Neurofibrillary tangles. Characteristic senile plaques and neurofibrillary tangles are seen in this microphotograph using a silver stain of the hippocampal cortex in a client with DAT.*

Source: Smock, T. K. (1999). *Physiological psychology: A neuroscience approach,* Figure 16–14, p. 408. Upper Saddle River, NJ: Prentice Hall.

- *Agnosia:* The loss of sensory ability to recognize objects. Initially, the person has difficulty recognizing everyday objects. In the later stages, people with agnosia recognize neither loved ones nor their own body parts.
- *Mnemonic disturbances:* Memory loss. The inability to remember recent events, especially in new or changing environments, extends to profound memory loss of both recent and past events (Grob et al., 2000).

Progression of Dementia of the Alzheimer's Type

There are three clinically distinct global stages of DAT based on functional and cognitive capacity: Stages 1, 2, and 3 (see Box 12–1). One assessment tool useful in assessing the cognitive capacity in DAT is the Mini-Mental State Exam (MMSE, see Chapter 9). Usually, a score of 18 or higher is seen in the early stages of DAT, moderate DAT between 12 and 18, and severe DAT scores are lower than 12. The average decline in MMSE scores is approximately three per year. Assessment guidelines for the three stages of the disease are outlined in the Assessment box on page 242. Functional disability can be assessed grossly through competence at activities of daily living (ADLs). Reisberg et al. (1989) formalized the Global Deterioration Scale (GDS), extending it to 16 levels of functional disability, which correspond to the 7 clinically identifiable global stages of central nervous system (CNS) aging and DAT, and formalized the Functional Assessment Stages (FAST). Both the GDS and FAST stages are summarized in ■ Table 12–2 (see page 243). The GDS notes the cognitive decline, and the FAST stages specify corresponding levels of functional disability.

DEMENTIA WITH LEWY BODIES

Dementia with Lewy bodies (DLB) is the second most common late-onset dementia after Dementia of the Alzheimer's type (DAT) accounting for 15% to 20% of the neurodegenerative dementias. The name of the dementia subtype comes from the histopathologic feature of Lewy inclusion bodies in the cerebral cortex. DLB has only lately been the subject of intense consideration and scrutiny. There is a distinct presentation of the dementia with **parkinsonism** (an adverse reaction that resembles Parkinson's disease, resulting from effects on the extrapyramidal tracts of the CNS), fluctuating confusion, disturbances of consciousness, falls, and psychiatric symptoms.

BOX 12–1 Stages of DAT

DAT has an average course of 5 to 10 years, with a range of 2 to 20 years. Early onset often leads to very rapid deterioration.

Stage 1 (2–4 Years)

Changes in behaviors include:

- Difficulty performing complex tasks related to a recent decline in memory.
- Concentration decreases while distractibility increases.
- Difficulty making accurate judgments.
- Disorientation about time occurs but memory about people and places remains.
- Difficulty balancing a checkbook or planning a meal.
- Personal appearance may decline and the person needs help in selecting appropriate clothing.
- Planning in general is seriously limited, so incomplete verbal or written reports are common at work sites.
- Verbal skills decline with word-finding and object-naming difficulty. Speech in noisy distracting environments is too difficult.
- May accuse others of wrongdoing because of transitory delusions of persecution ("You hid my keys"). People recognize their own confusion and are frightened by it. They cover up and rationalize symptoms.
- Poor driving skills because of misperceptions and errors in judgment can lead to accidents.
- *Hypertonia* (an increase in muscle tone) that can happen with dementia; it can result in muscle twitching.
- Anxiety and depression are common, as are frustration, helplessness, apathy, and shame.
- Psychotic symptoms are common in Stages 1 and 2.
- Depression worsens the symptoms of dementia and should be treated.

Stage 2 (Several Years)

Changes in behavior include:

- Progressive recent and remote memory loss.
- New information cannot be retained.
- Failure to recognize family members or past significant events signals loss of remote memory.
- Behavior deteriorates rapidly and is often socially unacceptable.
- Poor impulse control outbursts and tantrums.
- Emotional lability is common—from flat affect to marked irritability.
- Comprehension of language, interactions, and significance of objects is greatly diminished.
- Disorientation occurs to the three spheres of person, place, and time.
- Wandering occurs.
- Difficulty tracking the sequence of events especially for bathing, dressing, and toileting.
- Psychotic symptoms are common in Stages 1 and 2.
- *Misidentification syndrome* frequently occurs where familiar people are seen as unfamiliar and vice versa.
- Sleep cycle is impaired, with decrease in total sleep time and frequent awakenings.
- Accidents are common, especially falls and injuries because of difficulty in using sharp objects.

Stage 3 (1–2 Years)

Changes in behavior include:

- *Hyperorality* (placing everything within reach into the mouth) and periodic binge eating.
- *Hyperetamorphosis* occurs (the need to compulsively touch and examine every object in the environment).
- Motor skills seriously deteriorate such that the client cannot walk, sit up, or smile.
- Emotional responses dwindle to nonresponsiveness.

ASSESSMENT Early, Middle, and Late Stages of Dementia of the Alzheimer's Type (DAT)

Early Stage

Client complains of forgetfulness, as in remembering names and appointments.

Client covers up forgetfulness.

Client may blame others for forgetfulness.

Client acts confused, becomes irritable or quiet. Emotional lability is common.

Client begins to have problems in family, work, and social life.

Middle Stage

Memory problems become more pronounced. Recall of recent events is minimal.

Activities of daily living, including cooking, eating, bathing, and dressing, become increasingly problematic. Family and friends begin to take over for client.

Orientation and concentration are affected.

Client may become restless at night and may sleep only a few hours off and on throughout the day.

Client may become aggressive, even violent, when frustrated or when family attempts to help client.

Client may exhibit wandering and may call out and search for children or loved ones.

Client has increased aphasia, agnosia, and apraxia.

Hypertonia and unsteady gait are common.

Client may have insatiable appetite, yet lose weight.

Social habits are forgotten. Client may be socially inappropriate.

Late Stage

Client exhibits severe disorientation, including delusions, hallucinations, and paranoid ideation.

Client may lose all speech; may perseverate or echo sounds.

Client may touch self and objects frequently.

Client becomes bedridden, emaciated, and completely helpless.

Recent genetic studies have indicated potential candidate genes for DLB (Ballard, McLaren, & Morris, 2000).

One of the main concerns regarding DLB is accurate diagnosis prior to pharmacologic treatment. Neuroleptics typically used in dementia can cause a severe and even fatal sensitivity to the extrapyramidal side effects in DLB clients. The three core diagnostic features were defined by McKeith et al. (1996):

1. Spontaneous parkinsonism or extrapyramidal signs.
2. Persistent or recurrent visual hallucinations.
3. Fluctuating cognition.

Clients who will have DLB alone are much less common than those who will have a concomitant DAT. Neuropathologic studies have found that 20% to 30% of elderly clients with degenerative dementia have both (Lopez et al., 2000). It is difficult to differentiate DLB that is comorbid with DAT as a unique clinical syndrome from DAT alone. The number of studies on, and diagnoses of, DLB are increasing dramatically.

MediaLink EPSE: Parkinsonism Video / Tremor Videos

VASCULAR DEMENTIA

Vascular dementia, also known as ischemic vascular dementia (IVD) and formerly known in DSM-IV as multi-infarct dementia, accounts for about 19% of the dementias. Unlike Alzheimer's disease, vascular dementia is abrupt in onset and episodic, with multiple remissions. The client also demonstrates focal neurologic signs, such as one-sided weakness, emotional outbursts, and a stepwise rather than progressive decline in intellectual functioning, and has a history of hypertension, diabetes, or cardiovascular disease affecting other organs.

In vascular dementia the brain tissue is destroyed by intermittent emboli that can range from a few to over a dozen. Individual infarcts may vary by 1 cm in diameter. Symptoms are commonly absent until 100 to 200 cc of brain tissue have been destroyed.

PARKINSON'S DISEASE

Only recently has **Parkinson's disease** been associated with dementia. A minority of clients with dementia have Parkinson's disease. A subset of clients has both Parkinson's disease and DAT, and this diagnosis may be difficult. There are several different varieties of Parkinson's disease. The cause of classic Parkinson's disease is unknown. Another type, postencephalitic, has been linked to previous viral infection in the brain. An interesting feature of this type is the presence of neurofibrillary tangles similar to those found in clients with DAT (Farber et al., 2000).

HUNTINGTON'S DISEASE

Huntington's disease is a genetic, progressive, degenerative disorder characterized by both motor and cognitive changes, chorea, and dementia. This disease, one of the more frequently observed types of hereditary nervous system diseases, usually begins between the ages of 40 and 50. By the time of diagnosis, the client has usually reproduced, passing this inherited disease to another generation. The movement disorder is thought to be caused by vulnerability to damage and subsequent loss of nerve cells in the brain.

Mood disturbances, especially depression, are common early in the disease, followed by deterioration of cognitive function. Movement abnormalities slowly increase until all muscle groups are involved (Gottlieb, 2000). The motor dysfunction is characterized by *chorea:* quick, jerky, purposeless, involuntary movements. The average life span after an initial diagnosis is 15 years.

Supplementing with coenzyme Q10 (CoQ10) has been known to replace deficient levels of the enzyme in muscle and positively affect cerebellar ataxia. Recently, people with Huntington's disease were treated with CoQ10 in an effort to

TABLE 12–2 Global Deterioration Scale (GDS) Stages and Functional Assessment Stages (FAST) in Dementia of the Alzheimer's Type (DAT)

Stage	GDS Characteristics	FAST Characteristics
1	No subjective complaints of memory deficit and no memory deficit in clinical interview	No decrement
2	Subjective complaints of memory deficits with no objective deficits in employment or social situations	Subjective deficit in word finding
3	Earliest clear-cut deficit with objective evidence of deficit on interview and decreased performance in demanding employment and social setting	Deficits in demanding employment
4	Clear-cut deficit on clinical interview as evidenced by decreased knowledge of current and recent events and concentration deficits on serial subtractions and other complex tasks such as managing finances or preparing dinner for guests	Requires help in complex tasks, e.g., handling finances, planning a dinner party
5	Deficit sufficient to interfere with independent community survival with inability to recall a major relevant aspect of current and past life such as address or phone number, names of close family members, etc.	Requires help choosing proper attire
6a	Deficit sufficient to require assistance with basic activities of daily life such as dressing and bathing, etc.	Requires help dressing in severe DAT
6b		Requires help bathing properly
6c		Requires help with mechanics of toileting (e.g., flushing, wiping)
6d		Urinary incontinence
6e		Fecal incontinence
7a	Deficit sufficient to require help with toileting and feeding, urinary and fecal incontinence, etc.	Speech ability limited to about a half-dozen intelligible words
7b		Intelligible vocabulary limited to single word
7c		Ambulatory ability lost
7d		Ability to sit up lost
7e		Ability to smile lost
7f		Ability to hold up head lost

Source: Iqbal et al., Alzheimer's disease and related disorders (progress in clinical and biological research), copyright © 1989. This material is used by permission of John Wiley & Sons, Inc.

see if the enzyme could have an impact on the disease's progression (Huntington Study Group, 2001). The study's results showed some evidence of a trend toward a slower decline, but this slowing was not evident until after one year of treatment and the impact was not statistically significant. Interestingly, the CoQ10 was tolerated very well while other treatments were associated with several adverse effects. Rigorous research is required to explore this issue further and detect significant impacts. Associated concerns are the cost (from $60 to $150 U.S. dollars/month) and the fact that as a nutritional supplement, CoQ10 does not have the quality and control guarantees of a pharmaceutical product.

PICK'S DISEASE

Pick's disease is a rare disorder in which cerebral atrophy is present in the frontal and/or temporal lobes. These circumscribed pathologic changes are different from DAT, in which atrophy is mild and diffuse.

The two patterns of behavior evident in Pick's disease, representative of the temporal and frontal types, respectively, include talkativeness, lightheartedness, gaiety, anxiety and hyperattentiveness, or inertia, emotional dullness, and lack of initiative (Grob et al., 2000). As the disease progresses, the deterioration becomes more global, affecting memory and language. There is profound atrophy of the frontal and/or temporal lobes, with characteristic Pick inclusion bodies found on autopsy. The expected life span after the original diagnosis is seven years. A higher incidence is seen in some families, suggesting a genetic predisposition.

CREUTZFELDT–JAKOB DISEASE

Creutzfeldt–Jakob disease is a transmissible degenerative dementia affecting the cerebral cortex through cell destruction and overgrowth. It is marked clinically by a very rapid onset and involuntary movements. This profound dementia is evidenced by cerebellar ataxia, diffuse myoclonic jerks, and other visual and neurologic abnormalities. There are distinctive electroencephalographic changes with this disease. The infection is presumed to be caused by a *prion*, a small proteinaceous particle that is resistant to treatment and sterilization procedures. There may be a genetic susceptibility to infection; however, the only definitive spreading mechanism is iatrogenic, as seen after corneal transplantation, and after the injection of human growth hormone derived from the pituitary gland of cadavers with the disease (Grob et al., 2000).

NEW VARIANT CREUTZFELDT–JAKOB DISEASE

Once the disease known as mad cow disease (*bovine spongiform encephalopathy* [*BSE*]) became widespread, an unusual presentation of Creutzfeldt–Jakob disease was noted and since 1996 has been identified as **new variant Creutzfeldt–Jakob disease (nvCJD).** It appears to be caused by the same agent as BSE, although it is unclear how transmission to humans is taking place (Andrews et al., 2000). There is evidence suggesting that nvCJD in Europe is linked to eating contaminated beef. Usually, as noted above, Creutzfeldt–Jakob disease occurs in older clients and begins as dementia. This new variation can occur in younger clients and includes unusual spongiform changes in the cerebellum. nvCJD is currently more of a problem in Europe than in North America due to varying health codes and standards.

PSEUDODEMENTIA

Affective disorders, particularly depression, can be masked by symptoms suggestive of dementia. Clinical symptoms may include impaired attention and memory, apathy, self-neglect, and no complaints of depression. The term **pseudodementia** has been used to describe the reversible cognitive impairments seen in depression. It is essential to detect pseudodementia in clients because, with appropriate treatment, they can recover. Pseudodementia should be suspected when the onset is abrupt, the clinical course is rapid, and the client complains about cognitive failures (Elias et al., 2000). Clients with dementia often fail to perceive or attempt to cover up their deficits. Evidence of these deficits can be seen, such as in the clinical examples below.

CLINICAL EXAMPLE

Ms. Salerno, a 57-year-old woman, was having problems selecting the words she wanted to use and putting her thoughts on paper. She began to miss appointments and her scheduled workdays, and she could no longer handle her daily responsibilities.

Mr. Jorgensen, a 45-year-old man, was in the hospital in the final stages of AIDS. He would forget what day it was and whether or not his family had visited. Occasionally, he had visual hallucinations and on one occasion seemed to think he was at summer camp.

Amnestic Disorder

Amnestic disorder, a relatively uncommon cognitive disorder, is characterized by short- and long-term memory deficits, an inability to recall previously learned information or recall past events, an inability to learn new material, confabulation, apathy, and a bland affect. Impairment ranges from moderate to severe. Possible causes include head trauma, hypoxia, encephalitis, thiamine deficiency, and substance abuse. These causes shape the three main types of amnestic disorder, which are briefly described here: those due to (1) a medical condition, (2) a substance, or (3) other causes.

There must be a connection between the general medical condition (which includes physical trauma), and the amnestic disorder when this type is diagnosed. The timing of the onset of amnesia, an atypical presentation of a memory problem, and ruling out other explanations for the disorder support this diagnosis. Substance-induced amnesia persists beyond the immediate effects of the substance and the duration of intoxication or withdrawal from the substance. Deficits can worsen over the years despite abstinence from the substance. Amnestic disorder not otherwise specified (NOS) is the diagnosis used when the criteria are not met for the two other types described above, or when there is not enough supporting evidence to link a cause to the amnesia (Berlit, 2000; Sander et al., 2000).

Biopsychosocial Theories

Theories about the causes of cognitive disorders are as varied as the disorders themselves. Genetics, infection, and vascular insufficiency are all believed to be causative factors. Because delirium is usually caused by an underlying systemic illness, a prompt search is essential for treatable conditions such as dehydration, diabetes, hyponatremia, hypercalcemia, thyroid crisis, infection, silent myocardial infarction, drug intoxication, or liver or renal failure. If the cause is removed, complete recovery from delirium can be achieved.

The actual cause of dementia of the Alzheimer's type remains unknown, but several factors are believed to play a role. Dementia of the Alzheimer's type has been correlated with the loss of specific groups of nerve cells and the disruption of communication between nerve cells from acetylcholine and serotonin deficits. Research is being done to identify a slow-acting, virus-like causative agent. This work has been prompted by the findings of just such an agent in Creutzfeldt–Jakob disease.

To date, advanced age, family history of the illness, Down's syndrome, and a history of head trauma are risk factors for DAT (APA, 2000; White & Cummings, 1997). There are linkages between genetic markers and DAT made on a number of chromosomes, namely chromosomes 1, 14, and 21, and one or both alleles coding for the E4 variant of apolipoprotein on chromosome 19 (called apo E4). People with DAT have four times the family incidence of dementia. Yet in identical and fraternal twins, in only 40% of cases do both get DAT, suggesting that DAT cannot be due to a single autosomal dominant gene. The disease also appears in

CARING FOR THE SPIRIT

Is It Alzheimer's Disease or Vitamin B_{12} Deficiency?

Imagine what it must feel like to sense the deterioration of your cognitive abilities and the slow, but steady, loss of your sense of self. But what if your distress could have been prevented?

A deficiency of vitamin B_{12} can easily be mistaken for the dementia of Alzheimer's disease. Vitamin B_{12} depletion is common among older adults because of age-induced changes in the gastrointestinal tract. Many nursing and medical textbooks state that a lack of vitamin B_{12} first causes pernicious anemia, and clinicians look for a drop in hemoglobin and a variety of other hematologic markers. The same texts explain that, with time, anemia is accompanied by neurologic signs and symptoms, including diminished vibration and position senses and dementia. Unfortunately, it is rare for a clinician to suspect B_{12}-induced dementia when a client's complete blood count is normal. Older clients can suffer the psychiatric effects of vitamin B_{12} deficiency *without* developing anemia.

A few words of caution, however, are in order about B_{12} screening: Recognizing a deficiency in its early stage is possible but requires astute assessment skills and a willingness to act as a strong client advocate, even in the face of resistance from other health professionals. Special effort is needed because some health care providers may not know how to interpret the diagnostic markers used to pinpoint the disorder. Clinicians' ability to detect this common dietary disorder can prevent a great deal of misery and spiritual distress among elderly clients.

twins and in various family members at different times, making it difficult to interpret the markers found in genetic studies.

Other possible risk factors are environmental toxins, stroke, thyroid disorder, lower educational status, and female gender (Lyketsos et al., 2000). Ongoing research focuses on causes and drug treatment that can either protect or restore neurons, thereby combating memory loss. Additional drug studies focus on ameliorating behavioral symptoms. Vitamin B_{12} deficiency has been identified as a condition that mimics DAT, as explained in the Caring for the Spirit box.

THE NURSING PROCESS

Clients with Cognitive Disorders

The nursing process with all of these disorders revolves around similar principles of care used in dementia.

Assessment

Your skills in assessing for these disorders are important for developing and delivering competent client care. Use this information in each subsequent step of the nursing process.

SUBJECTIVE DATA

It is often difficult to gather data about clients with delirium, dementia, amnestic disorder, and other cognitive disorders. Such clients are sometimes anxious and defensive; confused clients give unreliable histories; and often there is no dependable secondary source of information. Gather all data in a milieu that is free from distraction and discomfort:

- Decibel levels of ambient noise must be low.
- Light should be sufficient to dispel shadows.
- Room temperature should be comfortable.

Pace the questions slowly to allow the client time to answer comfortably. Aging people can normally process information after receiving it but may have difficulty taking in information. Placing the client in a situation that interferes with an already compromised sensory apparatus only heightens the client's anxiety and seriously compromises the nurse's attempts to evaluate effectively.

Health History. When completing the client's health history, include all past and present medical conditions, paying special attention to chronic conditions for which the client is being treated and any recent changes in health status. Ask the client: "Are you seeing a physician at this time?" "Why did you seek medical help?" "What does the doctor say is the problem?" Infections may present as confusion and other symptoms of dementia before any change in temperature, pulse, and respirations is noted. The Assessment boxes on page 246 suggest instruments or tests that can be used to evaluate people with possible dementia or delirium.

Sensory Impairment. Older adults are particularly sensitive to the confusion associated with sensory deprivation. Physiologic changes in their sensory apparatus may be directly related to aging or to pathologic processes. Both diminish sensory receptive ability. The changes in sensory apparatus, however, are not clear-cut. The older adult may have difficulty hearing high-frequency sounds, such as consonants. Turning up the volume on the radio may help the person hear one range of sounds but may also cause sensory overload because the rest of the sounds are too loud. The overall result is deprivation and distortion.

Try to ascertain any possible sensory problems, especially in hearing and vision. To test hearing, stand so that the client can see your face, and ask a question in a normal tone of voice. The question should require more than a yes or no answer. Test vision with pictures that the client will easily recognize.

ASSESSMENT Assessment Instruments for Dementia

Cognitive
- Brief Cognitive Rating Scale
- Clinical Dementia Rating Scale
- Clock Completion Test
- Hamilton Depression Scale
- NINCDS/ADRDA Criteria (National Institute of Neurological and Communication Disorders and Stroke; Alzheimer's Disease and Related Disorders Association)
- SET Test
- Short Portable Mental Status Questionnaire
- Wechsler Adult Intelligence Scale
- Mini-Mental State Exam (MMSE)

Memory
- Blessed Orientation, Memory Concentration Test
- The Story Retell
- Procedural Memory Task
- Wechsler Memory Scale

Language
- Token Test
- Figural Fluency
- Proteus Mazes
- Verbal Fluency Task
- Wepman Aphasia Screening Test
- Western Aphasia Battery

Motor
- Manual Apraxia Battery
- Specific Activity Scale

Functional Level (Activities of Daily Living)
- Performance Test of Activities of Daily Living
- Physical Self-Maintenance Scale
- Refined ADL Assessment Scale (RADL)

Dietary History. When possible, obtain an estimate of the client's food intake. "What do you usually eat for breakfast? Lunch? Dinner?" Make special note of protein and vitamin intake. Avitaminosis, pellagra, anemia, and hypoglycemia have all been associated with reversible brain syndromes. Hydration is also an important factor, easily noted in the client's physical state (adequate hydration is indicated by a saliva pool below the tongue). Dehydration can also cause confusion. Anticholinergic side effects from any number of typically prescribed medications and over-the-counter (OTC) drugs can cause dehydration and confusion.

Head Trauma. Falls are common among elderly people. Misjudging distances and not being aware of obstructions also contribute to injuries. Cerebral contusions, midbrain hemorrhage, and subdural hematoma should all be considered. Confusion may be the primary result of such trauma.

Medication. Older adults are prone to adverse drug reactions as a result of age-related bodily changes. These factors are compounded by high consumption of many different drugs: 45% of all prescriptions are written for elderly clients. The aged are particularly susceptible to drugs with anticholinergic properties (major tranquilizers, antidepressants, barbiturates, adrenal steroids, atropine, antiparkinsonians, antihistamines, antihypertensives, and diuretics). Question the client about both prescription and over-the-counter drugs: "Are you now taking any medicines that your doctor prescribed?" "Do you take laxatives, cold pills, or other medicines that you buy at your drug store without a prescription?" "Have you tried some of the health foods or remedies they have at some of these stores?"

ASSESSMENT

Assessment Instruments for Delirium

- Delirium Symptom Interview (DSI)
- Confusion Rating Scale
- Clinical Assessment of Confusion—A NEECHAM Confusion Scale
- Visual Analogue Scale for Confusion

Alcohol Consumption. Ask the client about alcohol consumption. Beyond being another source of dehydration, alcohol is a CNS depressant, and intoxication may mimic symptoms of cognitive disorders. Alcohol also compromises nutritional status and may cause withdrawal effects. Ask questions such as "How much alcohol do you drink in one day/week?" and "Have you ever had periods of not remembering after you have been drinking?" Beer and wine coolers are sold in grocery stores with advertising and packaging that may be perceived as nonalcoholic or not "counting" as alcohol consumption. Questions about these substances could be asked separately from alcohol consumption questions, possibly when discussing diet and eating habits.

PSYCHOSOCIAL HISTORY

The psychosocial history should include an assessment of the client, the client's family, and their joint coping styles and level of intimacy. Some assessment of the client's functioning in the community should be included. Unlike cognitive testing, this assessment shows what clients are doing rather than what they might do.

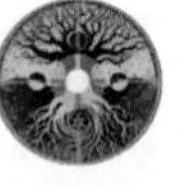

Family History. The families of impaired older adults can be a major source of information and support. In the United States, the majority of the elderly have seen one or more relatives the previous week, and many live within 30 minutes of their nearest child. Common living arrangements include living with a spouse, child, or sibling. Family assessment includes:

- Living arrangements.
- Care arrangements for the client (e.g., shopping assistance, daily visits, telephone calls).
- Family knowledge of the current illness.
- Family expectations for the future.
- Special family concerns about client care.
- Family style of coping with stress (e.g., death of a relative, illness).
- The identified spokesperson for the family.
- The family's perception of the client's coping abilities.

Throughout the interview, note the interactions between family members and the client. Do they support the client and respect what the client says? Do people listen to one another? What is the atmosphere in the group? What is the level of intimacy between family members? For a study about family caregiving needs of clients with DAT, see the Using Research Evidence box.

Activities of Daily Living. Assess the client carefully for level of self-care. This is often called a functional assessment. What can the client do without help? For which activities is help required? What type of help is needed? As cognitive deficits increase, the client becomes more dependent on others for assistance.

Community Functioning. The Comprehensive Functional Assessment (CFA) tool measures the ability to sustain oneself in the community. It covers the basic skills of living, working, relating to others, and recreating in community settings. Assess not only the ability to live independently in the community but also the degree of social involvement. Does the client belong to any clubs or groups? Do friends visit the client at home? Does the client belong to a particular church or temple? Ask about attendance at senior citizen programs and the level of participation in activities involving others.

OBJECTIVE DATA

Evaluating older adults with mental impairment is usually organized into three areas: physical assesment, laboratory assessment, and imaging techniques.

Physical Assessment. A thorough medical workup, including a complete neurologic exam (evaluation of cranial nerves, motor and sensory systems, and reflexes) and a psychiatric consultation for possible psychiatric illness is important for all elderly people with mental impairment. Because elderly people with organic illness frequently manifest confusion and depression, clinicians work from the assumption that reversible illness is present. Chest x-ray films and an electrocardiogram are taken.

USING RESEARCH EVIDENCE

You are a nurse in a combination treatment setting with long-term community care and short-term respite care. Abe, a 76-year-old client with dementia, is being treated at the long-term care section of the center. His daughter Esther is his caregiver and has been involved in both her father's care and in some program development at the clinic. Before building this treatment program for clients with DAT on this unit, it was important to find out more about what the caregivers of these clients want. Since individuals who have DAT cannot make these treatment decisions for themselves, staff must investigate the values and needs of the caregivers.

Esther regularly meets with the staff to inform them about how caregivers feel regarding certain aspects of care. This relationship empowers both the caregiver and your treatment plan. And when dealing with a frustrating and often disenfranchising caring experience such as DAT, empowerment is precious.

The main topics attended to in your program are all quality of life issues, such as:

1. Client mood.
2. Client ability to recognize and interact with caregiver.
3. Whether the disease can be delayed.
4. How much delay can be expected.
5. Whether behavioral interventions would be helpful.
6. Client ability to maintain basic care activities.
7. How important it is for the caregiver to delay putting the individual with DAT into a full-care facility.
8. What risks present themselves with pharmacologic treatment.

Your nursing knowledge of medications will be invaluable in all, particularly with the eighth point above. The level of risk caregivers are willing to take may be linked to a number of factors, such as disease stage and a family history of DAT. Current literature notes a difference in caregivers' tolerance of risks. Unlike other chronic and progressive diseases in which greater illness warrants the endorsement of riskier treatment protocols, caregivers of clients with DAT are actually less likely to take risks to treat the illness. It has been described as not wanting to expose an already vulnerable individual to harm. This unexpected value must be known prior to planning and implementation, otherwise the goals of the clinicians and the goals of the caregivers are at variance.

The planning and implementation stages of the nursing process yield a result based on the assessment and diagnosis stages. Incorporating these assessments of caregivers' needs and values into your plan and the implementation of that plan creates the potential for more insightful care. Your development of treatment protocols is a better product when borne of scientific discovery, such as in the following study, structured communication, and practical and relevant planning:

Karlawish, J. H. T., Klocinski, J. L., Merz, J., Clark, C. M., & Asch, D. A. (2000). Caregivers' preferences for the treatment of patients with Alzheimer's disease. *Neurology, 55*, 1008–1014.

MediaLink PET/SPECT Dementia Animation

Laboratory Assessment. The following tests are routinely ordered for elderly clients:

- Complete blood count, including folic acid and vitamin B_{12} levels to detect anemia.
- Erythrocyte sedimentation rate (ESR) to detect infection.
- SMA (Sequential Multiple Analyzer) to detect electrolyte imbalances.
- Syphilis tests (Venereal Disease Research Laboratory [VDRL]).
- Thyroid function studies.
- Serum levels of barbiturates, bromides, and digitalis.
- Liver function studies.
- Human immunodeficiency virus (HIV).
- Serology.
- Heavy metals.
- Toxicology.
- Urinalysis.

Imaging Techniques. Views of the brain's structure and function can be provided through a computed tomographic brain scan (CT scan), positron emission tomography (PET) and single-photon emission computed tomography (SPECT). These tests can be ordered for clients at high risk, that is, those having acute deterioration in cognitive functioning of recent onset. This deterioration is often associated with focal lesions and hydrocephalus (see Figure 12–3).

A number of elective procedures can also be used. However, their use should be limited unless indicated because of their intrusive nature and cost. These are:

- Lumbar puncture.
- Skull x-ray films.
- Electroencephalography (EEG).
- PET.
- SPECT.
- Magnetic resonance imaging (MRI).
- Cerebral angiography.
- Isotope cisternography.

COGNITIVE FUNCTIONING

Cognitive functioning includes memory, reasoning, abstraction, calculations, and judgment. Refer back to Box 12–1 on page 241 for detailed information on cognitive functioning during the various stages of DAT. Clients will not respond effectively unless they feel that the information requested is relevant, they see some purpose in the interview, and they are interested in the material. Choose testing materials carefully, and keep the endurance of the client in mind at all times. When assessing cognitive functioning, pay particular attention to the following clinical manifestations:

Appearance. Clients who appear disheveled, dirty, or unkempt may be experiencing problems with poor memory or a shortened attention span. This deficit may not be apparent if the client has a caregiver who helps with grooming.

Manner and Attitude. Some clients may exaggerate mannerisms to compensate for a perceived decline in functioning. For example, compulsive clients may become more set in their ways. An attitude of defensiveness, withdrawal, or paranoia may be a response to increasing anxiety about diminished abilities.

Communication. Assess communication in the areas of speech, gestures, facial expression, and writing. Difficulty in finding words and naming objects may suggest **expressive aphasia.** Difficulty grasping complex concepts may suggest **receptive aphasia.** Assess the client's ability to use gestures and

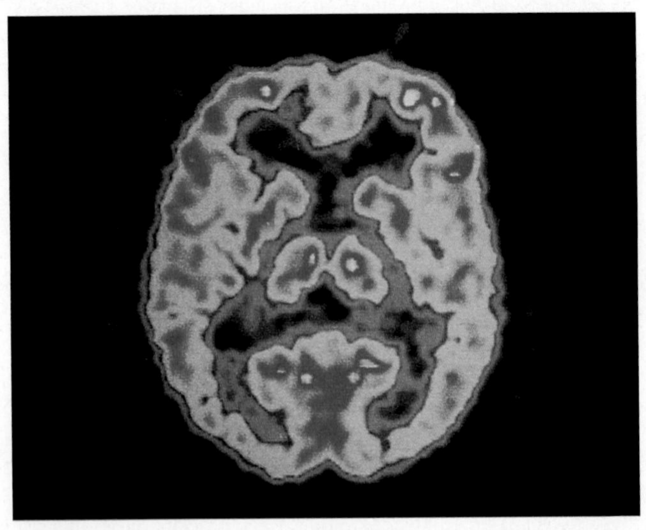
A

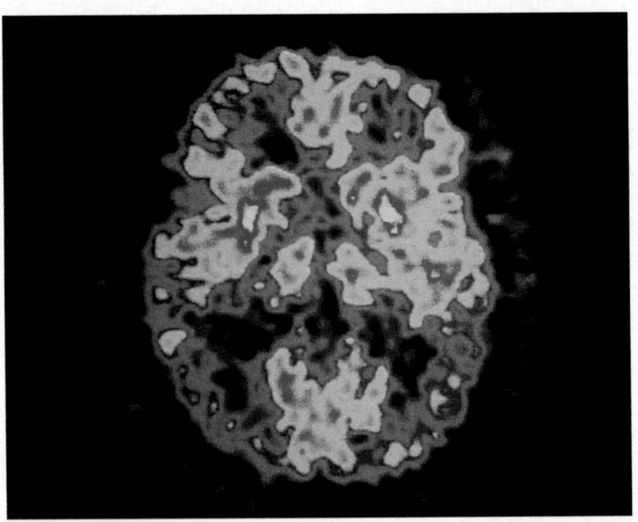
B

FIGURE 12–3 ■ *PET scan brain images in Alzheimer's disease. Compare a normal brain scan (A) with the brain of a person with Alzheimer's disease (B). (A) The red and yellow areas indicate normal metabolic rates. (B) Note the blue areas indicating abnormally low metabolism in the parietal and temporal lobes of the person with Alzheimer's disease.*

facial expressions to compensate for verbal aphasia. Not using facial expressions and gestures and speaking in a monotone may indicate depression. Also test written communication and reading ability, and assess the individual's language ability. Elderly individuals whose primary language is not English may revert to their native language; therefore, arrangements should be made for a translator.

Perception. Perception is the client's ability to recognize and integrate sensory information, including the conscious recognition of oneself in relation to the environment. Clients with asymmetric brain involvement of DAT may neglect one side of their body. These clients may also have difficulty recognizing objects (agnosia). Clients with perceptual difficulty may distort sensory information, with resulting hallucinations and delusions.

Attention and Wakefulness. Attention refers to alertness and the ability to attend selectively to stimuli and to direct one's focus. Can the client sustain or pay attention to the interview process, or is he or she easily distracted by the environment? Attention can be assessed by asking the client to spell a word backwards. Wakeful states range from hyperalertness to stupor. Stupor can be the result of medication intoxication or an acute systemic disease.

Motor Activity. Lethargy is often a symptom of depression, but it can also be the result of such medications as tranquilizers, antihypertensives, antidepressants, and antihistamines. Combinations of medications can also cause lethargy even when one of the medications alone may not be sedating. Lethargy can be caused by a number of disease processes, such as urinary tract infection, anemia, and meningitis. A shift between hypermotor and hypomotor activity is a sign of delirium. Agitation and physical striking out are occasionally demonstrated.

Mood and Affect. Depression may accompany the earlier stages of dementia. The more serious the dementia, however, the less depressed the client is. Clients with organic disease of the cerebral area are emotionally labile. Ask the client about any changes in eating or sleeping habits, and inquire about a recent loss of energy and interest in usual activities. If depression is suspected, evaluate the client for risk of suicide (see Chapter 22). Thoughts about dying and plans regarding self-harm or self-neglect to the point of harm or death need to be explored. Ask questions about suicide in a matter-of-fact manner, without hesitation, and record the findings carefully in the assessment notes.

Orientation. Disorientation to time, place, and person must be measured in an environment where the client has easy access to the information. Days in a hospital are all the same to clients housed without calendars and seasonal cues. Acute disorientation in all spheres is commonly found in people having toxic states and traumatic brain disease. Disorientation to place and person usually indicates a degenerative disorder.

Memory. People with dementias have difficulty acquiring recent memory or learning; this symptom may be a key to the early detection of dementia. At present there is no set of tests that can adequately measure the memory capacity of clients with dementia. Most tests measure episodic memory: the processing and storage of information, like recalling the events of the day. This type of memory is impaired in most clients with cognitive disorders, depression, and drug or alcohol intoxication. Semantic memory, or knowledge memory, is the ability to synthesize and think about events. It is used in language, abstraction, and logical operations. People with DAT have difficulty with semantic memory; however, depressed clients do not.

Test episodic memory by asking the client to repeat a series of words or recall a recent event, such as a meal. Test semantic memory by asking the client to develop a scenario, such as describing the events from dinner until bedtime. Episodic memory is also tested in relation to time and is usually divided into three spheres: recent, remote, and past.

Abstract Reasoning. Proverbs are the most common way of testing abstract reasoning. "What does it mean when we say, 'People who live in glass houses shouldn't throw stones'?" "What does 'A stitch in time saves nine' mean to you?" Clients with DAT often interpret these proverbs quite literally or concretely, for example replying to your question about the latter proverb with a statement such as "If you sew a single stitch you won't have to sew nine."

Calculations. The most common test of calculation ability is the serial sevens test: The person counts back from 100 in decrements of 7. This is a difficult process for the demented or delirious client. The test measures the client's ability to concentrate and focus thought. It may also be a measure of educational level.

Judgment. The test for judgment should predict whether a person will behave in a socially accepted manner, including the planning and carrying out of activities that require the client to discriminate reality from unrealistic situations. You might ask the client, "If you needed help during the night, how would you get it?" or "If you lost your wallet while doing errands, what would you do?".

Nursing Diagnoses: NANDA

A discussion of North American Nursing Diagnosis Association (NANDA) nursing diagnoses common to clients with cognitive disorders follows.

IMPAIRED PHYSICAL MOBILITY

Gait changes due to neurologic involvement are seen in people with a number of the dementias. These include DAT, Huntington's disease, Parkinson's disease, and Creutzfeldt–Jakob disease. Restlessness in the delirious client is reflected in hyperactive behavior. The client usually alternates between hyperactivity and hypoactivity.

SELF-CARE DEFICIT: BATHING/HYGIENE, DRESSING/GROOMING, FEEDING, TOILETING

Clients with delirium are unable to perceive, organize, or carry out the activities of daily living (e.g., bathing/hygiene, dress-

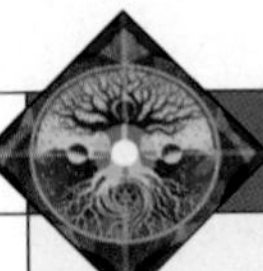

Case Study

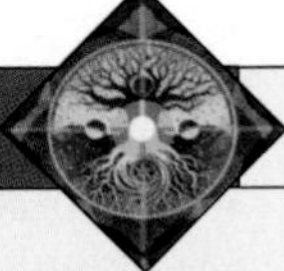

Client with Delirium

Identifying Information

Mr. Hennessey is a 70-year-old married man who entered the hospital to have colon surgery. His wife of 45 years stays with him and is extremely devoted. Mr. Hennessey has been hallucinating and is delusional. He struck a nurse and lashed out at his wife. He ripped out his IV and his nasogastric tube. Twenty-four hours after surgery Mr. Hennessey became disoriented and delusional.

History

Mr. Hennessey has no prior psychiatric history. His two grown children live nearby and are concerned, as is his wife. All are attentive to Mr. Hennessey, caring, and willing to help with his care.

Mr. Hennessey was a contractor and owned his own business. He retired 10 years ago to a garden apartment, where he and his wife have many friends and activities. He was diagnosed with a colon tumor one month ago and had a colon resection. The pathology report was positive for cancer. Mr. Hennessey had been healthy all his life until he noticed rectal bleeding a month ago.

Current Mental Status

Mr. Hennessey is disoriented the majority of time, and he is often aggressive. He has been having frightening visual hallucinations, especially at night. He is delusional that people are trying to hurt him.

Other Subjective or Objective Clinical Data

Mr. Hennessey is on morphine for pain management.

ing/grooming, feeding, toileting). They are far too distracted by stimuli and unable to focus. See the Case Study and Nursing Care Plan for a Client with Delirium for information. The DAT client has a distinct problem: apraxia, the loss of ability to perform formerly known skills. In the late stages of all the dementias, total care is a necessity as the client moves toward brain failure.

SLEEP PATTERN DISTURBANCE

Sundowning—commonly understood as confused behavior at night when environmental stimulation is low—can be seen in delirious and demented clients. The client catnaps during the day and wanders at night. Poor sensory processing can also be seen in demented clients who also wander at night. The client with DAT may not sleep for several days, moving about in a confused state.

ALTERED THOUGHT PROCESSES

Altered thought processes can occur as a variety of experiences. Clients will behave differently depending on their abilities to think as a result of these alterations.

Agnosia. Agnosia, the failure to recognize familiar objects, is a progressive problem that eventually renders the person unable to recognize or remember loved ones. Overall, in both delirium and dementia, the client's ability to use information in making judgments may be seriously impaired.

Memory. Episodic short-term memory is affected by delirium, dementia, and mood disorders. Long-term memory is diminished in the later stages of DAT and acute delirium. See ■ Figure 12–4 for a diagram of how short-term and long-term memory is established.

Orientation. Disorientation is seen in both demented and delirious clients. In the former it is related to progressive cerebral changes; in the latter, to an acute, usually identifiable causal agent.

MediaLink Care Plan: Delirium

Delusions

Delusions may be present in delirium and dementia. The client is prone to delusions as a result of reduced ability to distinguish and integrate sensory information. The problem is compounded by short- and long-term memory loss.

IMPAIRED VERBAL COMMUNICATION

Aphasia, both receptive and expressive, is one of the hallmarks of DAT. In the late stage of the illness, the client is completely mute. Confabulation is a common defense used by clients who cannot remember required information and therefore use fantasy to fill in the memory gaps. Confusion and paranoid ideation requires interacting in a nonthreatening manner. The Rx Communication box (A Client with Dementia) describes interactions with this in mind.

HIGH RISK FOR VIOLENCE: SELF-DIRECTED OR DIRECTED AT OTHERS

In clients with DAT and most of the other dementias, there is a gradual decline in the social acceptability of their behavior. Overstating distress and making threats are common, especially if this was the mode of coping when the client was more intact. See the Rx Communication box on page 252 (A Client with Dementia at Risk for Self-Harm) for an example of an interaction with a client making threats. High risk for violence is linked with impulsivity and unpredictability in these clients (see also Chapter 34). The client may also strike out at others while hallucinating or in a hyperactive phase. These behaviors are also seen in delirious clients, who are similarly unpredictable.

ALTERED ROLE PERFORMANCE

As a result of decreasing intellectual competence, the demented client moves from role of spouse, parent, employee, and community member to that of a dependent, regressed family member. The role loss and role change are anxiety provoking and at times overwhelming for the client and family. Characteristically, the family members

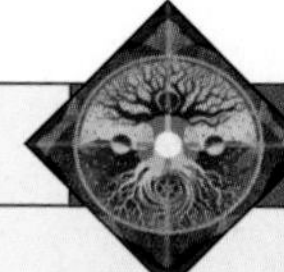

Nursing Care Plan

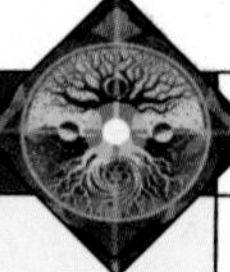

Nursing Diagnosis: High Risk for Violence related to confusion and fear inherent in delirium.

Expected Outcome: Mr. Hennessey does not attempt to harm self or others.

Short-Term Goals	*Interventions*	*Rationale*
Mr. Hennessey will maintain appropriate impulse control.	• Orient Mr. Hennessey whenever he is confused. • Move slowly, speak clearly, and explain all procedures. • Depending on neurologic examination, medicate Mr. Hennessey with a low-dose antipsychotic.	Decrease the stimuli that can exacerbate symptoms of confusion.

experience a period of acute grief after receiving the diagnosis. Their level of depression should be assessed. Feelings of isolation and being overwhelmed are also common.

SENSORY/PERCEPTUAL ALTERATIONS

The inability to attend and focus concentration is a hallmark of delirium. Decreased attention is also seen in the later stages of the dementias when the client loses the ability to encode. Delirium alters perception by reducing the client's ability to distinguish and integrate sensory information. As a result, the client has difficulty discriminating reality from hallucinations, dreams, illusions, and imagery. In the later stages of dementia, clients also experience hallucinations and delusions, which complicate delivery of care. The accompanying Rx Communication box (A Client with Dementia and Hallucinations, see page 253) shows an interaction with a client who experiences hallucinations.

SELF-ESTEEM DISTURBANCE

During the first stage of DAT and other dementias, the client is acutely aware of cognitive failure. This awareness and the resulting anxiety can be damaging to the self-esteem of a person living in a culture that does not tolerate or provide for dependence.

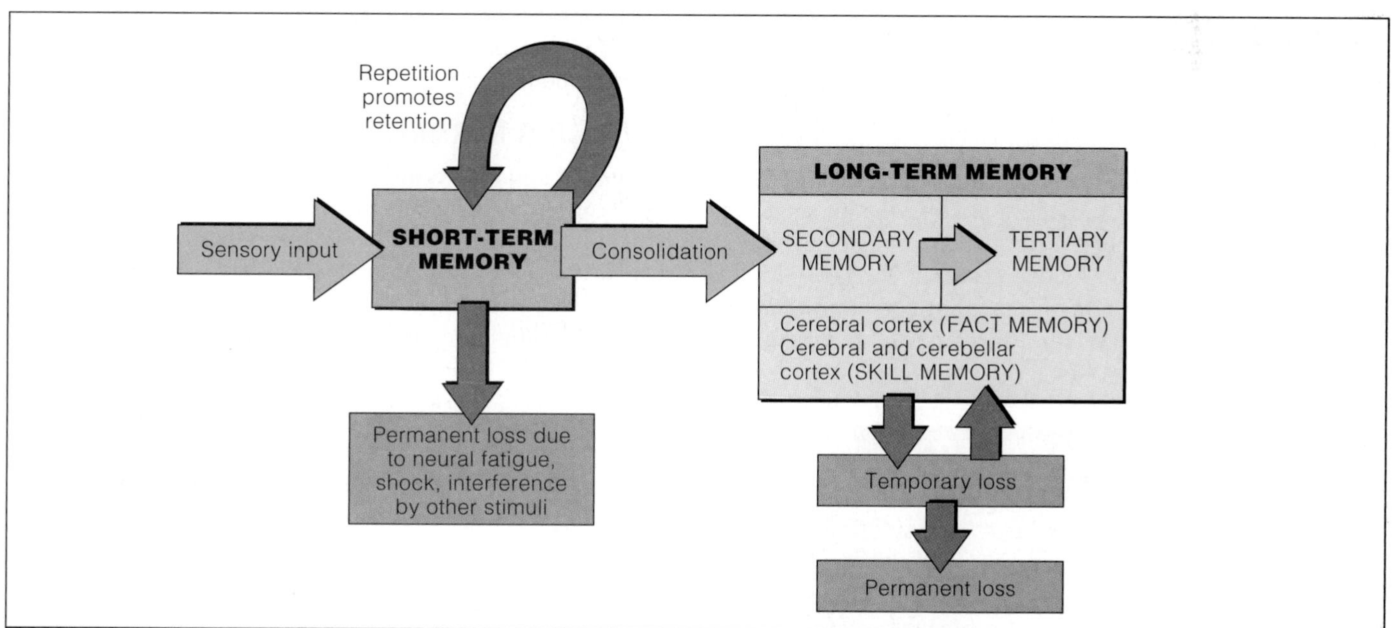

FIGURE 12–4 ■ *Memory storage. The steps needed for short-term and long-term memory and the process for transferring short-term into long-term memories.*

Source: Smock, T. K. (1999). *Physiological psychology: A neuroscience approach*. Upper Saddle River, NJ: Prentice Hall. Figure 15–19, p. 381.

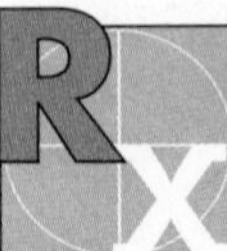

COMMUNICATION

Client with Dementia

CLIENT: "What are you doing here?"

NURSE RESPONSE 1: "Hello, my name is Betty and I would like to talk to you."

RATIONALE: This response helps you make contact with the client, establish what you are going to do to allay fears, and give an opportunity to interact in a non-threatening manner.

NURSE RESPONSE 2: "I'd like to talk with you. Can you tell me if anything is hurting you?"

RATIONALE: Many clients will be willing to talk about physical pain far easier than trying to articulate complex notions such as feelings and desires.

FUNCTIONAL URINARY INCONTINENCE, BOWEL INCONTINENCE

Incontinence of urine or feces is usually the result of confusion and failure to use the facilities. In the later stages of dementia, clients lose cortical control, but physiologic function remains. It is essential to ensure proper hygiene for clients; poor hygiene will result in infections and skin breakdown.

ALTERED NUTRITION, LESS/MORE THAN BODY REQUIREMENTS

Poor nutrition and some metabolic disorders can be the direct cause of confusion in elderly clients. The reverse can also be true; confusion and cerebral change can cause nutritional deficits. Without supervision, many older clients are not capable of providing for or ingesting adequate amounts of food. Clients who are in the later stages of DAT have symptoms of bulimia followed by total loss of appetite.

Outcome Identification: NOC

Nursing Outcomes Classification (NOC) organizes the expectations for this particular group of disorders. Clients with these disorders have varying outcomes; delirium in many cases is reversible, while dementia is not. Specific outcomes for clients experiencing cognitive disorders are listed in the nursing care plans. Clients' abilities to return to their previous lifestyles remain somewhat intact when disorders are reversible. However, in the deterioration of dementing conditions, careful scrutiny must be made of the expectations for outcomes. Family members and the client must have information about the illness and the ways that it will change lifestyle.

Planning and Implementation: NIC

Nursing interventions for clients with cognitive disorders can be divided into two broad groups: interventions for (1) clients with dementia and (2) clients with delirium. Sample nursing care plans for these clients are presented in this chapter. With few exceptions, the interventions are similar, although the overall goals are different as noted above in the Outcome Classifications. The goal with the dementia client is to minimize the loss of self-care capacity. Although functional loss is progressive, at every stage of the illness the nurse must assess and support the client's self-care capacity. Family members must also learn how to work with the client. See the Client/Family Teaching feature on page 253 for suggestions for families. With delirious clients, the overall goal for nursing intervention is to support existing sensory perception until the cognition stage can return to previous levels of functioning. Of course, in both conditions, keeping the client safe is the first priority.

PROMOTING NORMAL MOTOR BEHAVIOR

Because of impaired coordination in dementia, falls become a safety concern. Living areas must be well lit and furniture must remain in the same place. Remove any loose rugs and ensure that clients are wearing properly fitting shoes and shoes with a strap. Evaluate the client for visual and balance disturbances. Safety bars should be installed near toilets, showers, and tubs.

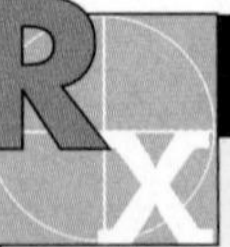

COMMUNICATION

Client with Dementia at Risk for Self-Harm

CLIENT: "I'm going to walk outside and get hit by a truck."

NURSE RESPONSE 1: "Tell me about why you are so upset."

RATIONALE: Client ventilates feelings in more constructive ways when discussing feeling states with the nurse.

NURSE RESPONSE 2: "Let's take a walk together."

RATIONALE: Client has the opportunity to use physical energy constructively by being distracted with empathic and supportive social interaction.

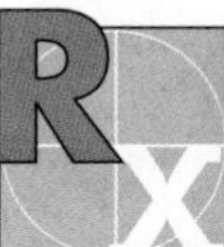

COMMUNICATION

Client with Dementia and Hallucinations

CLIENT: "Get those women out of here!"

NURSE RESPONSE 1: "Come with me. We'll go down the hall."

RATIONALE: Distracting the client from the internal stimuli, which may be transient, calms and addresses the emotional component of the client's experience.

NURSE RESPONSE 2: "You must be very nervous. Let's get you something to make you feel better."

RATIONALE: Client may need interventions (nonpharmacologic or pharmacologic) to control breakthrough symptomatology.

Teach clients who need assistance the safe use of walkers and wheelchairs. Evaluate all clients using tranquilizers and antidepressants for postural hypotension. A difference in blood pressures (BPs) taken supine and standing, wherein the standing BP is lower than the supine BP, is an indication of postural hypotension. Restlessness and wandering can be dealt with by allowing the demented client to wander in a closed milieu. Avoid crowds or large open spaces without boundaries.

In clients with delirium, hyperactivity can be decreased by controlling environmental stimuli. If this does not help, medications can be used judiciously. Take vital signs one hour before and after the administration of any medication, and observe the client carefully for signs of stupor. Interrupt prolonged periods of hypoactivity with range-of-motion exercises, frequent turning, and having the client stand up at bedside, as tolerated. During periods of fluctuating motor behavior, there is always concern for the client's safety. A staff member should be present at all times; keep the bed lowered and the side rails up. In DAT, wandering is a common and troublesome behavioral symptom. See the Intervention box on page 254 for guidelines for working with the wandering client.

MAINTAINING SELF-CARE

Allow the client to do as much as possible unassisted. The more the client can effectively control the daily routine, the less anxiety the client will experience. Remind the client about daily grooming and personal hygiene, and repeat instructions. If the client resists oral hygiene, use mouth swabs with dilute hydrogen peroxide. If the client resists this as well, having the client eat an apple may help to clean the mouth. If the client resists any routine procedures, wait a few moments and try again. The client often forgets to offer new resistance. Clients who are acutely delirious or in the last stages of dementia need total bed care.

PROMOTING ADEQUATE SLEEP

Clients with dementia and delirium respond poorly to hypnotics, which increase confusion and aggravate the disorientation that may be experienced in lowered light in older adults. A small amount of beer or wine at bedtime may produce enough relaxation without side effects. The most helpful measure may be to allow sleepless clients to wander in a confined area until they are tired. If the client is disoriented at night, make sure the room is light and without shadows. Possibly leave a radio on to provide more stimulation. Low doses of risperidone or an antianxiety agent may be prescribed. (Antianxiety medications should be used with caution and reevaluated regularly if used on a nightly basis.)

Mechanical restraints may be used to protect the client from injury or disrupting necessary medical treatments (e.g., a delirious client repeatedly tries to bear weight on a damaged limb or attempts to remove IV tubing or bandages). Use mechanical restraints according to established policy with effective and imaginative alternatives evaluated routinely to replace this method of restraint. Reassure clients who have been restrained that they are safe and that the restraints are there to protect and help them. See Chapter 34 for guidelines in the use of restraining techniques.

SUPPORTING KNOWLEDGE PROCESSES

The same interventions that are used to support memory and orientation are applied to the support of knowledge processes.

CLIENT/FAMILY TEACHING

Suggestions for Families Who Have Just Had a Family Member Diagnosed with DAT

- Have a family meeting and discuss strategies to care for the client at the present time and in the future, based on family responsibilities and resources.
- Contact the Alzheimer's Disease and Related Disorders Association (ADRDA) and request information. View their videotapes and read the available written material.
- Go to a support group for family caregivers.
- Contact an attorney and make decisions about power of attorney, and the control and distribution of client/family assets.
- Familiarize yourself with community resources such as day care treatment centers, nursing homes, and respite care for AD clients.
- Purchase a bracelet for the client identifying her/him as having AD.

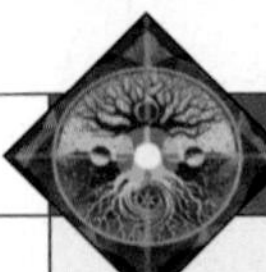

Case Study

Client with Dementia

Identifying Information

Mrs. Crownheart is an 83-year-old widow living alone in an apartment on her husband's retirement income and also receives Social Security. She was referred by her 72-year-old brother, who states, "She has been extremely forgetful lately," and brought her in for an evaluation.

She comes to the clinic stating, "I had nothing to do with coming here. My brother's daughter must have a friend here." She does admit to feeling confused with episodes of "not remembering things from one moment to the next." Mrs. Crownheart does not remember how long this has been going on but attributes it all to normal aging. Her brother describes her as "forgetful and just not herself." He has visited his sister and found the door unlocked and the stove burner on.

History

Mrs. Crownheart has no prior psychiatric history. Mrs. Crownheart states that her husband "dropped dead two years ago while watching TV." She has a 52-year old daughter who is married with three children and "lives in another state." Her brother and his daughter live nearby and are fairly active in their relationship with Mrs. Crownheart.

Mrs. Crownheart seems to have had a normal adulthood, passing through developmental milestones such as marriage, parenting, grandparenting, retirement, and widowhood without any problems. She had no formal occupational training. She reminisces at length and with great detail about her work at the theater as a dresser. Mrs. Crownheart married when she was 21. When asked how long she'd been married before her husband died, she replied, "Too many years." Her brother was able to report that she had been married for 60 years before her husband's death. Mrs. Crownheart described her marital relationship as "not very good." She routinely spends her days in her apartment.

Mrs. Crownheart has no history of major illness or injury. She states her appetite is "so-so," while her brother says she seems to have lost weight. When asked if she had any difficulty sleeping, she responded defensively, "No! No! No!"

Current Mental Status

Mrs. Crownheart is a cooperative elderly woman who appears somewhat unkempt with uncombed hair, wrinkled dress, and smelling of strong perfume. She is oriented to person and place, and she knows the year, but is unsure of the month and date. Her fund of general knowledge is poor, and she is unable to name the last five presidents. Mrs. Crownheart is alert, labile, superficial, sporadically anxious, and irritable. She denies having illusions, hallucinations, or delusions. She shows loose associations but can be redirected easily. She seems distractible and appears to have difficulty concentrating. She minimizes cognitive deficits, and confabulates and perserverates to hide them.

Other Subjective or Objective Clinical Data

Mrs. Crownheart is not on any medications; suicide/violence potential minimal.

Family education is imperative and can take the form of professional help and/or self-help groups. For a complete listing of professional help and/or self-help groups, refer to the Companion Website.

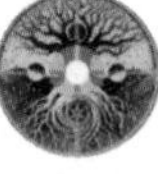

SUPPORTING OPTIMAL MEMORY FUNCTIONING

Gently orient the client. To allay anxiety, do not argue with the client about verbal discrepancies. Rather, direct the client toward areas of interest that are familiar and pleasurable. The environment should support whatever memory functions are still intact. Do not test the client for episodic memory unless it is absolutely necessary. If the client uses confabulation to fill in the memory gap, do not argue; note it as an ego-protective mechanism. Other strength-enhancing behavioral and psychotherapeutic treatment reminders are summarized in Box 12–2 on page 256.

Because of their episodic memory loss, DAT clients do not respond well to reality orientation classes. However, you can trigger semantic memory by initiating a procedure the client can then complete. In this leading technique, a combination of words and nonverbal cues are used. For instance, while handing the client a

INTERVENTION

Guidelines for Working with the Wandering Client

Strategy	Rationale
• Stay with the client, or be sure the client is in a safe, enclosed area.	• Wandering clients can get hurt. Safety is the first priority.
• Maintain a calm demeanor.	• Clients notice the feelings of others.
• Approach the client slowly and give her or him space. Use touch only if the client responds positively to it.	• The aim is to prevent aggressiveness, fear, and anxiety. Each client is different in response to touch, with specific people.
• Determine why the client is wandering. Is she or he upset? Thirsty? Hungry? Searching for family?	• When we understand why the client wanders, we can plan client-specific interventions.
• Meet the client's needs. If the client is searching, be supportive: "You are looking for X. . . . You must miss X. . . ."	• Support decreases anxiety, fear, and hostility.
• Attempt to engage the client in a repetitive activity such as rolling yarn or folding towels.	• Repetitive activities use energy and can be diversional

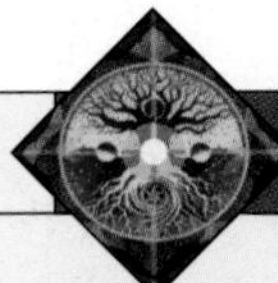

Nursing Care Plan

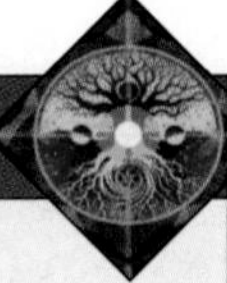

Nursing Diagnosis: Altered Thought Processes related to memory loss of dementia of the Alzheimer's type

Expected Outcome: Mrs. Crownheart will maintain optimal cognitive functioning.

Short-Term Goals	*Interventions*	*Rationale*
Mrs. Crownheart does not express delusions and appears less anxious.	• Structure environment to enhance memory (clock, calendar, orientation cues) • Label objects. • Provide consistent daily routine that does not overload her senses. • Validate the feelings expressed with delusional materials; do not argue with delusions. • Discuss psychopharmacologic interventions with other team members including acetylcholinesterase inhibitors and an atypical antipsychotic. • Teach family how to deal with delusions, confusion, and anger.	Dependable environment addresses Mrs. Crownheart's emotional health while supporting maximal functioning.

Nursing Diagnosis: Altered Nutrition: Less Than Body Requirements related to loss of memory in dementia of the Alzheimer's type (Mrs. Crownheart forgets to eat).

Expected Outcome: Mrs. Crownheart maintains or gains weight.

Short-term Goals	*Interventions*	*Rationale*
Mrs. Crownheart will have an adequate daily intake of food and fluids.	• Design home health care monitoring of food/fluid intake and include family in the effort. • Provide mealtime supervision and assistance if necessary. • High-protein and -carbohydrate diet in finger-food form with double portions. • Weigh weekly. • Assist family in developing strategies to ensure Mrs. Crownheart eats enough every day.	Enlisting family and health care providers in the effort to improve and maintain calorie intake assures a comprehensive and competent plan.

toothbrush and pointing toward the mouth with a brushing motion, say, "Brush your teeth." Constant repetition in a kind, firm manner is often necessary. See the Nursing Self-Awareness feature on page 256 to evaluate your skills in this area. Music therapy may also trigger past associations, aid the client's long-term memory, and help a normally aphasic client participate in a group.

MEDICATION MANAGEMENT

Drug therapy has also been proposed to assist the client in the early stages of DAT to maintain memory and orientation (see Chapter 31). Galantamine (Reminyl), donepezil (Aricept), rivastigmine (Exelon), and tacrine (Cognex), all potent acetylcholinesterase inhibitors, are available for treatment of DAT. Clinical trials and treatment outcome information for these drugs have resulted in both positive and negative results. The problems in demonstrating overall efficacy are believed to be due to the heterogeneity in DAT clients and the fact that these medications provide mild to moderate improvement.

PROMOTING OPTIMAL ORIENTATION

Structure the client's environment to support cognitive functions. The client should be wearing whatever aids (hearing, vision) are necessary to prevent sensory loss or distortion.

BOX 12–2 Reminders: Behavioral and Psychotherapeutic

- Calendars or other concrete reminders of what is going on by day of the week, date, and time.
- Objects or wall hangings that mirror the current season or holiday events; pictures that reflect seasonal events and people's actions and behaviors around those events (remember to be culturally sensitive).
- Photo album and sign-in book for visitors to remind clients of who visited and when.
- Discover a client's preferred avocational pursuits to add cues to the environment, which will be positively received (e.g., a team schedule for a sports fan).

Reminiscence

- Clients often need to talk, even repetitively, about important prior experiences as a part of the process of resolving feelings about these experiences and about difficulties in the recall of them.
- Encourage discussion of likely social and historical contexts operative during the earlier phases of the client's life (e.g., The Great Depression of the 1930s, World War II, and important events of the 1950s).

Positively Reinforcing and Providing Opportunities for Adaptive Functioning and Cognitive Preservation

Careful evaluation of remaining cognitive strengths through:

- Observation
- Psychological testing
- Diagnostic interviewing

When areas of strength are diagnosed:

- Provide opportunities for the client to exercise them.
- Give positive reinforcements such as praise, a pleasant experience such as listening to music, or a caring interaction when clients are exercising better preserved abilities.

When areas of deficit are diagnosed:

- Assist the client in coping with deficits (i.e., training and encouragement to use written reminders to compensate for failing memory).
- Give clients positive reinforcement for using such strategies.

MediaLink Case Study: Treating Clients with Alzheimer's Disease

Familiar objects from home, such as slippers, robe, and photographs, may also help orient the client. Easily read clocks, orientation boards, and a consistent daily routine that includes physical activity and socialization without sensory overload will also help orient the client. Verbally orient the client during conversation. Do not quiz the client about discrepancies.

SUPPORTING OPTIMAL VERBAL EXPRESSION

As communication skills decrease, the client's nonverbal communications become more important. Clients respond physically to the environment, especially if they feel threatened. Call the client by name, approach in clear view, and give simple directions.

SUPPORTING APPROPRIATE CONDUCT/IMPULSE CONTROL

All measures used to support perception and orientation are imperative here. The client may strike out in response to hallucinations or delusions. The client functions best in an environment where stimulation is controlled and sensory overload prevented. All changes, whether environmental or personal, need to be made slowly. Always approach the client in full view, calling his or her name, and refrain from touching the client. Requests should be simple and nondemanding. A client with short-term memory loss can often be distracted.

SUPPORTING OPTIMAL ROLE PERFORMANCE

To continue functioning in the family, the client must be viewed as an active member. Most clients with dementia remain at home until the caregiver can no longer manage the client's needs. The family needs support throughout this time such as home visits, day care, respite care, and support groups.

After the client is institutionalized, the family should be an integral part of the client's daily routine. Family members need extra emotional support as the rewards for maintaining involvement diminish. For the demented client, role maintenance involves supporting the client's need to be oriented.

MAINTAINING OPTIMAL ATTENTION SPAN

Repeat requests as needed. Speak in simple phrases, loud enough to be heard, and reinforce meaning with gestures. To decrease distractibility and hyperalertness, keep environmental stimulation at a minimum. Every effort should be made to lower the client's anxiety level by moving slowly, speaking clearly, and providing new information slowly.

PROMOTING OPTIMAL SELF-CONCEPT/SELF-ESTEEM

During the early stages of dementia, every effort should be made to maintain clients' self-esteem as they struggle with the personal awareness of cognitive loss. Encourage clients to

***Nursing* SELF-AWARENESS**

An Inventory for Nurses Who Care for Clients with Cognitive Disorders

- How do I feel about working with clients with cognitive disorders?
- What do I like about working with them?
- What frustrates me about working with them?
- What behavioral symptoms (e.g., wandering, agitation, hallucinations, delusions, hostility, eating problems, etc.) do I feel most competent to deal with? Least competent?
- What strategies have I used with clients that have been successful? Unsuccessful?
- Who are my favorite clients? Why? My least favorite clients? Why?
- What can I do to become more knowledgeable and/or skilled in dealing with clients with cognitive disorders?

express their fears and concerns, and listen attentively. Allow for the expression of anger and sadness.

Manipulate the environment to help the client with a failing memory. Helpful measures include labeling the bathroom and bedroom, posting notes to remind the client to turn off the stove and lock the door, and labeling the contents of drawers. Gently remind the client of forgotten events, and do not confront confabulations. Encourage the family to maintain the client as a productive member of this important group.

SUPPORTING OPTIMAL PERCEPTUAL FUNCTIONING

A quiet environment with soft music prevents the client from experiencing sensory overload. When speaking with the client, stand or sit so that you are in direct view. First giving a verbal warning and using touch with caution, touch the client's shoulder or hand, and slowly and clearly explain all procedures. Sometimes a very soothing touch can overexcite the client, who may respond by striking out. Make sure that the client is wearing hearing aids and eyeglasses if necessary.

In responding to hallucinations, simply state that you understand that these sensations can be very powerful and even disturbing. Do not argue or ask the client to elaborate. Take care of the emotional response (e.g., if the client is frightened, reassure) in your interactions. Give reassurance that these thoughts will go away. Say, "You are in a safe place." Do not leave the client alone or in an isolated room without some stimulation to help the client block out the hallucinations and support reality testing. The room should be well lit and without shadows or glare. If the client becomes combative, briefly intervene to redirect and prevent harm to self or others. Then attempt to distract, reassuring the client, "You are in a safe place."

PROMOTING OPTIMAL PATTERNS OF ELIMINATION

A regular toileting schedule helps demented clients control bowel and urinary incontinence. Clients are often not able to let the nurse know when they have to use the toilet or have soiled themselves.

During the early stage of dementia, a toileting routine is essential. As the disease progresses, the client no longer recognizes a toilet or its purpose. Such a client may resist sitting on the toilet. Forcing the client will only produce agitation and combativeness. Distract and try again. If all efforts at maintaining a routine fail, use disposable pants or diapers. The use of catheters and external drains is not recommended because of the possibility of infection and their certain removal by a confused client.

PROMOTING OPTIMAL NUTRITIONAL STATUS

Monitor the client's food and fluid intake. Give hyperactive clients a diet high in protein and carbohydrates, in finger-food form. Some clients may need double portions. Clients who chew constantly need to be reminded to swallow. Depending on the client's level of perception and motor activity, supervision and assistance at mealtimes may be necessary. Weigh the client routinely, and increase caloric intake as needed. In the final stages of the disease, the client loses all interest in food and must receive nasogastric, gastrostomy, or intravenous feedings.

Evaluation

Assess both the effectiveness of all interventions and the response to them of the client with a cognitive disorder. For guidance on self-assessment, see the Nursing Self-Awareness feature below.

DELIRIUM EVALUATION CRITERIA

The evaluation of nursing care for clients with delirium is based on the premise that clients are capable of returning to their previous level of functioning. During that process the goal is to help the client maintain optimal levels of sensory perception, participate in activities of daily living, and maintain physiologic homeostasis.

DEMENTIA EVALUATION CRITERIA

Dementia entails progressive intellectual, behavioral, and physiologic deterioration. The goal of nursing care is not to affect a cure but rather to sustain the client at the optimal level of self-care. Help the family sustain a personally rewarding relationship with their loved one throughout this terminal process.

Nursing SELF AWARENESS

Triggering Semantic Memory

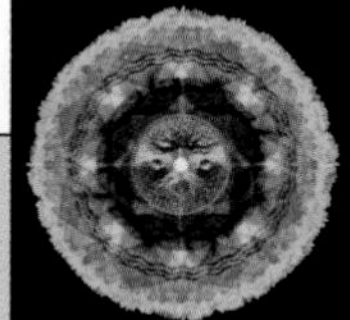

DAT clients experience episodic memory loss; therefore, interactions may not be retained, and repetition is necessary. Answer the following questions about your skill level when triggering semantic memory by initiating a procedure the client can then complete.

1. In this leading technique, a combination of words and nonverbal cues are used. Are your words and nonverbal cues
   Precise? ☐ Yes ☐ No
   Concise? ☐ Yes ☐ No
   Clear? ☐ Yes ☐ No
2. Constant repetition in a kind, firm manner is necessary. When you have to repeat yourself a number of times, are the following interaction impacts present?
   Is your tone on the third repetition identical to your tone the first time you said this? ☐ Yes ☐ No
   Is your affect kind the fourth time you've repeated yourself?
   ☐ Yes ☐ No
   Are your movements remaining the same even though you have to repeat them? ☐ Yes ☐ No
   Are you consistent? ☐ Yes ☐ No

   If you answered "Yes," you are doing very well and your communications with clients who have these disorders will be more effective. If any of these areas has a "No" response, you may need to improve the connection between your verbal and nonverbal cues as well as examine your emotional reactions to the need to repeat basic instructions.

Case Management

Case management of the client with dementia involves developing and organizing a program to address the symptoms present. It must be a flexible system to respond to the changing needs of the client as deterioration progresses. There is a great deal of contact with the caregiver(s). Provide regular monitoring and supervise the following:

- Regular physical examinations with a primary care provider.
- Prescription medications.
- Nutrition.
- OTC medications.
- Finances.
- Interpersonal relationships.

Community-Based Care

Community-based care for the client with dementia could involve appointments in a clinic setting, a day program designed for the current level of difficulties in functioning, medication clinic appointments, a supportive group, or some combination. Frequently, a family member or caregiver is involved, especially due to the need for transportation.

Counseling and face-to-face contacts are a way to decrease the social isolation inherent in a client with dementia. Psychotherapy can be useful to help mildly to moderately demented clients cope with loss of cognitive functions. The features of counseling or therapy would include:

- Empathic listening.
- Support.
- Working on coping methods.
- Providing the client with outlets for distress that might otherwise exacerbate disturbed behavior (e.g., talking over fears rather than acting out behaviorally).

Home Care

The most effective treatment for the client with dementia is a balance between stimulation/environmental demand and whatever internal resources remain for the client. The home would need to be evaluated for meeting the changing needs of the client. Some revisions are usually necessary so that safe wandering is available, dangers are minimized through safety devices, and activity can be controlled. A cycle of stimulation and rest is best so the client's abilities are engaged but not overwhelmed.

Supportive counseling is frequently helpful when providing home care for clients with dementia. You must understand the premorbid personality and developmental history of someone with dementia because the dementing process is superimposed on the preexisting personality. Get a picture for the role anxiety played in clients' lives, their previous self-view, and how conscious they were of themselves and their actions' impacts on others. Once anxiety is reduced for the client, the tendency toward better functioning will ensue.

Clients with mild to moderate dementia often go through stages of loss:

- Denial
- Emotion (Anger)
- Bargaining
- Depression
- Acceptance

For severely demented clients, the focus of treatment expands to include caregivers. Whether the caregivers are relatives, friends, or health care providers they may require explanations of symptoms and help in designing behavioral interventions. Caregivers working with severely demented clients may require help in coping with stress, countertransference (see Chapter 28), or issues with becoming discouraged.

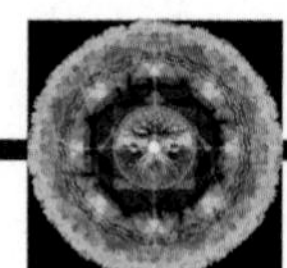

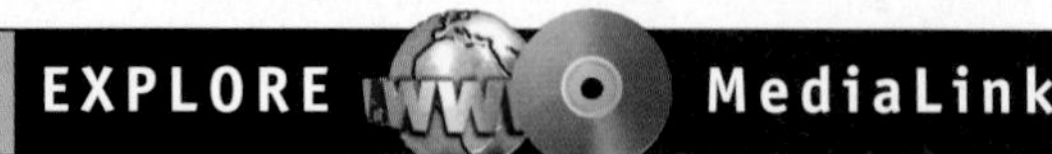

NCLEX review, case studies, and other interactive resources for this chapter can be found on the Companion Website at http://www.prenhall.com/kneisl. Click on Chapter 12 to select the activities for this chapter.

For animations, video tutorials, more NCLEX review questions, and an audio glossary, access the accompanying CD-ROM in this textbook.

BIBLIOGRAPHY

Alzheimer's Disease and Related Disorders Association. (2002). *Alzheimer's disease and related disorders*. Retrieved September 10, 2002, from the World Wide Web, www.alz.org.

Alzheimer, A. (1907). Uber eine eigenartige Erkraukung der Hirwrinde. *Allegmeine Zeitschrift für Psychiatrie, 64*, 146–148.

American Psychiatric Association. (2000). *Diagnostic and statistical manual of mental disorders* (4th ed., Text Revision) (DSM-IV-TR). Washington, DC: Author.

Andrews, N. J., Farrington, C. P., Cousens, S. N., Smith, P. G., Ward, H., Knight, R. S. G., et al. (2000). Incidence of variant Creutzfeldt–Jakob disease in the UK. *Lancet, 356,* 481–482.

Ballard, C., McLaren, A., & Morris, C. (2000). Non-Alzheimer dementias. *Current Opinion in Psychiatry, 13,* 409–414.

Berlit, P. (2000). Successful prophylaxis of recurrent transient global amnesia with metoprolol. *Neurology, 55,* 1937–1938.

Dijkstra, A., Brown, L., Havens, B., Romeren, T. I., Zanotti, R., Dassen, T., & van den Heuvel, W. (2000). An international psychometric testing of the Care Dependency Scale. *Journal of Advanced Nursing, 31,* 944–952.

Dresser, R. (2001). Advance directives in dementia research. *IRB: Ethics & Human Research 23,* 1-6.

Elias, M. F., Beiser, A., Wolf, P. A., Au, R., White, R. F., & D'Agostino, R. B. (2000). The preclinical phase of Alzheimer's disease: A 22-year prospective study of the Framingham cohort. *Archives of Neurology, 57,* 808–813.

Farber, N. B., Rubin, E. H., Newcomer, J. W., Kinscherf, D. A., Miller, J. P., Morris, J. C., et al. (2000). Increased neocortical neurofibrillary tangle density in subjects with Alzheimer Disease and psychosis. *Archives of General Psychiatry, 57,* 1165–1173.

Finkel, S. I., & Burns, A. (2000). Introduction. *International Psychogeriatrics, 12, (Suppl 1),* 9–12.

Folstein, M., Folstein, S., & McHugh, P. (1975). Mini-mental state: A practical method for grading the cognitive state of patients for the clinician. *Journal of Psychiatric Residency, 12,* 189–198.

Gottlieb, G. L. (2000). Geriatric psychiatry. In H. H. Goldman (Ed.), *Review of general psychiatry* (5th ed.). New York: Lange Medical Books/McGraw-Hill.

Grob, P., Lorreck, D., Binder, R., & Haller, E. (2000). Dementia, delirium, and amnestic disorders. In H. H. Goldman (Ed.), *Review of general psychiatry* (5th ed.). New York: Lange Medical Books/McGraw-Hill.

Grubb, N. R., Fox, K. A. A., Smith, K., Best, J., Blane, A., Ebmeier, K. P., Glabus, M. F., & O'Carroll, R. E. (2000). Memory impairment in out-of-hospital cardiac arrest survivors is associated with global reduction in brain volume, not focal hippocampal injury. *Stroke, 31,* 1509–1514.

Guttman, R. (1999). *Diagnosis, management and treatment of dementia: A practical guide for primary care physicians.* Chicago, IL: American Medical Association.

Hall, W. D., & Leipzig, R. M. (2000). Update in geriatrics. *Annals of Internal Medicine, 133,* 894–900.

Hansel, P. A. (1999). Mad cow disease—the OR connection. *AORN Journal, 70,* 224–238.

Hauber, A. B., Gnanasakthy, A., Snyder, E. H., Bala, M. V., Richter, A., & Mauskopf, J. A. (2000). Potential savings in the cost of caring for Alzheimer's disease: Treatment with rivastigmine. *Pharmacoeconomics, 17,* 351–360.

Huntington Study Group. (2001). A randomized, placebo-controlled trial of coenzyme Q_{10} and remacemide in Huntington's disease. *Neurology, 57,* 397–404.

Inouye, S. K., van Dyck, C. H., Alessi, C. A., Balkin, S., Siegal, A. P., & Horwitz, R. I. (1990). Clarifying confusion: The confusion assessment method: A new method for detection of delirium. *Annals of Internal Medicine, 113,* 941–948.

Lawlor, P. G., Fainsinger, R. L., & Bruera, E. D. (2000). Delirium at end of life: Critical issues in clinical practice and research. *Journal of the American Medical Association, 284,* 2427–2429.

Lopez, O. L., Hamilton, R. L., Becker, J. T., Wisniewski, S., Kaufer, D. I., & DeKosky, S. T. (2000). Severity of cognitive impairment and the clinical diagnosis of AD with Lewy bodies. *Neurology, 54,* 1780–1787.

Lyketsos, C. G., Steinberg, M., Tschanz, J. T., Norton, M. C., Steffens, D. C., & Breitner, J. C. S. (2000). Mental and behavioral disturbances in dementia: Findings from the Cache County Study on Memory in Aging. *American Journal of Psychiatry, 157,* 708–714.

McKeith, I. G., Galasko, D., Kosaka, K., Perry, E. K., Dickson D. W. Hansen L. A., et al. (1996). Consensus guidelines for the clinical and pathologic diagnosis of dementia with Lewy bodies (DLB): Report of the consortium on DLB international workshop. *Neurology, 47,* 1113–1124.

Meagher, D. J. (2001). Delirium: Optimising management. *British Medical Journal, 322,* 144–149.

Moudgil, S. S., Azzouz, M., Al-Azzaz, A., Haut, M., & Gutmann, L. (2000). Amnesia due to fornix infarction. *Stroke, 31,* 1418–1419.

Rabins, P. V., Black, B. S., Roca, R., et al. (2000). Effectiveness of a nurse-based outreach program for identifying and treating psychiatric illness in the elderly. *Journal of the American Medical Association, 283,* 2802–2809.

Reisberg, B., Ferris, S. H., Franssen, E., Jenkins, E. C., & Wisniewski, K. E. (1989). Clinical features of a neuropathologically verified familial Alzheimer's cohort with onset in the fourth decade: Comparison with senile onset Alzheimer's disease and etiopathogenic implications. *Progress in Clinical & Biological Research, 317,* 43–54.

Ritchie, K., & Touchon, J. (2000). Mild cognitive impairment: Conceptual basis and current nosological status. *Lancet, 355,* 225–228.

Sachdev, P. I., Smith, J. S, & Cathcart, S. (2001). Schizophrenia-like psychosis following traumatic brain injury: A chart-based descriptive and case-control study. *Psychological Medicine, 31,* 231–239.

Sander, D., Winbeck, K., Etgen, T., Knapp, R., Klingelhofer, J., & Conrad, B. (2000). Disturbance of venous flow patterns in patients with transient global amnesia. *Lancet, 356,* 1982–1984.

Tschanz, J. T., Welsh-Bohmer, K. A., Skoog, I., West, N., Norton, M. C., & Wyse, B. W., et al. (2000). Dementia diagnoses from clinical and neuropsychological data compared: The Cache County study. *Neurology, 54,* 1290–1296.

Walker, M. P., Ayre, G. A., Cummings, J. L., Wesnes, K., McKeith, I. G., O'Brien, J. T., & Ballard, C. G. (2000). The clinician assessment of fluctuation and the one day fluctuation assessment scale: Two methods to assess fluctuating confusion in dementia. *British Journal of Psychiatry, 177,* 252–256.

White, K. T., & Cummings, J. L. (1997). Neuropsychiatric aspects of Alzheimer's disease and other dementing illnesses. In S. C. Yudofsky & R. E. Hales (Eds.). *Textbook of Neuropsychiatry* (3rd ed.) (pp. 823–854). Washington, DC: American Psychiatric Press.

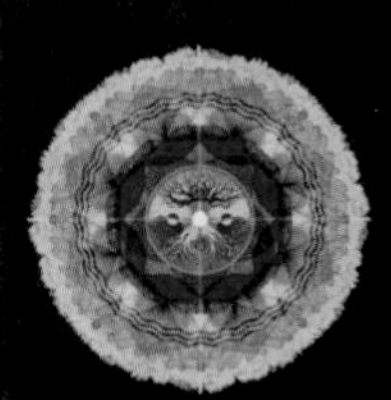

13

Chapter THIRTEEN

Substance-Related Disorders

EILEEN TRIGOBOFF
HOLLY SKODOL WILSON

KEY TERMS

alcohol-induced persisting amnestic disorder (Korsakoff's syndrome)
alcoholic encephalopathy (Wernicke's encephalopathy)
blackouts
codependent
delirium tremens (DTs)
enabler
fetal alcohol syndrome (FAS)
substance abuse
substance dependence
substance intoxication
substance withdrawal
substance withdrawal syndrome
tolerance
withdrawal

FOCUS QUESTIONS

- **What are the major theoretic explanations for substance-related disorders?**
- **Which groups are at risk for substance-related disorders?**
- **How do the physical, psychological, and withdrawal effects of the major categories of substances manifest themselves?**
- **How would you describe the variety of short-term and long-term nursing intervention strategies for clients with substance-related disorders?**
- **What are your outcome criteria for clients who have substance-related disorders?**
- **Have you examined your own feelings and attitudes about clients with substance-related disorders?**

MediaLink 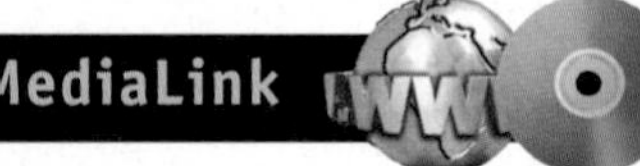 www.prenhall.com/kneisl

Additional resources for this chapter can be found on the Student CD-ROM accompanying this textbook, and on the Companion Website at www.prenhall.com/kneisl. Click on Chapter 13 to select the activities for this chapter.

CD-ROM
- Audio Glossary
- NCLEX Review
- Occupying a Receptor Site Animation
- Morphine (Astramorph PF, Duramorph, and Other Opioids) Drug Mechanism in Action Animation

Companion Website
- Additional NCLEX Review
- Care Plan: Alcohol Withdrawal
- Case Study: Teen Heroin Users

CHAPTER OUTLINE

CROSS REFERENCES

Other topics relevant to this content are: Anxiety and substance abuse, Chapter 16; Clients with a dual diagnosis of a mental disorder and substance abuse, Chapter 21; Cognitive disorders, Chapter 12; Depression, Chapter 15; Negative imagery, Chapter 30; Polydrug use among older adults, Chapter 27; Psychobiology, Chapter 4; Risk of HIV transmission for intravenous drug users, Chapter 24; Substance abuse with schizophrenia, Chapter 14; Substance use in adolescents, Chapter 26; Suicide assessment, Chapter 22.

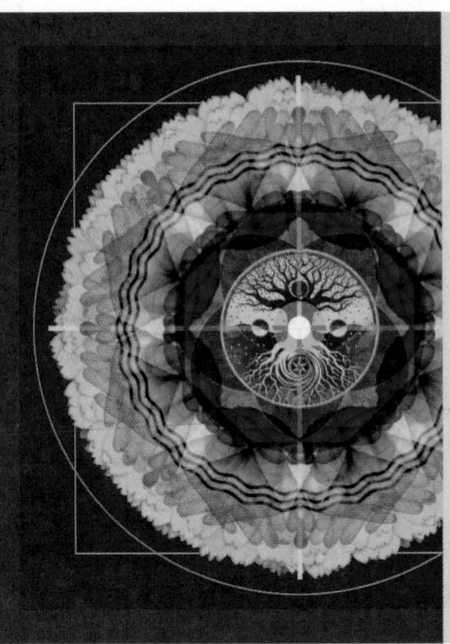

CRITICAL THINKING CHALLENGE

Billie is a 19-year-old homeless African-American woman pregnant with her third child and addicted to crack cocaine. When she appeared at your hospital's Family Practice Clinic for prenatal care one month before her delivery, she was referred to your team for assessment and treatment for her addiction. Billie is concerned about losing her children if she enters a drug treatment program, and she is fearful that her unborn baby is already damaged. She shuns Alcoholics Anonymous (AA) and Narcotics Anonymous (NA) because admitting "powerlessness" and "turning her life over to God the Father" is unacceptable to her; as a marginalized poor black woman, she's had it with powerlessness and would rather empower her daughters so that they "don't turn their lives over to men." Others on your treatment team initially refuse to accept her as an outpatient because she will not promise complete abstinence and is reluctant to commit to attending one NA or AA meeting per day. What are your options for her care? ■

Drug and alcohol abuse, already a widespread problem, is rapidly escalating. Substance abuse is a psychosocial and a biologic problem. Television and radio advertisements entice viewers with the hope of relief from pain and problems; they demonstrate that a life without stress is possible. The values portrayed are clear: Discomfort should be erased; drinking is vital to a stress-free life; drugs are acceptable mediators of emotions.

Substance abuse is a complex public health issue with grave ramifications. It increases the crime rate, auto accident deaths, number of teenage pregnancies, and the suicide rate. Individuals and families are destroyed. Every part of a substance abuser's life—social life, family life, work productivity and relationships, physical health—is affected. Substance abuse in the work environment increases accidents, workers' compensation claims, absenteeism, and theft while decreasing the quality of life for the other workers and potentially decreasing the quality of the work performed overall.

This chapter is a biopsychosocial exploration relevant to applying the nursing process with clients who have substance-related disorders. The significance of a knowledge base on this topic and the nurturing of caring attitudes as well as skills are underscored in the American Nurses Association Standards of Addictions Nursing Practice in Box 13–1.

Substance-Related Disorders

According to the DSM-IV-TR (APA, 2000), substance-related disorders are disorders that are: (1) a consequence of abusing a drug (such as alcohol), (2) the side effects of a medication (such as antihistamines), or (3) related to exposure to a toxin (fuel, paint, or other inhalants). Substance-related disorders are divided into two groups:

1. Substance use disorders that include substance dependence and substance abuse.
2. Substance-induced disorders (including substance intoxication and substance withdrawal as well as other substance-induced disorders such as substance-induced cognitive disorders, mood disorders, and the like).

This chapter focuses on substance dependence and substance abuse. The material refers to intoxication and withdrawal issues for those classes of substances that have traditionally been called psychoactive drugs. Substance-induced disorders are addressed in appropriate chapters elsewhere in this text. (See, for example, Chapters 12, 14, 15, and 16.)

Substance Dependence

Substance dependence is defined as a maladaptive pattern of substance use leading to clinically significant impairment or distress. The hallmarks of this pattern are:

- **Tolerance**, which is needing increased amounts of a substance to achieve the desired effect.
- **Withdrawal**, which is the uncomfortable and maladaptive physiologic and cognitive behavioral changes that are associated with lowered blood or tissue concentrations of a substance after an individual has been engaged in heavy use.
- Compulsive use.
- Needing larger amounts of the substance than intended.
- Making unsuccessful efforts to cut down or regulate substance use.
- Devoting a great deal of time trying to obtain the substance.
- Using the substance or recovering from the effects of the substance.
- Continuing to use the substance despite the recognition of associated adverse effects and difficulties.

BOX 13–1 ANA Standards of Addictions Nursing Practice

Standard I: Theory

The nurse uses appropriate knowledge from nursing theory and related disciplines in the practice of addictions nursing.

Standard II: Data Collection

Data collection is continual and systematic and is communicated effectively to the treatment team throughout each phase of the nursing process.

Standard III: Diagnosis

The nurse uses nursing diagnoses congruent with accepted nursing and interprofessional classification systems of addictions and associated physiological and psychological disorders to express conclusions supported by data obtained through the nursing process.

Standard IV: Planning

The nurse establishes a plan of care for the patient that is based on nursing diagnoses, addresses specific goals, defines expected outcomes, and delineates nursing actions unique to each patient's needs.

Standard V: Intervention

The nurse implements actions, independently and/or in collaboration with peers, members of other disciplines, and patients in prevention, intervention, and rehabilitation phases of the care of patients with health problems related to patterns of abuse and addiction.

Standard Va: Intervention: Therapeutic alliance
Standard Vb: Intervention: Education
Standard Vc: Intervention: Self-help groups
Standard Vd: Intervention: Pharmacological therapies
Standard Ve: Intervention: Therapeutic environment
Standard Vf: Intervention: Counseling

Standard VI: Evaluation

The nurse evaluates the responses of the patient and revises nursing diagnoses, interventions, and treatment plan accordingly.

Standard VII: Ethical Care

The nurse's decisions and activities on behalf of patients are in keeping with personal and professional codes of ethics and in accord with legal statutes.

Standard VIII: Quality Assurance

The nurse participates in peer review and other staff evaluation and quality assurance processes to assure that patients with abuse and addiction problems receive quality care.

Standard IX: Continuing Education

The nurse assumes responsibility for his or her own continuing education and professional development and contributes to the professional growth of others who work with or are learning about persons with abuse and addiction problems.

Standard X: Interdisciplinary Collaboration

The nurse collaborates with the interdisciplinary treatment team and consults with other health and evaluating programs and other activities related to addictions nursing.

Standard XI: Use of Community Health System

The nurse participates with other members of the community in assessing, planning and implementing, and evaluating community health services that attend to primary, secondary, and tertiary prevention of addictions.

Standard XII: Research

The nurse contributes to the nursing care of patients with addictions and to the addictions area of practice through innovations in theory and practice and participation in research, and communicates these contributions.

Source: Reprinted with permission from American Nurses Association, *Standards of Addictions Nursing Practice with Selected Diagnoses and Criteria,* © 1988 American Nurses Publishing, American Nurses Foundation/American Nurses Association.

This diagnosis can be made for every class of substance except caffeine. A summary of the DSM-IV-TR diagnostic criteria for substance dependence appears in the box on page 264. The latest information on substance abuse can be found at the Substance Abuse & Mental Health Services Administration (SAMHSA) Web site at www.sam hsa.gov/.

Substance Abuse

Substance abuse is characterized by a pattern of repeated use of substances that is maladaptive in that significant adverse consequences occur. Examples include the failure to fulfill major role obligations, using substances in physically hazardous situations, and recurrent social and relationship problems. A summary of the DSM-IV-TR diagnostic criteria for substance abuse is also in the box on page 264.

Substance Intoxication

Substance intoxication refers to a reversible syndrome of maladaptive physiologic and behavioral changes that are due to the effects of a substance on a person's central nervous system (CNS). The syndrome includes disturbances of mood (such as belligerence or mood lability), perception, the sleep–wake cycle, attention, thinking, judgment, and psychomotor as well as interpersonal behavior. The box on page 265 summarizes the DSM-IV-TR diagnostic criteria for substance intoxication.

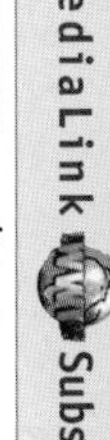

MediaLink Substance Abuse Administration

DSM-IV-TR **Diagnostic Criteria for Substance Abuse vs. Substance Dependence**

DIAGNOSTIC CRITERIA FOR SUBSTANCE ABUSE	DIAGNOSTIC CRITERIA FOR SUBSTANCE DEPENDENCE
A. A maladaptive pattern of substance use leading to clinically significant impairment or distress, as manifested by one (or more) of the following, occurring within a 12-month period: **1.** recurrent substance use resulting in a failure to fulfill major role obligations at work, school, or home **2.** recurrent substance use in situations in which it is physically hazardous **3.** recurrent substance-related legal problems **4.** continued substance use despite having persistent or recurrent social or interpersonal problems caused or exacerbated by the effects of the substance **B.** The symptoms have never met the criteria for substance dependence for this class of substance.	A maladaptive pattern of substance use, leading to clinically significant impairment or distress, as manifested by three (or more) of the following, occurring at any time in the same 12-month period: **1.** tolerance **2.** withdrawal **3.** the substance is often taken in larger amounts or over a longer period than was intended **4.** there is a persistent desire or unsuccessful efforts to cut down or control substance use **5.** a great deal of time is spent in activities necessary to obtain the substance **6.** important social, occupational, or recreational activities are given up or reduced **7.** the substance use is continued despite knowledge of having a persistent or recurrent physical or psychological problem that is likely to have been caused or exacerbated by the substance

Source: Reprinted with permission from American Psychiatric Association. (2000). *Diagnostic and statistical manual of mental disorders* (4th ed., Text Revision) (pp. 197–199). Washington, DC: Author.

Substance Withdrawal

Substance withdrawal refers to the development of maladaptive physiologic, behavioral, and cognitive changes that are due to reducing or stopping the heavy and regular use of a substance. Substance withdrawal syndrome is associated with distress and/or impairment in important areas of social functioning. The clinical example below describes the difficulties of withdrawing from long-term use of a substance. See the box on page 265 for the DSM-IV-TR diagnostic criteria for substance withdrawal.

CLINICAL EXAMPLE

Paul is a 40-year-old unemployed banker with a history of daily alcohol consumption that has gradually exceeded a quart of vodka per day for the past 25 years. He is estranged from his ex-wife and their two teenage children. He has tried unsuccessfully to cut back on his drinking on numerous occasions. His attempts to quit were particularly motivated when it became clear he would lose his job because of his declining performance and when he received a second arrest for driving while intoxicated. He is brought into the community crisis unit for medical detoxification and referral to Alcoholics Anonymous (AA) meetings and a mandatory outpatient recovery group program. He smokes at least a pack of cigarettes each day and drinks six cups of strong coffee as well. His physical exam reveals hypertension that is not responsive to medication, elevated liver enzymes, and ascites. He complains of dull abdominal pain, dry skin, diarrhea, and indigestion. He is sweaty, shaking, and irritable. He has been requesting that the physician write a prescription for pain to ease his current discomfort.

Biopsychosocial Theories

The theoretical frameworks for understanding substance problems include biologic, psychologic, sociocultural, and family systems theories.

BIOLOGIC/GENETIC THEORIES

The biologic explanation of alcoholism has assumed a great deal of importance in the last few years. Research to determine a genetic predisposition to alcoholism continues. Following are examples of research that is gaining respect in the scientific community.

- Classical research by Jellinek during the 1940s, 1950s, and 1960s, described as the Disease Model of Alcoholism, revealed that alcoholics proceed through phases, including the prealcoholic symptomatic phase, the prodromal phase, the crucial phase, and the chronic phase (Jellinek, 1946). He recognized "loss of control" in addictive alcoholics and hypothesized that it may have a biochemical basis. Building on this early work, researchers have recently associated low levels of dopamine (DA) neurotransmission, or an increased density of dopaminergic D2 receptors in the brain, to early relapse in alcohol-dependent clients (Guardia et al., 2000).
- Pharmacologic management, as opposed to psychosocial interventions, of alcoholism has advanced with the use of naltrexone, which is

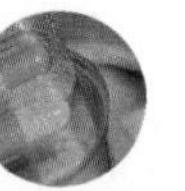

DSM-IV-TR **Diagnostic Criteria for Substance Intoxication and Withdrawal**

DIAGNOSTIC CRITERIA FOR SUBSTANCE INTOXICATION	DIAGNOSTIC CRITERIA FOR SUBSTANCE WITHDRAWAL
A. The development of a reversible substance-specific syndrome due to recent ingestion of (or exposure to) a substance. **Note:** Different substances may produce similar or identical syndromes. **B.** Clinically significant maladaptive behavioral or psychological changes that are due to the effect of the substance on the central nervous system (e.g., belligerence, mood lability, cognitive impairment, impaired judgment, impaired social or occupational functioning) and develop during or shortly after use of the substance. **C.** The symptoms are not due to a general medical condition and are not better accounted for by another mental disorder.	**A.** The development of a substance-specific syndrome due to the cessation of or reduction in substance use that has been heavy and prolonged. **B.** The substance-specific syndrome causes clinically significant distress or impairment in social, occupational, or other important areas of functioning. **C.** The symptoms are not due to a general medical condition and are not better accounted for by another mental disorder.

Source: Reprinted with permission from American Psychiatric Association (2000). *Diagnostic and statistical manual of mental disorders* (4th ed., Text Revision) (pp. 201–202). Washington, DC: Author.

believed to block the "high" associated with alcohol use and thus decrease cravings to continue to drink (Schneider, Levenson, & Schnoll, 2001).

- Between 1934 and 1974, Prescott, Aggen, and Kendler (1999) studied twins in the United States to determine genetic vulnerability to alcoholism. The scientists studied male and female twins for alcohol use disorders. Strong evidence suggests that genetic influences are equally important in the etiology of alcoholism in men and in women. However, there was little evidence to support the importance of shared environmental factors. In animals, alcohol is metabolized into tetrahydroisoquinolones (TIQs), opiate-like compounds that affect nerve receptors much as morphine and endorphins (the human body's naturally produced opiates) do. TIQ from alcohol has an opiate effect. In response, the body decreases or stops endorphin production. When the alcohol wears off, the endorphin level remains low, and the alcoholic cannot feel good without drinking.
- Alcoholics may have neurophysiologic defects. They may be vulnerable to intense sensory input and use alcohol as a protection from this heightened sensitivity.
- Research demonstrates that children of alcoholics are at fourfold risk of becoming alcoholics. Even if different families adopt them at birth, identical twins of alcoholic parents have more than a 60% chance of becoming alcoholics; fraternal twins have less than a 30% chance.
- Opiates have the highest rate of withdrawal symptoms (90.8%) and marijuana the lowest (40.9%). All except 13.1% of alcohol-dependent clients show physiologic signs of withdrawal (Schneider, Levenson, & Schnoll, 2001).
- Neurobiologic studies are clearly attesting that biologic factors such as genetics underpin vulnerability to substance-related disorders and also result from them. Furthermore, medications with anxiolytic and antidepressant effects are being used in both detoxification and relapse-prevention treatment.

PSYCHOLOGICAL THEORIES

From the psychologic perspective, the substance abuser is viewed as regressed and fixated at pregenital, oral levels of psychosexual development. Some writers relate the pattern of drug taking to parental inconsistency, self-centeredness, and inner dishonesty. The following personality traits are often associated with disruptive drug abuse:

- Dominant and critical behavior with underlying self-doubts and passivity.
- Overt extroversion.
- Tendency to describe own parents as self-reliant and efficient but not emotionally warm.
- Personal insecurity, with low self-esteem and self-criticism.
- Problems with sexual identification.
- Rebellious attitudes toward authority.
- Tendency to use defense mechanisms that are primarily escapist or sensation seeking.
- Difficulty with intimacy.
- Absence of a strong and efficient superego.
- Marked narcissistic trends.
- Difficulty with impulse control and feelings.

There is no real agreement about whether certain personality traits are sufficient to account for drug dependence, because the personality traits in question are studied after the diagnosis of substance abuse is made.

SOCIOCULTURAL THEORIES

Sociocultural models of substance abuse emphasize social forces, role models, and adaptive responses to stress in the sociocultural environment. Life's harsh realities come in many forms: the hopelessness and defeat of urban slum dwellers, the academic and social pressures generated by upper-middle-class families, the adolescent's feeling of impotence and alienation, the peer group pressure to join in and share experiences, the social vacuum of unloving families, in which meaningful attachments are dissolved or dissolving. All of these social conditions and contexts help create and sustain substance abuse. In addition, however, people who become addicts or alcoholics tend to live in environments where access to chemicals is easy and initiation into their use is widespread.

Substance abusers describe in interviews how they learned to drink or use drugs at high school and college parties or at home by watching their families. They recognized chemicals as a remedy for psychic and physical pain.

Gender researchers have suggested that in the case of abuse by the highly potent form of cocaine called crack, differences in how drug abuse begins and is maintained exist between women and men. Effective prevention and treatment programs depend on understanding such differences.

Studies clearly show that substance abuse is present in all cultures; however, which substance people abuse is often culturally determined. In Western culture, alcohol is the drug of choice. In Moslem countries, marijuana use is a problem because Islam prohibits alcohol use. Opium is used in China and other Eastern countries, whereas people in India and Africa use native herbs and chemicals. Native Americans use peyote (a cactus button with hallucinogenic properties) and alcohol more than other drugs.

FAMILY SYSTEMS THEORIES

A family systems explanation for substance abuse has gained increasing acceptance among health care professionals. When assessing substance abuse and the psychological impacts, ask yourself, "Is the addiction serving a purpose in this family?" The addiction may:

- Shift the family's focus.
- Give them a purpose or a challenge to distract them from other issues.
- Relieve one family member of a burden or provide a needed burden to one or several members.
- Provide a cohesive cause in which all family members can involve themselves.

The family systems perspective includes the phenomenon of codependence. A **codependent** is a person who allows another's behavior to affect him or her while being obsessed with controlling the other person's behavior. Codependents try to control events and people around them. A codependent is a family member who alternately rescues and blames (persecutes) the addict.

Although Alcoholics Anonymous (AA), a support group for alcoholics, does not openly endorse the family systems theory, they do recognize clearly that alcoholism is a family disease. Al-Anon and Ala-Teen are groups for spouses, parents, and teenage children of alcoholics. The focus is on helping these nonalcoholics learn to live and work effectively with alcoholics. The underlying belief is that family members often assume the role of **enablers**, or coalcoholics, perpetuating the alcoholic's drinking patterns.

CLINICAL EXAMPLE

Louise has been drinking for many years. She works full time as a secretary in a financial office setting. Adrienne, Louise's coworker for many years, routinely does Louise's work when Louise is too tired, confused, or otherwise unable to perform her duties. Adrienne believes she is helping Louise keep her job and her self-esteem. In reality, Adrienne is enabling Louise to continue to drink and not suffer the consequences of her drinking.

A cycle begins when the enablers do what they think is best in the situation. They begin to cover for the addict, such as by saying that he or she has a cold, is bruised because of stumbling in the dark, is asleep because of fatigue. Protected by the enabler, the addict is spared the consequences of his or her behavior and continues drinking or using drugs. The enabler, believing that the addict is coping with family, marital, or work problems "the best way he can," denies the disease of addiction. The addict blames the enabler; the enabler feels guilty and then attempts to control family life and the behaviors of the alcoholic/addict by throwing out liquor or taking the car keys. Of course, this behavior does not work. The enabler has tried the roles of protector, rescuer, controller, and blamer, but none is effective in altering the course of the disease. Consequently, enablers feel worthless and helpless because they are unsuccessful in terminating the addiction. Intervention and confrontation are necessary to break the cycle.

Dysfunctional Family Roles

When a family consists of one parent in the role of Addict, who is incapable of being emotionally present and fulfilling the parenting role adequately, and one parent in the role of Codependent or Enabler, who is trying to fix the Addict, children may be forced into dysfunctional family roles. Such children are consumed with meeting family needs and miss out on nurturing. Children's roles may consist of:

- The Hero or Martyr
- The Troublemaker or Scapegoat
- The Lost Child
- The Mascot

These defensive personalities represent survival strategies for children living in what they perceive to be a frightening family environment. Behaviors associated with each of these dysfunctional family roles appear in ■ Figure 13–1. Adult personalities are partially imprinted during childhood, and the roles that children take in order to cope in a family burdened by addiction can continue into adulthood if appropriate treatment is not provided.

Alcohol

Alcohol is a common, accessible substance that has just as much destructive power as any other substance of abuse. It is a liquid,

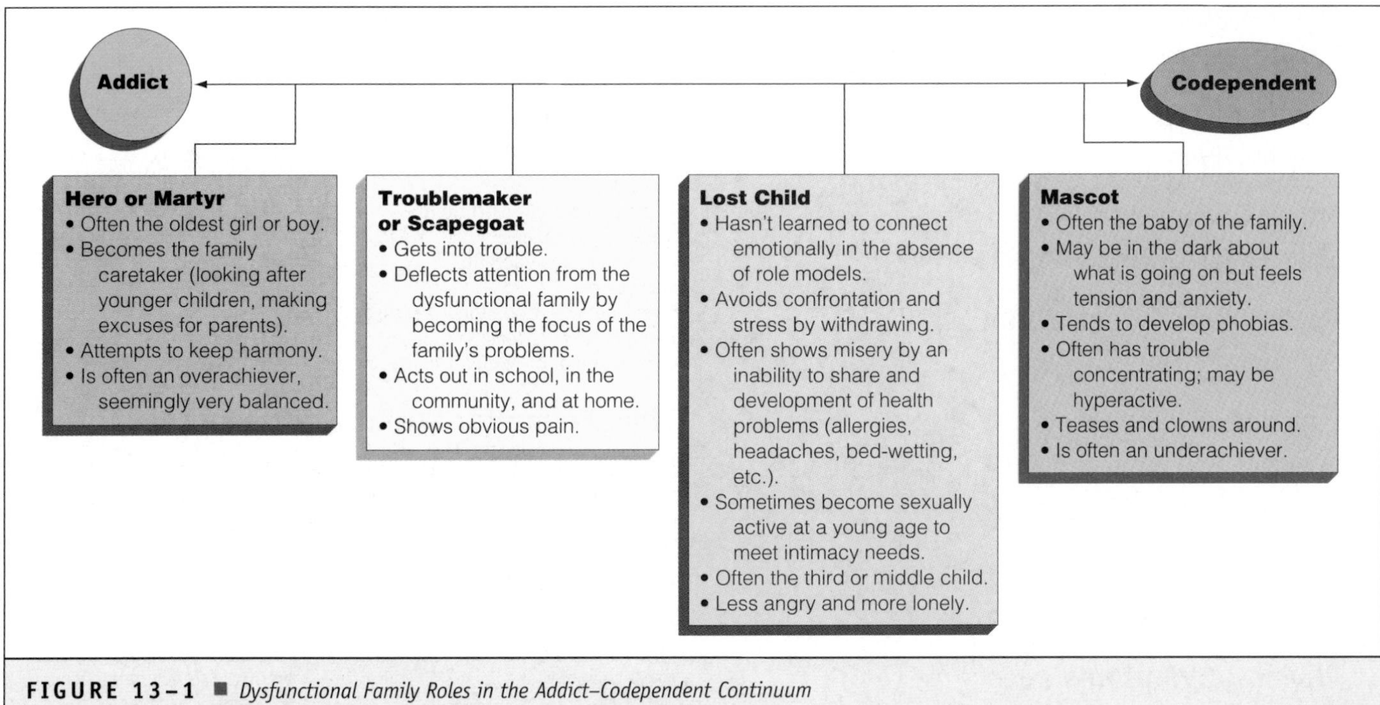

FIGURE 13–1 ■ *Dysfunctional Family Roles in the Addict–Codependent Continuum*

recreational drug that happens to be legal. Characteristic features with abuse of this drug are seen in the clinical example below.

CLINICAL EXAMPLE

Carol D, a 48-year-old woman, arrived at the hospital to be admitted for the fifth time. Her gait was unsteady and her speech slurred. Even though drunk, she avoided eye contact, appeared embarrassed, and apologized profusely for "getting into this mess again." She said, "I really don't need to be here. I can handle this problem."

Key facts about alcohol are presented in Box 13–2 (see page 268).

Several years ago, alcoholism was considered a neglected disease. Because of its increasing incidence and the highway carnage attributed to alcohol use, alcoholism is now the focus of magazine articles and radio and television programs. Perhaps this media blitz is in part a response to heightened awareness of the devastating effects of chronic alcoholism: depression; loss of self-respect; alienation from family, friends, and coworkers; malnutrition; infections; and damaging physiologic effects to most body systems. The physical effects of chronic alcoholism are listed in Box 13–3 (see page 269).

Although alcoholism was historically viewed as a moral problem, increased awareness played a part in the redefinition of alcoholism as a disease. As research about its biochemical aspects became known, earlier beliefs were challenged. The social stigma attached to alcoholism is decreasing, and more people are seeking help. Professionals, laypeople, alcoholics, and nonalcoholics are attending workshops and seminars on alcoholism; college courses at the graduate and undergraduate levels are offered. Recovery programs are reported widely in the popular media. See the latest research in treatment for alcohol and other drug abuse at the Web site for the National Institute on Drug Abuse (NIDA) at www.nida.nih.gov/.

MediaLink National Institute on Drug Abuse

THE EFFECTS OF ALCOHOL

A sedative anesthetic (CNS depressant), alcohol is absorbed in the mouth, stomach, and small intestine. Approximately 95% of alcohol is broken down by the liver; the rest is excreted through the lungs, kidneys, and skin. Generally, a person can metabolize 10 mL of alcohol (1 oz of whiskey) every 90 minutes. The rate of absorption varies based on many factors, such as weight, intake of food, and liver function. If taken in exceedingly high doses, alcohol can depress respiration and cause death. Intoxication occurs when a person's blood alcohol level (BAL) is 0.10% or more. This blood alcohol level is the legal definition of inebriation in most states, although there is a trend toward lowering the level to 0.08. ■ Figure 13–2 on page 269 illustrates the amount of alcohol that results in a BAL of 0.10 percent. See ■ Table 13–1 (page 270) which compares BALs and the behaviors exhibited at various levels.

PATTERNS OF USE

Alcoholics manifest one of three patterns of use: regular daily intake of large amounts of alcohol, regular heavy drinking limited to weekends, or long periods of sobriety interspersed with binges of heavy drinking lasting for weeks or months. Regardless of the preferred pattern, people who drink exces-

BOX 13-2 Key Facts About Alcohol (Ethyl Alcohol: C_2H_5OH or ETOH)

Examples

Liquor, wine, beer

Slang Terms

Hooch, booze, moonshine, sauce

Route of Administration

Oral (liquid)

Psychologic Symptoms

Irritability*
Mood swings*
Short attention span*
Loud and frequent talking*
Decreased judgment
Decreased inhibitions
Interference with memory

Physical Symptoms

Slurred speech*
Lack of coordination*
Unsteady gait*
Blackouts
Decreased REM sleep
Nystagmus*
Flushed face*
Decreased psychomotor functions

Withdrawal Symptoms

Nausea or vomiting
Anxiety
Depressed mood or irritability
Malaise or weakness
Autonomic hyperactivity
Tachycardia
Sweating; elevated blood pressure
Orthostatic hypotension
Coarse tremor of hands, tongue, eyelids

Time Frame for Withdrawal Symptoms

Mild withdrawal may begin within 12–24 hr following last drink. Symptoms may last 48–72 hr. Major withdrawal symptoms appear within 2–3 days following last drink and may last 3–5 days.

Dangers and Complications

Car accidents
Physical injury
Malnutrition
Hepatitis
Cirrhosis
Gastritis
Suicide
FAS (fetal alcohol syndrome)
Pancreatitis
GI bleeding
Wernicke's encephalopathy
Korsakoff's psychosis
Respiratory arrest
DTs

**Symptoms of intoxication noted in* DSM-IV-TR.

sively experience numerous negative physiologic and psychological symptoms.

ALCOHOL WITHDRAWAL SYNDROME

Alcohol withdrawal often includes the symptoms described below and in ■ Table 13–2 (see page 270).

Hangover

The term *hangover* is used to describe the unpleasant symptoms of mild alcohol withdrawal occurring approximately 4 to 6 hours after alcohol ingestion. These symptoms include:

- Nausea and vomiting
- Gastritis
- Headache
- Fatigue
- Sweating and thirst
- Restlessness
- Irritability
- The "shakes"
- Vasomotor instability

The cause of the symptoms is unclear, but they are attributed to dehydration, hypoglycemia, and the accumulation of lactic acid and acetaldehyde in the blood.

Alcoholic Hallucinosis

Alcoholic hallucinosis refers to auditory hallucinations reported by clients with alcohol dependence. The hallucinations occur approximately 24 to 48 hours after heavy drinking and may be vivid and frightening to the client.

Generalized Seizures

Generalized seizures ("rum fits") may occur 2 to 3 days after the person stops drinking. They can be prevented in a well-monitored medical withdrawal program.

Delirium Tremens

Delirium tremens (DTs), one symptom of withdrawal, is a condition of severe memory disturbance, agitation, anorexia, and hallucinations. Generally, DTs begin a few days after drinking stops and end within 1 to 5 days. They may, however, appear as late as the second week, especially when there is cross-addiction to other drugs. Additional medical illnesses may be present, such as pneumonia, pancreatitis, and hepatic decompensation.

Medical Detoxification

Medical treatment of alcoholism involves the management of withdrawal symptoms and the use of medication to deter the

BOX 13–3 Physical Effects of Chronic Alcoholism

Hepatic System

Alcoholic fatty liver syndrome
Alcoholic hepatitis
Laënnec's cirrhosis

Neurologic System

Wernicke–Korsakoff syndrome (related to thiamine deficiency)
Peripheral neuropathy (related to vitamin B deficiency)
Marchiafava disease*
Central pontine myelinosis*
Cerebellar degeneration*
Alcoholic amblyopia*

Cardiovascular System

Alcoholic cardiomyopathy
Hypokalemia
Hypomagnesemia
Hyperlipidemia
Altered fluid balance
Beriberi heart disease (related to thiamine deficiency)
Hematologic abnormalities

Musculoskeletal System

Acute alcoholic myopathy
Subclinical alcoholic myopathy
Chronic alcoholic myopathy

Gastrointestinal System

Gastritis
Esophagitis
Mallory–Weiss syndrome
Boerhaave's syndrome
Pancreatitis
Nutritional deficiency diseases
Nausea
Abdominal pain
Erratic bowel function (constipation and diarrhea)
Gastrointestinal hemorrhage
Jaundice
High incidence of digestive tract cancers
Glucose intolerance

Reproductive System

Impotence
Sterility
Gynecomastia
Anorgasmic (women)
FAS

*Very rare.

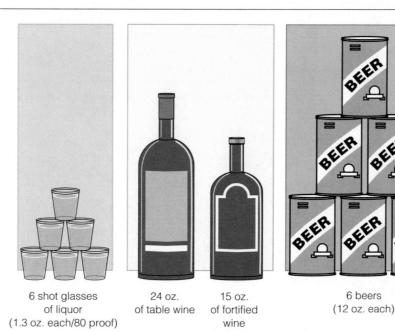

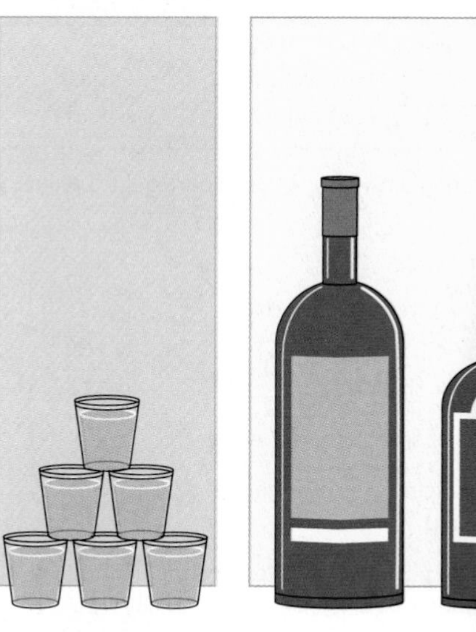
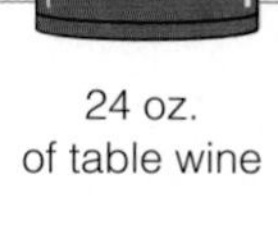
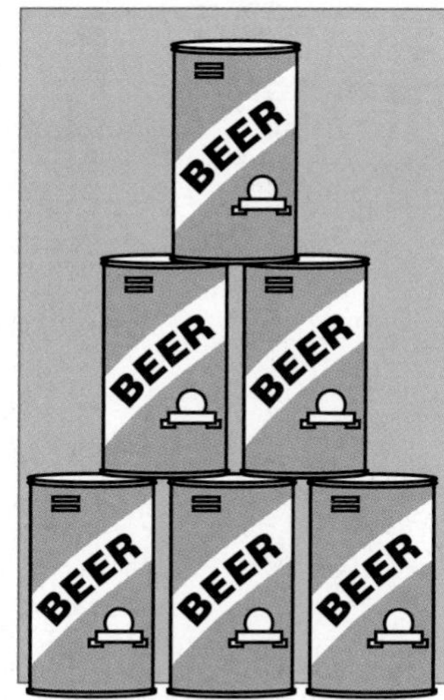

FIGURE 13–2 ■ *Intoxication. These amounts of alcoholic beverages, when consumed within a 2-hour period, will give a 160-pound person a BAL of 0.10.*

TABLE 13–1 Blood Alcohol Level (BAL) and Behaviors

Blood Alcohol Level (BAL)	Behavior
0.05 to 0.15 g/dL	Initial euphoria Mood lability Cognitive disturbances, including: • Decreased concentration • Impaired judgment • Sexual disinhibition
0.15 to 0.25 g/dL	Mood lability with outbursts Slurred speech Staggered gait or ataxia Diplopia Drowsiness
0.3 g/dL	Aggressive behavior Incoherent speech Labored breathing Vomiting Stupor
0.4 g/dL	Coma
0.5 g/dL	Severe respiratory depression Death

alcoholic from drinking. Alcohol withdrawal occurs after the addicted individual stops drinking. This syndrome is composed of a constellation of physiologic and behavioral symptoms that occur when the alcohol level drops.

Minor Withdrawal. A *minor withdrawal* from alcohol can occur within 6 to 12 hours after the alcoholic's last drink. Early symptoms include anxiety, agitation, and irritability. As the syndrome progresses, other symptoms occur. These include tremor, tachycardia, hypertension, diaphoresis, and hallucinations. Gastrointestinal symptoms of nausea, vomiting, diarrhea, and anorexia may also be present. The appearance of hallucinations (visual, auditory, olfactory, or tactile) and seizures marks the onset of a *major withdrawal.*

Major Withdrawal. A major withdrawal is the most advanced, potentially life-threatening stage of alcohol withdrawal. Symptoms associated with DTs usually develop 72 hours after the last drink. Physical symptoms of impending DTs include elevated temperature, severe diaphoresis, hypertension, and tachycardia. Behavioral symptoms include confusion and disorientation, agitation, tremors, and alterations in sensory perception (auditory and visual hallucinations). The best treatment for major alcohol withdrawal involves early detection. Medical treatment for withdrawal includes:

1. Monitoring the client's fluid status. Although some clients are overhydrated, many are dehydrated or have the potential for developing a fluid volume deficit. Fluids should be encouraged, up to 3,000 mL/day if no evidence exists to contraindicate this. If the client is unable to take fluids by mouth, fluids may be administered intravenously.

TABLE 13–2 Stages of Withdrawal from Alcohol

State	Peak Time of Onset After Last Drink	Symptoms	Potential Duration of Symptoms
Tremulousness	24 hours	At rest: slight tremors; during activities: gross and irregular tremors	1 week
		Diaphoresis	3–4 days
		Anorexia, nausea, vomiting	3–4 days
		Increased vital signs	3–4 days
		Sense of agitation and inner shakiness	2 weeks
		Insomnia with nightmares of seemingly real events	2 weeks or longer
Tremors and transitory hallucinosis	24 hours	Above cues plus visual hallucinations of events (e.g., having an accident while driving drunk)	3 days
Alcoholic hallucinosis	24 hours	Cues of tremulousness state plus vivid persecutory and auditory hallucinations, agitation, increased suicide and preassaultive potential	3 days–2 weeks
Delirium tremens	24–48 hours	Cues of tremulousness state plus delirium, generalized seizures, disorientation for time and place, visual hallucinations, agitation, panic level of anxiety	3–5 days
Rum fits	24–48 hours	2–6 generalized seizures; cues of delirium tremens	3–5 days

2. Administering magnesium sulfate to decrease the irritability caused by low magnesium levels and to prevent seizures.
3. Administering vitamins, especially thiamine (vitamin B_1) because alcohol interferes with the absorption of B vitamins.
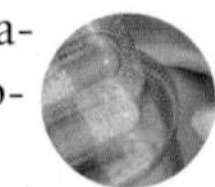
4. Prescribing benzodiazepines, such as diazepam (Valium) or chlordiazepoxide (Librium) to help prevent DTs. Seizures may be treated with IV diazepam, and the client may be placed on phenytoin (Dilantin).
5. Prescribing disulfiram (Antabuse, an agonist medication). The use of disulfiram may be prescribed in the treatment of alcoholic clients, although it is not used as often as it used to be. Disulfiram inhibits acetaldehyde dehydrogenase, which normally metabolizes acetaldehyde. As a result, acetaldehyde accumulates if alcohol is consumed. Acetaldehyde is highly toxic, producing nausea and hypotension. Hypotension leads to shock and may be fatal. If the client uses alcohol, a powerful *disulfiram reaction* may occur and last for up to 2 weeks. Reaction symptoms include nausea, vomiting, flushing, dizziness, and tachycardia. Because of the potential danger of disulfiram, instruct the client orally and in writing not to use alcohol in any form, including alcohol-based cough syrups or cold remedies such as those listed in ■ Table 13–3.
6. Prescribing naltrexone (ReVia, Trexan). Developed in 1984 for treatment of heroin abuse, this drug was approved in January 1994 for blocking the craving for alcohol and the pleasure derived from drinking it. It is the first new drug for alcoholism to be approved by the Food and Drug Administration (FDA) in 47 years. Rather than making the alcoholic sick, it blocks the need to ingest alcohol and thus may help prevent relapse when it is combined with long-term support groups and individual counseling. It has had more success as an active treatment mode than the punitive pharmacologic agent disulfiram.

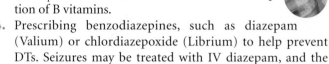

TABLE 13–3 Alcohol Content of Selected Over-the-Counter Cough and Cold Mixtures and Mouthwashes

Preparation	Amount of Alcohol (%)
Cough and Cold Mixtures	
Benylin Cough Syrup	5
Halls Mentho-Lyptus Decongestant Cough Formula	22
Nyquil Nighttime Cold Medicine	25
Robitussin Night Relief Cold Formula	25
Sudafed Cough Syrup	2.4
Vicks Formula 44 Cough Mixture	10
Mouthwashes	
ACT Fluoride	7
Cepacol	14
Listerine	26.9
Scope	18.5

Blackouts

Having **blackouts** is frequently confused with passing out. In fact, passing out refers to unconsciousness, whereas a blackout is anterograde amnesia: loss of short-term memories with retention of remote memories. A person can function effectively for up to several days—talking on the telephone, working, and shopping—yet have absolutely no memory of doing so. To others, the alcoholic may appear normal or "high." Interestingly, alcoholics appear unconcerned by the blackouts and eventually learn to cover them up. This appearance of unconcern may, in part, be due to euphoric recall: The alcoholic recalls feeling good but does not recall behavior. Reality is distorted. Some clients find blackouts very disturbing and seek treatment at that point.

Blackouts appearing later in the disease process may be indicative of physical dependence and are not related to the amount of alcohol consumed. They are unpredictable, and exactly how or why they occur is not clear. Some authorities believe blackouts are an acute syndrome caused by dehydration of brain tissue. When assessing an alcoholic client, determine whether blackouts are part of the symptoms.

ALCOHOL-INDUCED PERSISTING AMNESTIC DISORDER

Alcohol-induced persisting amnestic disorder (Korsakoff's syndrome) is a disturbance of short-term memory that occurs in people who have been drinking alcohol heavily for many years and have a thiamine deficiency. Korsakoff's syndrome is due to damage to the hippocampus and surrounding tissue from heavy alcohol ingestion.

If treated early, Korsakoff's syndrome may be avoided. Once this disorder is established, however, it has a chronic irreversible course, and impairment can become severe. It often follows an acute episode of **alcoholic encephalopathy (Wernicke's encephalopathy)**, a neurologic disease characterized by ataxia, sixth cranial nerve palsy, nystagmus, and confusion. Wernicke's encephalopathy may clear spontaneously in a few days or weeks and responds rapidly to large doses of parenteral thiamine in its acute, early stage.

FETAL ALCOHOL SYNDROME

Nurses need to be aware of the harmful effects of alcohol on pregnant women and unborn children. **Fetal alcohol syndrome (FAS)** is found in children of women who engage in heavy drinking of alcohol during pregnancy. Physical and mental defects include severe growth deficiency, heart defects, malformed facial features, mental retardation, low birth weight, learning problems, and hyperactivity. If a child has one or two of these characteristics, the con-

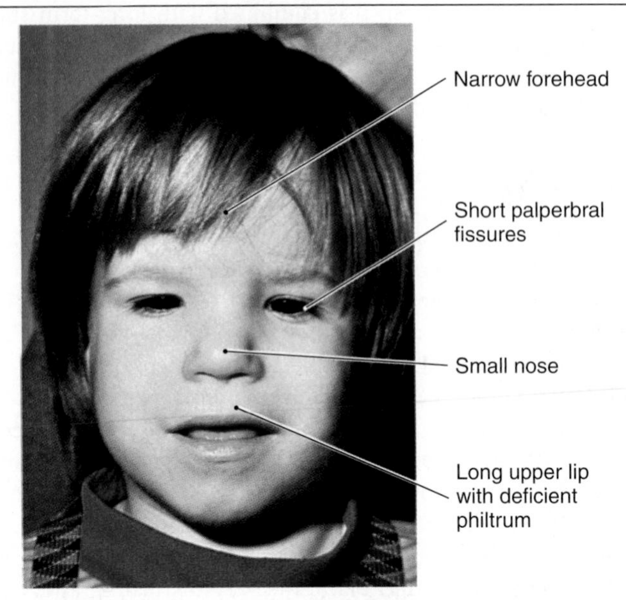

FIGURE 13–3 ■ *Fetal alcohol syndrome is the result of women consuming alcohol during pregnancy, and it can have many severe effects on the child; among them are physical malformations such as those shown here.*

Source: Fetal Alcohol & Drug Unit (FAS).

dition is called fetal alcohol effects. FAS affects 1 of every 750 babies born in the United States. A baby born to an alcoholic mother may need to be withdrawn gradually from alcohol immediately after birth. The characteristic physical features of a child with FAS are seen in ■ Figure 13–3.

SUICIDE AND ALCOHOLISM

Be alert to the possibility of suicide attempts by alcoholics. While 1% of the general population attempt suicide, 15% of alcoholics do. Watch for self-destructive behavior and for events in a client's life that represent a loss such as work, family, health, or legal problems. Such behavior and events put people in a high-risk category. Suicide is thoroughly discussed in Chapter 22.

Barbiturates or Similarly Acting Sedatives or Hypnotics

Barbiturates are overprescribed for anxiety, stress, and sleep difficulties. This is due to health care practitioners treating the symptom of anxiety, stress, or insomnia without determining and then appropriately eradicating the cause.

CLINICAL EXAMPLE

Elizabeth, a 45-year-old housewife, has been depressed and irritable over an impending divorce. Her physician prescribed diazepam (Valium) 5 mg for sleep and for anxiety (every 6 hours as needed). Because this dosage was not helping decrease her anxiety as much as she wanted, she increased her dosage and began taking 50 to 100 mg a day over a period of a few weeks. This evening Elizabeth's estranged husband found her mumbling incoherently. Her speech was slurred, she was bumping into furniture, and she was quite drowsy.

THE EFFECTS OF BARBITURATES, SEDATIVES, OR HYPNOTICS

Barbiturates are highly addictive drugs that cause people to feel euphoric, yet relaxed. They are frequently prescribed to relieve pain, reduce anxiety (sedative effects), and induce sleep (hypnotic effects). Barbiturates were the first drugs used to treat anxiety and insomnia. They were considered dangerous because of their ability to cause significant CNS depression and their lethality if used to overdose. Key facts about barbiturates are presented in Box 13–4.

Anxiolytic drugs, the benzodiazepines (BZDs), began to be widely used because of their ability to reduce anxiety without causing significant CNS depression. However, they also have the drawbacks of producing dependence and withdrawal syndromes. BZDs include many widely prescribed drugs, including diazepam (Valium), clorazepate (Tranxene), lorazepam (Ativan), and alprazolam (Xanax). These drugs are thought to modify anxiety by altering the balance of neurotransmitters, especially norepinephrine (NE) and gamma-aminobutyric acid (GABA) in the brain's limbic system. The limbic system is involved in the regulation of emotion. These drugs have a high risk for abuse and physical dependence. When the drug stops working and tolerance builds up, people tend to increase the dosage just "to cope." Even the nonbenzodiazepines such as zolpidem (Ambien) and zaleplon (Sonata) can be used to excess and have dependence issues associated with use (see Chapter 31).

PATTERNS OF USE

In party situations, teenagers and young adults take high doses of barbiturates, often in combination with alcohol, to get "high." The resultant CNS depression makes this practice especially dangerous. "Speed freaks" (amphetamine abusers) use barbiturates to "come down" from a high. Dependence, tolerance, and cross-tolerance to other depressant drugs develop rapidly.

ACTION

Barbiturates are metabolized in phases by the liver. When taken orally, they are initially absorbed and partially metabolized. However, the unmetabolized parts become active metabolites that are stored in the fatty tissues. Consequently, taking these drugs over a period of time results in a cumulative effect, unsuspected dependence, and possible overdose.

BOX 13-4 Key Facts About Barbiturates or Similarly Acting Sedatives or Hypnotics

Examples

Lorazepam (Ativan), alprazolam (Xanax), diazepam (Valium), chlordiazepoxide (Librium), chloral hydrate, methaqualone (Quaalude), secobarbital (Seconal), phenobarbital, pentobarbital (Nembutal)

Slang Terms

Downers, ludes, sopors, 714s, yellow jackets, reds, blues, rainbows, tranks

Route of Administration

Oral (pills or capsules), intravenous

Psychologic Symptoms

Euphoria
Mood lability*
Intoxication
Talkativeness*
Impaired attention and memory*
Irritability*
Anxiety
Sexual aggressiveness*

Physical Symptoms

Drowsiness
Slurred speech*
Long periods of sleep
Fever
Vomiting
Postural hypotension
Lack of coordination*
Unsteady gait

Withdrawal Symptoms

Nausea and vomiting
Malaise or weakness
Autonomic hyperactivity
Tachycardia
Sweating; elevated blood pressure
Anxiety
Depression or irritability
Orthostatic hypotension
Coarse tremor of hands, tongue, eyelids
Painful muscle contractions
Seizures
Status epilepticus (major epileptic attacks succeeding each other with little or no intermission)
Hallucinations

Time Frame for Withdrawal Symptoms

Short-acting barbiturates and BZDs are associated with withdrawal symptoms within the first 24 hr after discontinuation. Longer-acting barbiturates and BZDs are associated with withdrawal symptoms within 48–72 hr of discontinuation. Seizures may occur for up to 2 weeks after withdrawal.

Dangers and Complications

CNS depression
Possible overdose and death, especially if mixed with alcohol

Typical Users

Middle-class, middle-aged females
Teenagers
Young adults

**Symptoms of intoxication noted in* DSM-IV-TR.

More Americans die from barbiturate overdose than from opioid addiction. Many take alcohol and barbiturates together. While judgment is impaired, they take more pills, thereby unintentionally overdosing. Because alcohol and barbiturates are synergistic, an overdose can occur quickly. Barbiturates are often used in suicide attempts.

WITHDRAWAL

Barbiturate withdrawal is unpleasant and life threatening. A deep sleep is followed by decreased respiration, coma, and sometimes death. Babies born to mothers addicted to barbiturates are physically dependent and need to be helped through withdrawal.

Withdrawal from BZDs may produce symptoms similar to those of barbiturate withdrawal. Symptoms include autonomic hyperactivity (alterations in vital signs and diaphoresis), marked anxiety, agitation, insomnia, depression, and seizures. Medical detox can prevent a potentially serious emergency during withdrawal.

Opioids

The opioids include heroin and morphine, derived from the poppy plant, and synthetic drugs, such as oxycodone (Oxycontin), meperidine (Demerol), codeine, methadone, and others.

MediaLink 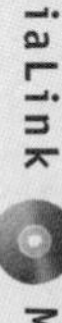 Morphine in Action Animation

CLINICAL EXAMPLE

Steven, a 20-year-old male, arrived at the hospital in an ambulance. He was unconscious. His respirations were slow, and his pupils were pinpoints. "Tracks" were visible on his arms and behind his knees. A source said Steven had just "shot up" heroin.

THE EFFECTS OF OPIOIDS

Opioids have analgesic qualities and are prescribed after surgery. They are quite potent and have the ability to remove painful stimuli. Depending on the person, the drugs may produce an euphoric high, as in drug addicts, but they generally cause people to feel drowsy and out of touch with the world. See Box 13–5 for more facts about opioids.

Heroin addiction by itself is not inherently dangerous. Unless there is an accidental overdose, heroin alone as a substance will not harm the individual. The ancillary issues of diluting agents (which are likely contaminated), needle cleanliness, and exposure to transmissible diseases such as hepatitis, tuberculosis, and HIV, along with typically criminal behaviors necessary to support the addiction, put the individual at great risk and make the addicted individual of concern to others. Methadone as a treatment option for these clients has been successful to a certain extent, but has had controversial aspects ethically and economically and is viewed as a public health concern.

PATTERNS OF USE

In 1898, heroin became widely available and initially was not believed to be addictive. Within a short time, its addictive properties became known, and the government intervened (Harrison Narcotics Act of 1914). Addiction to opiates has increased through the years. Because most opioid abusers take the drugs intravenously, they are at high risk for HIV/AIDS and hepatitis. Overdose, malnutrition, and infections spread by dirty drugs and needles are dangers. Dealers often add impurities to "cut" the heroin, thus increasing the quantity and their own profit. The impurities may cause poisoning and other problems.

Overdose

Constricted pupils, euphoria, psychomotor retardation, slurred speech, and/or drowsiness indicate opioid intoxication. If a client overdoses, naloxone (Narcan) (0.4 to 0.8 mg IV repeated in 5 to 15 minutes) is given. It is a fast-acting narcotic antagonist that counteracts respiratory depression. Abdominal cramps, rhinorrhea, and lacrimation may be treated with belladonna alkaloids or with phenobarbital.

WITHDRAWAL

Because opioids are physically addictive, withdrawal is a threat. People who use high doses of a drug and who "shoot up" or

BOX 13–5 Key Facts About Opioids

Examples

Heroin, morphine, hydromorphone (Dilaudid), codeine, methadone

Slang Terms

H, smack, junk, M, Miss Emma, Little D, School Boy, Horse

Route of Administration

Intravenous, oral, intramuscular, subcutaneous ("skin popping")

Psychologic Symptoms

Impaired attention/memory*
Euphoria*
Appearance of sedation ("nodding out")
Psychomotor retardation*
Insensitivity to pain
Agitation
Apathy*
Dysphoria*

Physical Symptoms

Pinpoint pupils
Drowsiness*
Slurred speech*
Nausea and vomiting
Hypothermia

Withdrawal Symptoms (Presents like Influenza)

Dilated pupils
Tearing
Runny nose
Piloerection
Sweating
Diarrhea
Fever
Yawning
Mild hypotension
Tachycardia
Insomnia
Restlessness and irritability
Muscle and joint pains
Increased respiration
Gastrointestinal symptoms
Loss of appetite

Time Frame for Withdrawal Symptoms

Withdrawal symptoms may appear within a few hours after the last dose of a short-acting opioid such as heroin. With longer acting opioids such as methadone, withdrawal symptoms may not appear for 2–3 days and may persist for 1–2 weeks.

Dangers and Complications

Death (especially if combined with barbiturates)
Pulmonary edema
Opioid poisoning (coma, shock, respiratory depression)
Malnutrition
Hepatitis; infections
AIDS

Typical Users

Teenagers
Young adults

**Symptoms of intoxication noted in* DSM-IV-TR.

"mainline" (use the drug intravenously) are at high risk for severe withdrawal symptoms. Withdrawal symptoms are usually evident within 12 hours after the last dose. The person experiences the most severe withdrawal within 36 to 48 hours, with the symptoms decreasing gradually over 2 weeks. During this stressful time, the person craves the drug. Clients in treatment may terminate against advice of health professionals. Babies who are born to addicted mothers must be treated for opioid withdrawal. These babies are irritable and have high-pitched crying, increased respirations, fever, sneezing, yawning, and tremors.

TREATMENT

In 1964, methadone was introduced to treat opiate addiction. By the late 1960s and early 1970s, when federal governments allocated money for treatment, methadone maintenance programs mushroomed all over North America. Methadone, a synthetic narcotic, was dispensed daily at clinics to narcotic addicts. Although addictive, methadone does not produce the "rush" (ecstatic feeling) associated with heroin. Methadone alleviates the addict's craving for narcotics and, therefore, was expected to decrease the illicit drug trafficking, theft, prostitution, and crime necessary to obtain money for the drugs, thereby allowing addicts to lead productive lives. Also, methadone therapy is far less expensive than residential programs or jail. Today, methadone maintenance programs remain a major treatment for opioid addicts.

Clients who are assessed to be not at risk for complications of the drug are first stabilized on methadone (3 to 5 days). Within 1 to 3 days after the methadone is discontinued, opiate withdrawal symptoms often appear. At this time, clonidine (Catapres) is begun and is given in increasing doses, until withdrawal symptoms are alleviated (up to 14 days). Clonidine (Catapres) blocks the withdrawal symptoms, making the detoxification process less painful and more rapid than with methadone. Psychologically, the client feels less anxious and depressed.

Recent legislation has shown that the effectiveness of Schedule III, IV, and V controlled substances including buprenorphine (Buprenex) are alternatives to methadone (U.S. Department of Health and Human Services, 2000). Buprenorphine (Buprenex) is an opioid mixed agonist and potent analgesic. It is also being investigated for its effectiveness in treating cocaine abuse. The issue of office-based treatment of opiate addictions is discussed in the Using Research Evidence feature below.

Amphetamines or Similarly Acting Sympathomimetics

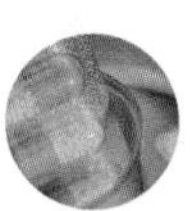

The sympathomimetics ("speed") include groups of synthetic drugs derived from ephedrine that stimulate the release of adrenaline.

THE EFFECTS OF AMPHETAMINES

In small doses, they cause a person to feel energetic, euphoric, and "turned on" to life. Users take these CNS stimulants to feel good. A growing number of people who do uppers and downers in a cyclic fashion take amphetamines to counteract the effects of barbiturates. Amphetamines are dangerous because they alter judgment and obscure feelings. Taken in high doses or intravenously, amphetamines can have dangerous side effects. Key facts about amphetamines are listed in Box 13–6 (see page 276).

Amphetamines act by mimicking the brain's most important neurotransmitters, dopamine (DA) and norepinephrine (NE). Any drug's ability to have an impact on a biological being must be able to do so at a receptor site or at a number of receptor sites. If the body does not have a specific amphetamine or cocaine receptor site, amphetamine and cocaine will take illegal control at existing receptor sites. As mentioned above, dopamine and dopamine receptor sites are intricately involved in the effects substances of abuse have on the nervous systems of clients. How specifically morphine, amphetamine, and cocaine are involved in this process is shown in ■ Figure 13–4 on page 277.

MediaLink Occupying a Receptor Site Animation

PATTERNS OF USE

In the 1950s and 1960s, amphetamines were heralded as wonder drugs for depression and lassitude. By the 1970s, their dangers became known, and today physicians prescribe them less frequently. Amphetamines are still used to control appetite and treat

USING RESEARCH EVIDENCE

Sekov is a 33-year-old native of Macedonia who has been in the United States since high school. Although bright and active in sports then, he began socializing with a group using alcohol and marijuana regularly and cocaine and heroin on occasion. After high school his activities dwindled and his opportunities shrank as he spent more and more time with these friends. Within a few years he was solely involved with marginal functioning and living to obtain heroin. Five years ago, Sekov agreed to enter treatment at the insistence and with the help of his large extended family.

Treatment at methadone clinics has been erratic for Sekov and others in his area as there are insufficient treatment slots available. This has been a significant barrier to his recovery. You are involved as the nurse in an office-based methadone maintenance treatment program that incorporates psychosocial treatments and education. Research shows that selected clients do well in this type of program in an office setting. As part of your position, you disseminate public information about access to these types of office-based programs, and you met Sekov and his mother at a community center presentation. As a result, you were able to assess his circumstances as paralleling research successes and provide this treatment access and option to Sekov, which may allow his recovery to proceed unimpeded.

These suggestions stem from the following research:

O'Connor, P. G. (2001). Treating opioid dependence. *New England Journal of Medicine, 344*, 530–531.

BOX 13-6 Key Facts About Amphetamines

Examples

Dexedrine, methamphetamine

Slang Terms

Bennies, dexies, uppers, black beauties, pep pills, crank, speed, diet pills

Route of Administration

Oral, intravenous

Psychologic Symptoms

Hypervigilance*
Irritability
Grandiosity*
Talkativeness*
Elation
Impaired judgment
Psychomotor agitation*
Aggressive, violent behavior
Paranoia
Hallucinations, delusions
Disorientation
Increased libido
Stereotypical compulsive behavior
Visual/auditory hallucinations

Physical Symptoms

Tachycardia*
Increased blood pressure*
Dilated pupils*
Perspiration or chills*
Nausea or vomiting*
Diarrhea
Headache
Dizziness
Cardiac arrhythmias
Hyperthermia
Decreased appetite
Delirium

Withdrawal Symptoms

Depression
Fatigue
Disturbed sleep
Dreaming
Restlessness
Disorientation

Dangers and Complications

Malnutrition
Cerebrovascular accident
Depression
Hyperpyrexia
Convulsions
Suicide attempt

Typical Users

Teenagers
Young adults

**Symptoms of intoxication noted in* DSM-IV-TR.

depression, narcolepsy, minimal brain dysfunctions, and attention-deficit disorders in children. Abusers are usually teenagers or people in their early twenties who are looking for a good time. Abusers are also using different types of speed than in years past. Truck drivers may use amphetamines to stay awake on long trips, and students may use them to study for exams. Athletes, hoping to improve their performance, may use amphetamines. Tolerance develops rapidly, and chronic abusers may suffer a toxic psychosis presenting with the symptoms of paranoid schizophrenia. Argumentativeness, delusions, hallucinations, stereotypic compulsive behavior, increased libido, interpersonal sensitivity, panic, and violence may occur (American Psychiatric Association [APA], 2000). This clinical example shows how an innocent reason and the best intentions can lead to dire consequences.

CLINICAL EXAMPLE

Laura, a 16-year-old high school girl, was on a diet so she could get into a favorite bathing suit. Her friend's brother, a pharmacist, gave her some Dexedrine "just until you lose the weight." Laura's mother initially noticed her rather unusual hyperactivity, her euphoria, and the fact that she refused dinner. Over a period of a few weeks, Laura's behavior changed. She appeared suspicious and irritable and continued to speak and move rapidly and her grades dropped significantly. Laura was rushed to the hospital after being found unconscious in the girls' locker room at school.

Clients who are chronic amphetamine abusers begin to crave the drugs and require higher and higher dosages. They are rowdy, paranoid, and irritable. A "crash" (depression), often with suicidal symptoms, may last for several weeks. Cyclical patterns of abuse and crashing may occur.

The most hypercharged form of speed is "crystal" or methamphetamine. Sold in small chunks as "glass" or "ice," it is a maximum stimulant with maximum risks. "Crank" is another nickname for street speed. The effects are similar to those produced by "crystal."

WITHDRAWAL

Chlorpromazine (Thorazine) may be ordered to combat the physiologic effects of amphetamines. Diazepam (Valium), given

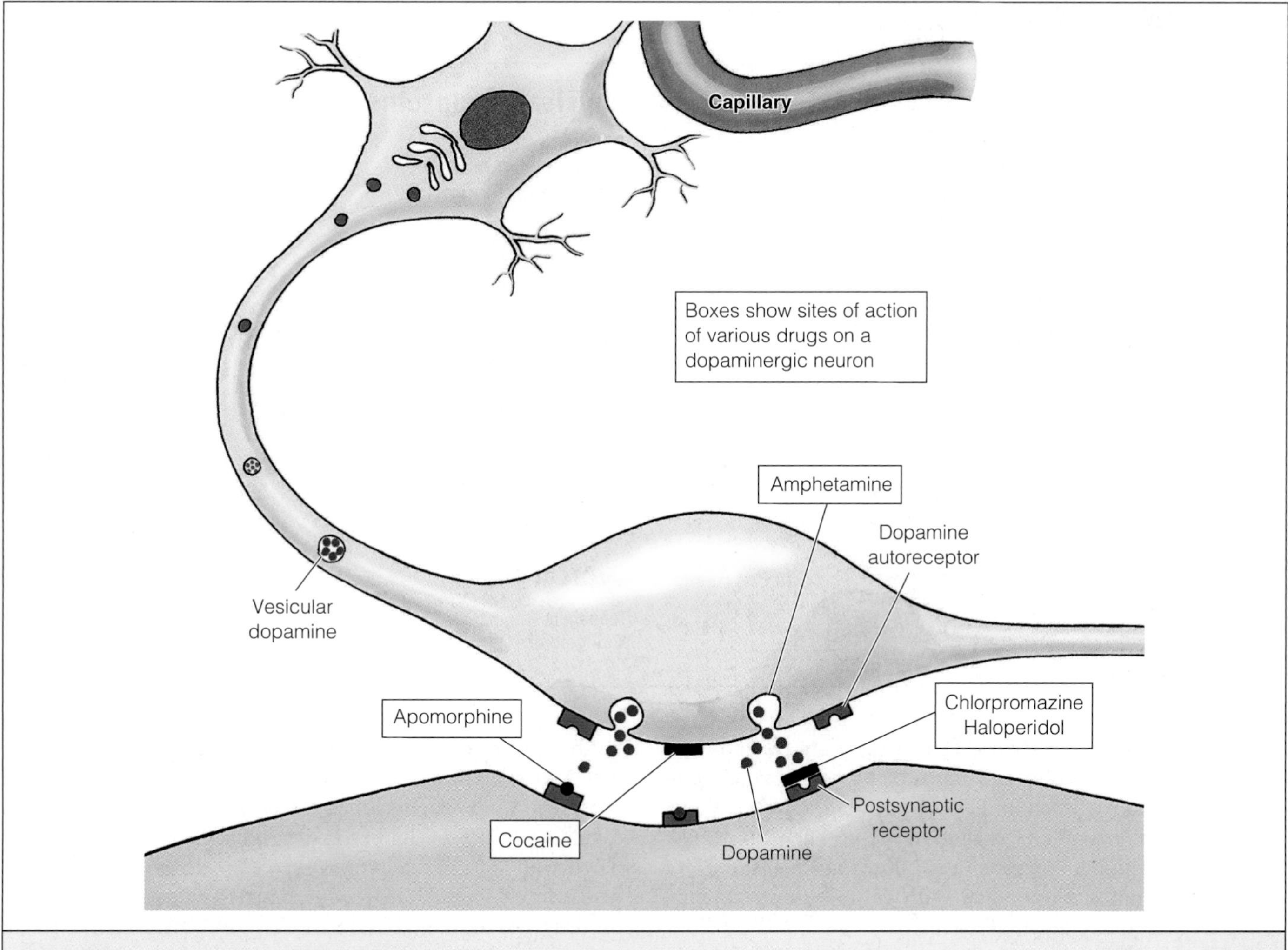

FIGURE 13–4 ■ *Action of Drugs on Dopaminergic Neurons*

Source: Smock, T. K. (1999). *Physiological psychology: A neuroscience approach*. Upper Saddle River, NJ: Prentice Hall.

intravenously, decreases tachycardia and the chance of convulsions. Depression and anxiety are the most common psychological pitfalls in recovering from the use of speed. Physiologically, the overuse of speed has been tied to stroke and even death.

Cannabis

Marijuana arrived in North America in the early 1900s. Although it has been illegal in the United States since 1937, marijuana is used more than any other chemical except tobacco, alcohol, and caffeine (see Box 13–7 on page 278).

CLINICAL EXAMPLE

Joe, a 35-year-old captain of a rescue squad, was having trouble at his job. He paid less and less attention to the accuracy of his patient reports; he was often late for work; he forgot to repair and replace his equipment, causing his unit to be unsafe and ill equipped. Joe told an emergency room nurse that he felt all the marijuana he was smoking was beginning to affect him. He revealed that he'd been a daily smoker for 5 years. At first, he felt there were no long-term effects, but lately he was concerned because "I never feel like doing anything." He has trouble concentrating, forgets what he is talking about in mid-sentence, and is unmotivated to make any positive changes in his life.

THE EFFECTS OF CANNABIS

Derived from an Indian hemp plant (*Cannabis sativa*), marijuana contains the psychoactive substance delta 6-3,4-tetrahydrocannabinol (THC). THC is found in the sticky yellow resin secreted by the tops and leaves of the ripe plants. Key facts about cannabis are presented in Box 13–7.

THC is transformed into metabolites in the body. Unlike alcohol, which is water soluble and leaves the body through

BOX 13–7 Key Facts About Cannabis

Examples

Marijuana, hashish, THC

Slang Terms

Pot, grass, bhang, hashish, ganja, joint, reefer, weed, "shit"

Route of Administration

Smoked in a pipe or cigarette, oral (mixed in food)

Psychologic Symptoms

Initial anxiety, then euphoria
Altered perceptions
Sensation of slowed time
Decreased concentration
Lack of motivation
Loss of short-term memory
Passivity
Abrupt mood changes
Paranoid ideation
Impaired judgment

Physical Symptoms

Dry mouth
Increased heart rate
Conjunctival irritation
Dilated pupils
Decreased coordination
Increased appetite, thirst
Craving for sweets
Fatigue
Impaired ovulation, impaired sperm count and motility, increase in abnormal sperm cells

Dangers and Complications

Lung damage
Psychologic dependence
Panic reaction
Impaired driving ability

Typical Users

Teenagers
Young adults

urine, breath, and perspiration, THC is stored in the fatty tissues (especially the brain and reproductive system). Consequently, it can be detected in the body for up to 6 weeks. From 1984 to 1986, marijuana increased in potency 10 times. Although marijuana contains over 400 chemicals, the THC content determines the potency. With an increase in potency comes an increase in health problems.

Researchers have found marijuana to produce a significant analgesic effect and to be modestly effective against the nausea and vomiting associated with chemotherapy. Although marijuana does decrease intraocular pressure, it requires high doses and has a short-lived effect, making it inappropriate for the treatment of glaucoma. Researchers are currently studying the effects of marijuana smoking by pregnant women on the fetus. The cannabinoids of marijuana cross the placental barrier and are distributed to fetal tissues. The risks of fetal death and abnormalities—CNS disturbances, low birth weight, decreased length, and smaller head circumference—increase when the mother uses marijuana. A suppressed prolactin level in the mother makes nursing impossible. If people with a history of schizophrenia or mood disorders use marijuana, they may have a relapse or their symptoms may worsen. Long-term marijuana smoking is associated with lung damage, increased risk of respiratory cancer, and poorer pregnancy outcomes (Watson, Benson, & Joy, 2000). The latest research about marijuana indicates there are dangers that were previously unexplored (Pacula et al. 2000; Zickler, 2000). See the list of marijuana facts in Box 13–8.

PATTERNS OF USE

Because marijuana smoking is so prevalent among teenagers and because its dangers are becoming increasingly known, some health care professionals advocate urine screening when teenagers have a checkup by a family doctor. Chemical dependence takes 10 to 15 years to develop in adults and only a few years to develop in a child. Only 25% of children in drug rehabilitation succeed, compared with 75% of adults who succeed. Because of this danger, pediatricians should initiate educational and treatment programs on drug and alcohol abuse. Likewise, psychiatric–mental health nurses need to respond to this vital public health issue.

BOX 13–8 Dangers of Marijuana

- Marijuana appears to lower testosterone levels in boys.
- In girls, hormone levels remain normal, but marijuana's chemicals may accumulate in the ovaries.
- Marijuana smoke has 50% more tar than regular cigarette smoke.
- Marijuana tar contains 70% more benzopyrene, a major cancer-causing chemical.
- Marijuana smoke produces greater cellular changes in the lungs than does tobacco smoke.
- Marijuana may cause emphysema twenty times faster than tobacco.
- Marijuana smoke increases airway resistance 25% under laboratory conditions in which a similar amount of tobacco smoke produces no significant increase in airway resistance.
- Brain wave tests show that teenagers who get high twice a week or more often have evidence of diffuse brain impairment for up to 2 months after the last time they use the drug. They experience disruptions in learning, short-term memory loss, problems concentrating, and amotivation syndrome (confusion, declining performance, and difficulty finishing tasks).
- After a person smokes marijuana, THC can be found in the blood and urine for up to 2 weeks; if the THC is radioactively labeled, it can be detected for up to a month.

For information on the efforts to prevent and treat youth drug abuse, see the Center for Treatment Research on Adolescent Drug Abuse (CTRADA) Web site at www.med.miami.edu/ctrada/ctrada.htm.

Marijuana use is endemic in the teenage culture. Therefore, nurses who work with teenagers must be knowledgeable about marijuana and its effects. When admitting a teenager to a psychiatric unit or interviewing a teenager as an outpatient, be aware of a variety of indicators of marijuana use. Parents should know these facts about marijuana and indications of its use:

- Marijuana smells like hemp or burning rope.
- Teenagers often burn incense or use perfumed sprays to mask its pungent odor.
- Teenagers may use eye drops (Murine) so that their eyes will not be red, and they may cough a lot.
- A teenager who uses marijuana may have smoking paraphernalia—plastic baggies filled with dried leaves, rolling papers, and "roach" clips (clips that hold the marijuana cigarette once it becomes too small to handle).

Cocaine

Over one third of the almost 600,000 people in drug treatment at any one time in the United States have cocaine as their primary drug.

CLINICAL EXAMPLE

Will, a 32-year-old male, was brought to the hospital by his father. Talkative and jumpy, his eyes darted around the examining room, and he repeatedly wiped his nose with his finger and rubbed the bottom of his face. He acted suspicious and kept saying someone was after him. His family stated he had a $400-a-day cocaine habit. He began casually snorting a few lines once in a while when he needed a sense of control over his full load of graduate school courses and full-time job. His use increased to every day, then every few hours.

Since cocaine abuse has been recognized as a widespread problem, government agencies have spent much money trying to block cocaine shipments from South America. Planes, boats, and "mules" (people who transport cocaine) have been seized, and tons of cocaine have been confiscated and destroyed. Yet it is still plentiful and is purer today than ever before. The cocaine industry is a multibillion-dollar enterprise involving bribery, corruption, and murder.

THE EFFECTS OF COCAINE

Cocaine is a stimulant extracted from the leaves of the coca plant found in Bolivia and Peru. It has long been known and used. For hundreds of years, South American Indians have chewed coca leaves, enjoying the effects of decreased appetite and increased ability to work at high altitudes. Slaves became more productive when given cocaine. Freud experimented with cocaine. It was an ingredient in Coca-Cola before federal regulations prohibited it in 1903. Today, cocaine is used as a local anesthetic in ear, nose, and throat surgery. When inhaled or injected, cocaine produces alertness and energy and makes users feel sociable, confident, and "in control." The drug blocks appetite and erases fatigue, which makes it appear to be an ideal performance booster.

Cocaine addicts develop a tolerance to the drug and use amounts that would have been lethal to them earlier. The euphoria diminishes. The development of new dendrites (branches of the nerve cells) to aid the uptake of the increased amount of DA accounts for the tolerance. Ultimately, the cocaine no longer produces pleasure, but not taking it feels even worse. Dopamine eventually becomes depleted, and the user becomes chronically fatigued, irritable, and anxious, even mentally confused and paranoid. Suicide attempts, accidents, and overdoses are common. The only effect of cocaine that is increased as tolerance develops is its ability to induce a convulsion or seizure. Nurses need to assess clients carefully to differentiate cocaine use from manic depression and chronic anxiety. ■ Figure 13–5 on page 280 illustrates the cocaine use cycle.

MediaLink Adolescent Drug Abuse

Cocaine Intoxication

Interestingly, low-level cocaine intoxication presents with symptoms similar to alcohol withdrawal: sweating, dilated pupils, psychomotor agitation, and increased blood pressure/ heart rate. With higher doses of cocaine, a person becomes increasingly intoxicated. Symptoms include high fever, cardiac arrhythmia, seizures, hallucinations, and a paranoid schizophrenic syndrome. Hallucinations typically involve "cocaine bugs," which feel like bugs under the skin. The client may scratch furiously in an attempt to get rid of them. Haloperidol (Haldol) is used to combat the psychotic symptoms; phenothiazines should not be used because they may decrease the seizure threshold.

The strength of the physiologic effects of cocaine is revealed by animal research. Monkeys work harder at pressing a bar to receive cocaine intravenously than to get any other drug. Even when starving to death or when confronted with a sexually receptive female, monkeys continue pressing the bar. Receiving an electric shock every time they touch the bar does not alter their behavior. Research with cocaine users indicates that the drug bromocriptine mesylate (Parlodel), a DA receptor agonist, eliminates the craving that users feel after they stop using cocaine. Cocaine initially increases DA neurotransmission. Over time, however, cocaine abuse depletes DA in the brain, and this depletion may be the basis for craving.

The "Post-Coke" Blues

It has not been proven that cocaine is physically addictive, but its ability to cause psychological dependence is clear. Cocaine users crave the drug. After a brief post–use euphoria (lasting approximately 5 to 10 minutes), they experience a strong desire to repeat the high. This high is followed by a crash—a terrible letdown called the "post-coke blues," or cocaine abstinence syndrome.

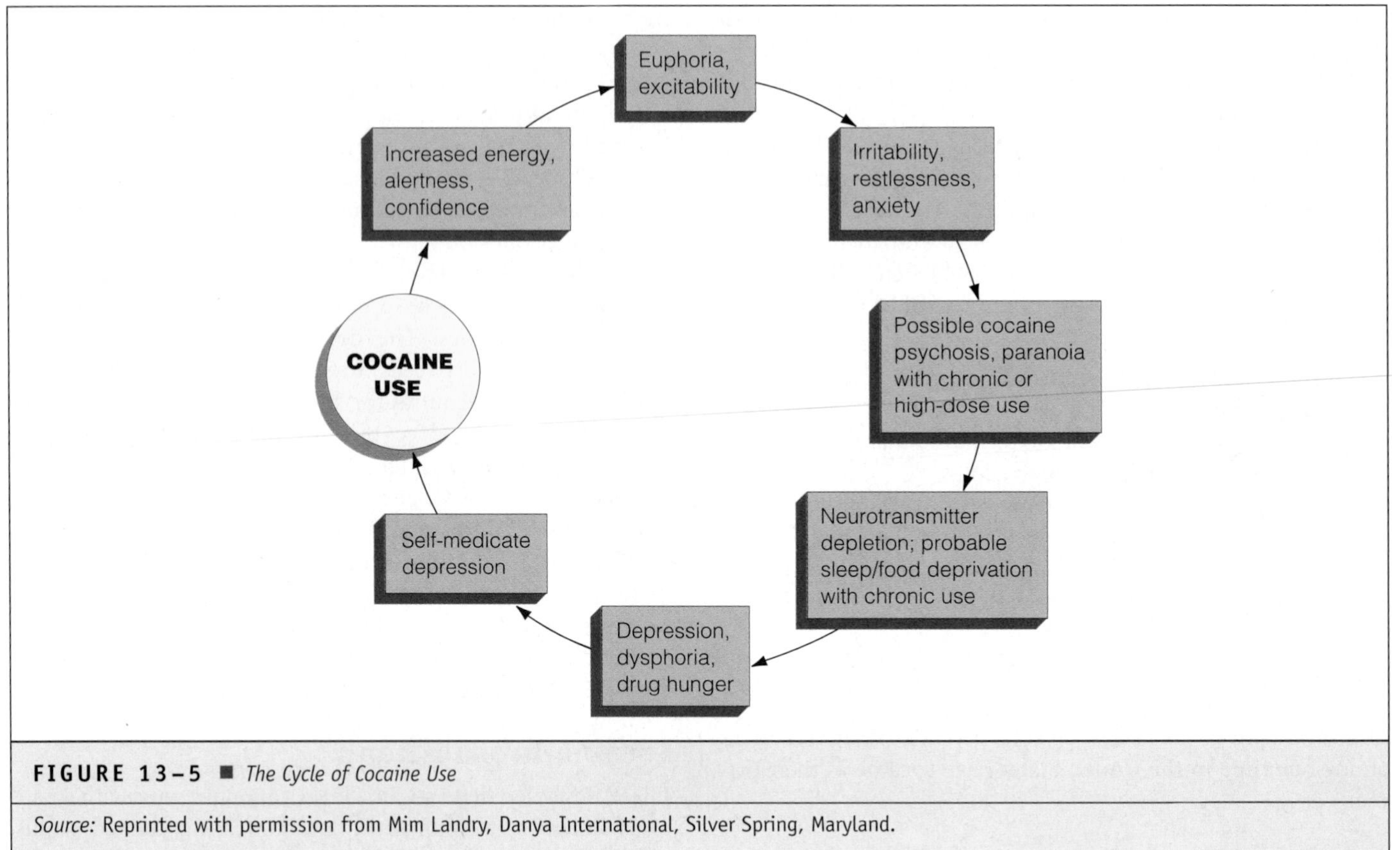

FIGURE 13–5 ■ *The Cycle of Cocaine Use*

Source: Reprinted with permission from Mim Landry, Danya International, Silver Spring, Maryland.

Anxiety, depression, and fatigue are part of this syndrome. The cocaine crash, lasting for approximately 30 to 60 minutes, results from depletion of DA, the neurotransmitter responsible for feelings of pleasure and well-being. The addict responds to the crash by feeling irritable, depressed, and tired. Although the brain needs to synthesize more DA, resulting from the chemical misprogramming from the addiction, it craves more cocaine, which offers immediate relief. The crash intensity appears to be related to the amount of cocaine used. Addicts often use other drugs, such as alcohol, marijuana, or sleeping pills, during the crash.

One addict described these post-coke blues as "pure hell, the most painful depression I have ever felt. I wanted to die from the pain." This painful depression, along with the memory of the cocaine high, causes people to want to use cocaine again and again to recapture the momentary ecstasy. The period of agitation, anxiety, and insomnia usually ceases within 2 weeks.

PATTERNS OF USE

Cocaine is no longer just the chic, expensive drug of choice (the champagne of drugs) of young upwardly mobile professionals and stars. In greater demand are smokable forms that have an effect similar to the injectable drug. Cocaine is now available to all cultural and socioeconomic groups; today, 50% of users are women. For some years, cocaine was believed to produce euphoria without addictive potential and without negative side effects. Lately, the horrors of cocaine abuse have been described in both lay and professional literature. Intranasal cocaine users place themselves at risk for hepatitis C. Key facts about cocaine are found in Box 13–9.

TREATMENT

Detoxification for cocaine abusers depends on the client's symptoms. Some hospitals use nothing; others administer diazepam (Valium) intravenously 1 to 20 mg at a slow rate (not more than 5 mg/min). In some hospitals, cocaine abusers are treated with a Valium protocol that lasts approximately 4 days; Valium is decreased from 10 mg q4hr PO/IM to 5 mg q8hr PO/IM, with additional doses as needed if the client has withdrawal symptoms. Other hospitals have PRN Valium orders only. Another protocol involves the use of phenobarbital in decreasing doses and imipramine hydrochloride (Tofranil). Because the depression is so great, Tofranil or other tricyclic antidepressants (TCAs) may be given for several weeks after detoxification. TCAs build up existing levels of neurotransmitters and make them available for transmission. Beta-adrenergic blockers such as propranolol (Inderal) may be used to counteract the tachycardia and hypertension that accompany acute cocaine intoxication, but their use may result in paroxysmal hypertension due to unopposed alpha-adrenergic stimulation. Therefore, they should be used cautiously and with constant blood pressure monitoring.

Use of TCAs to increase the number of neurotransmitters in the synapse is called synaptic treatment. Postsynaptic treatment for cocaine withdrawal and dependence includes the use of drugs such as bromocriptine (Parlodel) or amantadine (Symmetrel),

BOX 13–9 Key Facts About Cocaine

Slang Terms

Coke, lady, blow, snow, rabbits, C, powder

Route of Administration

Intranasal (flakes or powder sniffed), subcutaneous or intravenous, smoked in a pipe (freebasing)

Psychologic Symptoms

Psychomotor agitation*
Anxiety
Elation
Talkativeness*
Grandiosity*
Hypervigilance*
Impaired judgment
Ideas of reference; paranoia
Hallucinations
Formication (sensation of insects crawling on the skin)
Euphoria followed by depression and let-down (crash)
Violence
Insomnia
Anorexia

Physical Symptoms

Dilated pupils*
Tachycardia*
Elevated blood pressure*
Perspiration or chills*
Nausea or vomiting*
Anorexia
Dry mouth (characteristic bad breath)
Weight loss
Stuffy/runny nose
Burns and sores of nasal membranes
Tremors
Muscle cramping
Seizures

Withdrawal Symptoms

Severe craving
Fatigue
Psychomotor agitation
Hypersomnia
Irritability

Time Frame for Withdrawal Symptoms

Symptoms may appear within 24 hr after use; peak in 2–4 days. Depression may persist for months.

Dangers and Complications

Syncope
Fever
Chest pain
Depression
Death from convulsions
Cardiac/respiratory arrest

Typical Users

Teenagers
College students
Young urban professionals (yuppies)
Rock and movie stars
Executives

**Symptoms of intoxication noted in* DSM-IV-TR.

which increase dopaminergic activity in the synapse and enhance the effects of DA on the postsynaptic receptors. Presynaptic treatment with amino acids such as tryptophan was used until 1989, when tryptophan was removed from the market because of several deaths associated with its use. These amino acids were prescribed because the body converted them to neurotransmitters, which had been depleted by cocaine abuse.

CRACK

Crack, or "rock" cocaine, recently labeled "the most addictive drug known to man," is a potent form of hydrochloride cocaine that is mixed with baking soda and water, heated, allowed to harden, and then broken or "cracked" into little pieces and smoked in cigarettes or glass water pipes. Crack is more insidious, addictive, and toxic than cocaine. One user said, "I am worse in 3 weeks of using crack than in 6 years of using cocaine."

Crack is cheap and easily bought on the street, or in special crack houses where people congregate to smoke. A crack high has a rapid onset and is intensely euphoric, followed by a dramatic crash. Within seconds after "coming down," users feel compelled to smoke more crack. Because addiction is so rapid, many people are "hooked" and seek help when they can no longer support their habit. Crack users are flooding treatment centers, many of which have long waiting lists. Recidivism is estimated at over 90%. Key facts about crack are presented in Box 13–10 on page 382.

Symptoms of Crack Use

Symptoms of crack use include irritability, paranoia, depression, and physical symptoms that go along with the smoking of a toxic chemical, such as wheezing and coughing blood and black phlegm (see Box 13–10). Cardiac arrhythmias caused by crack use may lead to death. There is an increase in the number of babies being born to mothers who use crack. These babies are more likely to be premature or have low birth weights. They are irritable and have tremors and muscle rigidity.

FREEBASE

Freebase is a purified form of cocaine made by applying solvents to ordinary cocaine. Melting the cocaine with small butane torches helps in the purifying and delivery process. This

BOX 13–10 Key Facts About Crack (Hydrochloride Cocaine)

Slang Terms

Rock, crack

Route of Administration

Smoked

Psychologic Symptoms

Paranoia
Depression
Insomnia
Irritability
Deterioration of mental function
"Schizophrenia-like" psychosis
Appetite suppression

Physical Symptoms

Wheezing, shortness of breath
Black phlegm
Coughing blood
Parched throat and lips
Singed eyebrows and lashes
Increased heart rate and blood pressure
Weight loss

Withdrawal Symptoms

Severe craving
Depression
Fatigue
Hypersomnia
Irritability

Time Frame for Withdrawal Symptoms

Severe craving within minutes to hours. Depression appears within 3–7 days; may persist for weeks.

Dangers and Complications

Seizures
Cardiac arrhythmias
Respiratory paralysis
Paranoid psychoses
Pulmonary dysfunction

Typical Users

Teenagers
Young adults
All socioeconomic and cultural groups

action alone is dangerous due to the hazard of the solvent exploding. The effects of the freebase are brief but intense, and the short euphoria (3 to 5 minutes) immediately becomes a restless desire for more "base."

Phencyclidine (PCP)

PCP was originally used as an anesthetic for humans and as a tranquilizer for animals. Because of its dangerous side effects (see the key facts about phencyclidine in Box 13–11), it was removed from the market, except for veterinary use. However, by the mid-1960s, PCP was readily available as a street drug. PCP is inexpensive and easily synthesized by home chemists, making a supply always available.

CLINICAL EXAMPLE

Pete, an 18-year-old college student, was offered marijuana at a fraternity party. After smoking several joints, he was driving home with a friend when he became severely agitated. He insisted his friend stop the car near a pay phone; he jumped out and attempted to call the police, believing someone was trying to kill him. When the police arrived because of the disturbance he was causing (by then he was shouting and hallucinating), he rushed them, kicking at passersby and shooting at them as if he had a gun. During an assessment interview, the friend confessed to putting PCP in the marijuana.

THE EFFECTS OF PCP

People who use PCP frequently arrive at the emergency room in a psychotic, violent, and agitated state. The agitation and the sensations experienced by the user generate incredible power and strength where breaking heavy glass or fighting several people occurs even with a small, slight person. Some users fluctuate between coma and violence. Hallucinations are common. A differential diagnosis is important but difficult because the symptoms are similar to those of schizophrenia. It is believed that schizophrenics are particularly sensitive to PCP and that PCP may aggravate symptoms of schizophrenia.

A PCP high appears about 5 minutes after a person takes the drug and lasts 4 to 6 hours. Effects may last up to 48 hours. PCP may be recovered from the blood and urine for 7 to 10 days. While using PCP, a person experiences a wide variety of feelings, ranging from euphoria and utter peace to violence, confusion, and disorganization. Distorted sensory perceptions are common. During a bad "trip," anxiety, fear, and paranoia predominate. The dramatic physical and emotional effects of PCP may last for several weeks. Users may suffer from depression, fatigue, memory loss, concentration difficulty, and poor impulse control.

A substance very similar to PCP is Ketamine, a veterinary anesthesia agent also known as Special K, K, Vitamin K, and Cat Valium. It has a much shorter duration of action than PCP and is used recreationally because of its sedative and hallucinogenic properties (Schneider, Levenson, & Schnoll, 2001). It can cause delirium, amnesia, tachycardia, anxiety, and high blood pressure.

A vital problem with PCP is the question of its purity and its concentration. Because it is generally manufactured illegally,

BOX 13–11 Key Facts About Phencyclidine (PCP)

Slang Terms

PCP, angel dust, crystal, superjoint, hog, elephant tranquilizer, THC, rocket fuel, peace pill

Route of Administration

Oral, intravenous, smoked, inhaled

Psychologic Symptoms

Euphoria*
Psychomotor agitation*
Anxiety*
Grandiosity*
Disorientation swings
Emotional lability*
Sensation of slowed time*
Synesthesias (seeing sound or hearing colors)*
Facial grimacing
Muscle rigidity
Hallucinations
Paranoid ideation
Violent or bizarre behavior
Hostility, apathy
Depersonalization, isolation

Physical Symptoms

Vertical and horizontal nystagmus*
Increased blood pressure or heart rate*
Insensitivity to pain*
Dysarthria*
Ataxia*
Perspiration
Salivation
Vomiting

Dangers and Complications

Violence
Hypertension
Respiratory depression or arrest
Stupor
Coma
Convulsions
Death
Suicide

Typical Users

Adolescents
Young adults

**Symptoms of intoxication noted in* DSM-IV-TR.

users never really know what they are buying. Adulterants are often toxic to humans, causing a wide variety of responses, including death. Originally called the "peace pill," PCP is now recognized for its potential to cause violence, especially when the drug is taken in high dosages.

TREATMENT

Treatment of acute PCP intoxication may include the use of diazepam for muscle spasms, seizures, and agitation. Risperidone (Risperdal) or haloperidol (Haldol) may be used for severe psychotic behavior, but phenothiazines should not be used because PCP is anticholinergic. Calcium channel blockers such as verapamil (Depakote) may be given. These drugs are thought to prevent or reverse PCP-induced vasospasm, thereby decreasing the hallucinogenic effects of PCP. This treatment is controversial, however, because some clinicians feel that the use of verapamil (Depakote) may potentiate the effects of PCP. Nursing care during this period should focus on protecting the client and others from injury and reorienting the person to reality. Providing a quiet, safe environment and addressing the person in a calm, reassuring manner are important.

Hallucinogens

Hallucinogens are synthetic and natural drugs that cause hallucinations and unusual sensory experiences. Developed in 1938 for scientific research, LSD (lysergic acid diethylamide) became popular in the 1960s when Timothy Leary, a Harvard psychologist, described how it stimulated great insight and increased awareness. In the 1960s and 1970s, the U.S. Army experimented with LSD by giving it without informed consent to unsuspecting army employees. One dramatic and much publicized event concerned the army officer who leapt to his death from a window after unknowingly ingesting LSD. At this time the danger of LSD became publicized, as did the unethical research. Physician researchers also were interested in experimenting with the uses of LSD in the treatment of a variety of diseases; however, in 1966 LSD became illegal and could no longer be used in human research. Peyote, the active hallucinogen in cactus buttons, is still an integral part of religious rituals of Native Americans in the southwestern United States and Mexico. Psilocybin is the active hallucinogen in certain mushrooms. See the photographs of LSD and psilocybin in ■ Figure 13–6 on page 284.

CLINICAL EXAMPLE

Two high school seniors decided to take LSD. After 8 hours, one student was enjoying music, describing the varied colors he saw as the music changed in tempo. The other student was sweating profusely. His pupils were dilated, and he was trembling. He saw brightly colored dogs with huge teeth and claws changing into cats, snakes, and lions. He said he felt his gallbladder working with his liver and stomach. He eventually became so out of control that the other student took him to the emergency room.

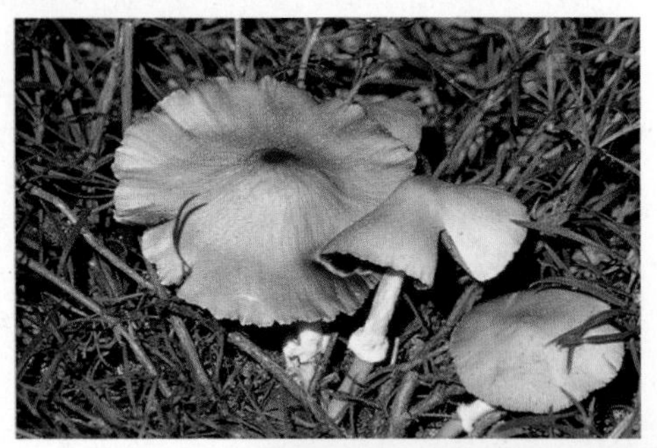

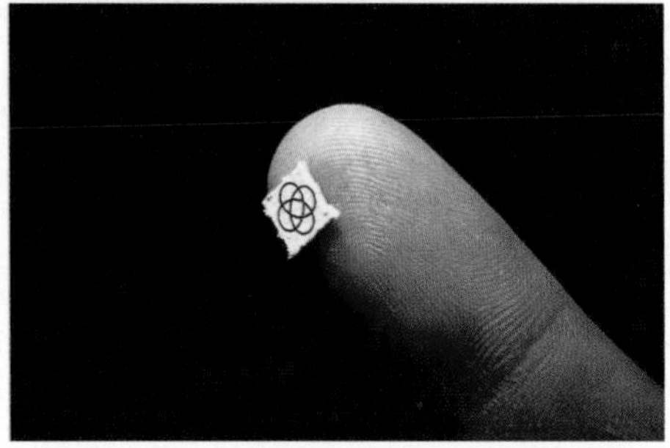

FIGURE 13–6 ■ *These photographs show psilocybin (A) and LSD (B). Both LSD and psilocybin induce psychedelic effects; however, LSD is much more potent than psilocybin (a product of various kinds of mushrooms).*

Source: **A)** James Beveridge/Visuals Unlimited. **B)** Custom Medical Stock Photo, Inc.

THE EFFECTS OF HALLUCINOGENS

After a lull in use, LSD ("acid") is again being used by teenagers because it is cheap ($2 to $5 a "hit") and causes an intense high that lasts 6 to 12 hours. Teenagers today are unacquainted with the horror stories of the 1960s. Today, people use LSD predominantly to get high rather than to expand consciousness. Psychological and physical dependence are unlikely because each experience with a hallucinogen is different. Increased creativity and brilliant personality revelations, presumed effects of the drugs, are short-lived at best. Key facts about hallucinogens are described in Box 13–12.

TREATMENT

The dangers of hallucinogens include "bad trips" and flashbacks.

Bad Trips

Users who experience *bad trips* may appear psychotic and extremely fearful. Reassuring the person and pointing out reality are helpful; occasionally, tranquilizers or antipsychotics are given. The symptoms usually disappear within 12 hours but may persist for months. People who are mentally ill or emotionally conflicted are more likely to have bad trips and flashbacks and to require hospitalization than are ordinary users.

Flashbacks

Flashbacks are a spontaneous reliving of the experiences the person felt while under the influence of the drug, although the

BOX 13–12 Key Facts About Hallucinogens

Examples

LSD, psilocybin, DMT, psilocin, mescaline, peyote, MDA

Slang Terms

Acid

Route of Administration

Oral

Psychologic Symptoms

Intensification of perceptions
Depersonalization
Derealization
Illusions, pseudohallucinations
Synesthesias (seeing sound or hearing colors)
Anxiety
Depression
Intense emotions
Body image changes
Ideas of reference
Paranoid ideation
Impaired judgment
Mood swings

Physical Symptoms

Dilated pupils
Tachycardia
Sweating
Palpitations
Blurred vision
Tremors
Lack of coordination

Dangers and Complications

Unpredictable behavior, resulting in harm to self or others
Flashbacks

Typical Users

Adolescents
Young adults

person is drug free. The experience may involve perceptual distortions, a variety of physical feelings, and strong emotions such as fear and pleasure. Flashbacks are generally brief, and they occur less frequently over time. Flashbacks may be induced by stress, fatigue, and drug or alcohol ingestion.

Some authorities believe hallucinogens pose a particular danger to adolescents in that they may precipitate a psychosis. Because teenagers' egos and defenses are weak, they may be especially susceptible to the effects of hallucinogens.

Inhalants

Inhalants are popular among teenagers and school-age children because they are cheap and easy to obtain. A new development in preferences for inhalants has been noted in an unusual area—embalming fluid.

CLINICAL EXAMPLE

Carlos is an 11-year-old homeless child from Brazil living on the streets in Miami, Florida. He comes to the attention of the clinic because he has been arrested for purse snatching. On clinical examination, Carlos appears giddy, dirty, disheveled, confused, and belligerent. His speech is slurred, he has an unsteady gait, and he smells like glue. His eyes are red and tearing, he is coughing, and he is nauseated. He has avoided attending school and has received no health care.

THE EFFECTS OF INHALANTS

The abuse of inhalants—glue, fuels, paints, aerosols, air fresheners, the substance used to resole shoes, and the propellants in canned whipped cream—is increasing at a frightening rate. Inhalants are inexpensive, easily available, and often legal. Their use causes euphoria, light-headedness, and excitement. Children are the most frequent users. Adult users often have a long history of polydrug abuse.

PATTERNS OF USE

Inhalants are sniffed or inhaled (called "huffing") in a variety of ways, such as from a rag soaked with the inhalant and placed in a plastic bag. Gas is frequently inhaled directly from a tank. Amyl and butyl nitrate (called "poppers") can be easily concealed and passed around a classroom, and paint thinner can be concealed in a soft drink can. Use of these inhalants and solvents can cause ventricular fibrillation, decreased cardiac output, serious brain damage, and sudden death.

TREATMENT

Although withdrawal must be managed as with the other substances covered in this chapter, careful assessment, early identification, detoxification, education, and prevention are particularly critical because so many inhalant abusers are children under the age of 12. Nurses need to be aware of the programs and resources available and should support legislation to make it more difficult for minors to obtain glue and paint products.

Nicotine

Nicotine is a psychoactive stimulating substance found in tobacco. It is associated with cancer, heart disease, emphysema, hypertension, and death. As a matter of fact, tobacco causes far more deaths than handguns during peacetime, more than 430,000 deaths each year in the United States—or one out of every five deaths (Cole, 2001; Schwartz, 2000). Nicotine is considered a substance of abuse. Our psychiatric–mental health clients have particular sensitivities to this substance—they become addicted much more easily and have greater difficulty quitting than those without a psychiatric–mental health diagnosis. Between 50% and 90% of clients with schizophrenia are regular cigarette smokers (Miotto, Preti, & Frezza, 2001). The behavioral and physiologic effects of nicotine frequently lead to addiction.

THE EFFECTS OF NICOTINE

Nicotine is a stimulant that acts in the central and peripheral nervous systems at cells that are normally acted upon by acetylcholine. The nicotinic receptor is a specific type of receptor for the neurotransmitter acetylcholine. In the CNS, nicotine binds to the cholinergic receptors in both DA and serotonin neural pathways. This causes the release of both DA and NE. The stimulant nicotine initially increases alertness and cognitive ability, and then has a depressant effect.

Research suggests a role for dopaminergic processes regulating the reinforcing effects of nicotine, making cessation of use more difficult. There is evidence that DA blockers can alter smoking behavior, but the human body compensates for this by then increasing the amount of smoking (Tomkins & Sellers, 2001). The usual impact of DA being turned over in the system at an increased rate is the reduction of hunger impulses. Once someone tries to quit smoking, hunger impulses return and the person may gain weight.

PATTERNS OF USE

Smoking cigarettes is an extremely common activity, despite smoke-free environments and restrictions on cigarette access. Approximately 47 million adults and 40% of adolescents in the United States smoke. There are also socioeconomic differences in smoking rates. The prevalence of smoking in Medicaid recipients is 44% compared to 19% with commercial HMO participants (Wadland, Soffelmayr, & Ives, 2001). As recipients of psychiatric services are at risk for socioeconomic downward drift, these statistics represent an alarming number of our clients.

Typically, people begin smoking at young ages, during peer pressure contacts, or during times of stress and thereafter find it very difficult to quit successfully. Use of tobacco products can be interrupted briefly during respiratory illnesses, hospitalizations, pregnancy, and following health care provider advice on smoking cessation. Return to tobacco use after a brief time is all too usual. Long-term quit rates range from 10% to 25% including pharmacologic cessation support (higher-dose nicotine gum, transdermal nicotine, psychopharmacology).

TREATMENT

The most commonly used approach for treating nicotine dependence is nicotine replacement therapies (patch, gum), which reduces craving by maintaining the blood level of nicotine. Multiple trials of bupropion (Zyban), an antidepressant, demonstrate its effectiveness in shorter-term abstinence. Office-based nursing and centralized telephone counseling services with an emphasis on relapse prevention has long-term abstinence effectiveness (Wadland, Soffelmayr, & Ives, 2001).

The transtheoretical model of behavior change (TTM) has been applied successfully to smoking cessation (Cole, 2001). TTM describes a continuum of five stages of behavior change (see ■ Table 13–4) and the underpinnings of movement from stage to stage.

Every person trying to make a change in behavior must go through stages before, during, and after the change is made. The beginning of this process is called assessing readiness to change. The entire model describes each of the stages in the process. There is a great deal to the theoretical model that can be useful to you in your nursing career and in your own health care behaviors.

Caffeine

Caffeine is available in a number of forms: coffee, tea, chocolate, and some pain relievers. It is a common and usual substance totally integrated into our social and occupational lives. In the United States more than half the population over the age of 10 drinks coffee. Like most other foodstuffs, an excessive intake of caffeine is not recommended, and around 300 mg is safe for most people. Over 600 mg caffeine per day is considered excessive.

The amount of caffeine in tea varies according to the plant variety it is made from and how long it is brewed—the longer it is brewed, the higher the caffeine level—but on average a 6-ounce cup of tea contains 40 mg of caffeine. Coffee also has variable amounts of caffeine; depending on its preparation method, 64 mg of caffeine are in a cup of instant coffee and 150 mg in a cup of filter coffee. A cup of coffee contains two or three times more caffeine than a cup of tea or chocolate. An average amount of caffeine ingested by a coffee-drinking adult each day is around 360 to 450 mg (Kleemola, Jousilahti, Pietinen, Vartiainen, & Tuomilehto, 2000). ■ Table 13–5 lists the caffeine content of selected beverages and drugs.

THE EFFECTS OF CAFFEINE

Caffeine acts as a stimulant, increasing the heart rate and stimulating the CNS. It is also a diuretic. There is evidence that a relationship exists between the amount of coffee consumption, total cholesterol, and low-density lipoprotein (LDL) cholesterol levels (Jee et al., 2001). The more caffeine ingested, the higher the total cholesterol and LDL cholesterol levels. Peak concentrations of caffeine are achieved 30 to 60 minutes after ingestion, and it takes around 3 hours to clear the system.

If coffee is withdrawn suddenly from people who drink large quantities of filtered coffee (six or more cups a day), they might become irritable and can even suffer from headaches. Given the stimulant effect of caffeine, it makes sense to advise those who complain of insomnia to switch to decaffeinated coffee or to have their last cup of coffee at least 3 hours before going to bed. Since tea has much less caffeine per cup than coffee, it does not have such a strong stimulating effect, but if there is a complaint

TABLE 13–4 The Transtheoretical Model of Behavior Change

TTM explains the stages of change and the processes of change. Features of change that occur throughout the stages, such as how decisional balance impacts on the process of change, an individual's vision of self-efficacy, and how temptation will likely be handled, make this perspective a useful one for promoting change.

Stage	Processes and Principles
1. Precontemplation	The client does not intend to change the health behavior in the near future, usually a 6-month period of time.
	Avoidance of communications designed to help change occur.
2. Contemplation	The client does intend to change the health behavior in the next 6 months.
	There is awareness of the benefits of change, but the barriers are being paid attention to and ambivalence is potent.
3. Preparation	The client intends to make the change in the next month.
	A plan of action is developed with small, important steps taken toward change.
4. Action	The client overtly modifies risky behavior and makes the change.
	Considerable time and energy are necessary in order to resist reverting to previous risky behaviors.
5. Maintenance	Work to prevent relapse occurs in this stage.
	Temptation gradually recedes over 6 months to 5 years. This stage is meant to extend through the client's life.

TABLE 13–5 Caffeine Content of Certain Beverages and Drugs

Source	Approximate Caffeine Content per 1 Cup (5 oz) or Tablet or Capsule
Beverages	
Drip coffee	56–176 mg (average 112)
Percolated coffee	39–168 (average 74)
Instant coffee	29–117 (average 66)
Decaffeinated coffee	1–8 mg (average 3)
Tea (bag or leaf)	30–91 mg (average 27)
Cocoa	2–7 mg (average 4)
Cola drinks (12 oz)	30–46 mg
Over-the-Counter Drugs	
Analgesics	
Aspirin (plain)	0 mg
Anacin, Bromo Seltzer, Cope, Empirin Compound, Midol	32 mg
Excedrin	65 mg
Vanquish	33 mg
Diuretics	
Aqua-Ban	100 mg
Stimulants	
NoDoz	100 mg
Vivarin	200 mg
Caffedrine	250 mg
Weight Control Aids	
Dexatrim	200 mg
Dietac	200 mg

of insomnia, it is worth not drinking large quantities of tea just before going to bed to address that problem. Strong coffee is capable of causing palpitations. Because of its stimulant properties, very young children should not drink coffee.

There is much concern about the negative physiologic effect of caffeine, especially related to cardiac risks. There have been variable research outcomes in this regard; however, it has become clear that some of the difficulty is the compound substance use of coffee and nicotine. The risk of congestive heart failure and death is much more competently explained by smoking and high serum cholesterol levels in combination with caffeine use than with caffeine ingestion alone (Kleemola et al., 2000).

PATTERNS OF USE

People who use caffeine use it for its stimulant properties. It is typically used upon awakening, during times of low energy or fatigue, and when an external source of comfort is required. Once a pattern of use has been established, individuals continue to use so that they do not suffer withdrawal symptoms. This is also seen in smoking behavior to obtain the substance nicotine.

TREATMENT

Reduction-of-harm modes of caffeine ingestion have been successful. The individual would decrease overall intake of the substance vehicle (such as coffee or tea), start using decaffeinated mixtures in increasing proportions, then complete the effort with cessation of caffeine ingestion. This process weans the individual from the substance without causing, or at least minimizing, jarring and uncomfortable withdrawal symptoms. Facilities frequently limit or restrict access to caffeinated beverages so that interference from the stimulating impacts does not complicate psychiatric treatment. Advance planning for alternative behaviors in social and occupational situations is helpful.

Polydrug Use

Most substance abusers today are polydrug users. This fact complicates diagnosis and treatment and increases the hazards associated with abuse. Synergistic or potentiating effects are possible; the effects of two or more drugs taken together are greater than the singular effects of each drug. Additive effects occur when two drugs that have similar effects are used together. Paradoxical effects occur if a drug causes a reaction opposite to that expected. Paradoxical effects may occur when only one drug is taken or when several drugs are taken. A pathologic reaction, too, may result from the ingestion of only one or several drugs: It is an unexpected and dramatic response to the drug. For example, the combination of alcohol and marijuana is especially dangerous because THC suppresses the nausea that results from an overdose of alcohol. Consequently, the person may continue to drink, risking respiratory depression, coma, and death.

Cocaine and alcohol are frequently used together; the cocaine gives the user a brief high, and the alcohol masks the ensuing depression. When the cocaine wears off, the person is intoxicated and unable to drive safely. Prescription drugs and alcohol are also a common combination. For up-to-date information on drugs of abuse, prevention, and treatment see the National Substance Abuse Web Index at nsawi.health.org/.

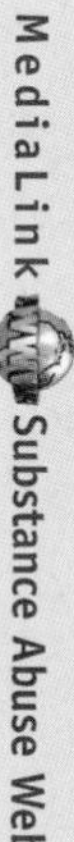

As illustrated in the clinical example on PCP, polydrug use can be inadvertent. Marijuana is often laced with PCP. In recent years dealers have also been putting heroin in marijuana. When heroin is smoked, it becomes a hidden addiction. The individual smokes more marijuana, increasing the amount of heroin needed to get the same high. The move from marijuana use to heroin use is then made.

Designer Drugs

Designer drugs, also called "club drugs," are chemical derivatives of controlled drugs. They are called analog drugs because they retain properties of controlled drugs, but one molecule is changed, making them initially not classifiable as controlled. According to the Controlled Substance Act of 1970, controlled substances (federally regulated substances) are classified from I (most regulated) through V, according to the potential for abuse and the current accepted medical use. As new information is made available, drugs may be reclassified.

Produced by underground chemists, analog drugs are initially legal until the government arranges for them to be analyzed and researched by chemists. Once a dangerous pattern of use is determined (often 3 to 6 months after police discover the drug), the drug may be classified as a controlled substance. Fentanyl citrate (Sublimaze), a synthetic anesthetic used as an anesthetic agent, is similar chemically to some designer drugs. Fentanyl is 100 times as strong as morphine and 20 to 40 times as strong as heroin. It provides a fast rush and an extraordinary high. A person can become addicted after one shot of fentanyl.

Methylenedioxymethamphetamine, also called Ecstasy, MDMA, Adam, XTC, X, Clarity, and Lover's Speed, has recently been classified as a Schedule I narcotic because research demonstrates that it causes structural damage to the brain. It is an amphetamine with hallucinogenic properties with effects lasting 3 to 6 hours. Currently, Ecstasy is the drug of choice for adolescents. It is easily and readily accessible.

In high doses, MDMA has been associated with malignant hyperthermia and rhabdomyolysis. MTPT (China white), an analog of meperidine (Demerol), has an adverse reaction similar to the rigidity caused by Parkinson's disease.

Flunitrazepam, also known as Rohypnol, Roofies, Rophies, Date-Rape Pill, and the Forget-Me Pill, is a fast acting benzodiazepine that causes anterograde amnesia (memory loss of events occurring while under the influence of the drug) and is tasteless, colorless, and odorless. Because it can be used to sexually victimize women by mixing it into drinks, it is the modern-day version of a Mickey Finn (alcohol and chloral hydrate). Another date-rape substance is gamma-hydroxybutyrate (called GHB, G, Liquid Ecstasy, Grievous Bodily Harm, and Georgia Home Boy). It produces euphoria and disinhibition, is used by body builders because of its anabolic properties, and is available on the Internet and in health food stores (Schneider, Levenson, & Schnoll, 2001).

Groups at Risk for Substance Abuse

People in a number of different circumstances can use and abuse a substance, however, there are those who are at greater risk for substance problems than others.

TEENAGERS

Drug abuse among teenagers is pervasive in our society. Although many adolescents experiment with drugs for only a brief time, many more who do so become addicted. Susceptibility to addiction seems to depend on several variables:

- Form and potency of the drug
- Dosage
- Frequency of use
- Pattern of use
- Stress
- Personality and genetic makeup of the user
- Family culture

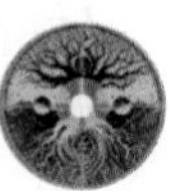

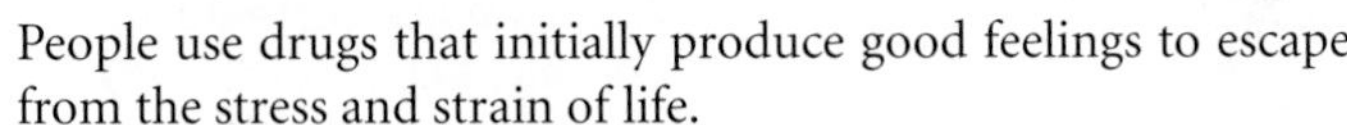

People use drugs that initially produce good feelings to escape from the stress and strain of life.

A teenager who relies on a quick "fix" (a drug) to ease mental pain does not learn healthy coping processes. If teenagers do not learn healthy coping mechanisms or work through the pains and mood swings associated with living, they never complete a necessary developmental stage. As a consequence, they remain fixated at a dependent level of development. They enter a dangerous cycle that is unlikely to be interrupted without professional intervention. Drug use, regardless of what drug is used, inevitably affects all areas of a teenager's life: school, work, social and family relationships, and sense of self-worth (see Chapter 26 for an assessment of teenage drug use).

Adolescent drug users manifest more psychopathologic conditions than nonusers do. Symptoms include feelings of depression, inadequacy, frustration, helplessness, and self-alienation. These teenagers also have ego structure deficiencies and poor impulse control. The earlier a child begins using a dependence-producing drug, the more likely the child is to use other dependence-producing drugs. Teenagers who use alcohol and drugs are likely to continue to use them in adulthood (Aarons, Brown, Hough, Garland, & Wood, 2001).

PSYCHIATRIC CLIENTS

Nurses need to be alert to possible, and sometimes likely, substance abuse by psychiatric clients. Problems may occur if clients take a combination of substances, and treatment is hindered if clients are under the influence of drugs or alcohol. There are a number of different ways to refer to psychiatric clients who use substances. Mentally ill chemical abusers (MICAs), chemically abusing mentally ill (CAMI), co-occurring mental and substance use disorders, and dual diagnosis (referring to both a mental illness and substance abuse diagnosis), among others, are phrases that try to explain the coexistence of these two demanding and divergent disorders. See Chapter 21 for further exploration of this population. The numerous problems facing clients make them both susceptible to substance use and as targets of drug dealers. Poor coping mechanisms, heightened stress, economic factors, and challenging and demoralizing illnesses influence a client's ability to steer clear of the escapism drugs offer.

It is estimated that between 16% and 60% of psychiatric clients have a substance use or abuse issue (American Public Health Association, 2001). Both of these disorders are chronic and clients tend to relapse. Close observation of teenagers and their visitors is useful, and the nurse should often ask clients directly if they are taking drugs. In most psychiatric hospitals, urine is routinely tested for the presence of drugs if there are any indications of use. Drug screening is usually done on admission and when the client returns from a pass.

Treatment programs for clients with psychiatric and substance use/abuse problems are best constructed with a reduction-of-harm perspective and built-in extensive psychosocial supports. Staff with credentials in psychiatry and substance treatment and rehabilitation work collaboratively with the client to manage the numerous chaotic upheavals seen with either one of the disorders at any time. When a client with these problems is treated in a setting designed for one or the other disorder, not both, the client is not likely to receive necessary specialized care.

WOMEN

Although alcoholism is a greater stigma for women than men, more women than ever before are drinking today. Many of these women are also using other drugs. Women respond to alcohol somewhat differently than men do because they metabolize alcohol less effectively than men. Research on women and alcohol makes it clear that treatment programs should be geared to women's needs. Such programs might include women-only groups, lesbian-only groups, female therapists, meetings with recovered women alcoholics/addicts, and help for the client families.

GENERAL HOSPITAL CLIENTS

Nurses who work in general hospitals must be alert to the possibility that clients with physical illnesses may be substance abusers and may be in danger of withdrawal. If you see symptoms that do not mesh with the condition under treatment, you may want to keep in mind that you may be seeing symptoms of substance withdrawal. Be alert and sensitive if physical assessment reveals any of the following:

- Debilitation out of proportion to the presenting health problem.
- Physical findings that do not correlate to the chief complaint.
- Unsteady gait, slurring of speech, dilated pupils, night sweats, chills, blackouts, tremors, skin tracks, abscesses, nasal septum perforation, or jaundice.
- Weight loss, poor hygiene, and poor nutrition.
- Symptoms of substance withdrawal.

Alert the primary health care provider and suggest appropriate laboratory studies (such as liver function tests). A nursing assessment may include questions about a client's drinking habits. If alcoholism is suspected, a helpful, matter-of-fact but nonjudgmental stance will facilitate the client's acceptance of treatment for possible withdrawal symptoms. Even among obviously intoxicated clients, responses to such direct questions may be angry and defensive.

THE ELDERLY

Elderly clients who are being treated for several chronic illnesses by different health care providers are at risk for drug problems from drug interactions and/or for drug dependence. For this reason, you should obtain a good history from the client, including a list of all the drugs taken, frequency of use, dosage, and duration of use. It is often useful to ask the family of an older client to bring all drugs to the hospital for review rather than relying on memory. Frequently, the confusion seen in elderly clients is a direct consequence of drug interactions or malabsorption.

In addition, substance abuse (especially alcoholism) is less likely to be detected and treated in older adults than in younger clients. It often goes unrecognized because the signs of substance abuse are difficult to distinguish from the changes associated with normal aging or degenerative brain disease. The difficulty in assessing drug abuse in older clients is further complicated by the paucity of elder-specific alcohol and drug treatment facilities, despite the fact that as much as 48% of the population over age 60 has an alcohol problem. This problem is likely to increase with the future graying of America. Both early- and late-onset elderly alcoholics have reported loneliness, losses, depression, and meager social support networks as antecedents of their alcohol abuse.

ADULT CHILDREN OF ALCOHOLICS

Adult children of alcoholics are at great risk of becoming alcoholics. If both parents are alcoholics, a child has a 70% chance of becoming an alcoholic; if one parent is an alcoholic, a child has a 40% chance. This type of alcoholism has been labeled familial. Research on familial alcoholism has shown that:

- A family history of alcoholism is present.
- Alcoholism develops early, usually by the time the person is in his or her late twenties.
- The alcoholism is generally severe and usually requires treatment.
- The risk of alcoholism is increased, but not the risk of other psychiatric disorders.

HEALTH CARE PROVIDERS

Many factors place health care providers at risk for developing chemical dependence. A primary risk factor is codependence. Many codependents, whether adult children of substance abusers or products of other dysfunctional family systems, choose careers in the health care professions, such as nursing. Codependent nurses often give more of themselves than is necessary for effective client care. They seek perfection and tend to ignore or repress problems and difficulties. Codependent nurses put supreme effort into taking care of everyone but themselves.

Health care workers in general work under a great deal of stress and have easy access to drugs. Every day, they give people medication to decrease pain. It is an easy leap to begin to self-medicate. However, such behavior is a violation of state practice acts and ethical standards of practice and, depending on the drug and method of obtaining it, may be a criminal offense.

Colleagues of chemically dependent health care workers need to be alert to behavior that suggests a problem. They should attempt to talk with the professional who is having difficulty before documenting and reporting such behavior to a supervisor. It is very common to cover up the behavior. Shielding such a health care provider—whatever the professional discipline—puts clients, the health care provider, and profession at risk and violates professional practice, the code of ethics, and the law in many states. Nurses, however, need to

BOX 13–13 Warning Signs of Chemically Dependent Health Care Providers

- Frequent absenteeism before and after days off; always working (in order to obtain supply)
- Irritability
- Abrupt mood changes; inappropriate affect
- Sloppy charting and client care
- Problems with drugs (missing drugs, frequent "wasting" of drugs, inaccurate records)
- Frequent errors in judgment
- Alcohol (stale or fresh) on breath
- Frequent disappearance from the assigned area
- Offering to give medication to clients
- Frequent night shift work
- Clients receiving medications from the health care provider complain of little or no pain relief

understand that their chemically dependent colleagues suffer from a disease, not a moral problem. This understanding empowers nurses to work together to help each other. See the warning signs in Box 13–13.

NURSING PROCESS

Clients with Substance-Related Disorders

As substance abuse becomes an increasing problem in society, more clients will be admitted to hospitals and clinics for help with intoxication and withdrawal. Substance abuse is a disease and not a weakness or flaw. A moralistic attitude always alienates the client. Recognizing and accepting that the disease is chronic, often with remissions and exacerbations, should keep you from succumbing to the frustration felt by many who treat substance abusers who relapse. At stressful times in life, anyone may develop a dependence on drugs or alcohol; however, certain people seem to be predisposed to the illness. Your expertise in the stages of the nursing process is vital to the care of clients with substance abuse problems. Your focus should be on helping clients work toward self-awareness, good health, and good interpersonal relationships so that they can lead productive, fulfilling, happy lives.

Drugs change rapidly, and nurses must keep up with the "drug scene" to assess and treat clients. Along with the knowledge acquired from reading, continuing education programs, and seminars, nurses need self-knowledge to be good therapists with substance abusers. Ongoing critical self-analysis of feelings, attitudes, and behavior toward clients is useful. See the Nursing Self-Awareness feature below for a list of questions to guide this self-analysis.

Assessment

Make an accurate assessment of the substances used and abused to anticipate potential toxic and withdrawal effects and to make nursing care plans as specific and relevant as possible. For example, a chronic alcoholic who is malnourished, exhausted, and depressed needs immediate diet regulation, rest, and gradual involvement in a treatment program. See the Case Study and Care Plan for the Client with Chronic Alcoholism on pages 292–293. Cocaine or crack abusers are likely to be resistant to treatment and need active staff intervention and a structured program to involve them in treatment. They should not be left alone or purposefully isolated, as might be done with an alcoholic.

Nursing SELF-AWARENESS — Your Stress Response and Susceptibility to Substance Use

Examine who you are when you are stressed by answering the following questions and attending to what this means about your coping mechanisms and your susceptibility to substance use. Make a connection between what you have experienced regarding substances and what your clients are experiencing.

Check the substances you choose to use when you seek comfort from stress:

- ☐ Food (carbohydrates)
- ☐ Food (noncarbohydrates)
- ☐ Cigarettes
- ☐ Coffee
- ☐ Wine
- ☐ Beer
- ☐ Liquor
- ☐ Chocolate
- ☐ Tea
- ☐ Pain relievers (ASA, acetaminophen, ibuprofen, other)
- ☐ Marijuana
- ☐ Recreational drugs

At what rate do you use any of the above?

- ☐ More than 5 times a day
- ☐ More than 2 times a day
- ☐ Daily
- ☐ Only at work/school
- ☐ Only on the weekends
- ☐ Only at dinner
- ☐ Only at parties
- ☐ Monthly
- ☐ Occasionally

At what rate would you use these if you had the money, time off, no weight concerns, or other release from responsibility?

- ☐ More than 5 times a day
- ☐ More than 2 times a day
- ☐ Daily
- ☐ Only at work/school
- ☐ Only on the weekends
- ☐ Only at dinner
- ☐ Only at parties
- ☐ Monthly
- ☐ Occasionally

SUBJECTIVE DATA

As part of the mental status exam and the psychiatric history, conduct a thorough, nonjudgmental substance use assessment.

Interview Questions

1. How many packs of cigarettes do you smoke?
2. Do you take any prescription drugs now?
3. Do you drink alcohol each day? If yes, do you drink a pint or about a quart? (Let the client correct you on your overstatement rather than fear shocking you with the truth.)
4. Do you drink a pint or quart of alcohol or more on occasion? When was your last drink?
5. Do you have a drug habit? What drugs do you use, and what is your daily cost?
6. When did you last drink more than you wanted to?

Simply asking, "How many drinks do you have at a time?" can be misleading and can minimize the problem if each drink exceeds standard bar amounts of about 2 ounces. The CAGE questions discussed in Box 13–14 are also helpful.

Accurate responses to these questions are most likely when they are part of an interview that includes general lifestyle inquiries about cigarette smoking, coffee consumption, and exercise habits. Experts agree that skillful assessment interviewing of clients and their family members remains the best source of data.

In an emergency situation the client may be unable to answer key questions like these:

- What did you take?
- How much did you take?
- When did you take it?
- What have you taken in the last 24 hours? In the last week?

When this happens, you must rely on family or friends as data sources, and then corroborate what you learn with the client once he or she is alert.

Common Defense Mechanisms in Client Responses. Denial and projection are two defense mechanisms common to substance abusers. These mechanisms, along with other behaviors—conning, bargaining, feigning—complicate all phases of the nursing assessment of subjective data. Alcoholics and other drug abusers tend to deny that they have a problem or minimize the problem: "I drink/use every day, but it rarely interferes with my work." Rationalization is common: "I know I shouldn't drink, and I'll stop as soon as I get through this problem. Drinking keeps me calm enough to function." A detailed assessment, along with family/coworker interviews, reveals that the problem is generally worse than the client says. Cocaine users tend to project and blame their difficulties on others, often a spouse. For instance, a man may bring up the issue of his wife's drinking and give a dozen reasons why he does not need treatment.

Substance abusers sometimes "con" (manipulate) people to get drugs. DSB, a term used in some treatment centers, refers to drug-seeking behaviors, such as feigning illness or an injury to get a drug. These people also bargain with themselves and staff members to get what they want. For example, an alcoholic/drug abuser is likely to think, "I know I shouldn't hang out with B and P since we all get loaded together, but I like them. I'll just be with them, I won't drink/use." Later on, the person may think, "I'll only use a gram of cocaine"; later, "I'll just do an eight-ball." This client might tell the nurse, "I'll be glad to go to group therapy next week; just let me rest for a few days. I'm really tired." Of course, substance abusers always con themselves first.

BOX 13–14 CAGE Questions

The CAGE is most frequently used for the detection of alcoholism in clinical settings. CAGE is a mnemonic for these four questions:

1. Have you ever felt like you should **C**ut down on your drinking?
2. Have people **A**nnoyed you by criticizing your drinking?
3. Have you ever felt bad or **G**uilty about your drinking?
4. Have you ever had a drink in the morning as an **E**ye-opener to get rid of a hangover?

Source: Ewing, J. A. (1999). Screening for alcoholism using CAGE. Cut down, Annoyed, Guilty, Eye opener. *JAMA,* February 17, 281(7), 611. Reprinted with permission from American Medical Association.

Motivation for Treatment. Nurses need to consider some important psychosocial issues when clients come for treatment. Clients may enter a treatment program voluntarily. This situation is best, because they are internally motivated and therefore have a better chance of success. However, they may be coerced by family, friends, physicians, or the police to undergo treatment. See the Web site for the National Center on Addiction and Substance Abuse at Columbia University at www.casa columbia.org/ for information on every form of substance abuse.

MediaLink National Center on Addiction

Coerced treatment inevitably causes anger and resentment. These clients may lash out at people, blame them (including you, the nurse), and demonstrate resistant or arrogant behavior. In these difficult situations, you must remain detached and nonjudgmental to avoid both power struggles and taking the role of persecutor or rescuer. At this time, you function as a data gatherer: "I know you are [uncomfortable, anxious, afraid, angry] now. To help you feel better, I need to ask you some questions about your drug use." A judgmental question is, "Don't you know that if you don't get help now you will only get worse?" Such questions prevent rapport and alienate the client.

The Importance of Language. Knowing the language of the drug world is important in obtaining an accurate nursing assessment of a substance abuser. Drug users have a language all their own; to understand them and the extent and nature of their habit, a nurse needs to learn this language. For example, "basing and balling" refer to freebasing (using ether to purify cocaine and make it more potent) and speed-balling (combining heroin and cocaine); "copping an eight-ball" means acquiring one-eighth ounce of cocaine; a "mission" is several days' use of crack; "drug of choice" is the client's favorite drug. Often, the clients themselves or a recovering addict can teach the nurse this language.

OBJECTIVE DATA

In addition to assessing subjective data, you should include a thorough consideration of relevant objective data. An assessment of behavioral changes can cue you to drug use.

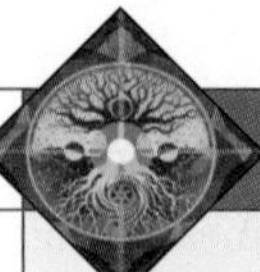

Case Study

Client with Chronic Alcoholism

Identifying Information

John Mills is a 54-year-old married civil servant. He is Catholic, has a high school education, and was referred from the Care Unit (a specialty hospital) where he has been for the last 28 days.

John states, "I've had a drinking problem for 35 years. My wife and boss told me if I don't shape up they'll kick me out of my home and my job. I want to feel better. It's been a living hell. But I'm not sure I can stop drinking; I've tried before." He describes his drinking as a way "to cope with my problems for most of my life." He "wants to stay dry." Fifteen years ago, his social drinking escalated and he began binge drinking on the weekends. Later, he began drinking throughout the week. He has been drinking daily for most of the last three years. He drank "enough to keep a buzz on" and occasionally "enough to pass out." John's problems with work include tardiness, absenteeism, and errors on the job. Marital problems are described as "she either yells at me or takes care of me." He describes years of his wife pouring out his hidden liquor and calling his boss to say John had the flu when he was really "hung over."

History

John has been in and out of AA groups and has seen three psychiatrists. He has been hospitalized three times for car accidents and injuries due to drinking (broken leg and ribs, contusions, concussion). After the last general hospital admission, he was admitted to the Care Unit for a 28-day alcohol treatment program.

Both of John's parents are deceased and both were alcoholics. His sister, aged 58, is a recovering alcoholic (has been "dry" for 10 years). The family has never been close. John feels he was "never allowed to be a normal, active kid." His sister cared for him when he was young and functioned as a surrogate mother.

John developed normally but always "felt different." He worked every summer and took a full-time job after high school graduation. He enjoyed "drinking buddies" from work, but has never had a close friend he could depend on. He smokes one pack of cigarettes daily and uses no other drugs. He spends his leisure time watching TV and at bars with friends.

John has cirrhosis of the liver. He is malnourished from chronic alcoholism and has a long history of insomnia.

Current Mental Status

John is well groomed, clean, and alert. His sensorium is within normal limits; affect appropriate yet apathetic. He appears depressed and he expresses feelings of self-reproach and guilt for his years of drinking and its effect on others. Speech is slow and spontaneous. Motor behavior, thought content, and thought processes are within normal limits. Insight questionable.

Other Subjective or Objective Clinical Data

Multivitamins qd; no indications of suicide or violence potential.

Physical Findings. Less dramatic physical findings may include dry skin, hangnails, malnutrition, ascites, elevated blood pressure, and the smell of alcohol or an inhalant on the client's breath. As alcoholism progresses, be alert to signs and symptoms of liver cirrhosis (see Box 13–15).

Standardized, Structured Questionnaires and Scales. The list of standardized, structured interviews; questionnaires; and scales used to assess substance abuse is long and includes the following, which are among the best known:

- DSM-IV-TR Structured Clinical Interview (SCID)
- Addiction Severity Index
- Chemical Use, Abuse, and Dependence Scale (CUAD)
- Millon Clinical Multiaxial Inventory
- Drinking Problems Index
- CAGE Questionnaire (in Box 13–14)

Laboratory Tests. For years, researchers and clinicians have been searching for an objective biologic marker that will reflect problem drinking and make assessment less challenging. Common laboratory tests in which elevated values are associated with excessive alcohol intake are:

- Blood alcohol concentration
- Gamma-glutamyl transferase (GGT)
- Alanine aminotransferase (ALT, formerly SGPT)
- Aspartate aminotransferase (AST, formerly SGOT)
- Lactate dehydrogenase
- Alkaline phosphatase
- Total bilirubin
- Cholesterol
- Triglycerides
- Uric acid
- Mean corpuscular volume (MCV)

BOX 13–15 Signs and Symptoms of Liver Cirrhosis

- *Skin.* Extremely dry skin; severe pruritus; abnormal pigmentation; spider angiomas on the face, neck, arms, and trunk; telangiectasis on the cheeks; prominent abdominal vessels; ecchymosis; palmar erythema; jaundice.
- *Gastrointestinal.* Abnormal nutrient absorption; anorexia; indigestion; nausea and vomiting; diarrhea or constipation; hemorrhoids; dull, aching abdominal pain; musty breath; ascites.
- *Central nervous system.* Lethargy; slurred speech; asterixis (flapping tremor of the hands); peripheral neuritis; confusion; coma.
- *Hematologic.* Bleeding tendencies (frequent nosebleeds, easy bruising, bleeding gums); anemia.
- *Hepatic.* Hepatomegaly. Replacement of lobules with fibrous tissue. In the early stages of cirrhosis, the liver will feel large and firm, with a sharp edge. Eventually it shrinks, and the edge feels nodular. There may also be pain in the right upper quadrant that intensifies when the client leans forward.

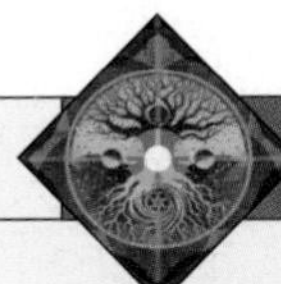

Nursing Care Plan

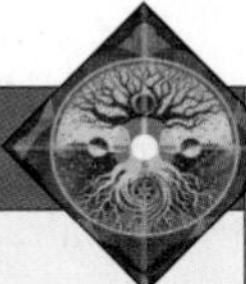

Nursing Diagnosis: Ineffective Individual Coping Related to Alcohol Abuse

Expected Outcome: Reduction of ineffective and self-destructive coping through alcohol abuse and regular use of more effective coping styles.

Short-Term Goals	*Interventions*	*Rationale*
Identification of two effective coping mechanisms	• John inventories those situations that challenge his abilities to cope. • John recognizes the automatic mechanisms involved in habitually responding to stress with alcohol. • John rehearses various coping strategies to prepare to select two for regular use. • John begins to substitute effective coping for alcohol use when stressed.	Revision of coping styles requires identification of the situations placing him at risk, typical problematic responses, and acknowledgment of needing to learn new coping styles.

Nursing Diagnosis: Sleep Pattern Disturbances Related to Alcohol Abuse

Expected Outcome: John will use sleep-inducing strategies nightly and report satisfaction with his quality of sleep.

Short-Term Goals	*Interventions*	*Rationale*
John will sleep a total of 6 hours/night	• Assess current pattern and effective strategies. • Respond to awakening with sleep hygiene: warm milk, reading, relaxation strategies. • Employ effective strategies regularly.	Reestablish a consistently healthy sleep routine.

Nursing Diagnosis: Altered Nutrition Related to Alcohol Abuse

Expected Outcome: John eats three meals every day plus snacks and takes a multivitamin as recommended.

Short-Term Goals	*Interventions*	*Rationale*
John identifies and discerns relationship between alcoholism and malnutrition. John gains weight through a balanced diet.	• Monitor intake of meals and snacks. • Initiate dietary consult. • Investigate dietary preferences to maximize John's abilities to expand his intake appropriately. • Educate regarding the impact of chronic alcohol ingestion on the digestive tract, metabolism, and overall health. • Offer frequent food and fluids throughout contacts.	Malnutrition from chronic alcoholism can be addressed with a comprehensive nutrition program.

These elevated laboratory test values are only one of the alerting factors for problem drinking. No single test or combination of tests alone to date is appropriate for clinical screening. Confirmation of the excessive use of alcohol in a sensitively conducted assessment interview remains the preferred assessment approach and is considered a prerequisite for successful intervention.

Nursing Diagnoses: NANDA

Because substance-related disorders are associated with biologic, psychosocial, and even spiritual distress, a wide variety of nursing diagnoses is likely to be fundamental to planning comprehensive care. Several diagnoses include:

- Ineffective Individual Coping
- Altered Family Processes: Alcoholism
- Impaired Adjustment
- Anxiety
- Nutrition: Less Than Body Requirements
- Decisional Conflict
- Pain
- Sensory/Perceptual Alterations
- Impaired Social Interaction
- Altered Thought Processes

Outcome Identification: NOC

When designing care for clients who have substance abuse disorders, outcomes must be specifically delineated. While the outcome of total and permanent abstinence may be achievable for some clients with some abuse disorders, for others it may be an unattainable goal. Each situation must be assessed individually. Make sure your outcomes can be measured so both you and your client are aware of progress and relapse. Outcome criteria for substance abusers include:

- Coping
- Decision making
- Impulse control

All of these outcomes impact on client sobriety, abstinence from drugs and alcohol, and "being clean." Further outcomes include risk reduction; improvement of work, family, and social relationships; and lifestyle changes that may include a growing sense of spirituality. Clients become more effective in using new attitudes and behaviors. Better feelings about themselves result. Although the fear of relapse is always present, over time the craving for chemicals diminishes, and the client establishes a new, healthy lifestyle.

Ask yourself, "Is the outcome one this client can relate to and invest energy into?" There is not a single addiction or abuse situation we've looked at in this chapter that is going to be easy for the client to abandon as a lifestyle. Imagine a habit you have that is not in your best interests (we all have such habits to one extent or another). Now imagine how you would best be able to work with a nurse to change that habit or eradicate it completely from your repertoire.

MediaLink Care Plan: Alcohol Withdrawal

Planning and Implementation: NIC

Nurses may hold positions in any of the following settings. Their roles may be slightly different in each setting, depending on the client's stage of illness and presenting symptoms. Interventions can address the wide range of nursing diagnoses relevant to substance-related disorders.

GENERAL HOSPITAL CARE

Substance abusers who are suicidal or acutely ill with DTs, hepatic coma, respiratory depression, or cardiac arrhythmias are often treated in a medical–surgical unit of a general hospital. Life-threatening physiologic symptoms are attended to first. When the client is out of danger, the alcoholism or drug addiction issues are addressed. In this setting, nurses:

- Monitor vital signs and respiratory and cardiovascular support.
- Administer prescribed medications.
- Apply ice packs for fever, such as fever caused by amphetamine intoxication or following cocaine use.
- Decrease stimulation; provide a darkened quiet room.
- Point out reality: "I know you are seeing things, and I know you are frightened. You are in the hospital, and we are caring for you. There are no bugs or monsters here. You are safe and will feel better soon."
- Make sure clients get adequate nutrition and fluids (they are disoriented and generally forget to eat and drink).
- Assess changes in level of consciousness.
- Monitor fluid intake and output.
- Protect skin integrity.
- Offer emotional support and encouragement to the client and his or her family.
- Refer clients to community resources for recovery programs.

SPECIALTY HOSPITAL CARE

Specialty hospital care is given in inpatient hospital units that are geared specifically for the treatment of substance abuse. If the hospital is equipped with trained personnel and appropriate resources, acutely ill clients, including those who are intoxicated may be admitted. The physical environment is modified to handle problems with substance abusers. For example, rooms devoid of furniture and potentially harmful materials offer a quiet, unstimulating environment that prevents convulsions and decreases anxiety. A primary nurse may be assigned to decrease confusion and stimulation. Members of the staff are experts in detoxification, education, and treatment. Clients also receive treatment for coexisting medical and psychiatric problems. Staff efforts are geared toward stabilization. The Rx Communication feature on page 295 focuses on intervening with the intoxicated client.

RESIDENTIAL REHABILITATION

Residential rehabilitation facilities offer inpatients expert care for substance abuse, but in some cases staff members are not skilled in treating medical or psychiatric problems.

EXTENDED RESIDENTIAL CARE

Extended care facilities provide services for people with physical impairments and a home for recovering alcoholics or drug addicts who have been rejected by their families. Apartments for independent living, a relatively new concept, are useful for these clients.

OUTPATIENT CARE

Outpatient care may consist of daily, weekly, or monthly individual, group, or family therapy in a variety of treatment centers. Daily care is usually given only in intensive programs of limited duration, usually one month. Employee assistance programs (EAPs) are now common in many industries and are one example of outpatient care given not in a clinic but in the workplace. Substance abuse outreach counselors work with chemically dependent employees.

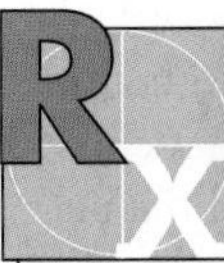

COMMUNICATION

Client with Alcoholism Who Is Intoxicated

CLIENT: "I'm so sorry I'm such a burden to you, and you're such a good nurse, and I never want to be the type of person who . . ."

NURSE RESPONSE 1: "I'm going to take your vital signs and then you will take some time to yourself."

RATIONALE: This interaction treats the event as an illness in which there are physical consequences to the behavior as well as sets limits on the interaction.

NURSE RESPONSE 2: "We will talk later when you are able to concentrate."

RATIONALE: An intoxicated client is not able to benefit from a detailed discussion.

Nurses who work with clients who have substance-related disorders in any of these settings need to recognize that addiction is a chronic, progressive disease. Each treatment setting calls for different skills. For example, in general or specialty hospitals, nurses need psychosocial skills along with technical skills to assess and monitor the physiologic components of abuse and withdrawal. In residential rehabilitation and extended residential care centers, the nurse may educate clients about the disease, help clients reenter the community as much as possible, and facilitate or lead support groups. At a student counseling center in a university or college, nurses are involved in treating the college student who has difficulty with drugs or alcohol (see ■ Figure 13–7).

SELF-HELP GROUPS

Self-help groups are also called mutual help groups where people with similar problems help one another. Groups composed of peers share experiences and knowledge of the problem to support and educate each other.

Twelve-Step Programs: AA and NA. In contrast to the previously described treatment programs, Alcoholics Anonymous (AA) and Narcotics Anonymous (NA) are not specifically treatment programs. They are spiritual programs based on the fellowship among its members. Both are successful self-help groups that meet daily or more often in different parts of large cities and weekly in smaller towns in places of worship, schools, town halls, and various mental health treatment facilities. Anyone who has a desire to stop drinking or taking drugs is welcome. This belief pervades both organizations: "Once an alcoholic/addict, always an alcoholic/addict." Members admit they are powerless over chemicals, live "one day at a time," recite the serenity prayer, and believe in "a power greater than man." Members learn to turn their problems over to "the God of my understanding." Their philosophy is revealed in part through their key slogans, "First things first," "Easy does it," and "Let go and let God." Alcoholics learn the "Twelve Steps of AA" (see Box 13–16).

FIGURE 13–7 ■ *Entrance to a student counseling center in a university or college.*

BOX 13–16 The Twelve Steps of Alcoholics Anonymous

1. We admitted we were powerless over alcohol—that our lives had become unmanageable.
2. Came to believe that a Power greater than ourselves could restore us to sanity.
3. Made a decision to turn our will and our lives over to the care of God, as we understood Him.
4. Made a searching and fearless moral inventory of ourselves.
5. Admitted to God, to ourselves, and to another human being the exact nature of our wrongs.
6. Were entirely ready to have God remove all these defects of character.
7. Humbly asked Him to remove our shortcomings.
8. Made a list of all people we had harmed, and became willing to make amends to them all.
9. Made direct amends to such people wherever possible, except when to do so would injure them or others.
10. Continued to take personal inventory and when we were wrong, promptly admitted it.
11. Sought through prayer and meditation to improve our conscious contact with God, as we understood Him, praying only for knowledge of His will for us and the power to carry that out.
12. Having had a spiritual awakening as the result of these steps, we tried to carry this message to alcoholics, and to practice these principles in all our affairs.

Source: The Twelve Steps are reprinted with permission of Alcoholics Anonymous World Services, Inc. (A.A.W.S.) Permission to reprint the Twelve Steps does not mean that A.A.W.S. has reviewed or approved the contents of this publication, or that A.A.W.S. necessarily agrees with the views expressed herein. A.A. is a program of recovery from alcoholism *only*—use of the Twelve Steps in connection with programs and activities which are patterned after A.A., but which address other problems, or in any other non–A.A. context, does not imply otherwise.

Through AA/NA, people learn to change negative attitudes and behaviors into positive ones. A key concept of AA/NA is that total abstinence is essential to recovery. As members become sober or drug free, they begin "sponsoring" (helping) other substance abusers. This offering of support is believed to be vital to recovery, as is regular attendance at AA/NA meetings. Twelve-step recovery programs also emphasize spirituality through meditation and prayer rather than will power as the means to recovery. Recognizing that AA's 12 steps were written in the 1930s by and for white Christian males (see Box 13–16) may require that the nurse adapt some of the language to a less patriarchal, less religious, and more generally spiritual and culturally relevant usage. The Caring for the Spirit feature below will help you to do so.

AA and NA, while excellent for clients with substance abuse problems, may cause some difficulties for the psychiatric client who has abuse or use problems. The AA/NA philosophy of complete abstinence from substances has been said to include psychiatric medications. This causes a rift between what clients are told by their psychiatric–mental health nurses and the path toward wellness according to AA/NA. Programs designed to provide the most effective treatment for the psychobiologic underpinnings of psychiatric disorders and accommodate the added stress of substances of abuse work best.

Women for Sobriety. Women for Sobriety (WFS) is another self-help group. Unlike AA/NA, WFS is not based on a spiritual philosophy; instead, the program is based on abstinence. WFS's 13 acceptance statements focus members on new ways of thinking. The women learn to cope and, over time, to change their daily lives. The group recognizes the differences of alcoholism in males and females.

CARING FOR THE SPIRIT

Twelve-Step Recovery

The twelve steps are grouped here into four categories: Surrender, Acceptance, Fellowship, and Bliss of Living. Each step is given a one-word description to indicate how the step works in the recovery process.

Surrender Steps

Step One: Honesty
Step Two: Hope
Step Three: Faith

Because many view surrender as a negative activity, using the words *honesty*, *hope*, and *faith* to describe each of the steps in the first category gives new meaning to the purpose of these steps. When seen from a patriarchal hierarchical view, the first step may appear to be a command. However, when it is a call to "get honest" with oneself, the step takes on new meaning without rewriting it or discounting the value it has had in helping others find recovery.

When seen as a way to expand one's spirituality through meditation and contemplation, the second step takes on new meaning as well. Hope comes from observation of others who have given up the need to control and be self-centered, who have found peace as a result of that action. The "came to believe" part of this step occurs over time as the client hears similar stories from multiple sources who share at twelve-step meetings. This is in part why a new member is urged to "Keep coming back . . . so more can be revealed."

The faith that results from taking the third step allows the client to move from ego-centered thinking to belief in a power greater than self, permitting that power to work on his or her behalf.

Acceptance Steps

Step Four: Courage
Step Five: Integrity
Step Six: Willingness

The next three steps follow from the change of attitude in the first three steps. These are action steps.

In the fourth step, clients use newly discovered courage to examine the specific aspects of their character they need to nurture and develop, as well as those that need to be eliminated because they are responsible for current discomfort and distress.

The fifth step works to restore integrity to the client's life and may be responsible for the euphoria reported by many during early recovery. The client may feel a growing spiritual connection, and the nurse may be in a position to support the client's awareness of how the steps have contributed to his or her improved condition.

The sixth step is a willingness activity in which clients must decide how to convert their growing spirituality into a change of behavior.

Fellowship Steps

Step Seven: Humility
Step Eight: Forgiveness
Step Nine: Discipline

The fellowship steps help clients progress in their spiritual awareness and recovery by developing qualities of humility, forgiveness, and discipline in their personal relationships and public lives.

Bliss of Living Steps

Step Ten: Perseverance
Step Eleven: Love of self
Step Twelve: Gratitude

The bliss of living steps bring clients back to a life with meaning. By developing perseverance clients gain a freedom from worry about when the accumulation of undesirable behavior will be discovered and how it will lead back to the pain of the past. In the eleventh step, clients learn through prayer and meditation the love of self, love of others and love of life. They come to feel that they are not in charge of the world and that trusting in a higher power who is in charge is "OK." In the twelfth step recovering addicts and alcoholics express their gratitude for what they have achieved and learn to value reaching out to other sufferers to share the hope of step two, the courage of step four, and the love of step eleven.

Nurses have the opportunity to assist with the unfolding of the process of twelve-step recovery. Clients do the work supported by their spiritual beliefs. Nurses can nourish the process of learning to live life in a new way.

Rational Recovery (RR). Alcoholics Anonymous is the most popular mutual-help recovery organization in the world, but it is not the only one. Alcoholics and addicts who failed to find a comfortable home in AA but were nevertheless determined to become sober have founded at least one other major organization to help others become clean and sober. This group, Rational Recovery (RR), rejects the spiritual approach of AA.

In addition, RR rejects the notion that alcoholics and addicts are powerless to stop their addictions, suggesting instead that until now they simply have not chosen to do so. Instead of reliance on a higher power (which RR considers another form of dependence), RR members are urged to build on strengths within themselves; the movement inspires independence whenever humanly possible. A constant theme is "Think yourself sober."

In RR, there are no steps, sponsors, moral inventories, making amends to others, or even caring about what others think of you. According to rational emotive therapy, on which RR is based, human beings should love themselves because they are human beings and not because others think well of them. The concept of staying sober one day at a time is rejected in favor of a decision to never drink or use again, period. Sobriety is not supposed to become the cornerstone of one's life. The goal is for members to wean themselves from dependence on alcohol, then from dependence on people, and finally from dependence on the group.

Meetings take place only twice a week, and most people attend for only one year, after which they may be pronounced "recovered." They can, however, return to meetings whenever the need arises. Discussions at meetings focus on the here and now rather than past history, and interactive discussion is encouraged.

Whereas AA relies totally on nonprofessionals helping one another, professional coordinators run RR, and each group has volunteer professional advisors available for advice and input. This is necessary because, unlike AA, there are no old timers around to help newcomers. Advisors attend meetings only occasionally. RR, like AA, offers written materials, the core of which is Rational Recovery from Alcoholism: The Small Book (meant to contrast with the Big Book of AA).

RR suggests looking within oneself for strength and direction. We all have within us an inner voice, says RR, that challenges us to go wrong. It is this voice, nicknamed "Beast," that urges one to drink or use drugs, takes over during blackouts, gets one to do terrible things, and speaks louder than one's rational self. It's the voice that tells one things like "You can stop anytime (but not now)" or "You're not really addicted (you just like the taste)" and that tears angrily into those who criticize or try to help. BEAST is an acronym used to help RR members avoid taking another drink or drug. See Box 13–17 for the specific aspects of the BEAST.

BOX 13–17 BEAST Acronym

- B is for Boozing Opportunities (weddings, parties, trips, etc.) RR says to be aware of the pitfalls but do not necessarily avoid them. You are not powerless in the face of temptations, and you can choose not to succumb.
- E is for Enemy Recognition. Distinguish those thoughts from the Enemy (Beast) that are positive about booze or drugs.
- A is for Accuse the Beast of Malice. You can be angry at the Beast for its evil deeds (trying to tempt you), or you can laugh at it. Either way, make clear to the Beast that you have the upper hand and you won't relinquish it.
- S is for Self-Control and Self-Worth Reminders. Find ways of showing the Beast that you have self-control (like moving your hands in front of your face and holding them there, totally in your control, until the Beast backs down). Find ways of telling yourself that you are a worthwhile person. Choose not to drink for the same reason you drank: to feel good about yourself.
- T is for Treasuring Your Sobriety. Focus on the pleasures of life that are attainable only in sobriety (a concept similar to that in AA).

RELAPSE

Relapse is common among substance abusers, and it seriously complicates treatment. Authorities in the field of alcoholism estimate that 60% to 75% of those who complete treatment programs drink again within the first 90 days. Data suggest that only 10% to 20% of alcoholics remain abstinent for one year following treatment, and that only 35% of these are abstinent five years later. In fact, recidivism rates are notoriously high across the spectrum of addictive behaviors.

Several common stages of the recovery process are:

1. Commitment to recovery and motivation for abstinence
2. Initiating change
3. Maintaining change

As a result of a successful initial change, the person experiences perceived control while remaining abstinent. This feeling of perceived control continues until the person encounters a high-risk situation involving negative emotional states, interpersonal conflict, or social pressure. The person can avoid relapse by using effective coping responses in the high-risk situation. If, however, the individual cannot cope successfully, an initial "lapse" occurs in which he or she resorts to the use of a chemical to control stress. The person then feels less able to exert control and develops a tendency to "give in" to the situation ("It's no use, I can't handle this"). In subsequent high-risk situations, the individual again resorts to the use of chemicals to relieve stress. Repeated lapses set the stage for a return to uncontrolled use (relapse).

Many treatment centers are now incorporating the concept of relapse prevention into their treatment programs. This concept is designed to teach clients how to anticipate relapse. By learning skills to use in high-risk situations, clients gain confidence and the expectation of being able to cope successfully, thus decreasing the probability of relapse. Box 13–18 on page 298 lists symptoms leading to relapse.

Research indicates that participation in a 12-step program can help prevent relapse. These programs focus on the individual being "in recovery" and maintaining sobriety, as opposed to having recovered or being cured.

BOX 13–18 A Checklist of Symptoms Leading to Relapse

1. *Exhaustion*. Don't allow yourself to become overly tired or to have poor health. Many chemically dependent people are also prone to work addictions. Perhaps they are in a hurry to make up for lost time or are overworking to compensate for feelings of guilt or personal inadequacy. Good health and enough rest are essential to recovery. Good feelings of physical well-being are associated with a healthy, optimistic mental outlook. Fatigue and feelings of physical illness often induce negative thinking and a pessimistic attitude. You may begin to think a drug or drink would help you return to a positive frame of mind.
2. *Dishonesty*. This symptom begins with a pattern of unnecessary little lies and deceits with fellow workers, friends, and family. Then come important lies to yourself. This is called rationalizing—making excuses for not doing what you do not want to do, or for doing what you know you should not do.
3. *Impatience*. Things are not happening fast enough, others are not doing what they should or what you want them to.
4. *Argumentativeness*. Arguing about small and ridiculous points of view indicates a need to always be right. Chemically dependent people need to learn an attitude of acceptance of their disease and the value of the tools of recovery.
5. *Depression*. Unreasonable and unaccountable melancholy and despair may occur from time to time as a *natural part of recovering* from chemical dependence. Periods of depression are times when the risk of relapse is very high. Deal with your negative feelings; talk about them.
6. *Frustration*. Remember, everything is not going to be just the way you want it.
7. *Self-pity*. "Why do these things happen to me?" "Why must I be chemically dependent?" "Nobody appreciates what I'm doing for them."
8. *Cockiness*. "I've got this problem licked; I have nothing to fear from drugs or booze." This dangerous attitude may lead to going into situations where friends are drinking and using drugs to prove to others that you don't have a problem. Do this often enough and your defenses against relapse will wear down. Don't *test* your recovery. You may lose!
9. *Complacency*. It is dangerous to let up on discipline because everything seems to be going so well. Always having a little fear is a good thing when it comes to maintaining abstinence. *More relapses occur when things are going well than when things are going badly*.
10. *Expecting too much from others*. "I've changed—why hasn't everybody else?" It's a plus if they do, but be prepared to deal with disappointment in your expectations of others. They may not trust you yet or they may be looking for more evidence of your improved physical and mental health. You may be setting yourself up for a lot of frustration and other negative feelings if you expect others to change their lifestyle just because you have.
11. *Letting up on discipline*. Continue with prayer, meditation, daily inventory, and twelve-step meeting attendance. This attitude may stem from complacency or from boredom. No chemically dependent person can afford to be bored with his or her recovery. The cost of relapse is too great.
12. *Use of mood-altering chemicals*. You may feel the need to ease things with a pill, and your doctor may agree with you. Perhaps you have had a problem only with alcohol or some other specific drug in the past. But you can easily lose hold of your recovery by starting to use mood changers. Different drugs may have unpredictable and treacherous reactions in chemically dependent people.
13. *Wanting too much*. Do not set goals you cannot reach with normal efforts.
14. *Forgetting gratitude*. You may be looking negatively on your life, concentrating on problems that still are not totally corrected. It is important to remember where you started from and how much better life is now.
15. *"It can't happen to me."* This kind of thinking is very dangerous. Almost anything can happen to you and is all the more likely to happen if you become careless with your recovery. Remember that you have a progressive disease and will be in even worse shape if you relapse.
16. *Omnipotence*. This is a feeling that results from a combination of many of the above attitudes. You may come to believe you have all the answers for yourself and for others. No one can tell you anything new. You may begin to ignore suggestions or advice from others. Relapse is probably imminent unless drastic change takes place.

Source: Anonymous.

GENERAL TREATMENT APPROACHES

Below are a number of general interventions for substance abuse.

Using Confrontation Strategies. For many years, it was believed that alcoholics and drug abusers needed to "hit bottom" before they could accept their problem and request help. Today, most people believe that intervention can occur as soon as the problem is identified. Group intervention/confrontation is one strategy that aims to break down the substance abuser's denial. Nurses are often "intervention specialists" and leaders in the process.

Several family members, friends, employers, coworkers, and an alcohol/drug intervention specialist confront the substance abuser in a private meeting. They list the evidence by going around the group, one by one. The family/friends/employer, following the leader's cues, speak calmly and slowly with minimal emotion. They are presenting the facts, the objective evidence, to the alcoholic/drug abuser. Yelling, blaming, and haranguing are avoided because the alcoholic/drug abuser will inevitably respond by denying the behavior or making excuses. However, confrontation by several people who really care and who persistently present the facts breaks through the denial. See the Intervention box on page 299 for examples of this.

The next step in group intervention/confrontation requires the family/friends/employer to make clear and direct statements to the alcoholic/drug abuser about the consequences of his or her behavior:

- "Either you get help now or you will have to leave your job."
- "Either you enter a treatment program now or I will move out with the kids."

If the client agrees to treatment, the caring people agree to remain involved.

Educating. Videotapes and talks by recovered substance abusers or experts in the effects of substance abuse are helpful. Education may take place in or out of the hospital, in one comprehensive session or several sessions over time. Nurse

INTERVENTION

Interacting with the Substance-Abusing Client During a Group Intervention

Use this series of steps to educate family or friends on how to interact with the substance-abusing client during a group intervention. Combine with the tone and style cues described in the chapter text.

Presentation of Facts

"You had slurred speech and didn't even respond when I told you I had to be hospitalized for surgery."

"You have not made your daughter's dinner all week. And you forgot to pick her up from school."

"You missed work for 3 days, and you have been late 8 days in the past month."

"You have alcohol on your breath (or needle marks on your arms)."

"I found two bottles (a syringe and empty vial) hidden in the bathroom."

Consequences

"Either you get help now or you will have to leave your job."

"Either you enter a treatment program now or I will move out with the kids."

educators should focus on the types of abused substances and their physical, psychological, and social effects. Families are often involved in these sessions because substance abuse is a family problem. The belief underlying such education is that knowledge and awareness may be useful in decreasing self-destructive behavior. But knowledge alone is never enough. Culturally sensitive and relevant educational resources should be used.

Referral and Self-Help Groups. Support and self-help groups are extremely useful in helping clients feel better about themselves and acquire new attitudes and behaviors. Merely being with many people who are suffering in similar ways is beneficial. By observing people who have been sober or drug free for long periods, clients can begin to learn similar behaviors. They can see that there is hope and that recovery is possible. Self-help groups also provide new friends, generally with healthy lifestyles. Clients may choose to attend support groups for the rest of their lives. Some clients who experiment with drugs or alcohol during one period of their lives and who succeed in stopping may attend only during the crisis.

Lifestyle Change. An emphasis on the requirement for a total lifestyle change is necessary. The Rx Communication feature below suggests communication techniques you can use to encourage lifestyle change. Nurses can help clients discuss ways to alter their destructive habits by suggesting different coping strategies and by encouraging clients to discover new interests and capabilities within themselves. Nurses and clients can role-play new responses to old situations. Recognizing that relapse is always a threat, nurses may set up contracts with clients. For example, clients may agree to contact the nurse or an AA/NA sponsor if and when they feel the urge to drink or do drugs. This agreement represents new behaviors that are necessary for a lifestyle change.

Clients must realize that spending time with friends who are substance abusers or hanging out at places where they used to take drugs or alcohol is not helpful. The mere sight or smell of paraphernalia or the desired substance is often enough to trigger a relapse. Old ties must be broken; new friends and activities must be pursued. See the Case Study and Nursing Care Plan on pages 300–301 for specifics on lifestyle changes with cocaine use.

HELPING THE FAMILY

Substance abuse affects not only the client but also the entire family system. Family members often engage in behaviors that enable clients to continue with their substance abuse by protecting them from the consequences of their substance abuse. Helping family members includes clarifying the problem and presenting possible solutions (treatment) and creating a support system for family members. Referring family members to Al-Anon can be a very helpful strategy.

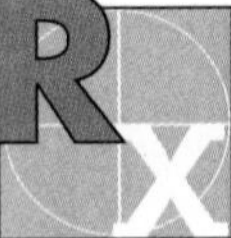

COMMUNICATION

Client Dependent on Substance, Not Currently Using

CLIENT: "I don't need to spend a lot of time talking to you about this stuff. I'm not going to take it anymore and you can bet on that."

NURSE RESPONSE 1: "I hear that you have no intention to use again, and that's good. I also want to make sure you have every support available to you when that time comes when your resolve gets shaky."

RATIONALE: This interaction provides direction around the eventual difficulties that face everyone dependent on a substance—temptation and relapse.

NURSE RESPONSE 2: "We don't have to do a lot of talking, but you have to make the changes in what you do and who you do it with."

RATIONALE: Clear statements about how the client is responsible for his or her behavior and the changes necessary interfere with urges to shift blame.

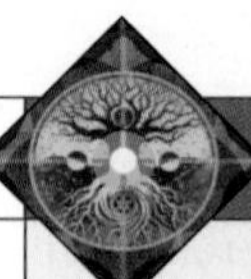

Case Study

Client with Cocaine Intoxication

Identifying Information

Leigh is a 29-year-old married woman. Her husband brought her to the hospital. Leigh is an advertising executive with Alrep & Niker (a large, local firm). She has a BA in business and an MBA in marketing. She is not and never has been in treatment or therapy.

Leigh does not feel she needs hospitalization, especially as she must return to work. She asserts she is extremely creative and productive and needs "to get my ideas down on paper." She is occasionally incoherent during the interview. Her only complaint is how much she is perspiring and feeling "sick to my stomach." Leigh admits to "working very hard," but does not feel she needs care right now. She feels she can handle this herself. She has been using cocaine intranasally for one year, spending most of her salary on it. Use has been four to five times a day for the last five days. Prior to that, her use was once or twice weekly. Leigh explains her recent increase in use as "helping me work harder and faster. I feel more productive." She is having trouble sitting still and sleeping. Leigh states she has not slept more than an hour or two for several days. Leigh's husband and one female colleague are her main support system.

History

Leigh has no prior psychiatric history. Her parents are both living and work together in their own business (retail shoe store). Her younger brother is a college senior. Although a close and loving family, Leigh's family is 2,000 miles away and they seldom see each other. Leigh's father is an alcoholic who has not been actively drinking for five years.

Leigh is a competitive woman who has always excelled at academics and at work. She "likes being number one." Leigh has few close friends and socializes with acquaintances from work. Cigarette smoking since age 17, Leigh admits to "moderate" drinking with occasional weekend alcohol binging. She has experimented with a variety of recreational drugs but states "cocaine really works for me." Leigh describes herself as a "the best kind of hard-driving, career-focused woman" but enjoys reading and tennis when time permits.

Leigh has no current or past medical problems. States she is in good health despite "feeling horrible now." BP 140/90, AP 110.

Current Mental Status

Leigh is attractive, disheveled, agitated, hyperalert, alternatively compliant and hostile, and occasionally incoherent. Sensorium impaired. Oriented to time, place, and person; judgment impaired. Affect labile; mood swings evident. Motor behavior notable for rapid and frequent movements. Thought content grandiose. Delusions present. Leigh reports seeing "signs" at work that are messages to her that she should "move onward and upward to take over the company." Thought processes occasionally incoherent, tangential, with difficulty concentrating and easy distraction. Little insight: "I can take care of myself. I know what I'm doing."

Other Subjective or Objective Clinical Data

Leigh is not taking any medications; suicide/violence potential is minimal.

In dysfunctional families, the substance abuser often becomes the "identified patient," focusing attention on that individual and away from the other problems in the family. Treatment for the substance abuser may require including some type of family therapy. Family members may need treatment for codependence through group or individual therapy or involvement in a twelve-step program such as Al-Anon or Codependents Anonymous (CODA). The Adult Children of Alcoholics (ACOA) support groups are also helpful.

Evaluation

Evaluating the recovery process when providing nursing services for substance-abusing clients includes an evaluation of the client's abilities to change. Is there evidence that the client is being honest, open, and willing to take responsibility for his or her own actions? Regardless of the substance of abuse, once a client stops the blaming of others for his or her use/abuse, treatment has made a positive impact. Another criterion is the amount of substance the client is placing in his or her body. Has it decreased? Other indications of positive treatment outcome are increased job stability, improvement in interpersonal relationships with others, and improved problem-solving techniques. Evaluating clients for emotional maturity and the ability to make the necessary changes in people, places, and things are critical for victory over substance dependence. Improvement in these areas is a good indication that the client is well on the road to recovery.

Case Management

Your career in case management services for clients with addictions has the potential to cover many areas. At any time for any client, you would be involved in:

- Arrangements for services at clinics.
- Responding to emergent and chronic health care needs.
- Designing access to educational resources.
- Living situation and residential movements.
- Revamping recreational options.

In fact, there are as many case management needs that you may encounter as there are different substance abuse clients.

Perhaps the most important task of the nurse case manager for a substance abuse client is availability and flexibility in response to client needs. These clients can experience a plethora of difficulties in their social, occupational, living, and familial/relationship arrangements. Any one of these has the potential to serve as a trigger for relapse into substance abuse or dependence. Assist the client in managing difficulties in these areas to lower the risk of a relapse. This must be done in

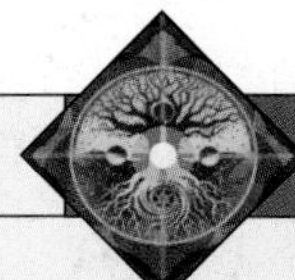

Nursing Care Plan

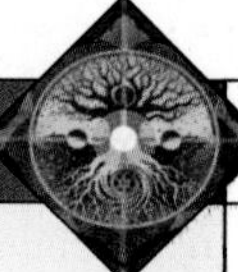

Nursing Diagnosis: Ineffective Individual Coping Related to Cocaine Abuse
Expected Outcome: Client will complete detox program and will remain free of cocaine.

Short-Term Goals	*Interventions*	*Rationale*
Meets with staff and attends group meetings according to schedule without prompting. "Clean" urine 72 hr after last use. Leigh discusses problems cocaine use has created. Replacement of destructive coping with two effective individual coping options.	• Individual meetings with Leigh regarding consequences of drug use in work, home, social, and physical arenas. • Convey agreement to work with Leigh on her problem areas. • Assign to daily individual and group therapy. • Observe every half hour. When drug-seeking behavior commences, interact about Leigh's feelings, educate about cravings and time frames for resolution. • Assist Leigh to recognize the automatic mechanisms involved in turning to cocaine. • Encourage Leigh to rehearse various coping strategies to prepare to select two for regular use. • Explore with Leigh how to substitute effective coping for cocaine use.	Improve Leigh's awareness of her behaviors, reduce denial, and educate about the addictions process. Monitor drug-seeking behavior as an inevitable aspect of her problem. Revision of coping styles requires learning and practice.

a manner that does not breach interpersonal boundaries and maintains the client's responsibilities for caring for him/herself.

Community-Based Care

In an outpatient treatment center, where the nurse functions in a community-based care environment, you may have the role of a counselor or a therapist. In all cases, the nurse must have psychosocial, physiologic, and spiritual skills. Such skills include interviewing, teaching clients about the disease process and alternative coping strategies, referring clients to appropriate sources and community support systems, and knowing how to conduct individual, group, or family therapy. You cannot give quality care without an in-depth understanding of the disease process—from the varying theoretic explanations to the varying methods of treatment at different stages.

Another feature of community-based care for substance abuse is that of court-mandated treatment. Addicts often exhibit poor judgment. For example, alcoholic clients may continue to drive while intoxicated. In most states, driving under the influence of alcohol or drugs is considered a crime for which the driver will face legal penalties. The law enforcement system may interact with the mental health system to force treatment on those found guilty of driving while intoxicated. A psychiatric–mental health nurse may care for those clients who have been "mandated for treatment."

Clients with poor judgment mandated to treatment may initially respond with minimal or superficial cooperation, although many clients do make positive changes as a result of mandated therapy. All clients mandated for treatment must be informed in writing of all policies inherent to the treatment process and the court mandate. Often, this mandate will include written evidence of participation in one-to-one therapy, family therapy, educational programming, and attending 12-step meetings. At times, random drug testing may be court ordered.

Clients may attempt to manipulate you into withholding information from the court. To allow the client to manipulate you will jeopardize the treatment process. Successful manipulation may decrease the client's feeling of responsibility for recovery. At no time can you consider violating the court mandate. The law enforcement system has the right to file charges against a nurse who fails to cooperate fully with court mandates.

When the state laws clearly mandate a treatment course, you must work within legal mandates. It is much more difficult to decide what to do when public opinion and legal mandate are less clear, or when the mandates seem to interfere with prudent treatment. For example, pregnant women who suffer from substance addiction potentially face conflict between the legal system and basic prenatal care. States vary in approach to the pregnant addict. Some states seek to incarcerate pregnant women who continue to use illegal drugs, and others mandate that health care workers report all women who have tested positive for drugs, determining such behavior to be child abuse.

Women face special obstacles to treatment for addictions. Some obstacles seem rooted within the opposing beliefs about the nature of addiction:

- Is addiction a bad behavior that should result in punishment?
- Is addiction an illness that should respond to treatment?

In mental health settings, addiction is perceived as an illness. Participation in the treatment process is a central responsibility of each nurse.

At times, you may need to interact with the legal system during mandated treatment. You may serve as an advocate who will facilitate treatment for the addict and her baby. This process of intervention can be complex. For example, it is difficult to identify active addiction, secondary use, and recreational use. While any drug use is potentially hazardous, regular use seen in addiction may be more damaging to mother and baby.

Home Care

Home care in addictions can involve a physiologic event resulting from substance use or abuse. Cerebral vascular accident from crack use, injury from driving while intoxicated, or brain damage from inhalant abuse are all likely scenarios requiring nursing home care services. In these circumstances, recovery from the physiologic threat is coupled with treatment for substance abuse.

One aspect of treatment for substance abuse that can be accomplished in the home is helping the client to develop drink- or drug-refusal skills. In many cases substance abuse clients who are sober relapse into using when they encounter commonly experienced events in their home lives that create stress with which they are poorly equipped to cope. Often, these events can include or lead to situations that include the offer of alcohol or drugs for personal use. The development of the interactional and social skills needed to negotiate refusals of these offers successfully can involve a home-based training component. You can play an instrumental role in designing and implementing this training.

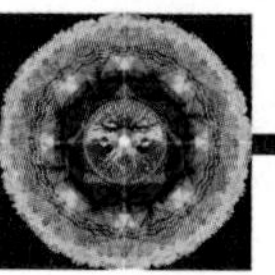

EXPLORE MediaLink

NCLEX review, case studies, and other interactive resources for this chapter can be found on the Companion Website at http://www.prenhall.com/kneisl. Click on Chapter 13 to select the activities for this chapter.

For animations, video tutorials, more NCLEX review questions, and an audio glossary, access the accompanying CD-ROM in this textbook.

BIBLIOGRAPHY

Aarons, G. A., Brown, S. A., Hough, R. L., Garland, A. F., & Wood, P. A. (2001). Prevalence of adolescent substance use disorders across five sectors of care. *Journal of the American Academy of Child and Adolescent Psychiatry, 40,* 419–426.

American Psychiatric Association (2000). *Diagnostic and statistical manual of mental disorders* (4th ed., Text Revision) (DSM-IV-TR). Washington, DC: Author.

American Public Health Association (2001). The need for mental health and substance abuse services for the incarcerated mentally ill. *American Journal of Public Health, 91,* 511–512.

Carroll, K. M., Sinha, R., Nich, C., Babuscio, T., & Rounsaville, B. J. (2002). Contingency management to enhance naltrexone treatment of opioid dependence: A randomized clinical trial of reinforcement magnitude. *Experimental & Clinical Psychopharmacology, 10,* 54–63.

Cole, T. (2001). Smoking cessation in the hospitalized patient using the transtheoretical model of behavior change. *Heart & Lung: The Journal of Acute and Critical Care, 30,* 148–158.

Guardia, J., Catafau, A. M., Battle, F., Martin, J. C., Segura, L., Gonzalvo, B., et al. (2000). Striatal dopaminergic D2 receptor density measured by [123I] Iodobenzamide SPECT in the prediction of treatment outcome of alcohol-dependent patients. *American Journal of Psychiatry, 157,* 127–129.

Jellinek, E. (1946). *Phases in the drinking history of alcoholics*. New Haven, CT: Hillhouse Press.

Jee, S. H., He, J., Appel, L. J., Whelton, P. K., Suh, I., & Klag, M. J. (2001). Coffee consumption and serum lipids: A meta-analysis of randomized controlled clinical trials. *American Journal of Epidemiology, 153,* 353–362.

Kleemola, P., Jousilahti, P., Pietinen, P., Vartiainen, E., & Tuomilehto, J. (2000). Coffee consumption and the risk of coronary heart disease and death. *Archives of Internal Medicine, 160,* 3393–3400.

Landry, M., & Smith, D. E. (1987). Crack: Anatomy of an addiction. *California Nursing Review,* March/April, 8–36.

Marlatt, G. A., & VandenBos, G. R. (1997). Addictive behaviors: Readings on etiology, prevention, and treatment. Washington, DC: American Psychological Association.

Martini, F. H. (2001). *Fundamentals of anatomy & physiology*. (5th ed.). Upper Saddle River, NJ: Prentice Hall.

Miotto, P., Preti, A., & Frezza, M. (2001). Heroin and schizophrenia: Subjective responses to abused drugs in dually diagnosed patients. *Journal of Clinical Psychopharmacology, 21,* 111–113.

O'Connor, P. G. (2001). Treating opioid dependence. *New England Journal of Medicine, 344,* 530–531.

Pacula, R. L., Grossman, M., Chaloupka, F. J., O'Malley, P. M., Johnston, L. D., & Farrelly, M. C. (2000). *Marijuana and youth*. ImpacTeen: Youth, Education, and Society.

Prescott, C. A., Aggen, S. H., & Kendler, K. S. (1999). Sex differences in the sources of genetic liability to alcohol abuse and dependence in a population-based sample of U.S. twins. *Alcohol Clinical Expertise in Research, 23,* 1136–1144.

Schneider, R. K., Levenson, J. L., & Schnoll, S. H. (2001). Update in addiction medicine. *Annals of Internal Medicine, 134,* 387–395.

Schwartz, T. (2000). Do you smoke? If so, stop. Please, stop. *American Journal of Nursing, 100,* 11.

Tanvetyanon, T., Dissin, J., & Selcer, U. (2001). Hyperthermia and chronic pancerebellar syndrome after cocaine abuse. *Archives of Internal Medicine, 161*, 608–610.

Tomkins, D. M., & Sellers, E. M. (2001). Addiction and the brain: The role of neurotransmitters in the cause and treatment of drug dependence. *Canadian Medical Association Journal, 164*, 817–821.

Wadland, W. C., Soffelmayr, B., & Ives, K. (2001). Enhancing smoking cessation of low-income smokers in managed care. *Journal of Family Practice, 50*, 138–144.

Watson, S. J., Benson, J. A., & Joy, J. E. (2000). Marijuana and medicine: Assessing the science base: A summary of the 1999 Institute of Medicine Report. *Archives of General Psychiatry, 57*, 547–552.

Zickler, P. (2000). Evidence accumulates that long-term marijuana users experience withdrawal. *National Institute on Drug Abuse*, 15.

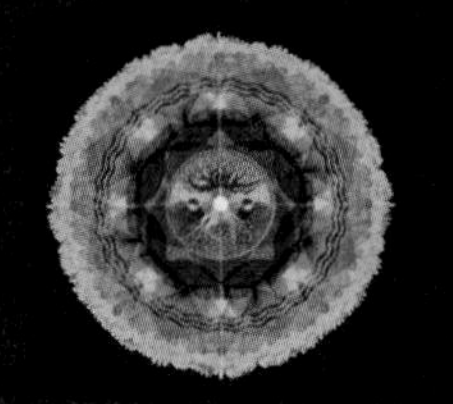

14

Chapter FOURTEEN

Schizophrenia and Other Psychotic Disorders

EILEEN TRIGOBOFF

KEY TERMS

anhedonia
blunted affect
delusional disorder
delusions
dopamine hypothesis
expressed emotion
flat affect
hallucination
illusions
negative symptoms of schizophrenia
positive symptoms of schizophrenia
relapse
schizoaffective disorder
schizophrenia
schizophrenia, catatonic type
schizophrenia, disorganized type
schizophrenia, paranoid type
schizophrenia, residual type
schizophrenia, undifferentiated type
schizophreniform disorder
thought blocking
thought disorganization
waxy flexibility

FOCUS QUESTIONS

- **What are the central features of schizophrenia?**
- **How can psychological and social pressures influence the course of schizophrenia?**
- **What are the major nursing implications in caring for clients with a difficult and chronic illness such as schizophrenia?**
- **What are the personal challenges you may encounter in working with clients who have interactional impairments?**
- **How would you prevent or minimize relapse in schizophrenia?**

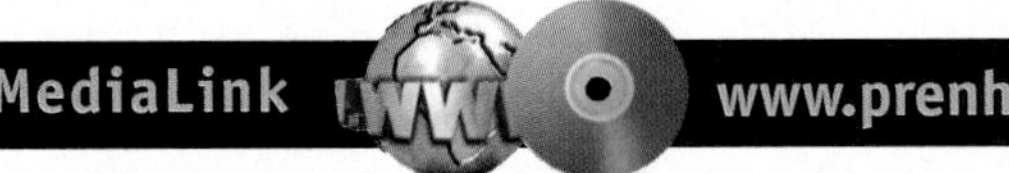

Additional resources for this chapter can be found on the Student CD-ROM accompanying this textbook, and on the Companion Website at www.prenhall.com/kneisl. Click on Chapter 14 to select the activities for this chapter.

CD-ROM
- Audio Glossary
- NCLEX Review
- PET/SPECT Schizophrenia Animation
- EPSE: Dystonia/Akathisia Video
- EPSE: Akinesia Video
- Extrapyramidal Side Effects:
  Dystonia (Blepharospasm, Cervical Torticollolis) Video
  Bradykinesia (Shuffling Gait) Video
  Akathisia (Legs) Video
  Akinesia & Pill Rolling Video
  Tardive Dyskinesia (Mouth, Trunk, Ambulation) Video

Companion Website
- Additional NCLEX Review
- Care Plan: Paranoid Schizophrenia
- Case Study: Schizophrenia with Auditory Hallucinations
- Learning from Clients: Schizophrenia Video

CHAPTER OUTLINE

CROSS REFERENCES

Other topics relevant to this content are: Cognitive-behavioral therapy, Chapter 30; Ethical and legal aspects of ECT and psychosurgery, Chapter 10; Family assessment, interventions, and psychoeducation groups, Chapter 29; History of ECT and psychosurgery, Chapter 2; Inpatient and outpatient settings for care, Chapter 11; NAMI family education program, Chapter 29; Nursing care of clients undergoing ECT, Chapter 15; Psychobiology, Chapter 4; Psychopharmacology, Chapter 31; Severely and persistently mentally ill, Chapter 11; Social skills training groups, Chapter 29; Therapeutic communication, Chapter 8; Treatment settings, Chapter 11.

CRITICAL THINKING CHALLENGE

Smithy, just like most individuals with schizophrenia, is extremely sensitive to her environment. When stressed, she often runs the risk of developing exacerbations of the symptoms of her illness. In the course of living in usual ways, everyone experiences stress related to conducting day-to-day activities. Smithy's nurse at the mental health clinic has been preparing her to be able to cope with working at a local store. Specific environmental features are particularly difficult for Smithy to deal with, such as noise and visual distractions. Why do mental health care providers advocate that people with schizophrenia interact with the larger community via treatment programs, jobs, and living in the community? Wouldn't they be better off in protected environments, like semistructured group homes or structured and sheltered workshops? ■

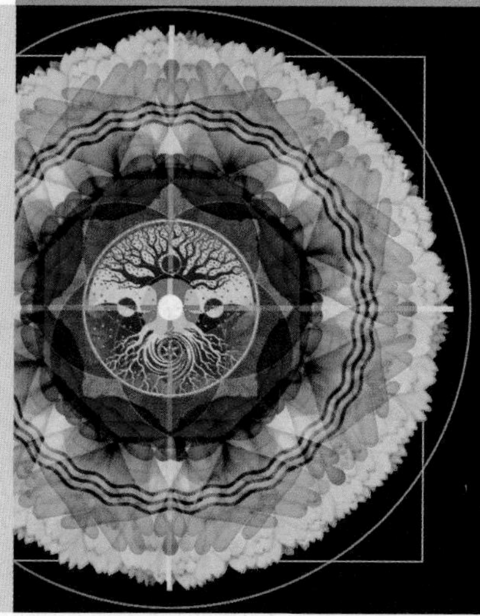

MediaLink Learning from Clients: Schizophrenia Video

Schizophrenia is a complex disorder with an extremely varied presentation of symptoms. You will see this disorder affect cognitive, emotional, and behavioral areas of functioning. Approximately 1% of the general population will have schizophrenia during their lifetime. Age of onset is typically between late teens and mid-thirties, although there are cases outside that range such as late-onset (after age 45) schizophrenia, which is seen more often in women, and a rare childhood schizophrenia. The illness is diagnosed most frequently in the early twenties for men and late twenties for women. The progression of the disease is as variable as its presentation. In some cases, the disease progresses through exacerbations and remissions; in other cases, it takes a chronic, stable course; while in still others, a chronic, progressively deteriorating course evolves.

Symptoms of Schizophrenia

The diagnosis of schizophrenia requires not only the presence of distinct symptoms but also the persistence of those symptoms over time. Symptoms must be present for at least 6 months, and active-phase symptoms (called Criterion A symptoms in the DSM-IV-TR) must be present for at least 1 month during that time, before schizophrenia can be diagnosed. The diagnostic criteria for schizophrenia are presented in the DSM-IV-TR feature below.

The symptoms of schizophrenia are conceptually separated into **positive symptoms,** which represent an excess or distortion of normal functioning, and **negative symptoms,** which represent a deficit in functioning. Another way to think about these symptoms is that positive symptoms are those that would not be present if the person is healthy. Negative symptoms are symptoms that are deficits; their presence means that the person is not healthy.

POSITIVE SYMPTOMS

Positive symptoms include the three most pronounced outward signs of the disorder: hallucinations, delusions, and disorganization in speech and behavior.

Hallucinations

Hallucinations are the most extreme and yet the most common perceptual disturbance in schizophrenia. A **hallucination** is a subjective perception of something that does not exist in the external environment. One or more of the five senses are involved in hallucinations. Hallucinations may be auditory (heard), visual (seen), olfactory (smelled), gustatory (tasted), or tactile (touched). ■ Figure 14–1 represents how someone with visual hallucinations may distort a scene.

The most common form of hallucination in schizophrenia is hearing voices or sounds that are distinct from the person's own

DSM-IV-TR Diagnostic Criteria for Schizophrenia

A. *Characteristic symptoms*: Two (or more) of the following, each present for a significant portion of time during a 1-month period (or less if successfully treated):

1. delusions
2. hallucinations
3. disorganized speech (e.g., frequent derailment or incoherence)
4. grossly disorganized or catatonic behavior
5. negative symptoms, i.e., affective flattening, alogia, or avolition

Note: Only one Criterion A symptom is required if delusions are bizarre or hallucinations consist of a voice keeping up a running commentary on the person's behavior or thoughts, or two or more voices conversing with each other.

B. *Social/occupational dysfunction*: For a significant portion of the time since the onset of the disturbance, one or more major areas of functioning such as work, interpersonal relations, or self-care are markedly below the level achieved prior to the onset (or when the onset is in childhood or adolescence, failure to achieve expected level of interpersonal, academic, or occupational achievement).

C. *Duration*: Continuous signs of the disturbance persist for at least 6 months. This 6-month period must include at least 1 month of symptoms (or less if successfully treated) that meet Criterion A (i.e., active-phase symptoms) and may include periods of prodromal or residual symptoms. During these prodromal or residual periods, the signs of the disturbance may be manifested by only negative symptoms or two or more symptoms listed in Criterion A present in an attenuated form (e.g., odd beliefs, unusual perceptual experiences).

D. *Schizoaffective and Mood Disorder exclusion:* Schizoaffective Disorder and Mood Disorder with Psychotic Features have been ruled out because either (1) no Major Depressive, Manic, or Mixed Episodes have occurred concurrently with the active-phase symptoms; or (2) if mood episodes have occurred during active-phase symptoms, their total duration has been brief relative to the duration of the active and residual periods.

E. *Substance/general medical condition exclusion*: The disturbance is not due to the direct physiological effects of a substance (e.g., a drug of abuse, a medication) or a general medical condition.

F. *Relationship to a Pervasive Developmental Disorder*: If there is a history of Autistic Disorder or another Pervasive Developmental Disorder, the additional diagnosis of Schizophrenia is made only if prominent delusions or hallucinations are also present for at least a month (or less if successfully treated).

Source: Reprinted with permission from American Psychiatric Association (2000). *Diagnostic and statistical manual of mental disorders* (4th ed., Text Revision) (pp. 312–313). Washington, DC: Author.

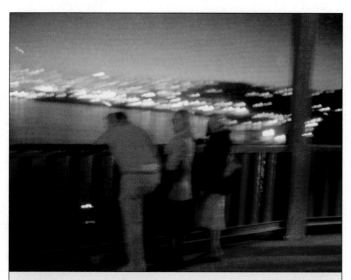

FIGURE 14–1 ■ *Distorted perceptions. The distorted visual perceptions indicated by this figure are what is experienced by someone during visual hallucinations.*

thoughts. If a voice is heard, it (or they) may be friendly or hostile and threatening. It is particularly significant if the person hears two or more voices conversing with each other, or hears a voice that provides continuous comments on the train of thought; reports of either of these symptoms have particular diagnostic significance (see DSM-IV-TR for details).

Having auditory hallucinations does not necessarily mean the individual is hearing human speech. (Table 14–3 on pages 309–310 lists examples). Do not confuse hallucinatory experiences with *synesthesia*, which is not a disease or disorder and involves the experience of having multiple senses involved in a single event. Distinguishing hallucinations can be accomplished by assuring that there is no external stimulation to the sensations. Examples of synesthesia include seeing sounds, seeing colors when in pain, and hearing smells. This knowledge must, necessarily, impact on the way you gather information during assessment.

Hallucinations are also seen in several other illnesses besides schizophrenia. See the chapters discussing dementia (Chapter 12), depression (Chapter 15), and substance abuse (Chapter 13) for more details. ■ Table 14–1 presents some of the associations made between hallucinations and other disease processes. Hallucinations can also be experienced when extreme physiologic stressors are present or as a side effect of medications.

TABLE 14–1 Types of Hallucinations

Perceptual Disturbance	Commonly Associated Disease Process
Auditory	Schizophrenia
Visual	Dementia
Tactile	Acute alcohol withdrawal
Olfactory	Seizure disorders
Gustatory	Seizure disorders
Somatic	Schizophrenia

Delusions

Delusions are mistaken or false beliefs about the self or the environment that are firmly held even in the face of disconfirming evidence. Delusions may take many forms. In *delusions of persecution*, the person may think that others are following him, spying on him, or trying to torment him (i. e., "They have misters in my apartment that spray LSD onto me when I walk around."). In another common form, *delusions of reference*, the person thinks that public expressions, like a story on the television or a newspaper article, are specifically addressed to him or her or happened because of his or her thoughts or actions (i. e., "When the newscaster wears navy blue, she is speaking my thoughts to the world."). Specific delusions are discussed in ■ Table 14–2 on page 308.

Disordered Speech and Behavior

Other positive symptoms represent "excesses" of language or behavior. Disorganized speech is the outward sign of disordered thoughts and may range from less severe forms, in which the person moves rapidly from one topic to another, to severe forms, in which the person's speech cannot be logically understood. Positive symptoms include disorganized behavior, such as agitated, nonpurposeful, or random movements, and catatonia, in which there is a low level of behavioral response to the environment. See ■ Table 14–3 on pages 309–310 for examples of positive symptoms of schizophrenia.

NEGATIVE SYMPTOMS

Negative symptoms of schizophrenia are less dramatic but just as debilitating as positive symptoms. See ■ Table 14–4 on page 310 for examples of negative symptoms of schizophrenia. Negative symptoms include the "four As" of schizophrenia:

1. Flat affect
2. Alogia
3. Avolition
4. Anhedonia

People with schizophrenia often appear to have nonemotional or very restricted emotional responses to their experiences. **Flat affect** "is the absence or near absence of any signs of affective expression" as well as poor eye contact (American Psychiatric Association [APA], 2000). To see how flat affect differs from a normal range of affect, imagine someone responding to winning a prize ("Yea, this is great and I'm so happy!"). Now imagine that same person with much less emotion in her response and no emotion showing on her face ("Oh."). The difference between the two responses is the flattening of affect.

Brief, empty verbal responses are known as *alogia*. Rather than saying a few sentences in response to a question, clients with alogia reply with a single word or a very limited number of

TABLE 14–2 Types of Delusions

Disturbances in Thinking	Definition	Example
Delusions of persecution	Belief that others are hostile or trying to harm the individual.	A woman notices a man looking at her and believes that he is trying to follow her.
Delusions of reference	False belief that public events or people are directly related to the individual.	A man hears a story on the evening news and believes it is about him.
Somatic delusions	Belief that one's body is altered from normal structure or function.	An elderly woman believes that her bowel is filled with cement and refuses to eat.
Thought broadcasting	Belief that one's unspoken thoughts can be heard.	A young client believes that everyone around him knows he's attracted to a nurse although he has said nothing.
Delusions of control	Belief that one's actions or thoughts are controlled by an external person or force.	A woman believes that her neighbor controls her thoughts by means of his home computer.

words. This *poverty of speech* is thought to be symptomatic of diminished thoughts and is different from a refusal to speak. Under these circumstances, the client does not use many words to express experiences or thoughts.

A symptom that is frequently misunderstood by families and members of the larger community is *avolition*, an inability to pursue and persist in goal-directed activities. You may see this negative symptom when a client fails to go for a job interview or does not become involved in an activity made easily available. The schizophrenic person's experience of avolition is often misinterpreted as laziness or an unwillingness to support him- or herself, rather than as a symptom of this chronic disorder. Frequently, this misunderstanding affects the ability of family members and friends to stay involved in relationships with the client due to the frustration of unfulfilled efforts and a sense of rejection from unheeded suggestions.

MediaLink National Institute of Mental Health

Anhedonia, the inability to experience pleasure, is an important symptom that challenges many nurses. It is difficult to imagine, and even more arduous to empathize with, someone who can't seem to enjoy even small aspects of life. It is important to remember that people who have schizophrenia cannot enjoy experiences for a physiologic reason over which they have no control.

Negative symptoms of schizophrenia are difficult to assess because they differ in degree but not in form from everyday experience. While few of us have experienced true hallucinations, many of us know what it is like to have a day without energy to pursue goal-directed activities. Another difficulty in recognizing negative symptoms is that people with schizophrenia often live in difficult situations that may lead to restricted emotional expression and disturbed goal-directed activities. Living in poverty or in unsettled circumstances like homelessness can induce feelings of desperation or despair, which may mimic the negative symptoms of schizophrenia. It is important to try to separate environmental influences on experience from the disease process, and to note the persistence of the symptoms over time across a variety of circumstances. For example, if a client is living in a rooming house where others around him are likely to steal, that client will not be safe talking in excited ways about having received a gift from his parents. If, however, the client is not excited when in his own home in front of his parents and trusted others, then you may be witnessing a negative symptom of schizophrenia.

Another important criterion for recognizing schizophrenia is detecting an impaired ability to perform and complete social and work obligations. It is diagnostic of schizophrenia that the person has difficulty performing in one or more areas of life including work, school, social relationships, and the maintenance of everyday activities such as dressing and providing food for oneself. Additional information can be accessed through a direct link to the National Institute of Mental Health Web site on schizophrenia (www.nlm.nih.gov/medlineplus/schizophrenia.html) through the Companion Website for this book.

SOMATIC TREATMENTS

Prior to the 1950s—which is referred to as the preneuroleptic age—insulin coma, drug or electrically induced shock treatments, and psychosurgery, including prefrontal lobotomies, were used. The impact of these extreme somatic treatments did make a difference, for a time, in symptomatology but were not durable or beneficial. Many hoped these treatments were the long-sought-after cure for schizophrenia because they were relatively quick and inexpensive treatments when compared to lengthy and costly analytic therapies. This hope was not realized. Contemporary psychosurgery has been refined from a gross assault on cranial tissue (the lobotomy of decades past) to procedures where specific involved areas of the brain are delicately shaped to reduce repetitive and destructive behaviors.

Electroconvulsive therapy (ECT) has been improved upon and crafted to an impressive degree in the last 20 years. Effective treatment with minimal risks has been offered mostly for mood-disordered clients.

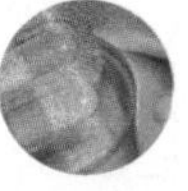

The introduction of psychoactive drugs in the 1950s provided new alternatives for the treatment of schizophrenia. Psychotropic medications, which influ-

TABLE 14–3 Positive Symptoms

Positive Symptom	Examples	
Auditory Hallucinations	Human speech (speaking clearly, mumbling, whispering, singing, yelling, screaming, one voice, several voices, voice speaking to client, voices speaking to each other, male, female, both, indistinguishable, imitating nonhuman sounds)	
	Mechanical sounds (clocks, metal clanging, clicking)	
	Music	
	Animal sounds	
	Insect sounds	
	Wind through the trees	
	Grating sounds made by sand under your feet	
	Crinkling sound from plastic or aluminum wraps	
	The sound of the earth moving or heaving as during an earthquake	
Visual	Blood	People
	Animals	Movement of large objects
	Distortions of everyday sights	Auras
Olfactory	Green peppers	Spices
	Blood	Fruit
	Onions	Burning materials
	Garlic	Paint
	Urine or feces	Rotting meat
	Semen	Sulfur
Gustatory	Metallic flavor	Urine or feces
	Blood	Semen
Tactile	Being pregnant	Being beaten
	Giving birth	Electrocution
	Being raped	Grease on hands
	Moving tumors	Band around head
	Internal movements	
Delusions		
Persecutory	"I cannot leave my apartment more than once a month. I have to have this cardboard in my pockets when I go so the CIA can't take photographs of me."	
Referential	"I was watching television and when the two reporters talked about the car explosion I knew they were talking specifically to me."	
Somatic	"I am going to be hemorrhaging, bleeding to death through my mouth." Or "I have an alien gestating in my belly. When he is mature he'll drip from my palms like sweat."	
Religious	"I can tell when someone is a false prophet, for I am the only Truth and Wisdom."	
Substitution	"It looks just like my wife but it's really a robot."	
Thought insertion	"These thoughts are being put in my head by the alien conspiracy." Or "When I get angry it's because the NSA is altering my brain waves."	
Nihilistic	"Everything is falling apart. My insides are rotting away and so is everything else."	
Grandiose	"There is a million dollars cemented up in my backyard barbecue that I'll share with you if you get me out of here." Or "I am the lost Russian princess, Anastasia, but I'm keeping this a secret until the Czar's guards can come and protect me."	

(continued)

TABLE 14–3 Positive Symptoms (continued)

Positive Symptom	Examples	
Disorganized Speech		
Loose associations	"I came here by bus, but bussing is kissing, I wasn't kissing but if you keep it simple that is a business tenet for KISS. That was a great group that played on and on but I'm not playing with you. You are ewe or youthful too."	
Word salad	"Whimple sitting purple which the twilighted cheshire, for then frames of silver ticking bubble and."	
Clanging	"I want to eat neat treat seat beat."	
	"I'm fine it's a sign fine whine wine pine dine."	
Echolalia	Client repeats pieces of what is said. Nurse asks "How are you today?" and the client states, "You today."	
Behavior		
Disorganized	Client walks around aimlessly picking up everything available to him and touching all surfaces.	
Catatonic	Excited catatonia	A client in the ER is repeatedly assaultive, hyperactive, or cannot sit still.
	Waxy flexibility	Client maintains a rigid position, allows you to move him or her into new positions and maintains the new position.
Thinking		
Lack of planning skills	Indecisiveness	Lack of problem-solving skills
Concrete thinking	Blocking	Difficulty initiating tasks

ence the thoughts, mood, and behavior of clients, made previously uncontrolled symptoms manageable. In the period following the introduction of psychotropic medications, the use of seclusion and restraints declined dramatically, as did the duration of hospital stays and numbers of clients in state hospitals.

TABLE 14–4 Negative Symptoms

Negative Symptom	Examples
Flat Affect	A client maintains the same emotional tone when told his mother has died as when he attends programs. "OK."
Apathy	Feelings of indifference toward people, events, activities, and learning.
Avolition	A client does not go to the dining room even when he is very hungry and dinner is being served.
Anhedonia	The client apparently derives no pleasure from bowling when, prior to getting sick, he used to enjoy it.
Alogia	Rather than using a series of sentences or several words, the client, when asked about his day, speaks sparsely in a limited, stilted manner saying, "Fine."

A new optimism arose regarding the possible outcomes of mental illness. Because they controlled the most difficult symptoms of psychosis, psychotropic medications made psychosocial or behavioral treatments possible for a much greater percentage of psychiatric clients. The major tranquilizers did not live up to their promise of providing a cure for schizophrenia and other chronic psychiatric illnesses. However, these drugs relieved the most debilitating symptoms for many clients and were the first step toward recovery or a higher level of functioning.

Refer to Chapters 2, 4, and 31 for more details on the history and the science behind somatic treatments. Ethical and legal aspects of somatic treatments are discussed in Chapter 10.

RELAPSE

A client with schizophrenia is vulnerable to a return to symptomatology after a period of stability, however brief or extended, partial or complete. This is referred to as a **relapse,** and the disease itself has a pattern of relapse and recovery. As a chronic disorder, schizophrenia is characterized by relapses alternating with periods of full or partial remission.

Although antipsychotic medication is effective in reducing relapse rates, 30% to 40% of clients relapse within 1 year after hospital discharge even if they are receiving maintenance medication. This is a tremendous difficulty for the client to overcome; therefore, acknowledge the sense of demoralization likely with such a recurrent and debilitating course that cannot be altered significantly. The need to improve methods for relapse prevention is clear (Goldstein & Shemansky, 2000). The following clinical examples detail how relapses can occur under certain circumstances.

CLINICAL EXAMPLE

Daryl, a 26-year-old with a diagnosis of paranoid schizophrenia, decided to stop taking his haloperidal (Haldol) because it made him feel heavy and too tired to get up in the morning. Within a few days of stopping the medication, he was unable to leave the house for fear of someone harming him. Although he liked his job at the local cannery and knew that he had the chance to earn more money in the near future, he refused to go to work for fear that he would be hit by a bus on his way there. He was eventually fired because of poor attendance. The loss of a structured schedule furthered his deterioration and Daryl relapsed, requiring hospitalization.

In this instance, a decrease in medication increased Daryl's biologic vulnerability, with marked behavioral, and eventually environmental, consequences. His relapse began with a medication issue and could have been prevented.

CLINICAL EXAMPLE

Jean, 22, lived with her divorced mother and younger sister Mary since her release from the hospital after her second psychotic episode. She found living alone too frightening and was more comfortable staying in her old room at home. When Mary began preparing to leave home for college, Jean became increasingly anxious, demanding to sleep in Mary's room at night and hiding Mary's belongings. As Mary's departure grew near, Jean began actively hallucinating and withdrew to her room, refusing to talk to her mother or sister.

In this case, the client did not have sufficient coping skills to deal with her sister's departure from the household, and her psychosis reemerged. Jean's relapse may have been averted had she been taught about coping skills and had the opportunity to practice them. However, learning is affected in schizophrenia, motivation and energy are problems, and even a competent program of teaching cannot remove all the stress from life.

SUBTYPES OF SCHIZOPHRENIA

Subtypes of schizophrenia are used to designate which symptoms are prominent. For more information, see the DSM-IV-TR Diagnostic Criteria feature below.

Paranoid Type

Prominent hallucinations and delusions are present in the **paranoid type** of schizophrenia. Delusions are often persecu-

DSM-IV-TR — **Diagnostic Criteria for Schizophrenia Subtypes**

PARANOID TYPE

A type of Schizophrenia in which the following criteria are met:

A. Preoccupation with one or more delusions or frequent auditory hallucinations.

B. None of the following is prominent: disorganized speech, disorganized or catatonic behavior, or flat or inappropriate affect.

DISORGANIZED TYPE

A type of Schizophrenia in which the following criteria are met:

A. All of the following are prominent:
1. disorganized speech
2. disorganized behavior
3. flat or inappropriate affect

B. The criteria are not met for Catatonic Type.

CATATONIC TYPE

A type of Schizophrenia in which the clinical picture is dominated by at least two of the following:

1. motoric immobility as evidenced by catalepsy (including waxy flexibility) or stupor
2. excessive motor activity (that is apparently purposeless and not influenced by external stimuli)
3. extreme negativism (an apparently motiveless resistance to all instructions or maintenance of a rigid posture against attempts to be moved) or mutism
4. peculiarities of voluntary movement as evidenced by posturing (voluntary assumption of inappropriate or bizarre postures), stereotyped movements, prominent mannerisms, or prominent grimacing
5. echolalia or echopraxia

UNDIFFERENTIATED TYPE

A type of Schizophrenia in which symptoms that meet Criterion A are present, but the criteria are not met for the Paranoid, Disorganized, or Catatonic Type.

RESIDUAL TYPE

A type of Schizophrenia in which the following criteria are met:

A. Absence of prominent delusions, hallucinations, disorganized speech, and grossly disorganized or catatonic behavior.

B. There is continuing evidence of the disturbance, as indicated by the presence of negative symptoms or two or more symptoms listed in Criterion A for Schizophrenia, present in an attenuated form (e.g., odd beliefs, unusual perceptual experiences).

Source: Reprinted with permission from American Psychiatric Association (2000). *Diagnostic and statistical manual of mental disorders* (4th ed., Text Revision) (pp. 313–317). Washington, DC: Author.

tory or grandiose, and they often connect into a somewhat organized story. Delusions may also be varied and include somatic or religious delusions. Hallucinations often link with the delusion, although this is not necessary. For example, a person who believes he is being monitored by the FBI may hear the voices of people he identifies as FBI agents laughing at him or talking with him when he goes out.

Disorganized Type

The central features present in the disorganized type of schizophrenia are disorganized speech and behavior and flat or inappropriate affect. The client appears disorganized and unkempt because basic everyday tasks like dressing oneself cannot be accomplished. The client may have all the necessary clothing on, but the order of putting each item of clothing in place or the steps required to accomplish dressing (e.g., buttoning, zipping, tying) may be too much to handle. Emotional expression may be either inappropriate to the content of what the client is saying (e.g., laughing when discussing being kicked out of the house) or restricted and flat. Hallucinations and delusions are typically more fragmentary and disorganized than in the paranoid type. This subtype has been referred to as potentially being the most severe form of the disease.

Catatonic Type

Although not seen frequently in the United States, the catatonic type of schizophrenia is a distinctive type characterized by extreme psychomotor disruption. The client may display substantially reduced movement accompanied by negativism and resistance to any intervention. A client could remain almost completely immobile in the same position for long stretches of time. This type of posturing is sometimes called waxy flexibility. Alternatively, extremely active and purposeless movement that is not influenced by what is going on around the person may be present. Additional signs of catatonic type are repeating what others say or mimicking their movements.

Undifferentiated Type

When a client is in an active psychotic state, meaning that Criterion A symptoms for schizophrenia are met and the client does not have prominent symptoms that match any of the prior subtypes, then undifferentiated type is diagnosed. Remember that a client's diagnosis may also change over the years as symptoms form and re-form. The particular subtype diagnosed at one point in time may not match what is currently happening to a client. The subtype of schizophrenia may have shifted, with the undifferentiated subtype now most representative of the course of the disease.

Residual Type

The residual type of schizophrenia is a subtype diagnosis reserved for a client who has had at least one documented episode of schizophrenia but now has no prominent positive symptoms of the illness. Negative symptoms such as flat affect and inability to work are present, but prominent hallucinations, delusions, and disorganized thoughts and behavior are not. When a client has these characteristics, the client is considered to have residual features of the illness and receives this subtype diagnosis.

Other Psychotic Disorders

Psychosis occurs in a number of disorders in addition to schizophrenia.

SCHIZOPHRENIFORM DISORDER

Schizophreniform disorder is very similar to schizophrenia except the person has not been ill for very long. The diagnostic criteria are the same as the Criterion A symptoms for schizophrenia. The main difference is that the client has experienced the symptoms for at least 1 month and either recovered from the symptoms before 6 months, or 6 months have not yet elapsed since the original symptoms began. Under the latter set of circumstances, the diagnosis of schizophreniform disorder is provisional until the 6 months have elapsed and then a diagnosis is set. A second difference, besides duration, is that the client may show no impairment in social and work functioning. Schizophreniform disorder may occur just prior to the onset of schizophrenia (i.e., be prodromal to [precede] schizophrenia), yet approximately one third of clients diagnosed with this disorder recover. The other two thirds go on to have either schizophrenia or schizoaffective disorder.

SCHIZOAFFECTIVE DISORDER

In schizoaffective disorder, two sets of symptoms are present concurrently in the same illness episode, not just at some time in a client's life: Criterion A symptoms in schizophrenia and symptoms of a mood disorder (either a major depressive or manic disorder; see Chapter 15). Schizoaffective disorder is less common than, and has a slightly better prognosis than, schizophrenia, but it has a substantially worse prognosis than mood disorders.

DELUSIONAL DISORDER

Delusional disorder is diagnosed when the client holds one or more nonbizarre delusions for a period of at least 1 month. The client must never have met the Criterion A symptoms for schizophrenia. Although it is sometimes difficult to differentiate bizarre from nonbizarre delusions, the key is that the nonbizarre delusions could conceivably arise in everyday life. An example of a nonbizarre delusion follows.

CLINICAL EXAMPLE

Martin holds the delusional belief that the police are trying to entrap him. He goes to extremes to protect his home with surveillance and security equipment. At the same time, he believes that the police won't bother him at work because his boss, with whom he works well, is the son of a policeman.

People with delusional disorders may function quite well in areas of their life not affected by the delusion, yet behave oddly in activities touched by the delusion. Delusional disorders are not common and arise predominantly during middle and late adulthood.

A subtype of delusional disorder, the erotomanic type, occurs when clients believe that another person is in love with them. Contacts, stalking, and displays to impress the imagined lover have involved celebrities, politicians, and even the man or woman next door.

BRIEF PSYCHOTIC DISORDER

In a brief psychotic disorder, at least one of the Criterion A symptoms for schizophrenia are present (hallucinations, delusions, disorganized speech or behavior) for at least 1 day, but for less than 1 month. Upon remission of these symptoms, clients return to their level of functioning prior to the onset of the illness. This disorder may be brought on by a particular stressful event in the person's life, including childbirth. In other instances, a stressful life event cannot be specifically identified. Brief psychotic disorder is an unusual and seldom seen phenomenon.

ADDITIONAL PSYCHOTIC DISORDERS

Several additional psychotic disorders are specified in the DSM-IV-TR:

- Shared psychotic disorder
- Psychotic disorder due to a general medical condition
- Substance-induced psychotic disorder
- Psychotic disorder not otherwise specified (NOS)

Consult the DSM-IV-TR for diagnostic criteria about these disorders. However, in diagnosing any psychotic disorder, the diagnostician must explore the alternative explanation that symptoms may be caused by an underlying medical disorder or by substance use.

Biopsychosocial Theories

Beliefs about the causes of schizophrenia have changed over the centuries since schizophrenia was equated with early senility. Theories about the treatment for schizophrenia have also undergone change. For example, at one point it was believed (based on the writings of Sigmund Freud) that people with schizophrenia could not be treated because they were unable to form a therapeutic relationship with a psychoanalyst. It is likely that several factors interrelate to cause schizophrenia and several forces influence the effectiveness of treatment.

BIOLOGIC THEORIES

It is unlikely that schizophrenia is caused by a specific biologic abnormality. Scientists have searched unsuccessfully for a unique biologic marker consistently present in people with schizophrenia but absent in healthy people. At the same time, scientific evidence suggests that the disorder is not merely psychological and that biologic alterations are present. Particularly convincing is the fact that the symptoms associated with schizophrenia, such as delusions or hallucinations, are found in healthy people only when they are in a state of metabolic imbalance or suffer from organic diseases. Individuals with brain tumors, or who have ingested certain drugs, for example, may experience hallucinations. Nutrition may also influence symptoms. See the Caring for the Spirit feature on nutrition and schizophrenia below.

Genetic Theories

People with schizophrenia inherit a genetic predisposition to the disease rather than the disease itself. Evidence supporting this theory is the fact that relatives of schizophrenics have a greater chance of developing the disease than do members of the general population. While

CARING FOR THE SPIRIT

Can Nutrition Influence Schizophrenia?

Schizophrenia is a distressing illness with many presentations. The distress people experience motivates the search for an explanation of the cause as well as a cure. We wonder:

1. Why are some people schizophrenic and others not?
2. Why does this illness have different faces in different people?
3. Why do some people have a serious version of the illness while others a mild one?

The search for answers has taken a variety of pathways, including the realm of food and nutrition.

Unconventional nutritional interventions have been proposed to treat schizophrenia. An example of a dietary intervention claimed to help is the gluten-free diet for schizophrenia. This is an elimination dieting format based on the principle that certain foods may contribute to chronic symptoms or disease when eaten in normal quantities by vulnerable people. Unlike classic allergy, these "food intolerances" do not involve a conventionally understood immune mechanism nor do they inevitably have a rapid onset.

Diagnosing food intolerance by an elimination diet consists of removing all but a few foods from the diet and then reintroducing foods one by one to see if they provoke the symptoms of concern. The theory also implies that after a period of complete exclusion, the problem substances can usually be gradually reintroduced without recurrence of symptoms. Although wheat and dairy "intolerance" is the most common determination, each client is said to be sensitive to a different set of foods.

The evidence for this as a nutritional intervention in treating schizophrenia is generally either negative or nonexistent. In addition, randomized trials have failed to show any benefit from vitamin megadose therapy for schizophrenia, Down syndrome, learning disability. Rigorous research on the naturopathic approach to chronic disease is needed.

1% of the population develops schizophrenia, 10% of the first-degree relatives (parents, siblings, children) of schizophrenics are diagnosed with the disease during their lifetimes (Cooper, 2001). The risk of developing schizophrenia increases with the closeness of relation to a diagnosed person. Siblings have a greater risk of developing the disease than do half-siblings or grandchildren, and these have a greater risk than more distant relatives, such as cousins.

There is no clear genetic marker for schizophrenia at this time, although several research projects are involved in the search for susceptibility genes (Malhotra, 2001). The most promising development has been the Human Genome Project. The Project's completion of the sequence of the human genome will guide the study of the genetic variations implicated in human disease. This is exciting news for psychiatric–mental health nurses.

The range of chromosomes showing modest linkage includes 1, 5, 6, 7, 8, 10, 13, 15, and 22 (Cowan & Kandel, 2001; Malhotra, 2001). It is becoming obvious that a single gene is not responsible for schizophrenia. This illness resists easy genetic codification due to its complexity and its variety of forms. It has been suggested that schizophrenia may be a collection of disorders rather than a single disease entity.

Research examining the occurrence of schizophrenia in twins indicates that both environmental and genetic factors are important. Concordance rates (which means both twins either express or do not express the trait) for schizophrenia are consistently higher for monozygotic twins than for dizygotic twins. Interestingly, monozygotic, or identical, twins need not both have schizophrenia but the chance of both twins being schizophrenic is 25% to 39%. This finding supports the hypothesis of some level of genetic transmission. The fact that both twins are not affected when they are genetically identical, however, indicates that environment plays a large part in the expression of the illness. If the disease were solely genetically determined, the concordance rates in this group would be close to 100%.

MediaLink PET/SPECT Schizophrenia Animation

Brain Structure Abnormalities

As a group, people with schizophrenia differ in their brain structure from people who do not have schizophrenia. People with chronic schizophrenia show changes to their frontotemporal cortical gray matter, among other areas. Greater clinical severity was associated with faster rates of frontotemporal brain volume changes in one study (Mathalon, Sullivan, Lim, & Pfefferbaum, 2001). These observations are consistent with other suppositions regarding brain structure abnormalities. As a check on why these brain changes might be present, several studies found no correlation between medication and brain changes over time. Thus, the hypothesis that psychosis or the illness itself causes neurologic damage and that medication is somehow neuroprotective remains speculative.

Altered brain structures may be genetically based and could represent a marker of vulnerability to schizophrenia that precedes any other symptomatology. How the brain structure abnormalities influence the progress of the disease is not well understood and requires further study. An example of PET scan differences between identical twins where one has schizophrenia and the other is unaffected is seen in ■ Figure 14–2.

Biochemical Theories

The biochemical basis of schizophrenia is captured in the **dopamine hypothesis**, which states that schizophrenic symp-

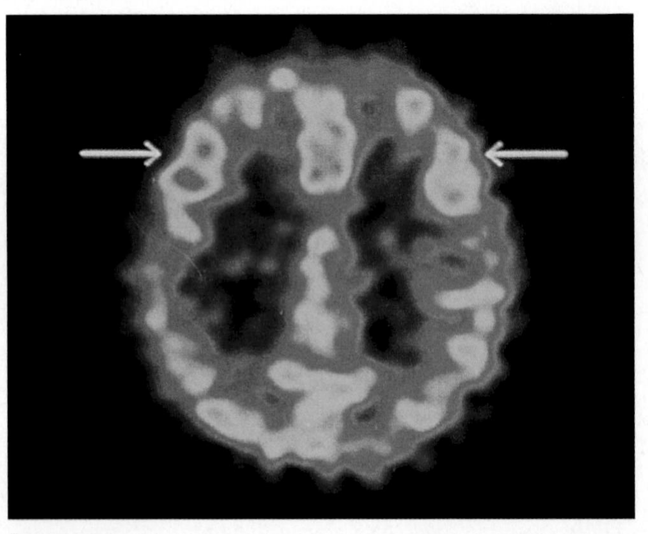
A

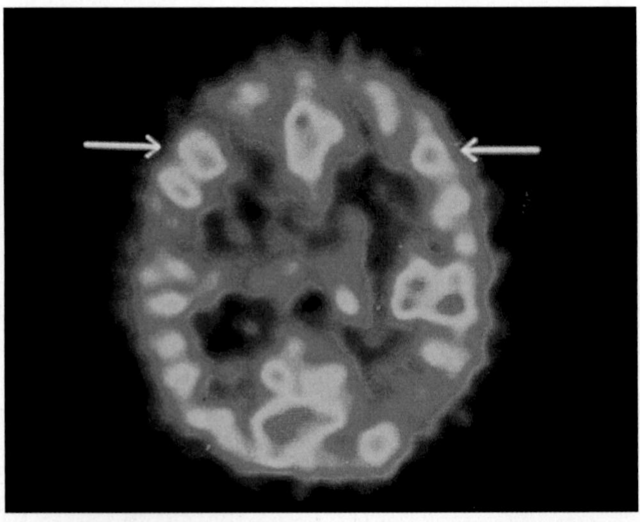
B

FIGURE 14–2 ■ *Schizophrenia scans. PET scans of discordant monozygotic twins taken during a test to provoke activity and measure regional cerebral blood flow.* ***(A)*** *Arrows indicate areas of normal blood flow and brain activity in the unaffected twin.* ***(B)*** *Arrows indicate areas of lower blood flow and brain activity in the twin with schizophrenia.*

Source: Courtesy of Dr. Karen F. Berman, *Clinical Brain Disorders Branch,* National Institute of Mental Health.

toms may be related to overactive neuronal activity that is dependent on dopamine (DA). In other words, positive psychotic symptoms are associated with excessive DA transmission.

The hypothesis was supported by numerous studies demonstrating that DA blockers, medications that decrease DA activity, alleviate symptoms. The traditional antipsychotic medications were shown to be effective because of their ability to antagonize DA receptors; however, this causes undesirable side effects such as extrapyramidal symptoms. The relief of positive symptoms with these traditional agents was not complete, and the negative symptoms of the disorder were much less responsive to DA blockers.

Research suggests that the relationships between DA activity and schizophrenic symptoms are much more complex than originally hypothesized. It is now known that there are multiple types of DA receptors, and different types of receptors are concentrated in different regions of the brain. The regulation of DA activity has been thoroughly studied as well, since DA dysregulation is recognized as being inherently involved in the pathology of schizophrenia (Schultz & Andreasen, 1999).

Further evidence that supports a biochemical theory is the physical impact that atypical antipsychotic agents have on clients with schizophrenia. These medications block DA as well as serotonin. This may help lessen extrapyramidal side effects such as dystonia and akathisia, and may be the reason why they are so useful in reducing negative symptoms.

PSYCHOLOGICAL THEORIES

Most psychological theories focus on the processing of information as well as attention and arousal states in schizophrenia.

Information Processing

Many schizophrenic clients have information-processing deficits. Two central types of information processing have been identified:

1. Automatic processing.
2. Controlled or effortful processing.

Automatic processing is the taking in of information unintentionally. Automatic processing can occur without the individual's being aware of it and it does not interfere with conscious thought processes occurring at the same time. An example of automatic information processing is being aware of the physical features of a new environment, such as a room being large and spacious as opposed to small and confined.

People with schizophrenia are deficient in controlled information processing. Their ability to perform directed, conscious, sequential thinking—for example, making comparisons between two stimuli or organizing a set of stimuli—is consistently inferior to that of healthy people. Someone with schizophrenia would not easily be able to perform the series of steps necessary to organize a classroom debate. See the Rx Communication feature for an example of an interaction with a client who is unfocused and having an information processing problem.

We do not know whether the schizophrenic person's inability to sustain conscious, directed thought is the primary problem or the result of a primary deficit in automatic thinking. If the primary deficit is in automatic processes, then the person is forced to complete automatic tasks at the conscious level, inhibiting and slowing controlled information processing. Sufficient evidence to resolve this question is not yet available.

Attention and Arousal

MediaLink EPSE: Dystonia/Akathisia Video

Attention and arousal are measured by physiologic states and alterations, such as galvanic skin response, heart rate, blood pressure, skin temperature, and pupillary response. Physiologic studies of attention and arousal in schizophrenic clients show promise in identifying clinically significant subgroups. One subgroup of clients exhibits abnormally low response levels to novel, or different, stimuli. This finding suggests that these clients are less adept than healthy people at attending to and responding to novel situations. An example of this state can be seen when a client with schizophrenia does not register that a ball is being thrown at him during a game of catch. The ball may even strike him, drop to the ground, and roll away before the client looks at it.

A second group of clients with schizophrenia demonstrates a state of hyperarousal evidenced by elevated electrodermal activity, heart rate, and blood pressure. Hyperarousal has been noted during both symptomatic and nonsymptomatic periods. These

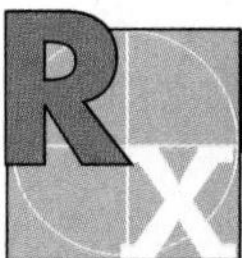

COMMUNICATION

Unfocused Client

CLIENT: "I went to the ballgame and I had great seats and I saw the whole game and I saw all the home runs and all the hits and all the strike outs and I saw the pitcher throw all the pitches, fast ball, curve ball, change up, and . . ."

NURSE RESPONSE 1: "Keith, tell me about this slower so I can keep up with you."

RATIONALE: This response is structured to be brief, focused, and to direct the client's attention to the speed with which he speaks.

NURSE RESPONSE 2: "How about if I ask you some questions about the game? If you give me a chance to ask questions I'll have a better idea of what you saw."

RATIONALE: This response defines the special skills required for a conversation.

clients demonstrate symptoms of irritability, excitement, and anxiety rather than apathy and withdrawal. An example of this state can be seen when a schizophrenic client angrily and loudly criticizes someone for using incorrect grammar in a sentence.

FAMILY THEORIES

Numerous theories implicating family interaction alone as a cause of schizophrenia have been proposed and unsupported. Research has failed to support the theory that dysfunctional family interaction alone causes the illness.

One theory suggests that disordered family communication (the inability to focus on and clearly share an observation or thought) causes schizophrenia only in the presence of a genetic predisposition to the disease. For example, the communication taking place at the dinner table may be chaotic and constant. No one finishes a sentence and nothing can be talked about to a logical conclusion. Living with this pattern of family communication during early development is thought to impair the schizophrenic person's ability to perceive the environment and communicate with others about it. People with schizophrenia are more likely to show symptoms of thought disorder when they are raised by people who have dysfunctional communication.

Schizophrenic individuals raised by adoptive mothers who themselves showed elevated levels of communication deviance show just as much thought disorder as those raised in birth families. In contrast, adoptees who were raised by adoptive parents with more functional communication were less likely to show thought disorder. In one study, this pattern was not evident in control adoptees—there was no discernible relationship between thought disorder in the adoptees and communication deviance in the adoptive parents. In other words, these findings did not detect the presence of a "schizophrenogenic environment" for individuals without a preexisting genetic liability. These examples support the view that genetic factors alone do not explain the development of schizophrenia, and that interactions with the environment are important (Tsuang, Stone, & Faraone, 2001).

A second theory is that the family's emotional tone can influence the course of schizophrenia over time. Researchers found that schizophrenic individuals from families who are highly critical, hostile, or overinvolved tend to relapse more often. Families exhibiting such characteristics have been described as having high **expressed emotion.** There is some evidence that family expressed emotion, life events, and biological factors combine with the individual's genetic liability to the disorder to cause schizophrenia (Tsuang, Stone, & Faraone, 2001). Recent research on schizophrenia can be found on the National Alliance for Research on Schizophrenia and Depression Web site at www.mhsource.com/narsad/ and through a direct link on the Companion Website for this book.

MediaLink National Alliance for Research

HUMANISTIC–INTERACTIONAL THEORIES

An interactional model of schizophrenia integrates many of the biologic and psychosocial theories already discussed. In this view, schizophrenia is due to the interaction of a genetic predisposition or biologic vulnerability, stress or change in the environment, and the individual's social skills and supports. In an interactional model, the influences are multidimensional. A biologic vulnerability may inhibit the individual's capacity to cope with even minor stressors such as the loss of a primary source of support. Similarly, schizophrenic people might grow worse upon entering an environment that demands coping skills they have not developed.

Stress–Vulnerability Model

An interactional model for understanding schizophrenia that has received wide acceptance is the stress–vulnerability model, which suggests that people with schizophrenia have a genetically based, biologically mediated vulnerability, to personal, family, and environmental stress. In this model, risk factors and protective factors interact in any of three ways:

1. Stressors, risk, and vulnerability factors combine additively and potentiate each other.
2. As long as stress is not excessive, it enhances competence.
3. Protective factors modulate or buffer the impact of stressors, by, for instance, improving coping, adaptation, and competence building (Fan & Eaton, 2001).

The stressors a client with schizophrenia experiences can overwhelm the resources available, and symptoms result. Psychobiologic stressors include the stress of living with schizophrenia itself. Altered attention and perception, as well as problems with motivation and energy, create stresses for people with schizophrenia. Environmental and interpersonal stressors include those that we all encounter, but a person with schizophrenia is particularly sensitive. These include stressful life events, environments that are highly demanding or stimulating, and family or living environments that are highly negative.

A quote that points to the validity of the stress–vulnerability concept, especially the protective qualities, was made by one client in the Angermeyer et al. study (2001), "I've got the impression, that the stuff [antipsychotic] shields me . . . that it shields my soul . . . because I'm not very well protected, and this medicine, Clozaril, is more capable of giving my soul some protection." A second client also conveyed this effect, "Therefore, it does help . . . well, because I don't experience these irritations as forcefully anymore . . . 'cause I am a little shielded."

Resources That Moderate Stress

Resources that can moderate stress (and are thought to affect the development of symptoms in schizophrenia) include:

- Skill in symptom recognition and management.
- Social support.
- Antipsychotic medication.

The capacities to self-monitor the waxing and waning of schizophrenia and to develop coping strategies to influence symptoms at the first sign of trouble show promise in influencing the longer-term course of the illness. An example of how you can help a client to self-monitor hallucinations and develop coping strategies is in the Using Research Evidence feature. This capacity to detect prodromal symptoms and acute symptoms is

USING RESEARCH EVIDENCE

Jane is a 33-year-old female with paranoid schizophrenia. She is one of the people with whom you work in an outpatient clinic for moderately ill people who have schizophrenia. Your education and experience have taught you that schizophrenia is a complex illness that requires more than just medications to address it adequately.

Jane is an excellent example. Her auditory hallucinations interfered greatly with her ability to function. It is important to carefully consider the meaning of the voices to her in order to help her develop relevant coping skills and implement effective care.

In contacts with your clients you may have noticed a certain connection between their coping styles and what the voices meant to them. For example, a client can effectively cope with benevolent voices through engaging the voices. Engaging is the process of the client talking to and interacting with the voices and making sure the client stays in charge of that conversation. In Jane's case, the voices were malevolent. A resistive coping style that allowed her to ignore or limit the impact of the voices worked best. Determining what the voices mean to each individual client can provide you with direction toward a coping skill that fits the client's beliefs.

Some people do believe their voices to be both malevolent and benevolent. This situation suggests the need to carefully and accurately assess and reassess what the voices mean to them and their ability to cope with the hallucinations as indicated in the following research:

Sayer, J., Ritter, S., & Gournay, K. (2000). Beliefs about voices and their effects on coping strategies. *Journal of Advanced Nursing, 31,* 1199–1205.

a resource that may work to mediate the stress that occurs in the person, family, or environment.

Social support has proven helpful in moderating stress for general populations and for people with schizophrenia in particular. Supportive others who provide empathy, contact, financial aid, problem solving, and other forms of support are capable of mitigating the difficulties of schizophrenia. Finally, antipsychotic medications moderate some, and sometimes most, symptoms of the disease, and thus some of the stressors induced by the disease (Birchwood, Meaden, Trower, Gilbert, & Plaistow, 2000).

NURSING PROCESS

Clients with Schizophrenia

Schizophrenia is a difficult and chronic illness requiring understanding and competent care in every facet of the client's life.

Assessment

Assessing clients who have schizophrenia occurs at individual, family, and environmental levels. Be aware of the client's status and of changes in the client's personal life, family situation, and environment in order to plan care and intervene effectively. In addition, care that addresses multiple levels of the client's life is consistent with the interactional theory of schizophrenia because it is assumed that changes in any aspect of the client's environment influence all other aspects of the personal environmental balance.

SUBJECTIVE DATA

These data describe the client's inner experience of schizophrenia.

Perceptual Changes. The perceptions of clients with schizophrenia may be either heightened or blunted. These changes may occur in all the senses or in just one or two. For example, a client may see colors as brighter than normal or may be acutely sensitive to sounds. Another may have a heightened sense of touch and therefore be extremely sensitive to any physical contact.

Illusions occur when the client misperceives or exaggerates stimuli in the external environment. A schizophrenic client may mistake a chair for a person or perceive that the walls of a hallway are closing in. The perceptual changes are sufficient to cause the client to mistake the stimulus for something that is not actually there.

Hallucinations are the most extreme and yet the most common perceptual disturbance in schizophrenia. Auditory hallucinations are the most common form of hallucination. Although hallucinations are a hallmark of schizophrenia, their presence alone does not establish the presence of the disorder. Table 14–1 on page 307, lists various types of hallucinations, along with a disease process commonly associated with the symptom.

Assess perceptual disturbances by asking the client about the experience and by observing for behaviors that indicate the client is frightened or attending to internal stimuli. Ask the client, "What are you seeing and hearing?" Note the degree to which this description differs from your perceptions of the environment.

Clients may be reluctant to discuss the extreme perceptual disturbance of hallucinations. A classic sign of auditory hallucinations is placing the hands over the ears when clients are frightened by the voices and attempt to block them out. Less obvious signs of hallucinations are inappropriate laughing or smiling, difficulty following a conversation, and difficulty attending to what is happening at the moment. Fleeting, rapid changes of expression that are not precipitated by events in the real world can be another sign. Finally, clients may talk to themselves, presumably in answer to the voices they hear. For more information, see the Assessment box on page 318.

OBJECTIVE DATA

These data are the observable symptoms and manifestations of schizophrenia that you, as a nurse, will be assessing.

ASSESSMENT

Hallucinating Client

A complete assessment of hallucinations should identify the following:

- Whether the hallucinations are solely auditory or include other senses.
- How long the client has experienced the hallucinations, what the initial hallucinations were like, and whether they have changed.
- Which situations are most likely to trigger hallucinations, and which times of day they occur most frequently.
- What the hallucinations are about. (Are they just sounds, or voices? If the client hears voices, what do they say?)
- How strongly the client believes in the reality of the hallucinations.
- Whether the hallucinations command the client to do something, and if so, how potentially destructive the commands are.
- Whether the client hears other voices contradicting commands received in hallucinations.
- How the client feels about the hallucinations.
- Which strategies the client has used to cope with the hallucinations and how effective the strategies were.

Disturbances in Thought and Expression. Clients with schizophrenia find that their thinking is muddled or unclear. Their thoughts are disconnected or disjointed, and the connections between one thought and another are vague.

The clarity of the client's communication often reflects the level of **thought disorganization.** Client responses may be simply inappropriate to the situation or conversation. They may have difficulty responding or stop in midsentence, as if they are stuck, a sign of **thought blocking.**

Note the rate and quality of the client's speech. Is it unusually loud, insistent, and continuous? Does the client wander from topic to topic (*tangential communication*) or bring up details that are irrelevant to the topic at hand (*circumstantial communication*)? Are the client's responses slow and hesitant, reflecting difficulty in taking in stimuli and responding to them?

Schizophrenic clients also have difficulty thinking abstractly. Their responses may be inappropriate because they interpret words literally rather than abstractly. For example, when told to prepare to have his blood drawn, a young man readied some paper and marking pens. Assess abstract thinking by asking clients the meaning of proverbs, a test requiring the client to abstract a general meaning from a specific or metaphysical statement, for example, "People who live in glass houses shouldn't throw stones." Schizophrenic clients are more likely to give concrete ("If you throw a stone the glass will break.") rather than abstract ("Don't criticize someone else if you behave the same way.") responses.

Disruptions in Emotional Responses. Tone of voice, rate of speech, content of speech, expressions, postures, and body movements indicate emotional tone. Disturbances in emotions commonly seen in schizophrenia are blunted or flattened affect or inappropriate expression of emotions. Assess the congruence between the content of the client's communication and the displayed emotion. For example, does the client laugh when describing a frightening or sad incident? The absence of emotion is also often indicative of schizophrenia.

Motor Behavior Changes. Disruptions seen in schizophrenia include disorganized behavior and catatonia. Disorganized behavior lacks a coherent goal, is aimless, or is disruptive. Catatonic behavior is manifested by unusual body movement or lack of movement. This activity disturbance includes *catatonic excitement* (the client moves excitedly but not in response to environmental influences), *catatonic posturing* (the client holds bizarre postures for periods of time), and *stupor* (the client holds the body still and is unresponsive to the environment).

Changes in Role Functioning. An important factor in predicting the course of schizophrenia is the client's level of functioning before the symptoms of the disease became pronounced. Assessment should therefore include a complete history of the client's success at completing developmental tasks. The prognosis is best if the client functioned at a high level prior to the onset of schizophrenic disturbance. Assess how well the client fulfilled role responsibilities in the family, in school, in relation to peers, and in work. Obtain a history of the rate of decline in these various roles. The onset of schizophrenia may be relatively acute, or degeneration may be slow.

Drug Use. Clients with drug toxicity or withdrawal may have behavior disturbances similar to those seen in schizophrenic clients. They may have auditory or visual hallucinations and may be confused, illogical, and highly anxious. For this reason, it is essential to obtain a detailed drug history. Assess both long-term and recent use of chemical substances. If the client is not a reliable historian, interview family or friends. In addition, both blood and urine should be tested for drugs if reliable information cannot be obtained.

Family Health History. Part of assessment is noting any history of mental disorder in the client's family. Of particular interest is a history of schizophrenia or any thought disorder, mood disorders (such as cyclical highs or depressions), or alcoholism in any family member. Note any report that family members had "nervous breakdowns" or any other colloquial descriptions of mental or emotional disorders.

Family Cohesion and Emotion. In families of people with schizophrenia, enmeshment (see Chapter 29), combined with a negative emotional tone, is thought to be detrimental to the ill member's well-being. However, the presence of acquaintances and family members showing emotional warmth in low expressed emotion (EE) situations can have a protective function.

Much of the nursing assessment of family cohesion and emotion can be carried out unobtrusively. Chapter 29 has specific guidelines for assessment of these and other family dynamics. The nursing staff, in conjunction with the interdisciplinary team can also arrange formal family assessment interviews (also discussed in Chapter 29).

Family Communication Problems. Unclear or incomplete communication is frequent in families of people with schizophrenia. This area requires nursing assessment. Unclear communication may result from continual interaction with the ill member or may contribute to the disorder. Clinicians must evaluate how effectively the family communicates to determine the potential need for intervention.

Assess these aspects of family communication:

- Ability to focus on a topic.
- Ability to discuss a topic in a meaningful way with other family members.
- Ability to maintain the discussion without wandering from the subject or becoming distracted.
- Use of language and explanations that are generally understandable (not peculiar to that family alone)

Also note who in the family seems to do the talking, who talks to whom, and whether members talk for, or interrupt one another. See Box 14–1 for types of communication problems that commonly occur with the diagnosis of schizophrenia and that interfere with all relationships, especially family communications.

Family Burden. Most families of schizophrenic individuals report that caring for the ill member places a burden on the family unit. Ask about the burdens the family is facing so that you can determine the information and support needs to be met. See Chapter 29 for examples of common family burdens.

Environmental Assessment. Assess the availability of support and services beyond the bounds of the family, including extended family and friends, as well as community groups and organizations that support schizophrenic clients. Mental health programs that address the specific needs of schizophrenic clients should be sought.

Nursing Diagnosis: NANDA

Nursing diagnoses with schizophrenic clients focus on alterations in the patterns of activity, cognition, emotion processes, interpersonal processes, and perception. Alterations in ecologic, physiologic, and valuation processes are assessed as well, but the central nursing problems relate to the former five processes.

IMPAIRED COMMUNICATION

Schizophrenia interferes with the ability to conduct complex and demanding communications.

Verbal. Schizophrenic clients communicate in a disorganized, sometimes incomprehensible fashion. Clients with less severe disorganization skip from topic to topic, making few if any logical links. When more severe thought disorganization is present, the client's statements may be totally incoherent. Some clients manifest thought disorganization by speaking very little, a characteristic labeled poverty of speech. Also note poverty of content in speech, in which the client converses but says very little.

Often, clients with schizophrenia communicate in ways that are overly concrete (a sign of an inability to think and communicate abstractly) or overly symbolic (a sign of preoccupation with unreal or delusional material). The symbols are usually difficult to decipher because their meanings are idiosyncratic.

Nonverbal. In schizophrenic clients, facial and body expressions that accompany verbal communication frequently do not match the content of the verbal message. This lack of congruence is primarily due to the blunting of emotions found in schizophrenia. Expected facial expressions—smiles, looks of concern or disgust—may not accompany the schizophrenic's statements. In addition, clients with motor or behavioral abnormalities—posturing, unusual movements, or grimacing—convey a confusing mix of verbal and nonverbal messages.

SELF-CARE DEFICITS

People with schizophrenia frequently appear indifferent to their personal appearance. They may neglect to bathe, change

BOX 14–1 Problematic Communication Patterns Common in Schizophrenia

Blocking

The client has trouble expressing a response or will stop in midsentence, as if he was stranded without a thought.

Clang Associations

Words that rhyme or sound alike are distributed throughout conversations without necessarily making sense.

Echolalia

Phrases, sentences, or entire conversations said to the client are repeated back by the client.

Neologisms

Words or meanings are invented by the client. This can include multisyllabic, pseudo-scientific words or simple words.

Perseveration

Maintaining a particular idea regardless of the topic being discussed or attempts to change the subject.

Word Salad

An incoherent medley of words emitted in conversation as if it was a sensible and articulate phrase.

clothes, or attend to minor grooming tasks such as combing their hair. Some show little awareness of current fashion styles, wearing clothing that makes them look out of place. Of greater concern are those who wear clothing that is inappropriate to the current season and weather conditions.

Lack of attention to grooming might be a simple annoyance to those who must live in close proximity to the person with schizophrenia. Health risks related to prolonged poor hygiene also arise. Assess immediate problems, such as inadequate nutrition, fluid intake, and elimination, as well as long-term problems, such as dental caries and increased susceptibility to infections.

Disregard for appearance and hygiene may extend to the client's environment. The client may fail to maintain a clean and safe living space. He or she may not take good care of personal belongings and may misplace them. Self-care deficiencies may result from consistently disturbed thought and perceptual processes. For example, a young man whose chronic hallucinations are only partly relieved by medication has difficulty concentrating for long periods and therefore demonstrates variable attention to grooming.

ACTIVITY INTOLERANCE

The emotional disturbances of ambivalence and apathy, common in schizophrenic disorders, can result in lack of interest and inactivity. Inactivity induced by ambivalence is associated with higher levels of emotion. Anxious about choosing one course of action and rejecting another, the client is immobilized. The following Clinical Examples describe the experience of intolerance to activity.

CLINICAL EXAMPLE

Jim is ambivalent about taking a pass out alone for the first time. He is undecided about taking the risk of leaving the hospital ward without a staff member, yet yearns for the freedom of walking the streets alone. Indecision leaves him standing, immobilized, by the doorway to the unit.

Extreme ambivalence can manifest itself in even the most automatic of behaviors.

CLINICAL EXAMPLE

Mary cannot eat because of ambivalence about where to sit or what to eat. She stands in the center of the dining room, turning first to one chair and then another, unable to choose and thus begin eating.

Clients who are inactive because of apathy demonstrate little emotional tone. Such clients may spend long hours lying in bed staring into space or listening to music. Often, but not always, apathetic individuals prefer isolation. The nurse might find several clients sitting in the same room, engaged in no apparent activities, and interacting with one another only when absolutely necessary.

SOCIAL ISOLATION

Extreme anxiety about relating to others often leads schizophrenic clients to withdraw from interaction and to isolate themselves. Some clients tolerate only a few moments of direct communication, whereas others can manage extended periods of contact. Assess the client's tolerance of brief periods of contact with nurses and other clients. Document patterns of relating and withdrawal, also noting which activities the client engages in when in contact with others and when alone.

DECISIONAL CONFLICT

Decisional conflict in schizophrenia is probably due to biochemical alterations in the brain that make it difficult for clients to take in, synthesize, and respond to information. Decisional conflict may be evident both in the mundane activities of daily life (e.g., selecting one's diet) and in major life decisions. This can be frustrating for caregivers and for clients. This clinical example shows how decisional conflict can remove even a pleasant aspect of life from the client. Education about the impacts this feature has upon clients' lives is helpful.

CLINICAL EXAMPLE

Murray refuses to take medications, even though not taking them means that he will be evicted from the residential treatment program he likes.

SENSORY/PERCEPTUAL ALTERATIONS

Alterations in the five senses (sound, sight, smell, taste, touch) creates an altered perception of the world.

Hallucinations. Hallucinations are both a clinical diagnostic sign of schizophrenia and a focus for nursing care. You need to know the extent and nature of clients' hallucinations. Monitoring a client's hallucinations over time provides information on stressors that precipitate hallucinations, the client's response to psychotropic medications, and nursing actions that may diminish this symptom.

Document many aspects of the client's hallucinatory experience. Discuss with the client, if able to, the details of his or her symptoms. Ask about and make note of situations or times of day that seem to trigger hallucinatory experiences. Record all sensory modes affected in the hallucination. The history of hallucinations and changes over time are important. Look for major themes in the content of the hallucinations, particularly whether the hallucinations command the client to do something.

The degree to which clients believe the hallucinatory experience is real and their ability to verify the reality of the experience by checking with others have important implications for interventions. Note the client's emotional response to hallucinations; some clients experience depression or despair about the continued presence of voices, others may be comforted or kept company by their voices. Client coping strategies, and their effectiveness or ineffectiveness, are also an important aspect of the diagnosis.

Illusions. Illusions make the client vulnerable to emotional and physical injury. The level of misperception may vary from day to day and even throughout the day. Misperceptions of the social environment make the client vulnerable to inappropriate responses and therefore ridicule. Misperceptions of the physical environment, such as misjudging the speed of an oncoming car, may lead to physical harm.

Body Image Disturbance. A body image disturbance is common in schizophrenic people. Clients may lose the sense of where their bodies leave off and where inanimate objects begin. They may become dissociated from various body parts and believe, for example, that their arms and legs belong to someone else. They may worry about the normalcy of their sexual organs. Clients often verbalize this altered sense of self directly, saying "I don't feel like myself" or "I feel like I am looking at my body from somewhere else in the room."

EXCESS FLUID VOLUME

Excess fluid volume, or water intoxication, is a problem that is observed primarily in clients who reside in institutions such as state mental hospitals. This physiologic state is brought on by excessive drinking, characterized by hyponatremia, confusion, and disorientation, and progresses to apathy and lethargy. In severe cases, seizures and death may result. This behavior can lead to irreversible brain damage and could be the cause of nearly a fifth of the deaths of schizophrenic clients below the age of 53 years. Polydipsia appears to be significantly associated with male gender, smoking, celibacy, and psychiatric chronicity. The polydipsic clients presented in one study also had a high prevalence of schizophrenia, mental retardation, pervasive developmental disorders, and high frequency of somatic disorders (Mercier-Guidez & Loas, 2000). For clients suspected to be at risk because of frequent drinking, preventive measures include regular measures of urine specific gravity, and regular weights designed to screen for increases in the body's fluid volume.

ALTERED THOUGHT PROCESSES

Schizophrenia changes the way thoughts are processed by distorting logic and organization.

Delusions. Clients express delusional thinking in direct interactions and, to a lesser extent, through behaviors. When asked, many clients willingly describe their delusional beliefs in detail. They seldom withhold this information because they believe firmly in the validity of the delusion, no matter how bizarre it seems to others. Clients' actions reflect the fixedness of their beliefs.

CLINICAL EXAMPLE

Gerry has the somatic delusion that her body is riddled with holes. She flatly refuses to drink, convinced that the fluid will flow directly out of the holes and soil her dress.

The content of delusions varies: delusions of persecution, reference, and so on (see Table 14–3). Reality-based delusions may seem plausible because they could, under some circumstances, actually occur. Bizarre delusions, more common among schizophrenic clients, have no possible basis in reality. The false belief that one's husband is having an affair with a neighbor is a reality-based delusion. In contrast, the belief that one's thoughts are directed by a television announcer, or that one's unspoken thoughts can be heard by others, are known as bizarre delusions.

Delusions often reflect the client's fears, particularly about personal inadequacies. For example, a man's grandiose delusion that he is the mayor of New York City is a defense against feelings of inferiority. Similarly, persecutory delusions defend against the person's own feelings of aggression. Aggressive feelings are projected onto a person or organization—for example, the police, whom the client then fears.

Magical Thinking. Magical thinking is the belief that events can happen simply because one wishes them to. Some people with schizophrenia claim they can exert their will to make people take certain actions or make specific events occur, like winning the lottery.

Thought Insertion, Withdrawal, and Broadcasting. Hallmarks of schizophrenic thought are the beliefs that others can put ideas into one's head (*thought insertion*) or take thoughts out of one's head (*thought withdrawal*). In addition, some clients believe that their thoughts are transmitted to others via radio, television, or other means but not directly by the client. This belief is known as *thought broadcasting*.

ALTERED EMOTIONAL RESPONSES

Clients who have schizophrenia respond emotionally in altered ways that can be difficult or frustrating for others.

Inappropriate Emotions. Many individuals with schizophrenia demonstrate inappropriate affect—emotional responses that are inappropriate to the situation. For example, a client may smile or laugh while relating a history of having been abused as a child. Or a client may become angry and anxious when asked to join a group of other clients for dinner. The degree to which a client's emotions are inappropriate is a prognostic indicator. Clients whose emotional response is preserved and generally appropriate have a more favorable prognosis than clients who demonstrate inappropriate affect.

A marked decrease in the variation or intensity of emotional expression is called **blunted affect.** The client may express joy, sorrow, or anger, but with little intensity. In flat affect, there is a total lack of emotional expression in verbal and nonverbal behavior; the face is impassive, and voice rate and tone are regular and monotonous.

Anhedonia. As already mentioned early in the chapter, anhedonia is the inability to experience pleasure or to imagine a pleasurable emotion. This inability is very distressing to clients, who are aware of how they differ from other people. One young man lamented, "How can it be possible to feel so many awful things and never feel happy?"

ALTERED FAMILY PROCESSES

Observe the family's interaction for notable signs of dysfunction.

Family Overinvolvement and Negativity. At present there are no clear-cut clinical markers of what constitutes overinvolvement and negative emotions in families. Nurses should note families who seem excessively bonded emotionally. Family members' inability to maintain emotional, social, or physical separateness is a clear sign of this problem. Also assess a high level of criticism among family members. Discuss families that seem seriously enmeshed or hypercritical with the treatment team.

ALTERED FAMILY FUNCTIONING

Families burdened with the long-term responsibility of caring for a schizophrenic relative may suffer disruptions in their household routine, work, social interactions, and physical well-being. The household may be disrupted by the client's insistence that the family act on and accommodate delusional beliefs. The family may bend to the client's wish, fearing an increase in the client's anxiety and possible fighting or shouting if they do not comply.

CLINICAL EXAMPLE

The Walker family built an extra bathroom rather than fight with Tim, their schizophrenic son, who spends hours in the bath completing elaborate washing rituals.

The Sherman family must eat out several times each week because Suzanne, their schizophrenic daughter, refuses to allow anyone in the room when she eats.

The family social life may be disrupted. For instance, the family may fear leaving the schizophrenic member home alone or they may fear that the ill person will embarrass visitors if friends are invited in. Some families are willing to be open about the adjustments they make in living with a schizophrenic loved one, whereas others choose to live isolated lives.

Family members' work can suffer because of the emotional strain of living with an ill member. They must take time off to accompany the schizophrenic person to doctors' appointments, make hospital visits, and help during interviews with social agencies or the police. Family health may suffer because of general inattention or because of prolonged stresses within the home.

Outcome Identification: NOC

The outcome criteria established for a schizophrenic client need to be flexible and include the option to acknowledge a partial behavior change as success. For example, the outcome for Body Image Distortion may include (a) recognizes symptom regularly, (b) speaks with important other person regarding body feelings often, and (c) often manages to function despite symptomatology. Setting realistic goals and continually reevaluating expectations based on your client's current status is imperative with outcomes development. Other issues for outcomes with this population are an awareness of the client's multiple functional deficits, your personal response to working with this population, and lethality factors.

Planning and Implementation: NIC

Nursing interventions are most effective when they focus on the needs of the client to maximize his or her functioning. In order to accomplish this, you must attend to the issues that are important to the client. The client's perspective is the most valuable tool you have to create competent and meaningful treatment interventions. See Box 14–2 for the issues most important to the client with schizophrenia, from the unique perspective of the client.

When planning care for any client with a chronic illness, nurses must be careful to set realistic goals for client change. Particular care must be taken with schizophrenic clients because they are extremely sensitive to change and failure. Deterioration in all aspects of functioning is characteristic of

BOX 14–2 Issues Important to the Client with Schizophrenia

People who have schizophrenia have to deal with an illness different from any other disease. Their perspectives are vital in developing meaningful treatment and conducting interventions. Remember these issues:

- Struggles to maintain and regain personal power and efficacy
- Difficulties with interpersonal relationships
- Pressures of social expectations
- Discrepancies between what one wished for oneself and what one is now
- Connecting with people
- Personal growth
- Self efficacy
- Stability
- Coping with relapses
- Spirituality
- Differentiating core beliefs and feelings from illness

Source: Adapted from Lester, H. (2000). Patients with schizophrenia valued self-empowerment, understanding how self related to illness, and coping with relapse. *Evidence-Based Nursing, 3*, 30. Reprinted with permission from the BMJ Publishing Group.

the disease. Nurses must focus upon the most troublesome areas of client functioning and set incremental, short-term goals that pave the way for successes in achieving long-term goals. See the Nursing Self-Awareness feature to increase your effectiveness in working with a psychotic client.

PREVENTING RELAPSE

Combining maintenance antipsychotic medication therapy with psychosocial approaches has been found to be more effective than pharmacotherapy alone in delaying or preventing relapse. It has been suggested that early intervention would be effective in preventing relapse in schizophrenic clients. This could be accomplished through close clinical or family monitoring for the client's particular *prodromal symptoms* (those symptoms that occur early in the relapse process for that client). Once identified, prompt clinical intervention with antipsychotic medication may reduce the overall frequency of the relapse event.

One program for relapse prevention (Herz et al., 2000) that combines standard doses of maintenance antipsychotic medication with psychosocial treatment results in the lowest relapse rate (30%) after 2 years. Weekly group therapy for clients is an opportunity to monitor prodromal symptoms and this clinical scrutiny may prevent or minimize relapse and rehospitalization in this population. A multifamily group component is helpful to support and educate the families along with providing peer contacts and in vivo experiences.

For clients residing with their families, educational and supportive family interventions have an important effect on relapse prevention. Those clients who live more independently and experience relapses could benefit from a community treatment contact. Prevention is more effective when clients and their families understand the likely triggers for relapse, as outlined in Box 14–3.

Nursing SELF AWARENESS

Working with Clients Who Have Schizophrenia

To increase self-awareness about working with a person with active psychosis, ask yourself:

- How do I feel about approaching a person who is having hallucinations?
- How do I feel about talking to someone who has delusions that frighten him?
- Have I ever encountered someone in public who was psychotic?
- Do I fear that I might do something that might make the person's illness worse?
- What kinds of understanding and knowledge do I need to feel comfortable working with clients with psychosis?

To increase self-awareness about working with clients with disrupted ability to care for themselves, ask yourself:

- Do I react negatively when I think about someone my age who has never worked?
- What goes through my mind when I see someone who is disheveled, unclear, or oddly dressed?
- How can I find a point of connection between myself and someone whose life is so dramatically different from my own?

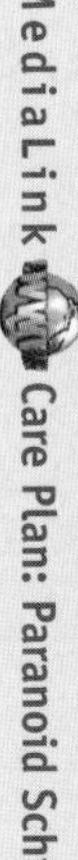

Other aspects of relapse prevention have been implemented clinically with good results. Clients with a psychosis that is not responsive to pharmacotherapy may benefit from specific modalities of cognitive–behavioral therapy (see Chapter 30), while persons with persistent negative symptoms and limited social competence may find social skills training useful. In addition, new programs of supported employment may enable some clients to maintain competitive employment (Bustillo, Lauriello, & Keith, 1999). The impacts of regularly scheduled employment and improved skills can be a helpful distracter from the onslaught of psychosis if it does not tax the client's coping abilities.

BOX 14–3 Causes of Relapse in Schizophrenia

Relapse can potentially occur as a result of any of the following:

Physiological Stressors

- Infection
- Acute illness
- Chronic illness
- Dehydration
- Insomnia
- Rape
- Pain
- Fatigue
- Side effects of medications
- Appetite changes
- Injury
- Surgery

Personal Stressors

- Exacerbation/relapse of illness
- Depression
- Negative symptoms of schizophrenia
- Spiritual distress
- Pet loss/illness/aging
- Financial difficulties
- An increase in responsibility
- A decrease in access to resources
- Recreational activity choice/access
- Maturational/developmental changes

Interpersonal Stressors

- Perceived rejection/abandonment
- Conflict, anger
- Loss of job or status within a job
- Altered contact with another or others
- Relationship changes (family, intimate relationships, friendships, etc.)
- Expressed emotion

Community Stressors

- Difficulties making living arrangements
- Roommate/family stressors
- Disruption of living situation
- Transportation
- Community disruption

PROMOTING ADEQUATE COMMUNICATION

Clients with schizophrenia try to communicate, even though their statements may be difficult to understand. Close attention to what the client is saying and honest attempts to understand the real and symbolic aspects of the message are important. The client will perceive nuances of your behavior. Therefore, one of the most direct and successful ways to demonstrate caring and respect is to attend seriously to the client.

Clients make valid observations about their environment, needs, and concerns. Some, if not all, of their observations and sensations exist in reality and are not to be treated as if they are all totally psychotic symptoms. And the sensitivity to the environment that can overwhelm someone with schizophrenia also clues him or her into aspects to which others may not have access. A client may make observations about events or situations that are beyond your awareness. For example, take seriously a client's communications about another client's drug use or suicidal threats. If a client complains of a physical symptom such as stomach distress, consider the symptom as real until there is evidence otherwise. It is easy to dismiss a client's statements, particularly those of a delusional client. Doing so, however, shows lack of respect for the client's intact capacities to see and respond to what is happening in the environment.

PROMOTING ADHERENCE WITH MEDICAL REGIMEN

Psychotropic medications play an important part in the treatment of schizophrenic disorders. Drugs that diminish focal symptoms (hallucinations and delusions) and yet produce relatively few untoward effects are now available. Complying with treatment, which for schizophrenia means medications, is a complex demand. You are going to have to be creative and ever mindful of your client's specific barriers to learning and maintaining certain behaviors. The disease itself causes difficulty in maintaining treatment adherence because of the lack of the ability to recognize the illness. This is called poor insight, but it has been compared to the unawareness or lack of insight into neurological deficits following a stroke. You must recognize that individuals respond to their illness, their circumstances, and their medications in different ways.

The idea of adherence can be expressed through a number of terms such as treatment adherence, role reliability, collaboration for health behaviors, and cooperation. Interviews and clinical contacts tell us that clients are able to participate in the treatment if they are included and made an integral part of the design of their care. See the accompanying Box 14–4 for a description of the barriers and challenges to treatment adherence.

Consistent adherence in taking medications as prescribed is not common among this client population. Researchers estimate that as few as 68% of psychiatric clients adhere to medication regimens while in the hospital. When these clients return to the community, 37% or fewer adhere to drug regimens. Clients may stop taking their medications for these reasons:

- They don't understand the administration instructions.
- They are too disorganized to follow the instructions.
- The side effects of major tranquilizers are too uncomfortable.
- They do not wish to be stigmatized as having schizophrenia and therefore reject treatment.
- They begin to feel better and believe the medication is no longer necessary.
- They don't have access to pharmacies easily because of transportation or interpersonal difficulties.

Clients who do not take medications are more vulnerable to stressors and risk more frequent relapse of symptoms than those who comply. Efforts to educate clients about their medications and to have them practice self-medication prior to discharge have increased the rate of adherence only marginally. Client attitudes toward the medications prescribed also influence their willingness to comply. You must be an active participant in assessing adherence and fostering a positive attitude toward medications. Commonly used antipsychotic medications and side effects are presented in Chapter 31.

Clients are often ambivalent about taking medications. Maintaining adequate blood levels of therapeutic medications is important for schizophrenic clients. To help them overcome ambivalence, give them time to think about taking the medications. Set a time limit. If the client fails to comply, come back later and try again. Two useful strategies are reminding clients of the positive effects of the medication and framing the action as a way for them to help themselves get better. Box 14–5, Adherence Enhancers, gives a compendium for increasing the effectiveness of your work with schizophrenic clients around treatment adherence issues.

BOX 14–4 Challenges to Adherence

- Difficulties with prescribed psychotropic medications
- Severe level of symptomatology
- Cognitive difficulties secondary to thought disorder
- Motivational problems secondary to negative symptoms
- Motivational problems secondary to flight into health (wanting to be "normal")
- Unpleasant side effects
- Persistence of positive symptoms (delusions) mitigating against adherence
- Financial issues
- Misperceptions and misunderstanding of the information presented in medication teaching
- Cursory or minimal medication teaching lacking relevance to all areas of the client's life
- Unresolved issues with treatment providers
- Cultural impacts

ASSISTING WITH GROOMING AND HYGIENE

Helping clients establish and maintain personal care habits is a complex process. If the client clearly lacks the skills, then teach the skills. If, however, the client has learned grooming skills but does not practice them, focus on ways to motivate the client. Intervention begins by establishing clear expectations about essential grooming habits. The frequency and timing of all aspects of grooming—including bathing, dressing, hair care,

MediaLink EPSE: Akinesia Video / Tardive Dyskinesia Videos

MediaLink Extrapyramidal Side Effects Video

BOX 14-5 Adherence Enhancers

- Involve client as a partner in medication-based treatment planning decisions.
- Change to another medication with a different neurotransmitter action with lower or different side effects that may be more tolerable. Atypical antipsychotic medications have a lower side effect profile and can increase adherence because they're not so hard to take.
- Teach client how to report side effects including the severity of it from dry mouth to priapism. May need role-play, assertiveness training.
- Teach client how to manage the side effects he does get—if possible, hard candy, rubber pillow case liner. It may make it tolerable to continue on the medication.
- Instruct, educate, and arrange for reminders well before discharge (especially with geriatric recipients) to maximize both knowledge and adherence (knowledge can be the number 1 factor determining adherence).
- Simplify the medication regimen.
- Match medication dosing strategy to client schedule, preferences, work situation, and recreational pursuits.
- Discuss the client's expectations of the medication—are they realistic?
- Take cultural impacts into account during comprehensive treatment planning.
- Use concrete educators—the tried and true cognition enhancers are: pamphlets, booklets, handbooks, workbooks, sheets, cards, videos, audiotapes, posters, magnets, logs, journals, etc.
- Perception of control over the treatment regimen.
- Self-administration of medications.
- Help the client take action to prevent untoward effects, such as maintaining fluid intake to avoid postural hypotension.
- Coping efforts involving planning for problem solving which increases adherence.
- Peer support is important. Hearing from *peers* how this new medication could help with symptoms, and asking the prescriber to consider it, improves adherence.
- Give hope—it pays to be well. It takes all the small steps to recovery in addition to medications to get better.
- Repetition—say the same thing over and over, with patience, especially with diagnostic groups of schizophrenia and depression.
- Develop reminders, cues to remembering (visual cues—when I see this I need to take my pills, when I eat lunch I take my pills, rubber band on wrist, calendars, to do lists; auditory cues—alarm clocks or watches).
- Depot medications given weekly, biweekly, or monthly can contribute to adherence by not having to remember to take pills. The marketing of an atypical antipsychotic in depot form (risperidone) adds to our choices.
- Pill boxes—come in many shapes, sizes, and organizational styles (multiple daily dose marked, layers for time of day, Braille markings, timers with small alarm clock feature that opens compartment). If the medication can't be taken out of its original container without an effect on potency, place small button or candy in pillbox to act as a reminder.
- Keep all medications and information about them in one dry, cool place. Plastic products such as containers and bags—*not* in bathroom or by a dishwasher in the kitchen.
- Involve the family.
- Match the degree of client autonomy in treatment to the needs of the individual client.
- Financial assistance might be available.
- Have client teach about their medications (after they have learned sufficiently) to other recipients or to significant others—nothing speeds learning as much as teaching others.

oral hygiene, and room care—can be specified in writing if that would be a useful learning device for your client.

Formal training programs for helping chronically mentally ill clients improve their grooming skills can be applied in inpatient settings. These programs are well developed and tested. They systematically help clients in all steps of personal grooming, including collecting grooming supplies, moving to the grooming area (a bathroom or bedroom with sink and mirror), completing each grooming step, completing appropriate dressing, and storing grooming materials. Nursing interventions at each step can progress from simple verbal coaching, to modeling, to gentle physical guidance. Acknowledge client efforts during each phase with realistic encouragement and praise. The success of these programs probably depends on daily staff attention to the client's training, along with consistent, meaningful rewards. Avoid power struggles regarding the completion of tasks. If initial prompts don't work, leave the client alone for a short period.

PROMOTING ORGANIZED BEHAVIOR

Clients whose behavior is disorganized require direction and limits to make their actions more effective and goal-directed. In working with a disorganized client, proceed slowly and remain calm. The client's perception of the environment may be distorted, but your calmness can help calm the client. Try to direct the client in simple, safe activities. Nursing goals and interventions for a disorganized client must focus on manageable steps. A case example of one such intervention follows.

CLINICAL EXAMPLE

George is moving quickly yet aimlessly from the refrigerator to the cupboard. He pulls a box of cereal from the cupboard, opens it, and then wanders away. Next he goes to the refrigerator, opens the door, peers in, and closes the door. Rummaging through all his pockets, he locates a comb, combs through his hair, sets the comb on the counter, and wanders back to the cupboard. This effortful yet unproductive behavior continues for several minutes when the nurse enters.

Nurse: *George, are you trying to get yourself some cereal?*

George: *Sort of. I was going to . . . brush . . . no . . . comb... no eat something. Yeah, I wanted something to eat.*

Nurse: *Try to concentrate on one thing. First, put the comb back in your pocket. (He does so.) Now, come over here and get the cereal box. Here's a bowl. Here's a spoon. (She*

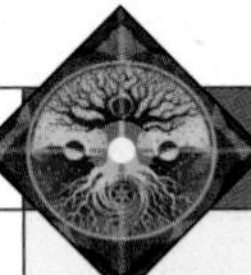

Case Study

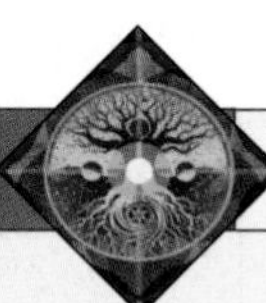

Client with Schizophrenia

Identifying Information

Jack May is a 24-year-old single male who lives with his mother and supports himself with SSI. He is brought to the psychiatric emergency service by his mother. He currently attends a structured work program 5 days a week, but stopped attending 8 days ago.

Jack says that he does not need to be hospitalized, but that his mother is the one with the problem. He wants to be left alone to work on his computer projects. He admits that he has been hearing multiple voices in his head for the past week. For the past 2 weeks, Jack has been increasingly isolated working on his personal computer in his room. While he will not tell anyone what the work is about, his mother has seen printouts that suggest it is a plan to soundproof and secure his room. Jack stopped attending his work program a week ago, saying that he had "more important work" to do at home. He refuses to eat or talk with his mother. His mother believes he stopped taking his medications. An identifiable stressor is that 2 weeks ago his father announced plans to remarry in the near future.

History

Two years ago, Jack had a serious psychosis precipitated by his move to a college out of state. He was diagnosed with schizophrenia, paranoid type. He was hospitalized for 2 weeks, stabilized on Haldol, and discharged home. Persecutory delusions, which shift with news events are always present at a low level. He has lived with his mother since diagnosis, attending day treatment and, for the last 8 months, a structured work program. He occasionally attends client support network meetings. His work attendance has been sporadic, and he has been on and off probation for nonattendance in this structured work environment. He receives medications and follow-up treatment at the community mental health center.

History

The Mays are both living and well. They were separated 3 years ago and divorced 2 years ago. Jack's father is an attorney, and Jack sees him approximately once a month. Their relationship is pleasant but not close. His mother runs her own crafts store and is agreeable to having Jack live with her. There are no other children.

History

Jack has completed high school and a few courses at the local community college. He was an above-average student and was always involved in school and extracurricular activities, until about 9 months before his first psychotic episode. Since that time, he has socialized primarily with his mother and rarely with a few acquaintances from the client support group. He smokes a pack of cigarettes a day and drinks beer occasionally. He denies any illicit drug use. Jack has a keen interest in computers. He took extensive coursework in computers in school and has collected considerable equipment and software, primarily gifts from his father. Other pastimes are listening to rock music and watching television.

History

No notable medical problems.

Current Mental Status

Jack is a healthy-looking 24-year-old who is anxious, somewhat guarded, but cooperative in the interview. He is oriented to person, time, and place, and demonstrates good memory and recall. Judgment is impaired. His affect is anxious. Speech is rapid, pressured, tangential. He is hyperalert to his environment and is notably startled by a siren outside. Persecutory delusions about people trying to take over his home and work are present, and he has hallucinations of unrecognizable voices and the voice of his father. No command hallucinations. Some loosening of associations present. Abstractions are concrete and self-referential. Insight poor; believes that his mother is "sick" and that she should not impede him in his important projects.

Other Subjective or Objective Clinical Data

Evidence that Jack may have stopped taking medications approximately 2 weeks ago. Suicide/violence potential minimal.

hands him the utensils.) Why don't you sit right here? (She seats him so that he has his back to the rest of the activity in the room.) Can you sit still for a bit?

George: *I think so.*

Nurse: *Pour yourself some cereal. I'll get the milk for you. (She does so.)*

George begins to eat his cereal quietly. The nurse stays with him for a few minutes and directs him to continue eating when he becomes distracted by others who come into the room.

PROMOTING SOCIAL INTERACTION AND ACTIVITY

The client's efforts to withdraw from social contact stem from past relationship failures and fear of rejection. Clients often find their internal world less risky and therefore more attractive than a world that requires interpersonal relating. When making efforts to help the client become less withdrawn, respect the client's sometimes overwhelming anxiety about human contact.

After establishing a basic level of trust, encourage the client to try out new behaviors within the relationship. The goal is to have the client experience success; therefore, encourage even small increments of change. If, for example, the client has difficulty initiating conversation, encourage the client to practice this skill once a day. Similarly, if the client avoids any activity in the environment because of fear of relating to groups, structure an activity involving the client, yourself, and one other client. Reinforce the client when he or she approaches you to communicate, even if that communication contains problematic patterns (see the Rx Communication feature on page 328).

PROMOTING SOCIAL SKILLS AND ACTIVITIES

Address social skills that are essential to functioning in the environment; introducing oneself, starting a conversation, ending a conversation, saying no, asking for assistance, and listening.

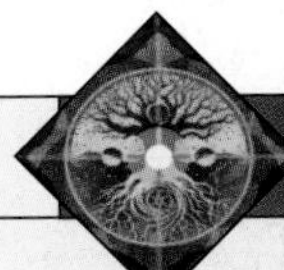

Nursing Care Plan

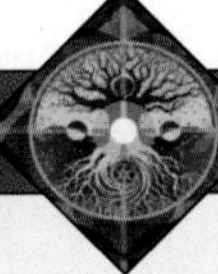

Nursing Diagnosis: Altered Thought Processes

Expected Outcome: Client will demonstrate the ability to cope competently with delusions.

Short-Term Goals	*Interventions*	*Rationale*
Client able to function in a variety of settings without intrusive delusional thought content.	• Make frequent, supportive, and brief contacts. • Allow description of delusional thoughts and acknowledge emotional impact of same. • Focus discussions on the client's feeling level concerning the delusions, and not the content. • Teach client how to cope with delusional thinking through engagement in activities for distraction, active self-talk promoting his efforts, support from others, treatment. • Reinforce adaptive efforts.	Some contacts can be overwhelming for a client with schizophrenia and need to be of a manageable length. The client must be taught how to cope with the symptoms of the illness in an effective manner.

Nursing Diagnosis: Anxiety related to delusions

Expected Outcome: Client will demonstrate decreased anxiety.

Short-Term Goals	*Interventions*	*Rationale*
Client able to describe a reduction in his anxiety. Client participates in his treatment.	• Make frequent, supportive, and brief contacts. • Reassure client verbally, with a structured routine, and by giving explanations congruent with client's abilities to understand. • Acknowledge anxiety. • Prompt client to interact with others when able to reduce feelings of isolation and alienation. • Provide an array of coping skills client may use when anxious.	Some contacts can be overwhelming for a client with schizophrenia and need to be of a manageable length. People with schizophrenia often do not have their feelings acknowledged. This validates the feeling. You must supply a variety of coping skills to choose from to suit various situations.

Staff members can model these skills and help clients role-play each skill. Focus discussion on situations in which clients might need the skill. If they see its applicability to dilemmas in their personal lives, they will be motivated to learn the skill. Praise and, if available, material rewards can also motivate clients. Social skills training can also be done in small groups (see Chapter 29).

Schizophrenia can disturb a person's will and capacity to accomplish meaningful activity. Clients with distorted perceptions and thinking expend considerable energy merely taking in and interpreting their immediate worlds. In addition, major tranquilizers, which control the positive symptoms of the disease, can further inhibit a client's active involvement and interest in activities. You must be aware of how much work it takes to cope with schizophrenic symptoms. Do not assume that periods of quiet or inactivity are due to laziness or lack of interest. Rather, assess each individual's need for quiet periods in which to organize perceptions and thoughts.

At the same time, clients with schizophrenia live in a culture in which action and accomplishment are highly prized and rewarded. They are not immune to the pressure for personal productivity as a measure of personal worth. For this reason, they feel better about themselves when they are involved in meaningful activities. Your task is to help clients find activities that are intrinsically rewarding or that bring some social or tangible reward, yet are within their capacities.

Learning clients' personal interests is a first step. Providing opportunities for the client to actively engage in an activity of

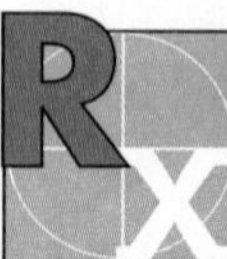

COMMUNICATION

Client with Clang Associations

CLIENT: "The dining room lining trying to eat forever."

NURSE RESPONSE 1: "Jack, are you having a problem getting your food?"

RATIONALE: Direct question allows the client with clang associations to answer with a "yes" or "no" response, models how the communication can be stated, and labels the situation as a problem.

NURSE RESPONSE 2: "Come with me and let's get you set up."

RATIONALE: This response reinforces the appropriateness of the client's coming to the nurse with a problem and concretely shows the client how to resolve the problem.

interest (by providing records, books, craft materials, or access to newspapers and television) is the next intervention. In addition, activities within the therapeutic milieu, such as attending groups and completing unit "jobs," can provide the external rewards of praise from staff and peers. These activities give clients confidence and develop and promote their work habits. Success in these activities can lead to success in volunteer or paid work in the community after discharge.

PROMOTING REALITY-BASED PERCEPTIONS

Delusions or hallucinations often frighten clients. Nurses can intervene by:

- Reassuring clients of their safety.
- Protecting them from physical harm as they respond to their altered perceptions.
- Validating reality.
- Helping clients distinguish reality from the hallucinatory experience.

Hallucinations are especially frightening if the client has never experienced them before or if their content is threatening or angry. Attempt to alleviate this anxiety by describing your perception of the frightened behavior and asking clients to discuss what they are experiencing. Make simple reassuring remarks, like "I hear what you're telling me. This sounds very frightening. No one means to harm you." See the Intervention box at right for intervention strategies that help a client manage hallucinations.

Protect clients from harm and reassure them about safety. A client may take impulsive action to escape the frightening experience or to obey voices in the hallucination. Prevent this by:

- Closely observing client behavior during active hallucinations.
- Use calming techniques and one–to–one interactions to shape and guide the situation.
- Reduce excess noise and distractions. One person speaks to the client at a time.
- Intervening quickly by giving additional doses of psychotropic medications or placing the client in a quiet room.
- If necessary, securing the unit so that the client cannot leave and take self-destructive or impulsive action.

Make every effort to help the client attend to real rather than internal stimuli, orient the client to the real situation, and encourage the client to focus on you rather than on the hallucination. "George, listen to me rather than to the sounds you hear. Remember, you are in the hospital and I am your nurse. I will help you find your shoes. Come with me." Active involvement in some activity, such as finding shoes, will help the client maintain a focus on real events and perceptions.

INTERVENING WITH DELUSIONS

General guidelines for working with delusional individuals are not to argue with their false beliefs, to focus on the reality-based aspects of their communications, and to protect them from acting on their delusions in a way that might harm themselves or others. See the Intervention box on page 329 for suggested nursing interventions that contain or manage psychotic symptoms such as delusions.

PROMOTING CONGRUENT EMOTIONAL RESPONSES

Working with clients who display blunted or flat affect can be confusing for nurses who are accustomed to reading emotional responses that fall within a more normal range. Be aware that these clients have feelings about events around them, including their interaction with you and other staff members, yet may have difficulty expressing those feelings.

Note any lack of congruence between the person's affect and the content of the message. If your relationship with the client is

INTERVENTION

Helping a Client Manage Hallucinations

- Determine the kind of hallucinations (auditory, visual, etc.).
- Is the symptom able to be managed with current coping?
- Access resources (advocacy groups, peers, staff, literature) for fresh ideas, better management techniques.
- Discuss options and success rate with professionals.
- Select options for coping with the stimuli:
  Distraction
  Resisting
  Calming
  Treatment (such as medication)
- Practice using an option to cope
- Use a technique based on the success you have with it.
- Be ready to replace coping styles when they don't work anymore.

INTERVENTION

Helping a Client Manage Delusions

- Determine if the client can tell the difference between the delusion ("I don't drink the water because it's poisoned.") and a personal preference ("I'm not drinking water because I prefer orange juice.").
- Work with advocacy groups, peers, and professional staff to clearly demarcate what constitutes delusional thinking.
- Suggest options to cope with delusional thoughts:
  Support from others
  Concrete tasks
  Caretaking activities
  Refocusing thoughts
  Determined efforts to steer thinking in another direction
- Make sure client understands how important it is to be surrounded with people who reinforce the client's efforts.
- Encourage clients to self-validate the struggle they are in and any level of effectiveness they achieve at coping.

well established, you might comment on the incongruity and explore it with the client. ("Malcolm, what you are telling me is sad but you are laughing. What shall I pay attention to?") Modeling clear, congruent communication is helpful. Little can be done to change the client's anhedonia, yet empathic listening might comfort the client.

Ambivalence, the simultaneous experience of contradictory feelings about a person, object, or action, can trouble schizophrenic clients. Ambivalence can even become great enough to immobilize a client. Such clients cannot express one emotion or the other, or choose one action over the other. You may be able to partially alleviate the client's unease by identifying aloud the emotions the client may be experiencing. ("Lily, I think you might be feeling both very happy to see your father and at the same time very angry.") Naming the conflicting emotions gives the client the opportunity to talk about them, although many times he or she may not be able to do so.

Immobility due to ambivalence is extremely uncomfortable. One way of intervening is to limit the number of choices the indecisive client has to make. For example, a man may be immobilized by his inability to decide whether to go out alone for the first time. You can help by telling him that it seems too soon for him to go out alone and that, for today, he must be accompanied. Another example is a young woman who is undecided about where to sit. You can remove extra chairs at the table in the dining room so that she has only one choice.

PROMOTING FAMILY UNDERSTANDING AND INVOLVEMENT

When a schizophrenic client is hospitalized, encourage the family and help them remain involved in the client's care. Except for unusual circumstances, share information on the client's status, treatment program, and future treatment plans, including discharge plans. Nurses may need to be active advocates for families' rights to information about, and involvement in, the care of the schizophrenic member. Of course, nurses need to comply with the client's wishes and with the laws governing disclosure of information, which vary by state and by institution.

Referral to Psychoeducation Programs. If assessment suggests that the family needs information about the disease and treatment, refer the family to education programs, if they are available. Family psychoeducation programs are preferable to direct teaching because they often combine education with mutual support. In such groups, families can meet others who share their life difficulties. These peers can provide informal support and information to help the family deal with the tasks that lie ahead. Nurses can reinforce the formal teaching that occurs in such programs when they meet with individual families. See the Client/Family Teaching feature on page 330.

Referral to NAMI. Without exception, families should know about a national family support group with many local and state affiliates. The National Alliance for the Mentally Ill (NAMI) serves families through educational programs, local support groups, and political activism. Most local organizations are listed in telephone directories or can be reached through the local community mental health agency responsible for information and referral. For a resource link to NAMI, go to the Companion Website for this book.

MediaLink National Alliance for the Mentally Ill

CLINICAL EXAMPLE

The Oddstads were worried about their daughter's failing grades at college for the last semester and were surprised to learn that she ended a relationship with her boyfriend. When she came home for spring break, she seemed disinterested and noncommunicative and wouldn't eat or socialize with the family. Her parents found her burning incense and chanting to herself in the mirror at 3:00 A.M. In a panic, they took her to the local emergency room. After a complete workup, they were shocked to learn that the probable diagnosis was schizophrenia. Furthermore, the physician wanted their daughter to start on medication.

The rapidity of the decline in their daughter's functioning, and the fact that she had hidden many of her symptoms from them, left the Oddstads feeling guilty, sad, and disbelieving. They could not fathom how this had happened to their beautiful daughter. A nurse at the emergency room had given them the number of a local NAMI support group and hotline. In their anguish, they called and were able to speak with other parents, who helped them begin to deal with their emotions and directed them to helpful books that explained schizophrenia and its treatment.

MediaLink Case Study: Schizophrenia with Auditory Hallucinations

The NAMI education program is discussed in detail in Chapter 29.

CLIENT / FAMILY TEACHING

Supporting Families of Clients with Schizophrenia

To assist families, you need to evaluate the family's current responses to living with and caring for a family member with schizophrenia. The following suggestions apply to the time period shortly after the disorder has been diagnosed.

Suggestions	Rationale
Discuss the basic nature of the disorder: Schizophrenia is a disease of the brain, like any other biologic disease.	Families misunderstand mental illness to be a personal failing and are comforted by the fact that it has a biologic basis.
Help families identify their responses to the early ambiguous signs of the illness and notice how their responses have changed now that the diagnosis has been made.	Families often misinterpret early signs of the disorder to be acting-out or developmentally appropriate behavior. On learning that these signs are part of the illness, they feel guilty for not seeking help sooner.
Reinforce families for supporting the ill member in seeking treatment.	Stigma about mental illness persists, and families need support for taking action and engaging with treatment systems.
Refer families to structured educational or psychoeducational programs in which they can learn about the disease and its treatment, as well as receive support.	Schizophrenia is extremely complex, and its treatment is multifaceted. Families can benefit by structured classes. Programs that offer support to families in addition to education have proven efficacy in improving the illness course for the ill member.
Inform families about how to reach the local National Alliance for the Mentally Ill. Hand out fliers that provide telephone numbers and people to contact.	NAMI is a nationwide family support organization that provides peer support, education, and advocacy for the seriously mentally ill and their families.

Provide families with access to information such as:

- Mueser, K. T., & Gingerich, S. (1994). *Schizophrenia: A guide for families*. New York: Harbinger.
- Torrey, E. F. (1995). *Surviving schizophrenia: A manual for families, consumers, and providers* (3rd ed.). New York: Harper Collins.

MediaLink National Library of Medicine

PROMOTING COMMUNITY CONTACTS

An awareness of a client's community supports and potential treatment programs can guide nurses in preparing clients for discharge. For example, the client's most important peer support group might be the clientele at a local day treatment program or social club. If so, several visits prior to discharge will help the client make the transition back to the community.

Preparing clients for the residence they will enter after hospital discharge is a central nursing task. Often, placement depends on how the client functions in the hospital. If the client is able to manage medications, participate in a variety of groups, and live cooperatively with other clients, then placement in a residential care facility that supports independent functioning is appropriate. In contrast, clients who need assistance with structuring free time, resist taking medications, or cannot be responsible for self-care require a more structured and supervised environment.

Nurses work with clients to help them achieve their highest level of functioning. They document clients' abilities to perform various tasks and make recommendations to the treatment team about appropriate placements.

Evaluation

To complete the nursing process, nurses evaluate changes in client status and behavior in response to nursing interventions. Evaluation criteria are linked to nursing goals and reflect an understanding of the limitations of schizophrenic clients. However, you must keep the concept of recovery in mind as every client can improve and recover to a certain extent. The National Library of Medicine MEDLINEplus Web site at www.nimh.nih.gov/publicat/schizmenu.cfm offers search options on schizophrenia and other topics.

COMMUNICATION

Clients will, with greater regularity, express their thoughts clearly and congruently. They will feel sufficient trust to talk to the nurse about troublesome symptoms or experiences. Because clients will probably continue to experience some symptoms even after medications have taken effect, this trust allows the client to express what has changed and what is still troublesome.

SELF-CARE

Clients will consistently appear clean and well groomed and will independently manage personal grooming and hygiene. Clients will have clean and reasonably appropriate clothes, in terms of both fashion and season. Individual styles of dress, which are the client's way of expressing or presenting the self, will be supported by nurses. The means for maintaining self-care after discharge from acute care are identified.

ACTIVITY INTOLERANCE

Clients will participate in goal-directed activities with minimal intervention. Clients will complete the activities they begin. Clients will demonstrate a broader range of interest and activities than they did on admission.

SOCIAL ISOLATION

Clients will demonstrate the capacity to interact, for at least brief periods, with nursing staff, with other clients, and in small groups. They will consistently demonstrate socially required interactions, such as greeting and starting a conversation with a stranger, asking for assistance, saying no, and listening to another's conversation. Clients will be inactive for shorter periods and spend more time engaged in interesting or meaningful activity. They will demonstrate the capacity to function outside the protective environment of acute or sheltered care.

SENSORY/PERCEPTUAL ALTERATIONS

Clients will have fewer episodes of attending to internal stimuli. If hallucinations persist, clients will begin to identify stressors or situations that precipitate them. Clients will identify and practice personal coping strategies that decrease the hallucination or its effects, such as going to a quiet room, engaging in social activities, and performing activities that demand concentration.

THOUGHT PROCESSES

Clients will engage in reality-based discussions. If delusions persist, clients will not act on delusions in ways that are harmful or detrimental to themselves or others. They will also identify significant others in their current living environment who can help them limit their hallucinations via distraction or social contact.

EMOTIONAL RESPONSES

Clients will have increased awareness that their emotional expressions at times do not match their verbal communications. They will monitor others' responses to them to learn cues about how they are varying their emotional expressions. Clients will experience fewer episodes of extreme discomfort due to ambivalence about people, events, or actions.

FAMILY FUNCTIONING

Families will be involved in all aspects of client care, including assessment, planning interventions, inpatient treatment choices, and planning for discharge. Family understanding of the illness trajectory and client capacities and limits will improve. Family difficulties with caring for clients will be considered in treatment and discharge planning, and adequate resources will be identified to support family needs. Families will report that their questions about the schizophrenic disease process, and about varying modes of treatment for the disorder, have been answered.

Case Management

Knowledge of the impact schizophrenia has on the way an individual thinks and functions is the underpinning of a competent case management program. In order to carry out any particular task, an individual with this illness must have specific tasks coupled with realistic expectations. The case management strategies that work best with schizophrenia and other psychotic disorders include:

1. Tasks broken into manageable steps.
2. Concrete actions.
3. Structured environment.
4. Routines and schedules.
5. Dependable professionals.
6. Flexibility to accommodate the shifts of the illness.

Intensive Case Management (ICM) assists people with schizophrenia in outpatient settings. While your caseload is smaller, you have greater involvement with clients who require more supervision and care. You would orchestrate appointments and daily functioning issues to enhance the client's abilities to remain in the community and to foster a more independent lifestyle. Whether your assignment involves case management or intensive case management, the difficulties with thought processing and communication mentioned earlier in the chapter will shape your management of the case.

Community-Based Care

People who have schizophrenia can have repetitive inpatient hospitalizations. The transition from inpatient back to the community setting must begin prior to the client's discharge from the inpatient setting, forming a bridge from inpatient to outpatient care (see Chapter 11).

There are a number of services necessary and available in the community to maximize both quality of life and more independent functioning for someone with schizophrenia and other psychotic disorders. Examples are:

1. Continuing day treatment programs.
2. Independent living centers.
3. Day hospitals.
4. Community mental health centers.
5. Social clubs.
6. Wellness centers.

These various settings are described in Chapter 11.

Counseling, psychotherapy, medication management, and other treatments are included in care delivered in the community. In addition, recreation must be remembered as a quality of life issue. Community-based care can be instrumental in providing the guidance needed for clients to integrate into community living with an illness that can be debilitating and difficult.

Home Care

You may play different roles in delivering clinical services and care to clients with schizophrenia in a home setting. For example, you may function as a case manager and make home visits. This can be particularly important for clients with schizophrenia who often have great difficulty successfully meeting daily responsibilities and maintaining independence in a healthy home environment.

An important function of the nurse, whether or not you are a case manager, is to assist clients who have schizophrenia with medication adherence. Clients with schizophrenia are at high risk for relapse because they may stop taking their antipsychotic medications. This can happen because of side effects (those reported and not reported to the prescriber), confusion about medication administration schedules, environmental factors that do not encourage adherence to a medication regimen, or any number of other factors. You can play an important role in reducing the likelihood of relapse during home care visits. The home is the environment in which most of the doses of their medications are taken and will shape adherence practices.

Home interventions by nurses, however, are not limited to case management or medication adherence issues. Some people with schizophrenia can benefit from supportive psychotherapeutic interventions delivered by you in the client's home. This can help generalize what treatment teaches them beyond the confines of the nurse's office or the clinic. When people who have schizophrenia live with significant others, it is sometimes possible for you to deliver psychoeducational interventions for everyone living as a unit. This allows the significant others and the client the opportunity to increase their skills in living together and coping with this serious illness in a way that lowers the probability of client relapse.

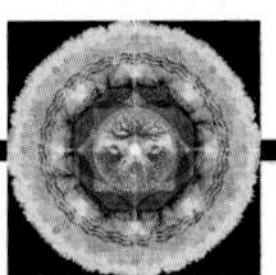

EXPLORE MediaLink

NCLEX review, case studies, and other interactive resources for this chapter can be found on the Companion Website at http://www.prenhall.com/kneisl. Click on Chapter 14 to select the activities for this chapter.

For animations, video tutorials, more NCLEX review questions, and an audio glossary, access the accompanying CD-ROM in this textbook.

BIBLIOGRAPHY

Angermeyer, M. C., Loffler, W., Muller, P., Schulze, B., & Priebe, S. (2001). Patients' and relatives' assessment of clozapine treatment. *Psychological Medicine, 31,* 509–517.

American Psychiatric Association (2000). *Diagnostic and statistical manual of mental disorders* (4th ed., Text Revision). Washington, DC: Author.

Birchwood, M., Meaden, A., Trower, P., Gilbert, P., & Plaistow, J. (2000). The power and omnipotence of voices: Subordination and entrapment by voices and significant others. *Psychological Medicine, 30,* 337–344.

Bustillo, J. R., Lauriello, J., & Keith, S. J. (1999). Schizophrenia: Improving outcome. *Harvard Review of Psychiatry, 6,* 229–240.

Coid, J., Kahtan, N., Gault, S., & Jarman, B. (2000). Ethnic differences in admissions to secure forensic psychiatry services. *British Journal of Psychiatry, 177,* 241–247.

Cooper, B. (2001). Nature, nurture, and mental disorder: Old concepts in the new millennium. *The British Journal of Psychiatry, 178, Supplement 40,* s91–s102.

Cowan, W. M., & Kandel, E. R. (2001). Prospects for neurology and psychiatry. *Journal of the American Medical Association, 285,* 594–600.

Egan, M. F., Goldberg, T. E., Gscheidle, T., Weirich, M., Bigelow, L. B., & Weinberger, D. R. (2000). Relative risk of attention deficits in siblings of patients with schizophrenia. *American Journal of Psychiatry, 157,* 1309–1316.

Fan, A. P., & Eaton, W. W. (2001). Longitudinal study assessing the joint effects of socio-economic status and birth risks on adult emotional and nervous conditions. *British Journal of Psychiatry, 178, Supplement 40,* s78–s83.

Fenton, W. S. (2001). Comorbid conditions in schizophrenia. *Current Opinion in Psychiatry, 14,* 17–23.

Goldstein, G., & Shemansky, W. J. (2000). Length and number of hospitalizations in two cohorts of veterans with chronic schizophrenia. *Psychiatric Services, 51,* 245–247.

Herz, M. I., Lamberti, J. S., Mintz, J., Scott, R., O'Dell, S. P., McCartan, L., & Nix, G. (2000). A program for relapse prevention in schizophrenia: A controlled study. *Archives of General Psychiatry, 57,* 277–283.

Jones, A. (2001). Hospital care pathways for patients with schizophrenia. *Journal of Clinical Nursing, 10,* 58–69.

Lester, H. (2000). Patients with schizophrenia valued self-empowerment, understanding how self related to illness, and coping with relapse. *Evidence-Based Nursing, 3,* 30.

Lewine, R. R. J., & Caudle, J. M. (2000). Racial effects on neuropsychological functioning in schizophrenia. *American Journal of Psychiatry, 157,* 2038–2040.

Malhotra, A. K. (2001). The genetics of schizophrenia. *Current Opinion in Psychiatry, 14,* 3–7.

Mathalon, D. H., Sullivan, E. V., Lim, K. O., & Pfefferbaum, A. (2001). Progressive brain volume changes and the clinical course of schizophrenia in men: A longitudinal magnetic resonance imaging study. *Archives of General Psychiatry, 58,* 148–157.

McKenna, P. J. (2001). Cognitive therapy in schizophrenia. *British Journal of Psychiatry, 178,* 379–380.

Mercier-Guidez, E., & Loas G. (2000). Polydipsia and water intoxication in 353 psychiatric inpatients: An epidemiological and psychopathological study. *Journal of the Association of European Psychiatrists, 15,* 306–311.

Mojtabai, R., Varma, V. K., Malhotra, S., Mattoo, S. K., Misra, A. K., Wig, N. N., & Susser, E. (2001). Mortality and long-term course in schizophrenia with a poor 2-year course: A study in a developing country. *British Journal of Psychiatry, 178,* 71–75.

Myin-Germeys, I., Nicolson, N. A., & Delespaul, P. A. E. G. (2001). The context of delusional experiences in the daily life of patients with schizophrenia. *Psychological Medicine, 31,* 489–498.

Sayer, J., Ritter, S., & Gournay, K. (2000). Beliefs about voices and their effects on coping strategies. *Journal of Advanced Nursing, 31,* 1199–1205.

Schultz, S. K. & Andreasen, N. C. (1999). Schizophrenia. *Lancet, 353,* 1425–1430.

Terry, L., & Cedar, S. H. (2001). An overview of education and "new genetics." *Nursing Standard, 15,* 38–40.

Tsuang, M. T., Stone, W. S., & Faraone, S. V. (2001). Genes, environment, and schizophrenia. *British Journal of Psychiatry, 178, Supplement 40,* s18–s24.

Vickers, A., & Zollman, C. (1999). Unconventional approaches to nutritional medicine. *British Medical Journal, 319,* 1419–1422.

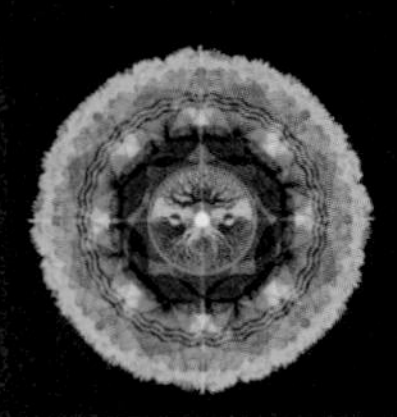

15

Chapter FIFTEEN

Mood Disorders

KAY K. CHITTY

KEY TERMS

affect
anhedonia
bipolar disorders
circadian rhythms
cyclothymic disorder
dysthymic disorder
electroconvulsive therapy (ECT)
flight of ideas
grand mal seizure
grandiosity
hypersomnia
hypomania
insomnia
major depressive disorder
major depressive episode
mania
monoamine oxidase inhibitors (MAOIs)
postpartum mood episode
psychomotor retardation
seasonal affective disorder (SAD)
selective serotonin reuptake inhibitors (SSRIs)
tricyclic antidepressants (TCAs)
vegetative symptoms

FOCUS QUESTIONS

- **What are the similarities and differences between major depressive disorder and bipolar disorder?**
- **Which elements of the biopsychosocial theories discussed here contribute most to understanding mood disorders?**
- **How would you conduct a nursing assessment of a client with a mood disorder?**
- **How would you describe your role in the appropriate nursing and biopsychologic therapies for clients with mood disorders?**
- **What are the nursing challenges that you associate with caring for clients with mood disorders?**

MediaLink 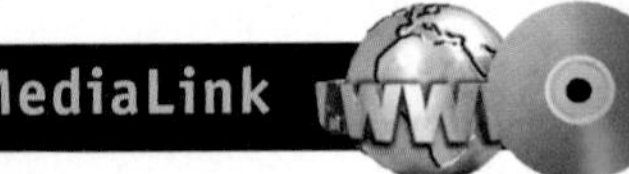 www.prenhall.com/kneisl

Additional resources for this chapter can be found on the Student CD-ROM accompanying this textbook, and on the Companion Website at www.prenhall.com/kneisl. Click on Chapter 15 to select the activities for this chapter.

CD-ROM
- Audio Glossary
- NCLEX Review

Companion Website
- Additional NCLEX Review
- Care Plan: Bipolar Disorder
- Case Study: Psychoeducation for Depression
- Learning from Clients: Depression Video
- Learning from Clients: Bipolar Disorder Video

CHAPTER OUTLINE

CROSS REFERENCES

Other topics related to this chapter are: Cognitive therapies for depression, Chapter 30; Cultural expressions of depression, Chapter 6; Insomnia and hypersomnia, Chapter 19; Medications in the treatment of depression and mania, Chapter 31; Psychobiology, Chapter 4; St. John's wort and other complementary and alternative therapies in the treatment of depression, Chapter 32; Suicide assessment, precautions, and intervention, Chapter 22.

CRITICAL THINKING CHALLENGE

Consuela R. is a severely manic 38-year-old woman who has not responded to psychopharmacologic interventions. The treatment team on her inpatient psychiatric unit has recommended electroconvulsive therapy (ECT) to Consuela and her family. Consuela is quite fearful of this procedure and believes that it will enable others to control her mind. She is adamantly opposed to it. What are the rights of severely ill psychiatric clients in determining their own treatment? Do they differ from other clients with physiologic disorders who now enjoy almost complete self-determination if they choose to exercise it? At what point does a client's right to autonomy and self-determination end? How might a treatment facility's philosophy on this issue be implemented to ensure consistency of care? ■

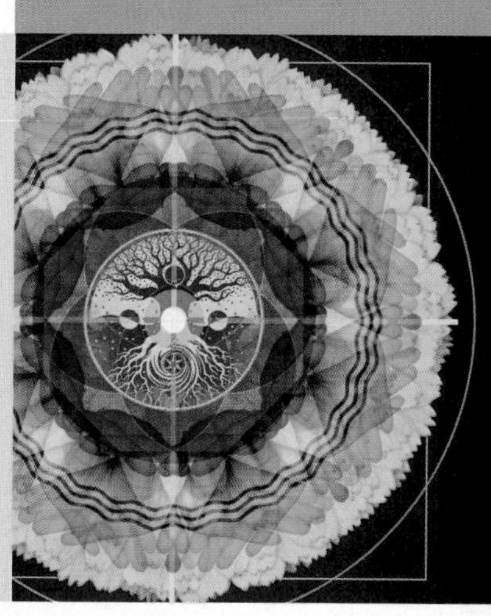

Approximately 7% of Americans suffer from mood disorders in any given year. Mood disorders are a group of psychiatric diagnoses characterized by disturbances in physical, emotional, and behavioral response patterns. These patterns of **affect** (mood) range from extreme elation and agitation to extreme depression with a serious potential for suicide. They are the most common of all mental disorders, largely due to the prevalence of depression. Other mood disorders that occur far less frequently than depression but can be severely incapacitating include dysthymic disorder and the bipolar disorders.

The symptoms of mood disorders—poor memory and concentration, fatigue, apathy, indecisiveness, and loss of self-confidence in depressed clients and grandiosity and unrealistic overconfidence in those with mania—all reduce the capacity to work and maintain the activities of daily living. Some mental health authorities believe that major depression is more disabling than many medical disorders, such as chronic lung disease, arthritis, and diabetes. It is the leading cause of lost workdays and diminished productivity on the job.

Many people with mood disorders are never seen in psychiatric settings. Because health care policy makers often consider insurance coverage for mental disorders to be a luxury, nearly two-thirds of depressed people in this country go undiagnosed and untreated. In addition, the symptoms of depression are often masked by physical complaints for which the client seeks help from primary health care providers, such as family physicians, who do not refer them for specialized treatment. As a nurse and a citizen, you will be in an excellent position to identify early signs of mood disorders and initiate treatment or action leading to early treatment.

Major Depressive Episode/Disorder

MediaLink Learning from Clients: Depression Video

A **major depressive episode** is characterized by either: (1) depressed mood not warranted by real circumstances in the individual's life that differs from the normal sadness and grief resulting from a personal loss or tragedy, or (2) loss of interest or pleasure in activities that were previously considered pleasurable—hobbies, social activities, sports, sex; along with four or more of the Diagnostic and Statistical Manual of Mental Disorders, 4th edition (Text Revision) (DSM-IV-TR) criteria listed in the DSM-IV-TR box on pages 337–338, during the same 2-week period (American Psychiatric Association [APA], 2000). **Major depressive disorder** may consist of a single episode or may recur as recurrent major depression at various points in life. The criteria for single episode and recurrent major depression are also listed in the DSM-IV-TR box on pages 337–338. Key facts about major depression are in Box 15–1.

Individuals with a history of a manic or hypomanic episode (discussed later in this chapter) are considered to have a bipolar disorder and are not classified under these categories.

Clients do not always describe their mood as "depressed." Instead, they may say that they are sad, discouraged, "down in the dumps," or feel helpless. Or they may complain of having no feelings or feeling "blah." In other cases, vague somatic complaints such as aches and pains are reported, while others report increased anger, frustration, and irritability, with uncharacteristic outbursts over minor matters.

When a person experiences a major depressive disorder, activities that previously gave pleasure, such as socializing, hobbies, sports, and sexual activities, often are no longer enjoyed. This condition is known as **anhedonia.**

Changes in physiologic functioning during depression are called **vegetative symptoms.** Changes in appetite, usually experienced as a reduction or loss of interest in food, is often seen, although increased appetite and cravings are also reported. Sleep disturbances are also common, particularly **insomnia** (the inability to fall asleep or to maintain sleep). Two types of insomnia are most often experienced by people having a major depressive episode. *Middle insomnia* refers to waking up during the night and having difficulty falling asleep again. *Terminal insomnia* refers to waking at the end of the night and being unable to return to sleep. Also reported is **hypersomnia,** in which the person sleeps for prolonged nighttime periods as well as during the day.

Fatigue and decreased energy are characteristic symptoms of depression, a condition known as *anergy*. Individuals report being tired upon awakening, regardless of how long they have slept. Even the smallest task seems insurmountable, and routine activities require substantial effort and take longer to accomplish. Decreased energy may be manifested in **psychomotor retardation,** in which thinking and body movements are noticeably slowed and speech is slowed or absent. Psychomotor agitation also may occur, in which the person cannot sit still, paces, wrings hands, and picks at the fingernails, skin, clothing, bedclothes, or other objects.

Other common symptoms in significantly depressed individuals include guilt or a sense of worthlessness, self-blame, impaired concentration and decision-making ability, even about trivial things, and suicidal ideation.

CLINICAL EXAMPLE

Becky is a 26-year-old insurance underwriter who was seen by the family planning nurse in a local Planned Parenthood clinic for a yearly checkup and Pap test. During the examination, she asked whether she might be anemic because she was "just exhausted all the time." Becky revealed that for the past month she had had difficulty getting out of bed in the morning. Getting dressed and ready for work left her drained. She described standing in front of her closet for long periods, unable to decide what to wear. She was also having extreme difficulty calling on potential clients. Whereas she was normally an assertive salesperson who called on perfect strangers with ease, she now described sitting at her desk for hours, trying to work up the motivation to pick up the phone. Coworkers, including her boss, had commented on her 15-lb weight gain, and these comments precipitated several uncharacteristic angry and tearful outbursts at work.

DSM-IV-TR Diagnostic Criteria for Depressive Disorders

MAJOR DEPRESSIVE EPISODE

A. Five (or more) of the following symptoms have been present during the same 2-week period and represent a change from previous functioning; at least one of the symptoms is either (1) depressed mood or (2) loss of interest or pleasure. **Note:** Do not include symptoms that are clearly due to a general medical condition, or mood-incongruent delusions or hallucinations.

1. depressed mood most of the day, nearly every day, as indicated by either subjective report (e.g., feels sad or empty) or observation made by others (e.g., appears tearful). **Note:** in children and adolescents, can be irritable mood.
2. markedly diminished interest or pleasure in all, or almost all, activities most of the day, nearly every day (as indicated by either subjective account or observation made by others)
3. significant weight loss when not dieting or weight gain (e.g., a change of more than 5% of body weight in a month), or decrease or increase in appetite nearly every day. **Note:** In children, consider failure to make expected weight gains.
4. insomnia or hypersomnia nearly every day
5. psychomotor agitation or retardation nearly every day (observable by others, not merely subjective feelings of restlessness or being slowed down)
6. fatigue or loss of energy nearly every day
7. feelings of worthlessness or excessive or inappropriate guilt (which may be delusional) nearly every day (not merely self-reproach or guilt about being sick)
8. diminished ability to think or concentrate, or indecisiveness, nearly every day (either by subjective account or as observed by others)
9. recurrent thoughts of death (not just fear of dying), recurrent suicidal ideation without a specific plan, or a suicide attempt or a specific plan for committing suicide

B. The symptoms do not meet criteria for a Mixed Episode.

C. The symptoms cause clinically significant distress or impairment in social, occupational, or other important areas of functioning.

D. The symptoms are not due to the direct physiological effects of a substance (e.g., a drug of abuse, a medication) or a general medical condition (e.g., hypothyroidism).

E. The symptoms are not better accounted for by bereavement, i.e., after the loss of a loved one, the symptoms persist for longer than 2 months or are characterized by marked functional impairment, morbid preoccupation with worthlessness, suicidal ideation, psychotic symptoms, or psychomotor retardation.

MAJOR DEPRESSIVE DISORDER, SINGLE EPISODE

A. Presence of a single Major Depressive Episode.

B. The Major Depressive Episode is not better accounted for by Schizoaffective Disorder and is not superimposed on Schizophrenia, Schizophreniform Disorder, Delusional Disorder, or Psychotic Disorder Not Otherwise Specified.

C. There has never been a Manic Episode, a Mixed Episode, or a Hypomanic Episode. **Note:** This exclusion does not apply if all of the manic-like, mixed-like, or hypomanic-like episodes are substance or treatment induced or are due to the direct physiological effects of a general medical condition.

MAJOR DEPRESSIVE DISORDER, RECURRENT

A. Presence of two or more Major Depressive Episodes.
Note: To be considered separate episodes, there must be an interval of at least 2 consecutive months in which criteria are not met for a Major Depressive Episode.

B. The Major Depressive Episodes are not better accounted for by Schizoaffective Disorder and are not superimposed on Schizophrenia, Schizophreniform Disorder, Delusional Disorder, or Psychotic Disorder Not Otherwise Specified.

C. There has never been a Manic Episode, a Mixed Episode, or a Hypomanic Episode. **Note:** This exclusion does not apply if all of the manic-like, mixed-like, or hypomanic-like episodes are substance or treatment induced or are due to the direct physiological effects of a general medical condition.

DYSTHYMIC DISORDER

A. Depressed mood for most of the day, for more days than not, as indicated either by subjective account or observation by others, for at least 2 years. **Note:** In children and adolescents, mood can be irritable and duration must be at least 1 year.

B. Presence, while depressed, of two (or more) of the following:

1. poor appetite or overeating
2. insomnia or hypersomnia
3. low energy or fatigue
4. low self-esteem
5. poor concentration or difficulty making decisions
6. feelings of hopelessness

C. During the 2-year period (1 year for children or adolescents) of the disturbance, the person has never been without the symptoms in Criteria A and B for more than 2 months at a time.

D. No Major Depressive Episode has been present during the first 2 years of the disturbance (1 year for children and adolescents); i.e., the disturbance is not better accounted for by chronic Major Depressive Disorder, or Major Depressive Disorder, in Partial Remission.
Note: There may have been a previous Major Depressive Episode provided there was a full remission (no significant signs or symptoms for 2 months) before development of the Dysthymic Disorder. In addition, after the initial 2 years (1 year in children or adolescents) of Dysthymic Disorder, there may be superimposed episodes of Major Depressive Disorder, in which case both diagnoses may be given when the criteria are met for a Major Depressive Episode.

E. There has never been a Manic Episode, a Mixed Episode, or a Hypomanic Episode, and criteria have never been met for Cyclothymic Disorder.

F. The disturbance does not occur exclusively during the course of a chronic Psychotic Disorder, such as Schizophrenia or Delusional Disorder.

G. The symptoms are not due to the direct physiological effects of a substance (e.g., a drug of abuse, a medication) or a general medical condition (e.g., hypothyroidism).

H. The symptoms cause clinically significant distress or impairment in social, occupational, or other important areas of functioning.

(continued)

DSM-IV-TR **Diagnostic Criteria for Depressive Disorders**

SEASONAL PATTERN SPECIFIER

Specify if:

With Seasonal Pattern (can be applied to the pattern of Major Depressive Episodes in Bipolar I Disorder, Bipolar II Disorder, or Major Depressive Disorder, Recurrent)

A. There has been a regular temporal relationship between the onset of Major Depressive Episodes in Bipolar I or Bipolar II Disorder or Major Depressive Disorder, Recurrent, and a particular time of the year (e.g., regular appearance of the Major Depressive Episode in the fall or winter).

Note: Do not include cases in which there is an obvious effect of seasonal-related psychosocial stressors (e.g., regularly being unemployed every winter).

B. Full remissions (or a change from depression to mania or hypomania) also occur at a characteristic time of the year (e.g., depression disappears in the spring).

C. In the last 2 years, two Major Depressive Episodes have occurred that demonstrate the temporal seasonal relationships defined in Criteria A and B, and no non-seasonal Major Depressive Episodes have occurred during that same period.

D. Seasonal Major Depressive Episodes (as described above) substantially outnumber the nonseasonal Major Depressive Episodes that may have occurred over the individual's lifetime.

Source: Reprinted with permission from the *Diagnostic and statistical manual of mental disorders,* 4th ed., Text Revision (pp. 375, 376, 380–381, 427). Copyright 2000 American Psychiatric Association.

The characteristics of a major depressive episode are illustrated in ■ Figure 15–1.

Dysthymic Disorder

A diagnosis of dysthymic disorder requires a chronically depressed mood for the majority of most days for at least 2 years (1 year for children and adolescents). There should have been no symptom-free interval of longer than 2 months. Symptoms in dysthymic disorder tend to be less severe than those in major depressive disorder, and there are fewer physiologic symptoms. The DSM-IV-TR criteria for dysthymic disorder are given in the DSM-IV-TR box on page 337.

BOX 15–1 **Key Facts About Major Depression**

- The average age of onset is the mid-twenties, although it can begin at any age and seems to be occurring in younger and younger people.
- The risk of developing major depressive disorder during a lifetime varies from 10% to 25% for females and from 5% to 12% for males, making depression twice as likely for women as for men.
- First-degree biologic relatives (parent or sibling) of people with major depressive disorder are up to three times as likely to develop depression as are members of the general population (APA, 2000).
- Symptoms usually develop over a period of time. The person may experience anxiety and mild depression for several days, weeks, or months before the onset of a full major depressive episode.
- Untreated, major depression lasts six or more months. In about 20% to 30% of cases, some depressive symptoms persist for longer periods, ranging from months to years. This is considered a partial remission and thought to be predictive of later depressive episodes and the development of chronic depression.

Dysthymic disorder tends to predispose people to the development of major depressive disorder. According to the DSM-IV-TR, 10% of individuals diagnosed with dysthymic disorder will develop major depressive disorder within the next year.

Dysthymic disorder often occurs in childhood, adolescence, or early adulthood and tends toward a chronic course. While both females and males are equally affected as children, in adults there are two to three times as many females as males with dysthymic disorder. The lifetime risk of developing dysthymic disorder is approximately 6% in the general population.

The symptoms of dysthymic disorder are similar to those of chronic major depressive disorder. This makes it difficult, even for experienced clinicians, to make an accurate differential diagnosis. Dysthymic disorder is mentioned here because you may read or hear of this diagnosis and should know what it means. In clinical practice, however, nursing care of the dysthymic client is similar to that of any depressed client.

CLINICAL EXAMPLE

Gregory G is a 14-year-old who was brought to a nurse psychotherapist by his mother upon the suggestion of the guidance counselor in his private school. In the letter of referral, the counselor stated that she was concerned because of Gregory's "persistent pessimistic outlook on life."

According to Mrs. G, who interviewed alone, Gregory has always been a cranky and irritable child. Since starting kindergarten, he has had difficulty relating to other children and is often left out of activities and social invitations. At home, he stays in his room much of the time, where he plays computer games and writes poetry. He does not do well in school, although testing has shown him to be far above average in intelligence. Despite their best efforts, his parents have never been able to interest him in scout-

Mood depressed; Memory problems
Anxious; Apathetic; Appetite changes
"**J**ust no fun"
Occupational impairment
Restlessness; Ruminative

Doubts self; Difficulty making decisions
Empty feeling
Pessimistic; Persistent sadness; Psychomotor retardation
Report vague pains
Energy gone
Suicidal thoughts and impulses
Sleep disturbances
Irritability; Inability to concentrate
Oppressive guilt
"**N**othing can help" (Hopelessness)

FIGURE 15–1 ■ *Characteristics of major depression.*

ing, sports, or other activities they deem appropriate for a boy his age. His parents reported that Gregory's weight, eating habits, and sleeping patterns were unchanged.

When Gregory was interviewed, he responded in monosyllables, made poor eye contact with the therapist, and sat slumped in his chair with no facial expression. He stated that he knew his parents were "disappointed" in him.

Seasonal Affective Disorder

Natural light is frequently taken for granted, but it influences the human experience in ways of which most people are unaware. As early as the days of Hippocrates, observers of human behavior noticed that some people suffer mood changes as the seasons change.

The relationships between light, biological rhythms, and mood are the subject of a great deal of current scientific study. This research focuses on the use of light in the treatment of **seasonal affective disorder (SAD)**, a depressive disorder that occurs in relation to the seasons, usually during winter months. Natural light may help modulate daily rhythms that influence sleep and activity patterns, neuroendocrine functions, and brain chemical systems. The criteria for specifying the occurrence of SAD are listed in the DSM-IV-TR box on page 338.

Research studies have explored the application of different forms of light to the skin and eyes at different times of day with mixed results (Birtwistle & Martin, 1999). The exact relationship between SAD and light, biologic rhythms, and events at the cellular level has not yet been determined. Information on SAD and the clinical application of light therapy is available through the Society for Light Treatment and Biological Rhythms (www.sltbr.org) and the Seasonal Affective Disorder Association (www.sada.org.uk) and can be accessed through the Companion Website for this book.

Bipolar Disorders

The **bipolar disorders** are a group of mood disorders that include manic episodes, hypomanic episodes, mixed episodes, depressed episodes, and cyclothymic disorder. The DSM-IV-TR criteria for these disorders are listed in the box on page 340.

A *bipolar I disorder* consists of one or more manic or mixed episodes, usually accompanied by major depressive episodes. A *bipolar II disorder* consists of one or more major depressive episodes accompanied by at least one hypomanic episode.

Bipolar disorders tend to be recurrent, decreasing in frequency as the individual ages. Most bipolar I disorder clients return to normal functioning during remissions, but approximately 20% to 30% have residual mood symptoms and as many as 60% have continuing interpersonal and occupational difficulties. Five to 10% of clients with bipolar II disorder have four or more mood episodes in a given year, and approximately 15% experience continuing mood lability and interpersonal and occupational difficulties (APA, 2000).

MediaLink Learning from Clients: Bipolar Disorder Video

MANIC AND HYPOMANIC EPISODES

Mania is characterized by an abnormal and persistently elevated, expansive, or irritable mood lasting at least one week, significantly impairing social or occupational functioning, and generally requiring hospitalization. This disturbance in mood must be accompanied by at least three additional symptoms such as "inflated self-esteem or **grandiosity**, decreased need for sleep, pressure of speech, **flight of ideas** (rapidly changing, fragmentary thoughts), distractibility, increased involvement in goal-directed activities or psychomotor agitation, and excessive involvement in pleasurable activities with a high potential for painful consequences" (APA, 2000, p. 377). Psychotic symptoms, such as delusions or hallucinations, may be a feature of severe mania. The DSM-IV-TR criteria for a manic episode are listed in the box on page 340.

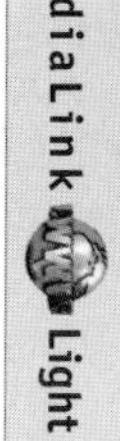

MediaLink Light Therapy

DSM-IV-TR Diagnostic Criteria for Bipolar Disorders

MANIC EPISODE

A. A distinct period of abnormally and persistently elevated, expansive, or irritable mood, lasting at least 1 week (or any duration if hospitalization is necessary).

B. During the period of mood disturbance, three (or more) of the following symptoms have persisted (four if the mood is only irritable) and have been present to a significant degree:

1. inflated self-esteem or grandiosity
2. decreased need for sleep (e.g., feels rested after only 3 hours of sleep)
3. more talkative than usual or pressure to keep talking
4. flight of ideas or subjective experience that thoughts are racing
5. distractibility (i.e., attention too easily drawn to unimportant or irrelevant external stimuli)
6. increase in goal-directed activity (either socially, at work or school, or sexually) or psychomotor agitation
7. excessive involvement in pleasurable activities that have a high potential for painful consequences (e.g., engaging in unrestrained buying sprees, sexual indiscretions, or foolish business investments)

C. The symptoms do not meet criteria for a Mixed Episode.

D. The mood disturbance is sufficiently severe to cause marked impairment in occupational functioning or in usual social activities or relationships with others, or to necessitate hospitalization to prevent harm to self or others, or there are psychotic features.

E. The symptoms are not due to the direct physiological effects of a substance (e.g., a drug of abuse, a medication, or other treatment) or a general medical condition (e.g., hyperthyroidism)

Note: Manic-like episodes that are clearly caused by somatic antidepressant treatment (e.g., medication, electroconvulsive therapy, light therapy) should not count toward a diagnosis of Bipolar I Disorder.

HYPOMANIC EPISODE

A. A distinct period of persistently elevated, expansive, or irritable mood, lasting throughout at least 4 days, that is clearly different from the usual nondepressed mood.

B. During the period of mood disturbance, three (or more) of the following symptoms have persisted (four if the mood is only irritable) and have been present to a significant degree:

1. inflated self-esteem or grandiosity
2. decreased need for sleep (e.g., feels rested after only 3 hours of sleep)
3. more talkative than usual or pressure to keep talking
4. flight of ideas or subjective experience that thoughts are racing
5. distractibility (i.e., attention too easily drawn to unimportant or irrelevant external stimuli)
6. increase in goal-directed activity (either socially, at work or school, or sexually) or psychomotor agitation
7. excessive involvement in pleasurable activities that have a high potential for painful consequences (e.g., the person engages in unrestrained buying sprees, sexual indiscretions, or foolish business investments)

C. The episode is associated with an unequivocal change in functioning that is uncharacteristic of the person when not symptomatic.

D. The disturbance in mood and the change in functioning are observable by others.

E. The episode is not severe enough to cause marked impairment in social or occupational functioning, or to necessitate hospitalization, and there are no psychotic features.

F. The symptoms are not due to the direct physiological effects of a substance (e.g., a drug of abuse, a medication, or other treatment) or a general medical condition (e.g., hyperthyroidism).

Note: Hypomanic-like episodes that are clearly caused by somatic antidepressant treatment (e.g., medication, electroconvulsive therapy, light therapy) should not count toward a diagnosis of Bipolar II Disorder.

MIXED EPISODE

A. The criteria are met both for a Manic Episode and for a Major Depressive Episode (except for duration) nearly every day during at least a 1-week period.

B. The mood disturbance is sufficiently severe to cause marked impairment in occupational functioning or in usual social activities or relationships with others, or to necessitate hospitalization to prevent harm to self or others, or there are psychotic features.

C. The symptoms are not due to the direct physiological effects of a substance (e.g., a drug of abuse, a medication, or other treatment) or a general medical condition (e.g., hyperthyroidism).

Note: Mixed-like episodes that are clearly caused by somatic antidepressant treatment (e.g., medication, electroconvulsive therapy, light therapy) should not count toward a diagnosis of Bipolar I Disorder.

CYCLOTHYMIC DISORDER

A. For at least 2 years, the presence of numerous periods with hypomanic symptoms and numerous periods with depressive symptoms that do not meet criteria for a Major Depressive Episode. **Note:** In children and adolescents, the duration must be at least 1 year.

B. During the above 2-year period (1 year in children and adolescents), the person has not been without the symptoms in Criterion A for more than 2 months at a time.

C. No Major Depressive Episode, Manic Episode, or Mixed Episode has been present during the first 2 years of the disturbance.

Note: After the initial 2 years (1 year in children and adolescents) of Cyclothymic Disorder, there may be superimposed Manic or Mixed Episodes (in which case both Bipolar I Disorder and Cyclothymic Disorder may be diagnosed) or Major Depressive Episodes (in which case both Bipolar II Disorder and Cyclothymic Disorder may be diagnosed).

D. The symptoms in Criterion A are not better accounted for by Schizoaffective Disorder and are not superimposed on Schizophrenia, Schizophreniform Disorder, Delusional Disorder, or Psychotic Disorder Not Otherwise Specified.

E. The symptoms are not due to the direct physiological effects of a substance (e.g., a drug of abuse, a medication) or a general medical condition (e.g., hyperthyroidism).

F. The symptoms cause clinically significant distress or impairment in social, occupational, or other important areas of functioning.

Source: Reprinted with permission from the *Diagnostic and statistical manual of mental disorders,* 4th ed., Text Revision (pp. 362, 365, 368, 400).

Hypomania is a less extreme form of mania that is not severe enough to markedly impair functioning or require hospitalization. Individuals experiencing hypomania will feel wonderful, "on top of the world," and will not recognize changes in themselves. Those who know the person well, however, will be aware of the changes in mood and behavior. There are no psychotic features in hypomania.

The onset of manic episodes is usually in the early twenties but may begin at any time. It often follows a severe disappointment, embarrassment, or other psychic stressor.

The mood of clients experiencing a manic episode is euphoric or "high." Their behavior is excessive and out of bounds. It is characterized by overly enthusiastic involvement in projects of an interpersonal, political, religious, or occupational nature. When thwarted, they become irritable, and their moods alternate between euphoria and irritability. Increased sexual behaviors are often seen. Women may dress in an uncharacteristically flashy or seductive manner and wear garish makeup. Speech is pressured, and racing thoughts or flight of ideas are often present. Grandiosity can reach delusional proportions. These clients rarely believe they are sick, even when they get into financial or legal trouble, and may vehemently protest treatment. The characteristics of a manic episode are illustrated in ■ Figure 15–2.

CLINICAL EXAMPLE

Mr. Gray, a 52-year-old engineer, was brought to the emergency psychiatric clinic by two adult sons at 2:00 AM. Their mother had called them to come help with their father, who had not slept in three days. When they arrived at their parents' home, they found their father working in the backyard on a large landscaping project involving stonework, a waterfall, fishpond, and extensive plantings of trees, shrubs, and flowers. According to the sons, Mr. Gray had three prior episodes of manic behavior, beginning when he was in the Army many years earlier. He was stabilized on lithium carbonate for years, but stopped taking it about a year ago because he felt so good. The current episode began about one week ago after he was passed over for a promotion at work. He then took a leave of absence from his job to create what he called "the world's first home-based theme park." Any attempt by his wife to talk him out of the project was met with anger and renewed resolve. Mr. Gray angrily told the admitting nurse, "I don't know why these boys brought me here. I need to get back to work! I'm going to get millions for this franchise."

DEPRESSED EPISODES

A diagnosis of bipolar disorder does not always mean that manic or hypomanic behaviors will be manifested in the current illness. There are several types of bipolar disorders in which manic or hypomanic episodes have occurred in the past, but the features of the current episode are purely depressive. This is termed a *depressed episode.* Treatment of depressed bipolar disorders is similar to treatment of any depression, with the possible exception of pharmacologic treatment.

MIXED EPISODES

In a *mixed episode,* symptoms of both mania and depression are present nearly every day in rapidly alternating succession over a period of at least a week. These clients are often agitated, suffering from insomnia and appetite disturbances, and may exhibit suicidal and psychotic thinking. They may have recently had a manic episode or a major depressive episode, although this is not always the case. Because the depressive symptoms are part of the clinical picture, they suffer more psychic pain than do

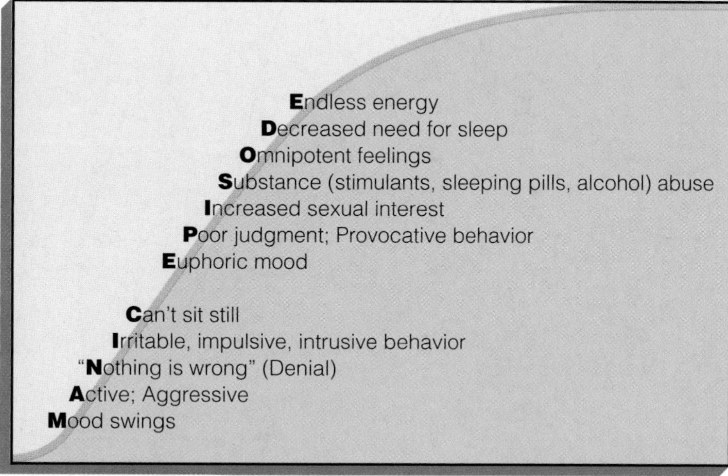

FIGURE 15–2 ■ *Characteristics of a manic episode.*

individuals who are in a state of mania and may seek help more readily.

CLINICAL EXAMPLE

Mrs. Kent is a 32-year-old high school teacher who was readmitted to the psychiatric unit 2 weeks after she was discharged following treatment for a major depressive episode. Her husband described her recent behavior as being extremely unstable, with rapidly alternating moods. "She is driving herself and me crazy, crying and talking about killing herself one day and out shopping for a new, glitzy wardrobe the next. She tried to go back to work right after she got out of the hospital the first time, but the principal put her on a leave of absence until the end of the year. He said she made a pass at him and was behaving flirtatiously toward the coaches and even some of her students."

CYCLOTHYMIC DISORDER

When clients have suffered for at least 2 years from "chronic, fluctuating mood disturbances involving numerous periods of hypomanic symptoms and numerous periods of depressive symptoms," they are diagnosed with **cyclothymic disorder** (APA 2000, p. 398). They must be free of severe symptoms that qualify for the diagnosis of manic disorder or major depressive disorder. These individuals are often considered to be moody, unpredictable, or temperamental, and they may go on to develop an overlay of symptoms that are of major depressive or manic intensity. ■ Figure 15–3 compares mood in major depressive disorder, bipolar disorders, dysthymia, and cyclothymia.

Cyclothymic disorder begins early, usually in adolescence or early adulthood. Although not common, with a lifetime risk of only 0.4% to 1% of the general population, it is thought to predispose the person to other mood disorders. The incidence is approximately equal between males and females.

Mood Disorders Due to Other Conditions

It is widely recognized that mood disorders may be manifestations of physiologic conditions (mood disorder due to a general medical condition) such as hepatitis or thyrotoxicosis. Mood disorders may also be induced by substance abuse, such as cocaine or amphetamines; prescribed medications, such as antihypertensives or oral contraceptives or toxins, such as lead or carbon monoxide. Practitioners should carefully evaluate the general medical condition of clients before making a diagnosis of mood disorder. The decision tree in ■ Figure 15–4 demonstrates the conditions under which mood disorders are differentiated from one another.

Postpartum Mood Episodes

Almost 70% of women experience the "baby blues"—transient mood changes, usually depression, that do not impair functioning—in the 10-day period after the birth of a baby (APA, 2000). However, when the symptoms meet the criteria for any of the DSM-IV-TR categories discussed earlier in this chapter, the

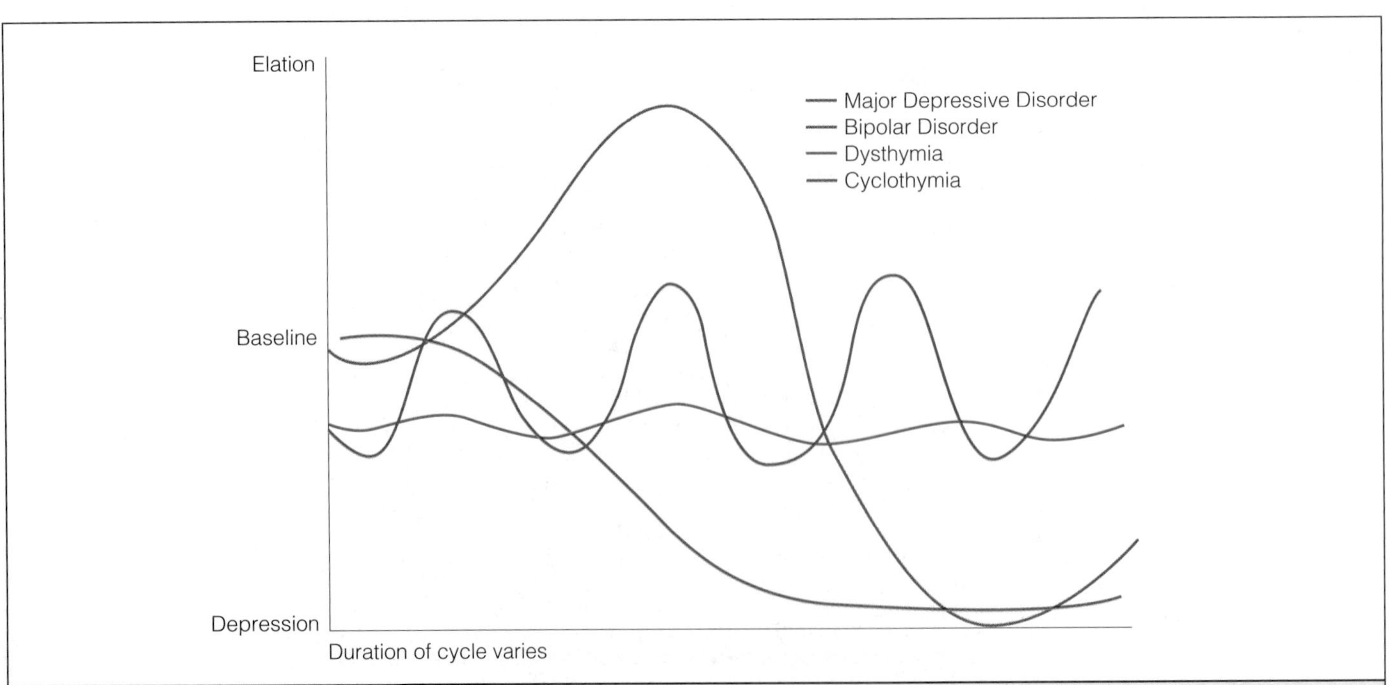

FIGURE 15–3 ■ *Comparison of affect (mood) in major depressive disorder, bipolar disorder, dysthymia and cyclothymia.*

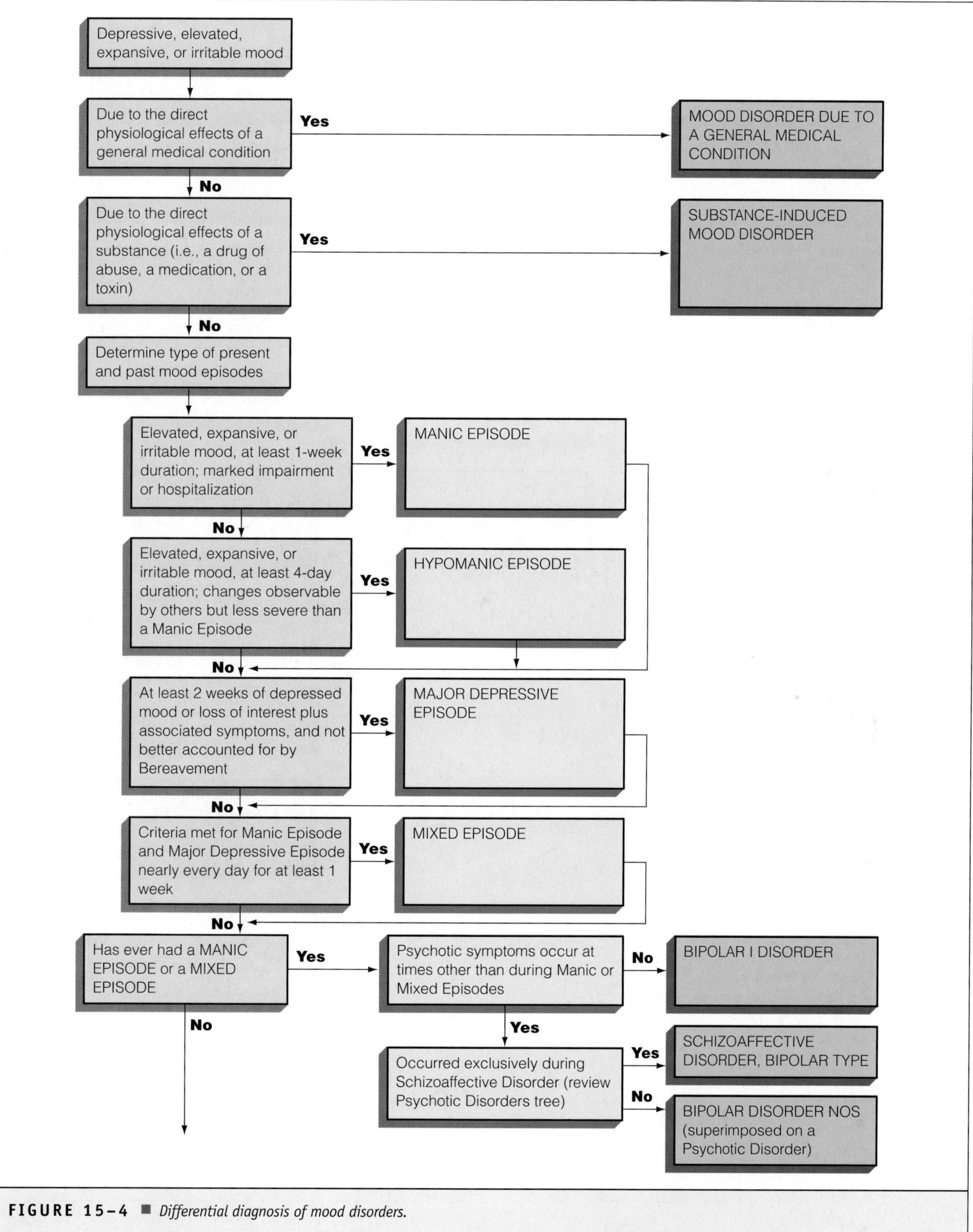

FIGURE 15–4 ■ *Differential diagnosis of mood disorders.*

(continues)

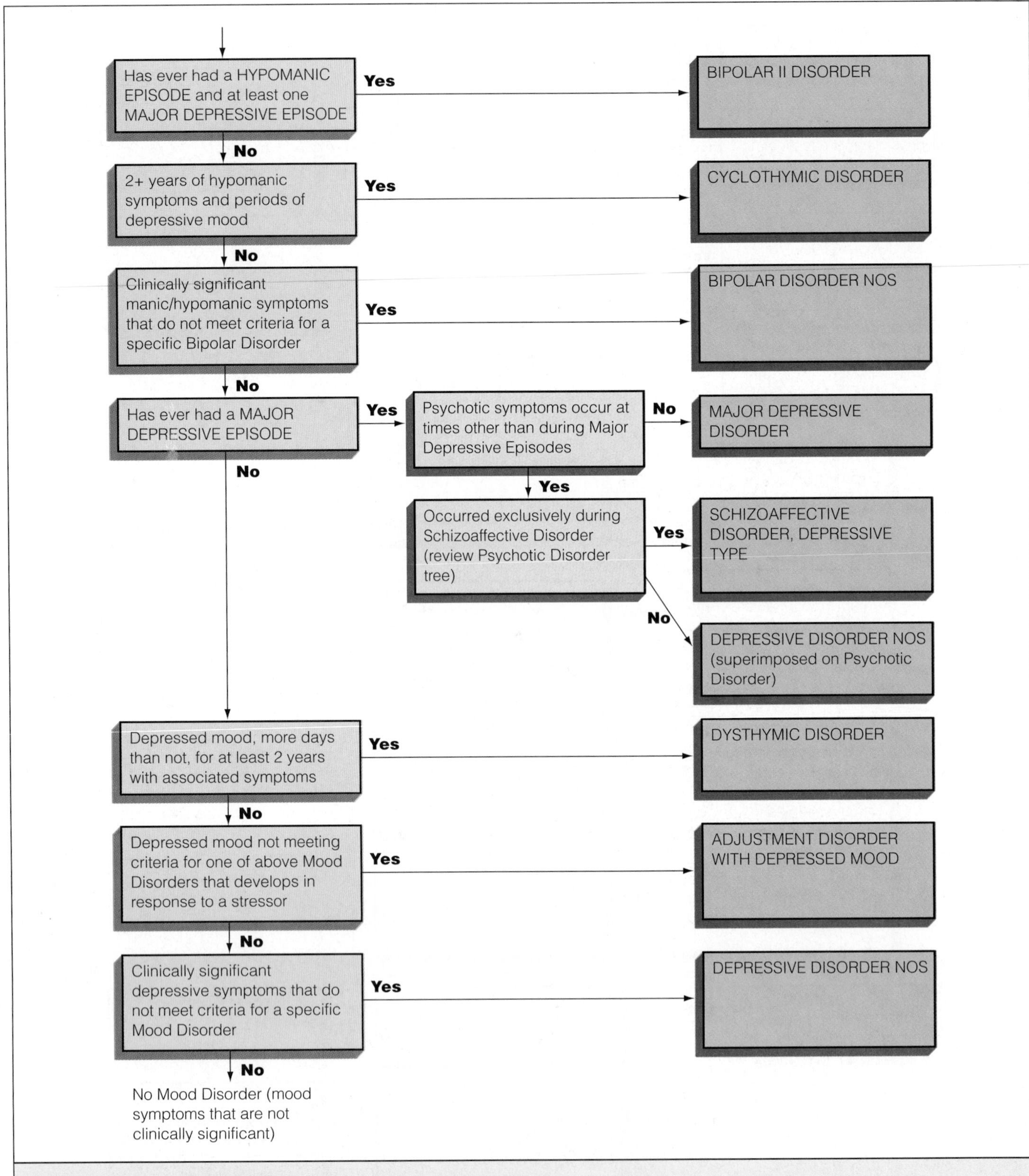

FIGURE 15–4 ■ *Differential diagnosis of mood disorders (continued).*

Source: Reprinted with permission from the *Diagnostic and statistical manual of mental disorders,* 4th ed., Text Revision (pp. 752–753). Copyright 2000 American Psychiatric Association.

client is diagnosed as having a mood disorder with postpartum onset or **postpartum mood episode.** The onset of a mood disorder with postpartum onset occurs within four weeks of giving birth but may occur anytime in the first year following childbirth (Beck, 2002).

The symptoms the client experiences are no different from the symptoms of other mood disorders except for a major one—preoccupation with infant well-being. This preoccupation can range from being overconcerned about the safety of her infant to severe ruminations about the infant's safety. Sometimes, but not always, psychotic features are evident. For example, the woman may have delusional thoughts about her infant (the infant is possessed by an evil presence) or command hallucinations (to kill or injure the infant).

CLINICAL EXAMPLE

A woman drowned her five children, believing that they were evil and that she was saving them from hell. Each of the five births, all within a period of seven years, was characterized by a postpartum mood episode, some with psychotic features that required hospitalization and psychotropic medications. She had attempted suicide at least twice. Despite the severity of her postpartum mood episodes, which occurred after each pregnancy, the couple did not modify their dream to have a large family.

The risk for a postpartum mood episode with psychotic features is increased for women who have had a prior mood disorder (especially bipolar I disorder) or a previous postpartum episode with psychotic features, or in women without a history of a prior mood disorder but with a family history of bipolar disorders. The risk for recurrence with a subsequent delivery is between 30% and 50% (APA, 2000).

You can refer depressed postpartum women to Postpartum Support International for a postpartum self-assessment test and help in locating a support group. Their Web site, www.chss.iup.edu/postpartum/, can be accessed through the Companion Website for this book.

Biopsychosocial Theories

People with certain personality types or temperaments are more prone than others to develop depressive and elated behaviors. Significant efforts have been devoted to identifying a single psychologic factor, trait, or mechanism that is unique to the development of mood disorders.

Research exploring the causative factors of mood disorders has focused on reactions to early separation from parents or parental loss, early mother-child relationships, errors in thinking, inherited tendencies, biologic factors, and other aspects of human development and experience. To date, no single personality type, biologic or psychological trait, or constellation of experiences has been established to account for all forms of mood disorders. There are multiple complex factors contributing to the development of mood disorders.

PSYCHOANALYTIC THEORY

The psychoanalytic theory of depression was originally formulated by Freud and later refined by others. It focuses on an unsatisfactory early mother–infant relationship as the primary factor predisposing individuals to later depression. If an infant's needs go unmet, a sense of loss occurs. Unresolved grief over the loss results in anger turned inward and the development of self-hate. The child's ego development is thereby adversely affected, resulting in a weak ego and an overdeveloped, punitive superego.

The psychoanalytic school of thought suggests a different etiology for bipolar disorder. This theory holds that the mother/primary caregiver derives pleasure from the infant's early dependence but feels threatened by increasing autonomy as the child develops. Independent behaviors are considered "bad," and the child must suppress his or her needs in order to sustain parental affection. Ambivalence resulting from the coexisting desires to please the parents and become more autonomous causes resentment and leads to a love–hate relationship with the parenting figures. Again, a weak ego and punitive superego create depression. Mania is seen as the denial of depression taken to the extreme.

Contemporary theorists and researchers criticize psychoanalytic theory for its tendency to blame mothers and the neglect of biologic factors.

COGNITIVE THEORY

Cognitive theorists, such as Clark and Beck (1999) believe that depression results from impaired cognition, or distorted thinking processes. People who think negative thoughts evaluate themselves critically and interpret stressful events as having a powerful, global impact on them. They feel guilty, inadequate, and hopeless about the future. Recent models of cognitive vulnerability to depression theorize that negative thoughts alone are not sufficient to cause depression unless the individual already suffers from a mildly depressed mood. In these instances, the combination of adverse life events (or the perception of adverse life events) and mildly depressed mood combine to create a downward spiral into depression (Mazure, Bruce, Maciejewski, & Jacobs, 2000). The Beck Depression Inventory is a clinical assessment tool. It asks clients to rate themselves on 21 groups of questions designed to detect negative thinking. Cognitive therapy seeks to teach individuals how to stop negative thinking and replace it with more positive self-appraisals. Cognitive therapies are discussed in detail in Chapter 32.

The theory of *learned helplessness* is a cognitive theory that proposes that learning plays an instrumental role in the development of depression. This theory holds that depression is based on the person's belief that he or she has no control over life situations. This conclusion is drawn from repeated failures, either real or perceived, to control life events. The result is that the individual gives up, stops trying to control, becomes dependent on others, and is thereby predisposed to depression.

MediaLink Postpartum Self-Assessment

OBJECT LOSS THEORY

In Bowlby's (1973) object loss theory of depression, the forced, often traumatic separation from, or abandonment of an infant by, the primary caregiver during the first 6 months of life plays a major role. Separation interrupts the bonding process that is so essential to the later development of relationships, and the child withdraws from other people and the environment. This establishes a pattern of anxiety, grief, helplessness, and hopelessness. Once the pattern is established, the individual uses these behaviors to deal with all subsequent losses, whether of major or minor magnitude. Such people feel helpless in coping effectively with the normal ups and downs of life and assume a hopeless, depressed attitude.

BIOLOGIC THEORIES

The most promising findings about the causes of mood disorders today are emerging from studies of biologic factors that alter brain function. Research on the physiologic basis for depression has been under way for more than 40 years and has generated a variety of hypotheses. Since mood disorders vary widely, it is unlikely that any single biologic causative factor can be isolated. This has led to a focus in current research on how various biologic factors already identified relate to one another, how they affect behavior, and how they respond to different therapies. In searching for biologic changes in mood disorders, it is important to remember that although a biologic abnormality may coexist with a mood disorder, it is not necessarily a causative factor. It could be a cause, a coexisting factor, or a consequence. See Box 15–2 for some abnormal findings on laboratory tests that may indicate the presence of a mood disorder.

BOX 15–2 Abnormal Biological Findings in Mood Disorders

While there are no laboratory studies that definitively diagnose mood disorders, some abnormal findings are noted more often in mood-disordered individuals when symptoms are present than in control subjects. These are:

- Sleep abnormalities in 40% to 60% of outpatients and up to 90% of inpatients with major depressive episode and in 25% to 50% of adults with dysthymic disorder; decreased need for sleep and abnormal polysomnographic findings in people with manic episode (sleep abnormalities may precede the onset of a mood disorder and may persist in the absence of other symptoms).
- Neurotransmitter and neuropeptide dysregulation in major depressive episode and manic episode.
- Hormonal disturbances (blunted growth hormone and thyroid-stimulating hormone); elevated urinary free cortisol; dexamethasone nonsuppression of prolactin; elevated plasma cortisol.
- Brain imaging studies may show increased blood flow in limbic and paralimbic regions and decreased blood flow in the lateral prefrontal cortex in depression; increased rates of right hemispheric lesions, or bilateral subcortical or preventricular lesions in persons with bipolar I disorder.
- Preventricular vascular changes when depression begins in late life.
- Urine and blood drug screens may indicate a substance-induced mood disorder.

Gender

Women are more prone to major depression and dysthymia than are men. This is true across cultures. Life stress, inadequate social support, inadequate economic power, and a tendency toward ruminative ways of coping (i.e. thinking and talking about a problem rather than taking action) all contribute to feeling trapped and helpless.

Endocrine and reproductive cycles may also play a role although menopause alone, contrary to popular belief, does not appear to be a risk factor for depression in women (Beck & Gable, 2001). It is also unclear whether prenatal and postpartum depression are hormonal in nature, result from increased stress of motherhood, or represent an interaction of these and other factors. See the Using Research Evidence feature for more information on the factors in postpartum depression. It is clear, however, that of all population groups, those at greatest risk for depression are young, poor women—white, black, and Hispanic—and that single mothers have double the risk of married women (Beck, 1999).

Recent findings by Bierut et al. (1999) indicate that while gender is important, environment and life experiences play a major role in the development of depression in both men and women.

Genetic Theories

Numerous studies have concentrated on the role heredity plays in depressive illness. Interest in this field of research was stimulated by the observation that the incidence of depression is higher among relatives of depressed individuals than in the general population. Studies of illness rates within and between generations of families, of monozygotic and dizygotic twins, of the general population, and those using known genetic markers such as blood type or color blindness all validate the increased incidence of depression in relatives of depressed individuals.

Studies have demonstrated that bipolar disorder is also increased among first-degree relatives of individuals with that disorder. Studies of identical twins reported an 80% concordance rate in bipolar disorder. This means that if one twin has the disorder, there is an 80% chance that the other twin will also develop it.

The role of genetics in the development of major mood disorders is complicated by the familiar question: Which plays the more important role, genes or environment? People who are biologically related tend to spend time together and influence one another's thinking. They share similar values and beliefs and are subjected to similar stressors, such as poverty or death of loved ones. It is therefore difficult to determine the relative weight of genetics, thinking patterns, family relationships, and learning in the development of mood disorders.

Biochemical Theories

Early biochemical studies established that an error in metabolism results in an electrolyte imbalance that seems to play a role in depression. The studies demonstrated that sodium and potassium were transposed in the neurons of depressed indi-

USING RESEARCH EVIDENCE

Eleanor M. is a 31-year-old woman who is hospitalized on an inpatient psychiatric unit for the treatment of postpartum depression following the birth of her first child 8 weeks ago. She has no previous psychiatric history. She reports becoming increasingly fatigued and despondent beginning when the baby was 3 weeks old. Her symptoms progressed until she was unable to care for the baby, cried most of the day, refused to bathe and groom herself, and expressed fears of harming the baby. Her husband John took all the vacation time he had accrued on his job but was reluctant to take family leave time for fear his career would be jeopardized. He has difficulty understanding why his wife, formerly an accountant with a responsible position in a large public accounting firm, cannot cope with the baby. "This is a woman who can keep six difficult clients happy and who supervises five other accountants," he exclaimed. "Staying home with the baby should be a piece of cake!"

While hospitalized, Eleanor has begun to respond to antidepressant medication but she is due to be discharged soon. As the time draws near, she again expresses concern about her ability to care for her son. The treatment team has referred Eleanor to a home health agency for twice-weekly home visits by a home health nurse. She will be seen weekly for medication follow-up at the local mental health center.

At her first home visit, the nurse finds John also at home, having taken yet another day off from work. He expresses irritation and impatiently paces the floor. The nurse assesses that Eleanor lacks partner support, which she knows has been shown to have a measurable effect on women experiencing postpartum depression. She decides to intervene by working with both marital partners.

After determining that John is usually home from work by 4:30 PM, the nurse sets up her twice-weekly appointments for that time. She begins by acknowledging that the birth of a child is typically marked by joy and that depression is a most unwelcome surprise that often causes dissension between partners. The demands of caring for the baby are new, and do not necessarily "come naturally" to all mothers. She also acknowledges that the husband goes through a difficult adjustment too, placing demands on the marriage that can create stress and tension.

During the next few visits the nurse assists the couple to identify essential tasks and to let go of certain things that were formerly important, such as a "neat-as-a-pin" house. She encourages Eleanor to include her husband in caring for the baby and participating in related tasks. In turn, she encourages John to see that Eleanor's disappointment in herself for not being a "superwoman" and her inability to care for the baby without help have been serious blows to her self-esteem. By reframing Eleanor's depression in this way, the nurse assists John to understand his wife's needs.

As communication between the couple improves, Eleanor is able to accept John's assistance with both the baby and some household tasks. She appreciates a take-out dinner he brought instead of interpreting it as a slap at her homemaking abilities. They both relax a bit about their roles in the family and work toward enjoying playtime together with the baby. By four weeks following her hospital discharge, Eleanor's mood is stable and her grooming improved, and she is able to care for the baby with no thoughts of harming him. Following a brief family leave, John has returned to work full time, but remembers to call home each morning and afternoon to listen to and encourage his wife. She has learned to express gratitude for his help and support.

These nursing interventions are based on the following research:

Misri, S., Kostaras, X., Fox, D. & Kostaras, D. (2000). The impact of partner support in the treatment of postpartum depression. *Canadian Journal of Psychiatry, 45*(6), 554–558.

viduals. This transposition alters the sensitivity of the neuronal cell membranes. Alterations in sensitivity of neuronal receptors are likely to lead to alterations in behavior. This may account for the efficacy of drugs, such as lithium carbonate and antidepressants, in the treatment of mood disorders.

Since then, scientific research has focused on the role of certain chemicals, the neurotransmitters, in the central nervous system. These are chemicals that transmit nervous impulses along neuronal pathways in the limbic area of the brain. Levels of certain monoamine neurotransmitters—norepinephrine, serotonin, epinephrine, and dopamine—were found to be deficient in many depressed people. Until the 1980s scientists believed that major depression resulted from norepinephrine or serotonin deficiencies, and the early antidepressants were formulated accordingly.

The monoamine hypothesis prevailed for years until it was found insufficient to explain fully the etiology of a complex disorder such as depression. Deficient levels of monoamine neurotransmitters have not been consistently found in depressed people and have not been able to relieve symptoms reliably. It is now believed that monoamine deficiencies are only one manifestation of depression. Many pharmacologic agents successfully used to treat depression and mania, however, do enhance monoamine activity. For example, study of the metabolism of serotonin and the discovery of the dysfunction of certain serotonergic neurons in depressed individuals led to the development of the selective serotonin reuptake inhibitors (SSRIs) and subsequent generations of these useful antidepressants.

Much current biochemical research focuses on the role of psychosocial stress in the pathophysiology of depression. The damaging effects of chronic stress, including its impact on limbic activity, are under extensive study. It is expected that interactive hypotheses of depression, that is, those that take into consideration a variety of biologic and psychosocial factors, are likely to be most useful in the future understanding of these complex disorders (Nemeroff, 1998).

Biologic Rhythms

It is widely recognized that we have self-sustained internal physiologic cycles that occur every 24 hours. These **circadian rhythms**, which include body temperature, sleep, and appetite, are activated, controlled, and integrated by the hypothalamus in the brain. The central controlling pacemaker is commonly known as the biological clock. A biological clock cell animation at www.cbt.virginia.edu/ can be accessed through the Companion Website for this look.

Researchers have described diurnal variations in mood, rest and activity cycles, EEG patterns, and neuroendocrine secretions. Circadian rhythm dysfunction can explain a number of mood disorder symptoms, such as insomnia, hypersomnia, early morning awakening, and variations in appetite, rest, and activity cycles (McEnany & Lee, 2000). Animal studies have demonstrated that alcohol and antimanic drugs, such as lithium, slow the biological clock, while estrogen and tricyclic antidepressants accelerate it or restore normal rhythms. The precise role biological rhythms play in mood disorders is yet to be determined.

PSYCHOLOGICAL FACTORS

All people, regardless of temperament and personality patterns, can and do become depressed. Mild depression is widely acknowledged as a part of the human experience.

Although most of us have had "the blues" from time to time, it is widely believed that certain people are more prone to developing true depression than others. Individuals who exhibit certain attitudes and beliefs—such as low self-esteem; lack of personal goals and direction; the tendency to avoid difficult situations rather than facing them directly; dependence and passivity in interpersonal relationships; acting and reacting impulsively; a limited ability to form enduring, mature relationships; and internalization of blame—are thought to be at risk for the development of depressive disorders.

SOCIOCULTURAL FACTORS

Most clinical investigators believe that life events and environmental stress play a role in mood disorders. There is less agreement, however, as to whether life events play a primary role or merely contribute to the onset of an inevitable episode of a mood disorder. Certain events, such as the death of a loved one, divorce, and other losses are widely recognized by both mental health professionals and the general public as precipitating events in depression. The unremitting stresses of living in poverty, and society's devaluation of the disadvantaged, also seem to predispose people to developing depression (Ruiz, 1998).

Culture exerts a powerful influence on how individuals experience and communicate psychic distress. Spiritual or religious concerns such as guilt may predominate and mask the underlying mood disorders. Some cultures experience depression largely in somatic terms. Be alert to complaints of headaches or "nerves" in Hispanic clients, of weakness or "imbalance" in Asian clients, and of bodily metaphors involving the heart in Middle Eastern and certain Native American clients. These may be culturally determined ways of expressing depression.

Be aware of the unique needs of clients who are likely to perceive the meaning and severity of psychiatric symptoms in relation to the norms of their cultural reference group. They include new immigrants to this country, individuals who are still heavily involved in the culture of origin, those who do not speak English, and those whose entire network of social and religious support remains embedded in the culture of origin.

Differences in culture and social status of clients and caregivers can create problems in diagnosis and treatment. Language differences, for example, create barriers in forming therapeutic relationships, while cultural differences in the expression of symptoms make it difficult to determine whether a behavior is normal or pathological. Culture also profoundly affects clients' attitudes toward and compliance with treatment (Ruiz, 1998).

NURSING PROCESS

Clients with Major Depressive Disorder

Nursing care of clients with mood disorders follows a problem solving model you are already accustomed to using, the nursing process.

Assessment

As already discussed, depression is characterized by low mood, often related to a loss. The loss may be concrete, such as the loss of a loved one or a job, or perceived, such as the loss of a cherished wish or disillusionment with a respected role model.

SUBJECTIVE DATA

Clients with depressive disorders may express some of the following:

- Feelings of sadness
- Fatigue
- Lack of interest in relationships and activities that were previously pleasurable
- Feelings of worthlessness
- Impaired concentration
- Impaired decision-making ability
- Sleep disturbances
- Loss of appetite; weight loss
- Excessive sleep
- Increased appetite; weight gain

Clients will often describe how long it takes them to complete activities that formerly were easily accomplished, such as preparing a simple meal. Tearfulness and emotional outbursts may also be a part of their description of the problem. They may or may not mention a loss or disappointment that they relate to the feelings.

Somatic Concerns. Somatic concerns are often the presenting complaint. Depressed clients may complain of abdominal pains, headaches, and vague bodily aches. A problem with sexual functioning or lack of desire may also be a presenting complaint. Constipation is a common result of the general slowing of metabolism due to inactivity.

Suicide Assessment. All clients who describe depressive symptoms should be assessed for suicide risk by direct questioning. Inquire about suicidal thinking, history of suicide attempts, and whether the client has a specific suicide plan. This aspect of assessment is reassuring, not alarming, to clients. Ask clients direct questions. You might ask, for example, "Tell me how you plan to kill yourself. Do you have the gun/pills/poison?" It is important to know whether the client has actually planned the suicide or if it is a vaguely formed thought. The more organized the plan is, the more concern it generates, particularly if the client has access to a lethal weapon, chemical, or other means of self-injury.

Other aspects of suicide will be discussed more fully later in this chapter under the heading "Preventing Suicide and Promoting Safety." Suicide lethality assessment is thoroughly discussed in Chapter 22.

OBJECTIVE DATA

Depressed clients are most likely to be females under the age of 40. They often have had prior episodes of depression and a family history of depression or bipolar disorder. A history of a recent stressful event and the lack of social support are also common features.

Objective signs and symptoms of depression are few. Psychomotor agitation or retardation may be observable if it is profound or if the nurse is familiar with the client's usual level of functioning. Family members may report observations of the client's agitation or apathy and lack of pleasure in usual activities. They may describe a pattern of social withdrawal and lack of social participation, combined with an intense preoccupation with the client's own feelings.

During assessment, many clinicians find it useful to provide a list of symptoms and ask clients to check the ones they are experiencing. A widely used and highly regarded self-reporting instrument designed to assess mood state is the Beck Depression Inventory. It has been in use for over 30 years and has been revised several times based on clinical research. There are several different types of Beck inventories now available (Beck, Steer, & Brown, 2000).

Other objective information to obtain during the nursing assessment includes concurrent general medical illnesses and concurrent substance use and abuse. Autoimmune, neurologic, metabolic, oncologic, and endocrine disorders often trigger depression. For example, hypothyroidism may be accompanied by depressive symptoms due to the underlying medical disease, while a client with AIDS or cancer may become depressed as a result of the diagnosis, prognosis, or disability connected with the disease.

Alcohol, which is a CNS depressant, and certain legal and illegal drugs can cause or complicate depression. A complete list of all substances and medications used by the client should be obtained through matter-of-fact questioning. A few prescription medications have depression as a side effect, and these should not be overlooked in the complete assessment. Birth control pills, sedatives, reserpine, glucocorticoids, and anabolic steroids have all been associated with the development of depression.

There are currently no laboratory tests specific for depression, but abnormal findings on several tests have been noted in depressed clients. They were discussed earlier in this chapter in Box 15–1.

Nursing Diagnosis: NANDA

The following sections discuss the implications of several nursing diagnoses commonly seen in depressed clients.

RISK FOR SELF-DIRECTED VIOLENCE

Thoughts about and impulses toward self-harm are related to feelings of worthlessness, feelings of guilt, repeated failure experiences, feelings of helplessness and hopelessness, or psychotic thinking. Suicidal clients should be hospitalized on either a general or a specialized hospital unit. Regardless of setting, whenever a client is at high risk for self-harm, that becomes *the* priority nursing diagnosis, and client safety becomes the most important aspect of nursing care.

SELF-ESTEEM DISTURBANCE

Depressed clients often express, either directly or indirectly, negative feelings about themselves and their abilities. Reduced self-esteem may be related to a variety of factors, including feeling abandoned by loved ones, experiencing repeated failures or losses, lacking positive feedback from others, thinking negative thoughts, engaging in negative "self-talk," or feeling guilty over real or perceived transgressions.

Evidence of low self-esteem is seen in clients who withdraw from social interaction; have difficulty accepting compliments or positive feedback; are harshly critical of themselves or others; are reluctant to try new activities because of fear of failure; express feelings of inferiority, worthlessness, and pessimism about the future; are overly sensitive to criticism; see social slights where none are intended; or set unrealistic goals and engage in grandiose thinking (denial of low self-esteem).

HOPELESSNESS

Individuals who have led lives characterized by hopelessness believe that their own actions cannot significantly influence an outcome. They believe there is no solution to their problems. They come to doubt their own abilities and are passive in response to others.

Evidence of hopelessness is seen in the behavior of clients who lack energy and initiative, refuse to engage in self-care, do not participate in decision making, verbally express a lack of control and doubts about their abilities, are reluctant to express feelings, avoid eye contact, generally lack involvement, and exhibit decreased affect.

SOCIAL ISOLATION

Low self-esteem and doubts about abilities lead many depressed clients to withdraw socially. Because inadequate social skills and self-absorption create impediments to positive interpersonal relationships, clients with low self-esteem frequently *are* avoided by others. This further reinforces their fears of undesirability and increases their social isolation. Evidence of social isolation and impaired social interaction is seen in behaviors such as spending inordinate amounts of time in bed, lack of verbalization, lack of eye contact, dull or monosyllabic responses to others' attempts at conversation, a preference for being alone, turning away or closing the eyes, and exhibiting discomfort in the presence of others.

Outcome Identification: NOC

For each NANDA diagnosis presented in the previous section, suggested outcomes for depressed clients with that diagnosis will now be discussed.

RISK FOR SELF-DIRECTED VIOLENCE

NOC outcomes have not yet been identified for this nursing diagnosis. Appropriate potential choices for depressed clients include Impulse Control: Ability to restrain compulsive or impulsive behavior, and Suicide Self-Restraint: Ability to refrain from gestures and attempts at killing self.

SELF-ESTEEM DISTURBANCE

The suggested NOC outcome for depressed clients with this nursing diagnosis is Self-Esteem: Personal judgment of self-worth.

HOPELESSNESS

Several NOC outcomes are relevant to depressed clients with this nursing diagnosis. They include Decision Making: Ability to choose between two or more alternatives, Hope: Presence of internal state of optimism that is personally satisfying and life supporting, Mood Equilibrium: Appropriate adjustment of prevailing emotional tone in response to circumstances, and Quality of Life: An individual's expressed satisfaction with current life circumstances.

SOCIAL ISOLATION

The depressed client with this nursing diagnosis has several potentially appropriate NOC outcomes. These outcomes include Loneliness: The extent of emotional, social, or existential isolation response; Social Interaction Skills: An individual's use of effective interaction behaviors; Social Involvement: Frequency of an individual's social interactions with persons, groups, or organizations; and Social Support: Perceived availability and actual provision of reliable assistance from other persons.

Planning and Implementation: NIC

When planning and implementing interventions designed to help depressed clients, keep two general principles in mind:

1. It is impossible to make depressed people feel better by being cheerful. In fact, an overly cheerful attitude tends to make them feel even worse because it belittles their feelings. Try to adopt a more emotionally neutral attitude while maintaining confidence that they will feel better.
2. Recognize that working with depressed people may eventually lower your mood and make you feel "down" yourself. Stay in touch with your own feelings. If you find yourself feeling down, assert yourself by asking to be assigned to a different type of client for a time.

PREVENTING SUICIDE AND PROMOTING SAFETY

There are few times when "always" and "never" are applicable. Client safety, however, *always* takes priority over other nursing care concerns. When the risk for self-directed violence is high, a number of actions call for immediate intervention. These actions are discussed in the Intervention box below. *Be aware that the risk of suicide increases as the severest stage of depression is alleviated, because clients then have sufficient energy and cognitive ability to plan and successfully implement a suicide plan.*

Encourage discussing all feelings. Clients need to know that all feelings are valid and that it benefits them to express their emotions, particularly anger and hopelessness, rather than acting them out through maladaptive behaviors. Use a calm, reassuring approach and teach calming measures, such as time-outs and controlled breathing. Provide safe physical outlets for expression of anger or increasing tension. Specific nursing interventions for anger are thoroughly discussed in Chapter 34. Assist in the transition from hospital to home by helping clients identify people in their usual environments to whom they can express feelings candidly without being judged.

Collaborate with clients to identify community resources to which they can turn if suicidal thoughts recur outside the hospital. Almost all communities have access to hotlines that are staffed around the clock with trained volunteers or professionals who are available to discuss feelings before they reach crisis proportions.

INTERVENTION

Preventing Inpatient Suicide and Promoting Safety

- Evaluate suicide level of intent regularly, and institute the appropriate level of staff supervision following unit protocol.
- Suicidal clients need to know that the environment is safe for them. Reassure them by removing sharp objects, razors, breakable glass items, mirrors, matches, and straps or belts, and explain why these objects are being removed. Monitor the use of scissors, razors, and other potential weapons.
- Place suicidal clients in a centrally located room near the nurses' station to facilitate ease of observation.
- Avoid establishing a predictable pattern of observation during the day and especially at night.
- Be particularly alert during change of shifts and on holidays or other times when staffing is limited, and during times of distraction, such as mealtimes and visiting hours.
- Examine items brought by visitors and monitor for safety.
- The no-suicide contract is a useful intervention, and it is discussed in detail in Chapter 22.

Encourage clients to seek you or another staff member when bothered by suicidal thoughts or impulses. Discussing these thoughts and impulses may be sufficient to diminish them and prevent a suicidal crisis from occurring. Avoid discussing suicidal ruminations in repetitious detail, however, since this may reinforce maladaptive behavior.

PROMOTING SELF-ESTEEM

While low self-esteem is a chronic problem, there are a number of things nurses can do to reduce negative thinking, thereby promoting improved self-esteem.

- Provide distraction from self-absorption by involving the client in recreational activities and pleasant pastimes. Simple conversation with a staff member or another client helps interrupt the pattern of negative thoughts. Use care to select activities that are not too complex for the client's current level of functioning. Experiences of success, not more failures, are needed. Increase complexity of activities as the client progresses.
- Dispel the notion clients often have that when they feel better, they will want to engage in activities. Explain that they must begin doing things *in order* to feel better. Be sure to acknowledge that it takes self-discipline and energy to do something when one doesn't really feel like it.
- Recognize accomplishment; do not use flattery or excessive praise. Give positive, matter-of-fact reinforcement, like "I notice that you have combed your hair," rather than overly enthusiastic compliments, such as "What a great hairstyle!" Appropriate recognition will increase the likelihood that the client will continue the positive behavior, while insincerity can be perceived as ridicule.
- Help clients identify their personal strengths. It may be useful to write these down. Recognize that it often takes some time for clients with low self-esteem to realize that they have any strengths. Avoid the temptation to point out characteristics you have noticed. It is far more useful for you to be supportively expectant of their ability to recognize their own positive qualities.
- Be accepting of clients' negative feelings, but set limits on the amount of time you will listen to accounts of past failures. Be alert for opportunities to interrupt the negative conversational patterns with more neutral ones.
- Teach assertiveness techniques, such as the ability to say "No" to protect one's own rights while respecting the rights of others. Clients with low self-esteem often allow others to take advantage of them. Defining passive, aggressive, and assertive behavior and giving examples of each are also helpful when teaching assertiveness (see the Client/Family Teaching feature on page 352.) Encourage clients and their family members to practice the new techniques in their relationship with you, so you can give feedback on how it feels to the recipient.

INSTILLING HOPE

Assisting depressed clients to develop a positive outlook is a priority nursing intervention. Clients who feel hopeless tend to form dependent relationships. Be aware of this tendency, and work from the first contact to minimize the likelihood that maladaptive dependence occurs in the nurse-client relationship. The list in the Nursing Self-Awareness feature on page 353 will give you direction on this.

Provide clients with responsibility and choices in the planning of their own care. For example, allow a client to choose whether to bathe in the morning or at night, or to choose from a short list of activities to attend.

Engage clients in setting goals they hope to achieve during hospitalization or outpatient therapy. Remember that unrealistically optimistic goals will ensure another failure experience and reinforce the client's sense of powerlessness. Make sure goals are attainable.

Clients who feel hopeless also need help in identifying ways to gain a sense of control in their relationships and lives outside the hospital. Collaborate with clients to identify changes they wish to make and action steps toward achieving them. Make the steps small and manageable. Accomplishing even small steps leads to a sense of mastery and optimism.

Teach clients coping measures such as problem-solving techniques, and encourage them to use them when confronting life situations. For example, if a client has difficulty paying rent, help him or her identify options, such as moving to a less expensive apartment or taking in a roommate. Explore the pros and cons of each option and the possible consequences. Emphasize confidence in the client's ability to identify, select, and carry out problem-solving activities that will result in a greater sense of involvement in his or her life.

Equally important is to help clients identify the aspects of their lives that are not within their control. The ability to accept what *cannot* be changed is just as essential as developing the ability to bring about positive change.

Planning for discharge should begin with the first client contact and is particularly important with hopeless, dependent clients. Help them and their families/significant others to identify resources in the community and to build support systems. Support groups, therapy groups, and social groups can all help clients separate from caregivers more readily when the time comes to end therapy.

ENHANCING SOCIALIZATION

When designing interventions for promoting social interactions, realize that both the quality and the quantity of a client's social behavior may be impaired. Early in the nurse–client relationship, make brief but frequent contacts with withdrawn clients, without making any demands. Your interest can increase a client's self-worth.

With extremely uncommunicative clients, simply spending time sitting quietly without any demand for interaction may be helpful. This approach communicates your belief that they are worth the investment of time. Nurses often find it difficult to be comfortable with silence, and they communicate that discomfort to clients. Remember that silence conveys acceptance and is a useful therapeutic communication technique.

When clients express feelings or cry, be nonjudgmental. Avoid showing surprise or disapproval. Two examples of how you can do this are in the Rx Communication: Major Depression feature on page 353. Recognize that ventilating feelings may provide temporary relief, particularly if anger is expressed. If clients are unable to verbalize feelings, they sometimes can act them out in safe and appropriate ways, such as tearing up an old magazine or beating on a pillow or bed. Provide privacy during these times.

CLIENT / FAMILY TEACHING

Assertive Communication

Assertiveness is learned behavior. Everyone has assertiveness potential, but we aren't born knowing how to be assertive. Children learn patterns of communicating from the adults around them. You can unlearn communication patterns if they aren't working and learn new ones and that is what assertiveness training is all about. The goal is helping people express themselves without fear of disapproval from others. Being assertive does not guarantee that others will always agree with you, but you do have the satisfaction of giving your opinion.

Definitions

Aggressive behavior is directed toward getting what one wants without considering the feelings of others. Aggressive communicators want to get their own way at any cost. They want others to "back off" and use intimidation to convey this message. An example of aggressive behavior is insisting on going to a certain movie even though you know your companion does not enjoy that type of movie. The outcome of aggressive behavior is that although you may get what you want in the short run, others feel discredited and tend to avoid you.

Passive behavior consists of avoiding conflict at any cost, even at the expense of one's own happiness. An example of passive behavior is agreeing to go to a movie you don't want to see because your friend pressures you to go. Passive communicators hold their feelings in and allow anger to build up. Anger can come out suddenly in an explosion or can be expressed in what is known as passive–aggressive behavior. An example of passive–aggressive behavior is taking a long time to get ready to go out while your friend is waiting because you are angry at him for insisting on seeing a movie you don't want to see. The outcome is that the passive person gives up control and is left with resentment, which usually emerges in other ways that damage relationships.

Assertive behavior consists of expressing one's wishes and opinions, or taking care of oneself, but not at the expense of others. An example of assertive communication is saying, "I really don't care for violent movies. Let's look at the movie listings and see if there is something playing that we can both enjoy." The outcome of assertive behavior is self-confidence and self-esteem.

Ways of Becoming More Assertive

1. Recognize your usual patterns. Are you passive, aggressive, or assertive in dealing with others?
2. Deliberately work on changing your pattern of thinking. Assertive people do not respond automatically; they take time to look at the situation and plan their responses. Don't be pressured into a quick decision. Instead say, "I want some time to think about it."
3. Don't feel guilty about your assertive behavior. Choose not to be responsible for others' feelings when you know your actions were reasonable.
4. Stand firm without precipitating an argument by using the "broken record" technique. This involves calmly repeating an assertive statement over and over. For example, you might say, "I really don't like violent movies," until your friend hears you.
5. Don't expect others to read your mind. This is an unrealistic expectation that ultimately will be destructive to your relationships. Instead, use assertive statements of feeling, such as, "Something is bothering me. I am feeling like my movie preferences don't matter."
6. Focus on remaining relaxed and calm. Breathe deeply, consciously relax your muscles, and speak in an even tone of voice. Make eye contact, and choose to remain in control of yourself.
7. Use "I" statements such as, "I am feeling on the spot. I want to have a nice evening with you, but I also want to see a movie I can enjoy." This expression of your own feelings and opinions helps the other person be nondefensive and listen to what you are saying instead of planning his response.
8. Use the "fogging" technique to respond to manipulative criticism. For example, if your friend says, "You're certainly being difficult tonight!" respond with, "I suppose I am." This sends a clear signal, "I'm not going to fight, and I'm not going to cave in, either."

Things to Keep in Mind

1. Don't expect too much too soon. Change comes slowly, with repeated practice. Be patient, and give yourself a chance.
2. Begin with small steps. What you need is a few successes to give you confidence. Go slowly and build a solid foundation.
3. Remember to give yourself credit when assertive behavior succeeds.
4. Ask for help when you need it. Seek qualified help, and state assertively what help you want. This may be an assertive friend, a teacher, or a counselor.
5. Remember that being assertive doesn't always work. Don't let setbacks stop you from trying.
6. Continue to learn about assertiveness. These books can be obtained through your local library: *Your Perfect Right*, 8th ed., by Robert E. Alberti and Michael L. Emmons, 2001; *The Assertiveness Workbook* by R. J. Patterson, 2000; and *The Disease to Please: Curing the People Pleasing Syndrome* by H. B. Braiker, 2000.

Encourage both verbal and nonverbal expressions of feelings by teaching clients that these are healthy behaviors. This intervention reinforces your acceptance of clients as unique and valuable individuals. Avoid disagreeing with, or otherwise belittling, a client's feelings by using overly cheerful reassurances like, "Now, now Mrs. Hamilton. You're feeling down right now but you'll feel better after a good night's sleep."

Once clients are comfortable interacting with one person, encourage group activities. Although this step may be difficult and frightening for clients, you can minimize their discomfort by attending activities with them at first. If their anxiety gets too uncomfortable, let them know that they can leave the situation without losing your approval. Give recognition for even small steps, gradually removing yourself and allowing them to stay in groups on their own.

Sometimes clients avoid social situations because they lack social skills and self-confidence. Create opportunities for clients to learn social skills and practice them in a protected environment. For example, teach them to read the newspaper or see a movie and select several items of interest to use in making "small talk." Demonstrate making small talk, and encourage them to practice with you. Give feedback on their progress. Make sure this is an enjoyable and nonthreatening activity.

Individuals who are either extremely passive or too aggressive in their social interactions are often avoided by others.

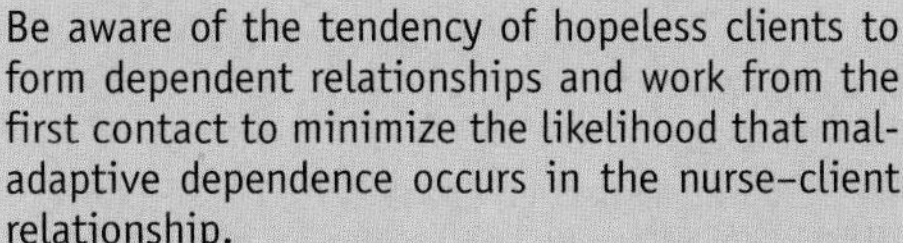

Nursing SELF-AWARENESS

Minimizing Maladaptive Dependence

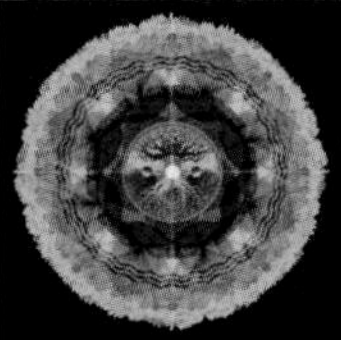

Be aware of the tendency of hopeless clients to form dependent relationships and work from the first contact to minimize the likelihood that maladaptive dependence occurs in the nurse–client relationship.

- Emphasizing the short-term nature of the relationship is essential.
- If the client singles out one staff member exclusively and refuses to relate to others, this is a clue that undue dependence is developing.
- Avoid giving dependent clients the hope that the nurse–client relationship can continue after the end of the therapy.
  1. Kindly, but firmly, refuse requests for your address or telephone number.
  2. Remind clients that social contact will not be allowed.
- If you find yourself wanting to continue relationships with certain clients, discuss these feelings with your instructor (if you are a student), or your supervisor or a respected professional peer (if you are a practicing nurse). It is essential that you separate your professional life from your social life.

Teaching such clients how to use assertive behavior can improve their interpersonal relationships. Use roleplaying to help them become comfortable with new skills. (Refer again to the Client/Family Teaching feature on page 352.

ADMINISTERING MEDICATIONS

The three main types of antidepressants nurses will administer to depressed clients are **tricyclic antidepressants (TCAs)**, **monoamine oxidase inhibitors (MAOIs)**, and newer antidepressants such as **selective serotonin reuptake inhibitors (SSRIs)**. The intended action of all antidepressants is to exert positive effects on mood and behavior. As some are sedating and others are energizing, the individual client's symptoms guide the choice of drug. None of the antidepressants is recommended for use during pregnancy.

Antidepressants are generally effective in alleviating most clients' symptoms and are helpful adjuncts to treatment. Because they do nothing to affect underlying psychosocial conflicts, they should not be used as the single treatment modality for depressed clients but should be used in conjunction with individual, family, and/or group therapy.

Responsibility for correct administration, monitoring for effects, and client education rests with nurses. See the Client/Family Teaching feature "Guidelines for Working with Clients on Antidepressant Therapy" and Chapter 31, Psychopharmacology, for additional information about antidepressant therapy and related nursing responsibilities.

MONITORING ELECTROCONVULSIVE THERAPY

Electroconvulsive therapy (ECT), a treatment procedure during which an electric current is passed through the brain, is useful in clients with severe depression, acute mania, some psychotic conditions, and those who are acutely suicidal. It is usually given several times a week until a course of 12 treatments is completed. Caution is advised when ECT is administered to clients with increased intracranial pressure, pregnant clients, and those who have had recent myocardial infarctions. Guidelines for working with clients receiving ECT are discussed in the Intervention box on page 355.

During a course of ECT, short-term memory loss is expected. This is distressing to some clients, and they need to be reassured that memory is usually completely restored. Since ECT is not curative, ongoing psychotherapy and pharmacotherapy are often continued to prevent relapse.

Evaluation

Specific client behaviors indicate that nursing interventions have been successful. Evaluation criteria answer the question, "How do we know that the depressed client's condition has improved?"

IMPULSE CONTROL AND SUICIDE SELF-RESTRAINT

The risk for self-directed violence is lessened when the client reports a decrease in suicidal thoughts and impulses and commits no acts of self-violence. Clients who are not suicidal can vent negative feelings appropriately and avoid high-risk environments or situations. They become more adept at identifying alternative ways of coping with problems and no longer depend on suicide as their primary coping skill.

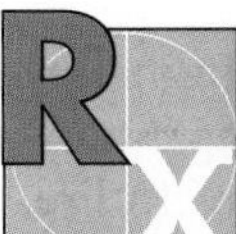

COMMUNICATION

Client with Major Depression

CLIENT: "I am upset and irritated all the time. All I do is yell at my kids and snap at my husband."

NURSE RESPONSE 1: "What can you tell me about what makes you feel so upset?"

RATIONALE: Open-ended questions elicit the client's perception of the problem and allow her to begin to explore her feelings where she can. Accepts the client where she now is without judging her.

NURSE RESPONSE 2: "It sounds like you are feeling out of control right now."

RATIONALE: Shows empathy and acceptance. By reflecting her expression of feelings, you validate the accuracy of your understanding and lay the groundwork for further exploration.

CLIENT / FAMILY TEACHING

Guidelines for Working with Clients on Antidepressant Therapy

Proper client education enhances the effectiveness of drug therapy. Good education can make the difference between client adherence and nonadherence with the drug regimen. It begins when drug therapy begins and is repeated during the course of the client's hospitalization. Give instructions orally and in writing. Include family members or significant others if they will supervise home administration.

Initiating Antidepressant Therapy

- Make sure the client knows the name and dose of the drug(s) being taken. *(Rationale: This is basic information every client should know.)*
- Advise the client to arise slowly from a sitting or lying position, and to sit on the side of the bed before standing up. *(Rationale: This allows the body time to compensate for postural hypotension.)*
- Encourage the use of ice chips, gum, hard candy, and increased fluids. *(Rationale: To alleviate dryness of mouth.)*
- Advise both client and family that it will take 2 to 4 weeks to see a therapeutic response to antidepressant therapy. *(Rationale: To prevent discouragement and impatience.)*
- Monitor for urinary retention or constipation, and take necessary actions. *(Rationale: These conditions may result from the anticholinergic effects of antidepressants.)*
- Give medication early in the day if insomnia occurs. *(Rationale: Some antidepressants have a stimulating effect.)*
- Monitor and record sleep patterns. *(Rationale: Normalization of sleep patterns should occur.)*
- Avoid giving TCAs and MAOIs concurrently. *(Rationale: To avoid hypertensive crisis, give 2 to 3 weeks apart.)*
- Observe the client for skin rashes, photosensitivity, weight gain, and signs of infection. *(Rationale: These are adverse side effects and should be evaluated.)*
- Advise the client that drowsiness, blurred vision, dry mouth, and jittery feelings will diminish after a few days on the drug. *(Rationale: Sedation and anticholinergic effects [except dry mouth] usually diminish over time. They will recur when dosage is raised, however.)*
- Monitor the client for suicide risk, particularly as depression begins to lift. *(Rationale: Profoundly depressed clients lack the energy to plan and implement suicide. As they begin to improve, risk increases.)*
- For clients on high doses of TCAs, observe closely for seizures. *(Rationale: High-dose tricyclics lower the seizure threshold.)*

Clients on MAOIs

- Supervise the client's intake, and make sure no tyramine-rich agents are offered. *(Rationale: Tyramine may precipitate hypertensive crisis.)*
- Monitor the client closely for headaches and elevated blood pressure. Withhold medication, and report these signs to the prescribing professional immediately. *(Rationale: These may be early signs of hypertensive crisis.)*
- Keep phentolamine mesylate (Regitine) on hand for treating hypertensive crisis. *(Rationale: This is an alpha-adrenergic blocker and potent antihypertensive agent.)*
- Observe diabetic clients closely for hypoglycemia. *(Rationale: MAOIs promote hypoglycemia.)*

Prior to Discharge

- In collaboration with the client, work out a time schedule that fits the client's lifestyle. *(Rationale: This will increase the likelihood that the client will actually take the medication.)*
- Advise the client to take the medication as ordered and to avoid using alcohol or other central nervous system depressants during therapy. *(Rationale: Varying the dosage impairs the maintenance of therapeutic blood levels. Alcohol and other central nervous system depressants have a potentiating effect on antidepressants and may cause stupor or coma.)*
- Teach the client and family about possible adverse reactions and measures to initiate if they occur. *(Rationale: To ensure maximum comfort and safety.)*
- Caution the client not to operate dangerous equipment, drive a car, or engage in tasks requiring mental alertness if drowsiness persists. *(Rationale: To ensure safety.)*
- Teach the client not to discontinue the drug abruptly. *(Rationale: Antidepressant dosage should be gradually decreased to avoid withdrawal symptoms of nausea, dizziness, insomnia, and headache.)*
- For clients on MAOIs, provide a list of tyramine-containing substances, (see Chapter 31) and make sure the client and family understand the consequences of consuming tyramine. *(Rationale: To ensure client safety.)*
- Record accurately and completely what drug education the client and family have received. *(Rationale: Documenting client education provides legal protection for the nurse and institution in the event of an adverse reaction.)*

SELF-ESTEEM

Clients who have improved self-esteem can verbalize self-acceptance and identify positive aspects of themselves. They can speak about increased feelings of self-worth. Their behaviors are consistent with increased self-esteem; for example, their posture is erect, and they groom and dress themselves with some care. They are able to accept a compliment, to express feelings directly and openly, and to communicate assertively with others, including maintaining eye contact. They express some optimism and hope for the future. Clients demonstrate self-esteem when they evaluate their own strengths realistically, set realistic, attainable goals for themselves, and work toward reaching them.

HOPELESSNESS

Depressed clients demonstrate progress toward eliminating hopelessness by consistently weighing and choosing among alternatives, expressing faith, the will to live, reasons to live, meaning in life, optimism, and belief in self or others. They can identify their own personal strengths, show interest in achieving life goals, and demonstrate satisfaction with life conditions or work to change them.

SOCIAL INVOLVEMENT

Improved social involvement is apparent when clients communicate and socialize with others. Voluntarily attending group activities is a measure of success. They can initiate interaction

INTERVENTION

Working with Clients Receiving ECT

- Prepare the client by explaining the procedure and answering all questions as fully as possible.
- A separate consent for treatment must be signed because ECT requires the administration of anesthesia. While informing clients and obtaining consent forms is legally a medical responsibility, in practice it is often shared by nurses.
- Clients are kept NPO for at least 4 hours before treatment.
- Just prior to treatment request the client to void and remove contact lenses, jewelry, hairpins, and dentures.
- Assess vital signs.
- The anesthetic preparation usually consists of the following:
  1. Generally, an atropine-like drug, such as glycopyrrolate (Robinul), is given to decrease secretions and block cardiac vagal reflexes during the seizure.
  2. A short-acting anesthetic, such as methohexital sodium (Brevital), is administered intravenously.
  3. Following induction, a skeletal muscle relaxant, such as succinylcholine chloride (Anectine), is administered to prevent injuries during the seizure.
  4. The client must be artificially ventilated until the muscle relaxant is fully metabolized, usually in 2 to 3 minutes. Oxygen is administered by positive pressure with a rubber bite block in place.
- An electrical current is passed through the brain by means of unilateral or bilateral electrodes placed on the temples. This causes a **grand mal** (or tonic–clonic) **seizure,** the effects of which are masked by the muscle relaxant. Often the only observable signs of seizure are a fluttering of the eyelids and carpopedal spasms.
- Clients are recovered in the lateral recumbent position to facilitate drainage and prevent aspiration. Upon awakening they will be confused and somewhat disoriented. After they are fully recovered and have been reoriented by the nurse, they may eat breakfast.

with another person appropriately and assume responsibility for dealing with feelings, including finding others with whom to talk. Clients can identify their own personal characteristics or behaviors that contribute to social isolation and accept responsibility for them. They report fewer experiences of feeling excluded.

For additional information about working with depressed clients, see the Case Study and Nursing Care Plan on pages 356–357. They plan for discharge by establishing or maintaining relationships, a social life, and a support system outside the hospital, and participating in leisure activities.

Case Management

Case management with depressed clients attempts to ensure that they receive needed services in a timely, flexible, cost-effective manner. This requires that the case manager understand risk factors and possible complicating factors of major depression, recognize symptoms early, anticipate possible complications, and understand effective case management outcomes. Depending on his or her educational preparation and experience, the case manager may or may not deliver direct psychotherapeutic care to depressed clients.

Risk factors include female gender, family history of depression, previous depression, lack of family/social support, stressful life events or losses, and substance abuse. Possible complicating factors include suicide attempt, substance abuse continuance or increase, presence of personality disorder, coexisting medical or psychiatric condition, resistance to treatment, and/or failure to respond to treatment (Smith & Bezon, 1997).

Symptoms that would alert the case manager to evaluate a client's need for treatment for major depression include the criteria in the DSM-IV-TR box on pages 337–338, suicidal thoughts, plan, or attempts, prior self-destructive violence, concurrent chronic or severe acute medical problem, prior medication-resistant depression, social withdrawal, and decline in work productivity (Walsh, 1998). Teach clients and family members to also be alert for symptoms that indicate the need for treatment.

Clients and families may find the following Web sites helpful:

- www.nimh.nih.gov/publicat/depresfact.htm (information presented by the National Institute for Mental Health is available in both English and Spanish)
- www.depression.org (the National Foundation for Depressive Illness)

These Web sites can be accessed through the Companion Website for this book.

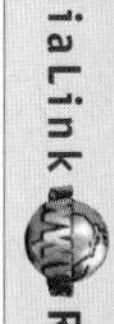

MediaLink Resources for Depression

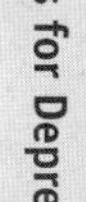

Desired case management outcomes include symptom remission, improvement in social, family, and occupational functioning, reduced risk for self-harm, and either avoidance of hospitalization or shortened hospital stay. Clients who lack financial resources and family, social, and employer support, and who resist or respond poorly to treatment, represent increased challenges for the case manager. The ultimate case management goal is earliest possible detection of symptoms, effective symptom reduction, and rapid return to maximal premorbid functioning.

Community-Based Care

A number of depressed clients can be effectively treated in community-based settings such as mental health centers, school and occupational health settings, doctors' offices, hospices, nursing homes, and others. Nurses in community settings play a major role by recognizing symptoms of depression, providing screening and assessment, providing emotional support and information, monitoring antidepressant therapy, and educating family members and significant others about depression. Severely depressed and/or suicidal clients, however, should be referred to inpatient treatment to ensure their safety.

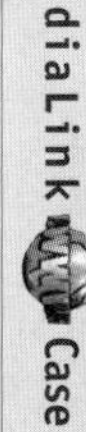

MediaLink Case Study: Psychoeducation for Depression

Nurses working in community health settings are generally not prepared as psychiatric–mental health nurses, but with minimal continuing education focused on the detection and treatment of depression, they can play a valuable role in the recovery of depressed clients while enabling them to stay in the community while in treatment (Armstrong, 1999).

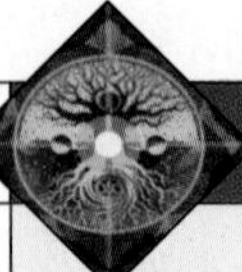

Case Study

Client with Depression

Identifying Information

Margaret M. is a 59-year-old, unmarried legal assistant who was admitted to the psychiatric unit following a gastric lavage in the emergency department. She had ingested 30 antidepressant tablets in a suicide attempt. Margaret stated that she had been home alone for 2 days, became increasingly depressed and hopeless, and took the antidepressants that her family doctor had prescribed for depression a few weeks ago. She became frightened almost immediately thereafter, was unable to make herself vomit, and called 911. Margaret stated, "I just don't have anything to look forward to anymore. No one would care if I died."

History

Margaret is the eldest of seven children from a small rural community. She had to leave school after the seventh grade to stay home and help with the younger children. At the age of 22 she returned to school and became a legal assistant. She moved to a large city over 100 miles from her home and built her life around her work. She never married. Because she works long hours in a large metropolitan law firm, she has virtually no social life and, except for a few coworkers, no friends. She stopped going to church recently, stating, "I just don't fit in anywhere and I never have."

Margaret reports that she has been concerned about her impending retirement at age 65 and her elderly mother's declining health. About a month ago, the health of her 86-year-old mother, who still lives in their small town, began to deteriorate. Margaret now fears that she will have to go care for her mother, with whom she has never gotten along. Her siblings are pressuring her to move back home, live with their mother, and serve as her caregiver. She fears that because she has no family of her own and no family ties in the city, she will eventually have to give in to their pressure.

She has no prior psychiatric history and no significant health problems. Vital signs: T, 98.4; P, 88; R, 18; Ht, 5'3"; Wt. 157 lb; BP, 138/78.

Current Mental Status

Margaret is somewhat disheveled and weeps occasionally during the interview. She is cooperative with the interviewer, even eager to talk. She reports being "exhausted" for the past three weeks. She has not slept well, has lost weight, had crying spells, has been irritable with coworkers, and had difficulty concentrating at work. She reports having had suicidal thoughts but did not have a specific plan until the weekend after the firm's senior partner told her to take a few days off to "get yourself together." She fears being fired, in which case she will have no reason to resist her siblings' pleas to "come take care of Mama."

Margaret is alert, responsive, and well oriented. There is no sign of a thought disorder, confusion, or impairment. She weeps as she discusses her situation, stating, "I have always been unattractive and nobody has ever loved me. If I died, all my family would lose is a nursemaid for Mama."

Other Significant Subjective or Objective Clinical Data

Margaret reports being in good health, although she is somewhat overweight. She has mild arthritis in her knees, which she treats symptomatically with aspirin. Until she was started on antidepressants, she took no other medicine.

Home Care

Nurses treating clients for major depressive disorder in the home setting require advanced preparation as psychiatric–mental health clinical nurse specialists (CNSs) at the master's or doctoral level. Nurses functioning in the role in the home serve as bridges between hospital, home, and community. Home care may substitute for inpatient care in carefully selected cases, or it may precede and follow the client's inpatient treatment. Home care aims to maximize the client's ability to stay in the family context and overlaps somewhat with the case management model discussed earlier. The advanced practice psychiatric–mental health nurse, however, is prepared to provide psychotherapeutic interventions directly to depressed clients and their families.

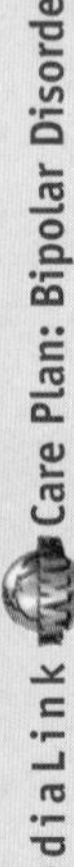

Working with depressed clients in the home and family contexts allows the CNS to observe the family dynamics and their impact on the family members, including the depressed client. These specialist nurses provide education to client and family about medications, side effects, desired effects, adverse effects, and possible drug and/or food interactions. In addition, advanced practice nurses educate clients and families about the nature of depression, the usual course of depression, what to expect, and when to seek help. They assist clients and families in establishing realistic goals, both short and long term. They collaborate with other professionals such as physicians, psychologists/psychiatrists, social workers, and others to improve communication and prevent gaps and overlaps in services. They also serve as client advocates, ensuring that depressed clients receive comprehensive, cost-effective care in the home setting (Hawranic & Strain, 2001).

NURSING PROCESS

Clients with Bipolar Disorders

Because the nursing care of clients experiencing depressive symptoms is the same whether the diagnosis is major depressive disorder, dysthymic disorder, or depressed episode bipolar disorder, this section will focus on hypomania and mania, which constitute the other half of the bipolar continuum of behaviors.

Assessment

The onset of a hypomanic or manic episode may be gradual or dramatic. Affect is euphoric or elated, but can change quickly to irritability or hostility if the person is confronted with limits or is otherwise frustrated. The signs and symptoms range in severity from mild in hypomania to extreme in a frank manic episode.

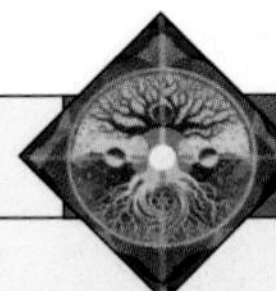

Nursing Care Plan

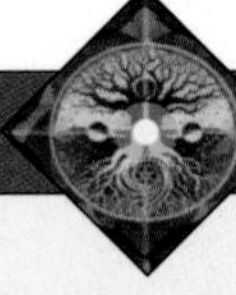

Nursing Diagnosis: Risk for Self-Directed Violence related to recent suicide attempt.

Expected Outcome: Impulse Control: Ability to restrain compulsive or impulsive behavior.
Suicide Self-Restraint: Ability to refrain from gestures and attempts at killing self.

Short-Term Goals	*Interventions*	*Rationale*
• Client will not harm self during hospitalization.	• Remove all dangerous articles from client's environment.	• To ensure safety; reassure client that she is in a safe place.
	• Observe client closely, using irregular schedule.	• Irregular schedule prevents her from predicting when she will be alone.
	• Adopt neutral, matter-of-fact attitude.	• To prevent dependency.
	• Evaluate suicidal intention at every shift and institute appropriate level of supervision.	• Suicidal thoughts and impulses may change rapidly.
	• Establish no-suicide contract.	• Nurse–client collaboration promotes self-responsibility.
	• Encourage client to seek nurse out when bothered by suicidal thoughts or impulses.	• To substitute talking it out for acting it out.
	• Limit repetitive discussion of suicidal ruminations.	• Repetition reinforces preoccupation with self-directed violence.
• Client will demonstrate alternative ways of dealing with stress, such as talking, exercise, relaxation techniques.	• Assist client to verbalize at least one reason for living.	• To counteract negative thinking.
	• Encourage the expression of feelings in one-to-one and group activities.	• Decreases isolation; elicits peer support.
	• Assist client to identify and practice alternative ways of dealing with stress.	• Increases client's coping behaviors.
• Client will identify resources where she can seek help if suicidal thoughts recur following discharge, such as crisis line, minister.	• Help client identify community resources and supports.	• Increases social support.
• Client will verbalize safe uses of antidepressant medication; describes potential drug/food interactions.	• Teach client safe use of antidepressant medication.	• This is information every client should know.

Nursing Diagnosis: Self-Esteem Disturbance related to impaired cognition fostering negative view of self.

Expected Outcome: Self-Esteem: Personal judgment of self-worth.

Short-Term Goals	*Interventions*	*Rationale*
• Client will sit and walk erectly; comb hair neatly; wear clean, matching clothes.	• Help client with hygiene and grooming as needed.	• Increases feelings of self-worth.
• Client will participate in unit activities.	• Teach client that activity helps decrease depression.	• This is information all depressed clients should know.
	• Involve client in simple, noncompetitive recreational activities.	• Provides for success experiences.
	• Increase the complexity of activities as client progresses.	• Reinforces growth and self-regard.
• Client will verbalize positive aspects of self and increased feelings of self-worth.	• Set limits on time spent reviewing past failures.	• To minimize negative self-view.
	• Help client enumerate her own personal strengths.	• To counteract negative self-view and increase self-worth.

(continues)

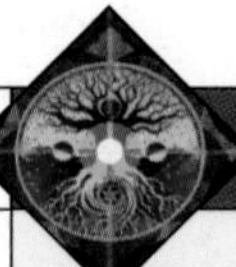

Nursing Care Plan (continued)

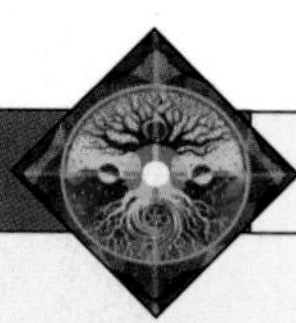

Short-Term Goals	*Interventions*	*Rationale*
• Client will communicate assertively with others; will explain to siblings that she will not give up her career to come home to care for mother.	• Teach client assertiveness techniques.	• Validates her right to take care of herself.
	• Practice (role play) client's direct expression of feelings.	• Gives permission to assert herself; promotes confidence.
	• Stay with client during difficult interactions, if desired.	• Provides support and reinforcement.
	• Give positive recognition when progress is shown.	• Reinforces healthy behaviors.

Nursing Diagnosis: Hopelessness related to inability to make and carry out decisions in her own behalf.

Expected Outcome: Decision making: Ability to choose between two or more alternatives.

Hope: Presence of internal state of optimism that is personally satisfying and life supporting.

Mood equilibrium: Appropriate adjustment of prevailing emotional tone in response to circumstances.

Quality of life: Expresses satisfaction with current life circumstances.

Short-Term Goals	*Interventions*	*Rationale*
• Client will verbalize feelings about situations over which she has no control; will realize that siblings' expectations do not control her responses.	• Assist client to identify situations over which she has no control	• Allows realistic appraisal of her situation.
	• Assist client to identify situations over which she can attain control.	• Focuses on areas in which she can effect change.
• Client will set realistic goals for self and work toward them.	• Engage client in goal setting for self.	• Supports concept of self-determination.
	• Provide options when possible.	• Validates concept of choice.
• Client will demonstrate a problem-solving system that she has used successfully.	• Explore problem-solving models with client and encourage her to select one.	• Information giving.
	• Practice problem-solving with small daily problems.	• To build confidence.
• Client will verbalize plans to attain control over life situations; works with siblings to find appropriate caretaker for mother.	• Role-play possible situations with siblings.	• Increases confidence.
	• Assist client to prepare for siblings' potential untoward responses.	• Promotes comfort and resourcefulness.
• Client expresses some hope for the future.	• Assist client to plan for retirement.	• To decrease fears of the unknown.
	• Identify community resources that assist individuals toward fulfilling retirement (e.g., AARP).	• To introduce new sources of support.
	• Involve client in identifying enjoyable leisure pastimes.	• To promote positive use of leisure time

Nursing Diagnosis: Social Isolation related to fear of rejection.

Expected Outcome: Social Interaction Skills: Use of effective interaction behavior.

Social Involvement: Social interactions with persons, groups, or organizations.

Social Support: Perception of availability of reliable assistance from other persons.

Short-Term Goals	*Interventions*	*Rationale*
• Client will communicate with nursing staff and socialize with other clients on the unit.	• Make brief, frequent contacts with client.	• Demonstrates availability.
	• Spend time with client with no demands.	• Demonstrates interest.
	• Use nonjudgmental attitude.	• Demonstrates acceptance.

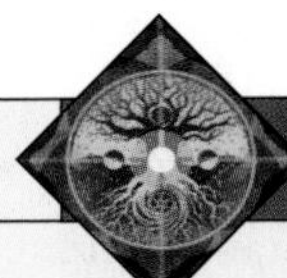

Nursing Care Plan *(continued)*

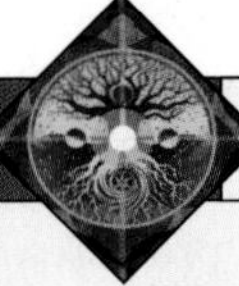

Short-Term Goals	*Intervention*	*Rationale*
	• Encourage client to ventilate verbally or through activity.	• Decreases internal tension; increases sociability and approachability.
• Client voluntarily attends group activities.	• Accompany client to group activities initially, withdrawing as tolerated.	• Provides support as needed; reinforces independence.
	• Teach social skills and assist client to practice them	• To increase confidence in social situations.
• Client assumes responsibility for dealing with feelings, including seeking others out; identifies key individuals outside hospital and initiates contact to renew relationships; makes concrete plans to go to church again.	• Teach assertive communication.	• Gives permission to take care of herself.
	• Encourage role-playing of phone calls, other contacts, anticipating others' possible responses.	• Decreases social anxiety; builds resourcefulness and flexibility.
	• Give positive feedback for all signs of progress.	• Validates efforts and reinforces growth

SUBJECTIVE DATA

Manic clients experience changes in their thought processes, sometimes stating that their "thoughts are racing." They often experience inflated self-esteem, sometimes to the extent of having delusions of grandeur. Delusions of persecution also may be a feature. They ignore fatigue and hunger, being too involved in activity to focus on physiologic sensations. Suffering from an inability to concentrate, they are easily distracted by the slightest stimulus in the environment. They may experience hallucinations. Hypomanic individuals and those early in manic episodes feel wonderful and do not understand why anyone is upset with their behavior.

OBJECTIVE DATA

Manic clients are most likely to be young people in their twenties, although adolescents are sometimes affected. Although bipolar disorder appears to have little gender specificity, the initial episode is likely to be manic in males and depressive in females (APA, 2000). To date, there is no documented evidence of the effect of race or ethnicity on bipolar disorder.

The hallmark of manic clients is constant motor activity. During a manic episode, they will not stop to eat. They do not rest, have disordered sleep patterns, and may go for days without sleep. Bruises and other injuries sometimes result from the constantly agitated behavior.

Flight of ideas is manifested in the manic client's communications, and pressured speech is an obvious symptom. Family members often report that they exhibit poor judgment, such as going on spending sprees and committing sexual and other indiscretions that are completely out of character with their usual behavior. Appearance may be unusual, such as inappropriate dress and garish makeup.

Impairment in occupational functioning may result in work layoff or being placed on a leave of absence because the behavior is disruptive in the workplace. Manic people cause interpersonal chaos by their manipulative behavior, testing of limits and playing off one person against another. If their manipulation attempts fail, they become irritable or hostile, and naturally such behavior alienates others (Cutler, 2001).

Just as they fail to settle down long enough to eat and sleep, they also neglect bathing. In time, the absence of personal hygiene further alienates them from other people.

There are no laboratory findings specific for the diagnosis of mania. Abnormal biologic findings were discussed earlier in this chapter in Box 15–2. Individuals experiencing manic episodes have been noted to have abnormal cortisol levels as well as abnormalities in neurotransmitter systems, but it is not known whether these abnormalities are a cause of or result from the disorder.

Manic clients are not usually able to cooperate fully in the assessment process. In many cases, you will find it necessary to rely on your own assessment skills and secondary sources, such as family members, in obtaining essential assessment data. Family members can often provide detailed information about the onset and progression of symptoms, as well as information about previous episodes, if any.

Nursing Diagnosis: (NANDA)

Several nursing diagnoses are common in the care of manic clients.

RISK FOR INJURY

Manic individuals are at risk for injury because their usual adaptive and defensive abilities are impaired. Because of their hyperactivity and agitation, they often lose control of their movements and bump into objects, fall, and otherwise injure themselves.

Their impulsivity, poor judgment, and propensity toward hostile outbursts also place them at risk for injury. Other clients are often extremely annoyed by inappropriate or unacceptable social behavior and may attack manic clients. As with self-directed violence, preventing injury becomes the nursing priority.

ALTERED THOUGHT PROCESSES

Manic clients experience disruption of their usual cognitive processes. This may be related to a variety of factors, including:

- Biochemical alteration
- Genetic predisposition
- Sleep deprivation
- A severe blow to self-esteem
- Massive denial of depression

Evidence of altered thought processes is seen in clients who cannot concentrate, have short attention spans, are easily distracted, and have impaired problem-solving abilities. They exhibit unwarranted optimism and poor judgment due to inaccurate interpretations of the environment. Delusional belief systems held by clients indicate a severe impairment of thought processes, as do hallucinations. Pressured speech, tangentiality, and flight of ideas are ample evidence of disrupted cognitive operations.

IMPAIRED SOCIAL INTERACTION

Unlike depressed clients who may isolate themselves and avoid social interaction, most manic clients are extremely gregarious and excessively social. But their social interactions are highly dysfunctional. Manipulating other people to meet their own wishes and needs is a major impediment to positive social interactions. Egocentrism, impulsiveness, lack of interest in the needs and concerns of others, and an unwillingness to accept responsibility for the impact of behavior on others all make manic clients difficult to tolerate. Poor personal hygiene aggravates the situation.

Nurses often have difficulty dealing with the unreasonable behavior of manic clients. The Nursing Self-Awareness feature below will help you determine how you may be affected by these behaviors.

SELF-CARE DEFICIT

Clients experiencing a manic episode have an impaired ability to perform the self-care activities of feeding, bathing, toileting, dressing, and grooming. This is related to hyperactivity, the inability to make accurate judgments about personal needs, alterations in thought processes, lack of awareness of personal needs, and fatigue. Self-care deficit is evidenced by inadequate food and fluid intake, an inability or refusal to bathe, a lack of interest in grooming and appropriateness of appearance, and an inability or unwillingness to toilet without assistance.

SLEEP PATTERN DISTURBANCE

The sleep pattern of manic clients is so disrupted that exhaustion and even death can result. Disrupted sleep is related to hyperactivity, agitation, and possibly to biochemical alterations. Sleep pattern disturbance includes the inability to fall asleep, roaming or pacing the halls during the night, awakening frequently during the night, and sleeping only for short naps with long periods of hyperactive, restless behavior in between.

Outcome Identification: NOC

Suggested outcomes for each NANDA diagnosis presented in the previous section are discussed below.

RISK FOR INJURY

NOC outcomes appropriate for the manic client include Risk Control: Actions to reduce or eliminate actual, potential, and modifiable health threats; and Safety Behavior: Fall prevention: Individual or caregiver actions to minimize risk factors that might precipitate falls.

ALTERED THOUGHT PROCESSES

Outcomes that address the manic client's altered thought processes include Cognitive Orientation: Ability to identify person, place, and time; Concentration: Ability to focus on a specific stimulus; Decision Making: Ability to choose between two or more alternatives; and Distorted Thought Control: Ability to self-restrain disruptions in perception, thought processes, and thought content.

IMPAIRED SOCIAL INTERACTION

Nursing outcomes relevant to the manic client's impaired social interaction include Social Interaction Skills: An individual's use of effective interaction behaviors; and Social Involvement: Frequency of an individual's social interactions with persons, groups, or organizations.

Nursing SELF-AWARENESS — **Potential Reactions to Working with Manic Clients**

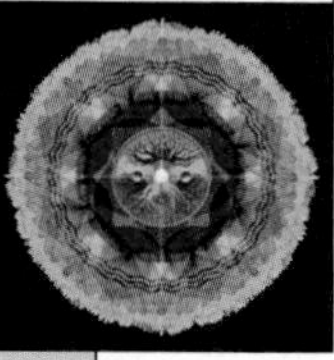

Working with manic clients will challenge your maturity, self-control, and professionalism. Listed below are some common reactions. When you work with manic clients, you may experience some of these feelings. Think about and discuss with classmates and your instructor how you might handle each of these reactions in order to maintain a positive nurse–client relationship.

- I feel annoyed by the client's demanding behavior.
- I feel outsmarted and outmaneuvered; I question whether my judgments and actions are appropriate.
- I develop rescue fantasies in response to a client's flattery and think I am the only one who understands this client.
- I become defensive and angry when colleagues point out a client's manipulative behavior.
- I feel anxious and insecure when a client turns on me, saying, "I'm not progressing because you're cold and mean."
- I have difficulty being objective about manic clients.
- I disagree emphatically with colleagues about how to handle a client's manipulative behavior; the client sits back and watches nurses fight with each other.
- I become angry and unsure of my judgment when a client consistently exceeds established limits.
- I withdraw and avoid manic clients to prevent embarrassment and self-doubt.

SELF-CARE DEFICIT

Manic clients' self-care deficits are addressed in the outcomes related to Self-Care: Feeding, bathing, toileting, dressing, and grooming. Some or all of these outcomes may be appropriate for a particular client.

SLEEP PATTERN DISTURBANCE

Outcomes that address the manic client's tendency to physical and mental exhaustion include Rest: Extent and pattern of diminished activity for mental and physical rejuvenation, and Sleep: Extent and pattern of sleep for mental and physical rejuvenation.

Planning and Implementation: NIC

With manic clients, your demeanor should be calm and relaxed but firm and matter-of-fact, particularly when communicating limits. Your own behavior serves as a model and is reassuring to out-of-control clients. As with all clients, building a trusting relationship is important. Therefore, make promises only when you are certain you can keep them.

PROMOTING CLIENT SAFETY

Provide a safe environment for manic clients by reducing environmental stimuli. This means providing a simply furnished private room that has had all unnecessary items removed. It should be in a quiet location to reduce noise stimulation. Low lighting can also be calming to the hyperactive client. Some hospitals have "quiet units." From there, clients can be transferred to milieu units when they are more able to deal with the distractions of community living.

Because manic clients have difficulty interacting appropriately with others, their participation in group activities should be limited until they are less agitated. Group settings tend to overstimulate these clients, and their behavior may antagonize others.

Smoking materials are particularly hazardous in the hands of agitated clients. They may burn themselves or leave burning cigarettes lying around when they become distracted by other stimuli. Allow them to smoke only under supervision.

Scheduling a program of appropriate activity, interspersed with rest periods, helps provide an outlet for tension while protecting clients from exhaustion. Appropriate activities include walks, exercising or dancing with the supervision of an activity therapist, and supervised vacuuming or sweeping chores. Avoid highly competitive activities that bring out hostility and overly aggressive behaviors.

Set and enforce limits on unsafe or socially inappropriate behavior with clients who are unable to control their impulses. Matter-of-fact intervention rather than angry scolding is the most effective approach. These clients may respond to verbal reminders, or you can use their distractibility to redirect them into safer and more appropriate activities. Remember to reward appropriate behavior with positive reinforcement such as, "I enjoyed our walk today because you were able to walk with me rather than running ahead."

ADMINISTERING MEDICATIONS

Hyperactive and agitated behavior usually responds fairly rapidly to antipsychotics such as chlorpromazine (Thorazine) or haloperidol (Haldol). These medications are often used to help manage manic clients who have started on lithium carbonate therapy, since lithium takes 1 to 3 weeks to become effective.

Nursing interventions include monitoring clients for adverse side effects of antipsychotic medications. Side effects include postural hypotension, dizziness, dry mouth, blurry vision, urinary retention, pseudoparkinsonism, and tardive dyskinesia. (See Chapter 31.) Several psychopharmacologic agents have proven effective in the long-term treatment of mania. The most effective and widely used of these agents is lithium carbonate.

Lithium Carbonate. Lithium carbonate is a potentially dangerous alkali metal that has been used in the treatment and prevention of acute manic episodes since the 1960s. It is now used in preventing the recurrence of bipolar disorder as well.

Lithium alters neurotransmission in the central nervous system. It is thought to interfere with the ionic pump mechanism in brain cells, but its exact mode of action is unknown. Its use is not recommended during pregnancy and breast-feeding or in clients with impaired renal function, congestive heart failure, sodium restricted diets, organic brain disease, and impaired central nervous system functioning.

Administered orally, the onset of action ranges from 1 to 3 weeks. The dosage is gradually increased until the recommended therapeutic blood level of 1.0 to 1.5 mEq/L is achieved. Once the desired effect is achieved, the dosage is adjusted downward to the maintenance blood level of 0.6 to 1.2 mEq/L.

Toxic symptoms begin appearing at blood levels above 1.5 mEq/L. Because there is such a narrow margin of safety, serum concentrations must be closely monitored until stabilized. The need for close monitoring means that clients are often hospitalized when lithium therapy is initiated. Before discharge, both clients and families must learn how to continue lithium therapy safely at home.

Include the following instructions in your teaching plan:

- The diet must include adequate salt and fluid intake, and the client should not take diuretics at any time.
- Regular testing of serum levels must be done, and the client's physician should be notified of any illness, especially if vomiting and diarrhea occur.
- The client should not vary the dosage and should continue to take the medicine even when feeling well, because discontinuing lithium therapy often precipitates a manic episode.
- If symptoms of lithium toxicity occur, such as nausea, vomiting, diarrhea, polyuria, muscle weakness, fine hand tremors, headache, blurred vision, slurred speech, dizziness, sluggishness, abdominal cramping, and tinnitus, the client should immediately discontinue the drug and contact the physician.

Alternative agents useful in mania therapy are the anticonvulsants carbamazepine (Tegretol) and valproic acid (Dalpro, Depakene). They seem to be useful to the 30% of manic clients who do not respond to lithium carbonate therapy. Their use in the prevention of unipolar depression is also under study.

Additional information about the pharmacology of mood disorders is found in Chapter 31.

PROMOTING REALITY-BASED THINKING

Present reality by spending time with clients; identify yourself, the time and day, location, and other orienting information as needed. Engage clients in reality-based, concrete activities, such as discussing a current event.

Consistency is reassuring to clients with altered thought processes. Establish consistency by having a schedule so clients understand what is expected of them. Consistency is also enhanced by assigning the same care-givers to work with the client whenever possible.

When dealing with delusional or hallucinating clients, communicate your acceptance of their need for false beliefs, while clearly stating that you do not share their perceptions. A statement such as, "I understand that you believe you are the Princess Anastasia, but I do not see it that way," conveys acceptance without supporting delusional thinking.

It is fruitless to argue or try to reason with delusional clients. This often serves to harden the belief system and can impair the development of trust. Instead, use statements such as, "I find that hard to believe" or "That is extremely unusual," to instill reasonable doubt as a therapeutic intervention.

When clients communicate altered reality perceptions, reflect their statements back to them for validation. For example, "Are you saying that your husband is trying to poison you with monosodium glutamate?" can help a client understand how her perceptions sound to others. You will recognize that clients are becoming less delusional when they make statements such as, "I know this sounds bizarre, but. . . ." Remember to give positive reinforcement when clients begin to focus on reality.

ENHANCING SOCIALIZATION

Nursing activities are designed to facilitate the manic client's ability to interact with others by identifying specific needed behavior changes and assigning tasks that will improve the client's interactions with others. This may require mediating between the client and others when the client exhibits negative behavior. Nursing actions should encourage and demonstrate honesty and respect for others' rights.

The major maladaptive behavior of manic clients that significantly impairs social interactions is manipulativeness. This may take a simple form, such as borrowing cigarettes from other clients rather than buying their own. Or it may be highly complex, such as pitting staff members against one another, as in the Rx Communication feature below, by giving them false information about each other.

Manipulativeness serves the purpose of increasing a client's sense of control and interpersonal power. Nursing interventions, such as setting limits, that promote client security often enable clients to curb their manipulative behavior or give it up entirely. Be aware of your own control needs, and provide opportunities for clients to be in control when appropriate (Hummelvoll & Severinsson, 2002).

Setting Limits. Out-of-control, manipulative behavior requires setting limits. All staff members must agree upon the established limits and must enforce them consistently. Violations of limits must have established consequences, also agreed upon by all staff. Clients must know what behaviors are expected and what consequences will result if limits are exceeded. Inconsistent application of consequences will cause failure in the efforts to decrease manipulative behavior.

You can expect clients to give charming explanations of why they had to exceed this or that limit, but do not be disarmed by these explanations. They are another form of manipulative behavior. Matter-of-fact limit enforcement and the consistent application of consequences are essential in promoting adaptive behaviors. The Intervention box on page 363 provides an overview of how to effectively set and enforce limits.

PROMOTING IMPROVED SELF-CARE

Well-being is compromised when clients do not receive sufficient nourishment and fluids for extended periods of time, par-

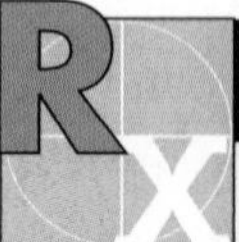

COMMUNICATION

Client with Bipolar Disorder

CLIENT: "I can't go to community group today! I'm expecting some top-level government officials to visit. The other nurse told me I didn't have to go."

NURSE RESPONSE 1: "I understand, Francis, but it is time for community group now and we expect everyone to attend. Let's walk over together."

RATIONALE: Acknowledges his need for the false belief without reinforcing or arguing with it. Maintains a consistent, routine schedule wherein this delusional client can feel safe. Clearly articulates what is expected of the client. Offers self.

NURSE RESPONSE 2: "All clients and staff members attend these meetings, Francis. You made some constructive comments last week. Let's go so we can get a good seat."

RATIONALE: Sets limits on manipulative behavior. Matter-of-fact enforcement of rules and expectations without allowing the client to involve you in a dispute with another staff member defuses the manipulative behavior and provides positive reinforcement of adaptive behavior.

INTERVENTION

Setting and Enforcing Limits

Effective limit setting requires that all members of the mental health team participate in establishing limits and determining and enforcing the consequences for exceeding them.

1. Establish limits only when and where there is a clear need. Limits must help client growth.
2. Establish reasonable and enforceable consequences for exceeding limits.
3. Explain the limits and consequences to clients in language they can understand. Explain why the limits are necessary, and allow clients to express their feelings about them.
4. Enforce the limits consistently. Written care plans help assure consistency.
5. Evaluate the continued need for limits frequently. Turn control over to clients as soon as behavior indicates the ability to exercise self-control.
6. Keep the client's dignity in mind at all times. Limit setting is not a punishment but a part of therapy.

ticularly during periods of hyperactivity. Monitoring intake and output is an important nursing activity. Frequent small snacks that can be eaten "on the go" are most likely to be consumed by the hyperactive client who is unable to sit down to eat. Work with a dietitian to ensure that high-calorie finger foods and nutritious liquids are available on the nursing unit until the client is able to attend regular meals.

A minimal level of personal hygiene is needed to ensure self-esteem and healthy social interactions. Assist hyperactive clients who are unwilling or unable to bathe, brush their teeth, shave, wash their hair, change clothes, or use the toilet. Autonomy is desirable, so allow clients to do as much for themselves as possible with verbal encouragement. Reinforce any attempts at self-care with recognition, for example, "I see you shaved today, Mr. Adams."

Incontinence of urine or feces is occasionally seen in severely regressed manic clients. This can be very disturbing to other clients and staff and insults the manic client's dignity. Nursing activities include establishing a schedule of frequent, regular toileting. Accompany the client to the bathroom every hour or half hour until "accidents" no longer occur.

A more common elimination problem is constipation. Hyperactive clients suppress the urge to defecate and may become severely constipated. The anticholinergic effect of some medications may also exacerbate constipation. Frequent fluid intake and a high-fiber diet can reduce constipation.

ENHANCING REST AND SLEEP

Clients in the manic phase of bipolar disorder appear deceptively energetic when they may actually be nearing the point of exhaustion. Design nursing activities to facilitate regular sleep–wake cycles. Monitor clients closely for signs of fatigue, and make provisions for rest periods. Promote nighttime sleeping by limiting extended daytime naps. Research findings indicate that sleep may promote the rapid resolution of first episodes of mania (Cutler, 2001).

Prior to bedtime, decrease light and noise and encourage quiet activities, and presleep routines, such as listening to soothing music. A warm bath and snack may aid relaxation, as may a backrub. Administer non-REM-sleep suppressing medications such as zolpidem tartrate (Ambien) as ordered.

If clients experience extended nighttime wakefulness, avoid engaging in long conversations or otherwise stimulating or giving extra attention during the night. Firmly encourage clients to stay in their darkened rooms with the expectation that they will fall asleep. If they will not stay in their rooms, assign a monotonous, repetitive task, such as folding towels or sorting papers to encourage drowsiness.

When manic clients are able to sleep, avoid waking them for nonessential care or activities. Allow for sleep cycles of at least 90 minutes.

Evaluation

Specific client behaviors indicate that nursing interventions have been successful. Evaluation and outcome criteria answer the question, "How do we know that the manic client's condition has improved?"

RISK FOR INJURY

If nursing interventions have been successful in promoting safety, clients will be free of accidental injuries. They will not engage in agitated or impulsive behaviors that can endanger them. Their social behaviors will no longer irritate or enrage other people, so they will no longer risk attacks from others. Clients will be able to enumerate safe ways of relieving excess tension when it occurs, such as verbal expression of feelings, writing feelings down in a diary or journal, or other adaptive methods. Clients will name their medications, understand the proper dosages, describe adverse effects, and explain lab monitoring needed, if any.

COGNITIVE ORIENTATION AND REALITY-BASED THINKING

Clients who base their thinking on reality will be oriented to time, place, and person. They will no longer experience delusional thinking or hallucinations. They will be able to establish trust relationships. Their attention spans will be increased. Their speech will be less pressured and will reflect diminished flight of ideas and tangentiality. Clients will recognize and verbalize errors in perception when they occur. Their thought processes and perceptions of environmental stimuli will be accurate and can be validated by others. They demonstrate logical, organized thought processes.

SOCIAL INTERACTION SKILLS

Improvements in social interaction skills will be demonstrated when clients can recognize and describe which of their interactions are successful and which are unsuccessful acknowledging the effect of their own behavior on social interactions. They demonstrate behaviors that may increase or improve social interactions. Clients acquire or improve skills such as cooperation, sensitivity, genuineness, and compromise. The absence of, or dramatic decrease in, the use of manipulation as a method of meeting their own needs also will signal improvement in social interaction. They now accept responsibility for their own behavior.

Other signs of improved social interaction include nondisruptive participation in activities, reestablishment of a social life, and identification of individuals with whom they can develop a social and support network.

SELF-CARE

Clients who have reestablished self-care will demonstrate this ability by performing the activities of daily living autonomously and willingly. This includes adequately bathing and grooming themselves, selecting appropriate clothing and makeup, establishing and maintaining adequate nutrition and fluid intake, and establishing and maintaining patterns of elimination without reminders or assistance.

REST AND SLEEP

The need for uninterrupted sleep varies from person to person depending on age, activity level, and usual pattern of sleep. Generally, clients who are able to sleep 6 or more hours per night without sleeping medication and awaken feeling refreshed will have demonstrated healthy sleep patterns. Being able to fall asleep within 30 minutes or less is another indicator. Recognizing fatigue and voluntarily resting or napping appropriately also indicates that clients are attending to their bodily sensations once again.

MediaLink Resources for Bipolar Disorder

Case Management, Community-Based Care, and Home Care

Case management and community-based care for clients with bipolar disorders, depressed phase, has been described earlier in the nursing process section discussing the care of depressed clients. Clients in the manic phase of bipolar disorders, however, often require hospitalization until stabilized on medication or through ECT.

Following discharge, goals for manic clients are the same as for others—high-quality, cost-effective treatment aimed at returning the client to full functioning as soon as feasible. Communication with family members, mental health professionals, employers, social workers, and others involved in the client's case is essential.

Monitoring the manic client's lithium level is an important aspect of the community-based nurse's role. Additional client and family teaching are often required to reinforce the information they received in the inpatient setting. ECT is increasingly used as an outpatient procedure, again calling on the community- and home-based nurse's teaching skills and sensitivity to concerns about safety, memory loss, and effectiveness.

Nurses in case management, community settings, and home care must be alert for "red flags" that signal exacerbation of the manic client's symptoms. These include nonadherence with treatment including refusal to take medications as ordered, escalating activity level that may include psychomotor excitement/agitation, spending sprees, shortening attention span, impaired occupational functioning, and grandiosity. Early recognition of red flags and mobilization of the treatment team can ward off rehospitalization and enable the client to stay at home while being treated and maintained in a community setting (Hawranik & Strain, 2001). Be sure that family members are also aware of behaviors that signal exacerbation of the client's symptoms.

Clients and their family members will find help from the Bipolar Disorder Information Center (www.mhsource.com/bipolar/index.html). A self-help resource for bipolar disorder and other mood disorders can be located at www.mental healtrecovery.com. Both Web sites can be accessed through the Companion Website for this book.

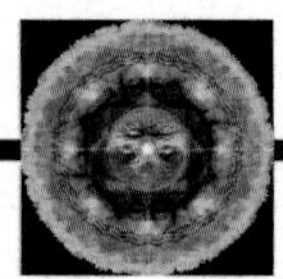

EXPLORE MediaLink

NCLEX review, case studies, and other interactive resources for this chapter can be found on the Companion Website at www.prenhall.com/kneisl. Click on Chapter 15 to select the activities for this chapter.

For animations, video tutorials, more NCLEX review questions, and an audio glossary, access the accompanying CD-ROM in this textbook.

BIBLIOGRAPHY

American Psychiatric Association (2000). *Diagnostic and statistical manual of mental disorders* (4th ed., Text Revision). Washington, DC: Author.

Armstrong, E. (1999). Role of the community nurse in caring for people with depression. *Nursing Standard, 13*(35), 40–43.

Beck, A. T., Steer, R. A., & Brown, G. K. (2000). *B-D-I-Fast Screen for medical patients*. San Antonio, TX: Psychological Corporation.

Beck, C. T. (1999). Postpartum depression: Stopping the thief that steals motherhood. *AWHONN Lifelines, 3*(4), 41–44.

Beck, C. T. (2002). Revision of the postpartum depression predictors inventory. *Journal of Obstetrical, Gynecological, and Neonatal nursing, 31*(4), 394–402.

Beck, C. T., & Gable, R. K. (2001). Further validation of the Postpartum Depression Screening Scale. *Nursing Research, 50*(3), 155–164.

Bierut, L. J., Heath, A. C., Bucholz, K. K., Dinwiddie, S. H., Madden, P. A., Statham, D. J., et al. (1999). Major depressive disorder in a community-based twin sample: Are there different genetic and environmental contributions for men and women? *Archives of General Psychiatry, 56*(6), 557–563.

Birtwistle, J., & Martin, N. (1999). Seasonal affective disorder: Its recognition and treatment. *British Journal of Nursing, 8*(15), 1004–1009.

Bowlby, J. (1973). *Attachment and loss: Separation, anxiety, and anger.* New York: Basic Books.

Clark, D. A., & Beck, A. T. (1999). *Scientific foundations of cognitive theory and therapy of depression*. New York: John Wiley & Sons.

Cutler, C. G. (2001). Self-care agency and symptom management in patients treated for mood disorder. *Archives of Psychiatric Nursing, 15*(1), 24–31.

Hawranik, P. G., & Strain, L. A. (2001). Cognitive impairment, disruptive behaviors, and home care utilization. *Western Journal of Nursing Research, 23*(2), 148–162.

Hummelvoll, J. K., & Severinsson, E. (2002). Nursing staffs' perceptions of persons suffering from mania in acute psychiatric care. *Journal of Advanced Nursing, 38*(4), 416–424.

Johnson, M., Maas, M., & Moorhead, S. (2000). *Nursing outcomes classification (NOC)* (2nd ed.). St. Louis, MO: Mosby.

Mazure, C. M., Bruce, M. L., Maciejewski, P. K., & Jacobs, S. C. (2000). Adverse life events and cognitive-personality characteristics in the prediction of major depression and antidepressant response. *American Journal of Psychiatry, 157*(6), 896–903.

McCloskey, J. C., & Bulechek, G. M. (1996). *Nursing interventions classification (NIC)* (2nd ed.). St. Louis, MO: Mosby.

McEnany, G. & Lee, K.A. (2000). Owls, larks and the significance of morningness/eveningness rhythm propensity in psychiatric–mental health nursing. *Issues in Mental Health Nursing, 21*(2), 203–216.

Misri, S., Kostaras, X., Fox, D. & Kostaras, D. (2000). The impact of partner support in the treatment of postpartum depression. *Canadian Journal of Psychiatry, 45*(6), 554–558.

Nemeroff, C.B. (1998). Psychopharmacology of affective disorders in the 21st century. *Biological Psychiatry, 44*(75), 517–525.

Ruiz, P. (1998). The role of culture in psychiatric care. *American Journal of Psychiatry, 155*(12), 1763–1765.

Smith, G., & Bezon, J. (1997). Case management guidelines: Major depression in adults and older adults. *Nursing Case Management, 2*(6), 246–254.

Walsh, J. (1998). The clinical case management of clients with major depression. *Journal of Case Management, 7*(2), 53–61.

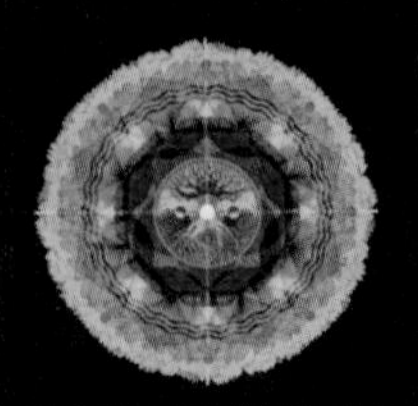

16

Chapter SIXTEEN

Anxiety, Somatoform, and Dissociative Disorders

SUE C. DeLAUNE

KEY TERMS

acute stress disorder
agoraphobia
alter
anxiety disorders
behavior modification
body dysmorphic disorder
compulsion
conversion disorder
depersonalization disorder
dissociative amnesia
dissociative disorders
dissociative fugue
dissociative identity disorder (DID)
factitious disorders
generalized anxiety disorder (GAD)
hypochondriasis
la belle indifférence
malingering
Munchausen by proxy syndrome (MBPS)
obsession
obsessive–compulsive disorder (OCD)
pain disorder
panic disorder
pediatric autoimmune neuropsychiatric disorders associated with streptococcal infections (PANDAS)

continued on next page

FOCUS QUESTIONS

- **Which theories do you find helpful in understanding anxiety disorders, somatoform disorders, and dissociative disorders?**
- **Although there are distinctive characteristics for each group of disorders, what are the common themes in the anxiety disorders? The somatoform disorders? The dissociative disorders?**
- **How is the concept of anxiety related to anxiety disorders, somatoform disorders, and dissociative disorders?**
- **Why is a thorough and comprehensive assessment especially important when caring for clients with these disorders?**
- **What nursing challenges do you anticipate in caring for clients with anxiety disorders, somatoform disorders, and dissociative disorders?**

MediaLink 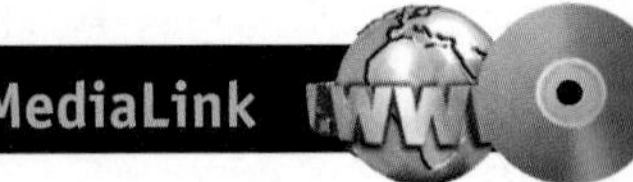 www.prenhall.com/kneisl

Additional resources for this chapter can be found on the Student CD-ROM accompanying this textbook, and on the Companion Website at www.prenhall.com/kneisl. Click on Chapter 16 to select the activities for this chapter.

CD-ROM
- Audio Glossary
- NCLEX Review

Companion Website
- Additional NCLEX Review
- Care Plan: PTSD
- Case Study: Compulsive Rituals
- Learning from Clients: Panic Disorder Video
- Learning from Clients: Obsessive-Compulsive Disorder Video

CHAPTER OUTLINE

Key Terms continued

phobia
posttraumatic stress disorder (PTSD)
primary gain
secondary gain
social phobia
somatization disorder
somatoform disorder
specific phobia
systematic desensitization
undifferentiated somatoform disorder

CROSS REFERENCES

Other topics relevant to this content are: Basics related to anxiety, stress, and coping, Chapter 5; Behavioral/cognitive approaches to the treatment of anxiety, phobic disorders, and obsessive compulsive disorder, Chapter 30; Crisis intervention for the acute stage of posttraumatic stress disorder, Chapter 33; Dissociative problems in victims of childhood sexual abuse, Chapter 23; Guidelines for teaching clients and families about antianxiety drugs, Chapter 31; Psychopharmacologic treatment of anxiety (the antianxiety drugs), Chapter 31; Relaxation and stress-management techniques, Chapter 32.

CRITICAL THINKING CHALLENGE

Barbara, a 32-year-old female diagnosed with dissociative identity disorder, has been admitted to the emergency department for attempting suicide by slashing her wrists. This is Barbara's fourth admission for self-induced wounds. You, the RN on duty, overhear another staff member referring to Barbara as someone who is "faking" her illness to seek attention. The other staff person says he does not believe in the existence of dissociative disorders and that "those people who say they have multiple personalities are making up their symptoms in attempts to receive sympathy." How would you respond to this staff member? ■

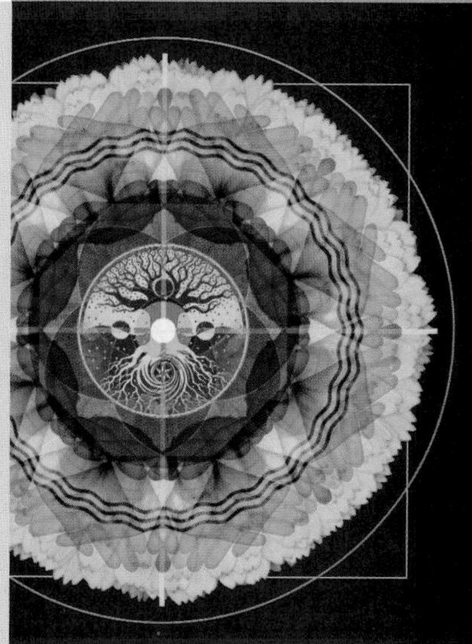

Although anxiety is a universal experience, people vary in their ability to tolerate anxiety and anxiety-producing situations. This chapter examines the experience of individuals with anxiety disorders, somatoform disorders, and dissociative disorders. People with these disorders all have one thing in common: Anxiety so disabling that they are unable to function. The functional disabilities may affect all dimensions of life including:

- Physical
- Emotional
- Cognitive
- Sociocultural
- Spiritual

Anxiety is a normal response that usually helps people cope with threatening situations. Common coping behaviors include withdrawal, acting out, avoidance, somatization, and problem solving. However, in people with anxiety disorders, the anxiety becomes disruptive and impairs functional abilities.

Anxiety disorders are the most common of all mental illnesses. Approximately 13 percent (19 million) of Americans aged 18 to 54 years have an anxiety disorder in any given year (National Institute of Mental Health [NIMH], 1999). It is not unusual for a person to have one anxiety disorder coexisting with another.

The high incidence of anxiety disorders results in much human suffering, as well as significant economic burden (Moreno & Delgado, 2000). Nurses encounter clients with anxiety disorders in every practice setting, not just mental health facilities. It is imperative that nurses perform accurate assessments in order to detect anxiety disorders and initiate appropriate treatment quickly.

Anxiety Disorders

Anxiety disorders are characterized by a mixture of physiologic, psychological, behavioral, and cognitive symptoms. The types of anxiety disorders are listed in ■ Table 16–1 . Each anxiety disorder has its own distinct characteristics, but they all have the common theme of excessive, irrational fear and dread. The physiologic, psychological, and cognitive symptoms of anxiety are outlined in the Assessment box on page 369.

In these disorders, anxiety is either the predominant disturbance, as in generalized anxiety disorder; or anxiety is experienced as avoidance behavior when the person attempts to master the symptoms, as in confronting the dreaded object or situation in a phobic disorder. When anxiety is not related to a specific stimulus, it may be called *free-floating anxiety*.

People in anxiety states experience anxiety both as a subjective emotion and as a variety of physical symptoms resulting from muscular tension and autonomic nervous system activity. (See Chapter 5 for a discussion of the symptoms of anxiety.) When acute, the anxiety drives the individual to seek help. When chronic, anxiety can lead to a number of somatic discomforts or disabilities (e.g., heartburn, epigastric distress, diarrhea, and constipation). Chronic muscular tension can lead to a variety of musculosketetal aches and pains.

Onset of anxiety may be sudden or gradual. Some people experience an unexpected, incapacitating outbreak of acute anxiety, as in panic disorder. In others, anxiety may express itself through relatively mild somatic symptoms in which the existence of underlying anxiety is overlooked unless specifically inquired about, as in generalized anxiety disorder.

TABLE 16–1 Anxiety Disorders: Types and Prevalence

Anxiety Disorder	Description	Prevalence[a]
Acute stress disorder	A condition similar to PTSD with a quicker onset and shorter duration	No statistics available
Generalized anxiety disorder (GAD)	Persistent, pervasive, and exaggerated sense of worry and anxiety	2.8% (4 million)
Obsessive–compulsive disorder (OCD)	A combination of intrusive, irrational thoughts and stereotypical behavioral rituals performed to dispel the unwanted thoughts	2.3% (3 million)
Panic disorder	Feelings of extreme fear that occur for no apparent reason and are accompanied by intense physical symptoms	2% (2.4 million)
Phobias	Intense fear of an object, event, or situation accompanied by CNS arousal symptoms *Social phobia*—fear of extreme embarrassment *Agoraphobia*—intense fear and avoidance of any situation in which escape might be difficult or help is unavailable *Specific phobia*—marked and persistent fear and compulsion to avoid the feared object or situation	Social phobia: 3–7% (5.3 million) Agoraphobia: 2.2% (3.2 million) Specific phobia: 4.4% (6.3 million)
Posttraumatic stress disorder (PTSD)	A reaction to a terrifying event; characterized by re-experiencing, avoidance/numbing, and hyperarousal	3–6% (5.2 million)

[a]Note that percentages and numbers refer to the estimated incidence of occurrences in American adults within a given year.

Source: National Institute of Mental Health (1999). The numbers count: Mental disorders in America. Retrieved September, 2000, from the World Wide Web, *www.nimh.nih.gov.*

ASSESSMENT — Guidelines for the Client with Anxiety Disorder

Physiologic	Psychological	Cognitive
Increased heart rate	Irritability	Forgetfulness
Elevated blood pressure	Angry outbursts	Preoccupation
Tightness in chest	Feelings of worthlessness	Rumination
Breathing difficulty	Depression	Mathematical and grammatical errors
Sweaty palms	Suspiciousness	Errors in judging distance
Trembling, tics, or twitching	Jealousy	Blocking
Tightness in neck or back muscles	Restlessness	Diminished fantasy life
Headache	Helplessness	Lack of concentration
Urinary frequency	Withdrawal	Lack of attention to details
Diarrhea	Diminished initiative	Past rather than present or future orientation
Nausea and/or vomiting	Tendency to cry	Lack of awareness of external stimuli
Sleep disturbance	Sobbing without tears	Reduced creativity
Anorexia	Reduced personal involvement with others	Diminished productivity
Sneezing	Tendency to blame others	Reduced interest
Constant state of fatigue	Excessive criticism of self and others	
Accident-proneness	Self-deprecation	
Susceptibility to minor illness	Lack of interest	
Slumped posture		

PANIC DISORDER

A common disorder, **panic disorder,** is characterized by recurrent attacks of severe anxiety lasting a few moments to an hour. These attacks are not associated with a stimulus but instead seem to occur suddenly and spontaneously. They may, however, become associated with certain situations, such as going to a shopping mall or driving a car. The person usually experiences physical symptoms such as palpitations, rapid pulse, nausea, diarrhea, dyspnea, and a feeling of choking or suffocation. The pupils are dilated, and the face is flushed. The person may feel dizzy or faint and often has a sense of impending doom or death. Restlessness is acute, and the person may make pleading, apprehensive appeals for help.

In its most advanced state, panic may create a symptom constellation mimicking myocardial infarction and mitral valve prolapse. Because these sensations often mimic symptoms of a life-threatening physical problem, such as a myocardial infarction, the diagnosis of panic disorder is often not made until expensive, extensive diagnostic and medical procedures fail to provide a correct diagnosis (NIMH, 2001).

CLINICAL EXAMPLE

Loretta has been to her primary care physician on two different occasions sure that she was having a heart attack. She got a clean bill of health both times. However, Loretta continued to experience palpitations, rapid pulse, and dizziness. Fearful that she would be labeled a hypochondriac, Loretta was reluctant to visit her physician again.

When the attacks occur frequently and when they interfere with the person's social functioning at work, school, or in the family, the condition is called panic disorder. People who have repeated attacks, or persistently worry about having another attack, are diagnosed with panic disorder.

Anticipatory fear of helplessness or of losing control during a panic attack is a common occurrence. The individual frequently avoids situations that induce the fear, sometimes developing a phobic avoidance reaction.

CLINICAL EXAMPLE

Loretta's panic attacks continued and gradually increased in frequency and severity. She noticed that her symptoms seemed to start every time she entered the elevator in the office building in which she worked. Loretta began to take frequent "sick days" rather than report for work and avoided all social activities with friends whenever a ride in an elevator was required.

MediaLink 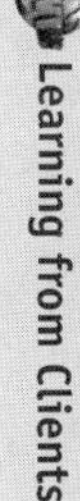 Learning from Clients: Panic Disorder Video

Agoraphobia, the marked fear of being alone or in public places from which escape might be difficult or in which help might not be available, is secondary to panic attacks. The DSM-IV-TR states that a diagnosis of panic disorder with agoraphobia is appropriate for an individual who experiences panic attacks and has phobic avoidance. In the absence of phobic avoidance, the condition is termed panic disorder without agoraphobia. Agoraphobia without panic attacks is uncommon. Agoraphobia with symptoms of panic attack is now treatable

DSM-IV-TR Diagnostic Criteria for Anxiety Disorders

DIAGNOSTIC CRITERIA FOR PANIC DISORDER WITHOUT AGORAPHOBIA AND PANIC DISORDER WITH AGORAPHOBIA

A. Both 1 and 2:
  1. Recurrent unexpected Panic Attacks
  2. At least one of the attacks has been followed by 1 month (or more) of one (or more) of the following:
    a. Persistent concern about having additional attacks
    b. Worry about the implications of the attack or its consequences (e.g., losing control, having a heart attack, "going crazy")
    c. A significant change in behavior related to the attacks

B. The presence of Agoraphobia (for 300.21 Panic Disorder With Agoraphobia)
OR
The absence of Agoraphobia (for 300.01 Panic Disorder Without Agoraphobia)

C. The Panic Attacks are not due to the direct physiological effects of a substance (e.g., a drug of abuse, a medication) or a general medical condition (e.g., hyperthyroidism).

D. The Panic Attacks are not better accounted for by another mental disorder, such as Social Phobia (e.g., occurring on exposure to feared social situations), Specific Phobia (e.g., on exposure to a specific phobic situation), Obsessive-Compulsive Disorder (e.g., on exposure to dirt in someone with an obsession about contamination), Posttraumatic Stress Disorder (e.g., in response to stimuli associated with a severe stressor), or Separation Anxiety Disorder (e.g., in response to being away from home or close relatives).

DIAGNOSTIC CRITERIA FOR OBSESSIVE-COMPULSIVE DISORDER

A. Either obsessions or compulsions:
Obsessions as defined by 1, 2, 3, and 4:
  1. recurrent and persistent thoughts, impulses, or images that are experienced, at some time during the disturbance, as intrusive and inappropriate and that cause marked anxiety or distress
  2. the thoughts, impulses, or images are not simply excessive worries about real-life problems
  3. the person attempts to ignore or suppress such thoughts, impulses, or images, or to neutralize them with some other thought or action
  4. the person recognizes that the obsessional thoughts, impulses, or images are a product of his or her own mind (not imposed from without as in thought insertion)

Compulsions as defined by 1 and 2:
  1. repetitive behaviors (e.g., hand washing, ordering, checking) or mental acts (e.g., praying, counting, repeating words silently) that the person feels driven to perform in response to an obsession, or according to rules that must be applied rigidly
  2. the behaviors or mental acts are aimed at preventing or reducing distress or preventing some dreaded event or situation; however, these behaviors or mental acts either are not connected in a realistic way with what they are designed to neutralize or prevent or are clearly excessive

B. At some point during the course of the disorder, the person has recognized that the obsessions or compulsions are excessive or unreasonable. **Note**: This does not apply to children.

C. The obsessions or compulsions cause marked distress, are time consuming (take more than 1 hour a day); or significantly interfere with the person's normal routine, occupational (or academic) functioning, or usual social activities or relationships.

D. If another Axis I disorder is present, the content of the obsessions or compulsions is not restricted to it (e.g., preoccupation with food in the presence of an Eating Disorder; hair pulling in the presence of Trichotillomania; concern with appearance in the presence of Body Dysmorphic Disorder; preoccupation with drugs in the presence of a Substance Use Disorder; preoccupation with having a serious illness in the presence of Hypochondriasis; preoccupation with sexual urges or fantasies in the presence of a Paraphilia; or guilty ruminations in the presence of Major Depressive Disorder).

E. The disturbance is not due to the direct physiological effects of a substance (e.g., a drug of abuse, a medication) or a general medical condition.

Specify if:

With Poor Insight: if, for most of the time during the current episode, the person does not recognize that the obsessions and compulsions are excessive or unreasonable

with some drugs (e.g., antidepressants). See the DSM-IV-TR box for diagnostic criteria for panic disorder.

Panic disorder is usually first noted in late adolescence or early adulthood. It may be limited to a single brief period lasting several weeks or months, recur several times, or become chronic. Panic disorder is diagnosed much more frequently in women than in men, and may be related to sudden object loss and separation anxiety in childhood. Physical disorders such as hypoglycemia, hyperthyroidism, and amphetamine or caffeine intoxication must be ruled out before a diagnosis of panic disorder can be made. The ways in which hypoglycemia mimics a panic attack are discussed in the Caring for the Spirit feature on page 372.

DSM-IV-TR | **Diagnostic Criteria for Anxiety Disorders**

DIAGNOSTIC CRITERIA FOR POSTTRAUMATIC STRESS DISORDER

A. The person has been exposed to a traumatic event in which both the following were present:
  1. the person experienced, witnessed, or was confronted with an event or events that involved actual or threatened death or serious injury, or a threat to the physical integrity of self or others
  2. the person's response involved intense fear, helplessness, or horror. **Note:** In children, this may be expressed instead by disorganized or agitated behavior

B. The traumatic event is persistently reexperienced in one (or more) of the following ways:
  1. recurrent and intrusive distressing recollections of the event, including images, thoughts, or perceptions. **Note:** In young children, repetitive play may occur in which themes or aspects of the trauma are expressed.
  2. recurrent distressing dreams of the event. **Note:** In children, there may be frightening dreams without recognizable content.
  3. acting or feeling as if the traumatic event were recurring (includes a sense of reliving the experience, illusions, hallucinations, and dissociative flashback episodes, including those that occur on awakening or when intoxicated). **Note:** In young children, trauma-specific reenactment may occur.
  4. intense psychological distress at exposure to internal or external cues that symbolize or resemble an aspect of the traumatic event
  5. physiological reactivity on exposure to internal or external cues that symbolize or resemble an aspect of the traumatic event

C. Persistent avoidance of stimuli associated with the trauma and numbing of general responsiveness (not present before the trauma), as indicated by three (or more) of the following:
  1. efforts to avoid thoughts, feelings, or conversations associated with the trauma
  2. efforts to avoid activities, places, or people that arouse recollections of the trauma
  3. inability to recall an important aspect of the trauma
  4. markedly diminished interest or participation in significant activities
  5. feeling of detachment or estrangement from others
  6. restricted range of affect (e.g., unable to have loving feelings)
  7. sense of a foreshortened future (e.g., does not expect to have a career, marriage, children, or a normal life span)

D. Persistent symptoms of increased arousal (not present before the trauma), as indicated by two (or more) of the following:
  1. difficulty falling or staying asleep
  2. irritability or outbursts of anger
  3. difficulty concentrating
  4. hypervigilance
  5. exaggerated startle response

E. Duration of the disturbance (symptoms in Criteria B, C, and D) is more than 1 month.

F. The disturbance causes clinically significant distress or impairment in social, occupational, or other important areas of functioning.

Specify if:
Acute: if duration of symptoms is less than 3 months
Chronic: if duration of symptoms is 3 months or more

Specify if:
With Delayed Onset: if onset of symptoms is at least 6 months after the stressor.

Source: American Psychiatric Association (2000). Diagnostic and statistical manual of mental disorders (4th ed., Text Revision) (pp. 440–441, 462, 463, 467–468). Washington, DC: Author.

PHOBIC DISORDERS

A **phobia** is a persistent and irrational fear of a specific object, activity, or situation that results in a compelling desire to avoid the dreaded object or situation. Nearly all phobic individuals experience panic when in contact with the phobic situation. The fear is recognized by adults or adolescents as unreasonable in proportion to the actual danger. However, children do not always identify their fears as unrealistic.

In the development of phobia, fear arises through a process of displacing an unconscious conflict onto an external object symbolically related to the conflict. Thus, in becoming phobic, the individual fears a specific external object rather than an

CARING FOR THE SPIRIT

Can Hypoglycemia Mimic an Anxiety Attack?

Much has been written in the lay press about the dangers of low blood sugar. Some popular authors claim it is a major scourge that afflicts millions of Americans, causing severe psychologic harm.

Postprandial hypoglycemia is a drop in plasma glucose following a carbohydrate load. It can occur after gastric surgery or in the very early stages of diabetes. However, when it has no clear-cut organic cause, it is called functional hypoglycemia.

Functional low blood sugar occurs in two major ways: Epinephrinelike signs and symptoms include nervousness, faintness, weakness, tremulousness, palpitations, sweating, and hunger. Central nervous system signs and symptoms include headache, confusion, visual disturbances, muscle weakness, ataxia, and marked personality changes.

Although there is little controlled clinical research to support the popular media view, psychiatric–mental health nurses should not dismiss hypoglycemia as a hypochondriac's invention. Negating a client's symptoms is akin to accusing the client of lying. Such insults wound the soul by dehumanizing the person. As holistic healers, nurses tend to the spirit by actively listening to the client and demonstrating support in all domains—physical, emotional, cognitive, and spiritual.

unknown internal source of distress. The phobic person can then control the intensity of the anxiety by avoiding the object with which the anxiety is associated.

A diagnosis of a phobic disorder is generally made when the avoidance behavior becomes so extreme or the problem so pervasive that it interferes with the person's normal functional ability. The DSM-IV-TR classifies the phobic disorders into three main types:

1. *Agoraphobia:* fear of being alone or in public places from which escape might be difficult or help might not be available.
2. *Social phobia:* fear of situations in which an individual may be exposed to scrutiny by others or that may be humiliating or embarrassing.
3. *Specific phobia:* fear of specific things.

Agoraphobia

Individuals with agoraphobia often fear leaving the safety of home, worrying that they might develop an incapacitating symptom, such as dizziness, loss of bowel or bladder control, or cardiac distress. Normal activities are increasingly curtailed as the fears dominate the person's life. Agoraphobic people often limit travel and need a companion when away from home. Those who endure the phobic situation experience intense anxiety. Other phobias associated with agoraphobia are listed in ■ Table 16–2.

Agoraphobia without panic attacks is relatively rare. More commonly, people with agoraphobia have spontaneous panic attacks. Most people with agoraphobia have a history of generalized anxiety or anxiety attacks at the onset of the phobic behavior. Onset of this disorder usually occurs in the middle to late twenties. Agoraphobia is more frequently diagnosed in women than in men. Separation anxiety in childhood and sudden object loss appear to be predisposing factors. Depression, anxiety, rituals, minor "checking" compulsions, and rumination are frequently associated features of agoraphobia.

The prognosis is variable. Some less severely disturbed individuals experience intermittent symptoms and may have periods of remission. Those who are more severely impaired may suffer lifelong disability.

Social Phobia

Social phobia is characterized by persistent fear and avoidance of situations in which the person may be exposed to scrutiny by others. The person especially fears being embarrassed. Examples of social phobias are extreme fear of performing or speaking in public, making complaints, or writing or eating in front of others. Other common phobias include fear of interacting with members of the opposite sex, superiors, or aggressive individuals. Usually a person has only one social phobia. This disorder is characterized by overwhelming anxiety and excessive self-consciousness in everyday situations; see the case study on social phobia later in this chapter.

According to the DSM-IV-TR, 10% to 20% of those who have anxiety disorders are also affected by social phobias. Generalized anxiety, agoraphobia, or specific phobia may also coexist with social phobia. Often appearing in late childhood or early adolescence, social phobia usually progresses to a chronic course. Some lessening of symptoms may occur in middle age,

TABLE 16–2 Common Phobias

Fear of	Name of Phobia
High places	Acrophobia
Closed places	Claustrophobia
Water	Hydrophobia
Dead bodies	Necrophobia
Strangers	Xenophobia
Animals	Zoophobia

but the disorder is usually lifelong with only occasional remissions. According to Lipsitz and Schneier (2000, p. 23), social phobia "entails significant economic costs in the form of educational underachievement, increased financial dependency, decreased work productivity, social impairment . . . it is often associated with increased prevalence of other psychiatric disorders including depression and alcohol dependence."

Familial pattern and predisposing factors are unknown and the incidence is evenly distributed between men and women.

Specific Phobia

More common than any other type of phobic disorder, a **specific phobia** is an isolated fear focused on one situation or object, such as darkness, heights, or animals. This category of phobic disorders encompasses all phobias not included in agoraphobia or social phobia. Many specific phobias begin in childhood and subsequently disappear. Those that persist into adulthood rarely go away without treatment. Specific phobia is more often diagnosed in females than in males.

Specific phobias generally cause minimal impairment if the phobic object is rarely encountered and easily avoided; for example, a fear of snakes does not seriously impair an individual living in a high-rise condominium. The phobia can, however, be incapacitating if the phobic situation is frequently encountered and not easily avoided. A fear of heights or elevators would seriously incapacitate a person living in a high-rise condominium. A specific phobia may lead to lifestyle restrictions varying in severity according to the degree of anxiety.

The object or situation avoided determines the subtype of specific phobia. The DSM-IV-TR identifies these subtypes:

- *Animal type:* fear related to animals, birds, or insects.
- *Natural environment type:* fear triggered by elements of nature, such as water, or weather.
- *Blood–injection–injury type:* fear caused by the sight of blood or an injury, or by receiving invasive medical procedures, such as an injection. The vasovagal response often occurs with this type of phobic reaction. There is a strong familial pattern with this subtype.
- *Situational type:* fear resulting from contact with enclosed places, bridges, and/or public transportation.

GENERALIZED ANXIETY DISORDER

Generalized anxiety disorder (GAD) is considered less specific and less debilitating than panic disorder and phobic disorder. GAD is characterized by pervasive, persistent anxiety of at least 6 months' duration but without phobias, panic attacks, or obsessions and compulsions. The person experiences chronic feelings of nervousness and apprehension for no apparent reason and is unable to control the worry. The worry is greatly exaggerated in relation to the probability that the event will actually occur.

People with GAD are unable to stop the worrying, even though they realize that their anxiety is more intense than the situation warrants. Overall, those with GAD are unable to relax. Their excessive worries usually lead to insomnia and are associated with physical symptoms such as muscle tension, headaches, sweating, hot flashes, headaches, shortness of breath, and dizziness. Irritability is a common psychological manifestation of GAD. Autonomic symptoms may be less frequent or less severe than in panic attacks. In order to accurately diagnose GAD, a thorough physical examination must be done to determine the presence of any medical conditions that lead to anxiety. Hyperthyroidism and Cushing's disease are the most common medical causes of anxiety (Gliatto, 2000).

There is little generally accepted information about age of onset, predisposing factors, cause of illness, prevalence, familial pattern, or sex ratio, although there appears to be a more equal sex ratio than in panic disorder. Associated mild depressive symptoms are not uncommon in individuals with generalized anxiety disorder. Although impairment in social or occupational functioning is rarely more than mild, the abuse of alcohol or other drugs may be a serious complication that interferes with effective motivation for treatment.

OBSESSIVE–COMPULSIVE DISORDER

Obsessive–compulsive disorder (OCD) is classified as an anxiety disorder because of the anxiety symptoms that develop when an individual tries to resist an obsession or compulsion.

An **obsession** is a recurring thought that cannot be dismissed from consciousness. These intrusive thoughts are sometimes trivial or ridiculous, often morbid or fearful, and always distressing and anxiety provoking.

CLINICAL EXAMPLE

Ernesto's inability to get the nursery rhyme "snips and snails and puppydog tails" out of his mind is an example of a strange but trivial obsession. Even though Ernesto tried to distract himself with activities, he found the rhyme running through his mind at work and at home, especially when he was trying to sleep at night.

Melinda's obsession was much more ominous. She could not stop thinking that she must kill her children to prevent a worldwide race war.

Other common obsessive thoughts have to do with violence or contamination.

A **compulsion** is an uncontrollable, persistent urge to perform certain acts or behaviors to relieve an otherwise unbearable tension. Most compulsive acts are attempts to control or modify obsessions because compulsive people either fear the consequences or are afraid that they will not be able to control the primary impulse. Although compulsions are attempts to reduce tension, they eventually increase tension because the individual becomes increasingly agitated, unable to decide whether to stop or to continue the compulsive actions.

Typical compulsive acts are endless hand washing, checking and rechecking doors to see if they have been locked, and elaborate dressing and undressing rituals. Such compulsive acts are defenses used to contain, neutralize, or ward off the anxiety related to the primary impulse.

CLINICAL EXAMPLE

Ernesto, the young man who could not dismiss the rhyme from his mind, developed a compulsion that involved ritualistic washing of his genitals to ward off the anxiety generated by his apparently silly obsession.

Melinda, obsessed with thoughts about killing her children, engaged in symbolic rituals of touching religious objects to repel evil influences through magical interventions by the saints.

MediaLink Learning from Clients: OCD Video

Such compulsive acts as counting and elaborately checking routine duties are frequently associated with the fear of failing or making a mistake, or with the need to be perfect.

Obsessive–compulsive people usually fear that they will harm someone or something. They rely heavily on avoidance and are best understood in terms of their control needs. Individuals who develop obsessive–compulsive symptoms have a great need to control themselves, others, and their environment. ■ Table 16–3 lists some common obsessions and compulsions. Obsessions and compulsions have the following features in common:

- An idea or impulse persistently intrudes into the person's awareness.
- A feeling of anxious dread accompanies the primary manifestation and often leads the person to take countermeasures against the forbidden thought or impulse.
- Both the obsessions and the compulsion are ego-alien—foreign to one's self-perception.
- No matter how compelling the obsession or compulsion, the person has enough insight to recognize it as irrational and experience it as a significant source of distress.

Many of the personality traits associated with obsession and compulsion are highly valued in American culture. Success in several professions and occupations demands cautiousness, deliberateness, and rationality. These traits are usually associated with the tendency toward obsession or compulsion. When these personality traits are carried to an extreme, or when the balance between control and impulse expression leads to paralysis, they become a liability. DSM-IV-TR diagnostic criteria for this disorder are listed in the box on pages 370–371.

OCD is equally common in both men and women. For many years, it was believed that OCD was extremely rare. However, a study by the National Institute of Mental Health (1999), discovered that OCD affects approximately 2% of the population, making it even more common than schizophrenia.

Children with Obsessive–Compulsive Disorder

Although OCD is usually diagnosed in older adolescents or young adults, there are some children affected with the disorder. Recently, the NIMH Pediatrics and Developmental Neuropsychiatry Branch (2000) has focused research efforts on **pediatric autoimmune neuropsychiatric disorders associated with streptococcal infections (PANDAS)**. PANDAS is used to describe a subset of children who have OCD and/or tic disorders, such as Tourette's syndrome, and in whom symptoms have exacerbated following streptococcal infections such as strep throat. It is theorized that, as part of the autoimmune response, the antibodies mistakenly affect the basal ganglia, which is believed to be responsible for movement and behavior. Children with PANDAS seem to have dramatic fluctuations in the OCD and/or tic severity; that is, the children have "good days" and "bad days." OCD does occur in children without PANDAS. However, when a child has a very episodic course of OCD/tic symptoms and seems to have strep throat right before or during a dramatic worsening of the symptoms, the possibility of PANDAS should be considered.

POSTTRAUMATIC STRESS DISORDER

Posttraumatic stress disorder (PTSD) is the experience of a significant stressor or trauma, outside the range of usual experience, that is followed by recurrent subjective reexperiencing of the trauma. PTSD includes traumatic stress reactions to military combat, and to criminal and natural catastrophes such as assault, rape, incest, skyjacking, and earthquake.

TABLE 16–3 Common Obsessive–Compulsive Behaviors

Behavior	Related Compulsion	Related Obsession
Repetitious hand washing	Urge to wash, scrub, or clean	Fear of disease or contamination
Returning home often to make sure appliances are turned off	Need to recheck related to self-doubt	Fear of disaster
Hoarding junk mail, receipts, and all types of papers	Need to keep everything	Fear of losing things
Ritualistic counting of number of stairs climbed	Urge to count repeatedly	Belief that counting will yield control and thus prevent making mistakes

CLINICAL EXAMPLE

Bill and Joe, both veterans of Desert Storm, are enrolled in a PTSD program at a veterans' hospital outpatient clinic. Upon returning home from combat, they essentially relived their experiences through recurrent nightmares about missile attacks with biological weapons. They both experienced insomnia and a loss of pleasure in previously enjoyed activities. Both men had trouble concentrating. Bill felt guilty about surviving when other men in his unit did not. Joe felt guilty about the actions he had to take in order to survive.

Children who have witnessed violence in their families, schools, or communities are also vulnerable to developing PTSD.

For a discussion of PTSD as it relates to the experience of rape or incest, see Chapter 21.

The course of PTSD is variable. Most people who have suffered a significant stressor tend to have an acute reaction from which they recover spontaneously. In others, however, the reaction may be delayed or prolonged and eventually become chronic.

PTSD is divided into categories according to onset and duration of symptoms:

- *Acute:* symptoms last less than 3 months.
- *Chronic:* symptoms last 3 months or more.
- *Delayed onset:* at least 6 months have lapsed between the trauma and the occurrence of symptoms.

PTSD can occur in people of any age, including children. Associated symptoms of depression, anxiety, and increased irritability are common, sometimes leading to unpredictable explosions of hostility with little or no provocation.

People with PTSD avoid the stimuli associated with the traumatic event. For example, a women who is raped in an elevator may very likely avoid using any elevator. This example shows how PTSD can restrict daily functioning. A significant complicating problem is the person's use of alcohol or other substances in an attempt to maintain control and soothe emotions. The DSM-IV-TR diagnostic criteria for PTSD are listed in the box on pages 370–371.

ACUTE STRESS DISORDER

A disorder recently defined in the DSM-IV-TR, **acute stress disorder** is the development of anxiety and dissociative symptoms occurring within 1 month of an extremely traumatic event.

CLINICAL EXAMPLE

Samuel worked for a large bond-trading firm located in Tower 1 of the World Trade Center. On September 11, 2001, when a hijacked airplane crashed into the tower, Samuel disregarded announcements over the public address system that the building was safe and to stay at his desk on the 82nd floor. While his coworkers remained on the job, Samuel began the long climb down to the first floor. He got out safely before the building collapsed. Samuel's symptoms of acute stress disorder began 1 week after the traumatic event.

The precipitating stressors are similar to those of PTSD. They include:

- Exposure to a traumatic event in which the individual experienced or witnessed event(s) that involved actual or threatened injury or death.
- A response involving intense helplessness, fear, or horror.
- Dissociative symptoms and avoidance of specific stimuli.
- Symptoms of hyperarousal.

Acute stress disorder is different from PTSD in the following ways:

- The duration is shorter.
- The interval from the trauma to the development of symptoms is shorter.
- The person has at least three of these dissociative manifestations: sense of detachment or numbing, depersonalization, derealization, dissociative amnesia, decreased awareness of surroundings (being in a "daze").
- The dissociative symptoms interfere with effective coping.

Individuals with acute stress disorder may experience depression accompanied by despair and helplessness. Thus, there is a very real danger of suicide. They may feel they are responsible for the outcome of the trauma. For example, if another person was killed in the traumatic event, survival guilt frequently occurs. They often neglect safety precautions and basic needs for daily living.

Biopsychosocial Theories

There are several schools of thought regarding the causes of anxiety disorders. Several theories are discussed below.

BIOLOGIC FACTORS

To understand the biologic basis of anxiety disorders, see ■ Figure 16–1, which summarizes the physiologic responses that occur with anxiety. See also Figure 5–5, which illustrates the sympathetic and parasympathetic divisions of the central nervous system. Notice that they are the same as the fight-or-flight response described in Chapter 5. A major research question that remains unanswered is: Are the physiologic imbalances a *cause* or a *result* of the anxiety disorder?

During the "Decade of the Brain" (the 1990s), research efforts were undertaken to determine a physiologic basis for mental disorders. Much of the research findings indicate biologic changes in the brains of individuals experiencing anxiety disorders. Some of those findings are:

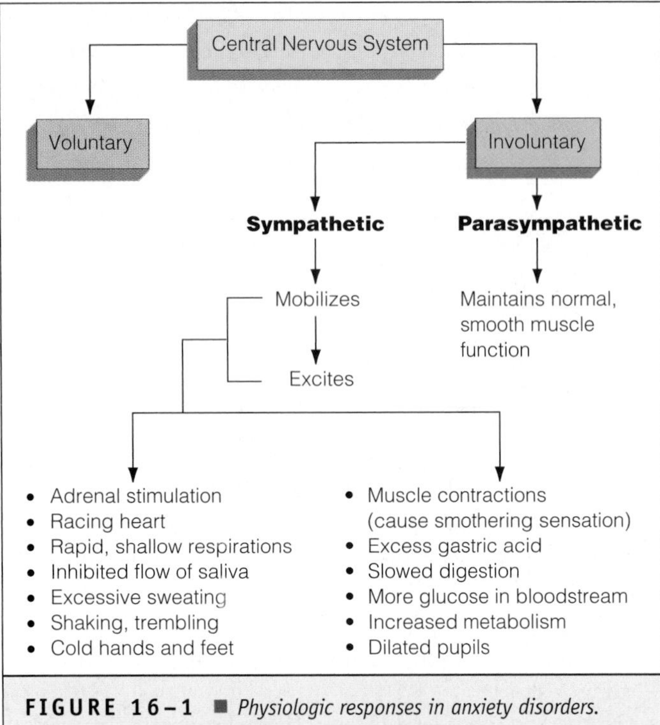

FIGURE 16–1 ■ *Physiologic responses in anxiety disorders.*

- The noradrenergic system in the brain is especially sensitive to the neurotransmitter norepinephrine (NE). One section of the noradrenergic system, called the locus ceruleus (located in the brain stem), appears to be involved in precipitating panic attacks. Drugs that increase the activity of the locus ceruleus have been found to cause panic attacks; drugs that inhibit the activity of the locus ceruleus block panic attacks (see ■ Figure 16–2). Tricyclic antidepressant medications stabilize the locus ceruleus and noradrenergic system; thus, they are sometimes useful in alleviating the symptoms associated with panic attack (Kaplan & Sadock 2000).
- The brain's benzodiazepine (BZD) receptor system is especially sensitive to BZD drugs. The BZDs enhance the action of gamma-aminobutyric acid (GABA), an inhibitory neurotransmitter. With the administration of GABA, or drugs that potentiate GABA, anxiety is reduced. On the other hand, drugs that inhibit the activity of GABA increase anxiety (Kaplan & Sadock 2000). GABA may have a slight tranquilizing effect (Bourne 2001).
- Structural changes have been discovered in the brains of people with PTSD. Specifically, atrophy of the hippocampus was shown in the brains of male Vietnam combat veterans (Sapolsky, 2000). The hippocampus is the area of the brain that regulates memory formulation and retention.
- Changes in another area of the brain, the amygdala, have been noted in people with OCD and other anxiety disorders (Szesko, et al., 1999). The amygdala is the site in the brain that controls fear responses.
- Magnetic resonance imaging (MRI) findings show that those subjects with panic disorder had significantly smaller temporal lobe volume than normal subjects (Vythilingam et al., 2000).
- The reason why females have higher rates than males in most anxiety disorders is unclear, although some theories have implicated the gonadal steroids (U.S. Public Health Service, 2000).
- Lactic acid levels are higher in some individuals experiencing panic attack. Lactic acid may actually precipitate anxiety in some people (Bourne, 2001).
- Many substances increase anxiety levels. Caffeine stimulates the central nervous system (CNS) and increases NE production. In fact, caffeine produces the same physiologic arousal response experienced with exposure to stress. The result is increased sympathetic nervous system activity and a release of adrenalin. Caffeine causes some people to remain in a chronically tense, aroused condition. Some researchers state that caffeine actually triggers panic attacks.
- Nicotine is another substance that is a suspected trigger for panic attacks. Nicotine, which is a strong stimulant, results in increased physiologic arousal, vasoconstriction, and increased blood pressure. Nicotine consumers tend to sleep less well than nonsmokers.

GENETIC THEORIES

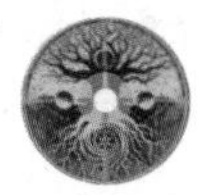

Research evidence indicates that a familial predisposition for anxiety disorders may exist. According to twin studies, there is a genetic factor is OCD and panic disorder (APA, 2000).

First-degree relatives of people with panic disorder are four to seven times more likely to develop panic disorder (APA, 2000). In approximately 25% of individuals with GAD, there is a family history of the disorder (Kaplan & Sadock, 2000).

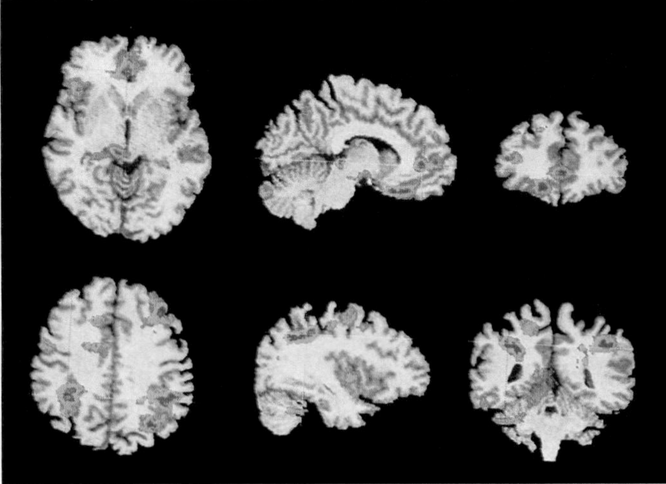

FIGURE 16–2 ■ *Pre- and post-treatment positron-emission tomography (PET) scans of the brain of a person with obsessive–compulsive disorder. This scan is of a client who was administered a selective serotonin reuptake inhibitor (SSRI), which decreased the activity of the caudate nucleus (rCD). LEGEND: Red = most activity, yellow = intermediate activity, blue = little activity.*

Source: Wellcome Dept. of Cognitive Neurology/Science Photo Library, Custom Medical Stock Photo, Inc.

PSYCHOSOCIAL THEORIES

Psychoanalytic theory views anxiety as a sign of psychologic conflict resulting from the threatened emergence into consciousness of forbidden or repressed ideas and/or emotions. The individual fears express the forbidden impulses, which occur in four forms, according to the nature of their consequences:

1. *Superego anxiety,* in which people suffer from anxious expectation of guilt if they break their inner code of ethics and standards.
2. *Castration anxiety,* or fear of fantasized danger or injuries to the body or genitals.
3. *Separation anxiety,* or fear of losing the love, esteem, and caring of significant people.
4. *Id or impulse anxiety,* or fear of the complete annihilation of self.

Other analytic views, sometimes referred to as neo-Freudian, evolved from the work of Freud and differ about the nature of anxiety. Rank (1952) believed that anxiety can be traced back to birth trauma. Sullivan (1953) stressed the importance of the early relationship between the mother and the child and the transmission of the mother's anxiety to the child.

According to the psychoanalytic model, the unconscious conflict must be brought into conscious awareness so that the real source of anxiety can be discovered and resolved. Treatment takes the form of analysis or the less time-consuming psychodynamic psychotherapy.

BEHAVIORAL THEORIES

Behaviorists (learning theorists) view anxiety as a learned response that can be unlearned. For example, behaviorists believe that the cause of phobias is traumatic exposure to the avoided object, situation, or activity. According to this theory, during the development of obsessions, an original neutral obsessive thought evokes anxiety because it becomes associated with an anxiety-provoking stimulus. In compulsions, a person discovers that a certain action relieves anxiety associated with the obsessive thought. The person repeats the action to achieve relief until eventually the act becomes a learned pattern of behavior. Compulsive behavior is viewed as a maladaptive attempt to alleviate anxiety.

Behavior modification is a treatment approach that teaches clients new ways to behave. "Conditioning" techniques—using positive and negative reinforcements—are examples of modification techniques. Another method of treatment is **systematic desensitization,** in which a client builds up tolerance to anxiety through gradual exposure to a series of anxiety-provoking stimuli.

Behavioral approaches are often effective in the treatment of anxiety and are widely used for modifying symptoms in phobic disorder and obsessive-compulsive disorder (see Chapter 30). Behavioral therapists believe it is unnecessary to use insight-oriented psychotherapy to induce clients to struggle with the anxiety. Instead, clients need only face the anxiety repeatedly until it becomes manageable. Behavioral treatment approaches are often used in treating phobic individuals because the methods are more efficient, less costly, and less time consuming than insight-oriented psychotherapy treatment. Like some psychodynamically and psychoanalytically oriented therapists, behavioral therapists tend to avoid the use of medication because they believe it may interfere with the client's ability to learn more appropriate behaviors.

HUMANISTIC THEORIES

The humanistic perspective is particularly important in understanding anxiety disorders. Environmental stressors, biologic factors, and intrapsychic fears or conflicts cannot be adequately dealt with separately but only as they interact with one another. For example, clients suffering from a phobic disorder experience shame and helplessness as they attempt to cope with fears of annihilation in the presence of the dreaded object or situation. The result may be interpersonal and functional withdrawal, creating long-lasting disability.

This perspective has given rise to a multifaceted approach to the care of clients with anxiety disorders. Humanistic treatment approaches are integrative and may include a range of psychotherapeutic interventions, including psychotherapy (cognitive, behavioral, and/or dynamic), measures to develop effective social support systems, measures to reduce environmental stress, and psychopharmacologic treatment.

NURSING PROCESS

Clients with Anxiety Disorders

Chapter 5 covers concepts of anxiety, stress, and coping that are relevant to the care of clients with anxiety disorders; it also covers the general anxiety continuum and the need to identify the client's level of anxiety. The subject of this section is the nurse's role with clients whose anxiety is severe enough to be classified as an anxiety disorder.

Assessment

Clients with anxiety disorders have impaired psychosocial and physiologic function. The emotional disturbances and physical and intellectual changes that take place as a result of extreme or chronic anxiety affect the client's work, school, and social functioning and frequently impair or threaten previously meaningful interpersonal relationships. The clinical manifestations are listed in the Assessment box on page 378. Clients can also review a variety of self-tests for GAD, OCD, PTSD, and other anxiety disorders on www.adaa.org. You can access these self-tests through the Companion Website for this book.

MediaLink Anxiety Disorders: Self-Tests

The occurrence of acute anxiety and its related symptoms is common to a number of physical conditions and acute medical emergencies. Therefore, a careful evaluation should always be conducted. A history and physical examination should rule out such conditions as hyperthyroidism and other endocrine problems, Ménière's syndrome, brain disorders, caffeine intoxication, mitral valve prolapse, and medical emergencies (such as myocardial infarction).

Differentiation from other psychiatric diagnoses is difficult when anxiety and depression are mixed. The question of which one predominates can puzzle many practitioners and necessitates ongoing thorough assessment. Some ways to differentiate anxiety and depression are listed in ■ Table 16–4. Anxiety is part of many other clinical syndromes, such as schizophrenia and mood disorders. The medical diagnosis may be made on the basis of the dominant, most debilitating symptom.

During assessment, determine not only whether the client is anxious (and, if so, to what extent) but also the possible source of the anxiety. Knowing the source will help you plan and implement effective care. For extremely anxious clients, suspend formal data gathering in favor of immediate, direct action to reduce anxiety. Common features of panic attack are listed in the Assessment box.

ASSESSMENT

Guidelines for the Client with Panic Attack

Psychological	Somatic
Sudden onset of:	Sudden onset of:
Intense nervousness or apprehension	Tachycardia or palpitations
Feeling of impending doom or death	Chest discomfort
Mental confusion	Dyspnea
Feelings of unreality	Unsteadiness, dizziness, vertigo
Fear of going crazy or doing something uncontrolled during an attack	Sweating
	Choking or smothering sensations
	Faintness
	Hot and cold flashes
	Paresthesias
	Trembling or shaking

SUBJECTIVE DATA

MediaLink Care Plan: PTSD

Clients with an anxiety disorder may report a variety of physical and emotional symptoms. It is important to encourage clients to describe symptoms in their own words and to explain how the symptoms affect their daily activities. They may report emotional distress, cognitive and perceptual changes, somatic discomforts, and/or role impairments.

Emotional Distress. Clients with anxiety disorders may reveal a number of distressing emotional feelings:

"I feel like something terrible is going to happen."

"I feel helpless; vulnerable for no reason at all!"

"I just can't seem to enjoy life—everything bothers me."

Anger, guilt, feelings of worthlessness, and anguish frequently accompany anxiety. When the anxiety is acute or extreme, as in panic disorder or PTSD, the client feels in immediate danger and may seek protection and reassurance from others. If the anxiety is too severe, however, clients may become immobilized and unable to report their terrifying feelings at all, or they may refuse assistance and run away or become physically aggressive.

Sometimes clients with anxiety disorders may deny the existence of anxious feelings. They try to protect themselves by dissociating these feelings. It is important to recognize clients' anxiety despite their denials. In such instances, assessment requires an especially careful observation of objective data.

Cognitive and Perceptual Changes. Anxious clients frequently have difficulty concentrating and making decisions. Some clients report feeling as if they are "going in circles," unable to think through a problem in order to make an effective decision. They may worry about their effectiveness at work and fear job loss as a result of attention and judgment problems.

In the clinical situation, clients may ask staff members to make decisions for them. At the same time, however, they may express difficulty following through with suggestions, finding many loopholes or possible problems with the plan of action. Other clients become forgetful or misinterpret what they hear.

In extreme anxiety, as in a panic attack, the client is unable to assess a situation accurately and realistically. The client needs immediate attention from and orientation by the nurse. The client may later report having had a frightening feeling of personality disintegration.

Somatic Discomfort. Clients with anxiety disorders may complain of nausea, indigestion, headache, decreased appetite, a constant feeling of fatigue, or other psychophysiologic conditions. They may relate these somatic disturbances to having "bad nerves," or they may be unaware of any psychologic component of their discomfort.

Clients with OCD who engage in repetitive activity, such as compulsive hand washing or hair pulling, may report special health problems (tissue breakdown or hair loss) as a result.

TABLE 16–4 Comparison of Anxiety and Depression

Clinical Manifestations	Anxiety	Depression
Affect	Fear and/or dread	Sadness, despair, helplessness, and/or hopelessness
Insomnia	Initial difficulty in falling asleep	Early morning awakening followed by difficulty returning to sleep
Motor activity	Agitation	Retardation (slowing)
Negativism	Limited to specific areas	Global

Clients with PTSD may report fitful sleep, terrifying nightmares, and a fear of returning to sleep. Common features of PTSD are listed in the Assessment box below.

Role Impairment. Clients may be aware of the impact that emotional, cognitive/perceptual, and somatic changes have on their social, family, and work roles. They report worry about losing their jobs or being unable to continue caring for their families.

CLINICAL EXAMPLE

Gisela despairs that she is unable to take her daughter out to the playground because her phobias prevent her leaving the house.

Abe, a middle-aged accountant, obsessed about tallying his firm's financial data, is unable to put his job aside for the weekend and misses his son's football game. He experiences anger, guilt, and self-recrimination as a result.

OBJECTIVE DATA

In addition to noting general signs and symptoms of anxiety as discussed in Chapter 5, other specific physical, emotional, cognitive, and role performance changes may be observed in very anxious clients.

Physical Findings. Clients with acute or extreme anxiety—clients with PTSD or panic disorder, and clients with phobic disorder who cannot avoid the phobic situation—may experience a panic reaction and show extreme discomfort. Look for acute physical changes, such as breathing difficulty, sweating, trembling, and/or vomiting, during these incidents. The client may be unable to verbalize, or verbalizations may be confused and incoherent. During a panic episode, clients may be so frightened that they refuse help at the moment and may require firm reassurance and protection until the episode subsides.

The client with an anxiety disorder may develop long-term physiologic effects, such as susceptibility to viral infections or the development of ulcers, hypertension, or asthma. Substance abuse may develop into a serious complicating problem when clients try to alleviate anxiety through chemical means. Substance abuse, which frequently occurs in individuals experiencing PTSD, may be the client's attempt to avoid traumatic memories. Other physical findings may be the effects of ritualistic or compulsive activity—skin lesions in a client who obsessively picks at the skin, for example.

Emotional Changes. Family and friends of a client with PTSD may report personality changes in the client including increased irritability, suspiciousness, angry outbursts, and a tendency to blame others and to withdraw emotionally. Remember to pay attention to your own feelings when interacting with highly anxious clients. Because anxiety can be transmitted interpersonally, use self-awareness to determine the source of your own anxiety.

Individuals with phobic disorder and obsessive-compulsive disorder show a lack of emotional distress as long as the phobic object or situation is avoided or alleviated with activity. There may be little spontaneity or active involvement by the client during assessment as rigid, stereotyped behavior patterns are common.

Cognitive Deficits. Unrealistic or distorted perception of a situation is common in anxiety states. During panic attacks, clients may distort or exaggerate details. They may complain about some seemingly insignificant detail. Clients may lose their ability to take in other pertinent data, and thus make errors in judgment. In assessment interviews, clients with an anxiety disorder are often forgetful and unable to concentrate or attend to details. Errors in calculation and grammar are common.

Impact on Role Function. The symptoms of anxiety disorder affect social, work, and family relationships (■ Figure 16–3 on page 380). It is important to understand the possible effects of anxiety symptoms on interpersonal relationships. Obsessive-compulsive acts, for instance, may become so pervasive that they take the place of relating to other people.

ASSESSMENT

Guidelines for the Client with PTSD

Aggressive behavior	Intrusive memories
Avoidance behavior	Memory impairment
Constricted affect	Nightmares
Depression	Panic attacks
Detachment	Phobic responses
Guilty rumination	Poor concentration
Hyperalertness	Repetitive dreams
Impulsiveness	Startle reactions
Insomnia	

CLINICAL EXAMPLE

Vanessa's house is so clean and orderly that you could literally "eat off the floor." Vanessa spends a large amount of her time after work and on weekends making sure that the house is sparkling clean. She prepares to-do cleaning lists for her young adult children to follow when they visit. When Vanessa's husband comes home after traveling on business, he is often met with his own to-do list. Family social activities are put on hold until Vanessa's lists have been accomplished. Vanessa's husband and children complain about having to clean an already clean house. Vanessa is upset that her children are visiting less often and that her husband seems to be spending more and more time traveling on business.

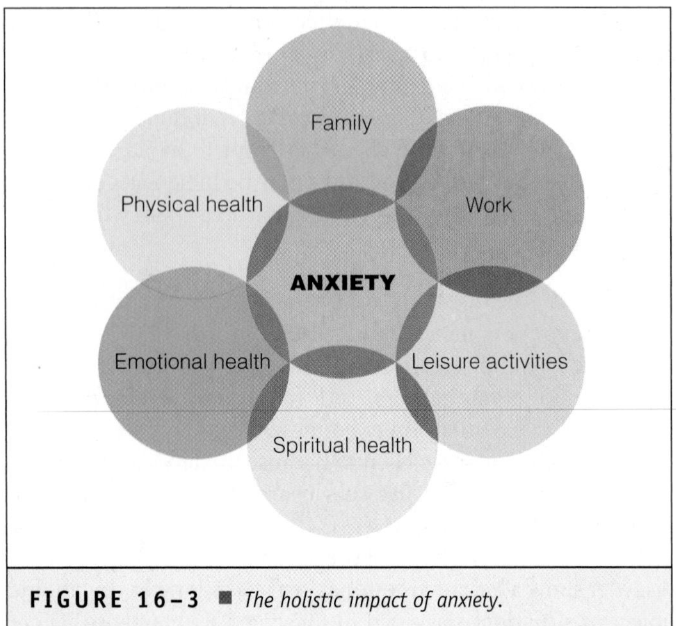

FIGURE 16–3 ■ *The holistic impact of anxiety.*

In other cases, clients may use obsessions and compulsions to negotiate social interactions and social roles. Nurses who plan intervention strategies for clients with anxiety disorders should first assess the impact on the family system.

Client or family member reports that the client is having trouble at work are additional evidence of role impairment. The client may be in jeopardy of losing a job because of poor performance. A person with PTSD, for example, may be fired for absences, drug or alcohol abuse, or for outbursts of temper.

Nursing Diagnosis: NANDA

It is impractical to try to identify all the nursing diagnoses that apply to clients experiencing anxiety disorders. However, there are three fundamental nursing diagnoses pertinent to clients experiencing anxiety disorders:

1. *Fear*—a response to a threat that is recognized as a danger.
2. *Anxiety*—a vague feeling of dread accompanied by an autonomic response; a feeling of apprehension in anticipation of danger.
3. *Ineffective coping*—an inability to form a reality-based appraisal of the stressors, inadequate selection of responses, and/or inability to use available adaptive resources (NANDA, 2001).

Following is a discussion of the three primary nursing diagnoses and other diagnoses that may apply to clients with anxiety disorders.

FEAR

Fearful responses to anxiety can occur on a continuum from slight apprehension to paralyzing terror. One anxious person may state, "I'm scared," whereas another may be filled with alarm and unable to verbalize feelings of panic. In extreme cases of anxiety, panic is communicated through behavioral responses rather than verbalizations.

ANXIETY

Apprehension and tension are emotional experiences common to clients with anxiety disorders.

Clients may worry excessively, ruminating about what might go wrong in the future. They may express anxiety through worry about their physical well-being; somatic preoccupation or hypochondriasis may develop. The potential for substance abuse is high, and suicidal potential is increased. Sexual drive or behavior may also be inhibited by anxiety.

INEFFECTIVE COPING

Excessive anxiety can cause alterations in conduct and impulse control. Some clients, such as those with PTSD or panic disorder, manifest unpredictable behaviors in an attempt to cope with their overwhelming fears. Individuals with OCD are unable to alter behavior, even though they may recognize it as harmful or irrational.

In an attempt to cope, clients with anxiety may turn to substance abuse, which results in disordered conduct and impaired impulse control.

INEFFECTIVE ROLE PERFORMANCE

Anxiety disorders impair performance in the family, at school, and at work. Anxious clients may become less efficient and accurate at work or school because of distractibility or other perceptual and cognitive difficulties. Clients may withdraw emotionally from formerly important and meaningful relationships, or they may become overly dependent on others for help. They may isolate themselves and avoid previously enjoyed activities and recreation. Excessive need for reassurance, decreased productivity, reduced creativity, impaired hygiene, and impaired home maintenance are all possible outcomes for the client with anxiety disorder.

IMPAIRED VERBAL COMMUNICATION

Clients with anxiety disorders often have difficulty communicating. They may speak too quickly, too loudly, may overelaborate, or talk about too many subjects at once. Easily distracted, anxious people may have trouble understanding explanations or retaining information. A client with severe anxiety may be incoherent, making verbal communication impossible. Written communication may also be impaired.

RISK FOR TRAUMA

Impairments in motor behavior are often related to hyperactivity and restlessness, which may place the client at risk for accidental injury. Wringing of the hands, poor coordination, and startle reaction are motor behaviors associated with anxiety disorders. Clients with OCD may perform bizarre repetitive acts, such as repeatedly washing the hands or counting, checking, and rechecking activity. These ritualistic acts often result in self-injury.

DISTURBED THOUGHT PROCESSES AND DISTURBED SENSORY PERCEPTION

Anxiety disorders affect perception, cognition, and reduce the client's ability to solve problems. Judgment, concentration, abstract thinking, and attention are impaired. The client is indecisive but at the same time may make decisions impulsively in an attempt to relieve tension. In panic disorder, the client may become disoriented, misinterpret reality, and distort the meaning of situations or events. Loss of self-esteem and a lowered self-concept often result as the client is unable to use previous skills.

INEFFECTIVE TISSUE PERFUSION

Alterations in circulation and elimination may occur as a result of stimulation of the autonomic nervous system. The client may experience increased blood pressure, rapid heart rate, dizziness, and palpitations as well as dry mouth, cold or clammy hands, sweating, shortness of breath, and a bad taste in the mouth. Diarrhea, enuresis, and slowed digestion may occur.

With extreme anxiety or panic, these symptoms are intensified, and the client may faint or vomit. A medical emergency may arise if the client has an additional major health problem such as cardiovascular disease.

DISTURBED SLEEP PATTERN

Insomnia is a frequent response to anxiety. Nearly all clients with anxiety disorders complain of trouble sleeping. Sleep may be further disturbed by nightmares or night terrors as experienced by people with PTSD.

Outcome Identification: NOC

In order to determine the effectiveness of nursing interventions, expected client outcomes need to clearly identified. When developing client outcomes, you must specifically state the outcomes in behavioral terms. For example, the statement "Mr. Atkins will be less anxious" is ambiguous and not easily measured. However, the statement "Mr. Atkins will participate in one relaxation session per day" is observable and measurable. Outcome identification depends on the client's clinical manifestations. Listed below are some outcomes that generally apply to clients experiencing anxiety disorders:

- Client will demonstrate absence of physical manifestations of anxiety.
- Client will identify indicators of own anxiety.
- Client will verbalize feelings of anxiety appropriately.
- Client will demonstrate the use of new coping skills.

Planning and Implementation: NIC

Planning and implementing care for anxious clients depends on a thorough assessment and determining the appropriate nursing diagnoses. Anxiety, which is communicated interpersonally, often affects the client's family and friends, other clients, and staff members as well. Refer to the Nursing Self-Awareness feature for help in reading your own bodily cues of anxiety.

Most mental health care professionals believe that clients who cope with the stress of anxiety disorders can grow and change with therapeutic intervention. Nursing interventions for clients with anxiety disorders should be geared toward effective coping. Refer to the Case Study and Nursing Care Plan on panic disorder with agoraphobia (see pages 382–383).

Nursing SELF-AWARENESS

Cues to Anxiety

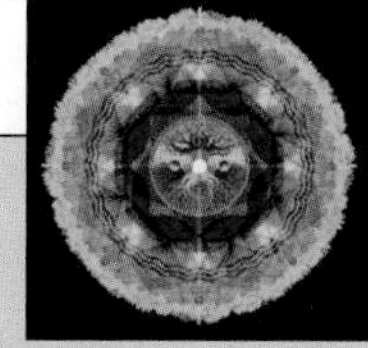

Since anxiety is communicated interpersonally, it is imperative that you are able to read your own somatic clues indicative of increasing anxiety. Which of the following are you most likely to experience when feeling anxious?

Physical Cues	Emotional Cues	Behavioral Cues
Dry mouth	Irritability	Forgetfulness
Profuse sweating	Fearfulness	Short attention span
Urinary frequency	Suspiciousness	Pacing and fidgeting
Nausea ("butterflies" in stomach)	Sadness	Withdrawal

REDUCING FEAR

Fear and anxiety usually coexist. A person who is fearful is generally anxious as well. The clinical manifestations of fear and anxiety are very similar. Thus, when dealing with a client who is afraid, nursing interventions for reducing anxiety (discussed below) are appropriate.

REDUCING ANXIETY

To help clients who are anxious, nurses must understand the operational definition of anxiety. The classic definition by Manaser and Werner (1964) includes the following:

- Expectations or needs are present.
- Expectations or needs are not met.
- Unexpected discomfort (anxiety) is felt.
- Anxiety is controlled and power is restored through some automatic behavior (anger, withdrawal, somatization) that has been effective in restoring control in the past.
- The relief behavior is rationalized or justified rather than explained or understood.

Because anxiety is such an uncomfortable feeling, we learn early in life to reduce it or diminish its effects as soon as possible. Although individuals use a variety of behaviors, the most common automatic responses to anxiety are anger, withdrawal, and somatization. Automatic responses are limiting, rigid, and inflexible and therefore prevent a creative response to the stressor.

Intervening with Clients in Panic. Clients who are extremely anxious or in a panic state require immediate, direct, and structured intervention. During an acute panic attack, perception and personality are disrupted to such a degree that the client cannot solve problems or discuss the source of anxiety. The first priority is to reduce the anxiety to more tolerable levels. The interventions for clients in panic listed in the Intervention box on page 384 can help to alleviate the client's panic. The goal is to reduce the client's immediate anxiety to more moderate and manageable levels. The family of the anxious person needs

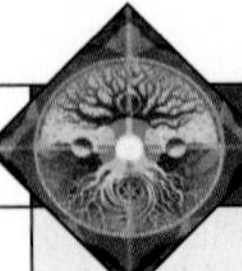

Case Study

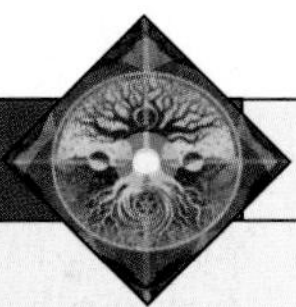

A Client with Panic Disorder with Agoraphobia

Identifying Information

Mrs. R is 43 years old, married and the mother of four daughters in their late teens and early twenties. She was referred to the psychiatric outpatient clinic for follow-up counseling by the emergency department of the local general hospital, where she had been rushed in acute distress the prior evening with symptoms of a panic attack.

Client's Description of the Problem

At the time of the panic attack, Mrs. R believed she was having a heart attack and feared she was dying. She reported racing heartbeat, sweating, and feeling faint. She could not identify any events, thoughts, or feelings that precipitated the incident; it seemed to her to occur "out of the blue." She felt unable to cope with the severity of the symptoms of the attack: "I tried to talk myself out of it; to tell myself it would go away, but it only got worse."

Mrs. R reported she had had similar attacks over the years and that she had always been reassured of her medical and cardiac health, but when these attacks occurred, she "feared the worst" and "lost all perspective." The attacks could last from 2 minutes to 2 hours. Her daily routine had become quite restricted, as she now sought to have one of her daughters or her husband with her when she went out of the home due to fear of an attack. She did not feel comfortable when alone in her home and could not go to sleep if the other family members were not home. She felt ashamed and angry about her growing disability and often tried to cover up her fears to friends and family.

By interviewing the family, the nurse was able to gather information about a number of significant recent life events preceding the panic episode:

- Recent major surgery. A hysterectomy occurred 4 weeks earlier.
- Loss of employment due to her hospitalization. She was abruptly terminated from her position at a new job due to too many absences.
- The upcoming anniversary date of her father's sudden death from a heart attack.

History

Mrs. R had never been hospitalized before for a psychiatric condition, although she had been to the emergency room on three prior occasions with symptoms of panic attack. She had seen a therapist years ago when the attacks first occurred, "about the time I left home to marry." She did not follow up with the therapist, however, saying she felt ashamed ("I've always been a strong and effective person!"), that the episodes were not so severe then, and that she found relief from panic attacks after she had the children.

Both Mrs. R's parents died within the past 6 years. She was especially close to her father, and the second anniversary of his death was approaching. Mrs. R's mother was considered a "homebody"; she rarely left the house and took part in social activities only if they occurred at the family home. Mrs. R wondered if her mother had "these fears" too.

She reported she had begun to curtail social and recreational activities, preferring to stay at home where she was most comfortable.

She described her relationship to her husband as emotionally warm and supportive. Although she sometimes resented his being away from her, she recognized this as part of her "problem" with being alone. Her primary relationships had been with her husband and children. She talked of facing the "empty nest" as her daughters, one by one, left for work or college.

With the exception of chronic gynecologic problems leading to the recent hysterectomy, Mrs. R reported a history of good health. She had no allergies or other chronic illnesses. Her only other hospitalizations were to have her children. The recent hospitalization had been more physically taxing than she expected, and the fact that she was not allowed to return to work after her recovery came as a blow.

Current Mental Status

Mrs. R is an attractive, carefully groomed woman who looks her stated age. She sits erect in the office chair, appearing somewhat tense. She answers questions cooperatively, but at times with some hesitation and as if expecting criticism or judgment from the interviewer.

She is oriented to time, place, and person. Her memory is intact and recall good. She has no difficulty with calculations. Her judgment is unimpaired. During times of panic, however, sensory and perceptive awareness are greatly impaired.

Affect appears normal, with occasional evidence of anger in the form of irritability and light sarcasm. Mood is within normal limits.

Speech is normal in flow and volume. It appears pressured at times when she attempts to correct an impression she believes the interviewer holds. Posture is at times rigid, but she relaxes as she becomes more comfortable with the interview.

There are no delusions, ideas of reference, or hallucinations. Obsessive worry about the occurrence of panic episodes and of her safety are present. Embarrassment and shame over her symptoms are apparent. Suicidal or homicidal thoughts are denied. Associations and abstractions are appropriate, and there is no evidence of thought process disorder or difficulty in concentration, except during acute panic, at which times concentration is impaired and thought processes are disorganized. Some guardedness toward the interviewer is noted. Insight into the meaning of the current situation is minimal.

Other Subjective or Objective Clinical Data

Mrs. R is considering the use of antianxiety medication, despite "hating the idea" of medication.

---

counseling about how to respond therapeutically because they are often present during a panic episode.

INTERVENING INTO LESS SEVERE ANXIETY

A nurse can frequently detect subtle indications of increasing anxiety and intervene to prevent escalation. Some clients are adept at covering up their anxiety, even though their behavior usually transmits cues to the sensitive observer. Often your own feeling of increased tension is a useful cue that the source of anxiety is in the client. Anxiety may make people excessively demanding. Your response to the demands must take into account the consequences for the course of the client's anxiety. In some cases, it may be reassuring to set limits and deny the request. In other cases, such a response may place further stress on the client.

You must know how to treat clients who suffer from prolonged anxiety. The intervention strategies are intended to help

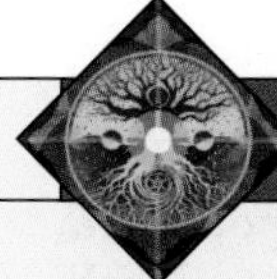

Nursing Care Plan

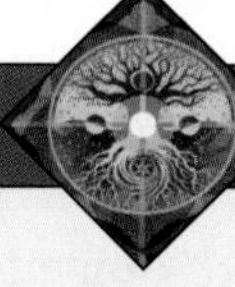

Nursing Diagnosis: Ineffective Role Performance related to fear and anxiety level.

Expected Outcome: Client will demonstrate role performance as evidenced by: ability to meet role expectations, knowledge of role transition periods, and reported strategies for role changes.

Short-Term Goals	*Interventions*	*Rationale*
• Describe specific changes in role function.	• Maintain a calm manner.	• Prevents escalation of anxiety.
	• Stay with the client.	• Promotes safety in client experiencing panic.
	• Use short, simple sentences.	• Facilitates anxious client's ability to concentrate and follow direction.
	• Direct client's attention to repetitive or physical task.	• Provides distraction and serves as an outlet for anxious energy.
	• Administer antianxiety medication.	• Reduces anxiety by altering brain chemistry.

Nursing Diagnosis: Disturbed thought processes related to high level of anxiety.

Expected Outcome: Client will demonstrate ability to choose between two or more alternatives.

Short-Term Goals	*Interventions*	*Rationale*
• Demonstrates appropriate decision making	• Teach relaxation exercises.	• Anxiety impairs the ability to concentrate and solve problems.
	• Encourage client to identify previous coping skills.	• Use of previously learned skills can be used to reduce anxiety level.

Nursing Diagnosis: Ineffective Coping related to overwhelming fears.

Expected Outcome: Client uses actions to manage stressors that tax personal resources.

Short-Term Goals	*Interventions*	*Rationale*
• Demonstrates effective coping as evidenced by employing behaviors to reduce stress; and reporting decreased negative feelings.	• Help client identify coping resources (including social supports).	• Helps client become aware of existing resources.
	• Teach client relaxation techniques.	• Relaxation counters the stress response.
	• Encourage client to verbalize feelings.	• Verbalization reduces stress through process of catharsis.

clients use their anxiety to learn about themselves and their coping strategies. This requires the client to endure the anxiety while searching out its causes. The client must then develop more effective and satisfying coping strategies to replace the old ones. To help clients learn to cope more effectively with anxiety, first detect the anxiety and then make thoughtful observations and responses that facilitate learning. Peplau's (1962) five-step plan of action, which includes the interventions listed in the Intervention box on page 384, is now considered a classic model for nursing intervention with anxious clients.

In working through this step-by-step intervention approach, avoid reinforcing the clients' justifications of their usual ways of coping. Often, clients try to give plausible explanations for their ineffective anger, withdrawal, or somatization. However, these rationalizations do not explain the relief in terms of the factors that caused the anxiety. The relief afforded by the usual coping patterns does not last long because the needs or expectations that originally caused the symptoms still exist. The needs may even become more intense. Clients can begin to change disturbed coping patterns only when they understand what their unmet needs are, what they did instead of fulfilling these needs, and their subsequent feelings.

Anxious clients have two alternatives. They can change their hopes and expectations, or they can try new tactics or resources

INTERVENTION

Guidelines for the Client in Panic

Strategy	Rationale
Stay with the client.	Being left alone may further increase the anxiety.
Maintain a calm, serene manner.	Knowing that the nurse is calm and in control may be calming to the client.
Use short, simple sentences.	Because the client's perceptual field is disrupted, the client will experience difficulty focusing.
Use a firm and authoritative voice.	Conveys the nurse's ability to provide external controls.
Move the client to a quieter, smaller, and less stimulating environment.	Prevents further disruption of the perceptual field by sensory stimuli.
Focus the client's diffuse energy on a repetitive or physically tiring task.	Repetitive tasks or physical exercise can help drain off excess energy.
Administer antianxiety medications if ordered.	Antianxiety medications may help reduce anxiety by altering brain chemistry.

MediaLink Anxiety Disorders: Medications

to get their needs met. Discuss these options with the client, and negotiate a contract to work on one or both goals. Acting on either option involves problem solving.

Simple physical activities often help reduce anxiety to more tolerable levels. Encourage adaptive mechanisms that work such as those in Box 16-1 (see page 385).

You can use a variety of techniques and skills in intervening with clients who experience anxiety. Progressive muscle relaxation, meditation, "thought-stopping" techniques, autogenic training, and guided imagery may help clients learn new ways to reduce the disturbing affect (see Chapters 30 and 32). Other methods include helping clients test reality, because their sense of danger is often out of proportion to actual danger. Developing goal-oriented contracts may help reduce a client's sense of inner chaos by providing structure and direction. The use of contracts also actively involves clients in their own healing process. This involvement increases a sense of control, thereby alleviating feelings of powerlessness.

TEACHING CLIENTS ABOUT MEDICATIONS

Educating clients about the use of medications is one of your essential responsibilities. Clients should be aware of the major drugs used to manage acute anxiety and their limitations and possible side effects. Anxiety that is secondary to major medical illness or acute trauma (such as the death of a child) requires a different dosage than that prescribed for the treatment of primary anxiety. A guide to medications is offered by the Anxiety Disorders Association of America (www.adaa. org) and can be accessed on the Companion Web site for this book.

Antianxiety medication should be used cautiously and sparingly. Certain antianxiety medications (diazepam, for one) are among the most overprescribed and abused drugs in the United States and Canada. Older adults are particularly sensitive to the effects of CNS depression associated with diazepam.

Benzodiazepines have proved effective and relatively safe in controlling situational anxiety for periods of 4 to 8 weeks. Antianxiety agents such as diazepam (Valium) and alprazolam (Xanax), or adrenergic blocking agents such as propranolol (Inderal) are sometimes used.

The last decade has seen significant progress in pharmacologic treatments for anxiety disorders. The selective serotonin reuptake inhibitors (SSRIs) are the class of drugs used most often in treating many types of anxiety disorders. The SSRIs are the

INTERVENTION

Guidelines for Clients with Anxiety

Step of Plan	Nursing Intervention
1. Observe the client for increased psychomotor activity, anger or withdrawal, excessive demands, and tearfulness.	Verbalizations intended to help client recognize and name his experience as anxiety.
2. Connect the feeling of anxiety with relief behavior. The client acknowledges, describes, and names feelings of nervousness or anxiety.	"Are you feeling uncomfortable?" "Are you anxious or nervous now?"
3. Investigate the situation that immediately preceded the feeling of anxiety.	When client says "Yes," he is ready for step 2.
4. Help the client observe, describe, and analyze connections between what led to the anxiety and what happened after. Only through seeing all parts of this experience can the client understand why the anxiety occurred.	Ask client what he does to feel more comfortable when he feels anxious.
5. Formulate the causes of the anxiety. Help the client state the causes. Help the client observe and recall similar instances of anxiety. Through such extensive discussions, the client will eventually be able to recognize and perhaps alter his or her pattern of handling anxiety.	When client understands that when he feels anxious he gets angry, withdraws, or somatizes, he is ready for step 3.
	Encourage client to recall and describe what he was experiencing immediately before he got anxious (including thoughts, actions, and other feelings).

Source: Adapted from Peplau H: Interpersonal techniques: The crux of nursing. The American Journal of Nursing Company. Vol 62, Issue 6, Copyright 1962. Reprinted with permission by Lippincott Williams & Wilkins.

BOX 16-1 Activities that Promote Relaxation

- Soaking in a warm bath.
- Listening to soothing music.
- Taking a walk or doing other exercise.
- Having a massage or back rub.
- Drinking a warm beverage.
- Taking slow, deep breaths to counteract the effects of hyperventilation.
- Doing progressive muscle relaxation

drugs of choice because they cause fewer side effects than the other antidepressants—tricyclics (TCAs) and monoamine oxidase inhibitors (MAOIs). Fluoxetine (Prozac), sertraline (Zoloft), fluvoxamine (Luvox), and paroxetine (Paxil) are some of the SSRIs used most often in treating panic disorder, social phobia, OCD, and PTSD. Venlafaxine (Effexor), a drug closely related to the SSRIs, is used in treating GAD. These medications are started at a low dosage level and gradually increased until a therapeutic level is achieved. Inform clients that it may take up to 2 to 4 weeks before they begin to feel better. This information is crucial in helping clients continue to take the medication. These medications are discussed more fully in Chapter 31.

Although medications may alleviate the symptoms of anxiety, they do nothing to help clients understand the source of their anxiety. These drugs should be used for the short-term treatment of anxiety—days, weeks, or months instead of years.

PROMOTING EFFECTIVE COPING

Coping skills can be taught to clients with every type of anxiety disorder.

Obsessive–Compulsive Disorders. Clients with OCD avoid anxiety by engaging in compulsive acts and rigid thinking. Nurses working in all practice areas will probably encounter an obsessive-compulsive client whose problem is severe enough to require hospitalization. Form a therapeutic alliance with your clients. One way to foster the bond is letting clients know that although their thoughts are irrational, they are rational beings.

Clients with OCD use compulsive rituals to control anxiety. Therefore, time any intervention to avoid increasing the client's anxiety. It is not usually fruitful, and may be countertherapeutic, to interfere prematurely with a ritual unless it is life threatening. Generally, the client needs plenty of time to complete the ritual. When the client is prohibited from, or interrupted when carrying out the compulsive behavior, anxiety escalates. It is best to time therapeutic activities to occur immediately following the ritual because the client's anxiety level is lowered by performing the ritual.

These clients often have a strong tendency toward negativism, which may cause them to become more firmly entrenched in their defenses if modifications are introduced prematurely or hurriedly. Attempt to develop an affirming, dependable relationship before suggesting that clients change their behavior patterns, gradually introducing a substitute behavior. Balance the value of intervening in behavior that protects clients from mental anguish against the need to prevent physical deterioration caused by the behavior.

Posttraumatic Stress Disorder. Clients with PTSD frequently experience behavioral disturbances as a result of the intense anxiety triggered by reexperiencing the trauma. Alcohol or other drugs, when used to relieve anxiety, may contribute to destructive and impulsive acts. Clients often experience disordered family relationships, physical disability, social and recreational disruptions, and impaired ability to work or attend school. They may experience symptoms and attitudes of demoralization that further hamper their functioning. In the acute stage, crisis counseling is essential. Because of the chronic course of PTSD and the many psychosocial problems associated with it, a comprehensive treatment approach is needed.

When planning care for the client with PTSD, determine the type and duration of trauma experienced. Was the trauma a single, brief incident? Several, ongoing incidents? A human trauma (combat or rape)? A natural trauma (hurricane or earthquake)? Natural disasters and human-induced traumatic events can have different effects. For example, a survivor of human-induced trauma (such as rape) frequently experiences more guilt and humiliation. After a natural disaster, a person may discuss feelings of survivor guilt. Clients with PTSD verbalize feelings of no longer being safe and will often exhibit passive and dependent behaviors.

The goal of therapy in treating clients with PTSD is to desensitize them to the memories of the traumatic event so that the ego can gain mastery over the anxiety. The techniques in the Intervention box below may be used singly or in combination.

Recent advances in psychopharmacology have led to the use of medication as an adjunct to the psychologic treatment of PTSD. As is true for the other anxiety disorders, however, you must be aware of the heightened potential for drug abuse among clients. The desire for immediate, total relief is powerful and may foster drug dependence and abuse.

INTERVENTION

Guidelines for Clients with PTSD

Abreaction: Process by which the client recalls painful repressed experiences.

Cognitive therapies: Cognitive restructuring provides new, less threatening interpretations of events. Includes techniques such as thought stopping and thought substitution.

Education: Provides an explanation of the dynamics of the disability and of treatment modalities.

Exercise and nutrition: Strengthens the body's adaptive efforts.

Family conferences: Seeks to provide support to client by encouraging the family to work on resolving the many psychosocial effects evoked by the trauma.

Group therapy: Provides support and reinforces new coping skills.

Hypnosis: Brings repressed materials to conscious awareness so it can be integrated into the ego structure.

Individual therapy: Provides important ego-supportive and/or cathartic benefits.

Relaxation training: Focuses on developing new skills that the client may use when faced with memories of the traumatic event.

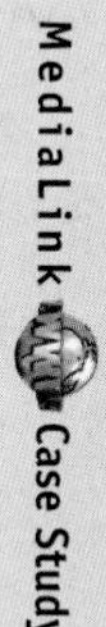

MediaLink Case Study: Compulsive Rituals

BZDs, TCAs, SSRIs, lithium, beta blockers, alpha-adrenergic antagonists, and neuroleptics have all been reported to relieve PTSD symptoms. During the initial stage (4 to 8 weeks), the use of benzodiazepines may be helpful in the treatment of anxiety, insomnia, and nightmares.

Sleeplessness, another common feature of PTSD, is best treated with a behavioral approach such as relaxation techniques, guided imagery, muscle relaxation, and exclusion of daytime naps. Sedatives are discouraged except for very brief use. Your goal is to help the client reestablish the ability to sleep naturally and cope more effectively without relying on the use of drugs.

Phobic Disorders. Clients with phobic disorders attempt to avoid anxiety by binding it to a specific object or situation. It is essential to recognize that forcing clients to come into contact with the feared object or the basic source of their anxiety can create an intense, disorganizing flood of panic.

Many clinicians agree that clients with phobic coping patterns are highly resistant to most insight-oriented therapies. These therapies require clients to confront and at least temporarily experience some of their originating anxiety. It is not surprising that insight-oriented therapists are ineffective with phobic clients, since the phobic's style is basically one of *avoidance*. Some symptomatic improvements have been made using techniques derived from behaviorist theory. The most commonly used interventions are desensitization, reciprocal inhibition, and cognitive restructuring. They are discussed in ■ Table 16–5 and in Chapter 30. Read the Using Research Evidence feature for an example of planning care for a client with social phobia.

Promoting Effective Communication. Nursing interventions that reduce anxiety are important measures to promote more effective communication and behavior. Many times, simply offering the opportunity to acknowledge and discuss feelings of anxiety helps the client regain control. At this point, clients are more likely to share their concerns because you have already taken the first steps in demonstrating genuine interest and concern. See the Rx Communication feature for the client with social phobia.

After encouraging the client to express feelings, listen. Clients may express fear, anger, sadness, disappointment, or alienation, and it may be difficult to hear about the client's pain. Some nurses feel helpless in the face of their client's catharsis and think they should be able to provide ready answers. Instead, ready answers are more likely to interfere with and thwart the client's communication. Genuine, concerned listening without judgment or giving advice is an effective intervention in itself.

Explanations should be simple, clear, and concise. Be careful not to overload severely anxious people with more information than they can handle. If anxiety has contributed to knowledge deficit, reduce the anxiety before trying to teach about health or provide information. If the client's perceptual field (see Chapter 5) is narrow or disrupted, the client will be unable to assimilate information.

Clients with OCD require patience and an unhurried attitude, especially in regard to details and ruminations. If you use the techniques of paraphrasing and reflecting, these clients will say you did not get the details right. They will then go on to correct, qualify, and clarify. This striving for accuracy produces greater vagueness and confusion. It is as if parallel conversations are going on. Clients hear only themselves repeating and correcting insignificant details and completely lose the overall meaning of the message. Developing patience in listening and skill in providing well-timed, simple direction is crucial to working effectively with clients with OCD.

PROMOTING SAFETY

Lack of coordination or tremors make anxious clients prone to accidents. Counsel clients not to perform potentially dangerous activities, such as driving a car, when anxiety is high. Advise them to move more slowly or to go over instructions carefully when they undertake new tasks or use tools and/or equipment.

TABLE 16–5 Cognitive–Behavioral Techniques for Treating PTSD

Technique	Description	Example
Systematic desensitization (exposure therapy)	Client is exposed to a series of increasingly anxiety-provoking situations, beginning with the least threatening. Client gradually becomes desensitized to each stimulus in the series until the stimulus that induced the most anxiety is no longer threatening.	A man who is terrified of earthworms might first talk about earthworms until the topic no longer evokes the same level of anxiety. Then he might be shown pictures of earthworms until he masters that level of closeness. Over time, he will progress to holding a live earthworm in his hand without experiencing severe or panic-level anxiety.
Reciprocal inhibition	The anxiety-provoking stimulus is paired with another stimulus associated with an opposite feeling strong enough to suppress the anxiety.	Through the use of meditation, yoga, biofeedback training, hypnosis, or antianxiety medications, clients learn how to induce a calm state.
Cognitive restructuring	This intervention is based on the belief that anxiety stems from erroneous interpretations of situations. The client learns to reframe (or relabel) a frightening situation, object, activity, or event so that it becomes less threatening.	A woman who feels she is going to die if she leaves her apartment learns to change her perception to one that is more reality based by saying, "I may feel uncomfortable but I will not die. I can do this."

USING RESEARCH EVIDENCE

Charlene is a 21-year-old female client at a community mental health center. During her initial session, she tells you, the admitting nurse, her story: "I couldn't go on dates or to parties. For a while, I couldn't even go to class. My sophomore year of college, I had to come home for a semester. My fear would happen in any social situation. I would be anxious before I even left the house, and it would escalate as I got closer to class, a party, or whatever. I would feel sick to my stomach—it almost felt like I had the flu. My heart would pound, my palms would get sweaty, and I would get this feeling of being removed from myself and from everybody else. When I would walk into a room full of people, I'd turn red and it would feel like everybody's eyes were on me. I was too embarrassed to stand off in a corner by myself, but I couldn't think of anything to say to anybody. I felt so clumsy, I couldn't wait to get out."

The mental health treatment team is meeting to develop a plan of care for Charlene. Treatment modalities will include the following:

1. A thorough assessment: To rule out underlying physiologic problems (i.e., cardiovascular or neurological impairments).
2. Relaxation training: To teach Charlene stress management techniques (i.e., imagery, deep breathing).
3. Cognitive-behavioral group therapy: To reduce anxiety and decrease the risk of potential depression.
4. SSRIs (especially paroxetine): To reduce the anxiety generated by social phobia.

These suggestions stem from the following research:

Baldwin, D., Bobes, J., Stein, D. J., Scharwachter, I., & Faure, M. (1999). Paroxetine in social phobia/social anxiety disorder. *British Journal of Psychiatry, 175*, 120–126.

Hayward, C., Varady, S., Albano, A. M., Thienemann, M., Henderson, L., & Schatzberg, F. (2000). Cognitive-behavioral group therapy for social phobia in female adolescents: Results of a pilot study. *Journal of the American Academy of Child and Adolescent Psychiatry, 39*, 721–726.

PROMOTING OPTIMAL TISSUE PERFUSION AND ELIMINATION

Like communication, circulation and elimination improve when anxiety is reduced. Focus on proper nutrition and adequate activity, because clients with anxiety frequently overlook self-care and their health needs. Walking, participating in sports, and/or developing new hobbies and interests promote healthy physiologic functioning and should be part of a comprehensive treatment plan for anxious clients.

PROMOTING EFFECTIVE SENSORY PERCEPTION AND THOUGHT PROCESSES

To function more effectively and independently, the client needs to know about normal anxiety and anxiety disorders. Providing accurate information at the right time and in an appropriate manner is an essential nursing responsibility. Other strategies to promote effective perception and cognition include the following:

- Use adjuncts to verbal communication, such as visual aids or role play, to stimulate the retention of information.
- Practice problem-solving vignettes to improve judgment and insight.
- Identify misperceptions that clients hold as a result of a narrowed perceptual field. Begin with comments such as "I wonder if you've considered this possibility?" or "Perhaps if we tried . . ."
- Help clients reality-test, that is, explore their opinions in the light of validated experience rather than emotional needs that block accurate perception.

PROMOTING SLEEP

Nonpharmacologic nursing measures to promote sleep should be used before medications. These may include a variety of relaxation techniques. A currently popular method is the use of music that promotes a relaxing atmosphere; listening to the sounds of nature is soothing and sleep-promoting to some people.

Suggest that the client read a boring book in bed, drink warm liquids, or take a warm tub bath before retiring. A client with PTSD may fear going to sleep because of nightmares. Having another member of the family nearby and aware of the client's fear may be reassuring. (Chapter 19 discusses other ways of promoting sleep).

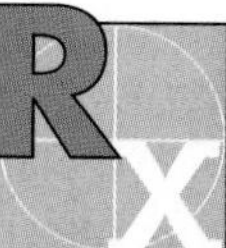

COMMUNICATION

Client with Social Phobia

CLIENT: I just had to get out of that room. I couldn't stand it with all those people looking at me. I thought I was going to die!

NURSE RESPONSE 1: That sounds very frightening. Tell me more about it.

RATIONALE: This response demonstrates reflection of the client's affect and encourages the client to verbalize more feelings.

NURSE RESPONSE 2: Think of other times when you've felt that way. What helped you feel less frightened?

RATIONALE: This response asks the client to identify specific coping methods that were helpful in a similar situation. Such methods can then be used in anticipatory planning for future anxiety-provoking situations.

Evaluation

It is important to evaluate clients in the following areas: anxiety, coping ability, role performance, communication, safety, thought processes, perception, tissue perfusion, and sleep.

ANXIETY

Clients will show no evidence of acute or intense anxiety and be able to perform activities of daily living independently when appropriate. Clients will verbalize feeling less anxious, and they will have fewer somatic complaints. They will state they feel more comfortable.

Clients will have fewer symptoms of physiologic distress, such as racing pulse, diaphoresis, and/or hyperventilation. Clients will be without signs of increased psychomotor activity. They will no longer complain of tearfulness, feelings of rage, or impatience. When appropriate, they will more readily engage in interactions with others. Phobic clients will tolerate the presence of the feared object, activity, or situation without experiencing panic or the need to flee.

INDIVIDUAL COPING

Clients will demonstrate the ability to continue with necessary activities even though some anxiety is present. They will be less likely to panic or flee. Family members will report that the client is "more like himself/herself" and appears less agitated, driven, or explosive in conduct.

The OCD client will limit or cease performing compulsive rituals; for example, a client with a hand-washing compulsion will wash hands no more than four times a day.

ROLE PERFORMANCE

The client will attend work or school on a regular basis. Family members will report that relationships at home have improved and that the client is once again participating in family activities.

Clients will report engaging in recreational or social activity and independently performing self-care. They will express feeling more comfortable about their performance at home, work, or school. Phobic clients will perform daily activities with less restriction or interference from any feared object, activity, or situation.

COMMUNICATION AND SAFETY

Clients will state satisfaction with their communication; they feel heard and understood. There will be open lines of communication between client and nurse and client and family. Clients will report no tremors and will not have accidents due to poor motor coordination. They will report being able to perform usual small motor tasks, such as writing, in a competent manner.

THOUGHT PROCESSES AND PERCEPTION

Clients will recall information taught by the nurse. They will begin to make decisions about their health care and ask questions about the anxiety process.

Clients will describe what led to their anxiety and what happened after they felt anxious. They will verbalize techniques to reduce anxiety.

Clients will correctly verbalize the use, side effects, and results of taking their medications. They will verbalize increased awareness of their environment.

TISSUE PERFUSION

Clients will report feeling energetic. Somatic complaints will decrease, and clients will report engaging in daily physical activity. Vital signs will be normal, and weight will be stable.

SLEEP

Clients will sleep through the night without medication or with appropriately prescribed medication. They will have fewer nightmares or wake less frequently during the night.

Community-Based Care/Case Management

Individuals with anxiety disorders and somatoform disorders are usually aware that their behaviors are problematic to themselves and others, whereas people with dissociative disorders usually lack this insight. However, insight alone does not necessarily result in behavioral changes. Or, when change does occur, it is a very gradual process. As a result, people with anxiety disorders, somatoform disorders, and dissociative disorders are often treated in the community—in mental health clinics, crisis centers, and therapists' offices.

The case manager plays an essential role by collaborating with clients and families and significant others by providing information on when to seek help and where to seek help. The case manager also monitors clients for adherence to the aftercare plan, including the client's medication usage. Issues to be considered during outpatient therapy include: identifying personal strengths, establishing realistic time frames for outcomes, identifying and strengthening support systems, and locating community support services.

Home Care

Nurses who provide psychiatric–mental health care in the home setting are significant in helping clients with anxiety, dissociative, and somatoform disorders to improve their social interactions and to help shape behavior. The following interventions are especially helpful for homebound clients experiencing these disorders:

- Meet with client and family member or significant other to discuss realistic expectations for the client.
- Teach the client home management skills necessary for independent living.
- Ask client if testing, placement services, or job skill retraining are desired.
- Refer to community agencies as needed.

Somatoform Disorders

The essential features of **somatoform disorders** are physical symptoms suggesting physical disorders for which there is no evidence of organic or physiologic causes.

CLINICAL EXAMPLE

Tom has a form of somatoform disorder called conversion disorder. He is unable to walk despite the absence of any medical evidence.

Somatoform disorders, formerly referred to as psychosomatic disorders, are sometimes confused with physical disorders. Educational information about somatoform disorders is available on www.psyweb.com and can be accessed through the Companion Website for this book.

FACTITIOUS DISORDER

Somatoform disorders may also be confused with **factitious disorders** in which clients consciously produce physical or psychological symptoms (APA, 2000).

CLINICAL EXAMPLE

Thelma takes anticoagulants to produce blood in her urine. Ron dislocates his shoulder on purpose. Both Thelma and Ron do this in order to assume a dependent role.

A rare form of factitious disorder is **Munchausen by proxy syndrome (MBPS)**, in which a caregiver fabricates or causes symptoms of an illness in another person. In MBPS, caregivers injure their victims in order to gain sympathy or attention for themselves. The DSM-IV-TR (APA, 2000) refers to MBPS as "factitious disorder by proxy" and designates four diagnostic criteria for the disorder:

1. The intentional production or feigning of signs or symptoms in another person.
2. The perpetrator's behavior is motivated by the need to assume the sick role by proxy.
3. There are no external rewards (such as monetary gain) for the behavior.
4. The behavior is not accounted for by another disorder.

CLINICAL EXAMPLE

A mother has been regularly and deliberately administering large doses of laxatives to her 15-month-old toddler over a period of several months. When the child has episodes of cramping, flatulence, and bloody diarrhea, the mother, appearing to be very concerned, takes her to the emergency department of a local hospital. Diagnostic studies show no medical reason for the toddler's symptoms.

According to Pasqualone and Fitzgerald (1999, p. 59), "The MPBS caretakers, especially mothers, have an insatiable need to bring attention to themselves . . . regardless of the harm that is caused to their children."

Malingering is a term that refers to deliberately faking symptoms in order to benefit. Malingering, like factitious disorder, is consciously motivated and usually results in secondary gain.

CLINICAL EXAMPLE

Joyce is a police officer. She fakes episodes of back pain in order to avoid street patrol.

The distinctions between somatoform disorder, factitious disorder, and malingering are listed in ■ Table 16–6.

SOMATIZATION DISORDER

The diagnosis of **somatization disorder** applies to clients who have sought medical attention for recurrent and multiple somatic complaints of several years' duration and seemingly without physiologic causes. Historically, somatization disorder has been referred to as "hysteria," "hysterical reaction," and "Briquet's syn-

TABLE 16–6 Comparison of Somatoform Disorder, Factitious Disorder, and Malingering

Somatoform Disorder	Factitious Disorder	Malingering
Symptoms are not under voluntary control	Symptoms are intentionally produced	Symptoms are feigned (consciously produced)
Unconscious motivation	Motivated to assume sick role in order to obtain medical treatment	Motivations are varied: avoiding duties, monetary gain, obtaining drugs
Primary gain: anxiety reduction	No obvious secondary gain	Obvious secondary gain(s) or payoffs

MediaLink Somatoform Disorders Resources

drome." This problem usually begins before the age of 30, has a chronic course, and is often accompanied by anxiety and depressed mood. Clients believe they have been sickly for a good part of their lives and report lengthy lists of symptoms, including blindness, paralysis, convulsions, dysmenorrhea, nausea and other gastrointestinal difficulties. These symptoms are not caused intentionally, nor are they feigned. The pain experienced by individuals with somatization disorder is real. Psychogenic pain hurts just as intensely as pain with a biologic basis.

Even though somatization is common in children, somatization disorder is rarely diagnosed in children and adolescents. Children who are diagnosed with somatization disorder tend to have caregivers who consistently overreact to the somatic complaints, thus reinforcing the complaints.

CONVERSION DISORDER

In conversion disorder, clients report impaired physical function that suggests a physical disorder that is related to the expression of a psychologic conflict. Symptoms in conversion disorder are not consciously produced. Two mechanisms are thought to explain what a person "gets" from having a conversion disorder. The first, primary gain, helps the person keep the psychologic need or conflict out of conscious awareness. For example, a woman may become "blind" to avoid acknowledging a traumatic event she has seen. In this instance, the symptom is a partial solution to the underlying conflict (not having to acknowledge witnessing the traumatic event because she has suddenly been struck blind). The second mechanism, secondary gain, helps the person avoid a distressing, uncomfortable, or repugnant activity while at the same time receiving support from others. For example, a soldier with a paralyzed arm could hardly be expected to fire a gun and is also likely to receive sympathy for his paralyzed condition.

The problem usually begins in adolescence or early adulthood, although a conversion disorder may appear at any time of life. Regardless of the time of onset, a conversion disorder can seriously impede normal life activities.

PAIN DISORDER

In pain disorder, clients experience pain in the absence of physiologic findings and the presence of possible psychological factors. The pain is usually severe enough to disrupt several functional areas. As a result of this dysfunction, the client often experiences unemployment, disability, and/or family problems. A person with Pain Disorder is often convinced that somewhere there is a health care provider who can "cure" the pain. Thus, the person may spend much time, money, and energy needlessly in pursuit of a "cure." The pain becomes the central issue of one's life; pain takes control of one's ability to function.

HYPOCHONDRIASIS

Clients with hypochondriasis are preoccupied with the fear or belief that they have a serious disease, which on physical evaluation is not present. The preoccupation may be built around any of the following:

- Bodily functions (peristalsis, heartbeat).
- Minor physical problems (an occasional headache, a slight cough).
- Ambiguous, vague physical feelings ("tired ovaries" or "aching veins").

The unrealistic fear or belief persists for a period of at least 6 months despite medical reassurance. This fear impairs the social or occupational functioning of the client.

BODY DYSMORPHIC DISORDER

Clients with body dysmorphic disorder are preoccupied with some imagined defect in physical appearance. The preoccupation is out of proportion to any actual abnormality. The belief, even though it may be extreme, is not of delusional proportion.

People with body dysmorphic disorder often use avoidance to cope with their perceived defect(s). The avoidance may result in extreme social isolation. For example, a man who tries to camouflage his "defect" of imaginary hair loss may leave his home only at night, and then only with a hat covering the "defective" part. The preoccupation with one's appearance is very time consuming; thus, it restricts activities.

UNDIFFERENTIATED SOMATOFORM DISORDER

In undifferentiated somatoform disorder, clients have multiple physical complaints lasting at least 6 months, and extensive evaluation reveals no organic problem. When there is related organic disease, the complaints or impairments are grossly excessive. Remember that the symptoms experienced by an individual with this disorder are not intentionally produced. The pain, which is psychogenic in nature, is real to the client.

Biopsychosocial Theories

Biologic, genetic, and psychosocial theories help to understand somatoform disorders.

BIOLOGIC FACTORS

In somatoform disorders, physical symptoms are present but evidence of physiologic disorder is not. The symptoms are thought to be linked to psychologic factors or emotional conflict. However, there is some evidence that brain abnormalities may lead to altered pain perception (Bourne, 2001; Kaplan & Sadock, 2000). Biochemical imbalances, such as decreased amounts of endorphins and serotonin, may cause some people to experience pain more intensely than those with normal brain chemistry.

GENETIC THEORIES

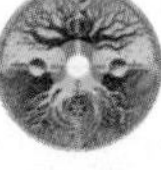

Somatization disorder occurs in 10% to 20% of female first-degree biologic relatives of women with somatization disorder (APA, 2000). The results of adoption studies indicate that both genetic and environmental factors contribute to the risk for somatization disorder (APA, 2000). Other studies with identical twins have shown an increased occurrence of hypochondriasis (Kaplan & Sadock, 2000). A genetic basis has not been determined.

PSYCHOSOCIAL THEORIES

Communication theorists believe that manifestations of somatization are really nonverbal body language intended to communicate a message to significant others. Sometimes the message is as general as "pay attention to me" or "take care of me." At other times the *conversion of anxiety* actually symbolizes the nature of the specific underlying conflict. For example, a woman who wants to strike her children may develop a paralysis of her arm. A girl who feels guilty about reading erotic books may become blind. Both experience the primary gain of protection from the anxiety-provoking impulses, and both get secondary gains of attention and sympathy as well. Such patterns are most likely to occur among clients who lack appropriate coping skills.

Many somatizing individuals were reared in chaotic families. The family dysfunction was usually marital discord, substance abuse, and/or personality disorders. Many somatizing people suffered physical or sexual abuse as children. For whatever reason, the child received inadequate nurturing.

Clients who deal with anxiety by converting it to physical symptoms usually show no other psychological symptoms, such as disturbed thoughts or depressed moods. However, they often exhibit subtle behavior patterns. For example, characteristics associated with conversion disorder clients are self-dramatization, exhibitionism, narcissism, emotionalism, seductiveness, dependence, manipulativeness, childishness, and suggestibility.

Pain is associated with a great many disease processes, including some of the organ-specific somatoform disorders. Pain can be adaptive or maladaptive. It often indicates real danger to the organism, but sometimes it interferes with functioning. Consciousness, attention, perception, and cognition are all necessary for the experience of pain. According to modern theories of pain perception, humans have a control system over pain that operates as a "gate." Pain stimuli can be "allowed in" or "shut out" from the cerebral cortex, depending essentially on the meaning the person attaches to the stimulus. This underscores the importance of meaning, symbol, and affect in the experience of pain sensation.

■ Figure 16–4 shows the basic mechanism for so-called idiopathic pain (pain of unknown origin). In psychoanalytic concepts, the unconscious conflicts are a result of traumatic or frustrating childhood experiences that are reawakened in adult life by a similar stress or frustration. According to this theory, the person cannot express the affect because of feelings of guilt, fear of loss of love, or fear of retribution. The affect is therefore repressed and transformed into physiologic correlates, such as pain.

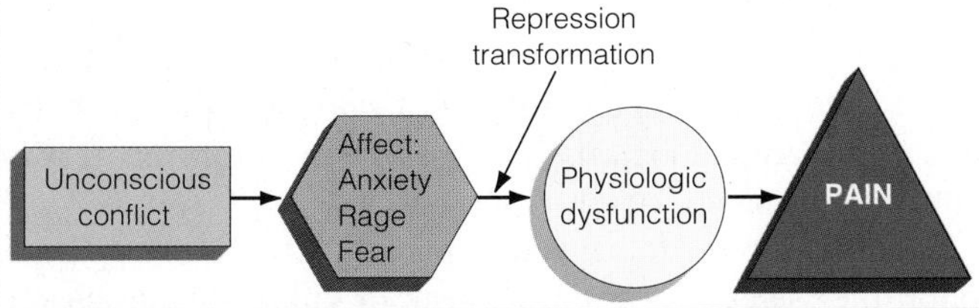

FIGURE 16–4 ■ *The mechanism of idiopathic pain.*

NURSING PROCESS

Clients with Somatoform Disorders

A thorough assessment carefully considers both subjective and objective data.

Assessment

Assessment of clients with somatoform disorders is complex because of the many psychobiologic factors involved. Careful and thorough assessment to rule out the possibility of a physical problem is crucial, as the following example suggests.

CLINICAL EXAMPLE

Magda was referred for treatment to a local mental health clinic by her primary care physician. She had weakness and numbness of her right arm. When her primary care physician could find no physiologic reason for Magda's symptoms, he diagnosed her problem as a conversion disorder. The psychiatric–mental health nurse who admitted Magda to the clinic performed a thorough physical assessment and history. The medical history revealed that Magda had surgery on her left kidney 3 months ago. The psychiatric–mental health nurse made the connection between the surgical position (on her right side) necessary to perform Magda's surgery and Magda's symptoms. The numbness and weakness were actually caused by pressure on the brachial plexus in her right arm during surgery. Magda was discharged from the mental health clinic and referred for physical rehabilitation.

In this instance, a careful assessment of all factors identified the treatment Magda needed and spared her from a stigmatizing psychiatric diagnosis.

SUBJECTIVE DATA

Clients with somatoform disorders report physical symptoms for which there is no positive evidence of organic or physiologic cause. Clients with hypochondriasis, for example, may return many times to the outpatient clinic or emergency department, demanding to be reexamined or retested. They feel they are suffering from some major illness that has been undetected. They are not reassured by the lack of physical findings and may go from doctor to doctor in an attempt to find someone who will validate their fears. This "doctor shopping" may lead to overmedication. Because the person is usually a poor historian, a complete medical history (including medications taken) is not always obtained. Although individuals with somatoform disorder usually describe their condition with colorful, exaggerated words, it is difficult to obtain specific facts about previous medical and surgical treatments.

In conversion disorder, the individual has loss of or an alteration in function.

CLINICAL EXAMPLE

Remember Tom, the client who is unable to walk? Although Tom stated, "I woke up this morning with no feeling in my legs; for some reason they won't move," he seems totally unconcerned about his problem despite its severity.

An inappropriate lack of concern about their disabilities—la belle indifférence—is characteristic of such clients. This nonchalant attitude toward physical problems indicates that the symptom is providing primary gain; that is, the anxiety is alleviated through the conversion process. The person is calmer as a result of the somatic symptom.

In contrast, clients with somatization disorder or hypochondriasis are overly dramatic and emotional in telling about their symptoms and pain. They report the history in vivid detail and colorful language but often pay more attention to how the symptoms have affected relationships in their lives than in giving careful description of the nature, character, location, onset, and duration of the symptoms.

Clients with body dysmorphic disorder may request unnecessary operations—for example, demanding cosmetic surgery for an imagined or greatly magnified defect in appearance.

Careful interviewing frequently reveals a stressful life situation with which the client is not coping, suggesting that the preoccupation with somatic disorder is a way of avoiding underlying conflict. Helping the client identify and express feelings is a crucial beginning to psychotherapeutic intervention.

OBJECTIVE DATA

Physical examination reveals no organic evidence for the symptoms of the client. Laboratory findings likewise do not substantiate organic or physiologic disorder. Despite this, the client may have undergone many exploratory procedures without relief or diagnosis.

Family members often report that the client is moody, self-centered, or demanding. They feel alienated from the client and are frustrated with the client's chronic preoccupation with physical symptoms. In a health care setting, these clients often create scenes that bring them the attention they need without regard for the needs of either fellow clients or staff. Nurses frequently find it difficult to be kind, understanding, and nonjudgmental with these clients. Nurses who do not cope with their own reactions to these clients cannot work with them effectively. Recognizing the client's somatization as part of the illness will help you to avoid personalizing the behavior. It may help to remember that these clients do not intentionally produce their symptoms, nor do they appreciate the effects of their behavior on other people. Nurses who understand the psychopathology of the disorder usually have more empathy for a client's coping style.

Nursing Diagnosis: NANDA

Five major nursing diagnoses applicable to individuals with somatoform disorders are discussed below.

IMPAIRED VERBAL COMMUNICATION

Clients with somatoform disorders have an impaired ability to communicate their needs. Though they may be highly verbal, careful listening reveals many gaps, oversimplifications, overdramatizations, and overgeneralizations in the clients' stories. Somatoform disorders are considered nonverbal substitutes for the expression of underlying conflicts.

INEFFECTIVE ROLE PERFORMANCE AND INTERRUPTED FAMILY PROCESSES

The manipulative and dependent behaviors of the client with a somatoform disorder lead to impairment in social, work, and family relationships and to diminished performance in these roles. Friends and relatives eventually tire of the demands and become less available for support. Clients become emotionally isolated because their self-absorption makes them unable to respond appropriately to the needs of others.

Work performance suffers from frequent absences due to imagined illness. Preoccupation with health status uses up creative energy that could otherwise be directed toward work.

INEFFECTIVE COPING

Clients with somatoform disorders experience anxiety, anger, and feelings of helplessness. They may feel these emotions acutely and demonstrate these feelings excessively, as in somatization disorder and hypochondriasis. Paradoxically, they may show an uncanny lack of feeling, as in the blithe reaction to loss of physical function in conversion disorder.

The client's emotions become increasingly restricted. The focus of emotional experience becomes somatic concerns, and clients no longer experience meaningful emotional connections with other people, activities, and events. Range of emotional expression may be limited to making demands, manipulation, and symbolic manifestations of anxiety.

DISTURBED THOUGHT PROCESSES AND DISTURBED SENSORY PERCEPTION

Clients with somatoform disorders show selective inattention; that is, they filter out stimuli as a response to anxiety. Judgment is often impaired. In a further effort to prove their ideas, they distort reality and tend to ramble. It is evident to the nurse that conclusions are not logical. Clients may also distort memory or show selective memory as well.

Clients with somatoform disorders have a body image disturbance; they sense that they are weak or vulnerable physically. They perceive sensory data incorrectly. For example, they may perceive abdominal discomfort as cancer rather than indigestion.

Outcome Identification: NOC

Expected outcomes are individualized for each client according to personal needs and the situation. Listed below, however, are some expected outcomes that are fairly common to those experiencing somatoform disorders. The client will:

- Demonstrate the ability to cope with anxiety through the use of a new stress management skill (i.e., deep breathing).
- Verbalize feelings instead of expressing them symbolically through physical symptoms.
- Express an increased degree of comfort regarding each physical symptom.

It is essential that the nurse and client work together in establishing expected outcomes. Significant others should also be included in the planning process to help assist the client in achieving the goals.

Planning and Implementation: NIC

Effective intervention involves the following:

1. Recognizing and understanding the life problem or adjustment the client is facing.
2. Recognizing and understanding the client's self-perception as being unable to cope.
3. Helping the client identify and learn more effective ways of adapting.

These steps may be accomplished by insight-oriented or supportive psychotherapy, behavior modification, hypnosis, or any of several other psychologic, as well as some physical, therapies. None can claim superior effectiveness, and new approaches and techniques are indicated when traditional ones prove inadequate.

It is important to recognize that many clients with somatoform disorders are highly resistant to change. Thus, progress may be slow and recovery partial.

PROMOTING EFFECTIVE COMMUNICATION

After assessing the meaning behind the client's communication patterns, plan intervention strategies that enhance the client's verbal communication and self-esteem to the point where the client feels ready to face problems. See the Rx Communication feature for the client with Somatoform Disorder.

Establishing a trusting relationship is key to effective therapy with a somatizing client. It is usually necessary to help these clients tone down their characteristic extravagances. Express respectful skepticism regarding their oversimplifications and overdramatizations. A communication group gives clients the opportunity to receive feedback about the effect of their behavior on others.

PROMOTING IMPROVED ROLE PERFORMANCE AND FAMILY PROCESSES

Working with the family is especially important for clients with somatoform disorders. Educate the family and the client about the disorder, stressing the importance of avoiding unnecessary surgical or medical procedures. Encourage independent functioning and reduce the possibility of secondary gain by not focusing on physical symptoms. Assume a matter-of-fact, supportive attitude, with the optimistic expectation that the client will return to functioning in work, family, and social roles.

PROMOTING EFFECTIVE COPING

The goal of counseling clients with somatoform disorders is to help them express their conflicts verbally rather than acting them out through symptomatic behaviors. The aim of long-term (insight) therapy is to promote effective emotional expression by exploring the sources of anxiety. It is a real challenge for nurses to help clients with somatoform disorders acknowledge the effects of psychosocial stress on symptoms. Supportive therapy seeks to improve self-esteem, perhaps through such measures as expanding clients' interest in their environment.

In general, try to avoid reinforcing the client's symptoms. A well-known psychiatric axiom that applies to clients in this general category is: Ignore the symptoms but never the client. Concentrating on the physical symptom by trying to get a "paralyzed" client to walk or a "blind" client to see again is giving the symptom more importance than it merits, thus increasing the secondary gain associated with it. Ultimately, this merely makes it harder for the client to relinquish the symptom.

PROMOTING IMPROVED PERCEPTION AND THOUGHT PROCESSES

Help clients improve their capacity for perception and thinking by supporting general measures to reduce anxiety. Maintain a

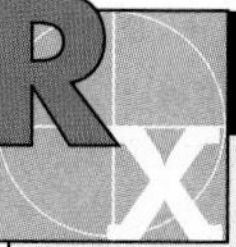

COMMUNICATION

Client with Somatoform Disorder

CLIENT: How can they help me get better if they can't even figure out what's wrong with me? I know I'm really sick.

NURSE RESPONSE 1: It sounds as if you are feeling hopeless.

RATIONALE: This response focuses on the client's feelings and encourages further exploration. It also is a way to determine suicidal ideation that may be related to the client's hopelessness.

NURSE RESPONSE 2: It must be very frustrating for you. All the exams and tests show no physical cause for your symptoms.

RATIONALE: This response demonstrates empathy while at the same time presenting reality. Reassurance that no organic pathology has been found helps dispute the client's delusions.

calm, unhurried attitude toward the client, listen carefully, and maintain an objective undistorted view of reality. Avoid a premature challenge to the client's symptoms and complaints. As clients gradually relinquish their defenses, propose other ways of understanding the condition, such as by suggesting a psychologic explanation for a physical complaint.

Evaluation

Consider communication, role performance, coping, perception, and thought processes when evaluating clients with somatoform disorder.

COMMUNICATION

Clients will more regularly express feelings and conflicts verbally. They will have fewer physical complaints and fewer somatic symptoms. Conversation with the client will "flow," with fewer monologues by the client and more natural dialogue between client and nurse. In other words, the client's communication will become spontaneous.

MediaLink Clinical Evidence for Dissociation

ROLE PERFORMANCE AND FAMILY PROCESSES

Clients will attend work regularly without frequent absences due to illness or worry about physical health. They will be more interested in outside activities and may begin to engage in socialization and recreation. Family and friends will report being more satisfied with their relationship with the client and will be more willing to interact with the client socially.

COPING

Clients will be less demanding, manipulative, and attention-seeking in interactions with others. They will appear less anxious and will talk about subjects other than their current physical status. They will appear less helpless and more able to participate in and make responsible decisions about their health care. For example, they may carry out a plan of treatment without voicing innumerable objections or worries. They will appear more interested and involved in the activities and attitudes of others and be more aware of the impact of their own behavior.

PERCEPTION AND THOUGHT PROCESSES

The client will distort and misinterpret reality less frequently. Judgment, insight, and memory will improve as a result of reduced defensiveness in perception and cognition. Clients may report feeling more positive about their bodies. They will be more assertive in physical activities because they no longer tend to feel so vulnerable.

Community-Based Care/Case Management/Home Care

Community-based care, case management, and home care for clients with somatoform disorders has been discussed earlier in this chapter. See page 388.

Dissociative Disorders

Dissociative disorders have, as their common denominator, the defense mechanism of dissociation, in which the client strips an idea, object, or situation of its emotional significance and affective content. Dissociative disorders are complex and are usually difficult to distinguish from one another. They share another characteristic: In any dissociative disorder, a cluster of related mental events is beyond the client's power of recall but can return spontaneously to conscious awareness. Dissociative disorders are not attributable to mental disorders that have an organic basis.

Dissociative disorders are commonly identified in adult survivors of childhood sexual abuse (Schwartz, 2000). See Chapter 21 for a discussion of dissociation and recovered memory in childhood sexual abuse.

DISSOCIATIVE IDENTITY DISORDER

Formerly known as multiple personality disorder, **dissociative identity disorder (DID)** is the presence of two or more distinct personalities within one individual. Each personality, at some time, takes full control of the person's behavior.

CLINICAL EXAMPLE

Anna is on trial for arson. She denies setting her employer's business on fire. Instead, Anna claims that Zoe, an evil personality that resides within her, is responsible.

There is much controversy about dissociative identity disorder. Many professionals are skeptical that such a phenomenon exists. However, clinical evidence of the existence of DID abounds. Refer to the Web site for the International Society for the Study of Dissociation (www. issd.org) which can be accessed through the Companion Website for this book.

DISSOCIATIVE FUGUE

A person with **dissociative fugue** wanders, usually far from home and for days at a time. During this period, clients completely forget their past life and associations; but unlike people with amnesia, they are unaware of having forgotten anything. When they return to their former consciousness, they do not remember the period of fugue. Clients experiencing dissociative fugue are generally reclusive and quiet, so their behavior rarely attracts attention. They may assume a completely new and apparently well-integrated identity during the fugue state.

DISSOCIATIVE AMNESIA

People with **dissociative amnesia** have one or more episodes of memory loss of important personal information. They suddenly become aware that they have a total loss of memory for events that occurred during a period that may range from a few hours to a whole lifetime. In *localized amnesia*, the most common form, a person forgets only specific and related past times, usually surrounding a disturbing event. *Selective amnesia* for some, but not all, of the events is less common. Least common are *generalized amnesia,* which encompasses the person's entire life, and *continuous amnesia,* in which the person cannot recall events up to a specific time, including the present. *Systematized amnesia* is the loss of memory for certain categories of information, such as all memories related to one's occupation, or all memories that are related to one's family.

DEPERSONALIZATION DISORDER

The essential feature of depersonalization disorder is one or more episodes of feeling detached from one's self so that the usual sense of personal reality is temporarily lost or changed. All the dissociated feelings are ego-dystonic.

CLINICAL EXAMPLE

Clyde feels as if he is living in a dream or a movie. It seems to him as if he can observe his own life. He explains his experiences by saying, "I don't feel real any more. It's like I can watch my life as if it's a TV show. I'm afraid I'm going crazy."

DISSOCIATIVE DISORDER, NOT OTHERWISE SPECIFIED (NOS)

This is a residual category used for disorders in which the predominant feature is a dissociative reaction that does not meet the diagnostic criteria of any specific dissociative disorder. An example is a person who enters a dissociated state following a period of brainwashing.

Biopsychosocial Theories

Although biologic and genetic factors are being studied, psychosocial theories are used most commonly to explain dissociative disorders.

BIOLOGIC FACTORS

At present, there is little documented evidence of a physiologic cause of dissociative disorders. However, certain physical illnesses (such as brain tumors and epilepsy) may lead to symptoms indicative of depersonalization disorder. Also, certain drugs may cause some people to experience depersonalization symptoms. These drugs include alcohol, scopolamine, barbiturates, benzodiazepines, and hallucinogens (Kaplan & Sadock, 2000).

GENETIC THEORIES

According to the DSM-IV-TR, dissociative identity disorder occurs more often in first-degree biologic relatives of people with the disorder (APA, 2000).

PSYCHOSOCIAL THEORIES

Pierre Janet (1859–1947) was the first to develop the concept of the "splitting off," or dissociation, of a part of consciousness. He believed that the individual needed to have a normal amount of "mental energy" to maintain integrative mental processes. When the level of energy was high, integration was maintained. When it became low, however, the personality might cease to function as a unit and split or dissociate.

Freud, in contrast, proposed the concept of repression to explain the loss of conscious awareness in dissociation. He then introduced the notion of the *dynamic unconscious,* a part of the mind in which emotions or ideas that were unacceptable to a person were pushed from awareness. Freud and other early analytic theorists accepted the basic concept of psychologic dissociation.

Current explanations of dissociation are based on Freud's dynamic concepts. The repression of ideas that leads to amnesia and other forms of dissociation is conceived as a way of protecting the individual from emotional pain. External circumstances or internal psychologic conflicts are viewed as precipitating factors. A dissociative reaction may be viewed as a flight from crisis or danger—a major psychologic route of escape from anxiety. Sometimes, as in states of dissociative fugue and dissociative identity disorder, the dissociated area takes over temporary direction and control of the entire personality. During such times, the person may appear to be functioning well.

Dissociative identity disorder originates in childhood as a result of chronic, unpredictable trauma. The trauma may be physical, psychological, or both. The major form of child abuse which contributes to the development of DID is sexual abuse. In attempts to cope with the horror of reality, the child's ego splits through the dissociative process. Each trauma-induced dissociative experience shapes the development of alternate (alter) personalities. Each alter has a unique identity, holds different feelings and memories, and performs different functions.

Chronic abuse leads to a fixation of the dissociated ego splits. ■ Figure 16–5 on page 396 illustrates this process. Through dissociation, the child may see the abuse as if it were occurring to someone else, as in a movie. This ability to remove the self from the abuse is a protective mechanism. Dissociation is the escape that allows survival (Schwartz, 2000).

Additional dynamic considerations relevant to dissociative disorders include the following ideas. In dissociative amnesia, the pattern is similar to conversion disorder except that the individual does not avoid some unpleasant situation by getting sick. Instead, the person does so by forgetting (repressing) certain traumatic events or stresses. In DID, there appears to be a deep-seated conflict between contradictory impulses and beliefs. A resolution is achieved by separating the conflicting parts and developing each into an autonomous personality (alter).

NURSING PROCESS

Clients with Dissociative Disorders

The nursing process is the framework for providing care to clients experiencing dissociative disorders.

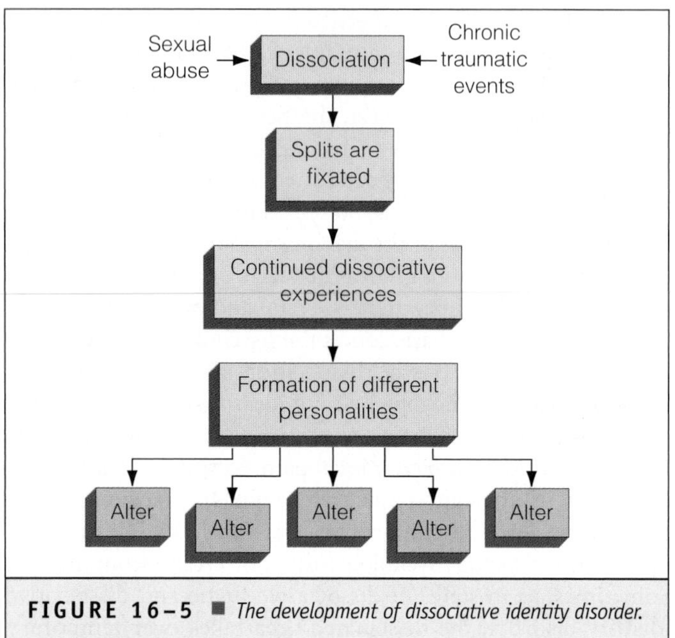

FIGURE 16–5 ■ *The development of dissociative identity disorder.*

Assessment

The major areas to focus on during assessment are identity, memory, and consciousness.

SUBJECTIVE DATA

Clients with dissociative disorders often report a sudden loss of memory of events. Clients may report, for example, that they cannot recall certain important personal events or information. They may not recall important aspects of their own identity, such as their age and where they reside.

Sometimes amnesia is only partial, and clients remain conscious of what happened, although they report that they feel no control over it. In cases of complete amnesia, the "lost" memories can be recovered under certain therapeutic circumstances (e.g., hypnosis), or they may return spontaneously. Clients who have sustained a loss of their own reality may have adopted a new identity.

If motor behavior is affected in dissociative disorders, clients or their families may report episodes during which clients physically traveled away from home. Clients with depersonalization disorder may report fears that they are going crazy and experience resulting anxiety. In clients with DID, the original personality typically is not aware of the existence of the secondary personalities. However, the secondary personalities may be aware of the original personality as well as of each other and may report this awareness to the staff.

OBJECTIVE DATA

Conduct a careful assessment of the client's physical condition to rule out the possibility of organic causes, such as a brain tumor. Many of the behaviors of clients with dissociative disorders resemble behaviors associated with organic conditions, including postconcussional amnesia and temporal lobe epilepsy. Your observations of the character, duration, frequency, and context of the dissociative disorder are crucial data. Physical examinations are not continued as part of the long-term intervention program, however, because they reinforce the symptoms and provide secondary gain. Therefore, the completeness and accuracy of the initial physical assessment are of the utmost importance.

A psychosocial assessment is conducted to discover the fundamental source of the anxiety as early as possible. Although many episodes of dissociation appear to occur spontaneously, there may be a history of a specific, shocking emotional trauma or a situation charged with painful emotions and psychological conflict. Family or friends may provide clues to the client's conflict and should be included in the psychosocial data gathering.

When assessing for the presence of DID, consider the clinical manifestations listed in the Assessment box below.

Events associated with the trauma can trigger memories that had been repressed. These stimuli can trigger a switch of alters. When interacting with the client, be alert for evidence of forgetfulness and fluctuations of voice tone, speech, and mannerisms.

Notice from session to session if there are uncharacteristic changes in behavior. Are there differences in hairstyles or dress?

To assess for amnesia, ask if the client has ever had blackouts, blank spells, lost time, or memory gaps.

To assess for dissociation, question whether the client ever "spaces out" or is unable to remember periods of time or events.

Nursing Diagnosis: NANDA

Three major nursing diagnoses are discussed below.

DISTURBED SENSORY PERCEPTION AND DISTURBED THOUGHT PROCESSES

Clients with dissociative disorders may experience sudden memory loss, disorientation, loss of personal identity, and alteration in state of consciousness. Clients with dissociative amnesia have a partial or total inability to recall or identify past expe-

ASSESSMENT

Guidelines for the Client with Dissociative Identity Disorder

- Amnesia, loss of time, time distortion
- Confabulation
- Multiple somatic complaints, including severe headaches
- Client's report of "hearing voices"
- Reports by others of uncharacteristic behavior that the client does not recall
- Client's discovery of unfamiliar objects, clothing, or writings in one's possession for which the client cannot account
- Client's use of "we" when speaking
- History of childhood abuse or trauma
- Frequent nightmares, insomnia

riences. In clients with depersonalization disorder, feelings of unreality and estrangement can affect their perception of the physical and psychologic self and of the world around them. Parts of the body or the entire body may seem foreign. Dizziness, anxiety, and distortion of time and space are common.

INEFFECTIVE ROLE PERFORMANCE

Unexplained disappearances, absences from work, unreliability, and unpredictability are common manifestations of dissociative disorders. Thus, the social or occupational functioning of the client is adversely affected.

Symptoms of depersonalization lead to limited or superficial involvement with others and to withdrawal or disengagement in work or social pursuits. As expected, relationships become highly complicated and disorganized when a client has multiple personalities.

INEFFECTIVE COPING

In addition to amnesia, a fugue state may occur in clients with dissociative disorders. In this state, clients defend against perceived danger by active flight. They may wander away from home. Days, weeks, or sometimes even years later they may suddenly find themselves in a strange place, not knowing how they got there. There is complete amnesia for the period of the fugue. Clients experiencing dissociative fugue may adopt a new identity and life pattern.

Outcome Identification: NOC

When developing expected outcomes, it is important to individualize plans for each client. For example, a client experiencing a dissociative identity disorder will probably need assistance in resolving issues related to self-concept. When planning outcomes, remember that they should be realistic and achievable. Some appropriate expected outcomes would include:

- The client will engage in a therapeutic alliance.
- The client will verbalize awareness of personality alters.

Following are some outcomes—written in NOC terminology (Johnson, Maas, & Moorhead, 2000, pp. 119–120)—for clients experiencing ineffective coping. The client will:

- Identify effective and ineffective coping patterns.
- Seek information about illness and treatment.
- Use stress-reduction behaviors.
- Report decrease in negative feelings.
- Demonstrate impulse control by consistently maintaining self-control without supervision.
- Identify personal strengths that may promote effective coping.

Planning and Implementation: NIC

In choosing intervention strategies for clients with dissociative disorders, the treatment team must decide whether to alleviate the troublesome symptoms or reintegrate the anxiety-producing conflict. Some teams emphasize the disruptions in day-to-day functioning precipitated by dissociative disorders. These include unexplained disappearances, absences from work, unreliability, and unpredictability. The dread associated with them justifies intervention strategies designed to change the disruptive behavior pattern. Others believe that new problems are created by removing the so-called symptoms without considering how they help the client control internal anxiety and maintain some balance in external social life.

Keep in mind that although clients may complain about the difficulties associated with their symptoms, the symptoms often form the basis of relationships with other significant people in their lives. Clients' roles in social groups are likewise built around their coping styles. Anyone who tries to change these coping styles must offer clients more effective and satisfying ways to handle anxiety and get support in their social network. Such a task usually requires long-term psychotherapy. However, behavior modification strategies can alleviate some of the problematic behaviors.

When planning care for a client with DID, you must remember that trust is a major issue. The basic building blocks of therapy with the dissociative individual are:

- Trust
- Safety
- Acceptance

For many individuals, receiving a diagnosis of DID is a relief. For years, they have been misdiagnosed and treated incorrectly. In addition to a sense of relief, another common reaction to the diagnosis is disbelief. The diagnosis itself may trigger the switching of alters. Thus, a safe, supportive environment is essential. The focus of treatment is to form a therapeutic alliance and work through the issues of each alternate identity.

The goal of integrating the alternate identities into one fused identity is difficult to achieve—but it is feasible. Integration occurs when there is no further need for separateness between identities. The integration process can be very painful for the client, as memories of previous trauma surface. However, it is important for the client to recall painful memories in order to work through unresolved conflicts.

When planning care for the client with DID, remember to:

- Trust the client to express his or her needs.
- Listen to each identity.
- Help the client accept the diagnosis.
- Provide support.
- Allow time.

PROMOTING IMPROVED SENSORY PERCEPTION AND THOUGHT PROCESSES

Strategies for identifying the underlying source of anxiety include those for recovering unconscious content, such as free association or dream description. At times, more active strategies are used. These may include projective psychometric tests (Rorschach, Thematic Apperception Test) and hypnosis, with or without intravenous administration of thiopental sodium (Pentothal).

Supportive insight therapy may be used with the goal of surfacing and integrating traumatic experiences in order to learn new ways of coping with future anxiety. This is especially relevant for those clients in whom the dissociative phenomena arise primarily against a background of intrapsychic conflict.

PROMOTING EFFECTIVE ROLE PERFORMANCE AND FAMILY PROCESSES

Including family members in a therapeutic counseling relationship helps them learn new ways of dealing with the client. As stated earlier, considerable secondary gain is often associated with dissociative behavior: The client can use the illness to escape responsibility and get special treatment. Families often need support in learning to avoid reinforcing dissociative behavior by acting as the source of secondary gain.

Environmental manipulation may be an indicated intervention. For example, it may be necessary to assist the client in problem solving with the goal of minimizing other stressful aspects of the environment. In learning to confront and become desensitized to the underlying conflict, the client will experience some anxiety and discomfort. This anxiety must be kept within manageable limits. Therefore, more obvious and alterable sources of stress and anxiety should be minimized.

PROMOTING EFFECTIVE COPING

The nurse may use measures such as psychotherapy (if prepared as a clinical specialist), environmental manipulation, and behavior modification to help the client cope more effectively with impairments of conduct and impulse, such as unpredictable and bizarre behavior. Treatment may prove to be long-term, and progress may be slow. Establishing a supportive therapeutic alliance with the client and the family is crucial in helping the family and client understand the periodic occurrence of symptoms and in supporting improved behaviors. See the Rx Communication feature, Client with Depersonalization Disorder.

Evaluation

Three major areas for evaluation are discussed below.

SENSORY PERCEPTION AND THOUGHT PROCESSES

Clients will no longer experience sudden memory loss, disorientation, loss of identity, or alteration in state of consciousness, or they will experience it less frequently. They will correctly recall and identify past experiences.

ROLE PERFORMANCE AND FAMILY PROCESSES

Clients will experience increased satisfaction with family and work relationships. Involvement with others will occur more often and will be more fulfilling. They will attend work or school regularly, without unexplained absences due to dissociative episodes.

INDIVIDUAL COPING

Clients will no longer exhibit bizarre or unpredictable behaviors, or they will experience them less frequently. For example, incidents of being missing from home without explanation will occur less frequently or not at all.

Community-Based Care/Case Management/Home Care

Community-based care, case management, and home care for clients with dissociative disorders has been discussed earlier in this chapter. See page 388.

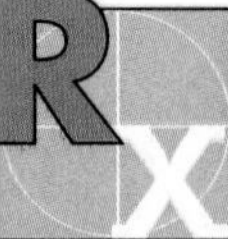

COMMUNICATION

Client with Depersonalization Disorder

CLIENT: I don't feel like myself; in fact, I don't even feel real.

NURSE RESPONSE 1: You sound as if you're afraid when those unreal episodes occur.

RATIONALE: This response demonstrates empathy and reassures the client that it is appropriate to discuss her feelings.

NURSE RESPONSE 2: When you are feeling this way, you look more anxious. We're here to help you learn to cope better with the anxiety.

RATIONALE: This response provides feedback on the congruence between the client's feelings and behavior. It also reassures the client that she can learn methods to decrease the anxiety associated with depersonalization.

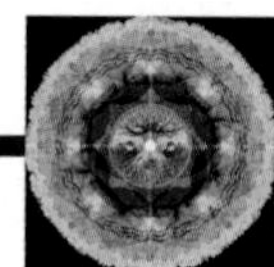

EXPLORE MediaLink

NCLEX review, case studies, and other interactive resources for this chapter can be found on the Companion Website at http://www.prenhall.com/kneisl. Click on Chapter 16 to select the activities for this chapter.

For animations, video tutorials, more NCLEX review questions, and an audio glossary, access the accompanying CD-ROM in this textbook.

BIBLIOGRAPHY

American Psychiatric Association (2000). *Diagnostic and statistical manual of mental disorders* (4th ed., Text Revision). Washington, DC: Author.

Baldwin, D., Bobes, J., Stein, D. J., Scharwachter, I., & Faure, M. (1999). *British Journal of Psychiatry, 175,* 120–126.

Bourne, E. J. (2001). *The anxiety and relaxation workbook* (3rd ed.). Oakland, CA: New Harbinger Publications.

Gliatto, M. F. (2000). Generalized anxiety disorder. *American Family Physician, 62*(7), 1591–1599.

Hayward, C., Varady, S., Albano, A. M., Thienemann, M., Henderson, L., & Schatzberg, F. (2000). Cognitive-behavioral group therapy for social phobia in female adolescents: Results of a pilot study. *Journal of the American Academy of Child and Adolescent Psychiatry, 39,* 721–726.

Johnson, M., Maas, M., & Moorhead, S. (2000). *Nursing outcomes classification (NOC)* (2nd ed.). St. Louis, MO: Mosby.

Kaplan, H. I., & Sadock, B. J. (2000). *Kaplan & Sadock's synopsis of psychiatry and study guide*. Philadelphia: Lippincott.

Lipsitz, J. D., & Schneier, F. R. (2000). Social phobia: Epidemiology and cost of illness. *Pharmacoeconomics, 18*(1), 23–32.

Manaser, J. C., & Werner, A. M. (1964). *Instruments for the study of nurse–patient interaction*. Hampshire, UK: Macmillan.

Moreno, F. A., & Delgado, P. L. (2000). Living with anxiety disorders: as good as it gets . . . ? *Bulletin of the Menninger Clinic, 64,* A4–21.

National Institute of Mental Health (1999). The numbers count: Mental disorders in America. Retrieved September, 2000, from the World Wide Web, *www.nimh.nih.gov*.

National Institute of Mental Health (2001). *When fear holds sway: Panic disorder*. Pub. No. 01-4596. Bethesda, MD: Author.

National Institute of Mental Health Pediatrics and Developmental Neuropsychiatry Branch (2000). Frequently asked questions about PANDAS. Retrieved January 31, 2001, from the World Wide Web, *www.intramural.nimh.nih.gov/research/pdn/faqs.htm*.

North American Nursing Diagnosis Association (2001). *Nursing diagnoses: Definitions & classification: 2001–2002*. Philadelphia: Author.

Pasqualone, G. A., & Fitzgerald, S. M. (1999). Munchausen by proxy syndrome: The forensic challenge of recognition, diagnosis, and reporting. *Critical Care Nursing Quarterly, 22,* 52–64.

Peplau, H. (1962). Interpersonal techniques: The crux of nursing. *American Journal of Nursing, 62,* 784–786.

Rank, O. (1952). *The trauma of birth*. Philadelphia: Robert Brunner.

Sapolsky, R. M. (2000). Glucocorticoids and hippocampal atrophy in neuropsychiatric disorders. *Archives of General Psychiatry, 57*(10), 925–937.

Schwartz, H. L. (2000). *Dialogues with forgotten voices: Relational perspectives on child abuse trauma and the treatment of severe dissociative disorders*. New York: Basic Books.

Sullivan, H. S. (1953). *The interpersonal theory of psychiatry*. New York: Norton.

Szesko, P. R., Robinson, D., Alvir, J. M., Bilder, R. M., Lencz, T., Ashtari, M., et al. (1999). Orbital frontal and amygdala volume reductions in obsessive-compulsive disorder. *Archives of General Psychiatry, 56,* 913–919.

U.S. Public Health Service (2000). Mental health: A report of the Surgeon General. Retrieved February 2, 2002, from the World Wide Web, *www.surgeongeneral.gov/library,mentalhealth/chapter4/sec2_1.html*.

Vythilingam, M., Anderson, E. R., Goddard, A., Woods, S. W., Staib, L. H., & Bremner, J. D. (2000). Temporal lobe volume in panic disorder—a quantitative magnetic resonance imaging study. *Psychiatry Research, 99*(2), 75–82.

Wisdom, C. S. (1999). Posttraumatic stress disorder in abused and neglected children grown up. *American Journal of Psychiatry, 156*(9), 1223–1229.

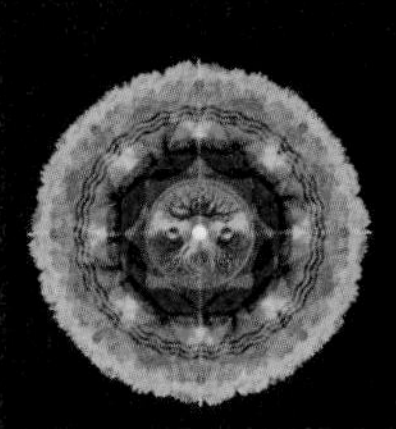

17

Gender Identity and Sexual Disorders

KAREN LEE FONTAINE

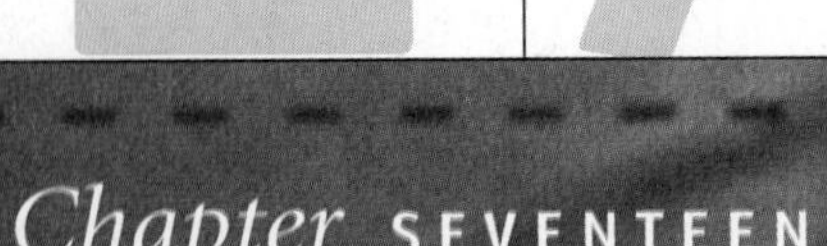

Chapter SEVENTEEN

KEY TERMS

androgyny
autoerotic asphyxia
cross-dressers
fetishism
gender identity
gender identity disorder
gender roles
paraphilias
sexual addiction
sexual dysfunctions
transgenderism
transsexuals

FOCUS QUESTIONS

- What values do you hold regarding sexuality?
- What are the ranges of transgendered identities and behaviors?
- What is the specific distinction between noncoercive and coercive paraphilias?
- Which biopsychosocial theories help to explain various sexual disorders and gender dysphoria?
- What principles are common to most treatment plans for persons with gender dysphoria or sexual disorders?
- How can you demonstrate sensitivity to the diversity of sexual values that exist in the world?

MediaLink 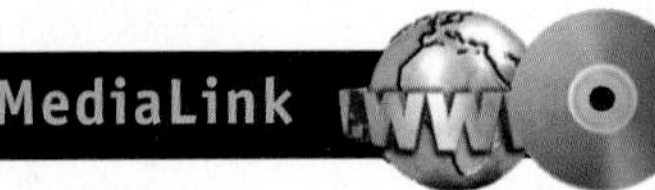 www.prenhall.com/kneisl

Additional resources for this chapter can be found on the Student CD-ROM accompanying this textbook, and on the Companion Website at www.prenhall.com/kneisl. Click on Chapter 17 to select the activities for this chapter.

CD-ROM
- Audio Glossary
- NCLEX Review

Companion Website
- Additional NCLEX Review
- Care Plan: Dyspareunia
- Case Study: Transsexual
- Learning from Clients: Transsexual Video

CHAPTER OUTLINE

CROSS REFERENCES

Other topics relevant to this content are: Codependence, Chapter 13; Family dynamics, Chapter 29; Generalist and specialist standards of practice, Chapter 1; HIV and high-risk sexual behaviors, Chapter 24; Hyperproteinemia and sexual side effects of drugs, Chapter 31; Incest and rape, Chapter 23.

CRITICAL THINKING CHALLENGE

Charles is a 54-year-old male being treated on the inpatient unit for depression. This is his first hospital stay for a psychiatric problem, although he has had difficulties with depression for months. He has been married for 25 years, has no children, and his relationship with his wife Claudia has been strained for some time.

One of the major problems Charles and Claudia are having is a sexual problem. His arousal was based on certain activities that Claudia no longer wanted to participate in; however, they were able to make some progress on this relationship problem with a specific plan designed for them by a sex therapist. Then Charles's symptoms of depression began affecting their sex life again and once he began treatment with an antidepressant he experienced significant sexual side effects.

When clients are admitted to inpatient settings for treatment of mental disorders, their sexual needs are very rarely addressed. Clients and their partners/spouses are expected to remain celibate throughout the hospital stay. There is no privacy provided for clients and their loved ones. In fact, visiting is often restricted to public areas. Do you agree with this practice? Are professionals imposing their values on clients? When clients are admitted, do they lose their right to consensual sexual activity with their partner? ■

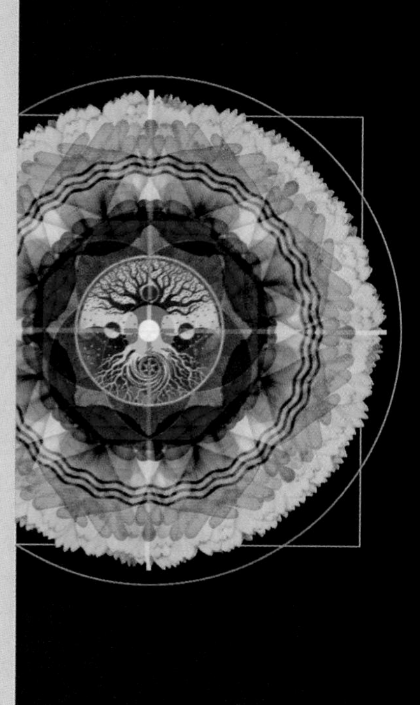

All humans are sexual beings. Regardless of gender, age, race, socioeconomic status, religious beliefs, physical and mental health, or other demographic factors, we express our sexuality in a variety of ways throughout our lives.

Human sexuality is difficult to define. Sexuality is an individually expressed and highly personal phenomenon whose meaning evolves from objective and subjective experiences. Physiologic, psychosocial, and cultural factors influence a person's sexuality and lead to the wide range of attitudes and behaviors seen in humans. There are no normal, universal sexual behaviors. Satisfying or "normal" sexual expression can generally be described as whatever behaviors give pleasure and satisfaction to those adults involved, without threat of coercion or injury to others. However, definitions of what constitutes "normal" sexual expression can vary among cultures and religions.

Sexual health is an individual and constantly changing phenomenon falling within the wide range of human sexual thoughts, feelings, needs, and desires. A person's degree of sexual health is best determined by that individual, sometimes with the assistance of a qualified professional.

Sexual health care is a relatively new area of involvement for psychiatric–mental health nurses. Until recently, sexuality has not been viewed as falling within the scope of treatment. Currently, sexuality is increasingly recognized as an important component of a holistic approach to our overall health status. Sexual health care is a legitimate and appropriate nursing concern. The close and often extended relationships that psychiatric–mental health nurses have with clients and families foster the rapport necessary to discuss this private area of clients' health status.

Nursing roles in the area of human sexuality are evolving gradually. Psychiatric–mental health nurses involved in nursing activities related to human sexual functioning need to have the following:

- Concrete and comprehensive knowledge about sexual function and dysfunction.
- Skill in communication techniques.
- Acceptance of, and comfort with, their own sexual values and expressions.
- A willingness to explore and separate personal values and attitudes from those of clients.
- The nurse generalist needs to be proficient in using the nursing process to assess the client's sexual health and sexual concerns, promote optimal sexual health, play a supportive role, and refer the client to an advanced practice nurse or other health care professional with expertise in this area.
- The advanced practice clinical nurse specialist or nurse practitioner with special training and interest in gender identity and sexual disorders can diagnose, intervene, and evaluate care to promote optimal sexual health.

Historically, human sexuality has been shrouded in myth and controversy. This history has hindered both the delivery and the receipt of services that promote sexual health and well-being. Although scientific knowledge has expanded immensely during the past several decades, modern North Americans continue to view sex and sexuality with discomfort. Our confusion is complicated by our traditional religious

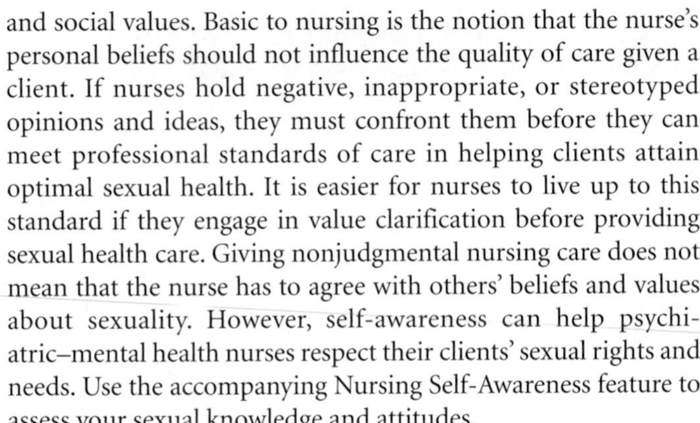

and social values. Basic to nursing is the notion that the nurse's personal beliefs should not influence the quality of care given a client. If nurses hold negative, inappropriate, or stereotyped opinions and ideas, they must confront them before they can meet professional standards of care in helping clients attain optimal sexual health. It is easier for nurses to live up to this standard if they engage in value clarification before providing sexual health care. Giving nonjudgmental nursing care does not mean that the nurse has to agree with others' beliefs and values about sexuality. However, self-awareness can help psychiatric–mental health nurses respect their clients' sexual rights and needs. Use the accompanying Nursing Self-Awareness feature to assess your sexual knowledge and attitudes.

Gender and Transgenderism

Western culture is deeply committed to the idea that there are only two sexes. Biologically speaking, however, there are many gradations running from female to male; this is known as **transgenderism.** In some cases gender is clear, in some it is unclear, and in other cases there is a blending of both genders within the same individual.

GENDER IDENTITY

Gender identity is an individual's personal or private sense of identity as female or male. Gender identity develops from an interaction of biology, identity imposed by others, and self-identity. A newborn is assigned a gender (identity imposed by others) according to the appearance of the external genitals (biology); by 3 years of age, the child says "I am a girl" or "I am a boy" (self-identity). Gender identity can be viewed as a continuum. At one end of the continuum are those whose gender identity is congruent with their anatomic sex. In the middle are *transvestites*, who have both male and female gender identities. At the other end of the continuum are *transsexuals*, whose gender identity conflicts with their anatomic sex.

GENDER ROLES

Gender roles are the roles a person is expected to perform as a result of being male or female in a particular culture. The expectation that people will exhibit certain behaviors because they are female or male is referred to as gender role stereotyping. Stereotypical images of people do not take into account individual differences. The danger of such stereotypes is that people take them seriously and act on them, turning a blind eye to the qualities and interests of individuals. In North American culture, gender roles are more strictly enforced for males than for females, and males are socially punished for female behavior.

ANDROGYNY

Androgyny, or flexibility in gender roles, is the belief that most characteristics and behaviors are human qualities that should not be limited to one specific gender or the other. Being androgynous does not mean being sexually neuter or imply anything about one's sexual orientation. Rather, it describes the

Nursing SELF-AWARENESS Check Your Knowledge and Attitudes About Sex

Use this checklist periodically to assess changes in your knowledge and attitudes.

Knowledge

Circle True or False for each statement.

T F Women can and do have orgasms while sleeping.
T F It is dangerous to engage in intercourse during menstruation.
T F Sex drive usually diminishes after a vasectomy.
T F The older male may actually have some advantages over the younger male in sexual activity.
T F Masturbation is a relatively common practice of both women and men.
T F Females have two kinds of orgasm: clitoral and vaginal.
T F Children raised by homosexual couples are very likely to become homosexual.
T F An adult male who has been castrated immediately loses his sex drive.
T F Intercourse should always be avoided during the last trimester of pregnancy.
T F Oral–genital stimulation is unhygienic.

Attitudes

Circle the letter corresponding to your level of agreement with each statement.

A: Strongly agree; B: Agree; C: Uncertain; D: Disagree; E: Strongly disagree

A B C D E Sex education has caused a rise in premarital intercourse.
A B C D E Extramarital relations are almost always harmful to a marriage.
A B C D E Relieving tension by masturbation is a healthy practice.
A B C D E Premarital intercourse is morally undesirable.
A B C D E Parents should stop their children from masturbating.
A B C D E Women should have sexual experience before marriage.
A B C D E Homosexual and bisexual behavior should be against the law.
A B C D E Seeing family members nude arouses undue curiosity in children.
A B C D E Promiscuity is widespread on college campuses today.
A B C D E Men should have sexual experience before marriage.

degree of flexibility a person has regarding gender-stereotypic behaviors. Adults who can behave flexibly regarding their sexual roles may be able to adapt better than those who adopt rigid stereotyped gender roles.

TRANSSEXUALS

The medical profession considers transsexuals to have a condition called *gender dysphoria* (strong and persistent feelings of discomfort with one's assigned sex) or gender identity disorder. For the transsexual person, sexual anatomy is not consistent with gender identity. Those who are born physically male but are emotionally and psychologically female are called Male to Female or MTFs. Those who are born female but are emotionally and psychologically male are called Female to Male or FTMs. There is some disagreement as to whether gender dysphoria is a physical condition, a psychological condition, or both. The DSM-IV-TR diagnostic criteria for gender identity disorder are in the box on page 404.

Most transsexuals report that they have felt gender dysphoria since earliest childhood. They often suffer for many years and try to hide the situation from family and friends from fear of being considered "crazy." Being transgendered puts women and men at extreme risk of being:

- Ridiculed and humiliated.
- In constant jeopardy over getting and keeping a job.
- Evicted without cause from restaurants and stores.
- Denied housing.
- Refused medical treatment, even to save a life (Lips, 2001).

As self-understanding and acceptance increase, many transsexuals live part time or full time as members of the other sex. *Cross-dressing* (dressing in the clothing of the opposite sex) not only makes their outward appearance consistent with their inner identity and gender role, but also increases their comfort with themselves. Their sexual orientation may be heterosexual, homosexual, or bisexual.

CROSS-DRESSERS

Cross-dressers are typically males who cross-dress to express the feminine side of their personality. In most instances cross-dressers are not interested in permanently altering their bodies through surgical means, especially since the majority of them are comfortable with their original birth gender. Most cross-dressers exhibit stereotypic masculine identity and behavior in their public and professional lives.

Cross-dressing is a conscious choice and may occur at home or in public settings. The frequency of the activity ranges from rarely to often. It is not unusual for cross-dressers to have a female name to go with the female personality and wardrobe. Cross-dressing occurs more frequently in cultures where males are expected to be strong, independent, and unemotional protectors. If the social climate is considered to be one with rigid gender roles, some men may need to express their gentleness and dependence by creating a separate world and female persona within that social climate (Richard, 2000).

Often, these individuals do not tell their spouses about the cross-dressing before their marriage. Some are embarrassed and do not know how to bring up the subject. Others view the need to cross-dress as a problem and hope that it will disappear after the marriage. Most wives eventually find out. For some women, the discovery raises doubts about their own sexuality and self-worth, and they may decide to terminate the relationship. Some women are not threatened by the cross-dressing but fear it will become public knowledge. Other women move on to full acceptance and understanding of their partner's cross-dressing.

MediaLink Case Study: Transsexual

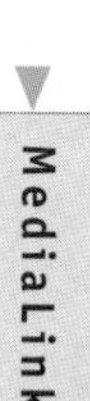

MediaLink Learning from Clients: Transsexual Video

DSM-IV-TR **Diagnostic Criteria for Gender Identity Disorder**

A. A strong and persistent cross-gender identification (not merely a desire for any perceived cultural advantages of being the other sex).

In children, the disturbance is manifested by four (or more) of the following:

1. repeatedly stated desire to be, or insistence that he or she is, the other sex
2. in boys, preference for cross-dressing or simulating female attire; in girls, insistence on wearing only stereotypical masculine clothing
3. strong and persistent preferences for cross-sex roles in make-believe play or persistent fantasies of being the other sex
4. intense desire to participate in the stereotypical games and pastimes of the other sex
5. strong preference for playmates of the other sex

In adolescents and adults, the disturbance is manifested by symptoms such as a stated desire to be the other sex, frequent passing as the other sex, desire to live or be treated as the other sex, or the conviction that he or she has the typical feelings and reactions of the other sex.

B. Persistent discomfort with his or her sex or sense of inappropriateness in the gender role of that sex.

In children, the disturbance is manifested by any of the following: in boys, assertion that his penis or testes are disgusting or will disappear or assertion that it would be better not to have a penis, or aversion toward rough-and-tumble play and rejection of male stereotypical toys, games, and activities; in girls, rejection of urinating in a sitting position, assertion that she has or will grow a penis, or assertion that she does not want to grow breasts or menstruate, or marked aversion toward normative feminine clothing.

In adolescents and adults, the disturbance is manifested by symptoms such as preoccupation with getting rid of primary and secondary sex characteristics (e.g., request for hormones, surgery, or other procedures to physically alter sexual characteristics to simulate the other sex) or belief that he or she was born the wrong sex.

C. The disturbance is not concurrent with a physical intersex condition.

D. The disturbance causes clinically significant distress or impairment in social, occupational, or other important areas of functioning.

Paraphilias

The DSM-IV-TR classifies **paraphilias** as a group of psychosexual disorders characterized by unconventional sexual behaviors. The person, usually a male, has learned to associate sexual arousal with some environmental stimulus, which triggers the unusual behavior.

Paraphilias have a strong obsessive–compulsive component. Affected individuals are often preoccupied with, and feel compelled to engage in, their particular sexual behaviors. One of the distinguishing characteristics of paraphilias is the person's inability to control or stop the behavior.

NONCOERCIVE PARAPHILIAS

Noncoercive paraphilias are unconventional sexual behaviors engaged in by oneself or with a consenting adult. Many people engage in mild forms of the noncoercive behaviors and consider them simply love play. The behavior becomes pathologic when it is severe, insistent, coercive, and harmful to self or others. The DSM-IV-TR diagnostic criteria for noncoercive paraphilias are in the box on page 405.

Fetishism

Humans respond to a wealth of sexual stimuli. Some people are aroused by the strident beat of rock music, while others are aroused by romantic music. Some people prefer making love in a brightly lit room; others, by candlelight; still others, in the dark. Everyone associates sexual arousal with an individual set of stimuli.

An association or stimulus that is not typical for the culture is called a fetish. A *fetish* is the sexualization of a body part, such as feet or hair, or an inanimate object, such as shoes, leather, or rubber. In **fetishism,** early associations of a particular object or body part with sexual arousal condition the person to respond sexually to that stimulus. Once the initial association is made, repeated viewing or use (fantasized or actual) of the part or object during sexual activity (usually masturbation) reinforces its arousing nature. For instance, a boy may get an erection after trying on his mother's panties. The erection is pleasurable. The next time the boy masturbates he puts the panties on or fantasizes about them. With repeated experiences, seeing the panties or putting them on becomes a sexual stimulus.

CLINICAL EXAMPLE

Ken, a 24-year-old college graduate with a major in accounting, was unable to hold a job because of his foot fetish. Ken spent a considerable amount of time fantasizing about feet—bare feet, pretty feet, long, narrow feet—and how they looked, they felt, they tasted, and they smelled. He fantasized at work, at the grocery store, and at the library (where he even went under tables to look at women's feet). Ken's fantasies made it impossible for him to work effectively or to maintain satisfactory interpersonal relationships with others. Ken refused therapy, preferring instead to pray that he would "get over it."

DSM-IV-TR — **Diagnostic Criteria for Noncoercive Paraphilias**

EXHIBITIONISM

A. Over a period of at least 6 months, recurrent, intense sexually arousing fantasies, sexual urges, or behaviors involving the exposure of one's genitals to an unsuspecting stranger.

B. The person has acted on these sexual urges, or the sexual urges or fantasies cause marked distress or interpersonal difficulty.

FETISHISM

A. Over a period of at least 6 months, recurrent, intense sexually arousing fantasies, sexual urges, or behaviors involving the use of nonliving objects (e.g., female undergarments).

B. The fantasies, sexual urges, or behaviors cause clinically significant distress or impairment in social, occupational or other important areas of functioning.

C. The fetish objects are not limited to articles of female clothing used in cross-dressing (as in Transvestic Fetishism) or devices designed for the purpose of tactile genital stimulation (e.g., a vibrator).

TRANSVESTIC FETISHISM

A. Over a period of at least 6 months, in a heterosexual male, recurrent, intense sexually arousing fantasies, sexual urges, or behaviors involving cross-dressing.

B. The fantasies, sexual urges, or behaviors cause clinically significant distress or impairment in social, occupational, or other important areas of functioning.

FROTTEURISM

A. Over a period of at least 6 months, recurrent, intense sexually arousing fantasies, sexual urges, or behaviors involving touching and rubbing against a nonconsenting person.

B. The person has acted on these sexual urges, or the sexual urges or fantasies cause marked distress or interpersonal difficulty.

Source: Reprinted with permission from the *Diagnostic and statistical manual of mental disorders,* 4th ed., Text Revision (pp. 569, 570, 575). Copyright 2000 American Psychiatric Association.

As with all people, fetishists' responses are highly individual. Fetishism is not considered a problem as long as it is not harmful and occurs in the context of consenting adult partners.

Transvestic Fetishism

In contrast with cross-dressers, men who become sexually aroused by dressing in women's clothing are considered *transvestic fetishists*. They may wear female underclothes or may cross-dress completely. Like other fetishists, they have often undergone conditioning, and female clothing is an intense sexual stimulus. Many report great emotional stress if they try to resist the urge to cross-dress. Like other fetishes, cross-dressing is not considered a problem among consenting adult partners.

Sexual Sadism and Sexual Masochism

Sexual sadism and sexual masochism (S/M) is highly stigmatized in North American culture, and few people admit to being sexually aroused by receiving or inflicting emotional or physical pain. As much as 10% of the population may participate in some form of S/M activity, and all groups—heterosexual, bisexual, homosexual—are represented. Physical behaviors include:

- Intense stimulation (scratching, biting, use of ice).
- Discipline (slapping, spanking, whipping).
- Bondage (holding down, tying down).
- Sensory deprivation (use of blindfolds, hoods, ear plugs).

Psychological behaviors include humiliation or degradation, such as verbally berating others or requiring them to perform menial acts. S/M behavior varies in intensity and in its significance in the lives of couples. Some couples engage in the behavior only during sex. Some integrate the roles throughout the relationship, but not at all times. Other couples attempt to live out the dominant/submissive roles continuously.

Thus, S/M may be only a part of foreplay, or it may be a significant component of lifestyle. Most sadomasochists do not engage in S/M behavior unless the partner is willing. Typically, both participants agree to safety "rules," and seldom is the behavior dangerous. Sadomasochists do not see the behavior as a problem and therefore do not wish to change (Wincze, 2000).

Autoerotic Asphyxia

A noncoercive but often fatal sexual behavior is **autoerotic asphyxia.** At present, it is not categorized as a paraphilia in the DSM-IV-TR but, like paraphilias, it is a compulsive and unconventional sexual behavior. Called head-rushing or scarfing, this behavior typically begins in adolescence and is primarily a male affliction. The person fashions a tourniquet-like device that constricts the neck, decreasing the blood and oxygen supply to the brain, masturbates, and, at the point of orgasm, releases the bonds to enhance the sensation or sexual high.

Tragically, this practice causes many deaths. The vagal nerve complex in the carotid artery is stimulated by pressure around the neck, slowing the heart rate and decreasing oxygen flow to the brain even further. The person becomes unconscious, slumps forward, and accidentally hangs himself. Many believe the cause of death is suicide, but family and friends cannot understand the reason for the suicide since these young men are not mentally ill or even troubled; the death is a tragic accident.

COERCIVE PARAPHILIAS

Coercive paraphiliacs become sexually aroused by including nonconsenting persons in their sexual acts. Coercive paraphilias are described in the legal code, and the sexual behavior is

DSM-IV-TR Diagnostic Criteria for Coercive Paraphilias

PEDOPHILIA

A. Over a period of at least 6 months, recurrent, intense sexually arousing fantasies, sexual urges, or behaviors involving sexual activity with a prepubescent child or children (generally age 13 years or younger).

B. The person has acted on these sexual urges, or the sexual urges or fantasies cause marked distress or interpersonal difficulty.

C. The person is at least age 16 years and at least 5 years older than the child or children in Criterion A.

SEXUAL MASOCHISM

A. Over a period of at least 6 months, recurrent intense sexually arousing fantasies, sexual urges, or behaviors involving the act (real, not simulated) of being humiliated, beaten, bound, or otherwise made to suffer.

B. The fantasies, sexual urges, or behaviors cause clinically significant distress or impairment in social, occupational, or other important areas of functioning.

SEXUAL SADISM

A. Over a period of at least 6 months, recurrent, intense sexually arousing fantasies, sexual urges, or behaviors involving act. (real, not simulated) in which the psychological or physical suffering (including humiliation) of the victim is sexually exciting to the person.

B. The person has acted on these sexual urges with a nonconsenting person, or the sexual urges or fantasies cause marked distress or interpersonal difficulty.

VOYEURISM

A. Over a period of at least 6 months, recurrent, intense sexually arousing fantasies, sexual urges, or behaviors involving the act of observing an unsuspecting person who is naked, in the process of disrobing, or engaging in sexual activity.

B. The person has acted on these sexual urges, or the sexual urges or fantasies cause marked distress or interpersonal difficulty.

Source: Reprinted with permission from the *Diagnostic and statistical manual of mental disorders,* 4th ed., Text Revision (pp. 572, 573, 574, 575). Copyright 2000 American Psychiatric Association.

considered a criminal act. The DSM-IV-TR diagnostic criteria for coercive paraphilias are in the box above.

Exhibitionism, Voyeurism, and Frotteurism

Exhibitionists and voyeurs, who are almost exclusively men, have powerful urges to display their genitals to strangers (exhibitionism) or peep at unsuspecting women involved in intimate behaviors (voyeurism). Frotteurs rub up against others, often in a crowded train or elevator, to achieve sexual arousal. The frotteur does not attempt to engage in sex with the victim and has no desire to form a relationship. Many describe the urge to peep, expose, or rub themselves against others as something that just "happens" to them and thus have difficulty assuming responsibility for their behavior (Strong, DeVault, & Sayad, 1999). Current information about sexual dysfunction and psychiatric care can be found in the Sexual Issues section of the *Psychiatric Times* Web site (www.mhsource.com/pt/disorder.html#Sex) or on the direct link to the Companion Website.

MediaLink Sexual Issues in Psychiatry

Obscene Phone Calling

A coercive sexual behavior, not categorized as a paraphilia in DSM-IV-TR, is obscene phone calling. Most women and many men have been victims of an obscene phone caller. The caller typically does not know the victim and becomes aroused when the victim reacts with disgust or shock or becomes upset. Some obscene callers breathe heavy, some make sexual noises, and some utter profanities. The caller may tell the victim that he is masturbating or may suggest they get together for sexual activity. Some pretend to have legitimate reasons for talking about sex (posing as researchers conducting a survey, for example) and continue until the victim is offended. The caller is sexually aroused by the combination of proximity (intimate conversation) and anonymity (Strong, DeVault, & Sayad, 1999).

Pedophilia

A *pedophile* is an adult who is sexually aroused by and engages in sexual activity with children. All sexual relationships between adults and children are criminal in North America. The courts consider these acts as nonconsensual because minors are presumed to have insufficient knowledge of the consequences of their acts to give meaningful consent. Pedophiliac activity can include exposure, voyeurism, explicit sex talk, touching, oral sex, intercourse, and anal sex. The child usually knows the pedophile, who may be a family member, neighbor, or friend. For a thorough discussion of the dynamics and consequences of the sexual abuse of children, see Chapter 23.

Sexual Dysfunctions

The DSM-IV-TR classifies problems or difficulties with sexual expression, referred to as **sexual dysfunctions,** according to the phase of the sexual response cycle that is affected. The DSM-IV-TR diagnostic criteria for sexual dysfunctions are in the box on page 408.

Sexual dysfunctions are generally acquired at some point in a relationship but may be lifelong in duration. They may be generalized to all sexual interactions and settings, or they may be situational, occurring in a specific setting or with specific types of sexual activity.

It is often difficult to sort out the multiple factors contributing to an individual's or a couple's sexual problems. Generally, a number of past and current factors are involved. Negative events or situations in the past include lack of sex education, internalization of the belief that sex is dirty or sinful, parental punishment for normally exploring one's genitals; or severe trauma, such as rape or childhood sexual abuse. Current situations or events contributing to sexual dysfunctions may include negative feelings, such as guilt, anxiety, or anger, that interfere with the ability to experience pleasure and joy. Fear of failure in sexual performance often becomes a vicious cycle; that is, fear of failure creates actual failure, which in turn produces more fear. *Spectatoring* is the detached appraisal of sexual performance or the body during a sexual act: "Am I going to lose my erection?" "Am I going to have an orgasm this time?" "My stomach is too flabby." "When did his thighs get that fat?"

Lack of intimacy and feeling like a sex object inhibit the feeling of communion and connection that is an important part of making love. Fear of intimacy prevents some people from truly entering into a trusting and loving relationship. Another factor in dysfunction is expecting one's partner to read one's mind about one's sexual needs. Lack of sex education and failure to communicate may result in one or both partners not knowing how to please the other.

Sexual dysfunction may also be symptomatic of relationship conflict. Until relationship issues are resolved, sex therapy is largely inappropriate. Even when couples are functioning well in all of these areas, physical changes brought on by illness, injury, or surgery may inhibit full sexual expression.

Sexual fulfillment is the result of the positive interaction of psychological, spiritual, sociologic, and physical factors, and dysfunctions are the result of a negative interaction. For an overview of past and current factors that may contribute to sexual dysfunctions, see ■ Table 17–1 (page 410). Male and female prevalence rates for sexual dysfunctions and problems are illustrated in ■ Figure 17–1 (page 411).

SEXUAL DESIRE DISORDERS

Sexual desire disorders are those that include a deficiency or absence of sexual fantasies and desire for sexual behavior or an aversion to and avoidance of genital sexual contact with a sex partner.

Hypoactive Sexual Desire Disorder

For most people, sexual desire varies from day to day as well as over the years. Some people, however, report a deficiency in or absence of sexual fantasies and persistently low interest or a total lack of interest in sexual activity; these clients suffer from *hypoactive sexual desire disorder*. The Rx Communication feature on page 410 illustrates an interaction with a client who has this type of sexual dysfunction. If both individuals in a relationship are similarly uninterested in sex, there really is no problem. More typically, there is a disparity of sexual needs, and the person with the greater desire becomes dissatisfied with the sexual relationship and often initiates seeking help. The key issue in the relationship is not frequency but rather the dovetailing of partners' needs.

Physiologic factors associated with lack of desire are fatigue, illness, pain, the use of medications, and substance abuse. Maturational factors such as menopause can also contribute to decreases in desire. See the Using Research Evidence feature on page 411 for a discussion of this topic. Intrapersonal factors may contribute to this dysfunction. Because vulnerability and intimacy are inherent in most sexual relationships, fear of these may lead to an avoidance of sex. Some people fear that if they allow themselves to experience sexual desire and pleasure, they will lose all control and continually act out sexually. Thus, these individuals may prefer to deny all desires rather than to try to fulfill them.

Relationship problems may be the source of inhibited sexual desire. Conflict and anger with one's partner are not conducive to positive sexual interaction. Some no longer feel physically attracted to one another or feel more attracted to someone else. Unless the partners experiment, sex may, in time, become boring. If there is a power imbalance in the relationship, the less powerful partner may lose interest in sex as a passive–aggressive way to achieve covert control. Typically, clients have little insight into the association between their lack of sexual desire and their negative feelings and relationship problems. Other, physiologically based reasons may exist for this problem.

SEXUAL AVERSION DISORDER

Sexual aversion disorder is a severe distaste for sexual activity or the thought of sexual activity, which then leads to a phobic avoidance of sex. It occurs in both women and men. Intense emotional dread of an impending sexual interaction also can trigger the physiologic symptoms of anxiety: sweating, increased heart rate, extreme muscle tension. The client then stops the sexual interaction or prevents it from even beginning. The most common cause of sexual aversion disorder is childhood sexual abuse or adult rape. This severe trauma can lead to a phobic response to sexual activity (Schnarch, 2000).

CLINICAL EXAMPLE

Linda and Mike, both 32 years of age, dated all through high school and have been married for 12 years. Linda has a strong aversion to body secretions. She spends hours in the bathtub before she and Mike have sex. Although Mike wears a condom, Linda jumps up and out of bed before he has finished ejaculating, and runs to the bathtub.

Linda can't identify any reasons for her feelings of disgust about body secretions and denies a history of sexual abuse. She does, however, talk about feeling violated by Mike when he "talked me into sex" at age 18. Sometimes she refers to this first sexual experience as date rape.

Despite this problem, Linda and Mike refer to themselves as best friends. Linda has suggested that their marriage be conducted as a platonic relationship. Mike's not sure he wants to live that way the rest of his life. They are in counseling and want to learn how to

DSM-IV-TR **Diagnostic Criteria for Sexual Dysfunctions**

SEXUAL DESIRE DISORDERS

Hypoactive Sexual Desire Disorder

A. Persistently or recurrently deficient (or absent) sexual fantasies and desire for sexual activity. The judgment of deficiency or absence is made by the clinician, taking into account factors that affect sexual functioning, such as age and the context of the person's life.
B. The disturbance causes marked distress or interpersonal difficulty.
C. The sexual dysfunction is not better accounted for by another Axis I disorder (except another Sexual Dysfunction) and is not due exclusively to the direct physiological effects of a substance (e.g., a drug of abuse, a medication) or a general medical condition.

Sexual Aversion Disorder

A. Persistent or recurrent extreme aversion to, and avoidance of, all (or almost all) genital sexual contact with a sexual partner.
B. The disturbance causes marked distress or interpersonal difficulty.
C. The sexual dysfunction is not better accounted for by another Axis I disorder (except another Sexual Dysfunction).

SEXUAL AROUSAL DISORDERS

Female Sexual Arousal Disorder

A. Persistent or recurrent inability to attain, or to maintain until completion of the sexual activity, an adequate lubrication-swelling response of sexual excitement.
B. The disturbance causes marked distress or interpersonal difficulty.
C. The sexual dysfunction is not better accounted for by another Axis I disorder (except another Sexual Dysfunction) and is not due exclusively to the direct physiological effects of a substance (e.g., a drug of abuse, a medication) or a general medical condition.

Male Erectile Disorder

A. Persistent or recurrent inability to attain, or to maintain until completion of the sexual activity, an adequate erection.
B. The disturbance causes marked distress or interpersonal difficulty.
C. The erectile dysfunction is not better accounted for by another Axis I disorder (other than a Sexual Dysfunction) and is not due exclusively to the direct physiological effects of a substance (e.g., a drug of abuse, a medication) or a general medical condition.

enjoy one another sexually. Currently, they are learning how to be less genitally focused and to spend more time cuddling, stroking, and touching.

SEXUAL AROUSAL DISORDERS

Sexual arousal refers to the physiologic responses and subjective sense of excitement experienced during sexual activity. Lack of lubrication and failure to attain or maintain an erection are the major disorders of the arousal phase. In *female sexual arousal disorder*, the lack of vaginal lubrication causes discomfort or pain during sexual intercourse. The diagnosis of *male erectile disorder* is usually made when the man has erection problems during 25% or more of his sexual interactions. Some men cannot attain a full erection, and others lose their erection prior to orgasm. The pejorative term commonly applied to this condition, *impotence*, implies that the man is feeble, inadequate, and incompetent. The accurate term is *erectile dysfunction (ED)*, which is objectively descriptive and not judgmental. Arousal disorder may also be diagnosed even when lubrication and erection are adequate if individuals report a persistent or recurring lack of subjective sexual excitement or pleasure.

Both male and female arousal can be inhibited by physiologic factors interfering with the vasocongestion necessary for lubrication or erection to occur. The absence of vasocongestion may result from disruption of the genital blood supply, from interference with innervation of the genitals, or, in women, from insufficient estrogen or testosterone levels. ED affects a significant proportion of men—at least 20% over the age of 50.

DSM-IV-TR Diagnostic Criteria for Sexual Dysfunctions

ORGASMIC DISORDERS

Female Orgasmic Disorder

A. Persistent or recurrent delay in, or absence of, orgasm following a normal sexual excitement phase. Women exhibit wide variability in the type or intensity of stimulation that triggers orgasm. The diagnosis of Female Orgasmic Disorder should be based on the clinician's judgment that the woman's orgasmic capacity is less than would be reasonable for her age, sexual experience, and the adequacy of sexual stimulation she receives.
B. The disturbance causes marked distress or interpersonal difficulty.
C. The orgasmic dysfunction is not better accounted for by another Axis I disorder (except another Sexual Dysfunction) and is not due exclusively to the direct physiological effects of a substance (e.g., a drug of abuse, a medication) or a general medical condition.

Male Orgasmic Disorder

A. Persistent or recurrent delay in, or absence of, orgasm following a normal sexual excitement phase during sexual activity that the clinician, taking into account the person's age, judges to be adequate in focus, intensity, and duration.
B. The disturbance causes marked distress or interpersonal difficulty.
C. The orgasmic dysfunction is not better accounted for by another Axis I disorder (except another Sexual Dysfunction) and is not due exclusively to the direct physiological effects of a substance (e.g., a drug of abuse, a medication) or a general medical condition.

Premature Ejaculation

A. Persistent or recurrent ejaculation with minimal sexual stimulation before, on, or shortly after penetration and before the person wishes it. The clinician must take into account factors that affect duration of the excitement phase, such as age, novelty of the sexual partner or situation, and recent frequency of sexual activity.
B. The disturbance causes marked distress or interpersonal difficulty.
C. The premature ejaculation is not due exclusively to the direct effects of a substance (e.g., withdrawal from opioids).

SEXUAL PAIN DISORDERS

Dyspareunia

A. Recurrent or persistent genital pain associated with sexual intercourse in either a male or a female.
B. The disturbance causes marked distress or interpersonal difficulty.
C. The disturbance is not caused exclusively by Vaginismus or lack of lubrication, is not better accounted for by another Axis I disorder (except another Sexual Dysfunction), and is not due exclusively to the direct physiological effects of a substance (e.g., a drug of abuse, a medication) or a general medical condition.

Vaginismus

A. Recurrent or persistent involuntary spasm of the musculature of the outer third of the vagina that interferes with sexual intercourse.
B. The disturbance causes marked distress or interpersonal difficulty.
C. The disturbance is not better accounted for by another Axis I disorder (e.g., Somatization Disorder) and is not due exclusively to the direct physiological effects of a general medical condition.

Source: Reprinted with permission from the *Diagnostic and statistical manual of mental disorders,* 4th ed., Text Revision (pp. 541, 542, 544, 547, 549, 552, 554, 556, 558).

In the majority of the cases, ED results from the additive and interactive nature of various diseases, medications, lifestyles, and affective and cognitive responses to these disruptions (Althof, 2000; Bartlik & Goldberg, 2000).

Psychological factors may also be a cause of arousal disorders. They include all the previously mentioned factors, such as fear of failure, anxiety, anger, spectatoring, poor communication, and relationship conflict. Insufficient vaginal lubrication is less likely than erectile inhibition to create severe distress for couples, because using saliva or a water-based lubricant such as KY Jelly or Astroglide can correct the immediate problem. Erectile problems may be threatening because the man often feels his whole sense of masculinity is at stake. Men tend to be dominated by a genital focus more than women are. Any difficulty in getting the penis to "perform" therefore results in feelings of humiliation and despair.

CLINICAL EXAMPLE

Ana and Jorge, both 45 years of age, sought counseling when Jorge found it impossible to achieve an erection. The first time Jorge was unable to achieve an erection was 6 years ago. This was an emotionally traumatic experience for Jorge, who spent a considerable amount of time worrying that it would happen again. Eventually it did, and Jorge found that he could not attain an erection more and more often. About 6 months ago he consulted a urologist. Nighttime penile tumescence studies showed normal functioning.

The couple was referred to a nurse sex therapist, who discovered that Jorge had believed, from an early age, that sexual functioning stopped once the man reached age 49. In working with the couple,

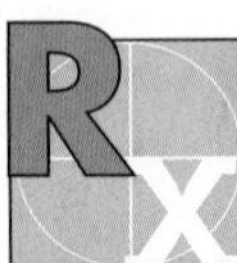

COMMUNICATION

Client with Sexual Dysfunction

CLIENT: "My husband always wants to have sex, and the more he wants, the less I'm interested."

NURSE RESPONSE 1: "Has there ever been a time in your relationship that you enjoyed sexual relations more?"

RATIONALE: Exploring the history of this problem's development in order to clarify whether the difficulty is interactional, intrapersonal, or perhaps medical in origin.

NURSE RESPONSE 2: "Have you spoken with your medical care provider about this problem?"

RATIONALE: Assessing any contributory medical factors.

the nurse focused on providing sex education and experiential/sensory awareness training. Once it didn't matter whether Jorge achieved an erection, his performance anxiety was decreased and he was able to do so.

ORGASMIC DISORDERS

Orgasmic disorders are those that occur at, or just before, the peaking of sexual pleasure. There are three types of orgasmic disorders: female orgasmic disorder, male orgasmic disorder, and premature ejaculation.

TABLE 17–1 Factors Contributing to Sexual Dysfunctions

Type	Past Factors	Current Factors
Psychologic	• Taught that sex is dirty • Childhood sexual abuse	• Performance anxiety • Spectatoring • Fear of failure • Guilt, anxiety, or anger • Negative thoughts
Spiritual	• Taught that sex is sinful • Childhood sexual abuse	• Not feeling connected to partner • Lack of intimacy • Fear of intimacy
Sociologic	• Punished as child for normal sex play • Lack of sex education	• Failure to communicate • Relationship conflict
Physical	• Trauma: abuse, rape	• Illness/injuries • Organic disorders • Medications • Substance abuse • Failure to engage in effective sexual behavior

Female Orgasmic Disorder

The pejorative term commonly applied in the past to women who did not experience orgasm, *frigid*, implies that the woman is totally incapable of responding sexually. The more accurate and objective term is *female orgasmic disorder*, which simply means that the sexual response stops before orgasm occurs. *Preorgasmic* women have never experienced an orgasm; *secondarily nonorgasmic* women have had orgasms in the past but do not currently experience them; and *situationally nonorgasmic* women have orgasms in some situations but not in others. Studies indicate that 10% to 15% of women are preorgasmic, and another 20% to 22% report irregular orgasms (Heiman, 2000). Compounding the orgasmic difficulty is the associated anxiety. In the preoccupation with orgasm, the real goal of being sexual—mutual pleasuring and intimacy—is lost, and the interchange becomes one of anxiety, frustration, and anger.

Physiologic factors related to inhibited female orgasm include fatigue, illness, neurologic or vascular damage, and drugs interfering with sexual response. In the physically healthy woman, lack of information or negative attitudes about female sexual response often contribute to orgasmic disorder. Women who were taught that masturbation is wrong or sinful may not have explored their own bodies. If so, they cannot teach a partner where, how, and when to touch.

Male Orgasmic Disorder

Some men suffer from *male orgasmic disorder*. Men with this disorder can maintain an erection for long periods (an hour or more) but have extreme difficulty ejaculating. In heterosexual intercourse, the difficulty may be limited to ejaculation in the vagina. Some men ejaculate after self-stimulation or manual or oral stimulation by the partner, whereas others have great difficulty ejaculating with any type of stimulation. This disorder is much less common than rapid ejaculation (Appelbaum, 2000).

Organic causes inhibiting orgasm include spinal cord injuries, multiple sclerosis, Parkinson's disease, and use of certain medications. Psychogenic factors include fear of pregnancy, performance pressure, fear of losing control, and anxiety and guilt about engaging in sexual activity. As with other dysfunctions, the difficulty can adversely affect the sexual relationship.

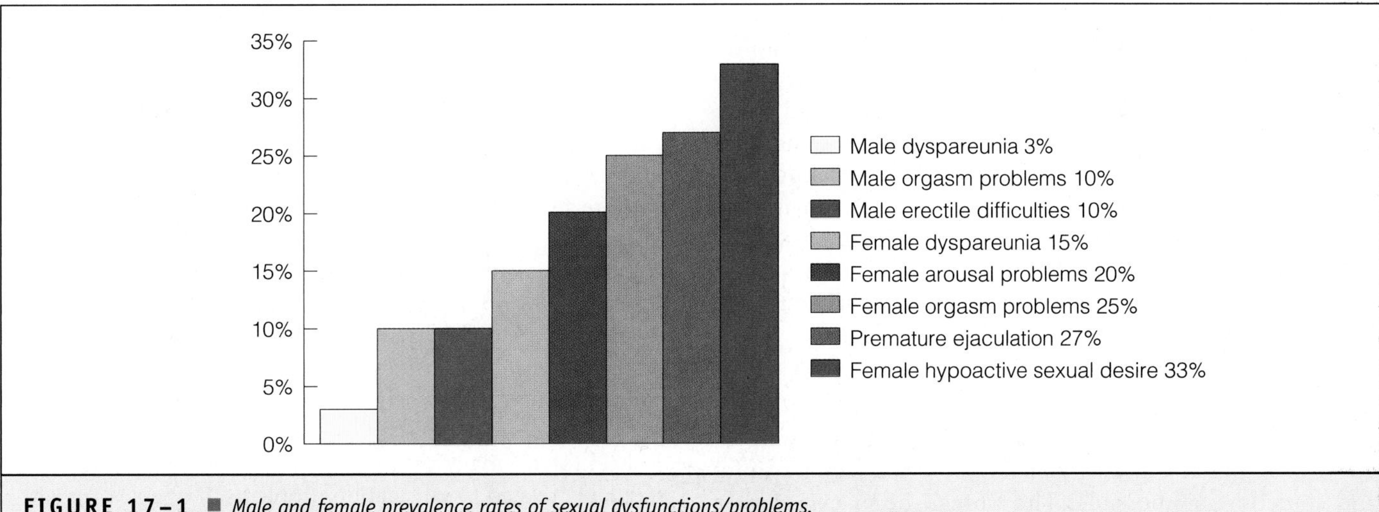

FIGURE 17–1 ■ *Male and female prevalence rates of sexual dysfunctions/problems.*

Premature Ejaculation

Premature ejaculation, or rapid ejaculation, is one of the most common sexual dysfunctions among men. There are many definitions, with descriptions ranging from ejaculating before being touched, ejaculating before penetration, ejaculating with one internal thrust, to ejaculating within a minute or two of penetration. A more helpful description is the absence of voluntary control of ejaculation. The problem is best self-defined: A man is concerned about his ejaculatory control, or the couple agrees that ejaculation is too rapid for mutual satisfaction.

There is very little information about the mechanisms causing rapid ejaculation. Possible influences include the man's:

- Inability to perceive his arousal level accurately.
- Lowered sensory threshold due to infrequent sexual activity.
- Early conditioning resulting from hurried masturbation or hurried sexual intercourse.
- Extreme anxiety during the sexual interaction, resulting in ejaculation triggered by sympathetic nervous system activity (Polonsky, 2000).

SEXUAL PAIN DISORDERS

A sexual pain disorder can be defined as genital pain occurring during sexual intercourse. The two types of sexual pain disorders are dyspareunia and vaginismus.

Dyspareunia

Both women and men can experience *dyspareunia*, pain during or immediately after intercourse. It is associated with many physiologic causes, especially those that inhibit lubrication. Thus, skin irritations, vaginal infections, estrogen deficiencies, and use of medications that dry vaginal secretions can cause women to experience discomfort with intercourse.

USING RESEARCH EVIDENCE

Peggy is a 57-year-old female who is postmenopausal and experiencing difficulties with how this life stage is affecting her sex life and her relationship with her partner. Her desire for sexual activity is particularly low and all other physical and psychologic sources for the problem have been ruled out. You work in the gynecology clinic where Peggy is being treated. Peggy asked the nurse practitioner about treatment with testosterone. You and the nurse practitioner were discussing testosterone's use in postmenopausal hormone replacement therapy following Peggy's appointment. Available data on its use is conflicting and confusing, but the practice is becoming more widespread. One of the problems with this choice of treatment is that women of Peggy's age group are routinely excluded from research examining effectiveness of treatment; therefore, specific information regarding benefits and risks are lacking.

Currently, there is extensive off-label use by women of a variety of testosterone preparations including implants, creams, and gels. Use of these products by men, especially those with muscle-building as well as sexuality concerns, has become a regular practice. There is reason for some concern as the use of this hormone is not without risk.

Further research is needed to determine the role of androgen insufficiency as a cause of low desire in premenopausal as well as postmenopausal women. The role androgens can play in female sexuality will become clearer once practitioners attend to the diurnal variation of testosterone in women and examine these impacts on sexual expression. Research that includes women as participants in testosterone treatment studies, such as the study cited below, can shed some light on risk before primary health care providers routinely prescribe testosterone to women experiencing low desire or to postmenopausal women:

Davis, S. (2000). Testosterone and sexual desire in women. *Journal of Sex Education and Therapy, 25*(1), 25–32.

Pelvic disorders, such as infections, small lesions, endometriosis, scar tissue, or tumors, can result in painful intercourse. Engaging in painful intercourse can lead to vaginismus because the body reflexively becomes guarded and tense. Similarly, in males, infection or inflammation of the glans penis or other genitourinary organs can cause pain with coitus. Also, some contraceptive foams, creams, or sponges can irritate either the vagina or the penis, causing pain. For both women and men, fear and anxiety in anticipation of pain can undermine the person's ability to feel pleasurable sexual responses and may lead to an avoidance of sexual activity.

Vaginismus

Vaginismus is an involuntary spasm of the outer one-third of the vaginal muscles, making penetration of the vagina painful and sometimes impossible. The woman often experiences desire, excitement, and orgasm with stimulation of the external sexual structures. Attempts at intercourse, however, elicit the involuntary spasm. She may have similar difficulty undergoing pelvic exams and inserting tampons or a diaphragm.

The partner often becomes fearful and anxious about hurting her or may become resentful and believe she is having the spasms on purpose. The partner may then develop secondary dysfunctions as a result of these negative feelings and interpretations of rejection.

The vaginismic response may develop initially as a protection against real or anticipated pain. It is often associated with sexual trauma, such as childhood sexual abuse or adult rape. Emotional conflict, such as extreme fear of pregnancy or intense guilt about engaging in sexual activity, may be additional contributing factors.

Other Sexual Concerns and Problems

Dissatisfaction problems, not mentioned in the DSM-IV-TR, which account for a significant group of individuals seeking sex therapy, are important to understand in order to provide effective sexual health care.

PROBLEMS WITH SATISFACTION

Some people experience sexual desire, arousal, and orgasm and yet feel dissatisfied with their sexual relationships. These sexual problems are more commonly related to the emotional tone of the relationship than to the physiologic response. Since giving and receiving pleasure in a mutually intimate relationship are the primary goals of sex for most people, dissatisfaction problems may be more disturbing than other types of sexual dysfunctions.

At times, satisfaction problems may be *situational*. For example, one partner may choose an inconvenient time, or a partner may feel anxious and therefore cannot experience much pleasure or joy. Some people describe their problems as related to lack of extragenital satisfaction. These people describe how much they miss and continue to need all the touching and caressing of their earlier lovemaking experiences. Unfortunately, people who have been relating sexually for a long time often become genitally focused and neglect the rest of the body. One or both partners may feel touch starved, long for more extragenital loving, and become dissatisfied with sex.

Satisfaction problems are often related to relationship difficulties. The inability to communicate effectively in other relationship areas frequently results in sexual frustration. Partners who are angry with each other and make love without resolving the conflict may feel unhappy about the relationship despite having experienced arousal and orgasm. Couples who define their relationship in terms of rigid, unequal power and gender roles may have difficulty negotiating and compromising about sexual issues. Not infrequently, the person with the least amount of power feels helpless and dissatisfied with the sexual interchanges.

Lack of intimacy or a feeling of connectedness is understandably related to satisfaction problems. If one has sex with a stranger, the body may function well, but there is often a sense of something missing after the sexual experience. Making love to one person while feeling more attracted to or in love with another person can result in feelings of emptiness or disconnection. Even couples in a committed relationship may complain of lack of intimacy. Dissatisfaction issues include lack of romance, love, tenderness, and nurturance. Fulfillment of sexuality, then, depends on the ability to relate with a partner in an intimate and mutually pleasing manner that is compatible with values and chosen lifestyle.

INCREASED SEXUAL INTEREST

An increased interest in sex and sexual activity is symptomatic of the manic phase of bipolar disorder. Elevated mood is accompanied by a corresponding rise in sexual activity, variety of activity, and often, number of partners. This behavior occurs despite contrary values and is out of the client's control. The end of the manic episode signals a return to the person's usual level of sexual interest and activity. Since memory is not impaired, the person may feel embarrassed and ashamed about uncontrolled sexual behavior during the manic episode.

Some adult survivors of childhood sexual abuse may go through periods of high sexual activity. This is often a desperate attempt to obtain the nurturance, love, care, and power they were denied in childhood. Having been sexualized at an inappropriately early age, some have learned to survive in a hostile environment by using their sexual availability to make contact with or control others.

SEXUAL ADDICTION

Frequency of sexual activity can be viewed on a continuum, with most people falling in the middle range. Some people have sex frequently in a way that enhances their lives; others have sex infrequently and report contentment and satisfaction. A sexual pattern that falls at either extreme of the continuum, however, can signal problems. At the low extreme is individuals who have great difficulty in choosing to be sexual; such people may have a sexual dysfunction. At the high extreme are people who have lost their ability to choose or control their sexual behavior; these people are sexual addicts.

Sexual addiction is a disorder in which the central focus of life is sex. People with this addiction spend 50% or more of all waking hours dealing with sex, from fantasy to acting-out behavior. Acting-out behavior is often victimless, as in having affairs; overindulging in masturbation, fetishism, pornography use, or commercial telephone sex; or visiting prostitutes. Victimizing behaviors (those with a nonconsenting partner) are less frequent. The incidence of sexual addiction is difficult to determine because of secrecy and shame, but it is estimated that 3% to 6% of the population may be affected. It is predominantly a male disorder with a gender ratio of 5:1 (Kafka, 2000).

It is unethical to label people who do not conform to conventional moral codes as sexual addicts. Sexual addiction is not simply the frequent enjoyment of sexual behaviors. Many people engage in those behaviors without becoming sexual addicts. Rather, sexual addiction is a progressive disorder in which sex is used to numb pain. The payoff is the same as in any other addiction: an intensely pleasurable high, a short-lived release from pain, and an escape from the problems of daily life. The consequences are also the same in that the addict's life eventually becomes unmanageable. The components of sexual addiction are discussed in Box 17–1.

Until their lives become totally unmanageable, sexual addicts may successfully live a double life. They work very hard to appear as normal, moral, and responsible individuals. Many people who have sexual addictions grew up in homes where they were emotionally, physically, or sexually abused. Most of them suffer from low self-esteem and believe themselves to be unlovable. Having a desperate need for love, they equate sex with proof of love. They are so fearful of rejection that they establish only superficial relationships, thus avoiding intimacy and potential abandonment. Often, there is a codependent in the family who is essentially addicted to the addict. The codependent enables the addict by denying the disease or obsessively trying to reform the addict. Codependents also suffer from low self-esteem, inability to express feelings, fear of abandonment, and resistance to change (Kafka, 2000). Codependency is discussed at greater length in Chapter 13.

BOX 17–1 Components of Sexual Addiction

The components of sexual addiction have the hallmarks of obsessive–compulsive behavior.

1. *Preoccupation*. The person spends hours thinking or obsessing about sex. Preoccupation, in itself, gives a sexual high and is so time consuming that the person cannot fulfill work, school, or family responsibilities.
2. *Ritualization*. The individual engages in specific behaviors done just the "right" way and in the same sequence each time. Ritual behaviors include wearing certain clothing, taking certain steps to get ready, driving certain routes, or looking for partners only in a certain area. The ritual seems to control anxiety; once addicts begin a ritual, they cannot stop until the cycle is completed.
3. *Compulsivity*. The person cannot control sexual behavior, and this behavior becomes the most important aspect of life. Some demonstrate sexually compulsive behavior in a regular pattern; others resist for a time and then have a binge cycle.
4. *Shame and despair*. At the end of the cycle, the person experiences guilt and shame at the loss of control. The pain of despair creates the need to begin the cycle all over again, because the addict seeks to relieve pain by getting high. Like other addicts, these individuals want to stop their behavior, promise to stop, try to stop, and are unable to stop without treatment.

SEXUAL DYSFUNCTION AMONG GAY MEN AND LESBIANS

Gay men and lesbians may have the same sexual dysfunctions that occur in the heterosexual population. Living in a culture that has fairly strict gender role expectations can be highly homophobic, however, gays and lesbians experience additional pressures, which may contribute to sexual dysfunctions.

Men, whether gay or straight, may accept stereotyped male gender roles that can lead to ambivalence about intimacy and dependence. Because social norms require that men be unemotional, competitive, and in control, two men in an intimate relationship are likely to experience conflict if both try to be "macho men." The success of the relationship often depends on the partners' ability to negotiate and compromise on issues of power, control, dependence, tenderness, and nurturance. Some gay men find it difficult to develop a positive sexual self-concept in a culture that does not positively model or reinforce a homosexual identity. Gays who internalize society's negative attitudes about homosexuality have low self-esteem and may have sexual problems as a result. It is not uncommon for gay men to interpret sexual problems in relationships as a sign that the relationship is over, as opposed to seeing the dysfunction as a problem to be solved (Nichols, 2000).

Not surprisingly, the reality of HIV infection and AIDS has increased the incidence of sexual dysfunction in the gay community. Anxiety about past exposure to HIV is not conducive to pleasurable and joyful sexual relations. Adapting sexual behavior to safer sex practices may be a source of temporary dysfunction for some gay men.

Not to be overlooked is the role of grief for gay men. A normal aspect of grief for all humans is a period of decreased sexual desire. With lovers and friends dying from AIDS, gay men begin to see the grief process as never ending, and some wonder if they will ever again be able to experience sexual desire. (For further discussion of HIV and AIDS, see Chapter 24.)

The most common sexual problem for lesbians in a committed relationship is one of low desire or low frequency of sexual activity. It is highly unusual for lesbian couples to have difficulty with arousal, orgasm, or satisfaction. The pattern of low desire is typically secondary; that is, it develops at a later point in an ongoing relationship. When sexual activity does occur, both partners feel a general sense of satisfaction.

There are several differences between lesbian couples and heterosexual couples experiencing low sexual desire. Unlike heterosexual couples, lesbian couples do not typically withdraw from sex because of a lack of intimacy, a power imbalance, or rigid gender roles in the relationship. A lesbian couple is more likely to report that the nonsexual areas of their relationship are pleasing and agreeable and that there is minimal conflict about sex. Decreasing sex drive may be related to the socialization of women as passive recipients rather than assertive initiators. Both lesbian and heterosexual women have been taught many sex-negative attitudes, experience more conflict about sex than men do, and may fail to develop their full potential as sexual beings. When two women in an intimate relationship each wait for the other to initiate sex, the result may be low frequency of activity. Thus, many lesbian couples must often make a conscious effort to make love regularly (Nichols, 2000).

Biopsychosocial Theories

Human sexual behavior has been studied from various theoretic perspectives. The most significant are intrapersonal, behavioral, sociocultural, and biologic theories.

A review of the various theoretic perspectives shows that human sexuality has been historically characterized by judgments and controversy that have inhibited sexual health care services. It is important for health care professionals to remember that *all* people to some extent deviate from some physical, social, behavioral, or emotional norm. Some are left-handed, some stutter, some are disabled, some are loners, and some are filled with fears. To achieve the highest level of professional practice, nurses must look beyond the characteristics and respond to the whole person.

Only in the past 40 years has human sexuality been scientifically studied from a multidisciplinary approach. With this knowledge came the beginnings of planned interventions for individuals suffering from a variety of sexual problems and disorders. Nursing has been an active participant in the evolution of treatment approaches and programs to provide sexual health care.

INTRAPERSONAL THEORY

Intrapersonal theorists view gender dysphoria, paraphilias, and sexual dysfunctions as problems occurring within the individual. Some view them as expressions of arrested psychosexual development, some seek an explanation in sexual guilt, and others see the issue as being one of self-punishment. People who grew up with rigid family and religious taboos about sex often experience guilt and anxiety about their adult sexual roles and behaviors. Performance anxiety, negative self-concept, and negative body image are all seen as contributing to sexual problems. Problems to be solved during the treatment process include fears of:

- Intimacy.
- Losing control.
- Pain.
- Pregnancy.
- Sexually transmitted diseases.

BEHAVIORAL THEORY

Behaviorists believe that gender dysphoria arises from social learning; that is, that the child was rewarded in some way for adopting behaviors of the other sex. They believe paraphilias are learned responses; the person is conditioned to respond erotically to nonsexual objects or particular sexual acts. In the area of sexual dysfunctions, contributing factors include poor communication skills, lack of sexual experience with oneself or a partner, concern with sexual performance, and ineffective stimulation. The dysfunctions, too, are seen as learned responses.

SOCIOCULTURAL THEORY

Ideas about sexuality and sexual behavior are based on cultural values and understanding. What is considered normal or abnormal depends on each group's specific viewpoint. The same behavior may be seen as positive in one culture and pathologic in another. Each culture tends to incorporate *ethnocentrism* in its beliefs; that is, its members believe their particular sexual values and behaviors are superior and preferable to those of any other culture. Ethnocentrism encourages people to view the sexual behavior of other people as eccentric, exotic, and bizarre.

Consider the diversity of sexual values throughout the world. The Mangaia of Polynesia believe that young adolescents of both genders have high sexual drives. However, as they leave young adulthood, they expect their desire to rapidly decline. In contrast, the Dani of New Guinea believe that neither women nor men have high sexual drives and that the primary purpose of sex is for reproduction. Following the birth of a child, the husband and wife remain celibate for the next 5 years. Among the Sambrans of New Guinea, young boys around age 7 or 8 have sex with older boys. It is believed that the ingestion of semen is required for physical growth. This pattern of behavior changes to heterosexual interaction as the young men become adults.

Cultures in some parts of Africa and the Middle East practice ritual mutilation of the clitoris, *female genital mutilation*, as a rite of initiation into womanhood. Because of serious medical complications and psychological trauma, the practice has been outlawed in many countries, although the laws are rarely enforced. Among many cultures throughout the world, there is a third gender. Among the Zuni of New Mexico, this person is called a *berdache*, a male who assumes female dress, gender role, and status. Individuals with this third gender are often considered to have great spiritual power (Strong, DeVault, & Sayad, 1999).

The sexual ethics of a culture reflect the culture's assumptions about the purpose of sex. In North American culture, sexual practices have been strongly influenced by the Judeo-Christian tradition, which historically considered procreation to be the primary purpose of sex. As a result, even modern North American culture is fairly sexually intolerant and harshly critical of those whose gender identity or sexual behavior is not in the mainstream.

How people communicate about sexuality is culturally determined. In general, North American culture reflects Euro-American values, which include a negative view of public sexual communication, as evidenced by censorship and sex as a taboo topic for general discussion. However, there are ethnic differ-

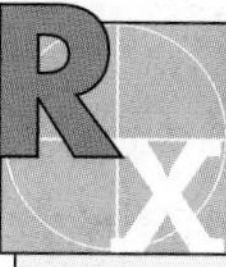

COMMUNICATION

Client Experiencing Homophobia

CLIENT: "The other day I overheard my brother saying to his friend that he'd like to kill me because I am gay. I was shocked and I'm still very upset."

NURSE RESPONSE 1: "In the past, how have you coped with hearing homophobic statements?"

RATIONALE: Building on the client's strengths previously used in other similar situations to help develop an adaptive response in this recurrent situation.

NURSE RESPONSE 2: "Has your brother ever physically hurt you?"

RATIONALE: Evaluating the client's safety and the possibility that the client may have been abused or traumatized.

ences in communication patterns. African-Americans tend to be very expressive and communicate directly about sexual topics. Latinos from the Caribbean and Central American cultures tend to use restraint in expressing their feelings while those from Argentina and some other Latin American countries are emotionally expressive. Asian-Americans are often less verbally expressive, so nonverbal communication assumes even more importance. The gay and lesbian subculture has developed private words and expressions in reaction to the homophobia of the dominant culture (Hecht, Collier, & Ribeau, 1993; Strong, Devault, & Sayad, 1999; Ting-Toomey & Chung, 2002). See the Rx Communication feature at the top of this page for an example of a client interaction around homophobia.

People with little tolerance for cross-gender behavior view transsexuals and cross-dressers as deviants. The sexual acts of noncoercive paraphiliacs conflict with the traditional value of sex for procreation, and they, too, are made to feel like outcasts. Sociocultural theories regarding sexual dysfunctions focus on disturbed relationships between partners, negative early learning, and past or present traumatic events.

BIOLOGIC THEORY

Those individuals who take a biologic approach are concerned with the physiologic aspects of gender identity and sexual behavior. Some believe there is a neurologic basis for gender differences and look to fetal exposure to sex hormones and adult levels of sex hormones as an explanation of gender dysphoria. They explore sexual dysfunctions to discover factors (e.g., organic disease, injury, medications, pain, and/or depression) that interfere with the physiologic reflexes during the sexual response cycle.

It is clear from research over the past several years that many problems of sexual function are physiologic in nature, initially. In middle age, for example, normal physiologic changes (such as decreased hormone production) may interfere with sexual pleasure and interest. Arteriosclerosis, diabetes, and other medical problems can interfere with the ability to have an erection. These biologic factors are discussed in two locations in this chapter—in the earlier section on sexual dysfunctions, and in the nursing process section that follows.

At this time there is no clear understanding of the etiology of transsexualism. Biologic theory is based on animal studies because experimental research cannot be conducted with humans. When exposed prenatally to increased male hormones, experimental animals exhibit increased male behavior. Decreasing the levels of male hormones prenatally increases female behavior in animals. In humans, the male gonads develop and begin secreting androgen during weeks 8 to 12 of gestation. Differentiation of the hypothalamus to a male pattern, which occurs in months 4 to 5 of gestation, requires high androgen levels. Thus, one explanation of transsexualism is that prenatal androgen levels were sufficient for the development of male anatomy but insufficient for differentiation in the brain. In transsexuals who are anatomically female, the androgenic influences may have been high at the critical time of hypothalamic development, although not at the time of genital formation (Lips, 2001).

NURSING PROCESS

Clients with Gender Identity and Sexual Disorders

MediaLink Care Plan: Dyspareunia

The nursing care of clients with gender identity and sexual disorders requires extensive background and experience. While nurses at all levels of practice should aim to develop a trusting relationship, assess clients for sexual concerns and refer clients to a health care provider with special expertise in dealing with these charged issues. The actual diagnoses and interventions of these clients are best left to the providers with special expertise. Keep the level of your professional skills and knowledge foremost in your mind when working with these clients and act appropriately and in tune with the standards of care discussed in Chapter 1. The Case Study and Nursing Care Plan on pages 416–417 can be useful to both the generalist and the specialist.

Assessment

You will find numerous opportunities to apply the nursing process to the promotion of sexual health. Assessment of sexual status is part of a thorough and comprehensive assessment of a client's general health.

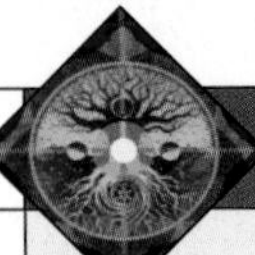

Case Study

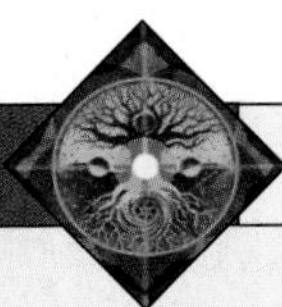

A Client with Low Sexual Desire and Orgasmic Disorder

Identifying Information

Susan is a 46-year-old married woman who has come with her 48-year-old husband, Brad, to the local mental health outpatient clinic. Neither of them has received mental health services prior to this time.

Client's Description of the Problem

Both Susan and Brad agree that there is a disparity of sexual needs. Susan is satisfied to have sex once a month, and Brad wants to have sex several times a week. Susan has never been orgasmic with Brad but does admit to achieving orgasms during masturbation, a fact she has never been able to tell Brad. Susan states that she would probably like to have sex more often if she would enjoy it. Her fear is that she will not become orgasmic. Brad thinks that entering therapy is the first big step, and he is hopeful that their sexual relationship will improve.

They both describe their sex life at the beginning of their marriage as fine for the first several years, although Susan states that she was never orgasmic during that time. They never talked about their sex life. Some years ago, after reading a "sex book," Susan experimented with masturbation for the first time and began to experience orgasms. She was never able to share this information with Brad because she felt guilty about touching herself when she was alone. They are verbally and physically affectionate with one another, but, they say, not as much as they used to be. Very seldom do they express their anger to one another, and they manage most relationship conflicts by avoiding the issue.

History

No prior psychiatric history. Both Susan and Brad are second-generation Americans of Eastern European descent. Both describe their parents as very modest and noncommunicative about any sexual issues. No sex education was given in the family. Susan and Brad have been married 25 years and have two children: a daughter, 19; and a son, 14. Brad has a good position in sales, and Susan is employed as a bookkeeper.

They both agree that Brad initiates sexual activity, primarily nonverbally. Sex typically occurs in the bedroom, after midnight, when they are both tired. Susan determines the length of foreplay, which usually lasts 5 to 10 minutes. The only position they use is man-on-top, but both agree they would like to try other positions. Brad has minimal verbal communication during sex, and Susan says she is too shy to say anything while they are making love. They both have difficulty talking about their sex life with one another. Susan states she is somewhat uncomfortable when Brad touches her body, except for her genitals and breasts. She is comfortable touching Brad's genitals but not touching her own genitals in front of him. She likes to receive oral sex but is uncomfortable giving it because she is afraid Brad will ejaculate in her mouth. Their mutual goals in therapy are to have sex more often, to feel freer to experiment, to discuss sex openly, and to have Susan experience pleasure and orgasms.

Brad has no current or past medical problems. Susan had a hysterectomy 5 years ago for endometriosis and is on hormone replacement therapy.

Current Mental Status

They are both quiet-spoken but articulate individuals. Eye contact is appropriate, mood is stable and appropriate, thought processes are logical, and there are no obvious symptoms of stress. Although they were both uncomfortable discussing sex, it became easier during a 2-hour history-taking time.

SUBJECTIVE DATA

The sexual history provides subjective assessment data needed for formulating nursing diagnoses. Elicit sexual information much as you elicit a general nursing history. Pay special attention, however, to planning a setting where privacy and uninterrupted time are available. Such a setting helps clients feel comfortable discussing these private aspects of their lives. It is helpful to begin the interview by explaining why you are asking about sexuality; for example: "Sexuality is a part of people's lives. People often have questions about sexual activity when they have changes in their health. I'd like to take this time to talk with you about your sex life."

Move from general to specific questions. This gradual focus on specific sexual behavior promotes trust and rapport. Initially, questions can relate sexuality to health status. Open-ended questions encourage clients to expand on their sexual experiences and concerns. Reassure clients that it is normal to have sexual concerns and questions, for instance: "It is common for many people to feel concerned about __________. Do you have any questions?" Restate clients' responses to encourage them to expand on feelings. The Assessment box on page 417 lists questions that can be part of a general nursing history. If clients do identify a sexual problem or if they take medications that affect sexual desire or sexual behavior, you can use the information in ■ Table 17–2 (page 418) to formulate your questions.

OBJECTIVE DATA

Objective data include observed nonverbal behaviors, laboratory data, test results, medical diagnoses, physical examination results, and other documented sources, such as the chart. Objective data may also include results of physiologic assessment of sexual function.

Erectile Capacity. The nocturnal penile tumescence (NPT) procedure provides a direct measure of erectile capacity. The device measures penile engorgement that occurs during sleep. NPT measurement is considered the best available method to determine if a man's erectile difficulties are physiologic. If so, there is minimal penile engorgement during sleep. Men whose erection difficulties appear to be psychological in origin have normal engorgement during sleep. Although the NPT procedure is an important source of objective data, its results are not always reliable. Research findings report a 28% to 42% error in accuracy (Rosen, 2000).

Female Sexual Function. Physiologic assessment of female sexual function is accomplished by the use of vaginal plethysmographs or probes. These devices are inserted into the vagina and measure vasocongestion of the vaginal wall tissue.

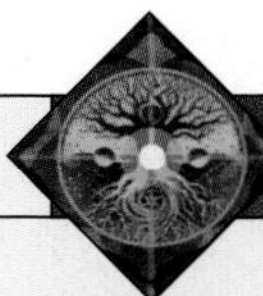

Nursing Care Plan

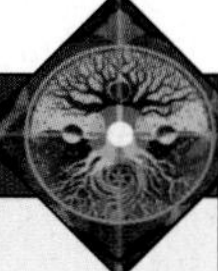

Nursing Diagnosis: Altered Sexuality Patterns related to disparity of needs.

Expected Outcome: Client will demonstrate an understanding of sexual anatomy, physiology, and openly communicate about sex.

Short-Term Goals	*Interventions*	*Rationale*
Susan will be able to discuss the frequency of sexual activity with Brad.	• Exploration of unspoken expectations and the potential for hurt feelings. • Discuss and train on the meaning of, and the process of, compromising. • Discuss alternative ways to meet sexual needs besides intercourse.	Sexual expectations are seldom similar and coming to a compromise regarding sex contributes to a healthy relationship.
The couple will agree on an average frequency for sex.	• Encourage communication during sex such as what they like and how they like things between them.	Masturbation and fantasy may not be readily accessible intercourse alternatives.
Susan will be able to achieve orgasm during sexual activity with Brad.	• Give homework assignments designed to address sexual communications.	Practice establishes behavior.
	• Discuss physiology of Susan's sexuality related to orgasmic functioning.	Information describes Susan's ability to achieve orgasm.
	• Encourage activities in which Susan has achieved orgasm.	

Laboratory Tests. Several sophisticated and expensive laboratory tests are designed to assess sexual function. For instance, testosterone and estrogen blood levels may be measured. However, laboratory data must be interpreted with caution because test results are not always reliable indicators of actual sexual behavior. Thus, clients' self-reports of sexual performance, feelings, and values (the subjective data) are of primary importance in assessment.

Nursing Diagnosis: NANDA

The following sections discuss the most likely nursing diagnoses and their implications for clients and nurses.

ANXIETY AND FEAR

Anxiety and fear inhibit the physiologic sexual response as well as the ability to experience pleasure and joy. People who grow

ASSESSMENT Sexual History: The ABCs

Affective Assessment

To whom do you feel most intimate and connected?
Describe the type of love and affection in this relationship.
In what way do you experience anxiety about sex?
In what way do you experience guilt about sex?
How depressed are you feeling?
In what way does anger interfere with your sexual functioning?
Do you dislike or feel an aversion to any parts of your body?

Behavioral Assessment

Describe your level of satisfaction with the frequency of your sexual activity.
Describe the positive aspects of your own sexual functioning.
Describe the negative aspects of your own sexual functioning.
What concerns do you have about your future sexual functioning?
What are your partner's concerns about current or future sexual functioning?

Cognitive Assessment

When you were growing up, how did you learn about sex?
How has your religion influenced your sexual values and behaviors?
What "shoulds/should nots," "musts/must nots" do you believe about your sexual behavior/relationships?
How rigidly were gender roles enforced in your family of origin?
How are gender roles enacted in your present relationship/family?
Describe the negative thoughts you have about sex.
Does the use of fantasy increase or decrease your sexual desire?

Sensation Assessment

Describe any physical discomfort you feel during sexual activity.
To what degree do you experience pleasure during sexual activity?

TABLE 17–2 Drugs and Related Sexual Side Effects

	Sexual Side Effects						
Drug	***Increased Sex Drive***	***Decreased Sex Drive***	***Decreased Arousal***	***Retrograde Ejaculation***	***Inhibited Ejaculation***	***Painful Ejaculation***	***Orgasm Problems***
Alcohol	small amts	large amts	yes		yes		
Amphetamines	yes		may		yes		yes
Antihypertensives		yes	yes		yes		
Antipsychotics (atypical)		yes	yes		yes		yes
Antipsychotics (conventional)		yes	yes	may	may		yes
Anxiolytics (very few side effects)							
Beta blockers		yes	yes				
Cocaine	yes				yes		yes
Diuretics		yes	yes				
Hallucinogens (unpredictable side effects)		may	may				may
Heroin		yes	yes		yes		yes
Lithium		yes	yes				
MAO inhibitors		may	may				may
Marijuana	small amts	large amts	chronic use				
Mood stabilizers		yes	yes				yes
SSRIs			yes				yes
Steroids		yes	yes				
Tricyclic antidepressants		yes	yes		yes	may	yes

up learning that sex is dirty and sinful often experience anxiety in an adult relationship or are so fearful that they develop a phobic avoidance of sex. Adults who have been emotionally, physically, or sexually abused as children often fear intimacy and find they cannot have a trusting relationship with another person. Even individuals with a positive sexual history may at some time feel anxious about their sexual performance and develop a secondary fear of failure as a sex partner.

SPIRITUAL DISTRESS

Lack of fulfillment in a sexual relationship may be related to a temporary feeling of distance from one's partner or an ongoing lack of intimacy in the relationship. Factors relating to lack of intimacy are relationship conflict, multiple fears, adult sexual abuse, or childhood sexual abuse.

INEFFECTIVE FAMILY COPING: COMPROMISED

It is difficult to experience sexual fulfillment when the relationship is in trouble in nonsexual spheres. The difficulty may be as straightforward as poor communication or as complex as conflict, anger, and unequal power. Other socioeconomic stressors include underemployment, unemployment, and lack of social network support. When one of the partners cross-dresses, the other partner must come to terms with the behavior if a healthy relationship is to be maintained. Being part of a family with a transsexual means finding ways to reintegrate the person as a member of the other sex, or else reject the transsexual person and distance the family from this particular member.

PERSONAL IDENTITY DISTURBANCE

In cultures with rigid gender roles, transsexuals and cross-dressers suffer a great deal of pain as they struggle with their gender identity. Transsexuals completely reject their anatomic sex, and cross-dressers alternate between their male and their female personas.

ALTERED ROLE PERFORMANCE

Sexual addicts often cannot maintain work, family, and social roles. The addiction is so time consuming that the addict cannot devote time or energy to work or relationships.

ALTERED SEXUALITY PATTERNS

Some people cannot achieve sexual arousal and orgasm without the stimulation of an unusual object or situation. These individuals are considered to have one of the paraphilias, which may be coercive or noncoercive. Most often they are preoccupied with, and feel compelled to engage in, their particular sexual behaviors.

RISK FOR VIOLENCE: SELF-DIRECTED OR DIRECTED AT OTHERS

Autoerotic asphyxia is noncoercive but often fatal. People with this sexual behavior are not suicidal and have no intention of harming themselves but may accidentally kill themselves during sexual activity. Coercive paraphilias are considered to be violent against others because the victim is nonconsenting and offended or hurt by the paraphiliac's sexual behavior.

PAIN

A nursing diagnosis of Pain applies to women who experience vaginismus. The origin may be past sexual trauma or current emotional conflict. The pain of dyspareunia may occur in both women and men and is typically related to organic factors.

KNOWLEDGE DEFICIT

People who grow up with no or very limited sex education may have difficulties in their adult sexual functioning. For people who don't know what to expect or how to touch themselves or their partners, sexual interactions can be frustrating rather than pleasurable. Lack of knowledge can contribute to ineffective sexual techniques and sexual dysfunctions.

SEXUAL DYSFUNCTION

Many of the above nursing diagnoses may be contributing factors to the development of sexual dysfunctions. In addition, illness, injury, surgery, medications, or substance abuse may contribute to sexual dysfunction. Problems with satisfaction may be described under either of these diagnoses: Sexual Dysfunction or Spiritual Distress.

Outcome Identification: NOC

The outcomes expected with this group of clients focuses on the specific problem interfering with normal functioning. If the client has been sexually abused or traumatized and this has affected sexual functioning, then the outcome expected is that the client will have sexual abuse recovery. Other issues, such as menopause and aging impacts, are addressed with physical aging status outcomes.

Risk control is important as an outcome for those with sexual addictions or an increase in sexual interest. Actions need to be taken to reduce or eliminate the behaviors associated with risky sexual behavior so that sexually transmitted diseases are avoided. Outcomes in this overall area of nursing are related to the likelihood of the disorder.

Planning and Implementation: NIC

Nurses play several roles in promoting sexual health. The Mims–Swensen Sexual Health Model (1980) identifies four levels (listed below) at which nurses can intervene, consistent with their comfort and knowledge. Determine the appropriate level for you and base your interventions accordingly.

LIFE EXPERIENCE LEVEL

This level of intervention is the minimal level of practice. Interventions are based solely on the nurse's own personal experiences. Interventions may be appropriate for clients who share similar life experiences. However, clients having different values or demonstrating different behaviors may perceive interventions based on the nurse's life experiences as irrelevant.

Despite increased openness regarding homosexuality, many nurses remain biased and unqualified to intervene with gay and lesbian clients. Much of their bias can be attributed to heterosexist or homophobic attitudes of the society in which we live. *Heterosexism* is a value system that assumes that heterosexuality is the only appropriate form of sexual interaction. *Homophobia* is discrimination, oppression, and violence against homosexuals and bisexuals. In order to be effective, nurses must learn to move beyond the life experience level of intervention.

BASIC LEVEL

This intervention level is grounded in the nurse's self-awareness combined with a nonjudgmental respect for others' sexual belief, practices, and concerns. Nurses at this level have some knowledge about human sexual function. The knowledgeable and nonjudgmental nurse can intervene as a facilitator for clients needing to talk about their sexuality.

INTERMEDIATE LEVEL

Nurses practicing at this level of intervention synthesize knowledge, self-awareness, communication skills, and the use of the nursing process. Nurses are validators of normal sexual behavior and accept the range of sexual expression in our society. Teaching about sexual response is another intervention to resolve client concerns. Teaching is often directed at helping clients understand their stage of sexual development. For instance, teenagers and young adults frequently require accurate information regarding anatomy and physiology, sexual desire, and contraception.

Counseling interventions are also implemented in the intermediate level. Counseling is not merely giving advice. The nurse counselor helps clients clarify their sexual problems and decide on alternatives to resolve the problems. Use only those techniques in which you have training and experience. Refer clients who require sex therapy to an advanced level practitioner.

ADVANCED LEVEL

At this level of intervention, nurses must have specialized preparation and knowledge of sexual and gender identity disorders. Nurses at the advanced level practice sex therapy, develop and present formal education programs, and do sex research.

Nurses who do function in the sex therapist role should meet the qualifications for practice identified by the American Association of Sex Educators, Counselors, and Therapists (AASECT), which differentiate sex counseling from sex therapy.

MediaLink Sex Therapy Resources

Sex counseling helps clients incorporate their sexual knowledge into satisfying lifestyles and socially responsible behavior. *Sex therapy* is a highly specialized, in-depth treatment to help clients resolve serious sexual problems, especially some sexual disorders. AASECT publishes a national directory of professionals, certified to provide sex education, counseling, or therapy. This directory is a sex therapy resource for nurses. A resource link to AASECT can be accessed through the Companion Website of this book.

Some specific sexual counseling strategies are listed in the Intervention box at right.

REDUCING ANXIETY AND FEAR

Accurate identification of feelings is the first step in the problem-solving process, and clients may need help labeling the feelings they are experiencing. Following this step, help clients identify one anxiety-producing situation within their sexual interactions. At this stage, it is productive to focus diffuse anxiety on a manageable single situation or event. With the client, analyze the situation or event to discover negative anticipatory thoughts that may be the source of the anxiety. Together, review how the client has handled anxiety in the past and evaluate the range and effectiveness of this past coping behavior. It may be appropriate to help the client redefine the sensations of anxiety as sensations of sexual excitement, which is more likely to result in positive expectations. Together, explore alternative coping behaviors, and have the client evaluate their effectiveness after implementing them.

MediaLink Support Groups

Many adult survivors of childhood sexual abuse are periodically overwhelmed by anxiety, fear, and panic (see Chapter 16). Refer adult survivors to support groups such as Incest Anonymous or VOICES, as well as individual therapy with a therapist who specializes in this field. Links to these resources are provided on the Companion Website for this book.

REDUCING SPIRITUAL DISTRESS

Because the origin of spiritual distress is a lack of intimacy or connection, the goal of nursing intervention is to help clients achieve and maintain a level of intimacy each partner finds comfortable. In the context of therapy, couples discuss their individual needs for closeness and identify barriers to intimacy. They are instructed to make three or four half-hour "dates" each week, during which they share warmth and intimacy. They spend some of the time discussing specific sexual issues; during other "dates," the couple explores intimate, nonsexual topics, such as hopes and expectations for the future. Couples should give these dates top priority, because a common way of avoiding intimacy is by not setting time aside for each other.

PROMOTING MORE EFFECTIVE FAMILY COPING

Good communication is an important part of a sexually fulfilling relationship. Apart from setting specific times to share feelings and beliefs, some couples need training in more effective communication skills. If they give ambiguous signals to indicate sexual interest, they need to learn how to state their interest clearly. Some people expect their partners to "read their minds" about sexual needs and desires; these people need encouragement to assert their needs tactfully. Teach couples to avoid "you" language, which evokes a

INTERVENTION

Guidelines for Working with Clients with Sexual Difficulties

Male Orgasmic Disorder

Reestablish a climate of comfort and acceptance for sexual interaction.

Encourage the client to masturbate and enjoy touch and body stimulation in general.

Premature Ejaculation

Instruct the client to stimulate the erect penis until the premonitory sensations of impending orgasm are felt. Then penile stimulation is abruptly stopped. This process is repeated to lower the threshold of excitability and make the client more tolerant of the stimuli. Sometimes the client uses the squeeze technique: At the point of orgasm, she squeezes the head of the penis with thumb and first two fingers for 3 to 4 seconds. This stops the urge to ejaculate.

The couple is also instructed in ways to reduce friction in the vagina by limiting the frequency of thrusts or the movement within the vagina.

Female Orgasmic Disorder

Instruct the client to avoid intercourse. Nongenital caressing exercises begin with man and woman alternating as the initiator of a session of caressing, thus sharing responsibility for sexual interaction.

Next, genital stimulation is added to provide positive sexual experiences without intercourse. When intercourse is attempted, the woman is instructed to assume the superior position and insert the man's penis into her vagina. When setbacks occur, the couple is advised to rely on sexual techniques that do not involve intercourse. The woman is to place her hand lightly on her partner's to indicate her preference for contact. The emphasis is not on achieving orgasm but on learning erotic preferences.

The couple is instructed to use the side-by-side position, which enables both partners to move freely with emphasis on slow, exploratory thrusting. The goal is to develop an ability to enjoy pelvic play with the penis inside the vagina.

Vaginismus

Begin with a physical demonstration to the woman of her involuntary vaginal spasm by inserting an examining finger into her vagina. Then Hegar dilators in graduated sizes are inserted by the man into the woman's vagina. At first she manually controls his insertion of the smallest dilator. Later he can insert larger dilators following her verbal instructions. After larger dilators are successfully inserted, she is instructed to retain the dilator for several hours each night. Most involuntary spasms can be relieved in 3 to 5 days with the daily use of dilators.

In addition to physical relief from spastic constriction, therapy is directed toward alleviating the fear that led to the onset of symptoms.

Sexual Acting-Out

After identifying increased levels of anxiety with clients, openly discuss the meanings of behaviors. Give feedback about inappropriate behavior, and discuss appropriate ways to meet sexual needs. Reassure clients that you are not rejecting them, but the behavior.

defensive response and results in arguments, and to use "I" language, which expresses personal thoughts, feelings, and needs. Some examples of accusatory "you" statements and answerable "I" statements are in the Intervention box below. If the relationship is in significant trouble, refer the couple for relationship or sex therapy.

If cross-dressing is a newly divulged secret, offer education and support. If the relationship is to continue, both partners need to agree on where and how cross-dressing will take place. Some couples compromise; for instance, a husband may agree never to cross-dress in front of his wife, and she may agree to give him privacy. Some agree to limit cross-dressing to the home; others are comfortable going out in public with the partner cross-dressed. The long-term success of the relationship depends on the couple's ability to negotiate these issues.

PROMOTING COMFORT WITH PERSONAL IDENTITY

People who experience gender dysphoria have many possible options to manage the transgendered part of themselves. Physically they may undergo hormonal treatment, genital reassignment surgery, electrolysis, breast surgery, or other cosmetic surgery. They may decide to live in the other gender role part time or full time, prefer to have sex as a woman or as a man with a female, male, both, or neither. They may view themselves as female, male, both, a third gender, or a transgendered person. Interventions focus on promoting comfort with the chosen gender role.

PROMOTING EFFECTIVE ROLE PERFORMANCE

Like other addicts, sexual addicts often do not seek help until they literally cannot manage their lives. They may lose their job, home, and relationships before admitting the consequences of the addiction. When that occurs, they may become severely depressed and even suicidal. Refer sexual addicts to self-help groups and specialized professional therapy. Recovery is a long-term process facilitated by individual, group, couple, family, and family-of-origin therapy.

INTERVENTION

Asserting Sexual Needs Tactfully

Couples involved in communications around emotionally difficult subjects such as sex convey messages more competently through "I" language than through the accusatory "you" language.

"You" Language

- "You only have sex on your mind. You're a pervert."
- "You keep grabbing at me like I'm always ready to go to bed with you."
- "You never pay attention to what turns me on. Are you dumb or hard of hearing?"

"I" Language

- "I'm concerned because we seem to have different expectations of how often we would like to make love."
- "I miss all the hugging and caressing we used to do even when we couldn't make love afterward."
- "I feel frustrated and hurt when it seems like I'm repeating myself. Maybe I'm not communicating my needs very clearly."

PROMOTING NONCOERCIVE SEXUALITY PATTERNS

Once paraphilias are a programmed part of arousal, they are very difficult to deprogram. The response to certain sexual or erotic stimuli tends to persist through life. A noncoercive, nonharmful paraphilia practiced with an adult, consenting partner requires no nursing intervention other than client and partner education and possible couple negotiation about the behavior.

REDUCING VIOLENCE AGAINST SELF AND OTHERS

The most important nursing intervention regarding autoerotic asphyxia is community education. Warnings about autoerotic asphyxia should be routinely included in adolescent sex-education programs. Teenagers who practice it must be encouraged to seek immediate professional help. Parents should be taught to look for physical signs of trauma to the neck such as bruising, abrasions, pressure marks, or rope burns. Ropes, knotted sheets, knotted T-shirts, or the like hidden in the bedroom may be warning signs.

Individuals who practice coercive paraphilias typically end up in the criminal justice system. The court may or may not mandate therapy. Therapy for sex offenders is a specialized area that should not be undertaken lightly. Although behavior-modification techniques, group therapy, and hypnosis are used, they are generally unsuccessful. In severe cases, male sex offenders are treated with the antiandrogen drug medroxyprogesterone acetate (Provera or Depo-Provera), which induces a reversible chemical castration. The drug reduces the male sex drive, erections, and ejaculation and decreases the obsessional focus on sex.

REDUCING PAIN

Whenever pain is associated with intercourse, a thorough physical examination is necessary to find and treat the organic cause of the pain. During vaginal exams, careful attention must be paid to tiny tears in the vaginal wall, which are often overlooked. Even very small tears can cause great pain during intercourse. Vaginismus is treated with education, dilators, and supportive psychotherapy. (See the Intervention box on page 420.)

INCREASING KNOWLEDGE

The lack of sex education is not unusual among people with sexual dysfunctions. Nurses can intervene by teaching clients about their sexual anatomy and the sexual response cycle. Encourage couples to talk with one another about their individual responses. Some people may be very uncomfortable with sexual language and need help learning sexual vocabulary and identifying which words are acceptable for intimate use. Part of the learning and desensitization process is having them repeat the words aloud to one another until they feel comfortable using them. Sexual disorders are explained in comfortable, lay terms on the Sexual Disorders Website at www. athealth.com/Consumer/disorders/Sexual.html.

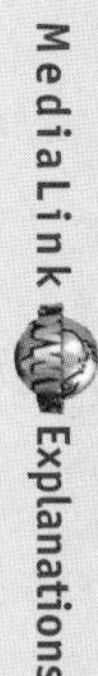

MANAGING SEXUAL DYSFUNCTIONS: SEX THERAPY

There are many approaches to the treatment of sexual dysfunctions, including individual, couple, and group treatment with one or two sex therapists. The duration of treatment varies. Treatment programs may be for heterosexual, homosexual, or bisexual individuals or couples. The effectiveness of these programs depends on the client's needs and the therapists' skill. The common components of sex therapy are discussed in Box 17–2.

Evaluation

Examining your care for effectiveness is especially important where discomfort and bias could interfere with treatment for a client's sexual dysfunction.

ANXIETY AND FEAR

Clients will be able to use the problem-solving process as one tool for decreasing anxiety and fear. They will implement effective coping measures and verbalize a decrease in anxiety. Adult survivors of childhood sexual abuse will participate in support groups and engage in psychotherapy to manage the fears and trauma of the past.

SPIRITUAL DISTRESS

Couples will report an acceptable and meaningful level of intimacy in their relationships. They will continue to set aside time for each other and engage in meaningful intimate time.

BOX 17–2 Common Components of Sex Therapy Programs

- **Information and education about sexual functions.** The therapist gives clients specific information about their particular needs. The therapist may assign books to read or discuss the information.
- **Experiential/sensory awareness.** The therapist helps clients recognize feelings of anxiety, anger, and pleasure by tuning into bodily cues. Clients focus on and describe feelings both in therapy sessions and at home. If they believe their genitals are ugly and unclean, the therapist assigns desensitization exercises at home for clients to explore and become familiar with their own bodies. Some clients need fantasy training if nonsexual thoughts interfere with sexual arousal.
- **Insight.** The therapist attempts to learn and understand what is causing and perpetuating the sexual problem. The goal is for clients to assume responsibility for their own behavior and recognize that change is possible.
- **Cognitive restructuring.** Clients identify and reevaluate their fears about sexual interaction. The therapist encourages them to identify and eliminate negative self-statements and irrational expectations.
- **Behavioral interventions.** Since the focus is on changing nonsexual behavior that contributes to sexual problems, the therapist may assign assertiveness training, communication training, stress-reduction exercises, and problem-solving techniques. Behavioral interventions include assigned pleasuring sessions to discover what is arousing and pleasing to the self and partner.

FAMILY COPING

Couples will increase the use of "I" language and decrease the use of blaming "you" language. They will express their sexual desires, needs, and preferences directly. If the relationship is in significant trouble, they will report a willingness to seek therapy. If one partner is a cross-dresser, the couple will negotiate the cross-dressing behavior, and both partners will report satisfaction with their relationship.

GENDER IDENTITY

Clients will report increasing comfort and satisfaction in their new gender role, which will be congruent with their gender identity. Each will be able to function socially and economically as a person of that gender.

ROLE PERFORMANCE

Clients will participate actively in self-help groups as well as professional therapy. If addicted they will be able to manage their addiction in such a way that they can maintain intimate relationships and be financially responsible. Family members will participate actively in the appropriate self-help groups.

NONCOERCIVE SEXUALITY PATTERNS

Clients and partners will verbalize an understanding that noncoercive paraphilias are lifelong patterns. Couples will be able to negotiate the behavior in a way that is mutually satisfying.

VIOLENCE

Community and family education programs will be established about the danger of autoerotic asphyxia. Victims of this disorder will be identified and referred for immediate treatment. Clients with this disorder will remain safe. Coercive paraphiliacs will curb their behavior, or society will set strict limits to protect potential victims.

PAIN

Individuals will report less pain or no pain during intercourse. Clients suffering from vaginismus will report success in using conscious control to relax vaginal muscles, allowing for pain-free intercourse.

KNOWLEDGE

Clients will describe sexual anatomy and the phases of the sexual response cycle. Couples will report increased communication about individual responses and preferences using a selected sexual vocabulary.

SEXUAL DYSFUNCTION

Clients will report a satisfying and fulfilling sex life. They will experience minimal difficulty with desire, arousal, or orgasm. They will be able to identify and label feelings and acknowledge responsibility for their own behavior. They will implement a chosen variety of sexual techniques.

Case Management

Case management services tend to revolve around the coercive paraphilias and autoerotic asphyxia. The criminal justice system is involved in the former, and may or may not be involved in the latter case. Case management consists mainly of making arrangements for services for the client, but the majority of effort is focused on protecting others. Treatment for coercive paraphilias has not been successful to any significant extent and recidivism is all too common.

Community-Based and Home Care

Transsexuals are usually referred to therapists who specialize in this area or to gender identity disorder clinics. Because gender identity is stable, the goal of treatment with transsexuals is to help them live and function in society in the cross-gender role. They need a great deal of support and assistance as they establish themselves in their new role. If the present job is not gender-role stereotyped, they may be able to remain in the same or similar position. Others may need retraining programs to find acceptable employment. A multidisciplinary approach is most effective in helping transsexuals adjust to their situation. Family and friends need support and counseling to reintegrate this person into their lives as a person of the other sex (Carroll, 2000).

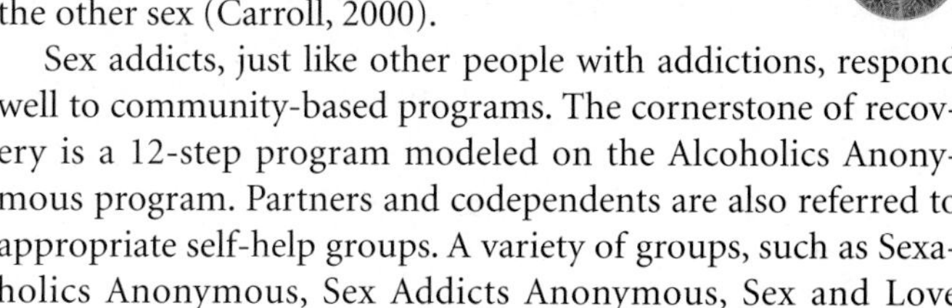

Sex addicts, just like other people with addictions, respond well to community-based programs. The cornerstone of recovery is a 12-step program modeled on the Alcoholics Anonymous program. Partners and codependents are also referred to appropriate self-help groups. A variety of groups, such as Sexaholics Anonymous, Sex Addicts Anonymous, Sex and Love Addicts Anonymous, S-Anon, and Co-Dependents of Sexual Addicts, have been formed throughout the country.

For cross-dressers, a community-based plan of care may include joining a club, such as Tri-Ess, where they can express their female personality in a safe social situation. Counseling for the individual or the couple at a community mental health clinic frequently focuses on the development of compromise within the relationship around cross-dressing issues.

Links to these resources can be found on the Companion Website for this book.

MediaLink Self-Help Groups

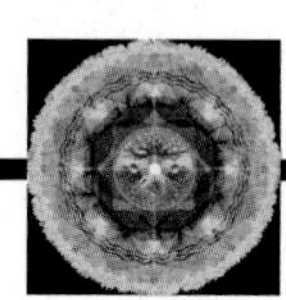

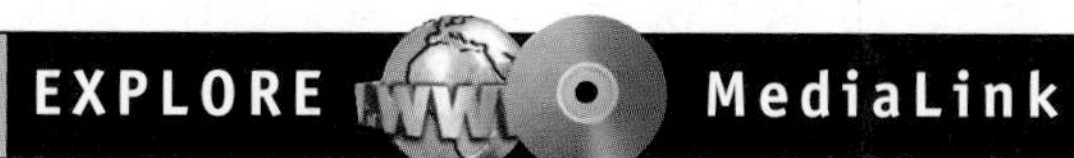

NCLEX review, case studies, and other interactive resources for this chapter can be found on the Companion Website at www.prenhall.com/kneisl. Click on Chapter 17 to select the activities for this chapter.

For animations, video tutorials, more NCLEX review questions, and an audio glossary, access the accompanying CD-ROM in this textbook.

BIBLIOGRAPHY

Althof, S. E. (2000). Erectile dysfunction. In S. R. Leiblum & R. C. Rosen (Eds.), *Principles and practice of sex therapy* (3rd ed.) (pp. 242–275). New York: Guilford Press.

American Psychiatric Association (2000). *Diagnostic and statistical manual of mental disorders* (4th ed., Text Revision). Washington, DC: Author.

Appelbaum, B. (2000). Retarded ejaculation. In S. R. Leiblum & R. C. Rosen (Eds.), *Principles and practice of sex therapy* (3rd ed.) (pp. 205–241). New York: Guilford Press.

Bartlik, B., & Goldberg, J. (2000). Female sexual arousal disorder. In S. R. Leiblum & R. C. Rosen (Eds.), *Principles and practice of sex therapy* (3rd ed.) (pp. 85–117). New York: Guilford Press.

Carroll, R. A. (2000). Assessment and treatment of gender dysphoria. In S. R. Leiblum & R. C. Rosen (Eds.), *Principles and practice of sex therapy* (3rd ed.) (pp. 368–397). New York: Guilford Press.

Hecht, M., Collier, M. J., & Ribeau, S. (1993). *African American Communication*. Thousand Oaks, CA: Sage.

Heiman, J. R. (2000). In S. R. Leiblum & R. C. Rosen (Eds.), *Principles and practice of sex therapy* (3rd ed.) (pp. 118–153). New York: Guilford Press.

Kafka, M. P. (2000). The paraphilia-related disorders. In S. R. Leiblum & R. C. Rosen (Eds.), *Principles and practice of sex therapy* (3rd ed.) (pp. 471–503). New York: Guilford Press.

Lips, H. M. (2001). *Sex and gender* (4th ed.). Mountain View, CA: Mayfield Publishing.

Mims, F. H., Swensen, M. (1980). *Sexuality: A nursing perspective.* McGraw-Hill.

Nichols, M. (2000). Therapy with sexual minorities. In S. R. Leiblum & R. C. Rosen (Eds.), *Principles and practice of sex therapy* (3rd ed.) (pp. 335-367). New York: Guilford Press.

Polonsky, D. C. (2000). Premature ejaculation. In S. R. Leiblum & R. C. Rosen (Eds.), *Principles and practice of sex therapy* (3rd ed.) (pp. 305–334). New York: Guilford Press.

Richard, D. (2000). Trans behind bars. *Contemporary Sexuality, 34*, 1–5.

Rosen, R. C. (2000). Medical and psychological interventions for erectile dysfunction. In S. R. Leiblum & R. C. Rosen (Eds.), *Principles and practice of sex therapy* (3rd ed.) (pp. 276–304). New York: Guilford Press.

Schnarch, D. (2000). Desire problems: A systemic perspective. In S. R. Leiblum & R. C. Rosen (Eds.), *Principles and practice of sex therapy* (3rd ed.) (pp. 1–16). New York: Guilford Press.

Strong, B., DeVault, C., & Sayad, B. W. (1999). *Human sexuality* (3rd ed.). Mountain View, CA: Mayfield Publishing.

Ting-Toomey, S., & Chung, L. (2002). *Understanding intercultural communication.* Los Angeles, CA: Roxbury.

Wincze, J. P. (2000). Assessment and treatment of atypical sexual behavior. In S. R. Leiblum & R. C. Rosen (Eds.), *Principles and practice of sex therapy* (3rd ed.) (pp. 449–470). New York: Guilford Press.

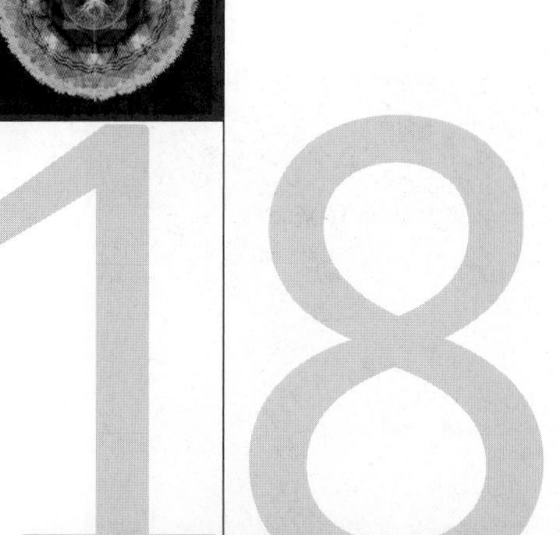

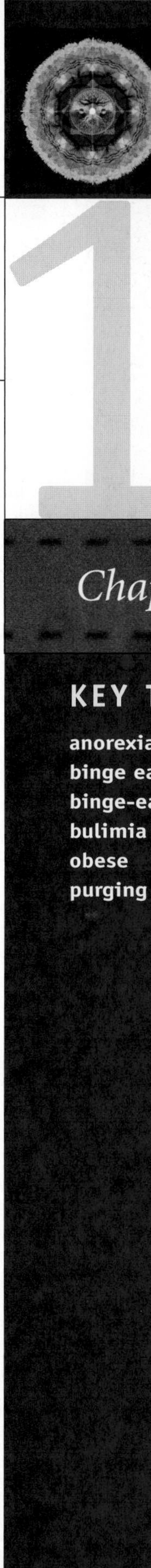

Eating Disorders

KAY K. CHITTY

18

Chapter EIGHTEEN

FOCUS QUESTIONS

- What roles do culture and biology play in the development of eating disorders?
- How would you go about assessing individual and family problems of clients with eating disorders?
- Why is psychoeducation important in both the prevention and treatment of eating disorders?
- How would you describe the nurse's role and appropriate nursing interventions for clients with eating disorders and their families?
- Why might you feel frustrated caring for clients with eating disorders?

KEY TERMS

anorexia nervosa
binge eating
binge-eating disorder
bulimia nervosa
obese
purging

MediaLink 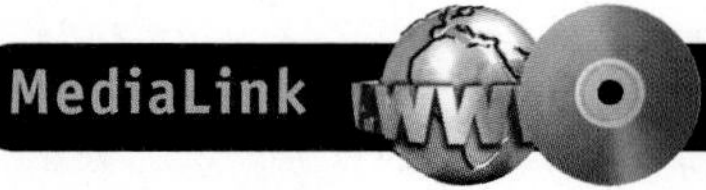 www.prenhall.com/kneisl

Additional resources for this chapter can be found on the Student CD-ROM accompanying this textbook, and on the Companion Website at www.prenhall.com/kneisl. Click on Chapter 18 to select the activities for this chapter.

CD-ROM

- Audio Glossary
- NCLEX Review

Companion Website

- Additional NCLEX Review
- Care Plan: Anorexia Nervosa
- Case Study: Bulimia Nervosa
- Learning from Clients: Anorexia Nervosa Video
- Learning from Clients: Bulimia Nervosa Video

CHAPTER OUTLINE

CROSS REFERENCES

Other topics relevant to this content are: Alternative and complementary therapies, Chapter 32; Cognitive restructuring techniques, Chapter 30; Dietary problems and eating disorders in adolescence, Chapter 26; Feeding and eating disorders in infancy or childhood, Chapter 25; Mood disorders, Chapter 15; Personality disorders, Chapter 20; Stress, anxiety, and coping, Chapter 5.

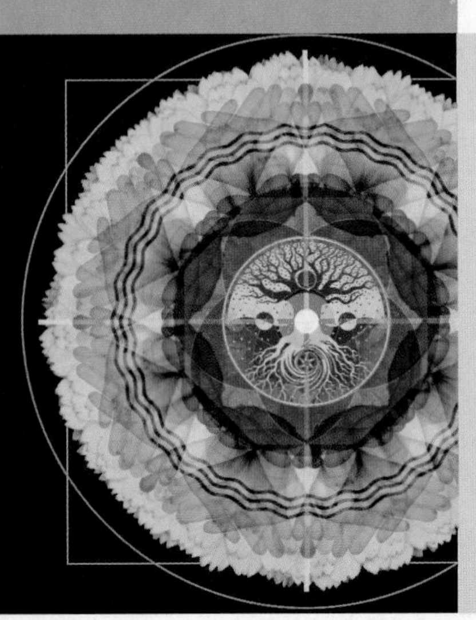

CRITICAL THINKING CHALLENGE

A school health nurse in a large public high school is aware that a number of girls diet constantly and throw up in the bathroom following lunch period. She also learns that boys on the wrestling team use vomiting as a means of "making weight." When the nurse takes her concerns to the principal to ask his support for an eating disorders educational program, he replies: "This is a health problem, not an educational problem. We just don't have time for this kind of thing. It's really up to the parents." In your opinion, what is the responsibility of nurses in educating the public about prevention of eating disorders? What kinds of information do people, particularly parents, teachers, and coaches, need to communicate about eating and health? What messages have you received that have helped or hindered you in developing healthy eating attitudes and behaviors? ■

Developed countries are experiencing what has been described as an epidemic of eating disorders. It has been estimated that 3% of women in industrialized nations will have an eating disorder over their lifetimes (Zhu & Walsh, 2002), and as many as 22% of young women regularly engage in eating-disordered behaviors (Botta & Dumlao, 2002). The emphasis on slimness has made increasing numbers of adolescents and young adults obsessively concerned about eating, weight, and body shape, size, and appearance. In a desperate attempt to achieve what may be perceived as perfection, some individuals go to extreme lengths to achieve thinness. While they starve themselves, sometimes to death, others apparently reject the cultural norms, overeat, and become obese.

For many, eating symbolizes parental nurturing—the love and care that are the prototype of, and basis for, all future intimate relationships. For some, however, eating creates anxiety because of its association with unsatisfactory and unpleasant parent–child interactions. Clearly, food and eating have greater individual and cultural meaning and importance than merely sustaining life. Disturbed eating patterns may develop as a means of coping with stress.

The three major eating disorders discussed in this chapter—anorexia nervosa, bulimia nervosa, and binge-eating disorder—create biologic, psychologic, and social imbalances that interfere with the individual's normal functioning. Changes in biochemistry, metabolic rate, emotional state, family relationships, and social status brought about by eating disorders can create depression, isolation, and sometimes self-destructive behavior.

Although estimates vary, it is believed that between one-quarter and one-half of people with eating disorders also suffer from major depressive disorder. Nearly all report feelings of low self-esteem, helplessness, and obsessions with food and weight (Harris, 1997). There is a high comorbidity of obssessive–compulsive disorder (29%) and eating disorders (Milos, Spindler, Ruggiero, Klaghofer, & Schnyder, 2002). In addition, the data from a longitudinal study showed that adolescents with eating disorders are at a substantially elevated risk for mental disorders—anxiety disorders, depressive disorders, and suicide (Johnson, Cohen, Kosen, & Brook, 2002). In this same study, only 22% of adolescents with current eating disorders had received treatment within the past year. Recent data also suggest that a possible concomitance may at times exist between eating disorders and posttraumatic stress disorder (Lating, O'Reilly, & Anderson, 2002). For example, disordered eating behaviors have been found to be associated with date violence and rape (Ackard & Neumark-Sztainer, 2002). The degree of hopelessness and anguish experienced by clients with these disorders is extreme and may be underestimated by caregivers.

Anorexia Nervosa

Anorexia nervosa is a potentially life-threatening disorder characterized by extreme perfectionism, weight fear, significant weight loss, body image disturbances, strenuous exercising, peculiar food-handling patterns, and reductions in heart rate, blood pressure, metabolic rate, and the production of estrogen or testosterone. A well-known pioneer in the treatment of eating-disordered clients, Hilde Bruch (1978), called it "the relentless pursuit of thinness." Anorexia nervosa is considered to have a particular relationship to perfectionism—that is, self-evaluation is dependent on the pursuit and attainment of personally demanding standards in the domain of control over eating, shape, and weight (Shafran, et. al., 2002). Anorexics equate weight gain with having failed and being self-indulgent, "bad," or "out of control."

Unchecked, the course of anorexia nervosa results in death in approximately 10% of those affected. They die from starvation, cardiac arrest, or other complications of malnutrition or during the refeeding process of recovery. This places anorexia nervosa among the most lethal of all psychiatric disorders (Walsh & Devlin, 1999). Outcomes for anorexia nervosa have not improved since Bruch wrote her classic work. A review of anorexia nervosa in the second half of the twentieth century found that less than one-half recovered, one-third improved, and 20% remained chronically ill (Steinhausen, 2002). The presence of vomiting, bulimia, purgative abuse, chronicity of illness, and obsessive-compulsive personality symptoms were all predictors of unfavorable outcomes. Outcomes are often poor because people with anorexia nervosa actively resist or refuse treatment (MacDonald, 2002).

It is estimated that 90% to 95% of anorexia nervosa clients are female, with the onset almost always occurring between 10 and 20 years of age (Scharer, 1999). The onset is sometimes associated with a stressful life event.

MediaLink Learning from Clients: Anorexia Nervosa Video

CLINICAL EXAMPLE

Simone is a tall, quiet girl who was considered polite, well-liked, and a good student. She was given responsibility beyond her years at both school and home because of her quiet competence and maturity. When she was 15, she entered a beauty contest at a local amusement park as a lark but did not win. She became convinced that she lost because her legs were too large and her abdomen protruded. She decided to diet. To radically control her own intake without arousing the family's suspicions, she began preparing all the family's meals. She herself did not eat, but played with her food during mealtimes.

Simone spent long hours alone in her room studying, dancing, and exercising vigorously. She began weighing herself several times daily, and if the scales showed an unacceptable number, she exercised even more frenziedly.

As she lost weight, Simone disguised her gauntness with loose, layered clothes. One day, when she and her mother were shopping, her mother saw her disrobed and was dismayed. She insisted that Simone see the family physician, who encouraged her to eat more and prescribed nutritional supplements.

When Simone collapsed at a shopping mall a few weeks later, her parents prevailed on the family doctor to admit her to the psychiatric unit of the community hospital. As an IV was started in the emergency room, Simone asked the nurse, "How many calories are in that bag?"

DSM-IV-TR **Diagnostic Criteria for Eating Disorders**

Anorexia Nervosa

A. Refusal to maintain body weight at or above a minimally normal weight for age and height (e.g., weight loss leading to maintenance of body weight less than 85% of that expected; or failure to make expected weight gain during period of growth, leading to body weight less than 85% of that expected).

B. Intense fear of gaining weight or becoming fat, even though underweight.

C. Disturbance in the way in which one's body image or shape is experienced, undue influence of body weight or shape on self-evaluation, or denial of the seriousness of the current low body weight.

D. In postmenarcheal females, amenorrhea, i.e., the absence of at least three consecutive menstrual cycles. (A woman is considered to have amenorrhea if her periods occur only following hormone, e.g., estrogen, administration.)

RESTRICTING TYPE

During the current episode of Anorexia Nervosa, the person has not regularly engaged in binge-eating or purging behavior (i.e., self-induced vomiting or the misuse of laxatives, diuretics, or enemas).

BINGE-EATING/PURGING TYPE

During the current episode of Anorexia Nervosa, the person has regularly engaged in binge-eating or purging behavior (i.e., self-induced vomiting or the misuse of laxatives, diuretics, or enemas).

Bulimia Nervosa

A. Recurrent episodes of binge eating. An episode of binge eating is characterized by both of the following:

1. Eating, in a discrete period of time (e.g., within any 2-hour period), an amount of food that is definitely larger than most people would eat during a similar period of time and under similar circumstances.

2. A sense of lack of control over eating during the episode (e.g., a feeling that one cannot stop eating or control what or how much one is eating).

B. Recurrent inappropriate compensatory behavior in order to prevent weight gain, such as self-induced vomiting; misuse of laxatives, diuretics, enemas, or other medications; fasting; or excessive exercise.

C. The binge eating and inappropriate compensatory behaviors both occur, on average, at least twice a week for 3 months.

D. Self-evaluation is unduly influenced by body shape and weight.

E. The disturbance does not occur exclusively during episodes of Anorexia Nervosa.

PURGING TYPE

During the current episode of Bulimia Nervosa, the person has regularly engaged in self-induced vomiting or the misuse of laxatives, diuretics, or enemas.

NONPURGING TYPE

During the current episode of Bulimia Nervosa, the person has used other inappropriate compensatory behaviors, such as fasting or excessive exercise, but has not regularly engaged in self-induced vomiting or the misuse of laxatives, diuretics, or enemas.

Research Criteria for Binge-Eating Disorder

A. Recurrent episodes of binge eating. An episode of binge eating is characterized by both of the following:

1. eating, in a discrete period of time (e.g., within any 2-hour period), an amount of food that is definitely larger than most people would eat in a similar period of time under similar circumstances

1. a sense of lack of control over eating during the episode (e.g., a feeling that one cannot stop eating or control what or how much one is eating)

B. The binge-eating episodes are associated with three (or more) of the following:

1. eating much more rapidly than normal

2. eating until feeling uncomfortably full

3. eating large amounts of food when not feeling physically hungry

4. eating alone because of being embarrassed by how much one is eating

5. feeling disgusted with oneself, depressed, or very guilty after overeating

C. Marked distress regarding binge eating is present.

D. The binge eating occurs, on average, at least 2 days a week for 6 months.

Note: The method of determining frequency differs from that used for Bulimia Nervosa; future research should address whether the preferred method of setting a frequency threshold is counting the number of days on which binges occur or counting the number of episodes of binge eating.

E. The binge eating is not associated with the regular use of inappropriate compensatory behaviors (e.g., purging, fasting, excessive exercise) and does not occur exclusively during the course of Anorexia Nervosa or Bulimia Nervosa.

MediaLink Learning from Clients: Bulimia Nervosa Video

For the DSM-IV-TR diagnostic criteria for anorexia nervosa, see the box above.

Bulimia Nervosa

Bulimia nervosa is a disorder characterized by **binge eating**, the frequent compulsion to eat large quantities of food in a short period of time followed by **purging**, self-induced vomiting and/or use of large doses of laxatives and diuretics. Enemas may also be used to rid the body of all traces of food consumed during a binge. Many anorexia nervosa clients also indulge in binge eating and purging. There must be a minimum average of two binge-eating episodes per week for at least 3 months to warrant this DSM-IV-TR diagnosis. Most bulimics are young females of high school or college age of normal or slightly above-average weight. Girls who have been physically or sexually abused are at high risk for developing eating disorders, particularly bulimia (Harris, 1997). Statistics show bulimia is escalating among older women and young men as well. Like anorexics, bulimics are preoccupied with body shape and size.

CLINICAL EXAMPLE

Beth is a 17-year-old high school student who had been binge eating and purging with vomiting and over-the-counter diuretics and laxatives for about 2 years. She was referred to the mental health center by her school nurse. Beth stated that her school friends became concerned about her increasing preoccupation with purging, even after eating very small amounts of food. She was spending a lot of time in the girls' restroom; after lengthy bouts of self-induced vomiting following lunch period, she was sometimes too exhausted to attend class. Her friends had been "covering" for her but had become frightened and went to the school nurse with their concerns.

Beth is of average weight for her height but admitted that she would be quite heavy if she didn't purge herself of the large amounts of food she consumes in her room at night after her parents have gone to bed. "I'm so embarrassed. My whole life is totally out of control," she told the intake worker.

Bulimia nervosa, a common secretive illness, poses a significant challenge to health care professionals; thus, the diagnosis is often missed (Dichter, Cohen, & Connolly, 2002).

For the DSM-IV-TR diagnostic criteria for bulimia nervosa, see the box on page 428.

Binge-Eating Disorder

Binge-eating disorder is a recently identified category of eating disorder characterized by repeated episodes of uncontrolled eating, sometimes called compulsive overeating. Because purging and excessive exercise are not features of binge-eating disorder, these individuals often become **obese,** which is defined as more than 20% above normal body weight. Some researchers believe that binge-eating disorder is the most common eating disorder, affecting 15% to 50% of people in weight control programs (American Psychiatric Association [APA], 2000). Nationwide estimates of obesity range from 1 to 2 million American adults.

Although obesity has adverse effects on both health and longevity, it also may adversely affect mental health. There is controversy as to whether obesity alone should be classified as an eating disorder. It is not included under that category in the DSM-IV-TR (APA, 2000), and many obese individuals are apparently quite well adjusted. Others, however, experience anxiety, depression, low self-esteem, and poor body image. People with binge eating disorder, in addition to health risks, experience feelings of guilt, depression, and self-disgust.

Whatever the diagnosis, people who overeat compulsively do so even when they are not physically hungry. They continue to eat even after they have had enough, ignoring their bodies' satiety cues (i.e., the sensation of being full after a meal). They eat for emotional rather than physical reasons, choosing food as a means of calming and nurturing themselves or to compensate for the love and nurturing they desire from others. They relieve stress by numbing themselves with food, often becoming obese, like the client discussed in the following Clinical Example.

MediaLink Case Study: Bulimia Nervosa

CLINICAL EXAMPLE

Joan is a 45-year-old secretary who is 5' 3" tall and weighs 167 lb. She came to the outpatient department of a private psychiatric hospital because of depression over her weight. She reported that she had always struggled with her weight but that it became a real problem after her husband left her 10 years ago. She experienced severe financial and emotional stress as a result of her divorce and had become dependent on her aging parents for companionship, financial help, and assistance in raising her son, now 18 years old.

Joan described herself as "tense and angry all the time." She had tried many diets but the problems remained, and eating seemed to be the only way to dull the pain. "When I look at myself in the mirror, I am so discouraged that I eat a whole bag of cookies just to feel better. Then I hate myself even more. I am trapped in a body and a life that I don't want."

Biopsychosocial Theories

Although many clinical studies have been published, the literature on eating disorders shows no theoretic consensus on etiology and treatment. Psychoanalytic theory, family systems theory, cognitive/behavioral theories, sociocultural theories, and biologic theories all contribute to an understanding of the development and dynamics of eating disorders.

PSYCHOANALYTIC THEORY

Since Freud first identified it as such, eating has been regarded as a critical aspect of psychological growth and development. An infant at the breast already is beginning to internalize a rudimentary understanding about life through the quality of the feeding experience.

Psychoanalytic theory considers eating disorders to be symptomatic of unconscious conflicts. Little attention is paid to biologic or cultural factors. Psychoanalytic theory relates eating disorders to regression to prepuberty and repudiation of developing sexuality. Anorexics are thought to fear sexual maturity; the anorexia is seen as a rejection of the feminine form and a desperate attempt to regain the contours and dimensions of a prepubertal child.

In psychoanalytic thinking, compulsive overeating represents overcompensation for unmet oral needs during infancy. In other words, people eat to compensate for emptiness in their lives. Obesity is also thought to represent a defense against intimacy with the opposite sex.

The basic treatment modality in the psychoanalytic model is long-term individual psychotherapy, sometimes accompanied by group therapy. The goal of therapy is the development of insight and subsequent "working through" of underlying issues to resolve the unconscious conflicts manifested by the eating disorder. There is little empirical evidence of the effectiveness of psychotherapy in the treatment of eating disorders (Kaplan, 2002). Promising new approaches include motivational enhancement therapy and psychotherapies aimed at relapse prevention.

FAMILY SYSTEMS THEORY

Hilde Bruch (1978) was a pioneer in the application of family systems theory in her work with clients with anorexia nervosa. Other therapists have incorporated family systems theory into their work with people who have other eating disorders as well. According to Bruch, the eating disorder itself expresses unconscious intrapersonal and interpersonal conflicts in the family. The symptom stabilizes the family by allowing them to focus on the family member's eating disorder, thus ignoring their own unresolved conflicts.

Bruch described the anorexic family as consisting of parents with overly rigid expectations of an overly compliant child. The child's conflict is between enslavement to parental expectations and the drive for autonomy. Anorexic adolescents sometimes see controlling their own body size as the only way to assert control in their lives.

The family systems approach to compulsive overeating includes a working theory that ambivalence of a parent or parents toward a child sets the stage for the child's obesity. Conflict between parents and subsequent scapegoating of a child are also seen as contributing factors.

Treatment in the family systems model, which focuses on defining the family conflicts for which the eating disorder compensates has been found useful in anorexia nervosa (Kaplan, 2002). Through both individual and family therapy, indirectly expressed conflicts are made overt. Healthier and more direct means of expressing family conflicts are identified and practiced until learned.

COGNITIVE/BEHAVIORAL THEORIES

Cognitive/behavioral theories view eating disorders as learned behaviors based on irrational thoughts and beliefs. They focus on changing cognitive and behavioral responses to physiologic, psychological, and social stimuli. Insight into the nature of the maladaptive behavior (the eating disorder) is integrated with new and healthier responses to emotional stimuli. Education about the psychology of compulsive behavior and the physiologic effects of starvation and purging behaviors is usually incorporated into the therapy. Other cognitive approaches include correction of perceptual disturbances of body size and elimination of irrational thoughts and beliefs linking weight to self-esteem, such as, "I've gained a pound; I must run 5 miles today and eat nothing," or "I'd rather be dead than fat."

Cognitive behavioral therapy has been a successful treatment method for reducing the symptomatology associated with bulimia nervosa (Anderson et al., 2002) and to result in more rapid treatment than with interpersonal psychotherapy (Wilson, Fairburn, Agras, Walsh, & Kraemer, 2002). These approaches are also useful in the treatment of binge-eating disorder (Wilfley et al., 2002).

SOCIOCULTURAL THEORY

Culture affects food preferences, attitudes, rituals, choices, and taboos. Eating behaviors are learned in the family and reflect its ethnic background. Culture also affects perceptions of beauty, which include cultural norms regarding body size and shape. In most cultures throughout history, women were considered desirable when they had plump breasts, hips, and thighs. Appearing well fed was fashionable, demonstrated that the male was a good provider, and symbolized sensuality and fertility. Portraits and photographs of famous beauties as recently as 40 years ago show rounded, curvaceous contours.

It is difficult to pinpoint exactly when this began to change. A 1992 study of Miss America contestants from the years 1979 to 1985 showed a steady downward trend in their weights and body measurements (Davis, Durnin, Dionne, & Gurevich, 1994). This change can be seen clearly by comparing photographs of a cultural model of feminine beauty and desirability from the 1950s, Marilyn Monroe, to today's gaunt supermodels and pop culture stars.

The cultural approach to understanding eating disorders assumes that although occasional cases of eating disorders have been documented for hundreds of years, Western society's current emphasis on thinness plays a major role in today's widespread development of eating disorders. People in developed countries are preoccupied with the importance of creating a body that "fits" norms of size and shape exemplified by fashion models, dancers, movie stars, and other cultural icons. Women are at greater risk than men for developing eating disorders, partly because of the cultural bias that large body size is acceptable, even desirable, for men but not for women. In television and magazine ads, women portrayed as successful, attractive, healthy, and popular are invariably slim. Becoming slim is a major pursuit in this country. The multimillion-dollar diet and exercise industry is based on the widespread desire to achieve that cultural norm.

In the past, most eating disordered clients who came to the attention of the psychiatric community were from middle-class or upper-middle-class white families. Recent studies show greater representation of all groups in this country and a spreading problem abroad, brought about by the globalization of Western culture and the export of American movies, music, and fashion. As a result, eating disorders are on the rise in all racial and ethnic groups in developed countries. The combination of acculturative stress with body dissatisfaction may render minority women more vulnerable to eating disorders (Perez, Voelz, Pettit, & Joiner, 2002).

A survey by Harris (1997) of adolescent girls in the United States found that both eating behaviors and acceptance of weight varied across racial and ethnic groups. While white, Hispanic, and Asian-American girls were more likely to believe they were overweight than were African-American girls, high percentages of all adolescent girls surveyed had dieted. Of the 3,586 girls surveyed in grades 5 through 12, 52% of white girls, 46% of Hispanic girls, 45% of Asian-American girls, and 38% of African-American girls reported dieting.

Regardless of their country, culture, or class, populations at higher risk for the development of weight-loss eating disorders are dancers, gymnasts, long-distance runners, flight attendants, high school and college wrestlers, and fashion models (Kann, Kinchen, & Williams, 1997). The cultural trend toward extreme thinness as a criterion of beauty, combined with the resurgence of interest in gourmet cooking and elaborate home entertaining centering on preparing and consuming foods, sets the stage for confusion and conflict, particularly in the young, who are just beginning to develop their own identities and are at high risk for developing eating disorders.

BIOLOGIC THEORY

The biologic forces that shape the behavior of people with eating disorders are receiving increased attention. Historically, it has been more common to explain eating disorders as based on cultural, family, cognitive, and intrapsychic phenomena. These explanations are incomplete, however, without further examination of the biologic factors influencing disordered eating behaviors.

Research has focused on several hypotheses, including disturbances of the gastrointestinal tract, the pituitary gland, the hypothalamic sites in the brain that control feeding, and the possible neurochemical basis of eating disorders. Several recent studies have examined the role of leptin, a hormone secreted by fat cells and thought to play an important role in the regulation of the fat stores of the body. Neurochemical models have been proposed for both anorexia nervosa and bulimia nervosa, and various neurochemical abnormalities have been demonstrated in both anorexic and bulimic individuals (Cowen & Smith, 1999). Studies of both anorexia and bulimia suggest possible central nervous system (CNS) abnormalities of the serotonergic (Monteleone, et al., 2000) and noradrenergic systems. Studies in animals have linked satiety to serotonin levels. Bulimics appear to have low levels of serotonin, which may predispose them to binge-eating behavior. Studies of twins support the hypothesis that genetic factors predispose to eating disorders, even when environmental factors are different (Cowen & Smith, 1999; Walsh & Devlin 1998). It is not clear whether these changes are a result of a starvation state or a cause of it, but nearly all the abnormalities disappear with weight restoration. Most researchers believe that a causal link between biological abnormalities and eating disorders has not been sufficiently demonstrated and that it is more likely that the identified changes are a result of the disorders rather than the cause (Walsh & Devlin, 1998). Pharmacotherapy has been found useful in reducing the binge and purge behaviors in bulimia nervosa (Rosenblum & Forman, 2002) and to decrease compulsive eating in binge-eating disorder (Appolinario, Fontanelle, Papelbaum, Bueno, & Coutinho, 2002).

In 1998, a panel of experts convened by the National Institute of Mental Health (NIMH) identified several areas of research that could prove promising in identifying the pathogenesis of eating disorders. They suggested using recent scientific and technological advances, including gene therapy to study the role of recently identified neuropeptides that regulate appetite. They also suggested the use of neuroimaging such as positron emission tomography (PET) studies and magnetic resonance imaging (MRI) to compare the brains of clients with eating disorders with the brains of individuals with other disorders, such as obsessive–compulsive disorder and depression.

In the future, research will undoubtedly reveal new knowledge about the biology of eating disorders. But biologic factors, sociocultural factors, and intrapsychic or interpersonal conflicts cannot—and should not—be dealt with separately. The interaction of these factors is extremely important. For example, clients suffering from severe obesity may experience shame and helplessness as they attempt to cope with fears of rejection and loss of love. These feelings can lead to compensatory overeating, which in turn can create interpersonal conflict with family members. The client may withdraw from others, thus reinforcing the feelings of rejection and increasing social isolation. Only by understanding the interrelatedness of the factors in eating disorders can psychiatric nurses take a holistic approach to the care of affected individuals and their families (see ■ Figure 18–1).

NURSING PROCESS

Clients with Anorexia Nervosa

The following section discusses the specific steps of the nursing process for clients with anorexia nervosa.

MediaLink Care Plan: Anorexia Nervosa

Assessment

When assessing clients with dramatic weight loss or gain, you must not lose sight of the fact that both can be caused by physical conditions. Certain illnesses must be ruled out before an eating disorder diagnosis can be made. Wasting conditions such as advanced cancer, tuberculosis, AIDS, hyperthyroidism, pyloric obstruction, and drug abuse must be considered when weight loss is a feature. Rapid weight gain can result from a brain tumor or an endocrine disorder. A good history and physical examination are often needed to provide information to eliminate the possibility of a physical basis for sudden weight loss or gain. After the presence of an eating disorder is established, you will assess the client using the following subjective and objective data.

SUBJECTIVE DATA

Clients with anorexia nervosa perceive themselves as overweight, no matter how thin they may be. However emaciated their bodies, they can always find some body part they believe is fat.

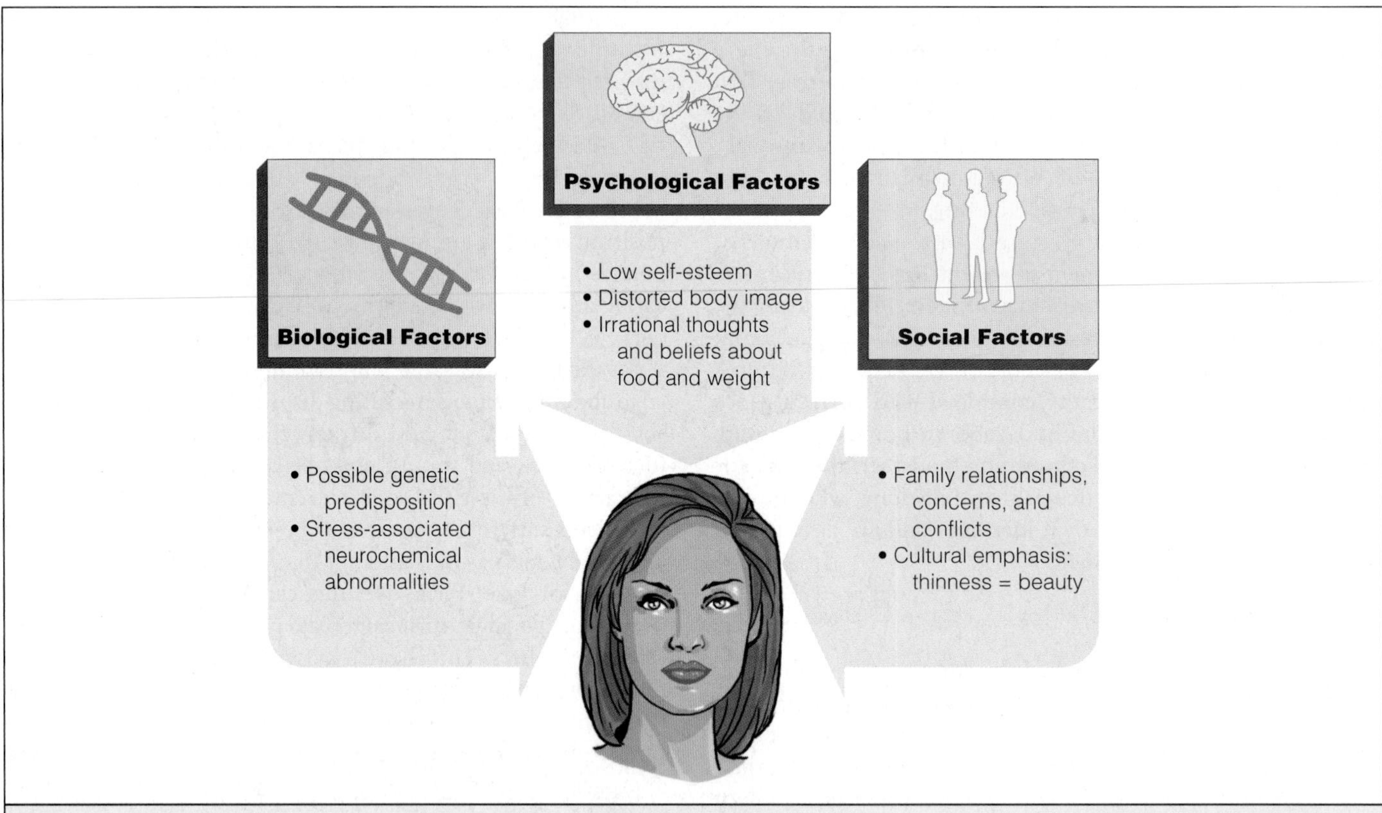

FIGURE 18–1 ■ *Biopsychosocial factors in eating disorders. Nurses who understand the interplay among biopsychosocial factors involved in eating disorders are able to take a holistic approach to client care.*

They are preoccupied with thoughts of food and simultaneously obsessed with rigidly controlling their own intake. They often collect cookbooks, cook prodigious amounts of food, and insist that others eat while not taking a morsel for themselves. They are fearful of even the slightest weight gain and view with suspicion anyone who encourages them to eat.

Another preoccupation is with exercise. It is not uncommon for anorexics to engage in extremely lengthy sessions of aerobics or calisthenics, or to run, bike, or walk to excess, even when in an emaciated condition. They push themselves to greater and greater levels of endurance and deprive themselves of sleep as a measure of self-control.

Anorexics frequently deny that they have a weight problem. They insist that they have never felt better and simply wish to be left alone about food. They report feeling strong, powerful, and good as a result of self-denial. They report feeling guilty, self-indulgent, and weak when they eat. They therefore resist treatment, although they may admit to feeling isolated and lonely and may even describe themselves as exhausted with the effort it takes to achieve the perfection they seek. They tend to have difficulty accepting nurturing behavior from others and therefore have difficulty forming therapeutic alliances. They report a loss of interest in sex but do not perceive this as a problem.

OBJECTIVE DATA

Anorexic clients, while often well-educated teenage females from middle-class and upper-middle-class families, may be from any racial, ethnic, or sociocultural background. There is evidence of extreme and/or rapid weight loss of at least 15% of original body weight. In women, amenorrhea is a cardinal sign. The client typically has extensive knowledge of the nutritional and caloric value of foods.

The anorexic client is emaciated, with sunken eyes and a skeletal appearence. In very young clients, growth failure may be present. Lanugo growth (babylike, fine hair) on the face, extremities, and trunk may occur. Other physical symptoms include bradycardia, hypotension, arrhythmias, delayed gastric motility, and a hypothyroid-like state manifested by dry skin, listlessness, and dry, falling hair. Peripheral edema may be a feature in advanced starvation.

Laboratory tests may reveal leukopenia, anemia, low serum potassium, and elevated blood urea nitrogen (BUN). High serum calcium levels indicate osteoporosis is occurring, and there is an increased risk of fracture (Walsh & Devlin, 1998).

Nursing Diagnosis: NANDA

Once the assessment process is completed, determine appropriate nursing diagnoses.

ALTERED NUTRITION: LESS THAN BODY REQUIREMENTS

By the time anorexic clients are seen in treatment, their physical condition is often so deteriorated from self-imposed starvation that it becomes the priority for nursing care. Life-threatening malnourishment is seen in 5% to 20% of these clients. Death may occur from malnutrition, infection, or cardiac abnormalities related to electrolyte imbalances. Intravenous therapy, tube feedings, and total parenteral hyperalimentation (TPH) are required in cases of medical emergency.

The client's preoccupation with food, evidenced by reading recipes, discussing food, and preparing food for others, is due to suppression and sublimation of the client's own hunger. Overexercising creates even more extreme nutritional deficits. In those anorexic clients who also purge by vomiting or using laxatives, nutritional status is further endangered.

Clients in a state of starvation experience hormonal, metabolic, and emotional changes. Some of those changes are manifested in amenorrhea or delay of onset of menses, ketosis, severe vitamin deficiencies, depressed immune response, lethargy, weakness, and irritability—conditions that vitally affect nurse–client relationships.

INEFFECTIVE INDIVIDUAL COPING

Clients experiencing anorexia nervosa demonstrate impairment of adaptive behaviors, such as self-care in activities of daily living. They have difficulty meeting daily demands, and role performance may be affected. Their preoccupation with the pursuit of thinness deprives them of the energy necessary for adaptive behavior and distracts them from interest in role fulfillment. The quest for thinness is the entire focus of their lives.

In addition, developmental issues such as the desire for independence and the longing for dependence combine with traditionally adolescent resentment of authority to influence the quality and character of the nurse–client relationship. Family overprotectiveness and unwillingness to allow the client to separate contribute to self-doubt and the inability to accept responsibility for self.

BODY IMAGE DISTURBANCE

Clients with anorexia nervosa are unable to make realistic appraisals of their own body size, although they can accurately evaluate the size of others. They drastically underestimate their own bodily needs, even in the face of overwhelming evidence of malnutrition. Profound disturbances in accurate perception of size and intense client denial indicate a poor prognosis. The client's body image disturbance is often the source of conflict in family and therapeutic relationships.

CHRONIC LOW SELF-ESTEEM

Anorexic clients' lack of confidence in themselves and feelings of inferiority are main factors in the disorder. Their self-deprivation and self-denial make them feel powerful and superior to others who cannot muster such profound self-control. The quest for perfection is never-ending, but they can never achieve a level of thinness that is satisfying; there are always a few more pounds to shed. They often present the picture of "model clients," in contrast to seemingly more disturbed clients. As a result, novice nurses may have difficulty assessing the severity of the illness accurately.

The low self-esteem of anorexic clients stems from unrealistic expectations by self and others, complicated by unmet dependency needs. The clinical picture is further complicated because cultural norms of thinness reinforce maladaptive behavior. The nurse–client relationship is affected by the extreme difficulty these clients have in accepting positive feedback and by their nonparticipation in self-care and therapeutic activities. Their preoccupation with their appearance and with others' perceptions of them may be irritating to other clients. The nurse–client relationship is also affected by the client's need to control, which often leads to manipulative behaviors. (See the Nursing Self-Awareness feature below for possible reactions of nurses working with clients with eating disorders.) Self-aware nurses recognize their own emotional reactions to clients and view clients' self-absorption and manipulativeness as symptoms of the disorder.

Outcome Identification: NOC

Suggested outcomes for each NANDA diagnosis in the previous section follow.

ALTERED NUTRITION: LESS THAN BODY REQUIREMENTS

This diagnosis inevitably leads to the desired outcome of improvement of Nutritional Status: Adequate nutrients taken into the body for height, frame, gender, and activity level.

INEFFECTIVE INDIVIDUAL COPING

Several NOC outcomes are relevant to anorexic clients with this nursing diagnosis. They include Coping: Actions to manage stressors that tax an individual's resources; Impulse Control:

Nursing SELF-AWARENESS

Possible Reactions to Working with Clients with Eating Disorders

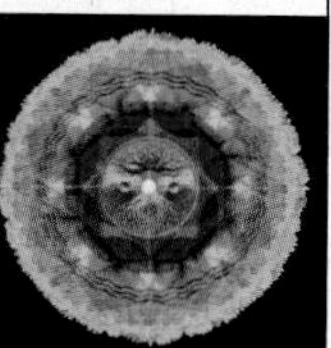

- You feel exhausted and defeated by the structured demands of the client's care plan.
- You feel resentment at the client's efforts to manipulate and attempts at "staff splitting."
- You identify with the client because of your own personal body image concerns.
- You feel overprotective of the client and allow a coalition between yourself and the client to form.
- You feel annoyance and anger toward the client and are unnecessarily rough during physical care.
- You have difficulty recognizing that the client's symptoms are as serious as those of a hallucinating or delusional client.
- You fail to monitor the client's mealtime and after-meal behaviors, allowing the client to continue maladaptive patterns of coping.
- You allow the client to reenact power struggles from home, such as those about food, weight, and exercising.
- You believe that the client is deliberately engaging in maladaptive coping behaviors to upset the staff and family.
- You feel repelled by the client's eating habits or the appearance of the client's body.
- You feel hopeless and are affected by the client's despondency.

Ability to self-restrain compulsive or impulsive behavior; and Information Processing: Ability to acquire, organize, and use information.

BODY IMAGE DISTURBANCE

For the anorexic client, who invariably has a distorted body image, NOC outcomes include Body Image: Positive perception of own appearance; and Distorted Thought Control: Ability to self-restrain altered perceptions.

CHRONIC LOW SELF-ESTEEM

As in many psychiatric disorders, low self-esteem plays a major role in anorexia nervosa, leading to the NOC outcome of Self-Esteem: Personal judgment of self-worth.

Planning and Implementation: NIC

When a client's behavior meets the criteria for a diagnosis of anorexia nervosa, effective nursing intervention is directed toward ensuring that the client will not die and helping the client learn more effective ways of coping with the demands of life. A variety of approaches, including behavioral, insight-oriented, and cognitive therapies may be useful; pharmacologic therapy may be used also. You must recognize that many, if not most, anorexic clients are extremely resistant to change. Progress may be slow, and recovery may be defined as the lessening of symptoms. For approximately 50% of clients with anorexia nervosa, the long-term outlook is not good (Walsh & Devlin 1998). In severely debilitated clients, inpatient treatment is indicated (see Box 18–1).

BOX 18–1 Criteria for Inpatient Admission

- Clients who are suicidal or severely out of control (self-mutilative; abusing large amounts of laxatives, emetics, and diuretics or street drugs).
- Severely emaciated clients (more than 30% below normal weight).
- Clients who have demonstrated a rapid, dramatic weight loss (in less than a 3-month period).
- Clients who have body temperature less than 96.8°F (36°C) from hypothermia due to loss of subcutaneous tissue.
- Clients who demonstrate fluid and electrolyte imbalance (K < 2.5 mEq/L).
- Clients in the first trimester of pregnancy with seriously disturbed eating habits.
- Clients who need extensive diagnostic evaluation to rule out comorbidities.
- Clients who develop somatic illnesses and are already compromised (as with infection).
- Clients who repeatedly fail to gain weight with outpatient treatment.

Source: Love, C. C., & Seaton, H. (1991). Eating disorders: Highlights of nursing assessment and therapeutics. *Nursing Clinics of North America, 26*(3), 687; and White, J. H., & Litovitz, G. (1998). A comparison of inpatient and outpatient women with eating disorders. *Archives of Psychiatric Nursing, 12*(4), 181–194. With permission from Elsevier Science.

MediaLink Anorexia: Self-Help Groups

MANAGING NUTRITION

To establish adequate eating patterns and fluid and electrolyte balance, assume a calm, matter-of-fact attitude and a positive expectation of the client. Meeting minimal nutritional goals, with the overall goal of gradual weight restoration, is nonnegotiable. A caloric intake of 1,200 to 1,500 cal/day is the usual range (see the Intervention box on page 435).

Nursing interventions may include tube feedings or intravenous therapy, which are administered in a nonjudgmental manner. Weighing the client daily, recording intake and output, observing the client during meals, and observing bathroom behavior may be necessary if you suspect the client is discarding food or inducing vomiting. Avoid discussing food, recipes, restaurants, and eating with the client because these conversations reinforce maladaptive behaviors. Providing a pleasant meal-time environment and adopting realistic expectations of how much the client will eat are critically important aspects of nursing care. Clients find frequent, small meals more acceptable than three large meals. Setting a time limit of about a half hour is a good way to forestall mealtime "marathons"—protracted meals during which the client eats little.

Acknowledge and recognize the efforts of clients who meet weight gain goals but avoid praise or flattery. Education about adequate eating patterns is a necessary part of discharge planning.

Consistency and coordination among staff members are essential to avoid manipulation by clients. Interdisciplinary planning conferences and adherence to written care plans promote effective care. Behavior modification programs, which base privileges on weight gain, may be useful for focusing on emotional issues, not just eating behaviors. You and the client may engage in a contract for weight gain, such as the one in ■ Figure 18–2 on page 436.

A target weight is usually chosen by the treatment team in collaboration with a dietitian. Target weight for discharge from treatment is usually 90% of average for age and height. Discharge planning can include referral to self-help groups such as the American Anorexia/Bulimia Association, Anorexia Nervosa and Related Eating Disorders, and Anorexia Nervosa and Associated Disorders. The Web sites for these self-help groups are included in the Client/Family Teaching special feature on page 443. These resources can be accessed through links on the Companion Website for this book.

FACILITATING COPING

The best way to promote individual coping is by involving clients in their own treatment planning. Self-determination fosters adaptive coping mechanisms in clients' day-to-day hospital experiences; this process carries over to daily life outside the hospital setting and helps clients meet its demands.

Although trust is difficult to establish with anorexic clients, it is the basis for all therapeutic relationships. Being honest, available, and matter-of-fact helps establish trust and encourages clients to express their feelings. If necessary, allow clients to assume a dependent role at first, but as trust is developed and physical condition improves, encourage them to take more responsibility for them-

INTERVENTION

Guidelines for Refeeding

Strategy	Rationale
• Validate the client's fears of weight gain.	• Reassures the client that fears are expected and not unique.
• Collaborate with the client and dietitian to plan a flexible refeeding program for gradual weight gain.	• Enlists the client as an active participant in treatment.
• Adopt a matter-of-fact, consistent, and nonjudgmental attitude.	• Conveys your confidence and acceptance of the client.
• Contract with the client for food and fluid intake adequate to meet the weight-restoration goal.	• Meets the clients need for structure and control.
• Support the client during refeeding sensations of fullness and bloating; teach that these are normal and transient feelings.	• The client's gastrointestinal tract must readjust to unaccustomed intake.
• Encourage the expression of feelings of loss of control.	• Upon resuming adequate intake, clients fear "losing control" and "becoming fat."
• Monitor fluid and electrolyte intake and output, vital signs, body temperature, and mood.	• Refeeding may precipitate both psychologic and metabolic emergencies. Monitor both physiologic and psychologic effects.

Source: Love, C. C., & Seaton, H. (1991). Eating Disorders: Highlights of nursing assessment and therapeutics. *Nursing Clinics of North America, 26*(3), 687. With permission from Elsevier Science.

selves. Participating in the planning of care gives clients opportunities to practice making decisions. Letting clients have input into their treatment plans also fosters compliance. Provide flexibility in activities of daily living, type and timing of exercise, and choice of occupational and recreational therapy activities. This autonomy increases clients' sense of responsibility for themselves.

Giving clients the opportunity to practice problem solving may lead to power struggles if you disagree with clients' choices. Demonstrate positive belief in their ability to regain healthy functioning and a willingness to tolerate "mistakes." The treatment team must set firm and clear limits, however, to provide the secure environment clients need to learn more effective coping behaviors. Also help clients identify ways to feel in control by other than anorexic and manipulative behaviors.

Clients need to explore their extreme fears of gaining weight before they can relinquish maladaptive behaviors. It is helpful to explore with clients their feelings about their family, their role in the family, and their autonomy within the family system (see the Using Research Evidence feature on page 437).

ENHANCING BODY IMAGE

To help clients regain an accurate perception of their body size and nutritional needs, first encourage clients to express feelings about body size. An example is shown in the Rx Communication feature on page 437. Reframe clients' misperceptions by using language that emphasizes health, strength, and evaluation. For example, if the client says "My thighs are huge," reply "Your thighs are becoming stronger now that you're gaining weight. Healthy muscles are rounded and firm, like yours." With practice, clients can replace negative thinking with positive self-talk. Teach and reinforce this skill, and help them practice it. For example, ask clients to make three positive statements (positive affirmations) about their bodies each day.

If clients are unable or unwilling to discuss their feelings about body size, ask them to draw themselves as they are now and as they desire to be. These drawings not only focus the discussion of body size and nutritional needs but also help you understand how clients view their bodies. Because clients with bulimia nervosa and compulsive overeating also have distorted body images, this activity can be incorporated into their plans of care as well. You could also use a more structured tool such as the one illustrated in ■ Figure 18–3. In addition, BodyImage, a software program for the assessment of body image disturbance, is available at www.homepage2.nifty.com/s_shibata/softwares/bodyimage.html at no cost and can be obtained through a link on the Companion Website for this book.

MediaLink Body Image Software

When clients share feelings honestly, show improvement in accurate perception of body image, or demonstrate healthier eating behaviors, reinforce their efforts through verbal recognition. It is also useful to examine with clients the ways in which the fashion and advertising industries support unrealistic cultural norms of excessive thinness incompatible with healthy functioning.

IMPROVING SELF-ESTEEM

Help clients reexamine negative feelings about themselves and identify their positive attributes. Encourage clients to record in a diary thoughts that are difficult to share directly. Be nonjudgmental in your acceptance of negative feelings and positively reinforce the honest expression of all feelings. Encouragement is particularly important when clients experiment with independently made decisions, even when outcomes are not entirely positive. The client needs to interpret each experience as worthwhile. Emphasize the feeling of control gained through independent decision making.

Together, you and the client explore the client's attempt to achieve perfection by controlling weight. The idea is for the client to realize that perfection is an unrealistic goal. You are a role model for the person who accepts imperfection yet retains self-esteem. One way to model strong self-esteem is to admit

Date: ______________________

Client's Name: ______________________________________ Age: ______________

Height: ____________ Weight: ____________ Goal Weight (range): ________________

1. You will be weighed: ____ daily ____twice a week ____weekly

upon arising and after voiding while wearing nightclothes. You should not eat or drink prior to weighing. Frequency of weights will change as you progress.

2. No exercising, jogging, or calisthenics are to be done without approval by your treatment team. As you progress, this privilege may be gradually reinstated.

3. Nutritional supplements will be required until made optional by your treatment team.

You will drink ____ cans of supplement per day if your weight gain is less than 1/4 pound over your last highest weight.

You will drink ____ cans of supplement per day if your weight gain is more than 1/4 pound over your last highest weight.

You will drink the nutritional supplement under nursing supervision at regular medication times of:

________________________________. You will consume each can within 15 minutes.

4. Your privilege status will depend upon your progress in weight gain. Your treatment team has determined weights to be attained for privilege status:

1:1 monitering status:	________ pounds		
Independent status:	________ pounds for	________	consecutive days
Buddy status:	________ pounds		
Pass status:	________ pounds for	________	consectuive days

5. Other issues:

I agree to abide by the provisions of this contract:

Signature of Client ____

Signature of Treatment Team Leader ______________________________

FIGURE 18–2 ■ *Sample contract for weight gain. A client contract for weight gain fosters client self-responsibility and nurse–client collaboration.*

errors willingly. Also model appropriate expressions of anger and teach clients the destructive effects of unexpressed anger.

Evaluation

Evaluation of the effectiveness of nursing interventions is an ongoing part of the nursing process.

NUTRITIONAL STATUS

Clients will regain and maintain at least 90% of normal weight for their height and age. Clients will follow eating patterns that demonstrate they recognize the importance of adequate nutrition. They will regain and maintain normal elimination patterns, vital signs, fluid and electrolyte balance, and muscle tone. Female clients will have normal menstrual cycles.

COPING

Clients will demonstrate effective coping when they participate actively in treatment planning and discharge planning using problem-solving skills. They will demonstrate interest and competence in self-care activities such as hygiene, sleep, activity,

USING RESEARCH EVIDENCE

Brittany M., age 15, was admitted to the eating disorders unit of a private psychiatric hospital by her family when her weight dropped to 77 pounds. She was immediately placed on a weight gain regimen and closely monitored for adverse reactions to refeeding. A nurse on the unit spent time with Brittany each evening but was unable to establish a relationship. Brittany kept to herself except for visits from her family, making charcoal sketches which she showed to no one. Most staff members and other clients left her alone, as she seemed to prefer.

One nurse, aware that family dynamics are thought to play a role in anorexia nervosa, decided to observe these interactions over several family visits. She noticed a pattern of irony and sarcasm in Brittany's parents toward each other as well as toward Brittany. Brittany consistently sat silently, saying as little as possible. Her mother became increasingly agitated, on one occasion complaining that Brittany "will be the death of me yet." Brittany's younger brother was heard to call her a "weirdo" before their father intervened. Following family visits, the nurse attempted to get Brittany to discuss what had happened but had little success. Brittany steadfastly refused to discuss her family, saying, "It wouldn't do any good."

One evening the nurse approached Brittany after her family left and said, "Could you draw what you are feeling right now?" After much encouragement, Brittany began a sketch, embarrassed and tentative at first, but soon becoming totally immersed in the drawing. After she finished, the nurse asked her to talk about her drawing. It was the first time Brittany had been able to voice any negative feelings. The nurse listened nonjudgmentally, making open-ended observations that encouraged Brittany to continue. She ended the conversation by pointing out Brittany's progress. After several such sessions Brittany was able to talk without sketching first, and she had much to say. "I have silenced myself for so long to keep peace in the family. It seemed the safest thing to do." The nurse shared the information that anorexic people often feel they must suppress negative emotions and that it often seems to make their eating disorder worse. They worked on how Brittany could express her feelings using "I" statements to prevent defensive responses, which she then could practice in group therapy and other "safe" interactions on the unit.

When family therapy was instituted, Brittany was able to use some of her new expressive techniques successfully. While this family had far to go in learning more effective communication techniques, the nurse knew that their sessions were helping prepare Brittany for the next steps in her therapy. These nursing interventions were influenced by data in the following research study:

Geller, J., Cockell, S. J., & Goldner, E. M. (2000). Inhibited expression of negative emotions and interpersonal orientation in anorexia nervosa. *International Journal of Eating Disorders, 28*(1), 8–19.

rest, diversional activities, and nutrition. They will accurately identify both maladaptive coping behaviors and adaptive coping behaviors that can be integrated into daily routines. Clients will express less anxiety about weight gain and will verbalize other means of feeling in control of their lives.

BODY IMAGE

Body image disturbance will have been alleviated when clients accurately assess their own body size and nutritional needs. They will use criteria such as strength and health, rather than appearance alone, to evaluate body size. They will verbalize less preoccupation with body size. Clients will verbalize positive statements about their own bodies.

SELF-ESTEEM

Clients will demonstrate self-esteem when they verbalize their own positive attributes. They will demonstrate less preoccupation with their own appearance and will focus increasingly on others. They will accept compliments and positive feedback and show greater interest in activities around them. They will verbalize that perfection is an unrealistic life goal. Clients will express anger appropriately without experiencing incapacitating guilt. They will demonstrate interpersonal relationships substantially free of manipulation. Clients will work toward success experiences in work, school, and or/social groups.

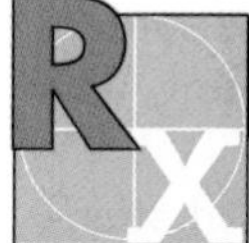

COMMUNICATION

Client with Anorexia Nervosa

CLIENT: [Tearfully] My doctor says I have to eat and gain weight but I still have this little fat tummy.

NURSE RESPONSE 1: I wonder if you can tell me what you are feeling right now.

RATIONALE: Asking the client to focus on her feelings assists her in becoming more self-aware. Obtaining additional subjective data from the client enables you to better understand her.

NURSE RESPONSE 2: It sounds as though you feel caught in the middle of the doctor's expectations and your own.

RATIONALE: Nonjudgmental acknowledgement of the client's conflict shows empathy and encourages her to clarify the dilemma from her doctor's point of view as well as her own. Avoids directly challenging the client's distorted perception of her body image.

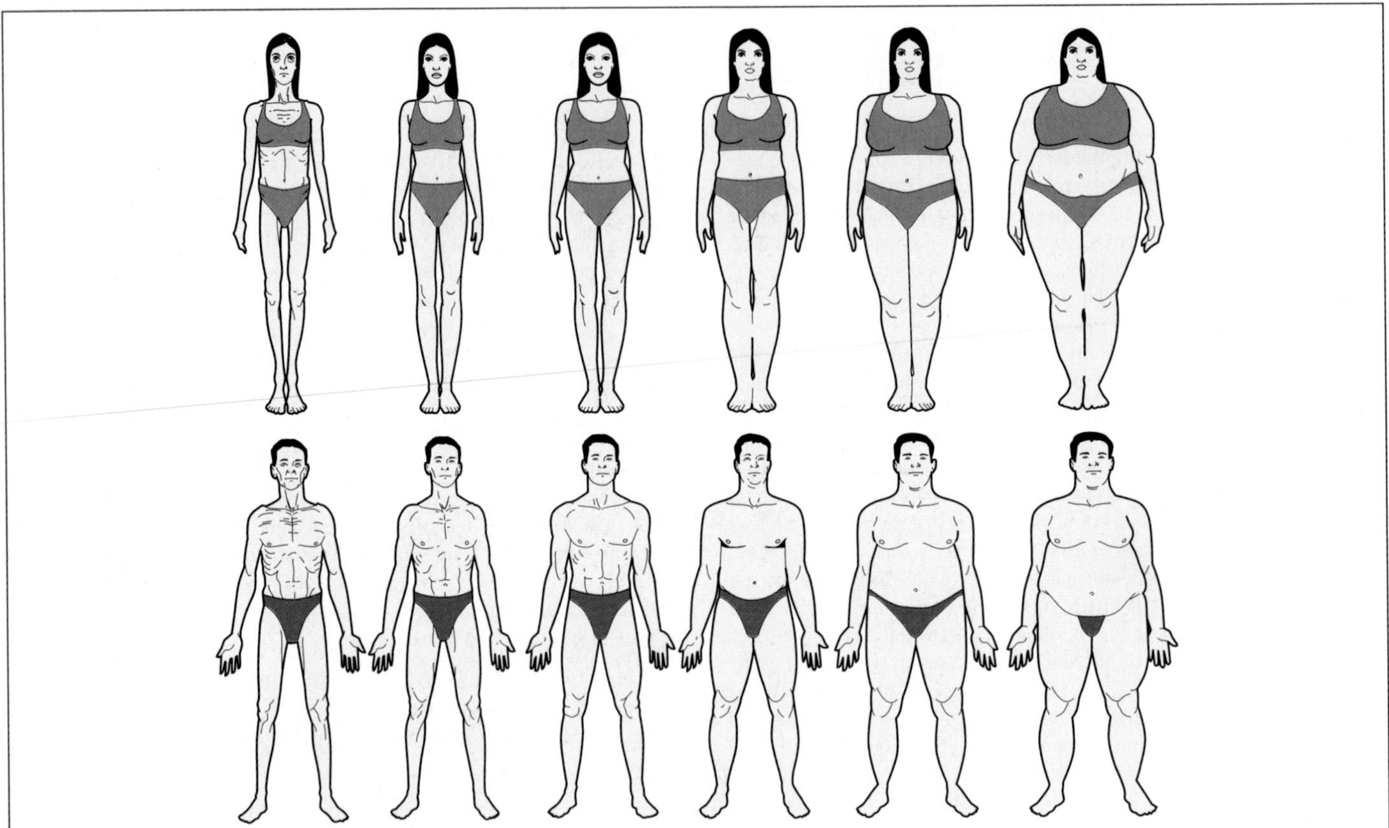

FIGURE 18–3 ■ *Assessing body image. A drawing such as this can be used in several ways: (1) Clients can be asked which image best represents them. This assesses the accuracy of the client's body image. Anorexic clients often believe themselves to be larger than they really are. (2) Clients can be asked which image best represents the ideal for them. This assesses whether a client has a positive (image is similar to the client's own body) or a negative (dissimilar image) body image.*

Case Management

Case managers working with clients who have eating disorders must understand the risk factors and possible complications of these disorders. This enables the case manager to recognize symptoms early, mobilize the treatment team and family resources, assure a smooth transition to inpatient therapy if needed, and ensure adequate follow-up.

Failure to respond to treatment occurs in about 50% of cases. Symptoms that would alert the case manager to evaluate a client's need for treatment include the DSM-IV-TR criteria in the box on page 428.

Desired case management outcomes include weight gain/loss, normalization of exercise periods, cessation of binge eating and purging behaviors, and decreased preoccupation with food and body size. Avoidance of hospitalization or the briefest possible hospital stay is a case management priority.

The ultimate case management goal is early detection of symptoms, effective symptom reduction, and rapid return to maximal premorbid function. Despite the best efforts, about half of clients with eating disorders progress from acute to chronic illness, which presents them, their families, and case managers with lifelong challenges.

Community-Based Care

While many, if not most, clients with bulimia nervosa and binge-eating disorder can be safely treated in community-based settings, severely anorexic clients usually are hospitalized. Criteria for hospitalization are found in Box 18–1. Nurses in community-based settings such as school nurses, occupational health nurses, and nurses in doctors' offices play a major role in recognizing symptoms of eating disorders, providing screening, information and support to clients and families, and referring clients for specialized treatment. Unlike some mental disorders such as depression, eating disorders are not self-limiting, and specialized care is required.

Prevention of eating disorders is receiving increased attention as an appropriate and much-needed focus for community-based nurses, particularly those in schools. Due to the early onset of anorexic thinking, education programs as early as grade school should be developed (Chally, 1998).

Nurses in community-based settings can play a valuable role in the education, support, and referral of clients and their families, often enabling clients to remain in the community while in treatment.

Home Care

Historically, clients with eating disorders were isolated from their families during treatment. It was thought that ongoing family conflict would jeopardize their recovery. This approach has been challenged, and changes in attitudes toward home-based care are gradually occurring. Even severely anorexic clients requiring TPH have been treated at home with the assistance of home health nurses on a professional team (Latzer, Eysen-Eylat, & Tabenkin, 2000). This requires that the client is motivated and can be relied on to self-administer the treatment. Anorexics are rarely motivated to regain weight, however, requiring that TPH and other refeeding programs indicated for severe anorexics be administered on an inpatient basis. Home care is rarely required for clients with bulimia nervosa and binge-eating disorder. They are most often seen in outpatient clinics and mental health centers.

NURSING PROCESS

Clients with Bulimia Nervosa

The following section discusses the nursing process for clients with bulimia nervosa. Since some clients with bulimia may also be anorexic, refer also to the earlier nursing process section on pages 431–437.

Assessment

Although the two disorders are described separately, the boundary between anorexia and bulimia is blurred. Many bulimics were formerly anorexic, while others may become anorexic in the future. As many as half of all anorexics are estimated to binge and purge at some time during their illnesses. During the assessment phase of the nursing process, keep in mind that these two conditions, although distinctly different, often coexist.

SUBJECTIVE DATA

Clients with bulimia nervosa have feelings of low self-esteem, worthlessness, inadequacy, and guilt. They experience shame and embarrassment over their secret binges (eating several quarts of ice cream, buckets of popcorn, or eight or more candy bars is not unusual) and subsequent purging activities. This shame may be manifested in self-deprecating remarks. Clients report feeling out of control, but at the same time they feel an excessive need to control. Unlike anorexics, clients with bulimia nervosa recognize that their eating behaviors are abnormal and bizarre.

Anxiety and unsatisfactory interpersonal relationships are features of this disorder. Anxiety is intensified when others see the bulimic as successful and in control, and they often appear so to others. They are impulsive and cannot delay gratification. Preoccupation with food, weight, and dieting is a prominent feature. Bulimic clients may report feeling weak and lethargic.

OBJECTIVE DATA

Like anorexic clients, bulimic clients tend to be young females. Bulimia first manifests itself later than anorexia, typically during late adolescence or young adulthood. Clients are likely to be white, middle-class females with a history of weight-control problems. They are usually of normal or slightly above-average weight. Appearance does not provide diagnostic clues, hence the term *normal-weight bulimic*. Weight tends to fluctuate but does not get dangerously low unless anorexia occurs concurrently.

Clients with bulimia nervosa are more outgoing than anorexics and tend to be more comfortable with sexual relationships. They sometimes manifest impulsive behaviors such as substance abuse, shoplifting, and self-in-flicted injury. In inpatient settings, they may steal others' food and hoard food in their rooms.

MediaLink Case Study: Bulimia Nervosa

Physical signs of bulimia nervosa include hoarseness and esophagitis, dental enamel erosion, enlarged parotid glands, abrasions or calluses on knuckles from inducing vomiting, and amenorrhea in about 40% of cases. The client may also have symptoms of fluid volume deficit: concentrated urine, decreased urine output, hypotension, elevated temperature, poor skin turgor, and weakness.

Laboratory tests may reveal electrolyte abnormalities, particularly low serum potassium. Potentially fatal cardiac arrythmias may result. The overuse of syrup of ipecac, an emetic agent, can create cumulative systemic toxicity affecting the gastrointestinal, neuromuscular, and cardiovascular systems, potentially leading to death from cardiotoxicity.

Another concern is the fact that the frequency of bulimia in diabetics is increasing, particularly among young women. This is a potentially deadly combination because binge eating and purging increase the risk for both hypoglycemic episodes and diabetic ketoacidosis (DKA). Closely monitoring blood glucose levels is indicated for these clients.

Nursing Diagnosis: NANDA

Four major nursing diagnoses for clients with bulimia are discussed below.

ANXIETY

Clients with bulimia nervosa experience anxiety: vague, uneasy feelings of moderate to intense severity related to preoccupation with body image. A rise in the client's anxiety level is usually a forerunner of binge/purge behaviors and may lead to purchasing or hoarding food in preparation for a binge.

FLUID VOLUME DEFICIT

Depletion of body fluids in clients with bulimia nervosa is usually related to self-induced vomiting and the excessive use of laxatives and diuretics, combined with decreased fluid intake. Extreme dehydration may lead to changes in electrolyte balance, causing altered mental status. Lethargy and confusion are symptoms of advanced dehydration. Edema may also be present.

INEFFECTIVE INDIVIDUAL COPING

Binge and purge behaviors are ineffective ways to cope with the stresses of life. Other impulse control problems, such as alcohol abuse, drug abuse, and shoplifting, are equally ineffective ways to reduce stress. The bulimic client's ineffective coping is related to issues such as independence/dependence, identity, and self-determination. Ineffective coping is manifested in the bulimic client's preoccupation with body size, poor self-esteem, distorted body image, and excessive overeating followed by purging.

INEFFECTIVE FAMILY COPING

The families of clients with bulimia nervosa perceive themselves as unable to deal effectively with the client's eating disorder related to the family's distorted perceptions of the problem. Parents may have difficulty allowing the client to grow up and may be overprotective; at the same time, they may have overly high expectations of the client. The bulimic client's behavior may become the family's focus, preventing the fulfillment of essential family roles. If disruption is extreme, the family may not be able to interact effectively with the larger community. Usual problem-solving methods are only partially adequate to deal with the stress of having a bulimic family member.

Outcome Identification: NOC

Suggested outcomes for each NANDA diagnosis in the previous section follow.

ANXIETY

Desired outcomes related to anxiety in bulimic clients may involve Coping: Actions to manage stressors that tax an individual's resources; and Impulse Control: Ability to self-restrain compulsive or impulsive behavior.

FLUID VOLUME DEFICIT

Two nursing outcomes that are useful with this nursing diagnosis are Electrolyte and Acid–Base Balance: Balance of electrolytes and nonelectrolytes in the intracellular and extracellular compartments of the body; and Hydration: Amount of water in the intracellular and extracellular compartments of the body.

INEFFECTIVE INDIVIDUAL COPING

Similar to the anorexic client, several NOC outcomes are relevant to bulimic clients with this nursing diagnosis. They include Coping: Actions to manage stressors that tax an individual's resources; Impulse Control: Ability to self-restrain compulsive or impulsive behavior; and Information Processing: Ability to acquire, organize, and use information.

INEFFECTIVE FAMILY COPING

NOC outcome statements relevant to the NANDA diagnosis of Ineffective Family Coping have not yet been developed. Appropriate outcomes might include those related to improving family communication, reducing family stress, learning developmental needs of family members, and seeking community resources.

Planning and Implementation: NIC

Several nursing interventions have been somewhat useful in treating bulimia nervosa.

MANAGING MEDICATION

Treatment is directed at symptoms or predisposing factors, particularly depression. Both anticonvulsant and antidepressant agents have been used. Some success has been reported with the tricyclic antidepressants (TCAs) desipramine (Norpramin) and amoxapine (Asendin). Although not a TCA, trazodone (Desyrel) has also been used (Walsh & Devlin, 1998).

Caution must be used when TCAs are given to clients with cardiac conditions because these medications may interfere with the conduction of electrical impulses in the heart. A baseline EKG and EKG monitoring until therapeutic blood levels are reached are safeguards. Teach clients to expect a delay of 2 to 5 weeks before seeing improvement of symptoms. They can also expect some unpleasant but temporary side effects, such as orthostatic hypotension, dry mouth, blurry vision, urinary retention, tachycardia, and palpitations.

Recent research on the effectiveness of fluoxetine hydrochloride (Prozac), a selective serotonin reuptake inhibitor (SSRI), has demonstrated some effectiveness in treating bulimia. Ongoing research offers hope for more effective pharmacologic treatment in the future.

REDUCING ANXIETY

The goal of nursing interventions with anxious bulimic clients is to help them recognize events that create anxiety and to avoid binge eating and purging in response to anxiety. Initially, being available to the anxious client is useful. Project a calm, reassuring attitude, and provide a quiet, nonstimulating environment. After trust is established, help the client identify anxiety-producing situations. Clients experience anxiety as occurring "out of the blue" and are often unaware that it is related to emotional issues and situations. Help clients identify previously used coping behaviors to determine whether they might be useful in current situations. How did the client handle anxiety before starting to binge and purge? Help bulimic clients identify feelings that precede binge/purge episodes such as those illustrated in ■ Figure 18–4, and explore healthier ways of dealing with those feelings.

Teach clients to recognize anxiety early, before it is severe, and to manage increasing anxiety. Energy-consuming activities, such as walking, running, and exercising, are useful but must be used very judiciously if the client's behavior includes overexercising. Clients can benefit from being taught progressive relaxation techniques and meditation (see Chapter 32). Administer antianxiety medications as ordered, but use caution because of the tendency to habituation. Also review the anxiety section of Chapter 16.

Client contracts are useful with bulimic clients. The contract is jointly developed with the client and renegotiated at periodic

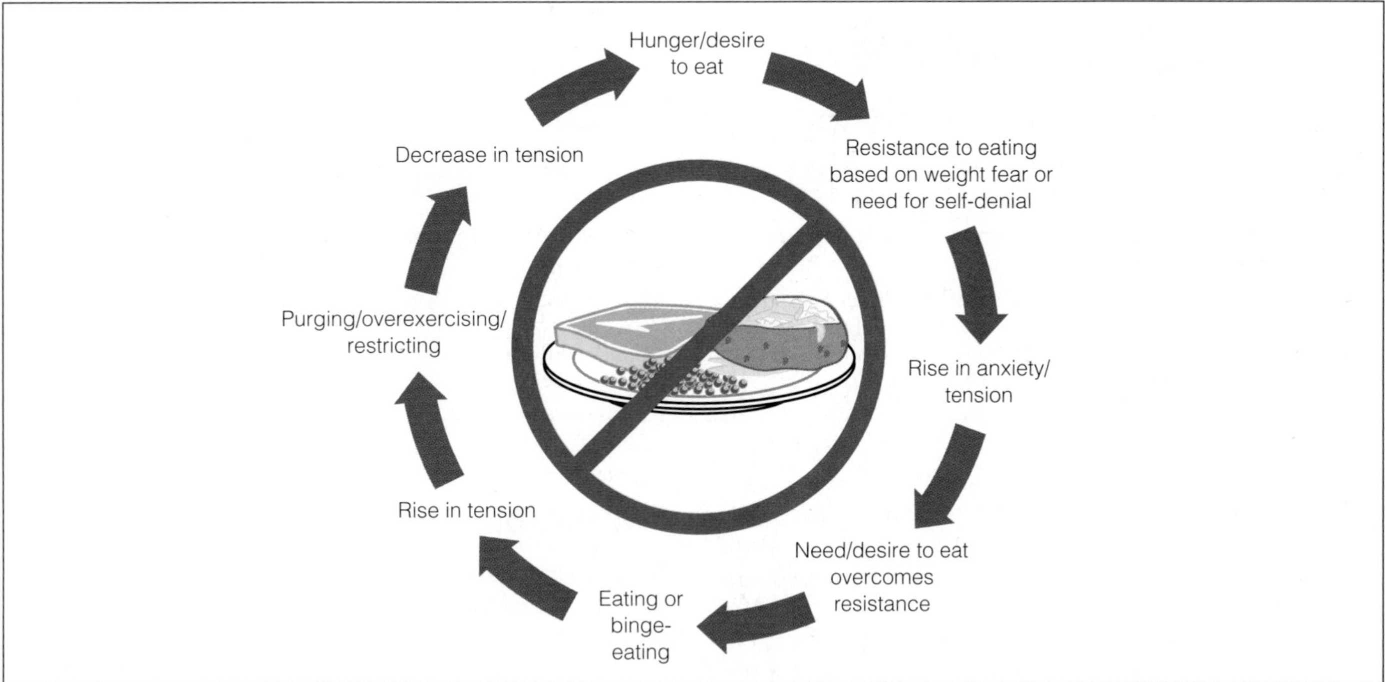

FIGURE 18–4 ■ *A disordered eating cycle. A nursing intervention to improve client self-awareness and anxiety reduction involves assisting clients to identify their personal eating cycle, which varies with the individual.*

intervals, depending on the client's goals, severity of symptoms, and compliance with the contract. Such a contract might include agreements about binge eating, vomiting, or hoarding food, such as those in Box 18–2.

Using a contract encourages clients to assume responsibility for themselves.

MANAGING FLUIDS AND ELECTROLYTES

The importance of accurate intake and output records cannot be overstated. Daily consumption of 2,000 to 3,000 mL of liquid promotes rehydration. Accurate daily weights are needed. Always weigh the client at the same time of day (immediately upon arising is preferred) and on the same scale. Assess and document the condition of the skin and oral mucous membranes as well as pulses and blood pressure daily, and monitor laboratory values, particularly urine specific gravity, reporting significant alterations to the physician. Observe clients for at least an hour after meals to prevent purging. To promote comfort in the dehydrated client, give frequent mouth care.

BOX 18–2 Sample Contract for a Client with Bulimia

- I will sit at the nurses' station for a half hour following my meals.
- I will not vomit after my meals.
- I will not take laxatives or diuretics.
- I will not bring any such substances onto the unit.
- I will tell the nursing staff if I feel like binge eating.
- I will stay away from the kitchen if I feel like going on a binge.

Client ______________________

Nurse ______________________

Date ______________________

FACILITATING COPING

Clients with bulimia nervosa can learn adaptive coping mechanisms to replace the out-of-control, binge/purge cycle. Once trust is developed, help the client plan and practice strategies for dealing effectively with intense feelings and the demands of daily living. It is important for clients to identify situations and patterns of events that precede binge/purge episodes. The Rx Communication feature on page 442 provides an example of how you might open up the discussion. Clients learn to identify, name, and express feelings that they formerly perceived only as "bad." Once this is accomplished, explore alternative ways for clients to express those feelings.

Help clients identify times when they are at risk for binge eating and lack impulse control, such as times when they are bored, frustrated, angry, lonely, or feeling unloved. Teach clients ways to nurture themselves during these times other than eating and purging. Suggest taking a warm bath, calling or visiting an old friend, or a hobby not involving food.

Clients with bulimia nervosa often perceive feelings of guilt and underlying resentment as overwhelming. They need to learn effective ways of expressing these feelings and assertiveness techniques to diminish guilty interactions in the future. Role-playing with the client helps the client practice assertiveness.

The worsening of both mood and bulimic symptoms during the winter has been reported in eating disorder literature

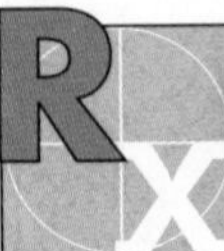

COMMUNICATION

Client with Bulimia Nervosa

CLIENT: Last night I made a pan of brownies and ate the whole thing. Then I had to throw up because I felt so miserable.

NURSE RESPONSE 1: Tell me about what was going on yesterday before you ate the brownies.

RATIONALE: Demonstrates nonjudgmental acceptance. Encourages the client to place events in time sequence. This enables her to connect the cause-and-effect relationship between her experiences, her feelings, and her subsequent behavior.

NURSE RESPONSE 2: That sounds uncomfortable. What are the miserable feelings about?

RATIONALE: Shows empathy for the client. Encourages her to focus on her feelings and their influence on her behavior, thereby promoting self-awareness.

with increasing frequency. Bright white light treatment has proven effective in treating bulimics with seasonal mood and symptom patterns. See Chapter 15 for a discussion of light treatment.

Involve the client in discharge planning. Topics covered in discharge planning include the productive use of time, identification of diversional activities not related to food, and participation in support groups.

MOBILIZING THE FAMILY

Certain family dynamics reinforce maladaptive eating behaviors; therefore, families must also develop effective coping mechanisms to support the client's healthier coping behaviors. Assess the family's feelings and perceptions of the client's bulimia, listening carefully for what is most stressful and threatening to family members. Correct misperceptions about the disorder. Encourage family members to explore together their usual coping strategies, and determine if any previously used strategies can be useful in the present situation.

Help the family identify their strengths and weaknesses. Encourage family members to share their thoughts and feelings, including feelings of guilt, blame, and resentment, with one another and with the client. Teach family members to use "I" statements, thereby acknowledging their feelings.

If the client's disorder impairs family functioning, help the family reorganize roles to reduce stress and ensure that members' needs continue to be met during the client's recovery. Help the family understand that two normal developmental needs of adolescents and young adults are to develop autonomy and to establish identities outside the family. Make appropriate referrals to community resources, such as the American Anorexia/Bulimia Association, Anorexia Nervosa and Related Eating Disorders, and Anorexia Nervosa and Associated Disorders groups (See Resources in the Client/Family Teaching feature "How You Can Help Someone with An Eating Disorder.").

Home visits for an evening or weekend can help both the client and the family learn to use their new coping behaviors. Planning before visits and evaluating the success of visits afterward are essential parts of nurse–client and nurse–family interventions.

Evaluation

The evaluation process determines the effectiveness of the nursing interventions.

ANXIETY

Clients will demonstrate anxiety control when they verbally identify situations and events that evoke anxiety. They will communicate needs and negative feelings appropriately. Clients will identify symptoms that indicate their own anxiety. They will identify ways of structuring the environment to prevent stressful situations that result in feeling out of control. Clients will eliminate binge/purge behaviors and demonstrate the use of anxiety-reduction strategies unrelated to eating. They will verbalize their acceptance of normal body weight without intense anxiety or will continue healthy eating patterns even though anxiety persists.

FLUID VOLUME

Dryness of oral mucosa and skin will not be evident. Skin turgor will be normal. Clients' vital signs and results of laboratory studies will be within normal limits. Input and output are balanced over 24-hour periods. Clients will verbalize their understanding of the relationship between dehydration and self-induced vomiting, laxative abuse, and diuretic abuse. Clients will verbalize understanding the physiologic and psychologic consequences of dehydration.

INDIVIDUAL COPING

Clients will demonstrate effective coping when they accurately assess maladaptive coping behaviors. They will demonstrate healthier ways to deal with stress and intense feelings. They will identify times of risk and verbalize alternative self-nurturing behaviors. They will demonstrate assertive communication techniques. Clients will demonstrate self-control in eating behaviors, gradually maintaining without supervision. They will verbalize increased self-confidence in the ability to handle the demands of daily life. They will follow through with recommended self-help or support groups and therapy following discharge.

CLIENT / FAMILY TEACHING

How You Can Help Someone with an Eating Disorder

Friends and family members of people with eating disorders are often at a loss as to how to help. Heather L. Howard, former administrator for the National Association of Anorexia Nervosa and Associated Disorders (ANAD), recommends the following guidelines:

- Accept that there are no quick and easy solutions. Attitudes and behaviors must change.
- Change takes time and requires the cooperation of the person with the disorder.
- Family and friends must also change to accommodate the person's growth.
- Cooperate fully with the person's therapist.
- Avoid arguments about weight and food.
- Express love and affection both verbally and physically.
- Admit your anger, frustration, helplessness, and powerlessness and help the person see these feelings do not mean you don't love him/her.
- Do things with the person that do not involve food.
- Don't diet yourself or talk about food, calories, fat grams, and the like.
- Avoid power struggles.
- Recognize that the person will make progress, then retreat into rituals for a time.
- Learn all you can about the disorder (see resource list).
- If the person will not seek help, CONFRONT in the following way:
  Concern—The reason you are confronting is that you care about the person.
  Organize—Decide who will be involved, when and where the confrontation will occur, what to say.
  Needs—What resources will be needed after the confrontation? Therapist or support group; other resources.
  Face—Face the actual confrontation. Be direct; do not back down if the person angrily denies having a problem.
  Respond—Respond after listening carefully.
  Offer—Offer help and suggestions; offer yourself as a sounding-board.
  Negotiate—Negotiate another time to talk and set a time frame for the person to seek professional help.
  Time—Time to begin work. Remember to stress that recovery takes time and patience but that it is time to begin the process. There is much to be gained by seeking help and much to lose if the behaviors continue.

RESOURCES*

Anorexia Nervosa and Related Disorders
P.O. Box 5102
Eugene OR 97405
503-344-1144
www.anred.com

National Association of Anorexia Nervosa and Associated Disorders
P.O. Box 7
Highland Park, IL 60035
847-831-3438
www.anad.org

National Eating Disorders Association
603 Stewart St., Suite 803
Seattle, WA 98101
206-382-3587
www.nationaleatingdisorders.org

Office on Women's Health
200 Independence Avenue SW, Room 730B
Washington, DC 20201
202-690-7650
www.4woman.gov/bodyimage

Weight-Control Information Network (WIN)
1 Win Way
Bethesda, MD 20892-3665
1-877-946-4627
www.niddk.nih.gov/health/nutrit/win.htm

Source: Heather L. Howard, former administrator, National Association for Anorexia Nervosa and Related Disorders (ANAD). Retrieved from the World Wide Web, www.anad.com.

*These resources can found on the Companion Website for this book.

MediaLink Eating Disorders Resources

FAMILY COPING

Families will verbalize accurate perceptions of their situation. They will verbalize their feelings about having a family member with an eating disorder. They will acknowledge the needs of both the client and the family unit. They will identify useful strategies for coping with the impact of bulimia nervosa on the family. They will use "I" statements during communication with one another, the client, and the nurse. They will verbalize an understanding of the developmental needs of family members. They will use more flexible problem-solving strategies. The family will reorganize family roles as necessary. They will identify community resources available to them and will follow through on referrals.

For additional information about the nursing process with clients with bulimia nervosa, see the accompanying Case Study and Nursing Care Plan feature.

Case Management/Community-Based Care/Home Care

Community based care, case management and home care for bulimia clients has been discussed earlier in this chapter. Refer to pages 438–439.

NURSING PROCESS

Clients with Binge-Eating Disorder

The nursing process for clients with binge-eating disorder is discussed in the following section.

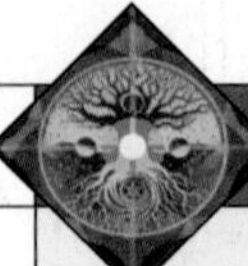

Case Study

Client with Bulimia Nervosa

Identifying Information

Lauren, a 28-year-old married woman, was admitted to the psychiatric unit from the emergency department where she was taken after collapsing during a marathon. She is a master's-prepared social worker who works in a drug abuse prevention program.

Lauren reports that she has been training for the marathon for about a year, running at least 35 miles a week. She believes that she had to be hospitalized because she did not ingest sufficient carbohydrates and fluids before the race.

Lauren states that she has been binge eating and purging for about 3 years, ever since she read about ballet dancers' and gymnasts' use of purging for weight control. On a typical day she arises at 5:00 AM, runs at least 5 miles, then gets ready for work. On the way to work she buys and consumes a dozen doughnuts. She arrives at work before anyone else and vomits in the employees' bathroom. She eats no lunch unless she can be sure of access to a "good" bathroom, which she describes as one with a single toilet and an outside door that locks. In the evening while preparing dinner she consumes a can of salted peanuts and four or five glasses of wine. She denies ever getting "high." After a large dinner she showers, vomiting while the shower is running. Her husband of 4 years is unaware of her "problem" but worries about her drinking and wonders how she can eat so much and never gain weight.

History

No prior psychiatric history. Lauren is the oldest of three children and the only girl. Her parents, both retired schoolteachers, live in a nearby town. She sees them infrequently because "they still treat me like I'm a little girl." She rarely sees her younger brothers and feels closer to her husband's family. There is no family history of eating disorders or substance abuse.

As the daughter of two schoolteachers, Lauren was expected to be the top student in her school. She had few friends because she was "the class geek." In college she excelled academically but was a "social failure." She states that she can drink an entire bottle of wine, vomit, and "sober up instantly." She has few friends or interests except running. She describes her job as "not fulfilling."

Lauren has no significant health problems. Vital signs: T, 98.2; P, 68; R, 14; Ht, 5' 7"; Wt, 110 lb; BP, 108/68.

Current Mental Status

Lauren is slim, neatly groomed, and cooperative, but reluctant. She is alert and oriented to time, place, and person. Her judgment is good and her ability to think abstractly is unimpaired. She is articulate; affect is appropriate to verbal content; no delusions, illusions, hallucinations, or other signs of thought disorder. She fidgets in her seat but makes good eye contact. She expresses embarrassment about hospitalization and shame about her behavior. She emphatically does not want her husband or office informed of the extent and details of her "problem." She maintains that she does not need to be hospitalized and can handle this herself.

Other Subjective or Objective Clinical Data

Lauren reports that she has not had a menstrual period in over 1 year. She takes no medications.

Assessment

The assessment of binge-eating disorder is not as straightforward as it might seem. Many obese individuals are apparently content and well adjusted. Do not assume that all obese people are emotionally distressed. The following discussion pertains to those clients who suffer psychologically from their excessive weight and who seek treatment for the resulting psychologic pain.

SUBJECTIVE DATA

Clients with binge-eating disorder report that a rise in tension usually leads to impaired control over eating and precipitates binges. Types and sources of the tension vary among individuals, but all report being significantly distressed by their binge eating. They describe eating large amounts of food rapidly, usually alone, due to embarrassment over their behavior (APA, 2000). They report feeling disgust, guilt, anger, depression, low self-esteem, and feelings of isolation during and after the binge. These feelings in turn create the desire to eat and the pathologic cycle begins again. Most clients with binge eating disorder report using food as a substitute for other forms of gratification such as companionship, attention from others, and emotional nurturing. They may also binge when happy or to reward themselves. Binge-eating disorder clients often report impaired social functioning, leading to withdrawal. Social isolation, however, only intensifies the obsessive preoccupation with food. Numerous attempts to lose weight are reported. Binge-eating disorder clients may describe a family history of marital conflict. Having one or more depressed parents is often reported.

OBJECTIVE DATA

Unlike anorexia and bulimia, which are found predominantly in women, binge-eating disorder is about equally prevalent in men and women. These clients are also older, averaging 40 years when seeking treatment, although they describe having started binge eating in their late teens or early twenties. Binge-eating disorder clients are almost universally obese, which is defined as body weight that exceeds by 20% the recommended weights on standard height and weight tables. The binge eating occurs, on average, at least 2 days a week for at least 6 months (APA, 2000). Clients tend to be sedentary and have one or more obesity-related disorders including hypertension, shortness of breath, and palpitations upon exertion.

Be sure to obtain a medication history during assessment. A number of medications, including birth control pills, some antipsychotics, steroids, antidepressants, and antacids, may contribute to weight gain. In addition, some perimenopausal women attribute increased appetite to hormone replacement therapy (HRT).

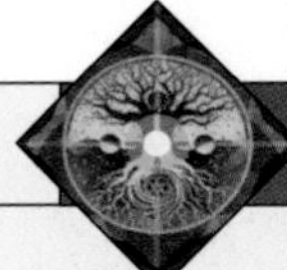

Nursing Care Plan

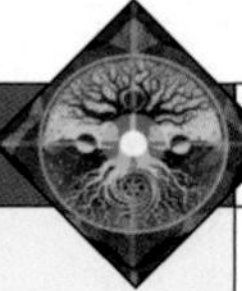

Nursing Diagnosis: Anxiety related to low self-esteem

Expected Outcome: Coping: Actions to manage stressors that tax an individual's resources.
Impulse Control: Ability to self-restrain compulsive or impulsive behavior.

Short-Term Goals	*Interventions*	*Rationale*
• Client will identify at least three sources of anxiety.	• Adopt a calm, reassuring attitude.	• Conveys safety and confidence.
	• Provide a quiet, nonstimulating environment.	• Minimizes anxiety-producing stimuli.
	• Help client recognize situations and events that create anxiety.	• Increases self-awareness.
	• Encourage client to identify previously used, successful coping behaviors.	• Promotes self-esteem.
	• Encourage client to identify alternatives to alcohol abuse, binge eating, and purging in response to anxiety.	• Increases coping skills.
	• Limit overexercising.	• Counteracts unhealthy preoccupations.
	• Negotiate a client contract to limit hoarding, vomiting, and other compulsive behaviors.	• Promotes self-responsibility and self-control.
• Client will demonstrate the use of relaxation techniques to manage anxiety.	• Teach progressive relaxation techniques and meditation.	• Gives useful information to improve coping skills.
	• Assist client to use techniques when feeling tension that would formerly lead to binge eating and purging.	• Provides reinforcement and support for effective coping.

Nursing Diagnosis: Fluid Volume Deficit related to self-induced vomiting and excessive exercising.

Expected Outcome: Electrolyte and Acid–Base Balance: Balance of electrolytes and nonelectrolytes in the intracellular and extracellular compartments of the body.
Hydration: Amount of water in the intracellular and extracellular compartments of the body.

Short-Term Goals	*Intervention*	*Rationale*
• Client will drink a minimum of 2 oz of fluids per hour.	• Teach client the importance of adequate fluid intake.	• Information every client should know.
	• Offer client her favorite beverages frequently during the day.	• Encourages fluid intake.
	• Weigh client daily to evaluate rehydration.	• Monitors hydration status.
	• Keep accurate intake and output records.	• Monitors hydration status.
	• Assess skin turgor and condition of mucous membranes daily and record.	• Monitors hydration status.
	• Encourage frequent mouth care to promote comfort.	• Comfort measure.
	• Monitor laboratory values, reporting significant alterations to the physician.	• Monitors electrolyte status.
• Client will not vomit following meals.	• Establish a no-purging contract with client.	• Promotes self-responsibility and self-control.
	• Observe client for at least 1 hour after meals to prevent purging.	• Provides support and reinforcement.
	• Give positive recognition when progress is shown.	• Reinforces healthy behaviors.

(continued)

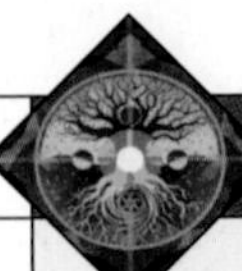

Nursing Care Plan (continued)

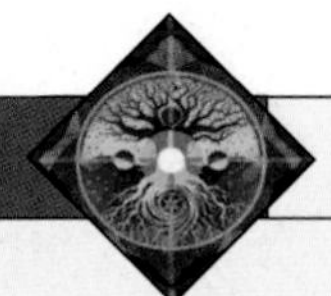

Nursing Diagnosis: Ineffective Individual Coping related to feelings of helplessness and lack of control in life situation.

Expected Outcome: Coping: Actions to manage stressors that tax an individual's resources.
Impulse Control: Ability to self-restrain compulsive or impulsive behavior.

Short-Term Goals	*Interventions*	*Rationale*
• Client will eat regularly within 1 week.	• Help client establish a trust relationship with you.	• Trust is basis for nurse–client relationship.
	• Assist client to plan for and practice how to deal with daily demands.	• Decreases helplessness; promotes self-responsibility and self-control.
	• Assist client to identify events preceding binge/purge episodes.	• Promotes self-awareness.
	• Encourage client to identify ways of nurturing herself without using food or alcohol.	• Validates concepts of choice, self-determination, and self-control.
• Client will refrain from discussing body image dissatisfactions within 1 week.	• Engage client in a process of identifying, naming, and expressing negative feelings.	• Promotes self-awareness and self-control.
	• Assist client to identify and practice alternative ways of expressing negative feelings.	• Increases coping skills; improves impulse control; decreases helplessness.

Nursing Diagnosis: NANDA

Several nursing diagnoses are appropriate for clients with binge-eating disorder.

KNOWLEDGE DEFICIT: DIET

Despite their preoccupation with food and eating, clients with binge-eating disorder often lack sufficient information about nutrition to make healthy decisions about diet. This knowledge deficit may be related to lack of interest, anxiety, denial of the need for information, confusion, misinformation, or other factors.

Evidence of nutritional knowledge deficit includes a history of noncompliance with dietary regimens, questions and statements indicating a lack of knowledge, misconceptions about the diet plan, and requests for information.

ALTERED NUTRITION: MORE THAN BODY REQUIREMENTS

The obese client's nutritional alteration is related to consuming more calories than required while expending few calories in exercise and activity. A sedentary lifestyle and occupation are common. Unhealthy eating patterns, such as night eating and binge eating, complicate the picture.

Recognize that the client's negative self-concept reinforces the desire for nurturance—that is, food—and that all negative feelings may be identified as hunger. These clients often ignore internal cues to hunger and eat in response to external cues, such as the time of day or stressful situations.

Obese binge-eating disorder clients are vulnerable to a variety of weight-loss fads such as appetite suppressants, fad diets, and expensive "get-thin-quick" programs at diet centers. Some 95% of dieters are unsuccessful, and in general, only 5% of obese individuals maintain a weight loss of at least 20 lb for 2 years or more. The failure of these efforts leads to guilt and a sense of hopelessness about ever losing weight. Depression and loss of faith in self are common in obese clients.

HOPELESSNESS

Clients who compulsively overeat frequently feel hopelessness related to their repeated failure to lose weight or to control their eating behavior. The inability to feel positive about the present life situation is manifested in a despondent and passive approach to living. Any effort seems too extreme; every task is too great. "What's the use?" is a question characteristically posed by hopeless clients.

Hopelessness is debilitating because clients cannot mobilize energy on their own behalf; nor do they believe that anyone else can help. Hopelessness is demonstrated by apathy and a lack of involvement in activities. Clients may lose interest in self-care activities. Oversleeping, decreased affect, and decreased response to stimuli are associated features. The speech of hopeless clients is filled with despondency. They may verbalize a loss of faith in God or another higher power.

SOCIAL ISOLATION

The social isolation reported by clients is related to rejection by others or self-imposed withdrawal from social interaction because of self-consciousness and fear of rejection. Regardless of the cause of social isolation, the resulting alienation and loneliness increase the client's depression and preoccupation with food. Obese clients want to participate in social situations, but their negative past experiences have conditioned them to expect ridicule and rejection.

Outcome Identification: NOC

Suggested outcomes for each NANDA diagnosis in the previous section follow.

KNOWLEDGE DEFICIT: DIET

The desired outcome related to this diagnosis involves the improvement of the binge-eating disorder client's extent of understanding conveyed about diet.

ALTERED NUTRITION: MORE THAN BODY REQUIREMENTS

Binge eating disorder clients are nearly universally obese and often binge on easily consumed, high-calorie foods such as cookies, chips, and doughnuts. Outcomes relevant to this nursing diagnosis therefore include modifications in Nutritional Status: Food and Fluid Intake: Amount of food and fluids taken in a 24-hour period; and Nutritional Status: Nutrient Intake: Adequacy of nutrients taken into the body.

HOPELESSNESS

Several outcomes are relevant to binge eating disorder clients with this nursing diagnosis. They include Hope: Presence of internal state of optimism that is personally satisfying and life supporting; Mood Equilibrium: Appropriate adjustment of prevailing emotional tone in response to circumstances; and Quality of Life: An individual's expressed satisfaction with current life circumstances.

SOCIAL ISOLATION

Isolation increases the preoccupation with food and the opportunities for binge eating. Therefore, NOC outcomes helpful to binge eating disorder clients include Social Involvement: Frequency of an individual's social interactions with persons, groups, or organizations; and Social Support: Perceived availability and actual provision of reliable assistance from other persons.

Planning and Implementation: NIC

Several important nursing interventions for clients with binge-eating disorder are discussed below.

PROVIDING NUTRITION EDUCATION

Providing basic nutritional education is the goal of interventions with clients who have a knowledge deficit in this area. First determine what knowledge or misconceptions the client has, and begin teaching at that level. Asking binge-eating disorder clients to write down and share with you the history of their numerous attempts to lose weight may be helpful. This provides an opportunity to establish rapport by demonstrating empathy for the anguish, helplessness, and hopelessness experienced by these clients.

The goal of this exercise is for the client to realize that dieting has not created a lasting change or sustained weight loss. If the client's information base of normal nutrition is minimal, begin by showing pictures of the basic food groups. Provide lists of foods in each group, and encourage the client to select favorite foods in each group. Discuss the body's need for proteins, carbohydrates, fats, vitamins, and minerals. Help the client plan a day's menus, keeping the client's food preferences in mind. Teach the client to analyze labels on prepared foods to determine foods with high nutrient value and reasonable caloric content. Supplement educational sessions with written materials the client can keep for later reference. Opportunities for teaching clients about nutrition can be used as a trust-building strategy.

ASSISTING WITH NUTRITION MANAGEMENT AND WEIGHT REDUCTION

In planning interventions to help binge-eating disorder clients improve their nutritional status, collaborative goal setting is essential. The client must set a personal goal of controlling eating behaviors and establish a realistic weight-loss goal. Help the client explore measures for changing eating habits. For instance, clients can keep a food diary to monitor the types and amounts of foods they eat. Slowing the rate of eating by chewing more thoroughly, placing implements on the plate between bites, conversing with table companions, and avoiding eating alone are helpful. Establishing a program of gradually increasing physical activity helps narrow the gap between caloric intake and energy expenditures.

Encourage clients to voice their feelings, maintaining a calm and accepting attitude as they do. Help clients develop new, nonfood-related coping strategies for dealing with troublesome feelings.

Cognitive restructuring techniques, such as correcting clients' irrational beliefs, are helpful. Help the client practice replacing negative self-talk with positive self-talk. Cognitive restructuring techniques are discussed in greater detail in Chapter 30.

Give positive reinforcement and recognition when clients achieve any small weight loss. Do not allow small "slips" to assume major importance or to impede steady progress. Teach the client how to select balanced, nutritionally sound meals when dining outside the home.

Provide information about community resources for exercise, such as the YMCA and YWCA. Make referrals to support groups and self-help groups, such as Overeaters Anonymous, Weight Watchers, and the National Association to Aid Fat Americans. Some support groups, such as Overeaters Anonymous, make use of sponsors for new members. Sponsors are individuals who are successfully coping with eating disorders and who can provide encouragement and support at difficult points in the recovery process. These individuals are a particularly valuable resource to people struggling to overcome reliance on compulsive overeating behaviors. Weight Watchers, an organization recommended by many health care professionals, provides healthful basic nutritional information, group support, and written educational materials that clients can use for reference. Resource links for these

MediaLink Binge-Eating: Self-Help Groups

organizations can be accessed through the Companion Website of this book.

INSTILLING HOPE

Personal hygiene and good grooming promote a sense of well-being. Spending time conversing with clients at mealtimes can slow the eating process and demonstrate that change is possible. Assume an unhurried and caring attitude.

Unresponsive, apathetic clients become more responsive when exercise becomes part of their daily routine. Encourage daily exercise or activity.

Also encourage clients to express both positive and negative feelings as an important step toward accepting their feelings as valid. The Rx Communication feature below demonstrates how to encourage expression of feelings. Adopt an empathic, nonjudgmental attitude, and over time, help clients move from expressing feelings to exploring ways of coping other than by eating. See Box 18–3 for affirming thoughts for compulsive overeaters.

Attaining an intellectual understanding of one's condition promotes hope and a sense of control. Helping compulsive overeaters learn to feel and respond to their internal body cues, particularly cues to hunger and satisfaction, is essential. This is a lengthy process that requires external support and inward self-examination. The purpose of the extra weight also must be explored. What protective function does being fat provide? The advantages and disadvantages of being both overweight and normal weight should be examined. Keeping a diary or journal may be helpful to clients as they struggle to experience and express their feelings without the numbing effect of overeating.

Visualization and guided imagery are useful with hopeless clients (see Chapter 32). Encourage them to focus on happy experiences from the past and to envision themselves as they wish to be—healthy, energetic, and filled with vitality. Reinforce any expression of hopefulness, no matter how tentative.

ENHANCING SOCIALIZATION

For the socially isolated client, the goal of nursing interventions is to increase time voluntarily spent in group settings. The first step is to offer companionship; just sitting quietly with the client while making no demands for interaction signifies your acceptance. Frequent, brief contacts indicate interest and foster the development of a therapeutic nurse–client relationship. Next, engage the socially isolated client in a noncompetitive one-to-one activity, such as working on a jigsaw puzzle. After the client feels comfortable during one-to-one activities, offer to accompany the client to a group activity. Help the client plan ahead, making sure the client realizes that leaving is okay if anxiety becomes too high. Positively reinforce any amount of time in groups, however brief.

As the client becomes more comfortable in groups, withdraw gradually, but remain available. Role playing social skills helps clients increase their repertoire of socially acceptable behaviors. Teach assertiveness techniques, because both passivity and aggressiveness invite rejection by others.

BOX 18–3 Affirmations for Compulsive Overeaters

1. My worth as a person is not diminished in *any* way by my body size or my eating patterns.
2. I will love myself no matter what my eating patterns are.
3. I will judge my days not by what or how much I eat, but by the accomplishments I have made and the love I have given.
4. My life is a gift, and I will not let my enjoyment of it be diminished by feeling guilty over my body size or how much I eat.
5. I am finished blaming others, situations, and myself for the way I eat. I will take action minute by minute, hour by hour, and day by day until I can eat normally again.
6. My eating disorder is a temporary condition in my life.
7. There is a normal eater within me. I will let him/her take over my life more and more each day as I am ready.
8. I *can* imagine a life without having an eating disorder.
9. When I feel stressed, I will close my eyes and picture how my all-powerful, normal eater would handle the situation.
10. I believe I will be a normal eater again. I know I will be a normal eater again!

Source: Reprinted with permission from Dusty Press, Copyright 2001, www.fatfairygodmother.com.

Evaluation

Evaluating the effectiveness of nursing interventions is an essential ongoing component of the nursing process.

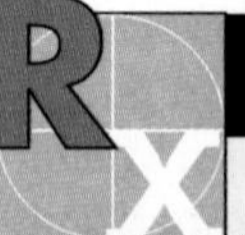

COMMUNICATION

Client with Binge-Eating Disorder

CLIENT: I hate the way I look now! I was a size 6 when I got married and now I wear a size 14!

NURSE RESPONSE 1: You sound upset. How are you feeling?

RATIONALE: Shows empathy and nonjudgmental acceptance. Assists the client to become aware of her feelings and how feelings influence her behavior.

NURSE RESPONSE 2: Give me an example of a time when you felt this way and what you did to feel better.

RATIONALE: Gathering more data from the client helps you understand her better. By asking her to describe a concrete incident you assist her to make connections between her feelings and her coping patterns. Fosters a nurse–client partnership to engage in problem-solving.

NUTRITION KNOWLEDGE

Clients will demonstrate knowledge of nutrition by identifying the correct food group for each food in a sample daily menu, recognizing missing food groups and identifying overrepresented groups. Clients will accurately assess the nutritional value of prepared foods, using label information. They will demonstrate the ability to select a nutritious, low-calorie, balanced daily diet for themselves. They will perform self-monitoring activities.

NUTRITIONAL STATUS

Clients will demonstrate improved nutritional status when they acknowledge their weight problems, verbalize the desire to lose weight, identify and verbalize feelings that trigger overeating, refrain from binge eating, and actively participate in a structured weight loss plan. They will verbalize feelings of increased self-control and greater self-esteem. Clients will progress steadily toward their personal weight-loss goals. They will demonstrate slower eating behaviors and avoid eating alone. They will describe how to order food in a restaurant yet adhere to their meal plans. They will participate in regular, structured exercise programs as well as self-help and/or support groups.

HOPEFULNESS

Clients will demonstrate hopefulness when they voluntarily assume responsibility for hygiene and grooming. They will demonstrate commitment to a program of daily exercise. Clients will verbalize both positive and negative feelings and recognize life events over which they have no control. Clients will verbalize an intellectual understanding of the meaning of their compulsive overeating and techniques for its management.

SOCIAL INVOLVEMENT

Clients will demonstrate social involvement when they willingly socialize with others. They will voluntarily attend and participate in client group activities. Clients will approach other people appropriately for one-to-one interactions and will report minimal anxiety during social interactions. They will participate in clubs or volunteer groups and will verbalize fewer feelings or experiences of being excluded.

Case Management/Community-Based Care/Home Care

Community based care, case management, and home care for clients with binge-eating disorder has been discussed earlier in this chapter. See pages 438–439.

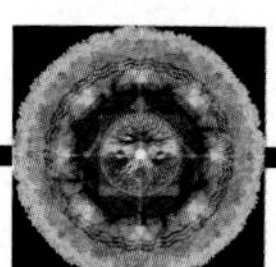

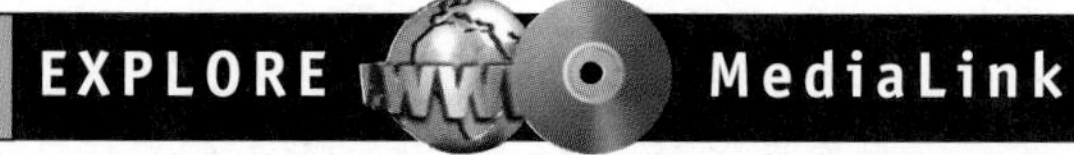

NCLEX review, case studies, and other interactive resources for this chapter can be found on the Companion Website at www.prenhall.com/kneisl. Click on Chapter 18 to select the activities for this chapter.

For animations, video tutorials, more NCLEX review questions, and an audio glossary, access the accompanying CD-ROM in this textbook.

BIBLIOGRAPHY

Ackard, D. M., & Neumark-Sztainer, D. (2002). Date violence and date rape among adolescents: Associations with disordered eating behaviors and psychological health. *Child Abuse and Neglect, 26*(5), 455–473.

American Psychiatric Association (2000). *Diagnostic and statistical manual of mental disorders* (4th ed., Text Revision). Washington, DC: Author.

Appolinario, J. C., Fontanelle, L. F., Papelbaum, M., Bueno, J. R., & Coutinho, W. (2002). Topiramate use in obese patients with binge eating disorder: An open study. *Canadian Journal of Psychiatry, 47*(3), 271–273.

Botta, R. A., & Dumlao, R. (2002). How do conflict and communication patterns between fathers and daughters contribute to or offset eating disorders? *Health Communication, 14*(2), 199–219.

Bruch, H. (1978). *The golden cage: The enigma of anorexia nervosa.* Cambridge, MA: Harvard University Press.

Chally, P. S. (1998). An eating disorders prevention program. *Journal of Child and Adolescent Psychiatric Nursing, 11*(2), 51–60.

Cowen, P. J. & Smith, K. A. (1999). Serotonin, dieting, and bulimia nervosa. *Advances in Experimental Medicine and Biology, 467*, 101–104.

Davis, C., Durnin, J., Dionne, M., & Durevich, M. (1994). The influence of body fat content and bone diameter measurements on body dissatisfaction in adult women. *International Journal of Mental Disorders, 15*(3), 257–263.

Dichter, J. R., Cohen, J., & Connolly, P. M. (2002). Bulimia nervosa: Knowledge, awareness, and skill levels among advanced practice nurses. *Journal of the American Academy of Nurse Practitioners, 14*(6), 269–275.

Doyle, M. M. (1995). Practical management of eating disorders. *Proceedings of the Nutritional Society (Ireland), 54*(3), 711–719.

Geller, J., Cockell, S. J., & Goldner, E. M. (2000). Inhibited expression of negative emotions and interpersonal orientation in anorexia nervosa. *International Journal of Eating Disorders, 28*(1), 8–19.

Harris, L. (1997). *The Commonwealth Fund survey of the health of adolescent girls*. New York: Louis Harris and Associates.

Howard, H. L. (2002). *How to confront*. National Association of Anorexia Nervosa and Associated Disorders. Retrieved from the World Wide Web at www.anad.org.

Johnson, J. G., Cohen, P., Kasen, S., & Brook, J. S. (2002). Eating disorders during adolescence and the risk for physical and mental disorders during early adulthood. *Archives of General Psychiatry, 59*(6), 545–552.

Kann, L., Kinchen, S. A., & Williams, B. I. (1997). *Youth risk behavior surveillance—United States*. Atlanta: Centers for Disease Control and Prevention, 47(SS-3), 1–89.

Kaplan, A. S. (2002). Psychological treatments for anorexia nervosa: A review of published studies and promising new directions. *Canadian Journal of Psychiatry, 47*(3), 235–242.

Lating, J. M., O'Reilly, M. A., & Anderson, K. P. (2002). Eating disorders and posttraumatic stress: Phenomenological and treatment considerations using the two-factor model. *International Journal of Emergency Mental Health, 4*(2), 113–118.

Latzer, Y., Eysen-Eylat, D., & Tabenkin, H. (2000). A case report: Treatment of severe anorexia nervosa with home total parenteral hyperalimentation. *International Journal of Eating Disorders, 27*(1), 115–118.

Love, C. C., & Seaton, H. (1991). Eating disorders: Highlights of nursing assessment and therapeutics. *Nursing Clinics of North America, 26*(3), 677–697.

MacDonald, C. (2002). Treatment resistance in anorexia nervosa and the pervasiveness of ethics in clinical decision making. *Canadian Journal of Psychiatry, 47*(3), 267–270.

Milos, G., Spindler, A., Ruggiero, G., Klaghofer, R., & Schnyder, U. (2002). Comorbidity of obsessive-compulsive disorders and duration of eating disorders. *International Journal of Eating Disorders, 31*(3), 284–289.

Monteleone, F., Brambilla, F., Bortolotti, F., & Maj, M. (2002). Serotonergic dysfunction across the eating disorders: Relationship to eating behaviour, purging behaviour, nutritional status and general psychopathology. *Psychological Medicine, 30*(5), 1099–1110.

National Institute of Mental Health. (1998). NIMH workshop on research in eating disorders, December 7–8. Retrieved from the World Wide Web at www.nimh.nih.gov/events/edsummary.cfm.

Perez, M., Voelz, Z. R., Pettit, J. W., & Joiner, T. E., Jr. (2002). The role of acculturative stress and body dissatisfaction in predicting bulimic symptomatology across ethnic groups. *International Journal of Eating Disorders, 31*(4), 442–454.

Rosenblum, J., & Forman, S. (2002). Evidence-based treatment of eating disorders. *Current Opinions in Pediatrics, 14*(4), 379–383.

Scharer, K. (1999). Eating disorder in a 10-year-old girl. *Journal of Child and Adolescent Psychiatric Nursing, 12*(2), 79–86.

Shafran, R., Cooper, Z., & Fairburn, C. G. (2002). Clinical perfectionism: A cognitive-behavioural analysis. *Behavioral Research and Therapy, 40*(7), 773–791.

Steinhausen, H. C. (2002). The outcome of anorexia nervosa in the 20th century. *American Journal of Psychiatry, 159*(8), 1284–1293.

Walsh, B. T., & Devlin, M. J. (1998). Eating disorders: Progress and problems. *Science, 280*(5368), 1387–1390.

White, J. H., & Litovitz, G. (1998). A comparison of inpatient and outpatient women with eating disorders. *Archives of Psychiatric Nursing, 12*(4), 181–194.

Wilfley, D. E., Welch, R. R., Stein, R. I., Spurrell, E. B., Cohen, L. R., Saelens, B. E., et. al. (2002). A randomized comparison of group cognitive-behavioral therapy and group interpersonal psychotherapy for the treatment of overweight individuals with binge-eating disorder. *Archives of General Psychiatry, 59*(8), 713–721.

Wilson, G. T., Fairburn, C. C., Agras, W. S., Walsh, B. T., & Kraemer, H. (2002). Cognitive-behavioral therapy for bulimia nervosa: Time course and mechanisms of change. *Journal of Consulting Clinical Psychology, 70*(2), 267–274.

Zhu, A. J., & Walsh, B. T. (2002). Pharmacologic treatment of eating disorders. *Canadian Journal of Psychiatry, 47*(3), 227–234.

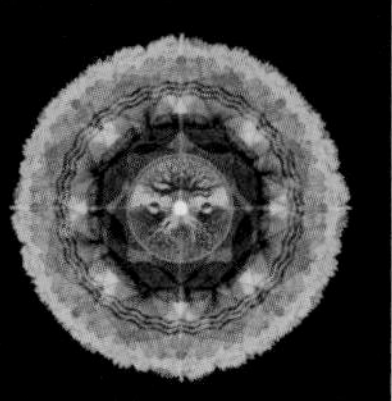

Sleep Disorders

MARLENE REIMER

19

Chapter NINETEEN

FOCUS QUESTIONS

- What sleep patterns are most commonly associated with major depressive disorder, manic episodes in bipolar disorder, schizophrenia, and substance abuse?
- How would you define the four major symptoms that characterize the different types of sleep disorders?
- Which three key assessments are pertinent to each of the major symptoms?
- How do the guidelines for good sleep hygiene compare and contrast with those for dealing with insomnia?
- Which of your beliefs about what constitutes normal sleep have been influenced by your family and your cultural background?

Media Link 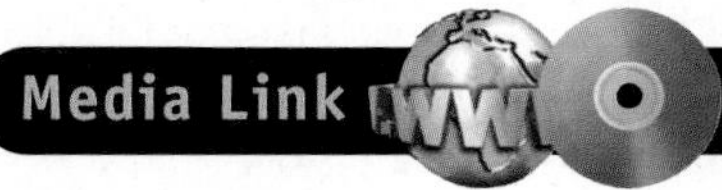 www.prenhall.com/kneisl

Additional resources for this chapter can be found on the Student CD-ROM accompanying this textbook, and on the Companion Website at www.prenhall.com/kneisl. Click on Chapter 19 to select the activities for this chapter.

CD-ROM
- Audio Glossary
- NCLEX Review

Companion Website
- Additional NCLEX Review
- Care Plan: Sleep Apnea
- Case Study: Insomnia

KEY TERMS

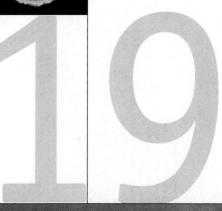

cataplexy
dyssomnia
hypersomnia
hypnagogic hallucinations
insomnia
parasomnia
polysomnography
REM rebound
sleep apnea
sleep bruxism
sleep enuresis
sleep paralysis
somnambulism

CHAPTER OUTLINE

CROSS REFERENCES

Other topics relevant to this content are: Assessing an individual's normal patterns and deviations, Chapter 9; Characteristic changes to sleep patterns in mood disorders, Chapter 15; Physiologic changes in sleep due to substances, Chapter 13; Psychobiology, Chapter 4; Psychopharmacologic sleep disorder causes and treatments, Chapter 31; Relaxation exercises, Chapter 32; Stress and its impact on sleep, Chapter 5.

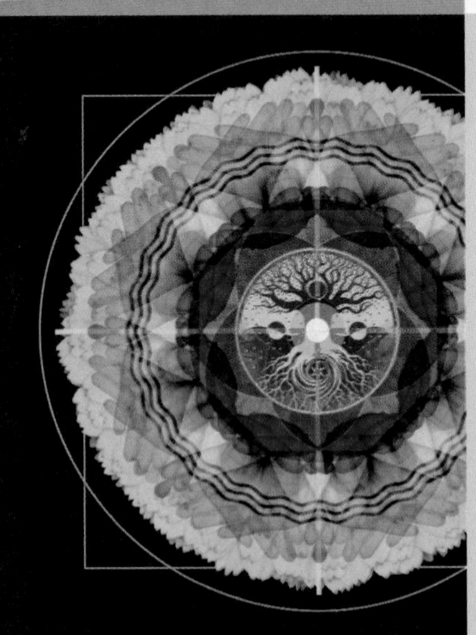

CRITICAL THINKING CHALLENGE

Jackie DeJong, a 24-year-old student being seen in the university counseling center, tells you that she has not had a good sleep in the last 2 months. She states, "The night I went to the sleep lab was particularly bad—I hardly slept a wink." However, you have read the sleep lab report on her health record. The polysomnogram showed a typical distribution of sleep stages for someone her age with sleep onset 15 minutes after lights out and three brief awakenings in a 7-hour period.

How can you reconcile her subjective report with the objective evidence? How might alternative explanations alter how you would apply the nursing process? Is any one view more correct than the other? ■

Sleep is a basic human need that affects, and is affected by, mental health. It is so much a part of the normal rhythm of our lives that it tends to be taken for granted until it is disrupted. Disrupted sleep is a particularly important consideration in mental health and illness because of its subtle but pervasive effects on mood, performance, and physical functioning (Hoy, Vennelle, Kingshott, Engleman, & Douglas, 1999). Lack of sleep tends to decrease our ability to cope, to deal with ambiguity, to make decisions, and to feel confident. Sleep pattern disturbance is often an early symptom of mental illness (Kaplan, Sadock, & Grebb, 2002). For example, a change in sleep patterns is among the diagnostic criteria for major depressive disorder, manic episode, and dysthymic disorder in the DSM-IV-TR (American Psychiatric Association [APA], 2000).

Sleep has been described as a neurobiologic window into the pathophysiology of psychiatric disorders (Gillin, 2000). An association between depression and **insomnia**—the chronic inability to get to sleep or to remain asleep during the usual sleep period—was observed as long ago as the time of Hippocrates. As a means of assessing the unconscious, Freud brought the study of dreams into the realm of science. The discovery of rapid eye movement (REM) sleep by Aserinsky and Kleitman in the early 1950s was a major breakthrough in the effort to understand the relationship between the mind and the body (Pivik, 2000). Until that time, sleep had been seen as a quiet state, as is characteristic of non-REM sleep. However, in REM sleep, the stage in which most dreaming occurs, brain waves show a level of cognitive activity comparable to the waking state, and physiologic functions are also in a heightened state of activity. The major difference between REM sleep and the awake state is the almost total paralysis of skeletal muscle during REM sleep, a factor that essentially prevents the acting out of dream states. More recent progress in the development of antidepressant medications, especially those that primarily target a particular neurotransmitter, has led to advances in our understanding of the physiologic aspects of mood disorders and sleep–wake states.

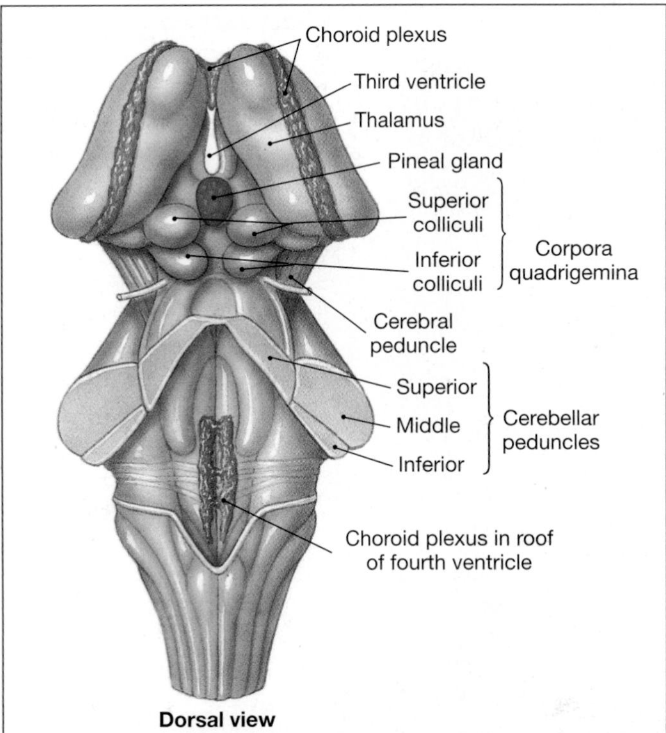

FIGURE 19–1 ■ *The pineal gland. Seasonal rhythms (such as hibernation) may be regulated by the pineal gland, which is located at the base of the brain between the lobes of the thalamus. The pineal gland secretes melatonin, which has been implicated in both types of biologic rhythms (seasonal and circadian), and is currently a subject of the investigation into the causes of aging.*

Source: Smock, T. K. (1999). *Physiological psychology: A neuroscience approach* (p. 307). Upper Saddle River, NJ: Prentice Hall.

Normal Sleep

This chapter begins with a brief summary of the range of normal sleep patterns across the life span. The key points are as follows:

- There is a wide range of sleep patterns among "good sleepers."
- Changes in sleep patterns normally occur as individuals progress through the life span.
- The pineal gland (see ■ Figure 19–1) provides the hormone melatonin that promotes drowsiness in lower light.
- Humans have considerable capacity to adapt to variations in sleep patterns.
- The functions of sleep are still poorly understood.

OPTIMAL SLEEP

A "good sleeper" can be identified in any of three ways: self-defined, behaviorally defined, or polysomnographically defined. Most people have a definite opinion about their sleep. Self-defined good sleepers generally describe themselves as getting enough sleep to feel refreshed in the morning, to have energy for the day, to fall asleep fairly quickly, and to wake up only briefly, if at all, during the night. To hypothesize that a client is a good sleeper from a subjective point of view, you would want to pay close attention to what he or she says about the quality of sleep.

For an objective assessment, observe alertness during sedentary, repetitive activity such as watching television or driving. You would note the ability to fall asleep in 10 to 30 minutes under usual circumstances, and final wakening at the habitual rising time, with or without an alarm clock. ■ Figure 19–2 on page 454 shows another type of sleep assessment—photographic serializing of movement during sleep. Assessment of sleep patterns should become part of your regular assessment with all clients (see the Assessment box on page 455). The depth with which you pursue potential problems will vary according to the presenting problems and context of care.

Polysomnography

Polysomnography is the simultaneous recording of several physical parameters during sleep, including brain wave activity,

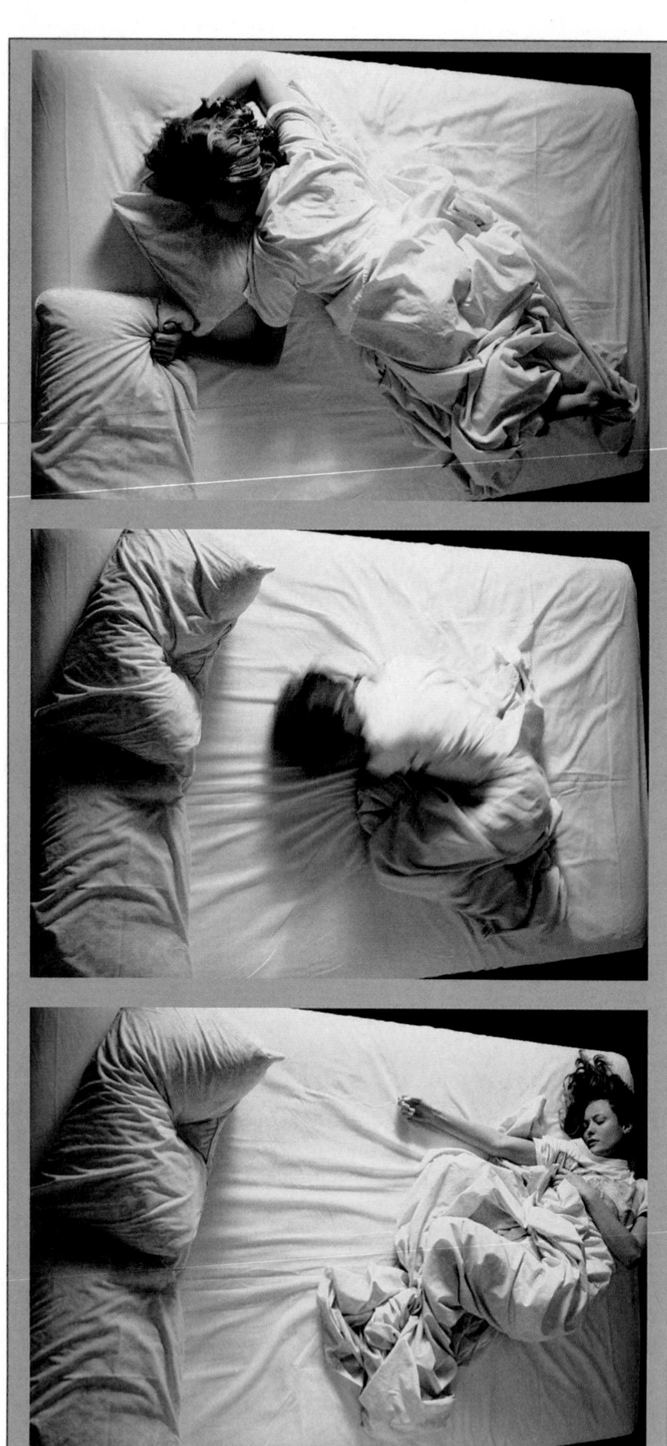

FIGURE 19–2 ■ *Overhead view of a woman sleeping.*

Source: Christopher Bissell, Getty Images Inc.-Stone.

eye movements, muscle tone, and respiration. The technique is useful in determining the type and stages of sleep, as well as number of arousals and total sleep time (see ■ Figure 19–3) on page 456. This electrophysiologic recording for a good sleeper would probably show recurrent sleep cycles about every 90 minutes, more slow-wave sleep (stages 3 and 4 of non-REM sleep) during the first part of the night combined with brief REM periods, changing to a greater percentage of REM sleep toward the end of the sleeping period (see ■ Figure 19–4) on page 457. Non-REM sleep consists of four stages, characterized by a progressive slowing of brain waves, decreasing muscle tone, and reduction in most physiologic functions. REM sleep is characterized by neurologic and physiologic activity that is similar to the waking state but with very low skeletal muscle tone.

Sleep Pattern Variations

The average amount of sleep required to feel rested varies widely from person to person. Requiring an average of 7 to 8 hours sleep per night is most common for adults. However, a small percentage of the population are short sleepers, requiring an average of 6 hours or less. Another small percentage are long sleepers, requiring an average of 9 or more hours each night (American Sleep Disorders Association [ASDA], 1997; Kaplan, Sadock, & Grebb, 2002).

The distinction between average hours needed and average hours obtained is important. Short or long sleepers by definition are good sleepers; that is, they habitually feel rested and alert after their normal sleep time. However, they may experience social pressure and/or even receive inappropriate pharmacologic intervention because they do not seem to conform to the norms of their family or peer group. More commonly, though, shortened sleep time is habitual, associated with the pressures of modern society.

There is growing concern that whole populations in developed countries are becoming chronically sleep deprived. As students, you are coping with pressures to study, to prepare for clinical experiences, and to complete assignments, as well as performing other roles that are important to you. Take the quiz in the Nursing Self-Awareness feature on page 456 to see whether you are getting enough sleep.

Behavioral Factors. You may also know of individuals who increase their habitual sleep time (or at least their total time in bed) as avoidance. In your psychiatric–mental health nursing practice, you may encounter clients who report the need for long periods of sleep and rest, often in association with depression. To distinguish normally long sleepers from clients who are trying to cope by spending more time in bed, it is useful to inquire about previous sleep patterns.

Situational and Developmental Factors. Sleep requirements also vary in relation to situational and developmental factors. With increased physical work, exercise, mental stress, or exposure to adverse weather conditions, total sleep requirements tend to increase. Specific needs for REM sleep increase in relation to periods of intense learning or other psychological stimuli.

Developmental changes in sleep patterns and requirements across the life span are not emphasized here because they are discussed in most fundamental nursing textbooks. The important point for the psychiatric–mental health nurse is to include

ASSESSMENT Sleep Patterns

Sleep–Wake Schedule

What time do you usually go to bed?

How long does it usually take you to fall asleep after you have turned off the light?

What time do you usually wake up?

What is different about your sleep–wake schedule on the week-end/days off?

How often do you take naps? (Be alert here for cultural influence, such as taking siestas, or occupational influence.) Under what circumstances?

Getting to Sleep

What helps you get to sleep?

What makes it difficult for you to get to sleep?

Staying Asleep

On average, how many times do you wake up during the night?

What seems to waken you?

How long does it usually take to get back to sleep?

What do you do if you are having trouble getting back to sleep?

Waking Up

How difficult is it for you to wake up?

How soon after waking up do you usually get up?

How do you feel when you first get up?

Daytime Functioning

At what time of day do you usually feel most energetic?

At what time of day do you feel most sleepy?

Would you call yourself a "morning person" or an "evening person"?

Satisfaction with Sleep; Potential Problems

How satisfied are you with the sleep you usually get?

Do you think you get enough sleep on average? How do you know?

How has your sleep been during the past 2 weeks in comparison to what is normal for you?

Are you concerned about any of the following things?

- Getting to sleep
- Waking up too many times during the night
- Waking up too early
- Having to fight sleepiness during the day
- Snoring, restlessness, talking or walking in your sleep
- Bad dreams
- Drinking too much coffee (or other caffeine/nicotine sources)

When do you enjoy sleep the most?

a consideration of the client's developmental stage as part of sleep pattern assessment. For example, the tendency of adolescents to sleep late and of older adults to get up earlier appears to have some physiologic basis from age-related shifts in circadian rhythms. The number of arousals tends to increase as adults get older. This change is often greeted with concern that something is wrong. However, if clients are able to get back to sleep without much distress, and/or the wakenings are mainly associated with the need to void, you can help them see the change as normal and become amenable to minor adjustments such as reducing fluid intake after the evening meal.

Physiologic Factors. We physiologically prioritize among types of sleep. Following periods of acute or chronic sleep deprivation, a rebound phenomenon occurs in which the recovery of REM sleep is given priority. You may have noticed how you seem to dream more after several nights of interrupted sleep. (Dreams can occur during non-REM as well as REM sleep, but dreams in non-REM sleep are usually more fragmentary and mundane, without much of a story line.)

Clients who have been taking medications or other substances that suppress REM sleep (tricyclic antidepressants, short-acting benzodiazepines) may notice increased dreaming with discontinuation. Through anticipatory teaching, you can help clients understand that this catching up on REM sleep, known as **REM rebound,** is a normal and passing experience. Such support is important because clients who have been relying on medication or other substances to induce sleep often interpret the reduced quality of their sleep as evidence that they should go back on the medication.

Recognition of the REM rebound phenomenon can be important with regard to physiologic function as well. Vital signs fluctuate during REM sleep, possibly putting added stress on weakened cardiovascular and respiratory systems. There is reduced stimulus to breathe, and ventilatory movement is limited to the diaphragm (because of very low skeletal muscle tone). Thus, clients who are already compromised (as from drug overdose, sleep apnea, chronic obstructive lung disease, or major trauma) may become hypoxic during REM sleep in the first night or two after REM-suppressing drugs are withdrawn.

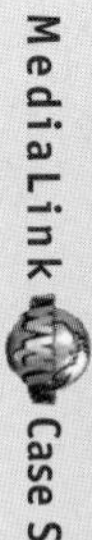

HEALTHY SLEEP BEHAVIORS

Sleep Pattern Disturbance is the appropriate North American Nursing Diagnosis Association (NANDA) diagnosis for any disruption of sleep time that causes discomfort or interferes with desired lifestyle. It should be differentiated from the nursing diagnoses of Fatigue and Activity Intolerance. *Fatigue* is described by clients as a lack of energy that persists regardless of the amount or quality of sleep. *Activity Intolerance* is a state of insufficient physical or psychological energy to complete daily activities without report of inadequate sleep.

Through sleep assessment, you may also create opportunities for teaching or reinforcing healthy sleep behaviors, such as

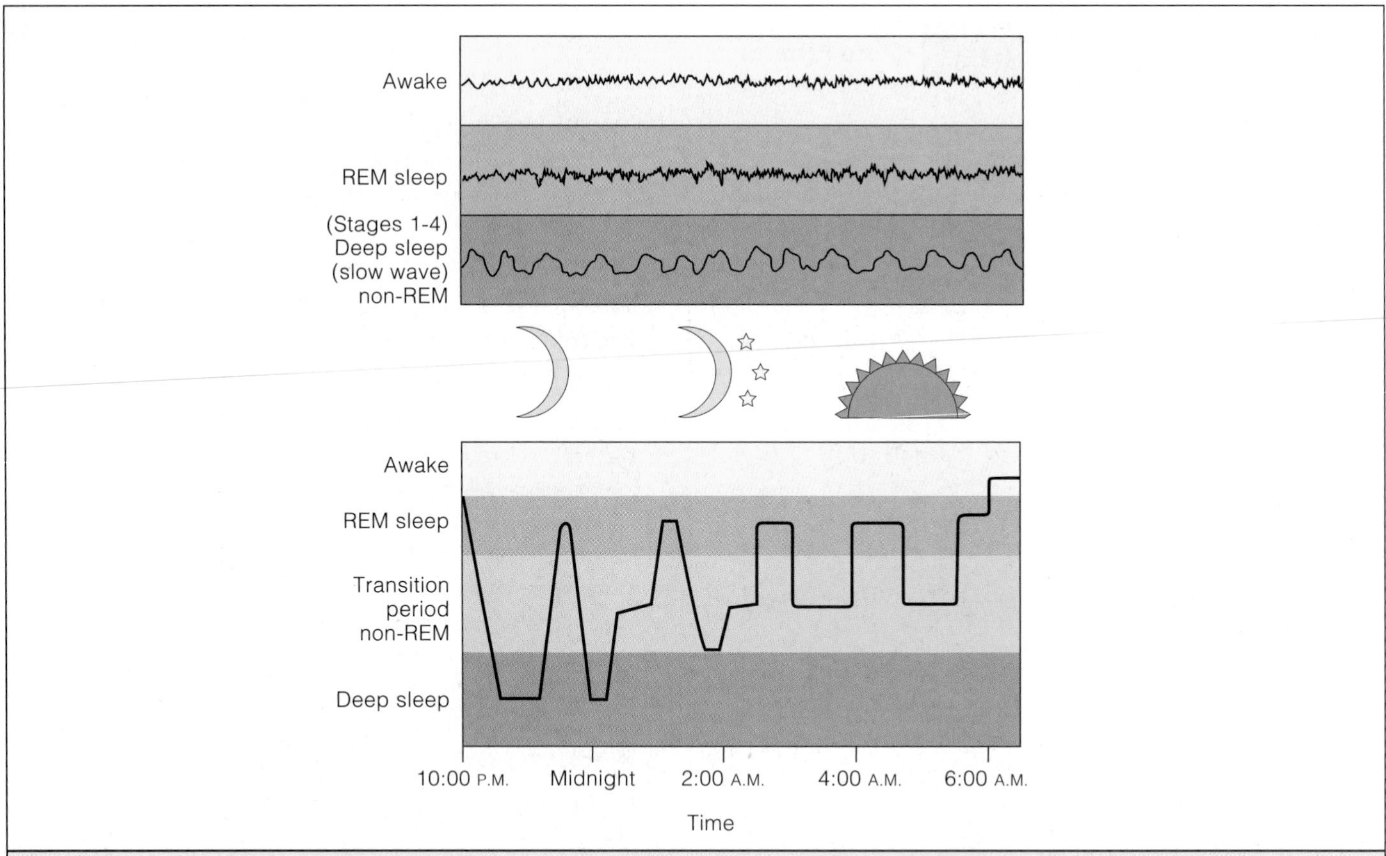

FIGURE 19–3 ■ *Cycles of sleep. During sleep, we move in cycles among several stages of non-REM sleep, ranging from light (stages 1 and 2) to deep sleep (stages 3 & 4). Approximately every 90 minutes we move from non-REM to REM sleep for a short time. REM sleep is also known as paradoxical sleep because the brain wave patterns resemble those of a wakeful or drowsy state.*

Source: Smock, T. K. (1999). *Physiological psychology: A neuroscience approach* (p. 308). Upper Saddle River, NJ: Prentice Hall.

sleep hygiene (see the Intervention box on page 457). There has been a tendency to be overprescriptive in terms of healthy behaviors. For example, a carefully designed English study provided evidence that people who usually have a snack before bedtime sleep better after a bedtime snack than without one; but people who usually do not have a snack before bedtime sleep better without a snack than with one (Adam, 1980). Likewise, guidelines intended for people with insomnia are often generalized to the rest of the population. For example, napping is not recommended for people with insomnia.

However, having a nap is common in some cultures, such as in countries where the siesta is part of the daily routine, in some farming communities, and among many retired and elderly people. Humans are biphasic, having a natural tendency for two sleep periods per 24-hour day, one major sleep period (commonly at night), and another shorter one (midafternoon) (Roehrs, Carskadon, Dement, & Roth, 2000).

Nursing SELF-AWARENESS

Are You Sleep Deprived?

- Do you usually fall asleep within 10 minutes after you turn off the lights?
- Do you struggle to stay awake in lectures?
- Do you "get by" all week and then try to catch up by sleeping in on the weekend?
- Do you do shift work?
- Do you often wake up with a headache?
- Do you have trouble getting going in the morning?
- Do you push yourself to keep going?

If you answered yes to more than two of these questions, you may not be getting as much sleep as you need.

Dyssomnias

There are two similar sets of diagnostic codes used to categorize sleep disorders. In psychiatric–mental health nursing, you may become more familiar with the DSM-IV-TR coding scheme for sleep disorders. However, you should also be aware of the more comprehensive International Classification of Sleep Disorders (ICSD) (ASDA, 1997). You may notice that the comparable ICSD coding is described in the DSM-IV-TR as the last point in each sleep disorder description. In this chapter, the commonal-

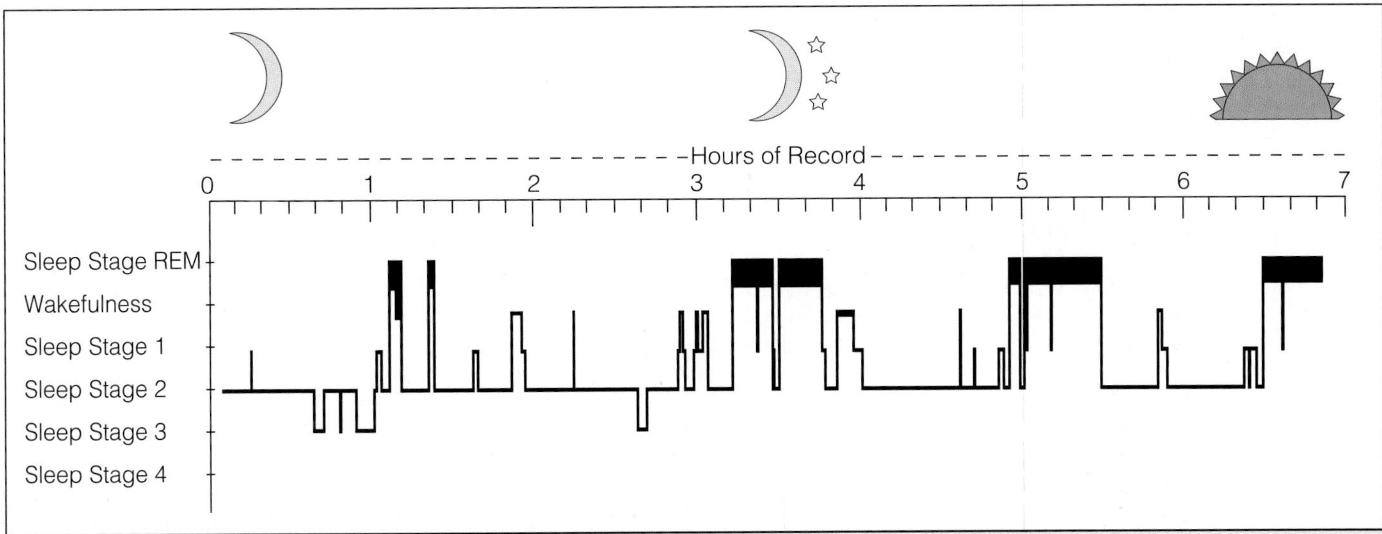

FIGURE 19–4 ■ *Sleep hypnogram summarizing pattern of sleep stages during an all-night polysomnograph recording on a young male. Note that sleep stage 2 (light non-REM sleep) was most common with several brief awakenings suggesting fragmented sleep. He entered some stage 3 (deep sleep) early in the night but did not have any stage 4 on the night of the recording. The solid bars represent periods of REM sleep. Note that the frequency and length of REM periods increased as the night progressed.*

ities rather than the differences will be emphasized. The DSM-IV-TR diagnostic criteria for sleep dyssomnias are in the box on page 458.

Sleep disorders fall into four main categories: the primary sleep disorders; sleep disorder related to another mental disorder, sleep disorder due to a general medical condition, and substance-induced sleep disorder. The primary sleep disorders are further divided into dyssomnias and parasomnias. **Dyssomnias** are sleep disorders characterized by difficulty initiating or maintaining sleep, or excessive sleepiness. **Parasomnias** are abnormal sleep disorders that intrude into sleep, including disorders of arousal and sleep stage transition (such as sleepwalking).

PRIMARY INSOMNIA

Insomnia, difficulty falling asleep or maintaining sleep, is a common complaint. Up to 15% of adults report severe or frequent insomnia, and another 15% report occasional episodes. It is important to try to distinguish between transitory insomnia,

INTERVENTION

Basic Principles of Sleep Hygiene

1. Maintain regularity in the sleep–wake schedule.
   - Avoid staying up too late or sleeping in too long on days off.
   - Enjoy an occasional nap, but stop taking naps if you notice that it is harder to get to sleep at night.
   - Be consistent in the time you get up, even if you have had less than usual sleep.
2. Go to bed only when you are reasonably sleepy and relaxed.
   - For a half-hour or so before you go to bed, engage in activities that are relaxing to you, even if you feel some pressure of things needing to be done.
   - If you are not drowsy when it is time to go to bed, engage in some activity that usually makes you drowsy, like reading something light.
   - Learn relaxation exercises (but practice them at other times of the day first).
   - Increase the physical exercise that you get during the day.
3. Maintain some sleep rituals as part of getting ready for bed.
   - Bring your day to a close with prayer or meditation if that is meaningful to you. Make this a time to focus on the good things that have happened, the accomplishments of the day, no matter how minor they may seem to be.
   - Get into a routine (brushing your teeth, winding the clock, opening the window, etc.).
4. Avoid the intake of stimulants or other substances that affect sleep patterns.
   - Instead of an alcoholic drink to induce sleep and relaxation, try a warm bath.
   - Experiment with decreasing the amount of coffee you drink, especially later in the day.
5. Enjoy what sleep you do get rather than thinking about what you think you need.
   - Move the clock so you cannot see what time it is every time you look in that direction.
   - Snuggle under the covers and think how nice it is that you can be resting in bed. If you are starting to feel restless or your mind is racing, get up and do some quiet activity such as reading until you feel drowsy again.

DSM-IV-TR Diagnostic Criteria for Sleep Dyssomnias

PRIMARY INSOMNIA	PRIMARY HYPERSOMNIA	BREATHING-RELATED SLEEP DISORDER
A. The predominant complaint is difficulty initiating or maintaining sleep, or nonrestorative sleep, for at least 1 month. **B.** The sleep disturbance (or associated daytime fatigue) causes clinically significant distress or impairment in social, occupational, or other important areas of functioning. **C.** The sleep disturbance does not occur exclusively during the course of Narcolepsy, Breathing-Related Sleep Disorder, Circadian Rhythm Sleep Disorder, or a Parasomnia. **D.** The disturbance does not occur exclusively during the course of another mental disorder (e.g., Major Depressive Disorder, Generalized Anxiety Disorder, a delirium). **E.** The disturbance is not due to the direct physiological effects of a substance (e.g., a drug of abuse, a medication) or a general medical condition.	**A.** The predominant complaint is excessive sleepiness for at least 1 month (or less if recurrent) as evidenced by either prolonged sleep episodes or daytime sleep episodes that occur almost daily. **B.** The excessive sleepiness causes clinically significant distress or impairment in social, occupational, or other important areas of functioning. **C.** The excessive sleepiness is not better accounted for by insomnia and does not occur exclusively during the course of another Sleep Disorder (e.g., Narcolepsy, Breathing-Related Sleep Disorder, Circadian Rhythm Sleep Disorder, or a Parasomnia) and cannot be accounted for by an inadequate amount of sleep. **D.** The disturbance does not occur exclusively during the course of another mental disorder. **E.** The disturbance is not due to the direct physiological effects of a substance (e.g., a drug of abuse, a medication) or a general medical condition.	**A.** Sleep disruption, leading to excessive sleepiness or insomnia, that is judged to be due to a sleep-related breathing condition (e.g., obstructive or central sleep apnea syndrome or central alveolar hypoventilation syndrome). **B.** The disturbance is not better accounted for by another mental disorder and is not due to the direct physiological effects of a substance (e.g., a drug of abuse, a medication) or another general medical condition (other than a breathing-related disorder).

commonly associated with change in environmental or situational stressors, and insomnia as a sleep disorder. Stress has a major impact on quality and duration of sleep (see ■ Figure 19–5) on page 460.

Primary insomnia is the term used in the DSM-IV-TR to describe difficulty initiating or maintaining sleep, or nonrestorative sleep that lasts for at least a month and does not occur exclusively in association with another sleep disorder or mental disorder. The most common type of insomnia is a pattern of delayed sleep onset and/or broken sleep that can be verified by polysomnography and that is perpetuated by an interaction between physically manifested tension (increased arousal) and learned associations that prevent sleep (negative conditioning). A careful history often identifies the onset of insomnia at the time of acute stress: The initial stressful event subsided, but the associations of frustration in trying to get to sleep persisted. A clinical example of a primary insomnia follows.

CLINICAL EXAMPLE

Peter Jacobi introduced himself to the other members of the insomnia group as someone who has always been a light sleeper. He has been having a lot more difficulty with sleeping though since he started working as a salesman about 3 months ago. He likes his job but finds it stressful, with lots of late nights entertaining customers. He denies excessive alcohol intake but admits he feels that he has to be sociable with the guys and is usually one of the last to leave the bar. On weekends he tries to catch up on sleep. He drinks 5 to 7 cups of coffee a day but never after dinner. He comments that for some reason he can usually sleep better when he is on out-of-town trips.

This case illustrates a fairly typical situation of what is sometimes termed *psychophysiological insomnia* (McCall & Reynolds, 2000). Peter's history as a light sleeper suggests that he may have been predisposed to insomnia. The anxiety and change of lifestyle associated with his new job may have precipitated this episode. Perpetuating factors would include an irregular schedule, frequent alcohol and caffeine intake, and a learned association of his bedroom with inability to sleep. See the Assessment box on page 461 for a structured exploration of insomnia's contributing factors.

PRIMARY HYPERSOMNIA

Hypersomnia refers to prolonged sleep and excessive sleepiness so severe as to interfere with function. Primary hypersomnia is

DSM-IV-TR Diagnostic Criteria for Sleep Dyssomnias

NARCOLEPSY

A. Irresistible attacks of refreshing sleep that occur daily over at least 3 months.

B. The presence of one or both of the following:
   1. cataplexy (i.e., brief episodes of sudden bilateral loss of muscle tone, most often in association with intense emotion).
   2. recurrent intrusions of elements of rapid eye movement (REM) sleep into the transition between sleep and wakefulness, as manifested by either hypnopompic or hypnagogic hallucinations or sleep paralysis at the beginning or end of sleep episodes.

C. The disturbance is not due to the direct physiological effects of a substance (e.g., a drug of abuse, a medication) or another general medical condition.

CIRCADIAN RHYTHM SLEEP DISORDER

A. A persistent or recurrent pattern of sleep disruption leading to excessive sleepiness or insomnia that is due to a mismatch between the sleep–wake schedule required by a person's environment and his or her circadian sleep–wake pattern.

B. The sleep disturbance causes clinically significant distress or impairment in social, occupational, or other important areas of functioning.

C. The disturbance does not occur exclusively during the course of another Sleep Disorder or other mental disorder.

D. The disturbance is not due to the direct physiological effects of a substance (e.g., a drug of abuse, a medication) or a general medical condition.

Specify type:

Delayed Sleep Phase Type: a persistent pattern of late sleep onset and late awakening times, with an inability to fall asleep and awaken at a desired earlier time.

Jet Lag Type: sleepiness and alertness that occur at inappropriate time of day relative to local time, occurring after repeated travel across more than one time zone.

Shift Work Type: insomnia during the major sleep period or excessive sleepiness during the major awake period associated with night shift work or frequently changing shift work.

Unspecified Type

Source: Reprinted with permission from the *Diagnostic and statistical manual of mental disorders*, 4th ed., Text Revision (pp. 604, 609, 622, 615, 629).

that which is not better explained by another sleep disorder (e.g., breathing-related sleep disorder or narcoplepsy, which also cause hypersomnia) or a mental disorder (e.g., depression). Such idiopathic hypersomnia is relatively uncommon, but the symptoms of hypersomnia are frequently seen in clients experiencing mental health challenges, and therefore the nursing process section will focus on the symptom more specifically.

BREATHING-RELATED SLEEP DISORDER

The most common form of breathing-related sleep disorder is **sleep apnea**. Apnea is the absence of breathing. The most common form of sleep apnea is the obstructive type, in which the upper airway partially or totally collapses in spite of repeated respiratory effort. Opening of the airway requires a partial arousal. With polysomnography, up to 200 to 300 arousals per night may be observed, even though the client may say he or she slept soundly. The outcome of the numerous arousals preceded by drops in oxygen saturation is hypersomnia, or excessive sleepiness. Clients with obstructive sleep apnea may report difficulty staying awake, even in social situations, at work, or driving in spite of a normal or longer nighttime sleep period, in addition to dozing off regularly when watching television.

People with obstructive sleep apnea are often obese middle-aged males with thick necks and a history of severe snoring. The loudness of the snoring, irregularity of nocturnal breathing, irritability, and constant sleepiness of the affected partner add strain to the interpersonal relationship. Bed partners often report that they, too, have a sleep pattern disturbance related to environmental noise and/or vigilance about breathing. Women may also develop obstructive sleep apnea, with incidence increasing after menopause. Elderly clients with obstructive sleep apnea may present with insomnia rather than hypersomnia. The explanation may be that they have more difficulty getting back to sleep after their frequent arousals. Clients suspected of sleep apnea should be seen by a sleep specialist. Overnight sleep monitoring is important for diagnosis and treatment. These clients often experience significant REM rebound when first treated.

The principle underlying the treatment of obstructive sleep apnea is reduction or removal of the obstruction. Conservative measures include weight loss, avoidance of alcohol and other central nervous system (CNS) depressants (which reduce muscle tone in the upper airway), and a change in habitual sleep positions (such as wearing something like a backpack to bed to prevent sleeping supine). Continuous positive airway pressure (CPAP) by nasal mask is the most common form of treatment. Surgical treatment includes removal of a portion of the soft palate, uvula,

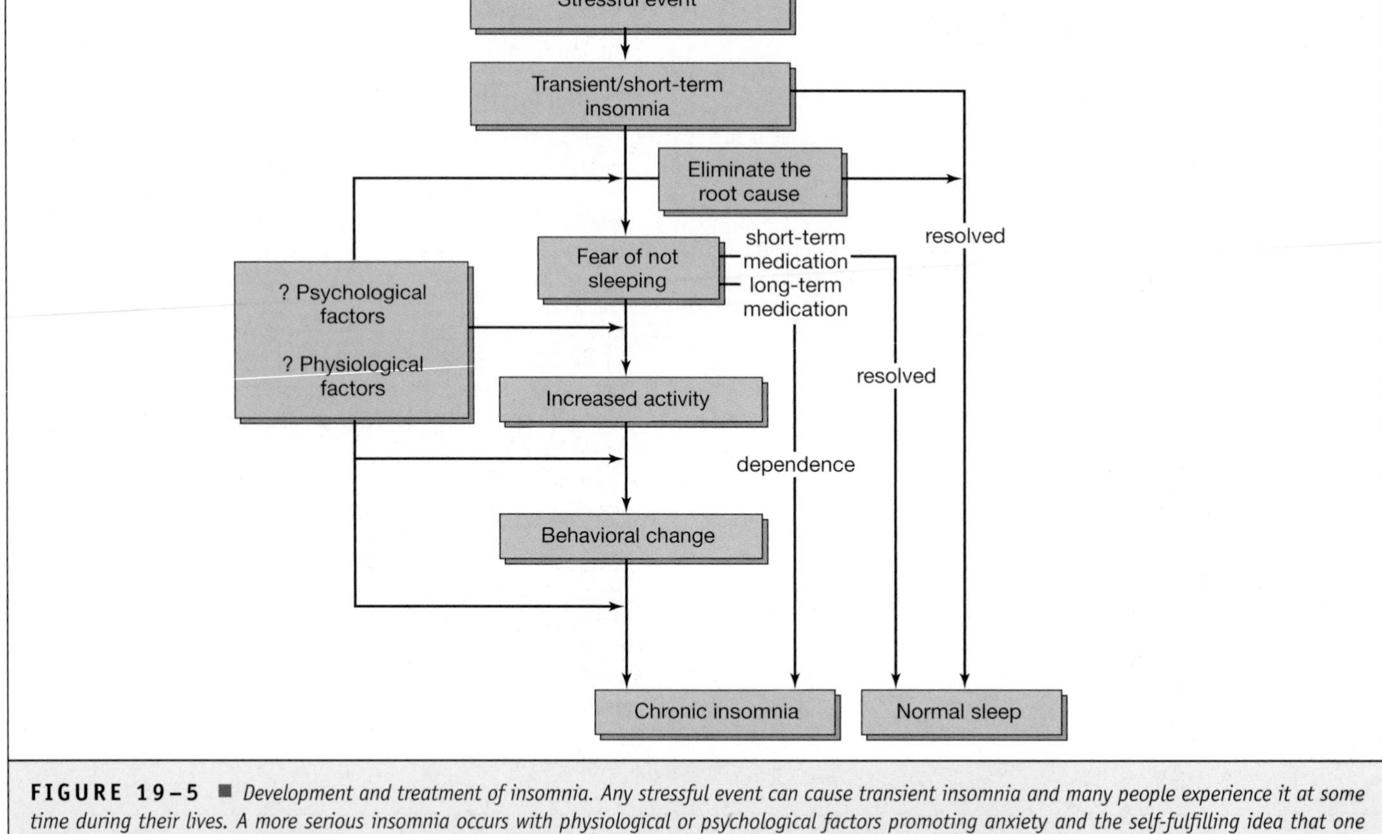

FIGURE 19–5 ■ *Development and treatment of insomnia. Any stressful event can cause transient insomnia and many people experience it at some time during their lives. A more serious insomnia occurs with physiological or psychological factors promoting anxiety and the self-fulfilling idea that one will not be able to sleep, leading to chronic insomnia. Treatments can include medications, but because insomnia is often a symptom of a larger problem, eliminating the root cause (the stressor) is generally the most successful solution.*

Source: Smock, T. K. (1999). Physiological psychology: A neuroscience approach (p. 321). Upper Saddle River, NJ: Prentice Hall.

and residual tonsillar tissue. Dental splints are the newest form of treatment for reducing apnea and the associated snoring.

In central sleep apnea, the airway remains open but the stimulus to breathe is missing or abnormal. This type of breathing-related sleep disorder is less common, except after some neurologic insults (such as brain stem lesions). Clients may present with hypersomnia or insomnia or be asymptomatic. It is not unusual to observe some central apneas mixed with obstructive episodes. Rather than actual apneas, there may be prolonged hypoventilation resulting in low oxygen saturation, a condition called central alveolar hypoventilation syndrome. The National Sleep Foundation site at www.sleepfoundation.org/default.html provides interesting information about these issues and has ample links to other sleep-related sites.

MediaLink National Sleep Foundation

As a psychiatric–mental health nurse, you must be vigilant for sleep apnea for several reasons. Clients may be unaware of a breathing-related sleep disorder and yet be concerned about hypersomnia, disrupted interpersonal relationships, or poor work performance. Depression secondary to obstructive sleep apnea is not uncommon. Other symptoms of mood disturbances, irritability, memory loss, and impaired concentration are similar to the presenting symptoms of various mental disorders. Furthermore, sleep apnea increases with aging, particularly with dementia (Phillips & Anconi-Israel, 2001). Thus, it is important to assess nocturnal breathing patterns in clients with dementia. Do not assume that their sleep pattern disturbance is the phenomenon called sundowning—increased restlessness and agitation during the evening and night hours.

NARCOLEPSY

Narcolepsy is brief episodes of deep sleep. But unlike sleep apnea, the sleep is followed by a sense of refreshment. The urge to sleep can be almost irresistible, and there is association with other symptoms such as cataplexy, sleep paralysis, and hypnagogic hallucinations. **Cataplexy,** which refers to the sudden collapse of muscle tone usually associated with intense emotion, occurs in about 70% of individuals with narcolepsy (APA, 2000). **Sleep paralysis,** a sense of being totally unable to move for a brief period after wakening or at sleep onset, occurs in 30% to 50% of those with narcolepsy. It may also occur occasionally in people who do not have narcolepsy or any other sleep disorder. **Hypnagogic hallucinations** are vivid dreamlike images that appear just before sleep onset and are reported by 20% to 40% of individuals with narcolepsy. All these symptoms are thought to be related to the recurrent intrusion of REM-like mechanisms into waking or the waking–sleep transition.

ASSESSMENT

Client with Sleep Pattern Disturbance (Insomnia)

Nature of the Insomnia

What do you have the most difficulty with?

- Getting to sleep?
- Waking up and then taking a long time to get back to sleep? or
- Waking up earlier than you want to and not being able to get back to sleep?

Possible Contributing Factors

- Does it help if you try to sleep somewhere else in your home?
- Is your sleep better or worse when you are away from home?
- Do you usually sleep with someone? If yes, does it make a difference if they are not with you? (Be alert here for possible disturbance by a partner, or poorer sleep when a habitual partner is not present. Note also that sharing the bed with infants and children varies across and within different cultures.)
- How many cups of coffee a day do you have? (Follow up regarding caffeinated or decaffeinated, timing, other caffeine-containing substances such as tea, chocolate, colas.)
- Do you smoke? How many packs a day?
- What medications and drugs are you using? (Note that many of the psychotropic medications alter sleep patterns, as do most substances of abuse.)
- What do you tend to think about while you are trying to get to sleep?
- What do you associate with sleep?
- What do you think is the single greatest factor affecting your ability to sleep?

As a psychiatric–mental nurse, be aware of narcolepsy because about 40% of people with this disorder also have a concurrent or prior-onset mental disorder. With onset typically occurring in adolescence, often exacerbated by an acute psychosocial stressor, these clients have experienced a life-changing and poorly accepted chronic illness during an important developmental stage. The frequency of daytime sleeping and cataplexy attacks is embarrassing and disruptive in relation to occupational and social activities (Douglas, 1998). Various theories have been offered about the association between narcolepsy and mental disorders, but no clear cause-and-effect explanation is anticipated. Stimulants such as amphetamines are the most common treatment for the hypersomnia. Tricyclic antidepressants (TCAs) are useful in controlling the associated symptoms of cataplexy, sleep paralysis, and hypnagogic hallucinations.

Nursing research has revealed numerous coping strategies used by persons with narcolepsy (Cohen, Nehring & Cloninger, 1996). These strategies include taking scheduled naps every day; avoiding stress, which may precipitate cataplexy; and maintaining a structured lifestyle.

Diagnostic Sleep Tests

Polysomnography in the form of a multiple sleep latency test (MSLT), preceded by an all-night sleep study, will confirm the diagnosis. The MSLT consists of five or six scheduled daytime naps at 2-hour intervals, during which the subject is monitored for 20 minutes in a quiet, darkened room with instructions to try to go to sleep. At the end of 20 minutes, subjects are wakened and not allowed to sleep until the next scheduled nap. One or more recordings of sleep latency less than 10 minutes, REM sleep latency (time from sleep onset to first REM period) less than 20 minutes, MSLT evidence of two or more sleep-onset REM periods, or a mean sleep latency of less than 5 minutes plus the associated symptoms are diagnostic of narcolepsy, according to ICSD diagnostic criteria (ASDA, 1997). For the DSM-IV-TR diagnostic criteria, see the box on page 459.

CIRCADIAN RHYTHM SLEEP DISORDERS

The circadian rhythm sleep disorders are those disorders in which the 24-hour sleep–wake schedule is disturbed through internal cues (e.g., phase delay is more common in teenagers and young adults; phase advance is more common in young children and older adults) or external cues (e.g., shift work, travel across time zones). The day–night cycle (as seen in ■ Figure 19–6 on page 462) determines much of our mammalian activity level. For the DSM-IV-TR diagnostic criteria for circadian rhythm sleep disorders, see the box on page 459.

Jet Lag Type

As a result of jet travel, a client's manic phase may be further exacerbated by jet lag and associated sleep deprivation.

CLINICAL EXAMPLE

Mr. Bernstein traveled from the United States to the Middle East on business. Upon his return to the United States, he made a series of irrational business decisions that he blamed on the stress of jet lag. However, it was subsequently determined that Mr. Bernstein had bipolar disorder.

Research, based on a chart review, suggests that first episodes of mania may be rapidly reversed in clients who are able to sleep (with haloperidol) during the first night of hospitalization (Nowlin-Finch, Altshuler, Szuba, & Mintz, 1994). The response was most evident in clients who also reported a known stressor, which may have precipitated the first manic episode. The stressor may have also contributed to sleep deprivation, like clients experiencing major sleep disruption through jet travel across seven time zones.

Shift Work Type

As you might expect, shift work is a major source of circadian rhythm disruption. If you choose hospital nursing, you may be concerned about this disorder for yourself as well as for clients.

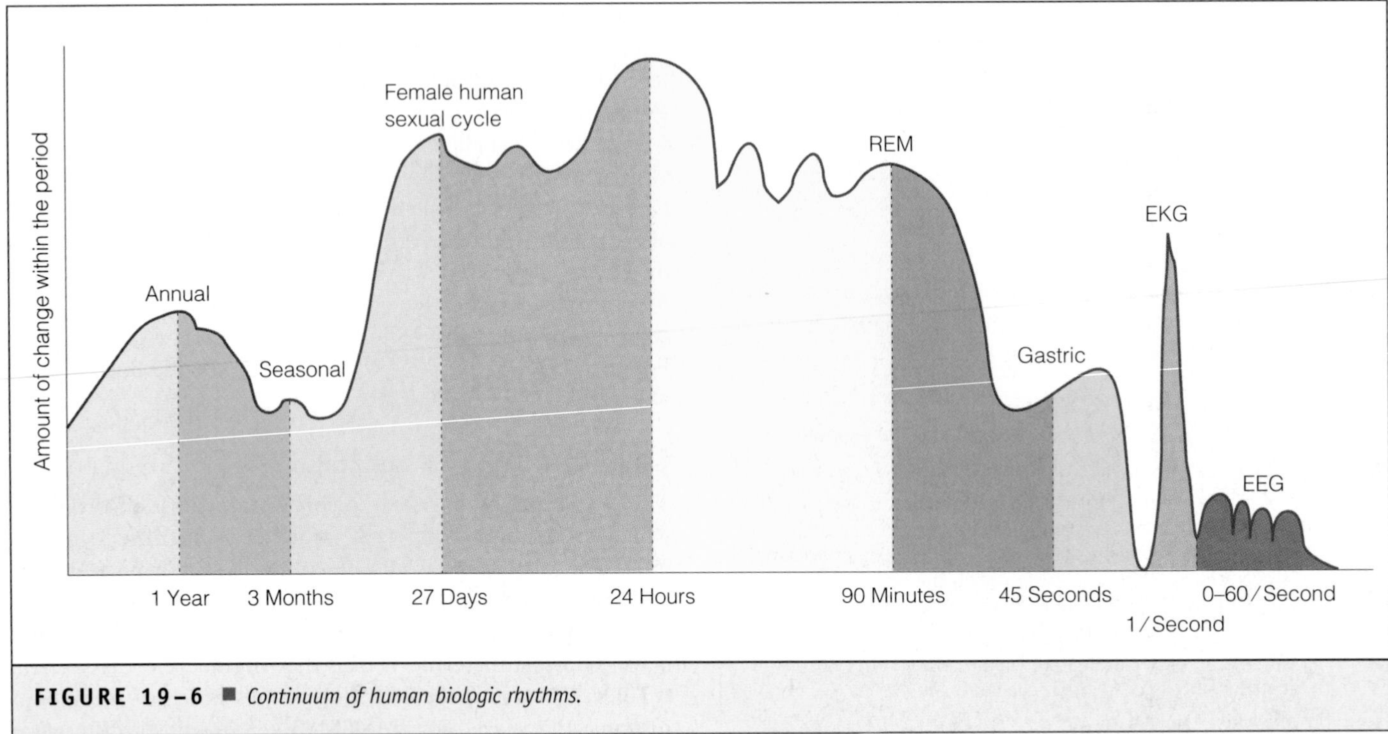

FIGURE 19–6 ■ *Continuum of human biologic rhythms.*

CLINICAL EXAMPLE

Jane was working rotating shifts in an intensive care unit. She noted that she had worsening insomnia and feared that her judgment would become affected by increasing sleep deprivation.

Chronobiology (the scientific study of the impact of time on the body) is rapidly expanding and has implications for coping with shift work. Inquiries about shift work should be a routine part of sleep assessment because the impact on sleep patterns and sleep disturbance often extends beyond the period of shift work.

CLINICAL EXAMPLE

Years after he had retired from his bakery business, Yürgen continued to awaken very early in the morning. This pattern further complicated a sleep disorder related to his medical condition of Parkinson's disease.

Delayed Sleep Phase Type

An abnormality in sleep phase can contribute to what may appear to be socially inappropriate or uncooperative behavior. Clients with this circadian rhythm disorder seem programmed to stay up late and sleep in late. This syndrome should not be confused with normal tendencies to be either a "night owl" or "morning lark." Delayed sleep phase syndrome is a persistent problem that is resistant to standard attempts to get up earlier. It is not unusual to encounter people with this disorder who have adapted by seeking types of employment and entertainment that are conducive to late nights and late rising. The disorder can also contribute to social isolation.

Advanced Sleep Phase Type

Advanced sleep phase syndrome is the reverse of delayed sleep phase syndrome in that early evening sleepiness regularly accompanies early wakening. A mildly advanced sleep phase is common among older adults and should not be confused with the early wakening associated with depression. With depression, other symptoms and sleep changes are evident.

The main consequences of delayed or advanced sleep phase syndrome are the disruption of family, work, and/or social activities. If the circadian pattern is problematic, phase shifting can be modified through chronotherapy or light therapy. Chronotherapy consists of systematically delaying bedtime, usually in 3-hour increments, over a period of several weeks until the client reaches the desired bedtime hour, after which the new schedule must be carefully maintained. Light therapy is timed to coincide with the time of day that sleepiness should be reduced. For people with advanced sleep phase syndrome, light therapy may be administered in the early evening.

PERIODIC LIMB MOVEMENT DISORDER

Periodic limb movement disorder (PLMD) usually involves the legs, which repeatedly move in a jerking, stereotypic manner during sleep, often causing partial arousals. This disorder can contribute to excessive sleepiness, unrefreshing sleep, and multiple awakenings. Prevalence tends to increase with age; it occurs in up to 34% of individuals over age 60 (ASDA, 1997).

Periodic limb movement disorder should be distinguished from restless legs syndrome (RLS), which may occur prior to sleep and is characterized by disagreeable sensations in the legs that are relieved only by movement. Persons with RLS usually have PLMD as well, but PLMD is not necessarily associated with RLS.

As a psychiatric–mental health nurse, it is important to know that TCAs and monamine oxidase inhibitors (MAOIs) can trigger or worsen periodic limb movement disorder (ASDA, 1997). Withdrawal of anticonvulsants, benzodiazepines, and other hypnotic drugs can also exacerbate the condition of periodic limb movement disorder.

NOCTURNAL EATING (DRINKING) SYNDROME

Nocturnal eating or drinking syndrome is characterized by repeated nighttime awakenings and the inability to get back to sleep without eating or drinking. Such a pattern is common among young children who have always been breast-fed or bottle-fed as a means of going to sleep. It is thought to be a learned behavior that can also occur in adults, and it can become obsessional (ASDA, 1997).

Parasomnias

The parasomnias include **somnambulism** (sleepwalking), sleep talking, nightmares, sleep terrors, **sleep bruxism** (teeth-grinding), and **sleep enuresis** (bed-wetting). They are characterized by CNS activation, including autonomic nervous system changes and skeletal muscle activity (ASDA,1997). The parasomnias will be discussed in relation to the sleep stages during which they typically occur.

Some parasomnias that emerge during slow-wave (non-REM) sleep include:

1. Sleepwalking.
2. Night terrors.

Certain medications used for psychiatric disorders, such as lithium (Lithane), desipramine (Norpramin), and thioridazine (Mellaril), may exacerbate or induce sleepwalking, as can fever or sleep deprivation (ASDA, 1997). Sleep terrors (also known as night terrors) are sudden arousals from slow-wave sleep, associated with intense autonomic and behavioral reactions characterized by fear. Unlike nightmares, which occur in REM sleep, there is little or no memory of the frightening episode. Both of these parasomnias are more common in children prior to puberty, but they may also occur in adults, particularly at times of intense stress (see the box on page 464 for diagnostic criteria for these disorders).

Parasomnias associated with REM sleep include:

1. Nightmares.
2. Sleep paralysis.
3. REM sleep behavior disorder.

REM sleep behavior disorder is a rare but potentially serious disorder in which motor activity occurs during REM sleep and may be associated with the apparent acting-out of dream sequences. Injuries to the individual or bed partner have been reported. It is thought to be more frequent during REM rebound following alcohol or sedative–hypnotic withdrawal. It has also been reported in association with the use of TCAs (ASDA, 1997).

Sleep bruxism, or teeth-grinding, is strongly associated with stress and anxiety. Sleep enuresis (bed-wetting) can occur during any sleep stage. A normal behavior in infancy, sleep enuresis may persist for some children into the early teens. The DSM-IV-TR diagnostic criteria for sleep parasomnias are in the box on page 464.

Sleep Disorder Related to Another Mental Disorder

The sleep disorders discussed prior to this point are those that any individual, with or without a mental disorder, may have. Sleep disorders are so common that you can expect that some of your psychiatric–mental health clients will have a sleep disorder. A psychiatric illness and/or its treatment may have an interactive effect on a preexisting or concurrent sleep pattern disturbance. Sleep disturbances that are symptomatic of underlying psychiatric illness are troublesome to clients. These symptoms are an important part of the experience of mental illness for clients, even though they may not meet the DSM-IV-TR criteria of being a predominant complaint (see the box on page 458 concerning insomnia and hypersomnia).

Sleep pattern disturbance may be related to psychoses, mood disorders, anxiety disorders, panic disorder, or alcohol use or abuse. Sleep disturbances associated with dementia and other cerebral degenerative disorders will also be considered.

Sleep disturbances that are secondary to psychiatric disorders generally fall into one of the four symptom categories mentioned above. While recognizing that a cyclical relationship is usually involved, it is helpful to try to differentiate primary sleep disorders from those that are secondary to a psychiatric disorder. Such differentiation can be particularly important for clients with depression, anxiety, and/or dementia. Sleep deprivation can lead to restlessness, reduced concentration, and, if prolonged, hallucinations and delusions (Kaplan, Sadock, & Grebb, 2002). Likewise, chronic sleep deprivation may exacerbate dementia behaviors.

CLINICAL EXAMPLE

Ellen, an elderly client, was recently hospitalized for acute management of a chronic medical condition. She was known to have early dementia of the Alzheimer's type but had been managing alone in her apartment up to this point. Over a period of several days, she became increasingly agitated, demanding cigarettes from nursing staff, other clients, and visitors. Attempts at distraction or providing unsolicited attention were unsuccessful. A nursing student began questioning how much sleep this woman had been getting. At that point the nurse's only cues were the lack of Ellen's

DSM-IV-TR Diagnostic Criteria for Sleep Parasomnia

SLEEPWALKING DISORDER

A. Repeated episodes of rising from bed during sleep and walking about, usually occurring during the first third of the major sleep episode.

B. While sleepwalking, the person has a blank, staring face, is relatively unresponsive to the efforts of others to communicate with him or her, and can be awakened only with great difficulty.

C. On awakening (either from the sleepwalking episode or the next morning), the person has amnesia for the episode.

D. Within several minutes after awakening from the sleepwalking episode, there is no impairment in mental activity or behavior (although there may initially be a short period of confusion or disorientation).

E. The sleepwalking causes clinically significant distress or impairment in social, occupational, or other important areas of functioning.

F. The disturbance is not due to the direct physiological effects of a substance (e.g., a drug of abuse, a medication) or a general medical condition.

SLEEP TERROR DISORDER

A. Recurrent episodes of abrupt wakening from sleep, usually occurring during the first third of the major sleep episode and beginning with a panicky scream.

B. Intense fear and signs of autonomic arousal, such as tachycardia, rapid breathing, and sweating, during each episode.

C. Relative unresponsiveness to efforts of others to comfort the person during the episode.

D. No detailed dream is recalled and there is amnesia for the episode.

E. The episodes cause clinically significant distress or impairment in social, occupational, or other important functioning.

F. The disturbance is not due to the direct physiological effects of a substance (e.g., a drug of abuse, a medication) or a general medical condition.

NIGHTMARE DISORDER

A. Repeated awakenings from the major sleep period or naps with detailed recall of extended and extremely frightening dreams, usually involving threats to survival, security, or self-esteem. The awakenings generally occur during the second half of the sleep period.

B. On awakening from the frightening dreams, the person rapidly becomes oriented and alert (in contrast to the confusion and disorientation seen in Sleep Terror Disorder and some forms of epilepsy).

C. The dream experience, or the sleep disturbance resulting from the awakening, causes clinically significant distress or impairment in social, occupational, or other important areas of functioning.

D. The nightmares do not occur exclusively during the course of another mental disorder (e.g., Delirium, Posttraumatic Stress Disorder) and are not due to the direct physiological effects of a substance (e.g., a drug of abuse, a medication) or a general medical condition.

Source: Reprinted with permission from the *Diagnostic and statistical manual of mental disorders,* 4th ed., Text Revision (pp. 644, 639, 634). Copyright 2000 American Psychiatric Association.

success with other interventions and her knowledge that sundowning is common in clients with dementia. The brief chart notes made by the night staff offered little information. From a neighbor who came to visit, she found out that prior to the hospitalization, Ellen had been phoning her a couple of times during the night in an agitated state. The night staff agreed to observe and record the amount of time the client spent sleeping. Day staff did the same. With this additional data it was soon apparent that Ellen was averaging no more than 4 hours of sleep per 24-hour period. Meanwhile, her agitated behavior was increasing.

After a client conference in which the nursing student offered her hypothesis of Sleep Pattern Disturbance, the physician agreed to try a mild short-acting hypnotic for the next three nights. Nursing staff continued to monitor Ellen's sleep patterns and behavior. By the end of the three nights, during which she did appear to sleep for longer periods, the agitated behavior and demands for cigarettes subsided considerably.

The use of hypnotics was not a long-term solution for the client in the above example, but it broke the escalating cycle of increasing agitation and decreasing sleep. Recognition of the role of sleep deprivation in contributing to a daytime behavior problem can facilitate effective short-term intervention and create a context for more comprehensive assessment of possible contributing factors, such as fear, relocation stress, powerlessness, or sensory and/or perceptual alterations.

Differentiation of sleep disorder secondary to psychiatric disorder from primary sleep disorder is a complex process that requires collaboration among clients, families, and health professionals. The sequence of onset may provide a clue. Many persons with unipolar depressive disorder initially present to family physicians or sleep clinics with insomnia. As in the example above, it may take a trial of an intervention known to be effective for one or the other type of disorder to help clarify the primary diagnosis.

As a psychiatric–mental health nurse, you will often need to be vigilant for the potential effects of a mismatched primary diagnosis with intervention. A depressed client misdiagnosed as having a primary sleep disorder of insomnia may be at risk of suicide if given a usual supply of hypnotic medication; likewise, obstructive sleep apnea with modest ingestion of alcohol can be mislabeled as alcohol abuse. As in any area of nursing practice, all components of the nursing process must be carefully and critically used. The DSM-IV-TR diagnostic criteria for sleep disorders due to another mental disorder are in the box on page 465.

DSM-IV-TR

Diagnostic Criteria for Sleep Disorders Related to Another Mental Disorder

INSOMNIA RELATED TO ANOTHER MENTAL DISORDER

A. The predominant complaint is difficulty initiating or maintaining sleep or nonrestorative sleep, for at least 1 month that is associated with daytime fatigue or impaired daytime functioning.
B. The sleep disturbance (or daytime sequelae) causes clinically significant distress or impairment in social, occupational, or other important areas of functioning.
C. The insomnia is judged to be related to another Axis I or Axis II disorder (e.g., Major Depressive Disorder, Generalized Anxiety Disorder, Adjustment Disorder with Anxiety), but is sufficiently severe to warrant independent clinical attention.
D. The disturbance is not better accounted for by another Sleep Disorder (e.g., Narcolepsy, Breathing-Related Sleep Disorder, a Parasomnia).
E. The disturbance is not due to the direct physiological effects of a substance (e.g., a drug of abuse, a medication) or a general medical condition.

HYPERSOMNIA RELATED TO ANOTHER MENTAL DISORDER

A. The predominant complaint is excessive sleepiness for at least 1 month as evidenced by either prolonged sleep episodes or daytime sleep episodes that occur almost daily.
B. The excessive sleepiness causes clinically significant distress or impairment in social, occupational, or other important areas of functioning.
C. The hypersomnia is judged to be related to another Axis I or Axis II disorder (e.g., Major Depressive Disorder, Dysthmic Disorder), but is sufficiently severe to warrant independent clinical attention.
D. The disturbance is not better accounted for by another Sleep Disorder (e.g., Narcolepsy, Breathing-Related Sleep Disorder, a Parasomnia) or by an inadequate amount of sleep.
E. The disturbance is not due to the direct physiological effects of a substance (e.g., a drug of abuse, a medication) or a general medical condition.

Source: Reprinted with permission from the *Diagnostic and statistical manual of mental disorders,* 4th ed., Text Revision (p. 650). Copyright 2000 American Psychiatric Association.

PSYCHOSES

Significant sleep disruption often occurs in conjunction with an exacerbation of schizophrenia (ASDA, 1997; Kaplan, Sadock, & Grebb, 2002). Great difficulty in getting to sleep may accompany extreme anxiety and concern about delusional and hallucinatory phenomena. The overall circadian cycle may also be disrupted. Clients with schizophrenia have reduced REM sleep and do not experience REM rebound. Deficit of slow-wave sleep, particularly stage 4, has been found in acute, chronic, and remitted schizophrenia (Benson & Zarcone, 2000). A link with serotonin, a neurotransmitter associated with non-REM sleep, has been hypothesized. Depressed, alcoholic, and elderly clients also have reduced stage 4 sleep.

MOOD DISORDERS

As discussed previously, insomnia of the maintenance or early wakening type commonly occurs in major depressive episodes. The sleep pattern disturbance may actually precede other symptoms of depression and likewise may respond to antidepressant medication more rapidly than the depression (ASDA, 1997). Partial sleep deprivation, particularly of REM sleep, has been associated with modest improvement in depression but the mechanism for this process is not well understood (Kaplan, Sadock, & Grebb, 2002). Most antidepressants suppress REM sleep and lengthen latency to the first REM period.

Seasonal affective disorder (SAD) is related to fluctuations in melatonin levels by variation in the hours of sunlight. The positive response of SAD to light therapy lends strength to the argument that its development is related to weakened circadian rhythmicity.

In the manic phase of bipolar disorder, sleep time is significantly reduced but clients do not complain of insomnia. They have reduced slow-wave sleep and reduced REM latency. During the depressive phase, these clients may experience excessive sleepiness, similar to clients with SAD (ASDA, 1997).

ANXIETY DISORDERS

Sleep onset or maintenance insomnia is commonly associated with heightened anxiety. The proportion of stages 1 and 2 non-REM sleep tends to increase as part of the overall state of hyperarousal.

PANIC DISORDER

Panic episodes may be associated with sudden awakenings, after which clients may find it very difficult to return to sleep. Sleep-associated panic episodes are most likely to occur during non-REM sleep, particularly stage 2. Current research and information about these problems can be found at the National Center on Sleep Disorders Research at www.nhlbi.nih.gov/about/ncsdr/.

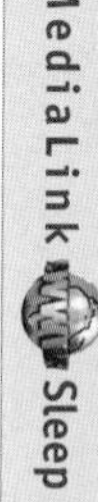

Sleep Disorder Due to a General Medical Condition

Many general medical conditions disturb sleep to some degree because of pain, discomfort, reduced mobility, itchiness, or gastrointestinal symptoms. However, in some cases the disturbance is so severe as to warrant identification as a sleep disorder. The symptoms may be those of insomnia, hypersomnia, parasomnia, or some combination thereof.

DEMENTIA AND OTHER CEREBRAL DEGENERATIVE CONDITIONS

The tendency for individuals with dementia to become more agitated, more verbal, and more restless as nighttime falls is known as sundowning. Unfortunately, definitions of this phenomenon have been vague, limiting the usefulness of much of the related research (Bliwise, 2000). However, it has been suggested that sundowning may be the most common trigger to the institutionalization of clients with dementia because of the additional demands on caregivers. In an exploratory nursing study, activity patterns of clients with dementia were found to increase between 4:00 and 6:00 PM, whereas cognitively healthy clients had decreased activity at that time, corresponding to general population norms. The most common causal assumption has been a temporal relationship to conditions of decreased light and other environmental stimulation. Apparent deterioration of circadian patterns may be associated with deterioration of the suprachiasmatic nucleus in the brain (Bliwise, 2000). Frequent arousals from sleep apnea, incontinence, or caregiver checks have also been implicated.

This population is particularly difficult to study because with increasing dementia, there is less and less tolerance of polysomnography. Other cerebral degenerative diseases that involve neurotransmitter imbalance such as Parkinson's disease and Huntington's chorea are also characterized by increasingly fragmented sleep. The DSM-IV-TR diagnostic criteria for sleep disorders due to a general medical condition are in the box on page 467.

Substance-Induced Sleep Disorder

Substances of abuse or by prescription (e.g., alcohol, cocaine, opioids, hypnotics, anxiolytics) may cause a severe sleep disorder during intoxication or withdrawal. Even after prolonged abstinence, the abuse of some substances such as alcohol and hallucinogens may affect sleep architecture.

Substance-induced sleep disorder is characterized by sustained use of stimulants for staying awake, or of alcohol to induce sleep. You will probably work with many clients who use stimulants or alcohol periodically for their effect on sleep. For example, the use of stimulants is not uncommon among long-distance truck drivers. Alcohol is and has been one of the most frequently used hypnotics. While a drink at bedtime reduces sleep latency, it usually induces wakening later in the night.

A wide range of biochemical substances can contribute to this sleep disorder by their presence in sufficient quantities (such as caffeine and prescription drugs), their unaccustomed absence (alcohol), or their abuse (street drugs). Clients with psychiatric disorders, especially schizophrenia or mania, or clients with a history of traumatic brain injury are particularly vulnerable to sleep disorders due to chemical imbalances.

CLINICAL EXAMPLE

Judith and Karina participate in a maintenance program for people with schizophrenia. They often meet for a drink together at the conclusion of a meeting. While they consume similar amounts of alcohol, Karina, who also has a history of minor brain injury, experiences much more disordered sleep.

The vulnerability may be twofold: direct effects of biochemical imbalance plus the use of alcohol or drugs as an attempted means to cope with a psychiatric disorder.

With acute alcohol intoxication, there is increased sleepiness for 3 to 4 hours. Sleep may be deep (increased stages 3 and 4) with REM suppression. However, after that, sleep tends to be fragmented, restless, and often accompanied by bizarre dreaming. During alcohol withdrawal, sleep tends to be very fragmented, with REM rebound. The vivid dreaming may be associated with alcohol withdrawal delirium (APA, 2000).

Sleep pattern disturbances persist even after a year or more of abstention. The pattern of prolonged sleep latency, increased number of arousals, higher proportion of stage 1 sleep at the expense of slow-wave sleep, and more interrupted REM sleep is thought to be due to a chronically high arousal (Monti et al., 1993).

Other abused drugs follow a similar pattern of exacerbation of their usual effect (sedation or stimulation) after excessive intake, along with rebound effects upon withdrawal (see Chapter 13). The DSM-IV-TR diagnostic criteria for substance induced sleep disorders are in the box on page 467.

Biopsychosocial Theories

Sleep is commonly believed to be restorative, but the evidence is actually quite conflicting. Arguments for sleep as a time of body restitution are based on the common observation that rest seems to promote healing; that growth hormone, which is anabolic, has its peak release during slow-wave sleep, whereas catabolic hormones such as the corticosteroids are at their lowest point of release during the night; and that conditions seem optimum for protein synthesis. However, protein synthesis is stimulated by amino acid absorption, little of which occurs during the nighttime fast; there is no sleep-related change in insulin release, a requirement for cell growth; and the release of growth hormone changes immediately with a change in sleep time, whereas change in corticosteroid release requires up to 2 weeks after a change in the sleep period.

Alternative theories about the function of sleep range from protective (there are fewer admissions to hospital emergency departments during the night) to adaptive (you cannot do much without light), from energy conservation, to sleep being somewhat optional. Horne (1988), the chief proponent of the latter view, suggests that there is a core amount of required sleep but that the excess sleep time is not really required. There is more agreement on the role REM sleep plays in memory storage, consolidation of experience, and learning.

The important point is although the functions of sleep are still poorly understood, client beliefs about the functions of sleep are important in psychiatric–mental health nursing prac-

DSM-IV-TR Diagnostic Criteria for Other Sleep Disorders

DIAGNOSTIC CRITERIA FOR SLEEP DISORDER DUE TO A GENERAL MEDICAL CONDITION

A. A prominent disturbance in sleep that is sufficiently severe to warrant independent clinical attention.
B. There is evidence from the history, physical examination, or laboratory findings that the sleep disturbance is the direct physiological consequence of a general medical condition.
C. The disturbance is not better accounted for by another mental disorder (e.g., an Adjustment Disorder in which the stressor is a serious medical illness).
D. The disturbance does not occur exclusively during the course of a delirium.
E. The disturbance does not meet the criteria for Breathing-Related Sleep Disorder or Narcolepsy.
F. The sleep disturbance causes clinically significant distress or impairment in social, occupational, or other important areas of functioning.

DIAGNOSTIC CRITERIA FOR SUBSTANCE-INDUCED SLEEP DISORDER

A. A prominent disturbance in sleep that is sufficiently severe to warrant independent clinical attention.
B. There is evidence from the history, physical examination, or laboratory findings of either (1) or (2):
  1. the symptoms in Criterion A developed during, or within a month of, Substance Intoxication or Withdrawal
  2. medication use is etiologically related to the sleep disturbance
C. The disturbance is not better accounted for by a Sleep Disorder that is not substance induced. Evidence that the symptoms are better accounted for by a Sleep Disorder that is not substance induced might include the following: the symptoms precede the onset of the substance use (or medication use); the symptoms persist for a substantial period of time (e.g., about a month) after the cessation of acute withdrawal or severe intoxication or are substantially in excess of what would be expected given the type or amount of the substance used or the duration of use; or there is other evidence that suggests the existence of an independent non-substance-induced Sleep Disorder (e.g., a history of recurrent non-substance-related episodes).
D. The disturbance does not occur exclusively during the course of a delirium.
E. The sleep disturbance causes clinically significant distress or impairment in social, occupational, or other important areas of functioning.

Source: Reprinted with permission from the *Diagnostic and statistical manual of mental disorders,* 4th ed., Text Revision (pp. 654, 660). Copyright 2000 American Psychiatric Association.

tice. Through recognition and an exploration of client beliefs about sleep, you may be able to reinforce healthy attitudes and offer alternative perspectives based on your knowledge of sleep and its disorders.

Insomnia has been associated with increased physiologic arousal, emotional arousal, cognitive arousal, and conditioning. Current theory suggests that primary insomnia occurs in the presence of a combination of predisposing, precipitating, and perpetuating factors.

PHYSIOLOGIC FACTORS

The evidence for a physiologic basis for insomnia comes from studies that have shown that people with chronic insomnia are more likely to have a higher core body temperature and increased vasoconstriction at bedtime than those without symptoms of insomnia (Stepanski, 2000). Poor sleepers also tend to have a higher and more variable heart rate and a higher metabolic rate. A family history of being light sleepers or being predisposed to depression suggests a possible genetic link, but this has not been confirmed. Heightened physiologic arousal is most frequently a predisposing factor. It could become a precipitating or perpetuating factor in the context of regularly increased core body temperature (e.g., with heavy regular exercise immediately before bedtime) or regular intake of stimulants (e.g., prescription or nonprescription medication). For examples of sleep-inducing and arousal-inducing substances, see ■ Table 19–1 on page 468.

PSYCHOSOCIAL FACTORS

Emotional arousal as in anxiety, or cognitive arousal as in worry and racing thoughts, can precipitate or perpetuate insomnia. There is some evidence to suggest that people who prefer a high degree of control or tend to internalize emotion may be more predisposed to insomnia. Grief and loss as through death or divorce may precipitate an episode of insomnia. Some clients report the onset of insomnia after the birth of their first baby because of their sense of needing to be more vigilant and adjusting to the new responsibilities.

ENVIRONMENTAL CONDITIONING

Association of the sleeping room with lying awake may become a powerful perpetuating factor. Other clients may associate the bedroom with marital discord and thus also be conditioned to have increased arousal in that environment.

TABLE 19–1 Substances Involved in Sleep and Wakefulness

Sleep-Inducing Substances	Arousal-Inducing Substances
1. Adenosine	1. Acetylcholine (ACh)
2. Antihistamines	2. Caffeine
3. Certain herbs (such as chamomile and valerian)	3. Dopamine (DA)
4. Endogenous melatonin (only that produced by your own pineal gland)	4. Histamine
5. Free calcium (as found in warm milk)	5. Nicotine
6. Serotonin (5-HT)	6. Norepinephrine (NE)

NURSING PROCESS

Clients with Primary Insomnia

The focus in this section will be on clients who present with insomnia. The common nature of this disorder will likely mean it will coexist with many other aspects of psychiatric–mental health nursing care and overall medical–surgical nursing care.

Assessment

Assessment is primarily subjective unless there are symptoms suggestive of other disorders. Building from the basic sleep pattern assessment, it is particularly useful to follow up on history of onset of insomnia, and possible contributing factors. An ability to sleep better away from the usual bedroom suggests a conditioned response to that setting from many sleepless nights. Explore potential environmental factors, from condition of the mattress to sounds heard from outside the personal dwelling. Inquiry into thought processes while trying to go to sleep may help detect fears, anxiety, or work/family/financial pressures. Listen for evidence of a perceived need for increased vigilance, either currently or at the time the problem developed. Explore beliefs about sleep and its importance. Particularly among individuals with a history of mental or physical disorders, there may be associated fears about death, disturbing dreams, or vulnerability to external threat (see the Rx Communication feature below).

Nursing Diagnosis: NANDA

Specify that insomnia is the type of sleep pattern disturbance, and further identify it as sleep onset, maintenance, or early wakening as appropriate. If the insomnia seems secondary to a mental disorder, that can be specified; but even for those clients, it is helpful to include other contributing factors. Even if environmental factors were not contributory initially, the client may begin to associate them with sleeplessness and/or they may become disturbing because of chronic hyperarousal.

Outcome Identification: NOC

The outcome expected from treatment of insomnia is improved sleep quality as reported by the client. Decreased sleep latency (time to fall asleep after lights out), fewer wakenings after sleep onset, and shorter time to get back to sleep after wakening can be estimated by the client through the use of a sleep diary.

Planning and Implementation: NIC

A few basic interventions for insomnia will be discussed in this section, but the overall treatment may be quite complex, requiring the skills of a specialist. If the insomnia is related primarily to a mental or physical disorder, management of that condition usually brings relief of associated symptoms. (See the Using Research Evidence feature on page 469 for a discussion of intervention strategies for insomnia.) Antidepressants are often effective in reducing sleep pattern disturbance before the antidepressant effect can be noticed (see ■ Table 19–2 on page 470).

The interventions that are discussed in this section may be appropriate with clients in a variety of settings. If the insomnia is relatively recent or mild, information on the basic principles of sleep hygiene may be adequate (refer back to Intervention

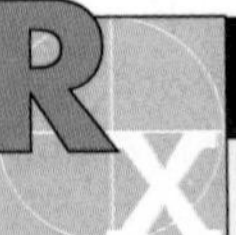

COMMUNICATION

Client with Primary Insomnia

CLIENT: "I'm having a lot of trouble falling asleep."

NURSE RESPONSE 1: "Tell me about your night's sleep and what it means to you."

RATIONALE: This response helps you detect aspects of the sleep pattern that indicate possible insomnia. There may be cultural differences between expectations and actual patterns of sleep.

NURSE RESPONSE 2: "Walk me through what a typical day is like for you."

RATIONALE: Evaluating the extent to which the client's daily distribution of activities may result in an agitated or nonrelaxed state at bedtime.

USING RESEARCH EVIDENCE

Rick Littlejohns is a 42-year-old businessman who has had recurrent episodes of depression and a history of chronic insomnia. He lives alone, except for two cats, having broken up with his wife 7 years ago. He describes himself as always being a light sleeper, but things got worse his second year of college when he started drinking heavily and sinking into his first major depression. Rick recently changed companies and since that time has been having increased difficulty getting to sleep and then with wakening again after a few hours. Recently, he missed work a couple of times because he finally managed to get into a sound sleep just as the alarm went off.

As a mental health counselor to whom he has come for help, you formulate a nursing care plan that addresses the following considerations:

1. Rick may have been predisposed to insomnia given his history of always being a light sleeper and history of depression. The current precipitating factor may be occupational stress associated with a new job. Perpetuating factors may include conditioned arousal to his own bedroom and an irregular sleep schedule.
2. Stimulus control therapy, by which the client is helped to reassociate his bedroom with sleep, and sleep restriction therapy (where the time the client can spend in bed is temporarily restricted to the usual amount of actual sleep he gets) are among the nonpharmacologic interventions that have been shown to be effective for insomnia.
3. Rick's history of recurrent depression and current sleep problems may be related, and thus you will monitor his progress closely.

Your plan of care is based on the research evidence summarized in the following journal article:

Morin, C. M., Hauri, P. J., Espie, C. A., Spielman, A. J., Buysse, D. J., & Bootzin, R. R. (1999). Nonpharmacologic treatment of chronic insomnia. *Sleep, 22,* 1134–1156.

box on page 457). If the insomnia is chronic and more severe, more rigorous intervention is warranted.

ENCOURAGING HOPE

Insomnia is such a discouraging and worrisome problem to clients that creating a sense of realistic hope that they will eventually learn to manage the problem is an important part of therapy (Morin et al., 1999). The goal is to change perception of the problem from something against which they are helpless to something over which they can gain control.

PROVIDING INFORMATION

Clients with severe insomnia are often well acquainted with the self-help literature. However, it is important to review what they have come to understand about managing insomnia. They may have misconceptions or difficulty applying some of the information to themselves. For example, some people are not aware that chocolate is also a source of caffeine. Others may not be aware of normal developmental changes in sleep patterns. Normalizing the experience of occasional times of prolonged sleep latency (more than 30 minutes) or awakenings during the night may be helpful as an intervention, as well as facilitating the setting of realistic goals. Clients with insomnia may also need some help in differentiating between myth and research-based evidence, between beliefs and facts. Of particular importance is recognizing that insomnia can be managed and that clients can continue to function adequately even on minimal sleep.

SHORTENING THE OVERALL SLEEP PERIOD WITH CONSISTENT RISING TIME

The time of rising is under voluntary control; the time of actually getting to sleep is not. With shorter total time in bed, sleep usually becomes more consolidated. These two principles are the basis for one of the most effective means of gaining control over insomnia:

1. Clients must not go to bed until they feel sleepy.
2. They must get up at the same time each morning.

Initially, this prescription may seem threatening to clients who have usually gotten into a pattern of getting sleep whenever and wherever they can. They will need support during this initial phase, possibly through a contracting process in which they go one week at a time. Reinforce that they will be able to get by and that their body will eventually begin to respond to the regularity of schedule, and that you believe in their ability to accomplish this goal. Clients with insomnia should not be permitted to nap. (For the very old or very ill, naps should be restricted to a brief, set time period.)

REDUCING KNOWN STIMULANTS AND OTHER SOURCES OF AROUSAL

Help clients with insomnia realize that they are susceptible to any stimulation, even though such stimulating factors may not have been contributory initially. Encourage them to avoid all sources of caffeine, nicotine, and other stimulants. However, in working with psychiatric clients, as with any client population, this intervention and all others must be considered in the context of the overall health problems, goals, and treatment plan as negotiated with the client, family, and other members of the health care team.

You may wish to collaborate with the client in making a list of possible contributing factors to the sleep pattern disturbance. For example, the client may identify interaction with a particular family member as generating a lot of emotion that is tough to deal with before going to bed. If fear or a perceived need for vigilance is a factor, it may be possible to modify the environment. The following clinical example discusses this aspect of sleep pattern disturbance.

TABLE 19–2 Drugs That Affect Sleep

Type	Examples	Comments
Antidepressants	Tricyclic antidepressants such as amitriptyline (Elavil)	Induce drowsiness to varying degrees, effect on insomnia associated with depression usually occurs earlier than antidepressant effect. Suppress REM.
	Selective serotonin reuptake inhibitors such as fluoxetine (Prozac)	Generally decrease total sleep time, increase wakefulness, may induce vivid dreaming.
Antiepileptics	Phenytoin (Dilantin) and phenobarbital	Sedation common, less so with newer seizure control drugs.
Antihistamines	Chlorpheniramine (Chlor-Trimeton) Pseudoephedrine compounds (Benylin cold capsules)	Induce drowsiness to varying degrees. Sometimes used as sleep-promoting agents because of their availability over the counter.
Antimanic drugs	Lithium (Lithane)	Improves sleep but may cause daytime sleepiness initially.
Antiparkinson drugs	Levodopa–carbidopa combinations (Sinemet), pergolide (Permax)	Low doses may improve sleep, but generally persons on medication for Parkinson's have poor sleep with insomnia, vivid dreaming.
Antipsychotics	Traditional antipsychotics such as chlorpromazine (Thorazine) and haloperidol (Haldol)	Chlorpromazine very sedating, haloperidol less so.
	Atypical antipsychotics such as clozapine (Clozaril), risperidone (Risperdal)	High incidence of sedation with clozapine, less so with risperidone.
Anxiolytics	Benzodiazepines such as temazepam (Restoril)	May be used as hypnotics to induce and sustain sleep (note differences between short- and long-acting types).
	Buspirone (BuSpar)	Little effect on sleep and alertness.
Caffeine	Additive to some pain and headache remedies, coffee, tea, colas	Increases wakefulness, effects may last 8–14 hours.
Cardiovascular drugs	Antihypertensives such as propranolol (Inderal), clonidine (Catapres), captopril (Capoten)	Insomnia, sedation, and nightmares, less so with captopril and other angiotensin-converting enzyme inhibitors.
Corticosteroids	Prednisone	Generally disturb sleep, especially if taken late in the day; suppress REM sleep.
Hypnotics	Zopiclone (Imovane) Zolpidem (Ambien)	Effective for sleep onset insomnia because of rapid absorption.
	Flurazepam (Dalmane)	Longer half-life, useful for sleep onset and maintenance insomnia.

CLINICAL EXAMPLE

An elderly widow, initially referred to a sleep clinic with possible obstructive sleep apnea, had become increasingly depressed. On a recent visit she confided that she had been sexually abused a few years prior and was extremely afraid to venture out of her apartment building. She felt especially vulnerable because of living in a basement suite, which could be readily broken into. Through the efforts of one of the nurse clinicians, the social welfare agency that was involved agreed to pay the slight additional cost involved in moving her to a second-story apartment, where she felt much safer. Through ongoing counseling with the nurse clinician, she began a modest exercise program in her own small apartment, and medical treatment for her sleep disturbance and depression resulted in clinically significant improvement over the next few months.

As discussed earlier, the state of arousal may be conditioned by objects in the bedroom environment or certain activities. Ways to alter these associations can be explored with the client. An assessment of the bedroom environment and its uses may call for relocating certain activities, such as paying bills or studying, to another part of the home. Rearranging furniture or even changing the color of pillowcases may help to reestablish associating the bedroom with sleep.

RELAXATION TRAINING

Relaxation exercises are discussed in Chapter 32. The important point in using them as an aid to sleep is that developing the skills should occur apart from the sleep period, so that they, too, do not become associated with the inability to sleep. See the Client/Family Teaching feature on page 471 for specific interventions regarding overall sleep improvement.

CLIENT/FAMILY TEACHING

Improving the Quality of Your Sleep

1. Think about the kind of sleep schedule that seems to fit you best.
2. Make a list of things that help you get to sleep (how dark you like it to be, what temperature, how you get ready for bed).
3. Jot down all the "rules" and "suggestions" you have heard about how to get better sleep. Cross out the ones that don't seem to fit. (Some people sleep better by not having a bedtime snack; other people sleep better after having a snack. Do what feels best for you. If you aren't sure, try an experiment doing it one way for a week and then the other way for the next week.) Put a question mark by the rules and suggestions you have never really tried, and underline the ones you think are important for you.
4. Consider what you could change to get an extra half-hour of sleep each night.
5. Keep a sleep diary for 2 weeks. For the first week just keep track of your usual pattern (time you went to bed and got up, number of hours of actual sleep, how you felt in the morning, etc.). At the end of the first week, review the diary and your responses to items 1 through 4 above. In the second week, experiment with one change you think would be helpful to you.
6. Carry on the process a bit longer if you like, but remember:
   - You can manage on very little sleep if you have to.
   - You know better than anyone else what works for you.
   - Your needs and preferences regarding sleep may change a bit as you get older or take on different roles and activities.

Evaluation

Early collaboration with the client in establishing realistic goals will help result in a satisfactory outcome. Regardless of behavioral or polysomnography-defined changes, it is important that the client can express some sense of mastery over his or her sleep problem. Whether that sense of control is achieved through reframing of essentially the same sleep patterns, a modest improvement in one or more parameters of sleep latency or number and length of awakenings, or an improved sense of energy for the day's activities is not important clinically. However, a better understanding of which interventions are most effective through carefully designed research studies would be a definite asset in helping nurses and others to choose among intervention alternatives.

Case Management

Case management of the client with primary insomnia would involve developing and organizing a program to address the problem. In this regard, you would help the client, to the extent necessary, with the following:

1. Making arrangements for a physical examiniation with a primary care provider.
2. Maintaining a log of sleep activities.
3. Keeping track of intake of stimulating substances such as caffeine.

It is important to rule out physical factors causing the difficulty as well as involving the client in an awareness of his or her activities that affect the quality and duration of sleep.

Community-Based Care

A large segment of the clients with insomnia will be treated in the community. Community-based care focuses on management of the problem area within the context of the client's life and activities. Stress, diet and nutrition, exercise, and environment all shape and influence sleep patterns, especially once that pattern becomes problematic. With this in mind, you would arrange for the client to attend nutrition and stress classes at the local community center.

Home Care

When you go into a client's home to provide care, you have the opportunity to directly observe the factors impacting on sleep. Direct observation is a powerful tool in addressing a sleep disorder. Evaluate the environment and the conditions in the client's bedroom or sleep area. Are the lighting and noise level factors of concern? Making observations of the exterior of the residence during a home visit at the usual sleep time can provide additional information. Gradual alterations can be made to resolve whatever issues are detected that cause or contribute to the insomnia.

NURSING PROCESS

Clients with Primary Hypersomnia

The focus in this section will be on clients with excessive sleepiness as part of their mental disorder. Basic assessments to identify clients who might benefit from referral to a sleep specialist are included. However, principles of treatment for most of the primary sleep disorders characterized by hypersomnia (obstructive sleep apnea, narcolepsy) were discussed earlier.

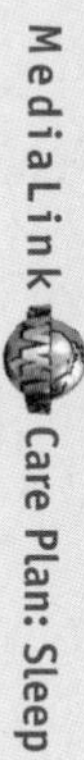

Assessment

Building from the basic sleep pattern assessment, explore potential contributing factors. With respect to the possibility of sleep apnea or periodic limb movement disorder:

- Try to interview the client's bed partner, or, if the client is institutionalized, to arrange for observation during sleep. If the bed partner describes recurrent periods of erratic breathing, including pauses of 20 seconds or longer interspersed between snoring, gasping, or snorting sounds, the client may have sleep apnea.

- Determine whether the problem disappears when the client is in a side-lying position, is worse after ingesting alcohol (even one or two drinks), is accompanied by morning headaches, or awakening with a feeling of still being tired.
- Ask the bed partner about the client's restlessness, repetitive jerking of one or more limbs, and/or gasping or choking noises.

An occasional apnea or myoclonic jerk about the time of sleep onset is not unusual. These are common occurrences as part of the normal wake–sleep transition. It is the recurrent episodes accompanied by some daytime somnolence that are of particular concern.

In the psychiatric context, you will encounter clients whose excessive sleepiness is associated with a coping mechanism, hopelessness, or an underlying mental disorder. Eliciting information about onset, patterns, and perceived causes may be difficult with these clients (see the Rx Communication feature below). Regular observation and recording of states of waking–sleeping in relation to clock time, activities, and environment may provide some clues about the pattern. For example, if the client is sleeping quite soundly whenever left undisturbed, chronic sleep deprivation or post-traumatic hypersomnia could be a factor (ASDA, 1997). Clients with secondary depression following a physical illness may also sleep more. In contrast, the lethargy that may accompany a major depressive episode or schizophrenia may be associated with lying with the eyes closed but not actually sleeping. (Such assessment will not be elaborated here, as it is best considered as part of the overall assessment for these clients.)

Nursing Diagnosis: NANDA

Specify that the type of Sleep Pattern Disturbance is hypersomnia, and describe contributing factors, if known. Frequently, contributing factors will be unknown or hypothetical at best. It is better to say unknown than to label a client in the absence of adequate evidence. See the Case Study and Care Plan for a client with hypersomnia and depression on pages 474–475.

Outcome Identification: NOC

Sleep efficiency (ratio of total sleep time/total time in bed) will be increased to at least 85%.

Planning and Implementation: NIC

The commonly observed interaction of aging, depression, and concurrent physical disease as contributors to excessive sleepiness illustrates the difficulty of planning and implementing specific interventions. Focus the interventions as follows:

1. Treat the underlying mental and physical disorders.
2. Ensure client safety, because of the frequently associated problems with loss of concentration and memory.
3. Regularize the client's schedule, alternating periods of activity and rest, to help gain a sense of control over the excessive sleepiness.
4. Expose the client to natural sunlight or light therapy in the morning; encourage walking outdoors.
5. Plan favorite events, such as a television program or visitor.
6. Maximize the use of environmental time cues, such as regular mealtimes and the visibility of a clock and windows.

Evaluation

The setting of short-term, achievable, and meaningful goals is important for clients with this condition. For them, time otherwise seems to become a blur of sleeping and eating.

Case Management and Community-Based Care

The case management services needed by the client with hypersomnia focuses on training for a healthier sleep pattern and safety. Participation in activities needs to be monitored to

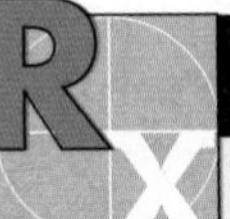

COMMUNICATION

Client with Primary Hypersomnia

CLIENT: "I seem to fall asleep at unusual times."

NURSE RESPONSE 1: "Tell me about what times you fall asleep."

RATIONALE: Determining if the pattern of symptoms is indeed unusual.

NURSE RESPONSE 2: "Tell me about your overall sleep pattern, both your usual sleeping at night and what happens during these unusual times."

RATIONALE: Determining whether the client's sleep disturbance can be attributed to fatigue.

assure that the client is not putting him- or herself in danger due to fatigue and hypersomnia. Times when the client feels most alert could be mapped and activities requiring attentiveness could be scheduled for those times. Arrange for appointments with health care providers specializing in sleep disorders to prioritize which factors play a role in generating fatigue for the client.

Community-based care has similar features and direction to case management services. The client's safety needs must be addressed. Does the hypersomnia interfere with transportation, relationships, nutrition, or the client's abilities to be aware of and respond to enviromental conditions? Do physical factors such as obesity or a sedentary lifestyle contribute to the hypersomnia? If so, and after obtaining medical clearance for the activity level, help the client arrange to attend an exercise class.

Home Care

Home care with a hypersomnic client will likely involve exploring the client's sleep environment firsthand. Numerous factors contribute to the sleep environment beyond the client's physiologic environment, or internal environment. You will be able to examine and incorporate the following external factors into your plan for how home care can be best maximized:

1. Who the client sleeps with—human and pets.
2. The room size, position within the traffic pattern in the home, and lighting.
3. Bed or sleeping surface.
4. Air circulation and ventilation.
5. Daily schedule—both client's and others in the environment.

Once these features of the external sleep environment have been examined, meet with the client and the entire family. A discussion about how the household functions in relation to sleep is helpful. Cultural features and expectations play a large role in determining sleep pattern expression in a home. A goal could be established with the help of all household members to help regulate the client's times of going to bed, going to sleep, and getting up.

NURSING PROCESS

Clients with Circadian Rhythm Sleep Disorder

This section will focus on clients with circadian rhythm sleep disorders expressed through disorganized sleep–wake patterns. The driving force behind the disorganization could be external events such as shift work or moving among different time zones (jet lag) or internal phenomena such as a mental disorder. Circadian rhythm sleep disorders are common difficulties among depressed and psychotic clients.

Assessment

Much of the information that you need will come from the basic sleep pattern assessment, if clients can participate and recall accurately. The next step is a combined assessment–intervention: a sleep diary. By keeping a diary, clients may confront their own irregularities and be more amenable to developing a regular schedule. Other psychiatric clients may be unable or unwilling to maintain a diary and may require help. See the accompanying Rx Communication feature for examples of assessing this problem with a client.

It is also useful to obtain information about previous patterns, tendencies toward being a morning or evening person, and the type of schedule to which they will most likely return as their condition improves. In that way, they will not have to cope with further schedule change upon discharge or resuming family and work roles.

Nursing Diagnosis: NANDA

The nursing diagnosis is Sleep Pattern Disturbance, but for this problem it is usually easier to identify contributing factors, at least to the immediate situation. For example, a client may live alone and be on an indefinite leave from work because of a major depressive episode. The mental disorder is an underlying cause, but the immediate and more rectifiable contributing factor is that there are few markers of time in the client's daily life, other than therapy appointments. Some clients, such as those with dementia, may have lost their ability to estimate time or even interpret cues. Other clients may live in such a chaotic environment that it is very difficult to achieve any regularity of schedule.

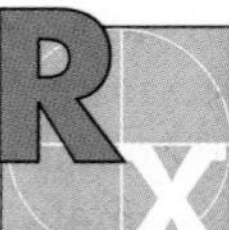

COMMUNICATION

Client with Circadian Rhythm Sleep Disorder

CLIENT: "For the last few weeks I wake up too soon and I can't get enough sleep."

NURSE RESPONSE 1: "How many hours of sleep a night are you getting?"

RATIONALE: Exploring the client's perceptions and definitions of symptoms to map out the exact nature of the difficulty.

NURSE RESPONSE 2: "Has anything changed in your schedule over that period of time?"

RATIONALE: Exploring whether any activities could be interfering with usual sleep patterns including birth of a child, intrusion of a chaotic element in the environment, or a change in work schedules of the client or sleep partner.

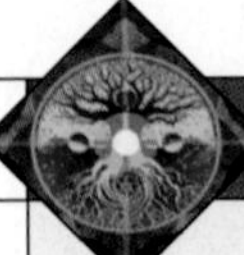

Case Study

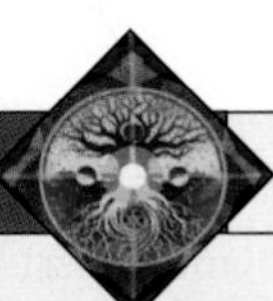

Depressed Client with Hypersomnia

Identifying Information

Maha is a 42-year-old woman presently living in a small apartment with her unmarried 22-year-old son. Maha states she has been having trouble with periodic wakenings and daytime sleepiness since before her divorce 2 years ago. She has been steadily gaining weight, feels that she has no energy, and says that the only thing she feels like doing is "watching my soaps on TV."

History

Never an energetic person, Maha feels that her present problems started years ago when she had to spend long hours with the children while her husband traveled. His homecomings usually included verbal abuse about her "slovenly" housekeeping and lack of discipline with the children. Having immigrated as a young wife she has deeply missed her family and made few friends here. Food has always been a source of comfort to her, particularly the traditional dishes of her homeland.

Maha was heavy even as an adolescent and has snored for as long as she can remember. When she was still married, her husband usually slept in another bedroom because of her snoring.

Her son describes her snoring as disruptive with periods of escalating noise culminating in a half minute or longer silence which ends abruptly with a gasp and gradual resumption of quiet breathing until the next episode. She goes to bed about 9:00 PM and stays there until 11:00 AM or later the next morning, sleeping most of the time. She often wakens with a headache, feeling as tired as she did the night before.

Maha's current depressive episode was diagnosed 6 months ago when her son insisted she see their family doctor. Treatment was initiated with fluoxetine (Prozac) 20 mg which has now been increased to 40 mg daily in the morning.

Current Mental Status

Maha appears somewhat drowsy, with a paucity of movement. Her speech is slow but coherent. She acknowledges some problems with short-term memory and concentration.

MediaLink Sleep Research Information

Outcome Identification: NOC

Wakeful at appropriate times is the NOC term that best describes the desired outcome for circadian rhythm disorders.

Planning and Implementation: NIC

Interventions will be highly individualized for each client. Establishing sleep regularity is a critical intervention.

ESTABLISHING REGULARITY AND CUES IN DAILY AND WEEKLY SCHEDULES

For the client who lives alone, external cues may be introduced through the help of family, friends, or social agencies. For example, a family member may agree to phone the client at the same time each day. A volunteer may agree to invite the client and two or three others to dinner every Wednesday evening. A service such as Meals on Wheels may be warranted, providing the combined benefit of better nutrition and another regular daily event. Scheduling morning appointments for these clients gives them a reason to get up early. As their condition gradually improves, they can take increasing responsibility for structuring their own schedule. Markers of the days of the week and even the season may further help them once again participate in life around them.

Clients who live in a chaotic environment and/or experience multiple role demands present a very different challenge. For example, a young single mother with a colicky baby and a toddler may find her days and nights have become a blur of child care. Sleep deprivation because of caregiving responsibilities may reduce her coping skills. Reliance on alcohol or drugs may further fragment sleep, as may memories of abuse or trauma. Crisis intervention may be necessary (see Chapter 33). However, a long-term plan of helping her reestablish control in her life will also be an important part of her overall therapy. The Talk About Sleep site at www.talkabout sleep.com/ has topical research and information for health care providers and clients.

Evaluation

A sleep diary, as suggested for assessment, is an excellent resource for evaluation. Reviewing the diary with the client suffering from sleep–wake disturbance can provide further opportunity for positive reinforcement on accomplishments and for revised goal setting.

Case Management

The case management of a client with circadian rhythm sleep disorder would depend on the nature of the cause of the disorder. If shift work was the cause, case management could include contacting the client's employee assistance program at work to determine if the work schedule can be made more flexible or different in any manner. With a client who has depressive symptomatology, interventions would focus on structuring the day and nighttime activities in such a way as to maximize sleep hygiene.

Community-Based Care

The structure of an outpatient's life may depend on community-based care appointments at first. Getting up for an appointment, a group activity, or a day program can shape the sleep schedule. Attention to a variety of activities can be

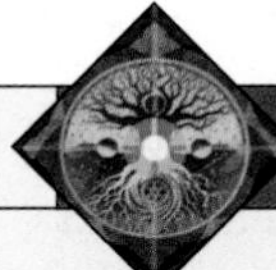

Nursing Care Plan

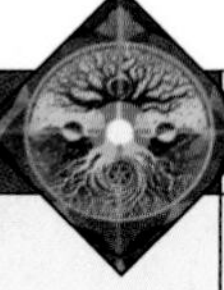

Nursing Diagnosis: Sleep Pattern Disturbance: Excessive somnolence related to inactivity secondary to depression, obstructive sleep apnea, and obesity

Expected Outcome: Sleep efficiency (ratio of total sleep time to total time in bed will improve to 85%)

Short-Term Goals	*Interventions*	*Rationale*
Client sees sleep specialist.	• Help client arrange for referral to sleep specialist.	Symptoms (snoring with apneas, daytime sleepiness, obesity) suggestive of obstructive sleep apnea.
Establish regular sleep.	• Negotiate with client to get up every morning at the same time.	Shorten time in bed to improve sleep efficiency.
Activity schedule.	• Encourage her to spend 30 minutes in outdoor activity every morning.	Exposure to natural sunlight early in the day improves sleep consolidation and reduces depression.
Increase activity and exercise.	• Explore previously enjoyed activities, involvement in exercise and sports.	Previously enjoyed activities make a good starting point.
	• Establish a contract based on what client believes she can manage.	Contracting can be effective in behavior change.

increased once symptomatology decreases and is more comfortably tolerated. If tension has been detected around sleep activities, you may arrange for the client to receive relaxation training in a local adult education program.

Home Care

Frequently these disorders occur with clients who experience psychotic symptoms or depression. Home care needs around sleep issues include interventions around these very real and disturbing sleep disruptions. Resolution of active symptoms of the psychiatric–mental health disorder contributes to resolution of many of the sleep difficulties. However, clients may live in circumstances that are chaotic. Make a series of visits to the client's residence at random times over several days during the part of the day the client is having trouble sleeping to determine if there are environmental factors interfering with the client's sleep that can be modified.

NURSING PROCESS

Clients with Parasomnias

Clients with parasomnias are often encountered in psychiatric settings because of the frequency of associated psychopathologic problems. The exception is young children, in whom parasomnias are considered a normal phenomenon or, at most, a transient sleep disorder (Broughton, 2000). In adults, parasomnias are often associated with major stressful events.

Assessment

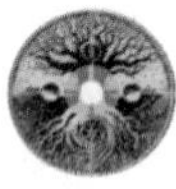

Besides the basic sleep pattern assessment, focus on the circumstances at the time of onset of the current and previous episodes and on family history.

- Clients with a single parasomnia may have a history of one or more other parasomnias, so ask about wakening with a sense of terror, vivid nightmares, and the like.
- Clients may be only partially aware of their parasomnias (they are usually amnesic about sleepwalking episodes), so question family members and sleep partners.
- The occurrence of subjective experiences like sleep terrors or sleep paralysis may never have been disclosed out of embarrassment or lack of adequate descriptive language; therefore, use normalizing statements followed by a question, such as, "Many people who have trouble with sleepwalking have also experienced times when they wake up feeling terribly frightened but aren't sure why. Has anything like that ever happened to you?"
- Inquiry about family history should not be limited to the same parasomnia, as there is some mixing of types among family members. The prevalence is higher among first-degree relatives than in the general population.
- Help clients explore stressors that might be associated with initial or recurrent episodes. "What else was happening in your life about then?"
- Ask about current and prior medications. Medication changes may also be a precipitator, particularly of the REM-related parasomnias such as nightmares. Remember that what was prescribed and what the client has actually taken may be different, so be sure to ask.

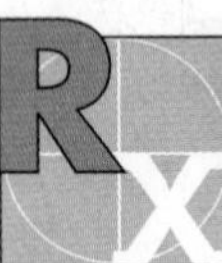

COMMUNICATION

Client with Parasomnia

CLIENT: "For the last couple of months I've been having nightmares."

NURSE RESPONSE 1: "Is there any pattern to the nightmares; for example, are they about one particular theme or subject?"

RATIONALE: Evaluating whether a specific stressor has played a role in precipitating the parasomnia.

NURSE RESPONSE 2: "How often do you get these nightmares and has anything else changed about the way in which you sleep?"

RATIONALE: Exploring the extent and topography of this sleep difficulty.

Nursing Diagnosis: NANDA

As with the other sleep pattern disturbances, specify the type(s), but the contributing factors may be unknown or hypothesized.

Outcome Identification: NOC

Reduction in frequency of parasomnias would be the desired outcome.

Planning and Implementation: NIC

Promoting client safety and administering medications are the two major nursing interventions.

PROMOTING CLIENT SAFETY

Physical and emotional safety is the major goal in planning and implementing interventions for clients with Sleep Pattern Disturbance related to parasomnias. Physically active parasomnias, such as somnambulism and REM sleep behavior disorder, pose the risk of injury to the client and/or others. At a children's camp, safety may be a matter of seeing that the affected child is assigned a lower bunk and that the cabin counselor is aware of the potential problem. Among older children or adults, the behaviors may be elaborate. Clients have been known to remove barricades, silence alarms, open exterior doors, and cross streets while sleepwalking. Protective intervention must be highly individualized and must involve close collaboration with the family. Caution family members to avoid wakening or arguing with the client.

Subjective parasomnias, such as sleep terrors and nightmares, can be extremely frightening to clients, particularly those who are already compromised by a mental disorder. The dreams of clients with posttraumatic stress disorder may likewise be one of the most frightening factors for them.

Clients who are aware that they have somnambulism or REM sleep behavior disorder also tend to carry some burden of fear as to what might happen during this phenomenon that seems beyond their control. Offer assistance by helping them explore these feelings and understand the physiologic basis. Clients can be guided in the decisions they make about taking their medication and other substances by understanding the possibility of REM rebound.

ADMINISTERING MEDICATIONS

Clients with REM sleep behavior disorder respond to the regular administration of clonazepam (Klonopin) (Mahowald & Schenck, 2000). However, there have been reports of breakthrough behavior even a year after beginning drug therapy. Somnambulism usually responds to clonazepam (Klonopin), diazepam (Valium), or imipramine (Tofranil) (Broughton, 2000). As noted earlier, many of the antidepressants suppress REM sleep and therefore offer some protection against nightmares. Caution clients against abruptly discontinuing the medication; REM rebound is less of a problem with gradual reduction of dosage.

Evaluation

Reducing the risk factors is the most important evaluation criterion. It is unrealistic to say you will prevent injury, because that is usually not within your realm of responsibility, nor is it realistic for any other care provider to guarantee injury prevention. In an environment of increasing litigation, the choice of words used in documentation is important.

Case Management and Community-Based Care

Case management can work to minimize some of the stressors associated with parasomnias. Initially, you may arrange for the client to spend a series of nights at a sleep laboratory to evaluate the sleep disturbance. Once those data have been analyzed, the case management focus will be to assist the client in moving through the system, getting the help he or she needs for the disorder, and assuring adherence to overall schedules.

Community-based care would be central in the long-term management of a parasomnia. An aspect of this care could concentrate on client access to an evaluation session with a psychiatric–mental health advanced practice nurse to determine whether there are any emotional issues contributing to the parasomnia. Following evaluations, careful examinations of the client's particular parasomnia and the sleep environment would direct the plan of care. Cooperation with the family and/or sleep partners is necessary to determine the effectiveness of treatment.

Home Care

Parasomnias such as sleepwalking have associated dangers that home care can evaluate and work to decrease. You will be in a unique position to answer the following questions:

1. What is the sleep environment like?
2. Are there stairs, outside doors, or obstacles in the immediate vicinity?
3. What are the distances involved in the sleepwalking?

Meet with the client and family to discuss these factors and to stress the importance of careful monitoring on the situation. It will be useful to have a conversation with the client and family or sleep partner to determine whether the response to the client's parasomnia may be positively reinforcing the parasomnia, making change more difficult to accomplish.

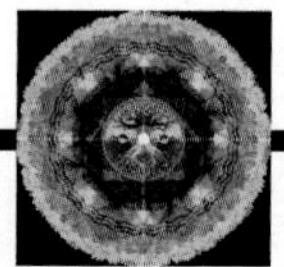

EXPLORE MediaLink

NCLEX review, case studies, and other interactive resources for this chapter can be found on the Companion Website at www.prenhall.com/kneisl. Click on Chapter 19 to select the activities for this chapter.

For animations, video tutorials, more NCLEX review questions, and an audio glossary, access the accompanying CD-ROM in this textbook.

BIBLIOGRAPHY

Adam, K. (1980). Dietary habits and sleep after bedtime food drinks. *Sleep, 3*, 47–58.

American Psychiatric Association. (2000). *Diagnostic and statistical manual of mental disorders* (4th ed., Text Revision). Washington, DC: Author.

American Sleep Disorders Association. (1997). The international classification of sleep disorders (revised): Diagnostic and coding manual. Rochester, MN: American Sleep Disorders Association.

Benson, K. L., & Zarcone, V. P. (2000). Schizophrenia. In M. H. Kryger, T. Roth, & W. C. Dement (Eds.), *Principles and practice of sleep medicine* (3rd ed.) (pp.1159–1167). Philadelphia: Saunders.

Bliwise, D. L. (2000). Dementia. In M. H. Kryger, T. Roth, & W. C. Dement (Eds.), *Principles and practice of sleep medicine* (3rd ed.) (pp.1058–1071). Philadelphia: Saunders.

Broughton, R. J. (2000). NREM arousal parasomnias. In M. H. Kryger, T. Roth, & W. C. Dement (Eds.), *Principles and practice of sleep medicine* (3rd ed.) (pp. 693–706). Philadelphia: Saunders.

Cohen, F. L., Nehring, W. M., & Cloninger, L. (1996). Symptom description and management in narcolepsy. *Holistic Nursing Practice, 10*(4), 44–53.

Douglas, N. J. (1998). The psychosocial aspects of narcolepsy. *Neurology, 50*(Suppl 1), S27–S30.

Gillin, J. C. (2000). Sleep and psychoactive drugs of abuse and dependence. In M. H. Kryger, T. Roth, & W. C. Dement (Eds.), *Principles and practice of sleep medicine* (3rd ed.). Philadelphia: Saunders.

Horne, J. A. (1988). *Why we sleep*. Oxford: Oxford University Press.

Hoy, C. J., Vennelle, M., Kingshott, R. N., Engleman, H. M., & Douglas, N. J. (1999). Can intensive support improve continuous positive airway pressure use in patients with the sleep apnea/hypopnea syndrome. *American Journal of Respiratory and Critical Care Medicine, 159*, 1096–1100.

Mahowald, M. W., & Schenck, C. H. (2000). REM sleep parasomnias. In M. H. Kryger, T. Roth, & W. C. Dement (Eds.), *Principles and practice of sleep medicine* (3rd ed.) (pp. 724–741). Philadelphia: Saunders.

McCall, W. V., & Reynolds, D. (2000). Psychiatric disorders and insomnia. In M. H. Kryger, T. Roth & W. C. Dement (Eds.), *Principles and practice of sleep medicine* (3rd ed.) (pp. 640–646). Philadelphia: Saunders.

Mendelson, W. B. (2000). Pharmacologic alteration of the perception of being awake or asleep. *Sleep, 16*(7), 641–646.

Monti, J. M., Alterwain, P., Estevez, F., Alvarino, F., Giusti, M., Olivera, S., et al. (1993). The effects of ritanserin on mood and sleep in abstinent alcoholic patients. *Sleep, 16*(7), 647–654.

Morin, C. M., Hauri, P. J., Espie, C. A., Spielman, A. J., Buysse, D. J. & Bootzin, R. R. (1999). Nonpharmacologic treatment of chronic insomnia. *Sleep, 22*(8), 1134–1156.

Nowlin-Finch, N. L., Altshuler, L. L., Szuba, M. P., & Mintz, J. (1994). Rapid resolution of first episodes of mania: Sleep related? *Journal of Clinical Psychiatry, 55*(1), 26–29.

Phillips, B., & Ancoli-Israel, S. (2001). Sleep disorders in the elderly. *Sleep Medicine, 2*, 99–114.

Pivik, R. T. (2000). Psychophysiology of dreams. In M. H. Kryger, T. Roth, & W. C. Dement (Eds.), *Principles and practice of sleep medicine* (3rd ed.) (pp. 491–501). Philadelphia: Saunders.

Roehrs, T., Carskadon, M. A., Dement, C., & Roth, T. (2000). Daytime sleepiness and alertness. In M. H. Kryger, T. Roth, & W. C. Dement (Eds.), *Principles and practice of sleep medicine* (3rd ed.) (pp. 43–52). Philadelphia: Saunders.

Sadock, B. J., & Sadock, V. A. (2002). *Kaplan and Sadock's synopsis of psychiatry* (9th ed.). Philadelphia: Lippincott Williams & Wilkins.

Shaver, J. L., Giblin, E. & Paulsen, V. (1991). Sleep quality subtypes in midlife women. *Sleep, 14*, 18–23.

Stepanski, E. J. (2000). Behavioral therapy for insomnia. In M. H. Kryger, T. Roth, & W. C. Dement (Eds.), *Principles and practice of sleep medicine* (3rd ed.) (pp. 647–656). Philadelphia: Saunders.

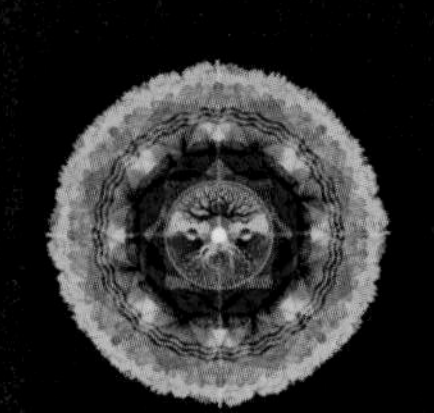

20

Chapter TWENTY

Personality Disorders

SUE C. DeLAUNE

KEY TERMS

abandonment
antisocial personality disorder
avoidant personality disorder
borderline personality disorder
countertransference
dependent personality disorder
enmeshment
histrionic personality disorder
hypervigilance
identity diffusion
narcissistic personality disorder
obsessive–compulsive personality disorder
paranoid personality disorder
personality
personality disorder (PD)
personality traits
schizoid personality disorder
schizotypal personality disorder
separation–individuation
splitting

FOCUS QUESTIONS

- How do you differentiate personality traits and styles from personality disorders?
- How do the biopsychosocial characteristics of various personality disorders compare and contrast with one another?
- What are the developmental and psychobiologic characteristics that distinguish the various personality disorders?
- Which key concepts would help you to apply the nursing process to the care of clients with personality disorders?
- What are the possible positive and negative effects of emotional responses to clients who have personality disorders?

MediaLink 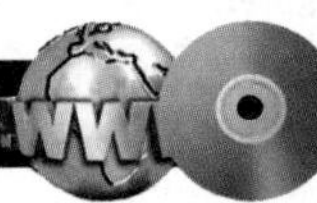 www.prenhall.com/kneisl

Additional resources for this chapter can be found on the Student CD-ROM accompanying this textbook, and on the Companion Website at www.prenhall.com/kneisl. Click on Chapter 20 to select the activities for this chapter.

CD-ROM
- Audio Glossary
- NCLEX Review

Companion Website
- Additional NCLEX Review
- Care Plan: Self-Destructive Behavior
- Case Study: Self-Mutilation
- Learning from Clients: Antisocial PD Video

CHAPTER OUTLINE

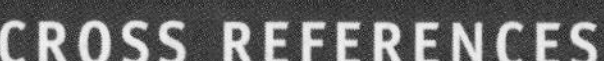

CROSS REFERENCES

Other topics relevant to this content are: Assertiveness training, Chapter 1; Cognitive treatment, Chapter 30; Forensic nursing, Chapter 35; Group interventions, Chapter 29; Relaxation skills, Chapter 32; One-to-one relationship skills, Chapter 28; Stress and coping, Chapter 5; Structuring the therapeutic environment, Chapter 11; Substance abuse and mental illness, Chapter 21; Suicide and self-destructive behavior, Chapter 22; Violent clients, Chapter 34.

CRITICAL THINKING CHALLENGE

As a newly employed nurse on a crisis unit, you get a request from a client to bend the rules for her by extending her pass for two hours longer in order that she may meet her boyfriend for dinner before her return to the unit. When you question the legitimacy of this request and suggest that she get approval from the treatment team, the client becomes angry and accuses you of "not being the caring nurse" she thought you were. She states that she will remember this incident and warn her friends about the unfeeling nurses at this facility. How would you handle this situation with the client? What is your rationale? ■

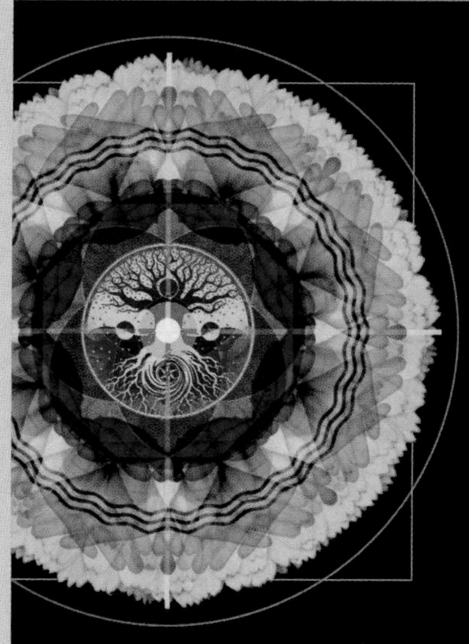

At times, every individual demonstrates behavior that challenges others. However, working with clients who consistently demonstrate impatient, manipulative, self-centered, or overly suspicious behaviors can be especially challenging.

What distinguishes an individual is referred to as **personality**, which is defined as the individual qualities, including habitual behavior patterns, that make a person unique. **Personality traits** are persistent behavioral patterns that do not significantly interfere with one's life, even though the behaviors may be annoying or frustrating to others. Both personality and personality traits tend to be stable over time. A **personality disorder (PD)** is a rigid, stereotyped behavioral pattern that persists throughout a person's life. A PD is a lifelong maladaptive pattern of perceiving, thinking, and relating that impairs social or occupational functioning. Individuals who have a PD lack insight; that is, they lack understanding of the impact of their behavior on the environment. They fail to accept the consequences of their own behavior and, when feeling threatened, they attempt to ease the stress by changing the environment rather than changing their own behavior. Personality-disordered individuals' relationships are characterized by superficiality. The box below lists the diagnostic criteria for PD as defined by the American Psychiatric Association (APA).

This chapter discusses the various types of PDs and the major characteristics of each. Nursing responses to individuals with PDs are explained. The goal of therapeutic approaches is not restructuring the client's basic personality. Instead, the interventions are implemented to help those with PDs learn to deal with others in more productive, less stressful ways.

Personality Disorders

There are three major categories of PDs, referred to as *clusters* by the APA. The diagnostic criteria box on pages 481–483 provides a description of each cluster. Even though there are some differences among the three clusters, three traits are common to people with all types of PDs:

- Lack of insight—individuals lack understanding of the impact of their behavior on others.
- External response to stress—when feeling threatened, individuals try to change the environment instead of changing themselves.
- Failure to accept the consequences of their own behavior.

The essential characteristics of PDs are chronicity, pervasiveness, and maladaptation. The individual with a PD often goes through life repeating the same dysfunctional pattern. The PD affects every dimension of life and seriously impairs interpersonal and functional abilities.

Other problematic behaviors that are characteristic of people with PDs include manipulation, narcissism, and impulsiveness. Manipulation is control behavior; the manipulative individual uses and exploits others for personal gain. Narcissism is self-centered behavior in which the individual feels entitled to special favors due to a mistaken perception of oneself as the "center of the universe." Impulsiveness describes the actions of those who act without considering the consequences of their behavior.

The DSM-IV-TR delineates diagnostic criteria for PDs on Axis II. Essential features of these disorders include significant distress or impairment in at least two of the following areas of functioning:

- Cognition
- Affect
- Interpersonal relationships
- Impulse control

The DSM-IV-TR points out that these behavior patterns must be evident by early adulthood and not accounted for by other mental disorders or the effects of substance use (APA, 2000). It is important to distinguish the behaviors that define personality disorders from responses that may emerge from specific situational stressors or transient mental states. Therefore, it is often necessary and important to conduct more than one interview with the client, over a period of time. While person-

DSM-IV-TR — **Diagnostic Criteria for a Personality Disorder**

A. An enduring pattern of inner experience and behavior that deviates markedly from the expectations of the individual's culture. This pattern is manifested in two (or more) of the following areas:

1. Cognition (i.e., ways of perceiving and interpreting self, other people, and events).
1. Affectivity (i.e., the range, intensity, lability, and appropriateness of emotional response).
2. Interpersonal functioning.
3. Impulse control.

B. The enduring pattern is inflexible and pervasive across a broad range of personal and social situations.

C. The enduring pattern leads to clinically significant distress or impairment in social, occupational, or other important areas of functioning.

D. The pattern is stable and of long duration and its onset can be traced back at least to adolescence or early adulthood.

E. The enduring pattern is not better accounted for as a manifestation or consequence of another mental disorder.

F. The enduring pattern is not due to the direct physiological effects of a substance (e.g., a drug of abuse, a medication) or a general medical condition (e.g., head trauma).

Source: Reprinted with permission from the *Diagnostic and statistical manual of mental disorders,* 4th ed., Text Revision (p. 689). Copyright 2000 American Psychiatric Association.

DSM-IV-TR — Diagnostic Criteria for Personality Disorders: Clusters A, B, C

CLUSTER A (ODD–ECCENTRIC)	CLUSTER B (DRAMATIC–EMOTIONAL)	CLUSTER C (FEARFUL–ANXIOUS)
Paranoid Personality Disorder A pervasive distrust and suspiciousness of others such that their motives are interpreted as malevolent, beginning by early adulthood and present in a variety of contexts, as indicated by four (or more) of the following: **1.** Suspects, without sufficient basis, that others are exploiting, harming, or deceiving him or her. **2.** Is preoccupied with unjustified doubts about the loyalty or trustworthiness of friends or associates. **3.** Is reluctant to confide in others because of unwarranted fear that the information will be used maliciously against him or her. **4.** Reads hidden demeaning or threatening meanings into benign remarks or events. **5.** Persistently bears grudges, i.e., is unforgiving of insults, injuries, or slights. **6.** Perceives attacks on his or her character or reputation that are not apparent to others and is quick to react angrily or to counter-attack. **7.** Has recurrent suspicions, without justification, regarding fidelity of spouse or sexual partner.	*Borderline Personality Disorder* A pervasive pattern of instability of interpersonal relationships, self-image, and affects, and marked impulsivity beginning by early adulthood and present in a variety of contexts, as indicated by five (or more) of the following: **1.** Frantic efforts to avoid real or imagined abandonment. **Note:** Do not include suicidal or self-mutilating behavior covered in Criterion 5. **2.** A pattern of unstable and intense interpersonal relationships characterized by alternating between extremes of idealization and devaluation. **3.** Identity disturbance: markedly and persistently unstable self-image or sense of self. **4.** Impulsivity in at least two areas that are potentially self-damaging (e.g., spending, sex, substance abuse, reckless driving, binge eating). **5.** Recurrent suicidal behavior, gestures, or threats, or self-mutilating behavior. **6.** Affective instability due to a marked reactivity of mood (e.g., intense episodic dysphoria, irritability, or anxiety usually lasting a few hours and only rarely more than a few days). **7.** Chronic feelings of emptiness. **8.** Inappropriate, intense anger or difficulty controlling anger (e.g., frequent displays of temper, constant anger, recurrent physical fights). **9.** Transient, stress-related paranoid ideation or severe dissociative symptoms.	*Avoidant Personality Disorder* A pervasive pattern of social inhibition, feelings of inadequacy, and hypersensitivity to negative evaluation, beginning by early adulthood and present in a variety of contexts, as indicated by four (or more) of the following: **1.** Avoids occupational activities that involve significant interpersonal contact, because of fears of criticism, disapproval, or rejection. **2.** Is unwilling to get involved with people unless certain of being liked **3.** Shows restraint within intimate relationships because of the fear of being shamed or ridiculed. **4.** Is preoccupied with being criticized or rejected in social situations. **Note:** Do not include suicidal or self-mutilating behavior covered in Criterion 5. **5.** Is inhibited in new interpersonal situations because of feelings of inadequacy. **6.** Views self as socially inept, personally unappealing, or inferior to others. **7.** Is unusually reluctant to take personal risks or to engage in any new activities because they may prove embarrassing.
Schizoid Personality Disorder A pervasive pattern of detachment from social relationships and a restricted range of expression of emotions in interpersonal settings, beginning by early adulthood and present in a variety of contexts, as indicated by four (or more) of the following: **1.** Neither desires nor enjoys close relationships, including being part of a family. **2.** Almost always chooses solitary activities. **3.** Has little, if any, interest in having sexual experiences with another person. **4.** Takes pleasure in few, if any, activities. **5.** Lacks close friends or confidants other than first-degree relatives.	*Histrionic Personality Disorder* A pervasive pattern of excessive emotionality and attention seeking, beginning by early adulthood and present in a variety of contexts, as indicated by five (or more) of the following: **1.** Is uncomfortable in situations in which he or she is not the center of attention. **2.** Interaction with others is often characterized by inappropriate sexually seductive or provocative behavior. **3.** Displays rapidly shifting and shallow expression of emotions. **4.** Consistently uses physical appearance to draw attention to self. **5.** Has a style of speech that is excessively impressionistic and lacking in detail.	*Dependent Personality Disorder* A pervasive and excessive need to be taken care of that leads to submissive and clinging behavior and fears of separation, beginning by early adulthood and present in a variety of contexts, as indicated by five (or more) of the following: **1.** Has difficulty making everyday decisions without an excessive amount of advice and reassurance from others. **2.** Needs others to assume responsibility for most major areas of his or her life. **3.** Has difficulty expressing disagreement with others because of fear of loss of support or approval. **Note:** Do not include realistic fears of retribution. *(continued)*

DSM-IV-TR Diagnostic Criteria for Personality Disorders: Clusters A, B, C

CLUSTER A (ODD–ECCENTRIC)

Schizoid Personality Disorder

6. Appears indifferent to the praise or criticism of others.
7. Shows emotional coldness, detachment, or flattened affectivity.
8. Considers relationships to be more intimate than they actually are.

Schizotypal Personality Disorder

A pervasive pattern of social and interpersonal deficits marked by acute discomfort with, and reduced capacity for, close relationships as well as by cognitive or perceptual distortions and eccentricities of behavior, beginning by early adulthood and present in a variety of contexts, as indicated by five (or more) of the following:

1. Ideas of reference (excluding delusions of reference).
2. Odd beliefs or magical thinking that influences behavior and is inconsistent with subcultural norms (e.g., superstitiousness, belief in clairvoyance, telepathy, or "sixth sense"; in children and adolescents, bizarre fantasies or preoccupations).
3. Unusual perceptual experiences, including bodily illusions.
4. Odd thinking and speech (e.g., vague, circumstantial, metaphorical, overelaborate, or stereotyped).
5. Suspiciousness or paranoid ideation.
6. Inappropriate or constricted affect.
7. Behavior or appearance that is odd, eccentric, or peculiar.
8. Lack of close friends or confidants other than first-degree relatives.
9. Excessive social anxiety that does not diminish with familiarity and tends to be associated with paranoid fears rather than negative judgments about self.

CLUSTER B (DRAMATIC–EMOTIONAL)

Histrionic Personality Disorder

6. Shows self-dramatization, theatricality, and exaggerated expression of emotion.
7. Is suggestible, i.e., easily influenced by others or circumstances.

Narcissistic Personality Disorder

A pervasive pattern of grandiosity (in fantasy or behavior), need for admiration, and lack of empathy, beginning by early adulthood and present in a variety of contexts, as indicated by five (or more) of the following:

1. Has a grandiose sense of self-importance (e.g., exaggerates achievements and talents, expects to be recognized as superior without commensurate achievements).
2. Is preoccupied with fantasies of unlimited success, power, brilliance, beauty, or ideal love.
3. Believes that he or she is "special" and unique and can only be understood by, or should associate with, other special or high-status people (or institutions).
4. Requires excessive admiration.
5. Has a sense of entitlement, i.e., unreasonable expectations of especially favorable treatment or automatic compliance with his or her expectations.
6. Is interpersonally exploitative, i.e., takes advantage of others to achieve his or her own ends.
7. Lacks empathy: is unwilling to recognize or identify with the feelings and needs of others.
8. Is often envious of others or believes that others are envious of him or her.

CLUSTER C (FEARFUL–ANXIOUS)

Dependent Personality Disorder

4. Has difficulty initiating projects or doing things on his or her own (because of a lack of self-confidence in judgment or abilities rather than a lack of motivation or energy).
5. Goes to excessive lengths to obtain nurturance and support from others, to the point of volunteering to do things that are unpleasant.
6. Feels uncomfortable or helpless when alone because of exaggerated fears of being unable to care for himself or herself.
7. Urgently seeks another relationship as a source of care and support when a close relationship ends.
8. Is unrealistically preoccupied with fears of being left to take care of himself or herself.

Obsessive–Compulsive Personality Disorder

A pervasive pattern of preoccupation with orderliness, perfectionism, and mental and interpersonal control, at the expense of flexibility, openness, and efficiency, beginning by early adulthood and present in a variety of contexts, as indicated by four (or more) of the following:

1. Is preoccupied with details, rules, lists, order, organization, or schedules to the extent that the major point of the activity is lost.
2. Shows perfectionism that interferes with task completion (e.g., is unable to complete a project because his or her own overly strict standards are not met).
3. Is excessively devoted to work and productivity to the exclusion of leisure activities and friendships (not accounted for by obvious economic necessity).
4. Is overconscientious, scrupulous, and inflexible about matters of morality, ethics, or values (not accounted for by cultural or religious identification).
5. Is unable to discard worn-out or worthless objects even when they have no sentimental value.
6. Is reluctant to delegate tasks or to work with others unless they submit to exactly his or her way of doing things.
7. Adopts a miserly spending style toward both self and others; money is viewed as something to be hoarded for future catastrophes.

DSM-IV-TR	Diagnostic Criteria for Personality Disorders: Clusters A, B, C	
	CLUSTER B (DRAMATIC–EMOTIONAL) *Narcissistic Personality Disorder* **9.** Shows arrogant, haughty behaviors or attitudes.	**CLUSTER C (FEARFUL–ANXIOUS)** *Obsessive–Compulsive Personality Disorder* **8.** Shows rigidity and stubbornness.
	Antisocial Personality Disorder There is a pervasive pattern of disregard for and violation of the rights of others occurring since age 15 years, as indicated by three (or more) of the following: **1.** Failure to conform to social norms with respect to lawful behaviors as indicated by repeatedly performing acts that are grounds for arrest. **2.** Deceitfulness, as indicated by repeated lying, use of aliases, or conning others for personal profit or pleasure. **3.** Impulsivity or failure to plan ahead. **4.** Irritability and aggressiveness, as indicated by repeated physical fights or assaults. **5.** Reckless disregard for safety of self or others. **6.** Consistent irresponsibility, as indicated by repeated failure to sustain consistent work behavior or honor financial obligations. **7.** Lack of remorse, as indicated by being indifferent to or rationalizing having hurt, mistreated, or stolen from another.	

Source: Reprinted with permission from the *Diagnostic and statistical manual of mental disorders,* 4th ed., Text Revision (pp. 694, 697, 701, 706, 710, 714, 717, 721, 723, 725, 729). Copyright 2000 American Psychiatric Association.

ality-disordered people display enduring, inflexible, and pervasive maladaptive behaviors in a broad variety of personal, occupational, and social situations, they may or may not view their lifestyles as abnormal or intrusive. They may not seek professional help unless there is extreme external stress and/or internal distress (APA, 2000).

Personality disorders may coexist with extreme psychopathology, considered under DSM-IV-TR Axis I groupings. In addition, under stress, the individual with a personality disorder may progressively deteriorate even to the point of psychosis.

Biopsychosocial Theories

As the individual experiences life, adaptive-defensive operations solidify, ultimately resulting in an automatic response style. When the response style is based on misperceived or distorted object relations, a personality disorder may develop. Given these premises, the psychiatric nurse using a biopsychosocial model views clients with personality disorders as people whose communication and behavior are greatly influenced by past experiences, a need to maintain self-direction and control, and a unique style of interpreting their world.

BIOLOGIC FACTORS

Recent literature points to genetic and biologic factors in the development of some personality disorders.

Biologic factors associated with personality-disordered individuals as reported by Kaplan and Sadock (2000) include alterations in hormone levels and platelet monoamine oxidase (MAO) levels, smooth-pursuit eye movements, levels of endorphin and 5-HIAA (a metabolite of serotonin), and electroencephalographic (EEG) changes. Listed below are key research findings regarding biologic factors that may influence the development of various PDs:

- Magnetic resonance imaging (MRI) in female clients with borderline personality disorder (BPD) showed a reduction in the volume of the hippocampus and the amygdala (Driessen et al., 2000).

- Bohus, Landwehrmeyer, and Stiglmayr (1999) hypothesize that an increased activity of the opioid system contributes to dissociative symptoms, such as flashbacks, in BPD.
- Goodman and New (2000) state that the underlying biologic basis for impulsive aggression is related to serotonin levels. They hypothesize that impulsive aggressive behaviors (including physical aggression toward others, suicide attempts, self-mutilation, and substance abuse) exhibited by individuals with BPD are affected by serotonin. The positive response of some individuals with BPD to selective serotonin reuptake inhibitors (SSRIs) seems to validate this hypothesis.
- People with schizotypal personality disorder show reductions in temporal lobe volume with resultant cognitive impairment in areas of memory, verbal learning, and attention (Kirrane & Siever, 2000).
- Kaylor (1999) questions whether biologic differences are the cause or the effect of problematic behaviors associated with antisocial personality disorder.

Recent literature addresses the role of biologic factors in the genesis of BPD. Hormones are being implicated to the extent that increased levels of testosterone, 17-estradiol, and estrone have been observed in people with impulse control problems. Dexamethasone suppression test (DST) findings have also been abnormal in some people with depressive symptoms, who are diagnosed with BPD. The serotonin metabolite 5-HIAA has been shown to be low in people who attempt suicide and in those with aggression and impulse control problems (Kaplan & Sadock, 2000).

GENETIC THEORIES

Riso, Klein, Anderson, and Ouimette (2000) indicate that there are increased rates of mood disorders and PDs in relatives of those with similar disorders.

Using studies from 15,000 pairs of monozygotic and dizygotic twins in the United States, Kaplan and Sadock (2000) identified significant familial correlations of schizotypal personality disorder (Cluster A) among people with family members who are schizophrenic. Cluster B illnesses (borderline, histrionic, narcissistic, and antisocial) are often correlated with histories of mood disorders, alcoholism, and somatization disorders among family members.

Parental deprivation; inadequate, excessive, or inconsistent discipline; and failure of the child to develop integrated cognitive, affective, and behavioral modes in early life may lead to Cluster B disorders. Clients have generalized feelings of low self-esteem, need to control people and situations, and are unable to delay gratification. In response, dramatic–emotional clients tend to interact by negatively manipulating others. Although manipulation is a standard response in the repertoire of people with these PDs, its occurrence escalates with increased stress.

Schizoid and schizotypal PDs are significantly more common among first-degree relatives of schizophrenic clients. At this time, however, there is no substantial evidence that these PDs are early indicators of a future schizophrenic process (Kaplan & Sadock, 2000).

Research indicates strong familial tendencies toward antisocial PD. It is more common among first-degree relatives; having a female biologic relative with the disorder tends to increase the risk. While adoption studies show that more genetic and environmental factors contribute to the risk, adopted children are at a higher risk for development of this psychopathology (APA, 2000).

PSYCHOSOCIAL THEORIES

Psychological fixations in the genital stage of development may account for many of the behaviors noted in some PDs. For example, it is developmentally appropriate for a toddler to expect immediate gratification of needs. However, many adults with PDs display developmental immaturity through an inability to postpone immediate gratification of needs and wants. Impulsive and self-centered behaviors are examples of this type of developmental fixation.

Separation–individuation is part of the psychodynamic basis of borderline personality disorder. Normal autism and symbiosis must occur before the separation–individuation process, referred to as "psychological birth," can begin. The inability to unify the "good and bad" objects into one whole is demonstrated by the inability to integrate the self as both "good and bad" or to separate or individuate from the maternal object.

The sense of self originates with the earliest parent–child interactions. If parents are not sensitive and attuned to the child's needs, they will fail to confirm the child's emerging sense of reality. Consequently, the child distorts reality and develops an unreal "as-if" personality that shifts to meet the demands of cues in the outer world.

Individuals with PDs have serious impairments related to establishing and maintaining healthy interpersonal boundaries. Intimacy is characterized by the ability to be close to another while maintaining a sense of separateness. Those with PDs generally have issues related to enmeshment and/or abandonment, which interfere with intimacy. **Enmeshment** refers to a feeling of being engulfed by others or of being overpowered by dominant others. Common signs of enmeshment include speaking for another person, answering for someone else, or responding to an event as another person would. **Abandonment** refers to feelings of being left alone; many people with PDs are vulnerable to feelings of abandonment as their sometimes bizarre, demanding behaviors push others away, resulting in alienation and isolation. Due to a fear of intimacy, some individuals will sabotage relationships by provoking rejection while simultaneously fearing rejection.

Erikson (1964) coined the term **identity diffusion** to describe the failure to integrate various childhood identifications into a harmonious adult psychosocial identity. Kernberg (1975) suggests that when, as infants, borderline clients perceive the parenting figure as both nurturing and punishing, the child learns to reduce anxiety and resolve resulting conflicts by the use of primitive defensive strategies including splitting, projective identification, primitive idealization, omnipotence, devaluation, and denial.

Another psychosocial factor influencing the development of PDs is chronic trauma. Extensive research has indicated that children who are sexually abused are vulnerable to developing

PDs in adulthood. According to Painter and Howell (1999), the child who is sexually abused experiences a pervasive anxiety that cannot be alleviated by coping methods usually employed by children. Such children often engage in self-destructive behavior in an attempt to feel better. Sexual abuse is significantly related to borderline personality symptomatology (Timmermann & Emmelkamp, 2001). A diagnosis of BPD is associated with early onset of abuse and high rates of physical and verbal abuse (Heffernan & Cloitre, 2000).

HUMANISTIC THEORIES

Individuals need to feel that they are a part of something greater. In their search for meaning, some individuals with personality disorder often engage in self-damaging acts. For example, after slitting her wrists with a razor, a client may state, "When I feel hurt, I feel real." While attempting to negate existential emptiness, the client actually threatens his or her own well-being.

NURSING PROCESS

Clients with Personality Disorders

Clinical manifestations of each PD are described in separate assessment sections (see the Nursing Self-Awareness feature). The remaining steps of the nursing process address all the PDs together.

Assessment: Odd–Eccentric Personality Disorders (Cluster A)

This cluster consists of the **paranoid, schizoid,** and **schizotypal personality disorders.** The major features of these disorders are pervasive distrust, social detachment, and subsequent impairment in social and occupational functioning.

People with odd–eccentric personality disorders have more cognitive style impairments, are the most peculiar, and reflect the most maladaptive defensive styles than do people with other types of PDs. See ■ Table 20–1 on page 486 for a description of characteristics of odd–eccentric personality disorders.

Nursing SELF-AWARENESS

Assessing Clients with PDs

When assessing clients with PDs, it is imperative that nurses:

- Remain aware of personal feelings.
- Maintain congruency between words and actions.
- Examine their own feelings and beliefs about helplessness, anger, and criminality.
- Be alert for personal susceptibility to flattery and compliments.
- Maintain professional distance by employing empathy.

PARANOID PERSONALITY DISORDER

Of the disorders in this group, the one most commonly seen in inpatient psychiatric settings is paranoid personality disorder (APA, 2000).

When conducting interviews with clients with paranoid personality disorder, it is very important to remember that behavior is culturally defined. Many individuals, particularly those from minority and/or immigrant groups, are erroneously labeled mentally ill because their behaviors are not congruent with the expected standards of the health care team. Indeed, the clinical evaluation may reinforce suspiciousness, hostility, and acting-out behavior because the client is unfamiliar with and frightened by the process. It is also important to remember that paranoid traits may be adaptive in threatening situations. The diagnosis of paranoid personality disorder should be made only when the behavior is long-standing, maladaptive, and causes significant distress (APA, 2000).

When interviewing a client who has paranoid personality disorder, maintain an open, nonthreatening style of questioning. Do not argue with or interpret the client's responses. Because these clients may hold grudges and are quick to attack, consider safety provisions for the staff as well as the clients.

Paranoid clients often report that others plot against them or attempt to use or deceive them. They will talk about disloyal friends and coworkers and the irreversible harm others' actions have caused. They may be surprised and mistrustful of loyalty shown to them. They may refuse to answer questions, saying, "This is no one's business." A frequent theme in client interviews is one of pathologic suspicion of spousal or partner infidelity. During the interview, grandiose, unrealistic fantasies often emerge; clients may discuss activities with others who share their beliefs, such as special interest groups or cults. Client affect may be labile with hostile, stubborn sarcasm predominant.

Suspiciousness and Mistrust. Suspiciousness and mistrust reflect an attitude of doubt toward the trustworthiness of objects or people. The suspicious person is usually preoccupied with being maneuvered, tricked, or framed. Suspiciousness is also a way of thinking and includes such manifestations as expectations of trickery or harm, guardedness, secretiveness, pathologic jealousy, and overconcern with hidden motives and special meanings. For example, the suspicious person may perceive a birthday gift as a trick to create an obligation. Legal disputes may arise from the client's response to perceived threats.

Rigidity. Paranoid people are inflexible in their perception of the world. They are preoccupied with their expectations of others and relentlessly try to confirm these expectations, often through argumentation. They closely examine arguments and information, with prejudice. The paranoid person justifies a position by excessive rationalization, rejecting any evidence that refutes the original notion. It is not unusual for a paranoid person to suspect people with opposing ideas. Paranoid clients go to great lengths to prove a point. The need to be in control is another characteristic, as is a preoccupation with one's rank

TABLE 20–1 Characteristics of Personality Disorders

Odd–Eccentric (Cluster A)	Dramatic-Emotional (Cluster B)	Fearful-Anxious (Cluster C)
Paranoid Personality Disorder	***Borderline Personality Disorder***	***Avoidant Personality Disorder***
Is pervasively and unjustifiably suspicious and mistrustful, as evidenced by jealousy, accusations of infidelity, and guardedness. Is hypersensitive and usually feels mistreated and misjudged. Restricts feelings, as evidenced by lack of humor, absence of sentimental or tender feelings, and pride in being cold and unemotional. Bears grudges and is quick to counterattack.	Is impulsive and unpredictable in areas of life that are self-damaging. Has unstable but intense interpersonal relationships involving manipulation of others. Displays temper inappropriately. Has unstable moods (including rage); is uncertain about identity, and may experience severe dissociative symptoms. May inflict physical damage on self. Has chronic feelings of boredom and emptiness. Fears abandonment.	Is hypersensitive to rejection and interprets innocuous events as ridicule. Is unwilling to become involved with others unless given a guarantee of acceptance. Withdraws socially in interpersonal and work roles; avoids new situations. Desires affection and acceptance, yet shows restraint in intimate situations for fear of ridicule. Feels inept and infuriated.
Schizoid Personality Disorder	***Histrionic Personality Disorder***	***Dependent Personality Disorder***
Is emotionally cold and aloof. Shows indifference to the praise or criticism of others. Has little or no desire for social or sexual involvement. Does not desire or enjoy close relationships. Has few friends.	Is overly dramatic and reactive, and responds intensely. Engages in attention seeking, self-dramatization, sexual provocation, and irrational outbursts of emotion. Is perceived by others as shallow, self-indulgent, and demanding. Uses appearance and style of speech to draw attention to self. Is suggestible and overrates the intimacy of relationships.	Passively allows others to assume responsibility for major areas of life. Subordinates own needs. Lacks self-confidence and initiative. Has difficulty disagreeing with others. Fears being alone so urgently seeks a close relationship.
Schizotypal Personality Disorder	***Narcissistic Personality Disorder***	***Obsessive–Compulsive Personality Disorder***
Manifests various oddities of thought, perceptions, speech, affect, and behavior, such as ideas of reference, bizarre fantasies, and preoccupations. Is suspicious and hypersensitive to real or imagined criticism. Isolates self from society because of acute discomfort.	Has grandiose sense of self-importance. Is preoccupied with fantasies of unlimited success, power, beauty, brilliance, etc. Needs attention and admiration. Shows an arrogant attitude based on feelings of entitlement and envy. In relationships with others, expects special favors. Takes advantage of others; shifts between overidealizing others to disregarding them. Lacks ability for empathy.	Is overconscientious, overmeticulous, and perfectionistic. Is excessively concerned with conformity. Adheres rigidly to strict standards of morality and values. Is preoccupied with trivial details, rules, schedules, and lists. Keeps worthless objects. Is unable to delegate without control. Is miserly and stubborn.
	Antisocial Personality Disorder	
	Engages in behavior that causes conflict with society, such as theft, vandalism, fighting, delinquency, truancy, lying. Is unable to sustain consistent work or to function as a responsible parent or spouse. Cannot maintain an enduring attachment to a sex partner. Lacks respect and loyalty; is irritable and aggressive. Manipulates others for personal gain, does not plan ahead, lacks guilt, does not learn from past experiences, blames others. Disregards the safety of self and others.	

and status. The need to be self-sufficient may result in difficulty working with others.

Hypervigilance. Hypervigilance is an increased state of watchfulness in which the person is always on guard and unable to relax. Constant sensitivity to nuances in social relations, interpretation of both open and hidden attitudes of others, and scrutiny are modes of operation.

Distortions of Reality. Although paranoid people perceive facts accurately, they may attribute a special significance to the events. In this way, they create a private reality. They have a special interest in hidden motives, underlying purposes, and special meanings. They do not necessarily disagree with the average observer about the existence of any given fact, only about its meaning and significance. Therefore, even severely paranoid people can recognize various essential facts well enough to achieve a limited adjustment to the normal social world. They often have difficulty distinguishing real from imagined offenses (see the Rx Communication feature). The individual's distorted attitudes antagonize others and may lead to real discrimination.

CLINICAL EXAMPLE

Ellen is a paranoid woman who is quick to detect signs of anger, jealousy, and rejection in the actions of her coworkers. She magnifies these negative aspects and overlooks such positive behaviors as humor, support, and empathy. Eventually, Ellen's coworkers begin to snicker when she makes public statements, and they gossip about her.

Projection. People who are paranoid attribute their own intolerable motivations, drives, or feelings to others. Projection is used to attribute to others the evil intentions that they themselves feel. In this way, the idea that one may be harmed really reflects the individual's own wish to harm others.

CLINICAL EXAMPLE

Nancy's idea that her boyfriend is seeing another woman may reflect her wish to terminate their relationship.

Restricted Affect. Labile emotional expressiveness and a lack of spontaneity characterize people with paranoid personality disorder. They often appear cold, humorless, and devoid of tender, sensitive feelings. Although they may demonstrate temper outbursts, they pride themselves on remaining objective and reasonable and frequently use intellectualization and rationalization to avoid affective experiences. Some paranoid people may appear friendly, but in fact this friendliness is a "script" that helps them adapt to social situations or achieve their goals.

Exclusion. Because of the paranoid person's antagonism and suspiciousness, tension develops between the person and significant others. The persistent strain on relationships causes others to define the paranoid person as more than simply "different." Instead, they see the individual as unreliable or untrustworthy, and others begin to interact according to their perceptions. These behaviors reinforce the suspicions and beliefs of the paranoid person. The effects of this process include:

- Blocked communication, which increases the process of exclusion.
- Emergence of a crisis, which formally excludes the paranoid person.
- Reinforcement of the paranoid person's beliefs, interpretations, or ideas of reference.

Because paranoid people are generally intelligent, persuasive, and creative in justifying their beliefs, these clients may adapt in one of two ways. They may join quasi-political groups, esoteric religions, cults, or quasi-scientific organizations that reinforce their interpretations of reality. Or they may join organizations that challenge societal norms and trends in an effort to direct and thus control hostile feelings.

CLINICAL EXAMPLE

Jim, a 39-year-old engineer, suspects that his employer is withholding significant data from him pertaining to an important job assignment. Jim began to question others about the reliability and integrity of his boss. Jim went to the plant one Sunday morning without authorization. A security guard found him going through the filing cabinets of his employer, who confronted him the following day and sent him to the employee assistance program nurse. During the interview, Jim states, "I knew he [the employer] was dishonest from the start. He never could give me a straight answer. As soon as I was almost on him, he sets me up to lose face and maybe my job."

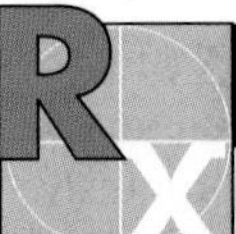

COMMUNICATION

Client with Paranoid Personality Disorder

CLIENT: "What did you mean by that remark? People are always making fun of me."

NURSE RESPONSE 1: "That remark was not meant for you, Jerry. It was directed at everyone in the group."

RATIONALE: This response provides a simple explanation without being argumentative or overly detailed in explanation. It is also reinforces reality for the client.

NURSE RESPONSE 2: "You feel others are laughing at you . . ."

RATIONALE: Encourages the client to verbalize feelings of mistrust. Is stated in a nonjudgmental manner by the nurse who maintains appropriate eye contact, which is a behavior that promotes trust.

MediaLink NIMH

Other behaviors characteristic of paranoid individuals are described at www.nimh.gov which can be accessed through the Companion Website for this book.

SCHIZOID AND SCHIZOTYPAL PERSONALITY DISORDERS

When assessing both schizoid and schizotypal clients, it is imperative to consider the person's ethnicity, cultural milieu, and spiritual belief system. Within many cultures, speaking in tongues, rooting, voodoo, and psychic phenomena are natural experiences and should not be deemed pathologic. People who are making a transition from one environment to another—from a rural to an urban setting, for instance—may seem different because of their constricted affect and solitary activities. Immigrants must be assessed from a multicultural viewpoint in order to differentiate between lack of understanding and indifference. What may seem odd in Parker, Georgia, may be commonplace in New York City.

Individuals who are diagnosed with schizoid personality disorder are rarely seen in clinical settings, but schizotypal personality disorder is found in about 3% of the population. These clients are frequently treated for symptoms associated with anxiety, depression, or dysphoric affect. Clients in both categories may experience transient psychotic episodes which may last a few minutes to several hours (APA, 2000).

Clients with schizoid personality disorder claim to enjoy being alone and to prefer occupations where there is minimal social interaction. They may decline job promotions because social demands (i.e., meetings, supervisory responsibilities) accompany the change. When asked if they think this loner-type behavior is unusual, a typical response is, "I never thought about it much . . . it doesn't much matter to me." Accompanying disclaimers about social needs, schizoid clients acknowledge that they rarely become excited, angry, upset, or joyful.

In contrast, clients with schizotypal personality disorder report a great deal of subjective anxiety in social situations. They report bizarre fantasies, especially of paranormal events. During an interview, they may remark, "I know what you're going to ask me before you say it," believing they are endowed with special powers or have the ability to control others' behavior by simply "willing it to happen." Often, these clients have speech patterns that are so loose, digressive, or vague that an interview is difficult to conduct. The client may acknowledge this behavior by stating, "I was never talkable" (APA, 2000).

While indifference is a hallmark of the schizoid personality, suspicion, including paranoid ideation, is noted in the schizotypal client. Maintaining eye contact may be difficult during the interview, and interviewing strategies such as humor to defuse anxiety may be met with a stare and questions about the meaning of or purpose for the joking.

Onset of schizotypal PD is believed to be in childhood or early adolescence, as clients report poor academic achievement and peer relationships as well as social anxiety, even as children. When questioned about sexual activity, clients with both types of PDs usually deny interest in or involvement in intimate relationships.

People with schizoid and schizotypal personality disorders generally have a detached and aloof social style. The schizotypal personality, however, has more cognitive impairments than the schizoid personality does. There is a range of adjustment in clients with these personality disorders. Some are fairly well-adjusted individuals who are loners; others live out their lives in protective environments, such as group homes, mental hospitals, and prisons.

Social Isolation. Clients with schizoid and schizotypal PDs show a preference for solitary interests and occupations. They have a history of being loners and neither desire nor enjoy close relationships. Friends and confidants are not part of their lifestyle. They are indifferent to feedback and insensitive to others. These clients will choose solitary hobbies such as solitaire and computer games, and jobs such as night security guard or bridge worker. The detachment from social relationships is also noted in the schizoid or schizotypal personality-disordered client's lack of interest in having intimate or sexual relationships.

Blunted Affective Response. Clients may appear cool, aloof, humorless, "in a fog," or bored, and may seem to be cognitively impaired. These individuals appear "joyless" and are slow to anger.

Detachment. Clients with schizoid and schizotypal PDs appear absent-minded: They daydream, are vague about goals, are indecisive, and lack social skills. They do not respond in a usual manner to social cues and may seem like social misfits.

The schizotypal personality-disordered client demonstrates eccentricities in communication and behavior not seen in a person with schizoid personality. Examples include such oddities of thought as magical thinking and ideas of reference; altered perceptions, such as illusions, depersonalization, and derealization; speech alterations, including circumstantiality (giving detailed, factual but nonessential information), digression, metaphoric speech patterns, and overly concrete or abstract responses; and an odd or unkempt manner of dress, which includes ill-fitting, stained, and mismatched clothing.

Assessment: Dramatic–Emotional Personality Disorders (Cluster B)

The DSM-IV-TR identifies the **borderline, histrionic, narcissistic,** and **antisocial personality disorders** as dramatic, emotional, erratic dysfunctions. Individuals with these disorders are often in conflict with society because of their impulsive behavior. Impulsivity is the common factor in all four Cluster B disorders (Looper & Paris, 2000). Impulsive people view the world as a discontinuous, fragmented collection of opportunities, frustrations, and affective experiences. They live only in the present moment and lack the ability to formulate long-range plans. They act decisively without critical evaluation of consequences. The focus of their intellectual and emotional goals is to achieve immediate gain and satisfaction. This lack of impulse control and inability to delay gratification often result in both verbal and nonverbal outbursts of anger, which may be self-directed or other-directed. Indeed, clients with dramatic–emotional personality disorders may experience rapid escalation of anxiety when their own angry impulses are not controlled by others. Table 20–1 on page 486 provides a description of the Cluster B personality disorders. Also see the Assessment box below.

Traditionally, individuals with BPD have been considered to be bordering between reality and psychosis. It is common for such clients to experience psychotic breaks from reality when severe stress is experienced. Often, individuals with BPD will also have other coexisting mental disorders (i.e., depression, anxiety disorders). According to Schneidt (2000), most clients who have BPD have had a diagnosis of at least one Axis I disorder and an average of three PDs. Prevalence of this disorder is about 2% of the general population (APA, 2000).

Instability or Unpredictability. Impulsiveness may be expressed in self-damaging ways, demonstrating a lack of responsibility and disregard for the consequences of the behavior. "I just told my boss to take this job and shove it" may be the response to a work situation that is perceived as intolerable. "I just got another credit card with a $5,000 limit, so I don't have to worry about going over the limit on my other three cards." "I only drink wine when I'm driving, so I don't worry about DUIs." "I don't worry about AIDS; all my partners come from the high-rent districts, so they are clean and safe." Responses such as "I did it; I don't know why I did it, I just did" are common when clients are questioned about the reasons for particular actions.

The individual with BPD has fluctuating responses in situations that are subjectively interpreted and often distorted. Impulsiveness is manifested in spending habits, sexual promiscuity, substance use, abnormal eating habits, shoplifting, and frequent job changes.

ASSESSMENT

Guidelines for the Client with Dramatic–Emotional Personality Disorders

- Labile affective responses
- Intense episodes of anger/rage
- Self-centeredness/egocentricity
- Unstable personal relationships
- Superficiality, exploitiveness, and manipulativeness
- Lack of empathy for others
- Inability to postpone gratification
- Boredom or need for constant attention
- Poor judgment
- Failure to learn by experience
- Failure to assume responsibility for behavior
- Poorly integrated sexual identity
- Ability to test reality and absence of major thought or affective disorders

Unstable Interpersonal Relationships. Clients relate stories of "one-night stands" in search of the perfect partner. Any real or perceived threat of abandonment results in the client's "switching" to another partner. "He's never there when I need him" may be used in conjunction with "I always see to it that his shirts are ironed and his dinner is ready when he gets home from work." These clients need a payback in return for any giving they do. The failure to resolve the separation–individuation process described by Mahler, Pine, and Bergman (1975) is reflected in the person's attitudes toward self and others.

Interpersonal relationships may include such behaviors as:

- Manipulation of others.
- Pitting individuals against one another.
- Intense attachment.
- Explosive separations.
- Sudden shifts in attitude toward others perceived as good or bad.
- Clinging, demanding.
- Controlling, exploitative.
- Sadism or masochism in close relationships.
- Relationships motivated by a need to avoid being alone rather than the need to be with others.
- Lack of empathy.
- Diminished capacity to evaluate others realistically.
- Transient, superficial relationships.

Intense Anger. Borderline clients tend to instigate problems as they become involved in therapeutic relationships. The anger may manifest itself in accusations, frequent displays of temper, inability to control anger (acting-out), irritability, sarcasm, argumentativeness, devaluing others, and overreaction to minor irritants.

These clients are unable to tolerate their own "bad" image and project it onto others, often raging at the perceived attributes of the other. Anger tends to be greatest toward those people who remind them of a nurturing/frustrating parent. "I can't stand that fat slob of a nurse. She acts like God went on vacation and appointed her to substitute for Him." "So what if I yell when I get angry; I'm paying a lot of money to be here. If you don't like it, leave."

Identity Diffusion. Clients with BPD display behaviors that show confusion about values and goals in life. These clients are described as chameleon-like because they are constantly changing their behavior to match the behavior of those around them. An intense fear of rejection causes borderline individuals to say what they think others want to hear and to behave in a manner that they believe will win them popularity or special favors (see the Rx Communication feature on page 490). It is difficult to determine what the borderline individual really thinks or feels. These clients cannot genuinely experience feelings and emotions; their core personality is hollow. They do not assume responsibility for their actions but project blame and credit onto others.

Problems of identity diffusion are also apparent in the areas of sexual intimacy and gender identity. Sexual intimacy is disturbed as a result of the person's fears of being engulfed and

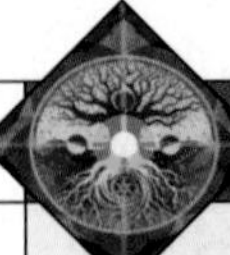

Case Study

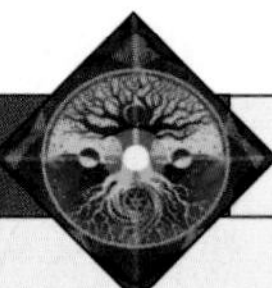

Client with Borderline Personality Disorder

Identifying Information

Wendy is a 27-year-old divorced woman who was admitted to the hospital after threatening to commit suicide. Wendy is a dental hygienist who has been employed for 6 months. Her employer confronted her 1 week ago about her rapid mood swings, irritability, and absenteeism related to chemical dependence.

Wendy states that she does not need to be on a psychiatric unit because she really was not going to kill herself; she was merely looking for some attention. She states that her employer is jealous that the male patients are attracted to her. She thinks it is unfair that her employer asked her not to see patients socially after hours. She also stated that her employer was jealous of Wendy's physical appearance and decided to have her treated for an alcohol problem that Wendy denies having. Wendy states that she only drinks to unwind.

History

Wendy reports a history of being unable to relate well with previous female employers. She prefers the company of men, even though she states she was abused physically and sexually as a child. Wendy does state that she began drinking more often after her second abortion.

Current Mental Status

The mental status assessment shows Wendy to be hyperactive. She is oriented to time, place, and person. Her judgment is impaired, and her affect is labile. Mood swings alternate between crying and excessive smiling. She denies delusions or hallucinations. Her speech is clear and coherent, though pressured at times. Wendy states she is being treated unjustly and blames others for her hospitalization.

destroyed or abandoned by another. An approach–avoidance conflict emerges as a consequence of the parent having thwarted independence and rewarded dependent behavior. As a result, the borderline client develops two major fears: the fear of abandonment, which leads to clinging behavior, and fear of engulfment, which leads to distancing from others. The client desperately wants intimate relationships but is terrified of losing the self. These fears are reminiscent of the early choice between parent's love and autonomy, which is the core of the borderline conflict. This conflict is managed by using the primitive dissociation defense, also called **splitting**, which can best be described as the inability to integrate contradictory experiences. Splitting is based on dichotomous thinking, a cognitive distortion in which the person has an "all-or-none" mentality about others; people are viewed as either all "good" or all "bad."

Gender identity disturbance may be manifested by the selection of rejecting or abusive partners, the preference for homosexual relationships while maintaining a heterosexual lifestyle and bizarre fantasies.

Another area of identity diffusion is temporal discontinuity, which is manifested by a searching for one's origins or keeping detailed chronologic journals. Borderline individuals seem unable to integrate past, present, and future into a continuum. They may frantically plan for the future while reminiscing about past events. These behaviors often lead to difficulty in choosing long-term goals, making career choices, and reassessing personal values. "I can't make up my mind if I should stay in nursing or try interior design" (after completing 1 year in a 2-year nursing program). "I feel so totally empty inside. I burned my wrist with the cigarette just to see if I could still feel."

Affective Instability. The failure to resolve object permanence issues is also related to the inability of the borderline person to maintain a consistent, satisfying, affective state. Characteristic of this individual are intense fluctuations of mood, normally of short duration (a few hours or a few days); intense, discrete episodes of depression with accompanying suicidal ideation and gestures; and hypomanic or elated episodes. "Of course I knew I wouldn't kill myself when I took those pills—do you think I'm stupid or something?" "I only told him [partner] I was HIV-positive to see if he really cared for me as much as he said."

Feelings of Emptiness and Aloneness. Individuals with borderline personality disorder report hollow, empty feelings, lack of peaceful solitude, a sense of being disconnected, and anhedonia (absence of pleasure in performing ordinarily plea-

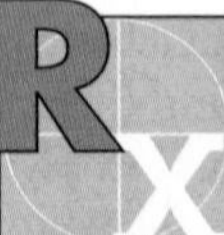

COMMUNICATION

Client with Borderline Personality Disorder

CLIENT: "You're the sweetest nurse on the unit. I know you can help me get a pass for next Friday."

NURSE RESPONSE 1: "Darlene, whenever you compliment me, you usually want something from me."

RATIONALE: Confronting the client on her manipulative behavior will help the client identify maladaptive approaches. If the nurse fails to confront the behavior consistently, the clients will assume the behavior is tolerated and acceptable.

NURSE RESPONSE 2: "Darlene, when you compliment people because you want something from them, they are not likely to trust anything you say."

RATIONALE: This response points out the negative consequences of the manipulative behavior. It encourages the client to consider other ways of interacting.

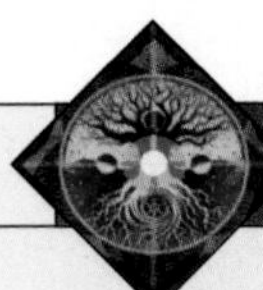

Nursing Care Plan

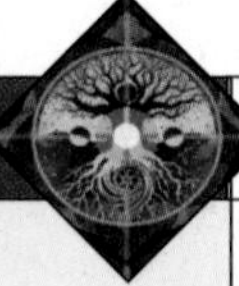

Nursing Diagnosis: Ineffective Coping related to inadequate level of confidence in ability to cope

Expected Outcome: Client will demonstrate the ability to self-control impulsive behaviors.

Short-Term Goals	*Interventions*	*Rationale*
• Client will verbalize decreased need to act impulsively.	• Point out incidences of impulsive behavior to client.	• Confrontation makes the client more aware of problematic behaviors.
	• Use active listening during all interactions with client.	• Active listening promotes expression of feelings
	• Assign nonjudgmental staff to work with client.	• A nonjudgmental approach helps client feel accepted and more willing to express feelings.
• Client will use relaxation techniques to control impulsive behaviors.	• Teach relaxation techniques (e.g., deep breathing, visualization).	• Anxiety interferes with the ability to plan ahead.
	• Have client demonstrate newly learned techniques.	• Demonstration and repetition reinforce learning.
• Client will demonstrate lower incidence of impulsive acts.	• Encourage client to state negative outcomes of impulsive behavior.	• Considering the negative consequences of behavior is an incentive to change.
	• Allow time for the client to modify old patterns of behavior.	• It takes time to change ingrained behaviors.
	• Set limits on client behavior to maintain safety.	• Setting external limits establishes boundaries for behavior that is appropriate and safe.

Nursing Diagnosis: Ineffective Coping related to manipulative attempts to control others.

Expected Outcome: Client will state needs directly and engage in active problem solving independently.

Short-Term Goals	*Interventions*	*Rationale*
• Client will demonstrate a decreased incidence of manipulative behaviors.	• Inform client of acceptable behaviors.	• Knowledge of expectations increases the likelihood of compliance.
	• Consistently enforce limits when client attempts to manipulate.	• Consistency reduces the effectiveness of manipulative attempts.
	• Avoid seeking client's approval.	• People-pleasing behavior provides opportunity for manipulation to occur.
	• Remain neutral to client's comments, being neither flattered nor offended.	• Flattery is a form of manipulation; using a matter-of-fact approach removes the effect of manipulative attempts.
	• Use group techniques to teach self-responsibility.	• Peer feedback is often effective in shaping behavior.
	• Avoid rescuing or rejecting client.	• Rescuing behaviors reinforce the client's sense of powerlessness and inadequacy; rejecting behaviors increase client's perception of threat. Both these behaviors lead to escalation of manipulation.
	• Provide feedback to client about the effects of his or her behavior on others.	• Awareness of consequences of behavior may serve as a catalyst to change.
• Client will demonstrate independence in daily activities.	• Encourage client to be independent while being available to help only when necessary.	• Providing assistance only when absolutely necessary encourages the client's self-reliance.

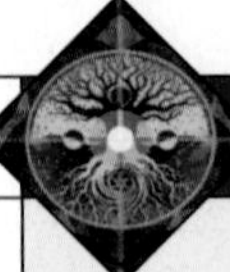

Nursing Care Plan

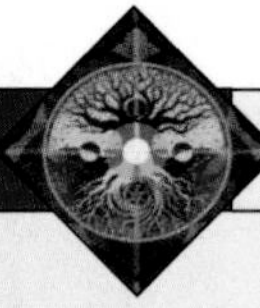

Short-Term Goals	Interventions	Rationale
	• Give positive reinforcement for achievement of goals.	• Encourages the development of a sense of mastery and boosts self-esteem.
	• Help client evaluate personal progress (e.g., through 1:1, group, journaling)	• Seeing progress encourages independence and success

Nursing Diagnosis: Potential for Self-Directed Violence related to intense rage.

Expected Outcome: Client will remain free from self-inflicted injury.

Short-Term Goals	*Interventions*	*Rationale*
• Client will verbalize feelings of anger and self-destructive ideation.	• Establish a trusting relationship with client.	• Encourages the expression of feelings.
	• Use a nonjudgmental attitude when client discusses suicidal/self-destructive thoughts.	• Promotes continued dialogue.
	• Assess history of previous suicidal/self-mutilating thoughts.	• Previous self-damaging acts increases the potential for such behavior to be repeated.
• Client will remain safe from harm.	• Inform clients that they are in a safe place and will be protected from self-harm.	• Decreases anxiety by providing reassurance.
	• Set limits on destructive behavior.	• External limits will maintain safety until the client learns inner control of impulses.
	• Implement safety precautions (e.g., close observation of behavior, searching client belongings for contraband, suicide precautions).	• To maintain client safety at all times.

surable acts). The person may attempt to combat these feelings by compulsive eating, drinking, drug abuse, sexual encounters, and self-mutilation. "I get depressed and I think about taking some pills, but then my boyfriend calls and we'll go out and I won't be depressed anymore."

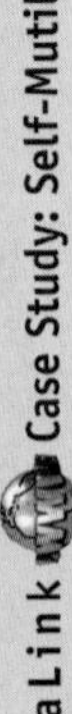

Self-Damaging Acts. Impulsiveness, together with identity disturbances, often leads to self-destructive behaviors. People with BPD are often depressed, but they may make self-destructive gestures to affirm their reality and relieve tension rather than to express a wish to die (see the Using Research Evidence feature). Self-damaging behaviors include self-mutilation (cigarette burns, cutting, taking drug overdoses), recurrent accidents, and physical fights. Self-mutilating clients are more likely to have severe boundary disturbances and use splitting than are other personality-disordered individuals (Fowler, Hilsenroth, & Nolan, 2000). "I don't see what's the big deal, so I tried to cut my wrists a couple of times—doesn't everybody?" "Yeah, I vomit after I eat; it keeps my weight down and I still get to have all the desserts I want."

Distortions of Reality. When identity diffusion reaches panic proportions, the borderline individual may experience the following:

- *Depersonalization:* feeling of strangeness or unreality about one's self.
- *Derealization:* feeling of disconnectedness from the environment.

CLINICAL EXAMPLE

Steve has multiple cigarette burns but reports no pain or discomfort and smiles when the lesions are being cleaned and dressed.

HISTRIONIC PERSONALITY DISORDER

People with histrionic personality disorder (HPD) show a lifelong tendency for dramatic, egocentric, attention-seeking response patterns. Their seeming lack of sincerity and emotional commitment contributes to disturbances in interpersonal relationships. These people appear to be continually "on stage" and acting a role. Their extensive use of coping patterns based on repression, denial, and dissociation leads them to deal with problems as though they do not exist. More females than males are diagnosed with this condition.

As with other PDs, it is important to consider cultural and ethnic background. Approximately 3% of the general population are diagnosed with this disorder (APA, 2000).

USING RESEARCH EVIDENCE

Darlene is a 28-year-old woman admitted to an inpatient psychiatric unit from the emergency department where she was treated for a fractured arm, black eye, and multiple bruises as a reported result of being beaten by her boyfriend. She also had several superficial slashes on her wrists that she stated she made herself in order to "feel real." On this admission, Darlene is screaming hysterically, "Leave me alone. Just let me die because no one loves me." Darlene has been married three times and is currently in an abusive relationship with a man who sells drugs. "I hope you go to prison this time," Darlene yelled; however, she refuses to file criminal charges against him.

This is Darlene's fourth admission to the unit, where staff members are very familiar with her history. On the last admission, Darlene manipulated the staff through splitting. She told three nurses that they were "special" and the "only ones who ever really cared about me."

The treatment team has developed a plan of care for Darlene using the following approaches:

1. Staff members need to examine their own responses in order to confront any prejudice toward Darlene.
2. Priority will be given to preventing self-destructive behavior; this will involve one-to-one sessions, close observation, and the use of no-harm contracts.
3. The primary nurse will focus on establishing rapport with Darlene in order to improve opportunities for dialogue.
4. All staff will guard against the initiative to rescue Darlene from her problems.

This plan of care for Darlene is based on the following research:

Gunderson, J. G., & Ridolfi, M. E. (2001). Borderline personality disorder: Suicidality and self-mutilation. *Annals of New York Academy of Science, 932*, 73–77; Nehls, N. (1999). Borderline personality disorder: The voice of patients. *Research in Nursing & Health, 22*, 285–293.

CLINICAL EXAMPLE

Linda, a 33-year-old woman who is twice divorced, was observed at the outpatient clinic responding flirtatiously to male staff members. She was neatly groomed but dressed in a low-cut peasant blouse, a tight miniskirt, and bright red knee-high boots. When called by the female therapist for her appointment, Linda screamed that she had waited too long, complaining loudly about patients' rights to rapid treatment. She quickly captured the attention of others in the waiting room. Then Linda feigned dizziness and "fell" as she arose from her chair. During the ensuing session, Linda complained that several men had made passes at her on the bus. When the therapist failed to share her outrage, Linda accused her of being jealous. Linda terminated the interview at that point and left the office, slamming the door behind her and stating, "My problems are physical, and no one cares whether I live or die. You'll be sorry for treating me this way!"

Dramatic, Exhibitionistic, and Egocentric Responses. Responses are characterized by exaggerated emotional expression; craving for attention, activity, and excitement; overreaction to minor stessors; irrational emotional outbursts; and temper tantrums. "I need someone to see me right now. . . . What kind of physicians staff this emergency room—sadists?"

Dysfunctional Interpersonal Relationships. Histrionic clients constantly need love, reassurance, and validation of their existence because of their feelings of dependence and helplessness. For this reason, they have problems with significant relationships. These individuals are likely to manipulate others to hold on to a love object while being highly inconsiderate and lacking empathy.

CLINICAL EXAMPLE

Calling her current boyfriend at 3:00 in the morning, Mary says, "Oh, Jim, I couldn't sleep and I knew you would want to be with me, at least in spirit."

Impaired Sexual Expression. People with HPD are generally provocative and seductive and use sexual expression to manipulate and control others in relationships. Clients are often unaware of this flamboyance and how others perceive it. Individuals are often competitive with those of the same sex and seductive with members of the opposite sex. This personality disorder is more frequent in women than men, although men may express themselves in terms of their athletic prowess (APA, 2000). A potential problem is promiscuous sexual activity and risk of HIV transmission.

Disregard for the welfare and safety of others may be noted in sexual acting-out, including having intimate relationships with others on the unit. "I've been talking to the social worker about the need for conjugal visits; maybe now you'll understand how important it is to meet our biologic as well as our psychological needs."

Dysphoric Mood. Dysphoria is a sense of disquiet or restlessness. Histrionic clients may experience depression when their demands for attention and affection are not met. They may act out in a suicidal fashion in order to manipulate or coerce others. Often, these individuals behave frivolously, acting silly and making nuisances of themselves.

CLINICAL EXAMPLE

Client to spouse who is threatening to leave him: "If you won't stay with me, there's no point in living. You'll be very sorry you are doing this."

Cognitive Alterations. Clients with HPD are much more interested in creative or imaginative pursuits than in analytic or academic achievements. They tend to be impressionable and highly suggestible and tend to look to authority figures for magical solutions to problems.

Impaired Health Patterns. Regression and the development of somatic and/or dissociative disorders are frequent among histrionic people. These disabling symptoms may serve the purpose of calling attention to the person. Generally, the symptoms occur when an audience is present or when an unpleasant situation is anticipated. Substance use, depression, seizure-like activity, blackouts, falling, dizziness, or reactive psychoses may lead to hospitalization.

NARCISSISTIC PERSONALITY DISORDER

People with narcissistic personality disorder (NPD) have difficulty regulating self-esteem and, therefore, demand attention from others. Their self-evaluation is dependent on admiration and devotion from others. The constant desire to be the center of attention is based on a strong sense of entitlement; narcissistic people feel that they deserve to be treated in a special manner. When these needs for constant attention are unmet, the narcissistic person feels rejected and may retaliate through acting-out behavior. Characteristics most frequently observed include a sense of entitlement, interpersonal manipulations, lack of empathy, and indifference toward others.

About 1% of the general population has NPD, and it is increasing steadily. Of those diagnosed, 50% to 75% are male (APA, 2000). There may be a higher than usual risk in children of narcissistic parents who impart to them an unrealistic sense of omnipotence, grandiosity, beauty, and talent (Kaplan & Sadock, 2000). While narcissistic traits are quite common (and developmentally appropriate) in adolescents, they do not necessarily go on to develop NPD (APA, 2000).

Grandiosity. Grandiosity is evidenced by expressions of exaggerated self-importance, self-absorption, and egocentricity. This inflated self-concept may be a compensation for feelings of diminished self-worth. Isolating a child from the feedback of others and the parents' failing to mirror the child's behavior may contribute to this disorder. Mirroring or "mirror images" reflect what the parents think of and how they treat the child. When coming in contact with people outside the home, the child may discover a discrepancy between the way others treat him or her and the mirror images developed at home. Excessive boasting may result from this inconsistency in self-concept. Humility is not a characteristic of people with NPD.

Exhibitionism. Exhibitionistic behavior is evidenced by the constant seeking of support and admiration from others. Because of their limited interests, these clients boast about themselves to the point of boring others. Concern over declining physical attractiveness and occupational limitations may lead them to seek cosmetic surgery.

Labile Affective Response. In spite of the narcissistic individual's extensive use of rationalization for failures, there is an underlying sense of rage, shame, and diminished self-esteem. The perceptive nurse may observe cool indifference, emptiness, humiliation, uncontrolled anger, or desire for revenge. They lack empathy for others, especially those who are perceived to be of lower status.

Dysfunctional Interpersonal Relationships. Clients with NPD feel entitled to special favors and attention. Further, they refuse to assume mutual responsibilities in relationships. They tend to exploit others and disregard their rights. Kernberg (1975) emphasizes that chronic, intense envy and defenses against envy lead to idealization or devaluation of others. Responses to others may include lack of concern, mistrust, lack of intimacy, accusations of incompetence, and demand for unattainable perfection. They see interpersonal relationships as a means of enhancing their own self-esteem. A narcissistic person often will select a spouse or a mate who will be dutiful and subservient in return for assurances of security and faithfulness.

Impaired Sexual Expression. Perverse sexual fantasies and promiscuity may be associated with this disorder. There may be confusion regarding sex-role behavior.

CLINICAL EXAMPLE

Alicia is a 40-year-old teacher who seeks professional counseling after dropping out of a graduate program. Alicia makes it clear on initial contact that she has a wide circle of friends. Indeed, she devotes the first 30 minutes of the session to recounting sexual encounters and venting anger that concern about AIDS is limiting her sex partners. She states she had a live-in relationship with one partner for 15 years but that recently this partner became discontented with her need to "party." Consequently, the two are not "communicating." Alicia defends her desire to seek out a variety of partners by focusing on her personal needs and the "lack of consideration" of her significant other.

When questioned about dropping out of graduate school, Alicia rationalizes her failure by blaming it on a "hostile major professor" and further proclaiming "I know more than he does." She describes herself as the "leader" in her group of six graduate students and interprets this to mean that they have great respect for her.

She tells the therapist that she attempted to call two friends following her withdrawal from school. She dramatically and self-righteously expresses anger and disappointment that they were not available to her. (One was vacationing out of state and the other was hospitalized for major surgery.) When the therapist inquired how her friend was doing following surgery, Alicia responded, "How in the world should I know? That's not my problem. She never even bothered to call me back."

Alicia requests that the therapist set up Saturday morning appointments (no office hours were normally scheduled on this day) because she becomes very tired in the afternoons and always takes a nap. When the therapist refuses to meet this request, Alicia becomes angry and shouts, "You're just like all the rest of them. No one considers my needs! I'll see to it that your supervisor hears about this, and I'll let all my friends know how incompetent you are as a therapist."

ANTISOCIAL PERSONALITY DISORDER

Antisocial personality disorder (ASPD) was one of the earliest to be identified. It has been labeled *psychopathy*, *sociopathy*, *dyssocial disorder*, and *moral insanity*. Most people with ASPD do not seek medical help but often come to the attention of authorities because of criminal activity that leads to judicial commitment to psychiatric facilities or incarceration in correctional facilities for treatment.

Manipulation, which is a hallmark of the antisocial client's behavior, may be a normal, nondestructive mode of meeting one's needs. However, when used to control others, manipulation interferes with interpersonal relationships. In antisocial clients, the drive to manipulate others is paramount, because these clients feel a need to be "number one" at all times.

In clinical settings, 3% to 30% of the population may have this disorder. Higher prevalence rates are found in substance abuse treatment centers and forensic settings (APA, 2000).

In contacts with antisocial people, you may find them initially charming. They are often intellectually bright, conversationally glib, and they will tell you what you want to hear. Because they are so astute in identifying others' vulnerabilities, nurses are frequently amazed at the "empathy" they show for others. These behaviors are manipulative and are used to create a situation which the antisocial person can control.

During the initial interview, it is common for the person diagnosed with ASPD to refuse responsibility for admission to the mental health or forensic facility. In fact, this individual will probably claim that the victim of his or her actions is at fault; in addition no remorse will be shown. "Well, you know, the only reason I'm here is because those cops made a mistake and thought I was the one who was assaulting that woman. Actually I stopped to help her and she told them I was trying to rape her. You know if she hadn't parked her car in the mall garage, then she wouldn't have been at risk for an assault in the first place."

Manipulation may be evident in the client's attempt to form alliances with the staff. Once alliances are formed, splitting occurs and the client is in control. "You know, you are the only nurse on this unit who knows anything about the meds that we get. I always feel so safe when you are at the med station. You know when I really need my tranquilizers. The other nurses look at me suspiciously like I'm some kind of criminal. Thank God you're on duty tonight." This same client may tell the nurse on the following shift, "That night nurse does nothing but pass pills all night long; she never spends time with the patients or even tries to talk to them before she drugs them up. I think something should be done about her."

Impulsiveness is manifested in the client's making quick decisions without any regard for the consequences. "I'm going on pass right now; it doesn't matter if you discharge me AMA." Aggression may be shown in picking fights with other clients, often when the antisocial person feels a need for excitement or has not received sufficient attention from the staff. "Hey, if you guys would get more sports going for us here, we wouldn't be getting on each other's nerves so much."

Disregard for the welfare and safety of others may be noted in sexual acting-out, including having intimate relationships with others on the unit. "I've been talking to the social worker about the need for conjugal visits; maybe now you'll understand how important it is to meet our biologic as well as our psychological needs."

Lack of anxiety is notable with these clients, unless there is extreme external stress, in which case they may act out in ways that put them at high risk for accidents, physical injury, or suicidal acts. History of violence toward others is very common, including sex offenses (i.e., rape, child pornography, child molestation) and murder. These clients have histories of drug dealing and substance abuse, prostitution, homelessness, erratic job histories, and exploitive sexual relationships. While these individuals can identify correct and appropriate behavior, they do not believe that rules apply to them, only to others.

People with ASPD need immediate gratification in most situations but can delay rewards to the extent that they need planning time to achieve what they want. They are often admitted to mental health facilities for depressive symptoms, suicidal attempts, substance abuse, somatic disorders, and/or anxiety disorders.

MediaLink Learning from Clients: Antisocial PD Video

Assessment: Anxious–Fearful Personality Disorders (Cluster C)

According to the DSM-IV-TR, individuals who present primarily as anxious or fearful may be diagnosed with **avoidant**, **dependent**, or **obsessive–compulsive personality disorder**. Anxious–fearful people generally experience both social and occupational impairments as a result of their restricted affect, nonassertiveness, problems expressing feelings, unrealistic expectations of others, and impaired decision making and problem solving. The lifestyle of the anxious–fearful person is characterized by intense emotional repression and behaviors that are socially isolating and self-defeating. The behaviors of anxious–fearful personalities tend to overlap, and common features are described in Table 20–1 on page 486.

AVOIDANT PERSONALITY DISORDER

The essential feature of people with avoidant personality disorder (APD) is a pattern of social withdrawal along with a sense of inadequacy, and fear and hypersensitivity to potential rejection and shame. These people withdraw socially even though they avidly desire affection and acceptance. Their avoidant behavior results in visiting public places (movies, museums, and ballparks) simply to experience the presence of other people because they do not enjoy being alone. When in public places, however, they maintain a safe distance from others. For example, in a movie theater, one can be physically close to people without feeling that one's personal space is being invaded.

Avoidant people devalue their own achievements. They appear overly serious, humorless, and painfully shy. Speech is often slow, and they do not readily express feelings. Thought content is generally serious.

CLINICAL EXAMPLE

Mary Jane is a 27-year-old single female who sought counseling because of her feelings of loneliness and lack of friends. She describes herself as having grown up on a mid-western farm where she was "pretty much a homebody." In high school she made good grades but did not participate in any extracurricular activities. She studied library science in college and admits to receiving second-hand pleasure from reading about others' experiences. She is currently employed as a reference librarian in a large computer software company where she has minimal contact with other people. She says she wants to establish both male and female friendships but feels afraid that people will laugh at her. Mary Jane joined the company bowling team at the suggestion of a coworker but quit after the first evening because she felt she would "hold them back." Mary Jane rationalized her decision by stating, "I think I would be more comfortable pursuing an intellectual hobby."

DEPENDENT PERSONALITY DISORDER

The essential features of dependent personality disorder (DPD) include a pervasive, excessive, and unrealistic need to be cared for; fear of separation; lack of self-confidence; an inability to make decisions; and an inability to function independently. In sharp contrast to the avoidant person, dependent people cling to others and passively accept their dictates and leadership. Dependent people view themselves as "helpless" or "stupid" and seek out dominant others or objects to lean on for guidance, control, and support as well as for "permission" to behave (see the Rx Communication feature). They have difficulty initiating projects and function adequately only when assured of approval and supervision.

In dependent people, the normal symbiotic parent-child relationship has been excessively prolonged, impairing their capacity for thinking, feeling, and responding on their own. They believe they must be taken care of and consequently rely on others to mirror their feelings to them.

Dependent people subordinate their desires and needs to the wishes of others in order to maintain relationships. They often appear friendly, helpful, and indispensable. Indeed, they will volunteer for unpleasant tasks if they think it will be reciprocated with nurturing. When the dominant other or object is unavailable, or perceived as unavailable, dependent people experience intense anxiety. This may lead to feelings of unhappiness, anger, resentment, or depression. It is also noteworthy that significant others may eventually respond to dependent people with anger and resentment because of their continuous clinging and ingratiating behaviors.

Like people with other personality disorders, the dependent person may have multiple DSM-IV-TR Axis II diagnoses. DPD is among the most frequently reported of the personality disorders (APA, 2000).

The following example illustrates how a dependent client might behave.

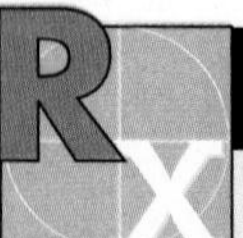

COMMUNICATION

Client with Dependent Personality Disorder

CLIENT: "You must help me right now! It's too hard for me to do by myself."

NURSE RESPONSE 1: "Nancy, in the past you have made your appointments very well on your own."

RATIONALE: This response reinforces the clients' sense of mastery by pointing out previous success.

NURSE RESPONSE 2: "Nancy, demanding help with tasks you can do for yourself will cause others to leave you alone. It's more effective to ask for help only with tasks that are really difficult for you."

RATIONALE: This response confronts the client with the clinging, demanding behavior and points out the results of such behavior.

CLINICAL EXAMPLE

Marie is a 40-year-old single parent of two teenage daughters. She has gained 70 lbs since her divorce 2 years ago. Currently, Marie is sporadically attending a group for displaced homemakers, where she has shared a great deal of information about herself. She states that she is essentially a "home-body" and feels most satisfied when baking, cooking, and sewing for her daughters. Marie describes her secondhand pleasure in their activities, including ballet, gymnastics, and modeling. In fact, Marie becomes visibly saddened when she discusses her daughters' eventual departure for college. When her daughters expressed concern about Marie's weight gain and general health, Marie giggled and said, "Better to be fat and jolly than skinny and mean."

Marie has made no attempt to develop new friendships or social outlets since her divorce. She is poorly groomed and haphazardly dressed, in contrast to her impeccably groomed daughters. When confronted by group members about setting priorities and the need to direct some energy toward herself, Marie responded, "My life is devoted to my daughters; their needs are more important than mine, and that's why I agreed to make the 30 costumes for their dance recital next week."

Nurses frequently avoid or voice dislike for dependent clients because of their cloying, clinging, and demanding behaviors. This avoidance response tends to reinforce the clients' perceptions that other people are unwilling to help and that they are unable to help themselves. As a result, clients increase their clinging responses because they know no other way to behave. This increased clinging only leads to further avoidance by others.

OBSESSIVE–COMPULSIVE PERSONALITY DISORDER

People with obsessive–compulsive personality disorder (OCPD) demonstrate anxiety and fearfulness by behavior that shows fear of losing control over situations, objects, or people. The obsessive-compulsive personality strives at all times to keep the world predictable and organized. The major features of this disorder are an excessive dedication to work, productivity, and perfectionism to the exclusion of feelings and pleasure. A person with OCPD may be likened to a drill sergeant in the military who is rigid, serious, detail-oriented, and stingy with emotions.

They tend to focus on trivial details. Although these people may be highly praised for their organizational skills and work ethic, eventually their rigidity causes them to fear making mistakes. Because they repeatedly check their work, they are not good time managers. Projects may not get completed. They are self-critical and adhere strictly and concretely to rules. Consequently, they postpone making decisions. They tend to resent authority but rarely express this resentment openly. Instead, they may engage in passive–aggressive behavior, such as procrastination and stubbornness.

Interestingly, excessively conscientious, rigid people often exhibit a contradictory pattern of slovenliness, which is also compulsive. Thus, a compulsive housewife may scrub her kitchen floor daily but allow bags of garbage to accumulate and become infested.

Because many cultures emphasize and positively reinforce adherence to a work ethic, it is important to consider cultural factors when assessing clients with OCPD. This disorder appears in males more often than females and in about 1% of the general population (APA, 2000). Nurses often experience a range of responses to obsessive–compulsive clients, including pity, disgust, anger, frustration, anxiety, and intense discomfort. Because anxiety may be contagious, it is wise to limit the duration of one-to-one sessions and make contracts with clients to avoid spending an entire session on obsessional material.

When clients with OCPD describe their lifestyle, you will quickly become aware of their rigidity, concreteness, and need for order and perfection.

CLINICAL EXAMPLE

John explained, "I have all my clothes hanging in the closet according to the day of the week, including my socks and underwear, so I know if it's a Tuesday after a long weekend with a Monday holiday that I need to wear the clothing on the hanger marked Tuesday."

To manage their procrastination, obsessive–compulsive people often initiate work on a project far in advance of the due date.

CLINICAL EXAMPLE

Peter set himself a deadline in early fall for ordering his family's Christmas gifts. His family found this deadline something of an annoyance. Yet Peter persisted in his attempts to get commitments from everyone about what they wanted. Often, he would mislay his early purchases by the time Christmas arrived, and he would rush out to do last-minute shopping anyway.

In the above example, Peter appears to be concerned with his family and interpersonal relationships, but he is really more concerned with meeting the Christmas deadline and checking off his list than in his relatives' enjoyment of their gifts. Although Peter suffers under the pressure of his deadlines, he sets them for himself. He functions as his own overseer, issuing commands, directives, reminders, warnings, and admonitions about what should be done.

People with OCPD are also keenly aware of other people's expectations, of the threat of possible criticism, of the weight and direction of authority, of rules, regulations, and conventions, and of a great collection of moral or quasimoral principles. They feel required to fulfill unending duties, responsibilities, and tasks that are, in their view, not chosen, but simply there.

Obsessive–compulsive people do not view taking work home and working long hours as an imposition, since work organizes their lives and binds their anxiety. Indeed, they will manage to make work out of pleasurable activities.

CLINICAL EXAMPLE

Jennifer planned her European vacation in meticulous detail. She scheduled exhausting daily tours and activities from 6:30 AM until 12:00 PM. Jennifer planned to visit every attraction available as quickly as possible. So as not to waste time, she wrote her postcards to her family while she rode tour buses. The cards were crammed with information about weather, prices of goods and services, menus, and daily time tables. She wrote nothing about how she felt or what she was experiencing. Upon returning home, she spent two weeks cataloging all her photographs and typing short paragraphs to accompany each photo. She passed her album around at work during lunch hour expecting that her coworkers would read all the captions. She became insulted and irate when several coworkers flipped through the album quickly. Jennifer found it difficult to forgive them for "slighting" her in this way.

Always consider how clients will react to the realization that years of denying themselves satisfaction, working hard, saving, and restricting the quality of life have not produced the expected rewards (e.g., career advancement, status, promotions). This realization often leads to the potential for depression, especially during middle life.

Nursing Diagnosis: NANDA

Effective nursing diagnosis depends on collection of accurate data in a thorough, organized assessment. There is much overlap of the problematic behaviors in the various types of PD. Nursing diagnoses are focused on the client's response to a disorder rather than on a specific diagnostic category. Since nursing is client centered rather than disease oriented, this section will describe the primary diagnoses for each type PD. There is frequent overlap in that individuals may have more than one PD at the same time.

The major nursing diagnoses for clients with odd–eccentric (Cluster A) PDs are:

- Ineffective coping.
- Impaired social interaction.

Individuals with dramatic–emotional (Cluster B) personality disorders are likely to experience:

- Chronic low self-esteem.
- Risk for self-directed violence.
- Risk for other-directed violence.

People with anxious–fearful (Cluster C) personality disorders often demonstrate:

- Social isolation.
- Defensive coping.

Note that the nursing diagnoses listed above may apply to a client with any type PD. They may also have several other diagnoses, based on their unique situations.

Outcome Identification: NOC

Expected outcomes must be individualized for each client considering the unique situations and cultural context. The major goal is that clients with odd–eccentric (Cluster A) PDs will interact with others in a socially appropriate manner. Specific outcomes that indicate progress toward achievement of this goal include:

- Participates in activity groups.
- Approaches staff and other clients without encouragement.
- Verbalizes thoughts and feelings that interfere with socialization.
- Identifies behaviors that maximize social interaction.
- Verbalizes trust in clients, staff, and family.

Wilkinson (2000, p. 93) has identified the following as appropriate expected outcomes for a client with odd–eccentric (Cluster A) type PD:

- Modifies lifestyle as needed.
- Seeks information concerning illness and treatment.
- Seeks professional help, as appropriate.
- Uses effective coping strategies.

Clients with dramatic–emotional (Cluster B) personality disorders have several issues that need to be resolved, such as improving self-esteem, controlling aggressive behavior, and learning to act in a less impulsive manner. Decreased impulsivity can be measured by the following expected outcomes:

- Identifies consequences of impulsive behavior.
- Verbalizes need to act less impulsively.
- Uses techniques to control impulsive behavior (e.g., deep breathing, counting to 10 before acting, taking a "time out" for decision making).
- Verbalizes control of impulses.
- Demonstrates a decreased incidence of impulsive acts (e.g., criminal acts, substance abuse, sexual promiscuity).

The following expected outcomes help measure the client's potential for violence directed at self and/or others:

- Identifies when feeling angry, frustrated, or aggressive.
- Verbalizes negative feelings appropriately.

- Formulates a contract in which the nurse is informed of the desire to act out destructively.
- Uses coping strategies to gain a sense of control over negative feelings.
- Demonstrates no abuse of self or others (Wilkinson, 2000, p. 515).

Expected outcomes that are relevant to self-esteem include the following:

- Acknowledges personal strengths.
- Identifies specific situations that evoke negative feelings or fears (e.g., failure, inadequacy).
- Verbalizes acceptance of self.
- Accepts compliments from others.
- Participates in decision-making and problem-solving activities.
- Demonstrates erect posture, eye contact, and grooming/hygiene (Copel, 2000, p 273; Wilkinson, 2000, p. 397)

Clients with anxious–fearful (Cluster C) PDs primarily need to develop more appropriate interpersonal relationships and learn to cope with stressors in a functional manner. Suggested expected outcomes include:

- Identifies feelings about threatening events and situations.
- Identifies the consequences of perfectionistic tendencies on relationships.
- Identifies feelings and beliefs that interfere with asking for help in an appropriate manner.
- Makes decisions independently.
- Demonstrates ability for self-care.

Planning and Implementation: NIC

This section describes interventions for specific behaviors that are prevalent in most people with PDs. The problematic behaviors addressed include manipulation, impulsiveness, impaired social interaction, aggression, self-destructive behavior, and chronic low self-esteem. See the Client/Family Teaching Guidelines feature.

MANIPULATION

Manipulation is pervasive in the life of someone with a PD. Therefore, it is difficult for most clients to change behaviors that are so ingrained. Learning to meet one's needs directly is the major challenge for those who demonstrate manipulative behavior. By establishing an interpersonal relationship with the personality-disordered client, the nurse will be better able to role-model appropriate behavior.

Splitting (playing one staff member against another) is a common manipulative ploy used by clients with PDs. A team approach is the only way to successfully counter this behavior. Ongoing communication with colleagues individually and in team meetings is imperative in order to know what the manipulative client is telling each staff member. Consistently responding to the manipulative behavior will gradually help it lessen in intensity.

A major intervention in dealing with manipulative behavior is limit setting. It is important to remember that limits are set on the behavior that is most dysfunctional and problematic. If limits are imposed globally, the client will only be more likely to rebel and the dysfunctional behavior will escalate. Limit setting is done for three fundamental reasons: (1) to prevent escalation of negative behavior, (2) to establish boundaries, and (3) to counteract resistance. Establishment of boundaries is done by providing consistent expectations and guidelines for self-control. Nursing interventions that provide structure encourage a sense of security in the client; thus, the need to manipulate is decreased. Trying to coerce a client to change is nontherapeutic and counterproductive. The use of confrontation and appropriate self-disclosure are techniques that may help reduce the client's resistance.

In addition to consistency and limit-setting, other strategies for dealing with manipulative behavior are teaching the client relaxation skills and encouraging the client to ask directly for what is needed instead of demonstrating the need through acting-out behavior. All of these approaches require commitment and patience from staff members, whether they are working on inpatient psychiatric or forensic units or in outpatient settings. See the Intervention box on page 500.

IMPULSIVENESS

Clients with PDs often act before thinking about the potential consequences of their actions. As a result, many clients find themselves in dangerous situations that could have been prevented with forethought and planning. Safety maintenance is a primary concern for health care providers working with impulsive clients. Helping clients learn to face the consequences of their own actions is difficult for some nurses who want to always protect clients. Implementation of consequences must

CLIENT / FAMILY **TEACHING**

Psychoeducation Guidelines for Clients with Personality Disorders

- Role-model assertive behavior.
- Teach client to develop strategies for confronting others in acceptable ways.
- Provide social skills training (cooking, money management) as needed.
- Teach problem-solving techniques, including goal setting, identifying alternative responses, and evaluating consequences.
- Teach stress-reduction techniques (i.e., guided imagery, relaxation).
- Provide instruction in cognitive behavioral techniques (i.e., thought stopping).
- Teach client how to use humor to reduce stress.
- Practice and/or role-play newly acquired skills.

INTERVENTION

Guidelines for Clients with Manipulative Behaviors

Nursing Intervention	Rationale
• Assign one staff member as primary resource person.	• Consistency prevents opportunities for splitting staff.
• Make limits realistic with enforceable consequences	• Unpleasant consequences may help decrease negative behavior.
• Give reasons for limits and consequences.	• Helps client make appropriate choices.
• Model respect, honesty, openness, and assertiveness	• Demonstrates expected behavior.
• Interact with client when client is not acting out.	• Reinforces positive behavior.
• Confront client each time manipulation occurs.	• Consequences must follow behavior closely.
• Discuss with the client alternative ways of dealing with people or situations.	• Promotes personal responsibility.
• Help client identify assets.	• Promotes self-esteem.
• Remove limits from treatment plan when client adheres to objectives consistently.	• Rewards appropriate behavior.
• Evaluate effectiveness of limit setting.	• Clarifies discharge planning goals.
• Jointly develop contracts for behavioral change.	• Establishes client responsibility.
• Offer support to other clients who may be targets of manipulation.	• Ensures safety of all clients.
• Teach stress-reduction techniques (guided imagery, relaxation, thought stopping; see Chapters 30 and 32).	• Defuses anxiety and reinforces ability for self-control.
• Involve client in assertiveness training and problem solving (see Chapter 1).	• Teaches assertion as opposed to aggression.

MediaLink Care Plan: Self-Destructive Behavior

be done consistently by all staff. Behavioral contracts can be useful for some clients in curbing their impulsive urges. The group setting is often a safe place for impulsive clients to learn to increase their capacity to tolerate frustration.

IMPAIRED SOCIAL INTERACTION

Whether it is the paranoid individual who mistrusts others, the borderline person who makes numerous demands, the antisocial person who exploits others, the obsessive–compulsive person who orders others about, or the dependent person with an excessive and unrealistic need to be cared for (see the Intervention box on page 501), dysfunctional interpersonal relationships are typical of persons with PDs. Confront the client's illogical perceptions of others as the first step in helping them to increase their capacity for intimacy. Establishing a therapeutic relationship with personality-disordered individuals is challenging as it goes against the basic nature of most personality-disordered clients to trust others and express their true feelings. It is helpful to start with a one-to-one interaction (see Chapter 28), then encourage the client to interact in a group setting (see Chapter 29). Assertiveness training is appropriate for helping clients differentiate aggressive, dependent, and healthy functional behaviors. Assertiveness involves learning how to say no and how to get one's needs met without violating others' rights. Remember to use a matter-of-fact approach when responding to the client. It is also important to provide feedback to the client about emotional cues sent to others (i.e., suspiciousness, contempt, intimidation). Role-play and group process are tools that are often useful in helping clients understand the impact of their behavior on others.

SELF-DESTRUCTIVE BEHAVIOR

As a result of impulsiveness and low self-esteem, many clients with PDs inflict harm on themselves. Such behavior is upsetting to some care providers. "Psychiatric patients who engage in self-destructive behavior by cutting, burning, or abrading their skin are currently one of the most difficult-to-treat groups in both inpatient and outpatient settings" (Fowler, Hilsenroth, & Nolan, 2000, p. 365). Never dismiss or negate a suicidal gesture as "just" attention-seeking behavior. All verbalizations of intent to harm oneself must be thoroughly assessed.

Milieu maintenance is one of the most effective nursing interventions in preventing client self-destructive behaviors. Physical safety precautions (i.e., locking doors, removing sharp objects) are some basic measures to ensure client safety. Establishing an environment that is psychologically safe is equally important. Nurses who demonstrate trustworthiness help clients feel more secure. Clearly explaining expectations and consequences for inappropriate behavior also adds to a sense of stability. Letting clients know that they are in a safe environment and will not be allowed to harm themselves is especially crucial for people with BPD. The use of no-harm contracts is therapeutic for some clients. This is an agreement between client and nurse that the client will contact the nurse whenever the feeling to hurt oneself is experienced. See Chapter 22 for more information on intervening with those engaged in self-destructive behavior.

AGGRESSIVE BEHAVIOR

Clients with paranoid personality disorder, antisocial personality disorder, and borderline disorder are those most likely to demonstrate aggressive behavior. Cluster B symptoms experienced during adolescence may increase the risk for violent behavior that persists into early adulthood (Johnson et al., 2000). It is important to help clients learn to differentiate anger and aggression. Anger is an emotion, and aggression is a behavior. Everyone is entitled to feel the way they feel; however, the way in which those feelings are expressed must be modified if harm is caused to others. Limit setting and assertiveness training are important interventions for helping clients learn to change aggressive acts to behavior that is appropriate. Another important facet of treatment is helping clients understand and appreciate the rights and needs of others; these concepts can be effectively taught in group settings.

INTERVENTION

Guidelines for the Client with Dependent Personality Disorder

Nursing Intervention	Rationale
• Evaluate client's ability to perform self-care activities; encourage grooming and personal hygiene.	• Fosters independent living skills.
• Avoid doing for the client those things the client is capable of doing without help.	• Promotes independence.
• Schedule regular sessions as a way to anticipate client needs *before* the client demands attention through inappropriate responses.	• Anticipatory guidance minimizes anxiety and acting-out.
• Help client identify assets and liabilities, including plans for change; emphasize strengths and potential.	• Self-assessment can enhance a positive self-concept.
• Encourage client to take responsibility for own opinions; point out when client negates own feelings or opinions.	• Fosters independence.
• Share with client your observations of client's manipulative behavior.	• Feedback from staff and peers fosters self-awareness.
• Set realistic limits on what should and should not be done for the client.	• Minimizes client dependence on others.
• Explore with client the consequences of behavior (e.g., clinging tends to result in avoidance by others).	• Increases client's self-awareness.
• Discuss personal responsibilities and the fact that client has choices.	• Choices optimize independent functioning.
• Give positive reinforcement for successful achievements.	• Reinforces client's ability to succeed.

It is important to avoid personalizing the client's aggression. "Taking it personally" increases the nurse's defensiveness, which in turn increases the client's perception of threat and can result in escalation of inappropriate behavior. Nurses who personalize clients' behavior lose their professional credibility. It is helpful to look at clients' inappropriate behavior as a clinical manifestation of a disorder instead of an act deliberately intended to harm the nurse.

When working with aggressive clients, safety is of utmost importance. Clients with PDs are at high risk of hurting themselves or others. See the Intervention box on page 502. See also Chapter 34.

CHRONIC LOW SELF-ESTEEM

A common thread in PDs is a pervasive sense of inferiority. Nursing interventions aimed at helping clients develop higher levels of self-esteem is appropriate for all those with PDs. It is important to confront clients' negative beliefs about themselves and help clients learn to replace the thoughts with more realistic ones. Cognitive behavioral techniques (such as thought stopping) are useful in countering the irrational thoughts. They are discussed in detail in Chapter 30. Another way to help clients develop a more positive self-esteem is to encourage them to identify their strengths. Once identified, these assets are the tools for building a better view of oneself. Applying the concept of unconditional positive regard (Rogers, 1957) with every client, regardless of behaviors, helps clients feel more valued. Other techniques that can help clients improve self-esteem include journaling, exercise, and relaxation skills (see Chapter 32). See also the Intervention box on page 503.

Because of their charm, air of superiority, and persuasiveness, antisocial people sometimes manipulate nurses to assume the roles of nurturers and rescuers (see the Intervention box on page 503). Never give out your telephone number, assign special privileges, or make yourself available to these clients outside the therapeutic relationship. These clients have lifelong patterns of victimizing and exploiting others.

Incorporate clear, concise, and consistent limit setting and directions into all intervention strategies. Develop these strategies using a team approach, and contract with the client. When infractions of the rules or manipulations occur, apply consequences immediately.

Evaluation

When evaluating any client with a PD, consider the potential for major psychiatric conditions such as depression and anxiety-related disturbances. Even though people with obsessive–compulsive personalities often seek treatment for subjective distress, the course of treatment may be drawn out and ineffective as a result of the rigidity of their defensive operations. If the behavior is confronted directly, the client might develop acute psychiatric conditions because of intense anxiety.

Evaluation focuses on both client expected outcomes and the process of nursing care delivery. When assessing personality-disordered clients for progress, it is essential that the outcome criteria focus on resolution of short-term crises rather than global changes in the client's lifestyle. Keep in mind that PDs are lifelong traits and behaviors, so it is unrealistic to expect a client to change easily or in a short period of time. Using specific outcome criteria for measurement is necessary for evaluation to be meaningful. It is also important to include the client and significant others in evaluating the response to treatment.

When evaluating the delivery of nursing care, it is necessary that nurses not judge their effectiveness only by the client's progress or lack thereof. Instead, evaluation of nursing interventions should consider how nurses responded to the client, what milieu was maintained for the client, and whether nurses consistently set appropriate limits in an attempt to teach the client skills necessary for living as an independent adult. A determination of whether stability and safety were maintained is just as important as considering the client's response to the treatment plan.

Whenever possible, include family members or significant others in some aspects of therapy. Clients should be able to

INTERVENTION

Guidelines for Clients with Aggressive Behavior

Nursing Intervention	Rationale
• Use a calm, unhurried approach.	• Calmness promotes security.
• Do not touch indiscriminately.	• Touch may be misinterpreted as aggressive or sexual.
• Respect personal space.	• Space provides insulation/protection.
• Use active listening skills.	• Attention and direct eye contact promote trust.
• Remain aware of own personal feelings.	• Helps to avoid countertransference reactions.
• Use statements to provide feedback and identify sources of anger: "I notice your fists are clenched . . . what's happening?"	• Feedback on feelings increases client awareness.
• Assure client that staff will not allow the client to hurt self or others.	• Conveys the presence of external controls.
• Observe for escalation of anger (increased activity, verbal and nonverbal acting-out).	• Early awareness prevents crisis.
• Institute precautions against suicide, homicide, assault, or escape, as indicated.	• Ensures safety of client and others.
• Discuss alternate means of releasing tension and physical energy.	• Increases self-esteem through adaptive oulets.
• Provide physical outlets to reduce tension, such as exercise, gardening, clay, music, art (avoid competitive or contact sports).	• Exercise releases anxiety/tension.
• Protect other clients from verbal/physical abuse.	• Ensures safety of all clients.
• Clearly communicate and enforce agency regulations concerning acting-out behavior.	• People behave according to expectations.
• Postpone discussion of consequences of acting-out until client is in control.	• Avoids triggering aggressive behavior.
• Role-model appropriate assertions of angry feelings: "I dislike it when. . ."	• New behaviors can be learned by watching others.
• Communicate desire to help client maintain/regain control.	• Offering self helps to establish trust.
• Hold client responsible for behavior; remind client of the ability to make choices.	• Promotes internal control.
• Use contracts for behavioral control, including seeking out staff people when feelings emerge.	• Reinforces personal responsibility.
• Teach assertiveness skills, relaxation, imagery, thought stopping, thought control (see Chapters 1, 30, and 32).	• Defuses anxiety and reinforces ability for self-control

identify and verbalize their fears and some specific areas where change is indicated. The following are among the factors that influence the likelihood of successful change:

- The severity of the client's emotional deprivation.
- The rigidity of the client's personality structure.
- The client's ego strengths.
- The client's motivation to change.
- The nurse's skill and commitment.
- Social support systems in the client's family or milieu that favor the desired change.

Community-Based Care and Case Management

Individuals with PDs lack insight about their behavior; that is, they are generally unaware that their behaviors are problematic to themselves and others. As a result, few people with PDs voluntarily seek inpatient treatment unless they are experiencing a crisis. Many people with PDs are, therefore, treated in the community—in mental health clinics, crisis centers, and through routine visits to therapists' offices. The case manager plays an essential role by collaborating with clients and families/significant others by providing information on when and where to seek help. The case manager also monitors clients for compliance to the aftercare plan, including the client's medication usage.

When working with personality-disordered clients on an outpatient basis, it is especially important to help clients identify their personal strengths to use as building blocks for therapy. Also, nurses need to help clients develop a realistic time frame in which to achieve expected outcomes. Clients usually need help in identifying community support services and in developing a support system. This can be facilitated by asking the client to identify one family member or friend he or she would trust to help with personal needs. Role play can be an effective tool for helping clients learn to detect social cues given by others.

INTERVENTION

Guidelines for the Client with Paranoid Personality Disorder

Nursing Intervention	Rationale
• Respect personal space.	• Promotes a sense of security.
• Respect client's privacy and preferences as much as is reasonable.	• Predictable environments (schedules, consistent caregivers, etc.) decrease anxiety and foster trust.
• Give feedback to client based on observed nonverbal cues of responsiveness, such as eye movement, posturing, voice tones.	• Improves interpersonal effectiveness.
• Provide client with a daily schedule of activities and inform client of changes.	• Activity schedules will diminish anxiety about social interactions and may help ensure participation.
• Help client identify adaptive diversionary activities (leisure, recreation) in one-to-one sessions and groups.	• Participation in groups may increase client's support system.
• Use role-playing to help client identify feelings, thoughts, and responses brought on by stressful situations.	• Rehearsing social behaviors in a safe environment provides immediate feedback and time for altering responses.
• Encourage client to evaluate how client behaviors led to the current crisis.	• Points out cause-and-effect aspects of interaction.
• Use an objective, matter-of-fact approach with client.	• Client will identify the nurse as a reliable person who gives respect without argument.
• Use concrete, specific words rather than global abstractions.	• Keeps intended message clear.
• Respond to suspicious ideas by focusing on feelings: "It must be distressing. . ." "You see him as vindictive. . ."	• Communicates empathy.
• Conduct brief one-to-one sessions daily (avoid lengthy sessions).	• Shortened sessions decrease fear and anxiety.
• Gradually introduce client to group situations.	• Trust-building is a slow process.

Home Care

Nurses who provide psychiatric–mental health care in the home setting are significant in helping clients with PDs to improve their social interactions and to help shape behavior. The following interventions are especially helpful for homebound clients experiencing PD:

- Meet with client and family member or significant other to discuss realistic expectations for the client.
- Teach the client home management skills necessary for independent living.
- Ask client if testing, placement services, or job skill retraining are desired.
- Refer to community agencies as needed. A list of resources for people who care about someone with BPD is available at www.bpdcentral.com that can be accessed through the Companion Website for this book.

MediaLink 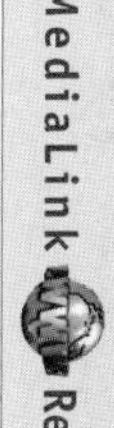 Resources for Borderline PD

INTERVENTION

Guidelines for the Client with Antisocial Personality Disorder

Nursing Intervention	Rationale
• Use a concerned, matter-of-fact approach.	• Appropriate distance must be given all clients.
• Set, communicate, and maintain consistent rules and regulations for all clients.	• Provides a sense of security.
• Do not argue, bargain, or rationalize.	• Decreases power struggles.
• Confront inappropriate behaviors without anger, punitiveness, or personalization.	• The behavior, not the person, should be addressed.
• Do not seek approval, or coax; use choices and consequences.	• A professional relationship increases client self-control.
• Be alert for flattery or verbal attacks.	• Being prepared decreases the chance of being manipulated.
• Using contracts and relaxation techniques, teach client to delay immediate gratification and impulsiveness.	• Provides other outlets for anger and aggression.
• Use peer pressure (groups, buddy systems) to modify manipulative behaviors.	• Peer feedback is a better reinforcer than staff input.
• Role-model self-discipline.	• New behaviors can be patterned after those of others.

Nurses' Self-Awareness

Self-awareness is the first step in developing therapeutic approaches to clients with any personality disorder. By examining one's own responses and feelings toward the client, the nurse is better able to prevent **countertransference** from occurring (see Chapter 28). The behaviors demonstrated by personality-disordered clients often evoke strong negative feelings and responses in nurses. Nurses often stigmatize individuals with PDs, especially those with borderline personality disorder (Nehls, 2000). Clients may be labeled and stereotyped, which leads to depersonalization and inadequate treatment.

Nurses' responses to clients who have Cluster B personality disorders may be similar to the behaviors displayed by the clients—anger, helplessness, increased anxiety, rescuer notions, defensiveness, and guilt from a sense of powerlessness.

You must be attuned to your own feelings and reactions when working with clients with NPD. Do not criticize their haughty, uncaring attitude, but demonstrate by actions that they are accepted regardless of wealth, position, or status.

The arousal of feelings of anger, powerlessness, a sense of having been "conned," disappointment, and even guilt and shame is common among nurses who work with PD clients.

Nurses are often unaware of the beliefs which may be countertherapeutic. By using introspection and supervision, nurses can become more aware of the impact of their own feelings and behaviors on others. Only then are nurses able to respond more appropriately to all clients.

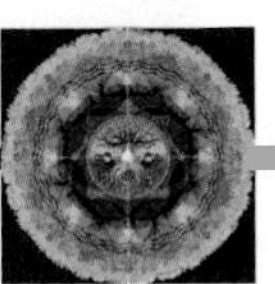

EXPLORE MediaLink

NCLEX review, case studies, and other interactive resources for this chapter can be found on the Companion Website at http://www.prenhall.com/kneisl. Click on Chapter 20 to select the activities for this chapter.

For animations, video tutorials, more NCLEX review questions, and an audio glossary, access the accompanying CD-ROM in this textbook.

BIBLIOGRAPHY

American Psychiatric Association (2000). *Diagnostic and statistical manual of mental disorders* (4th ed., Text Revision). Washington, DC: Author.

Bohus, M. J., Landwehrmeyer, B., & Stiglmayr, C. E. (1999). Naltrexone in the treatment of dissociative symptoms in patients with borderline personality disorder: An open-label trial. *Journal of Clinical Psychiatry, 60*, 598–603.

Copel, L. C. (2000). *Psychiatric and mental health nurses' clinical guide* (2nd ed.). Springhouse, PA: Springhouse.

Driessen, M., Herrmann, J., Stahl, K., Zwaan, M., Meier, S., Hill, A., et al. (2000). Magnetic resonance imaging volume of the hippocampus and the amygdala in women with borderline personality disorder and early traumatization. *Archives of General Psychiatry, 57*, 1115–1127.

Erikson, E. H. (1964). *Childhood and society*. New York: Norton.

Fowler, J. C., Hilsenroth, M. J., & Nolan, E. (2000). Exploring the inner world of self-mutilating borderline patients: A Rorschach investigation. *Bulletin of the Menninger Clinic, 64*, 365–385.

Goodman, M., & New, M. (2000). Impulsive aggression in borderline personality disorder. *Current Psychiatry Report, 2*, 56–61.

Gunderson, J. G., & Ridolfi, M. E. (2001). Borderline personality disorder: Suicidality and self-mutilation. *Annals of New York Academy of Science, 932*, 73–77.

Heffernan, K., & Cloitre, M. (2000). A comparison of posttraumatic stress disorder with and without borderline personality disorder among women with a history of childhood sexual abuse: Etiological and clinical characteristics. *Journal of Nervous and Mental Disorders, 188*, 589–595.

Johnson, J. G., Cohen, P., Smailes, E., Kasen, S., Oldham, J. M., Skodol, A. E., et al. (2000). Adolescent personality disorders associated with violence and criminal behavior during adolescence and early adulthood. *American Journal of Psychiatry, 157*, 1406–1412.

Kaplan, H. I., & Sadock, B. J. (2000). *Kaplan & Sadock's synopsis of psychiatry and study guide*. Philadelphia: Lippincott.

Kaylor, L. (1999). Antisocial personality disorder: Ethical and treatment issues. *Issues in Mental Health Nursing, 20*, 247–258.

Kernberg, O. (1975). *Borderline conditions and pathological narcissism*. New York: Aronson.

Kirrane, R. M., & Siever, L. J. (2000). New perspectives on schizotypal personality disorder. *Current Psychiatry Report, 2*, 62–66.

Looper, K. J., & Paris, J. (2000). What dimensions underlie Cluster B personality disorders? *Comprehensive Psychiatry, 41*, 432–437.

Mahler, M. S., Pine, F., & Bergman, A. (1975). *The psychological birth of the human infant: Symbiosis and individuation*. New York: Basic Books.

Nehls, N. (2000). Recovering: A process of empowerment. *Advances in Nursing Science, 22*, 62–70.

Nehls, N. (1999). Borderline personality disorder: The voice of patients. *Research in Nursing & Health, 22*, 285–293.

North American Nursing Diagnosis Association. (2001). *Nursing diagnoses: Definitions & classification: 2001–2002*. Philadelphia: Author.

Painter, S. G., & Howell, C. C. (1999). Rage and women's sexuality after childhood sexual abuse: A phenomenological study. *Perspectives in Psychiatric Care, 35*, 5–20.

Riso, L. P., Klein, D. N., Anderson, R. I., & Ouimette, P. C. (2000). A family study of outpatients with borderline personality disorder with no history of mood disorders. *Journal of Personality Disorders, 14*, 208–217.

Rogers, C. (1957). The necessary and sufficient conditions for therapeutic personality change. *Journal of Consulting Psychology, 21*, 95–103.

Schneidt, K. S. (2000). Borderline personality disorder in primary care. *Journal of the American Academy of Physicians Assistants, 13*, 19–28.

Timmermann, I. G., & Emmelkamp, P. M. (2001). The relationship between traumatic experiences, dissociation, and borderline personality pathology among male forensic patients and prisoners. *Journal of Personality Disorders, 15*, 136–149.

Wilkinson, J. M. (2000). *Nursing diagnosis handbook with NIC interventions and NOC outcomes*. Upper Saddle River, NJ: Prentice Hall.

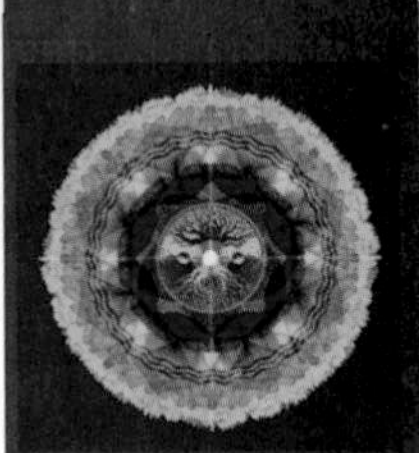

21

Chapter TWENTY-ONE

Coexisting Psychiatric and Substance Use Disorders

BETHANY J. PHOENIX
KIMBERLY PELISH

KEY TERMS

comorbidity
craving
drug of choice
dual diagnosis
high-risk situations
lapse
mentally ill chemical abuser (MICA)
polysubstance abuse
psychoactive
relapse
self-medication
sobriety
triggers

FOCUS QUESTIONS

- **Why do people with mental illnesses have such a high rate of substance use disorders?**
- **How can the use of alcohol or drugs complicate the course of a psychiatric disorder?**
- **What are the components of an effective substance use assessment for a mentally ill client?**
- **What are some of the ways that the mental health and substance abuse treatment systems may fail to meet the needs of clients with coexisting psychiatric and substance use disorders?**
- **What kinds of interventions are most likely to be effective in working with clients with coexisting disorders?**

MediaLink 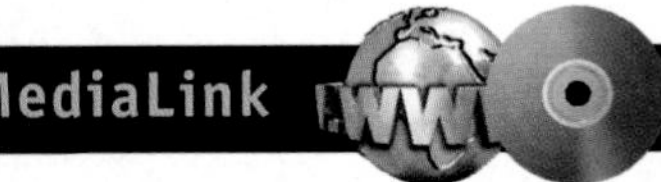 www.prenhall.com/kneisl

Additional resources for this chapter can be found on the Student CD-ROM accompanying this textbook, and on the Companion Website at www.prenhall.com/kneisl. Click on Chapter 21 to select the activities for this chapter.

CD-ROM
- Audio Glossary
- NCLEX Review

Companion Website
- Additional NCLEX Review
- Care Plan: Emergency Treatment
- Case Study: PTSD and Substance Abuse

CHAPTER OUTLINE

CROSS REFERENCES

Other topics relevant to this content are: Assessment of clients taking psychiatric medications, Chapter 31; HIV risk with substance abuse, Chapter 24; Major mood disorders, Chapter 15; Personality disorders, Chapter 20; Persons at risk for violence, Chapter 23; Psychobiologic basis of psychiatric illness, Chapter 4; Schizophrenia, Chapter 14; Substance abuse and dependence and harm reduction, Chapter 13; Self-help groups and family enmeshment, Chapter 29; Suicide risk, Chapter 22.

CRITICAL THINKING CHALLENGE

Jerry Jenkins, one of your clients at a psychiatric day treatment program, tells you he's confused about what to do. A friend of Jerry's in Alcoholics Anonymous has told Jerry that the medications he takes to treat schizoaffective disorder are "just more mind-altering substances" and that he can't proceed with his recovery if he continues to use medication as a "crutch." Jerry feels that going to AA meetings "saved my life" by providing him with support to stop drinking and using amphetamines, and he wants to continue to live a life free from drugs and alcohol. He is fearful, however, that he will have a psychotic relapse if he stops taking his antipsychotic and antidepressant medications.

How would you advise Jerry to deal with this situation? What information or resources do you think might be helpful to Jerry in deciding what to do? ■

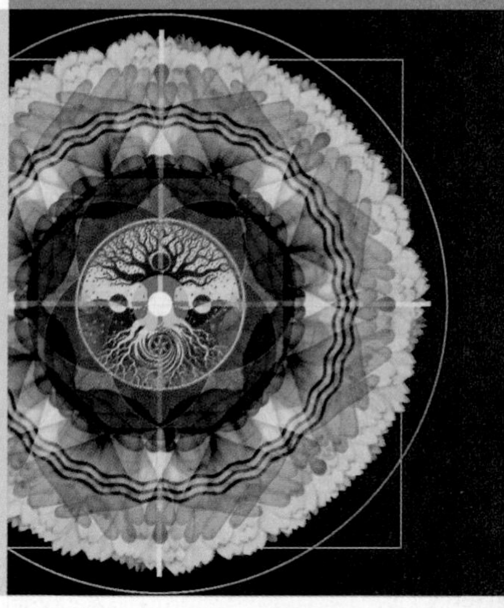

In the deinstitutionalization movement of the 1970s, the care of people with severe mental illness moved from state hospitals into the community. Along with new freedoms, mental health consumers encountered a new threat to their quality of life—abuse of alcohol and drugs. This chapter will focus on the impact of substance abuse on people with coexisting mental illness.

The terms **dual diagnosis** and "dual disorder," as well as **mentally ill chemical abuser (MICA)** and substance abusing mentally ill (SAMI), have been used to refer to mentally ill people who have problems with drug and alcohol use (see Chapter 13 for descriptions of substance abuse and substance dependence and the many issues associated with drinking and drug use). These terms are problematic—"dual diagnosis" is not specific to the combination of psychiatric and substance use disorders, and terms such as MICA have been criticized by mental health consumers for identifying a person by a disorder. This chapter will use "coexisting disorders" as a shorthand term to refer to the combination of mental illness and substance use disorders.

Prevalence of Coexisting Psychiatric and Substance Use Disorders

People with psychiatric illness are at high risk for substance use disorders. The Epidemiological Catchment Area (ECA) study, which surveyed over 20,000 people to identify the prevalence of mental health problems, found that substance use disorders were significantly more common in people with any psychiatric disorder than in others in the population (see ■ Figure 21–1). People with the most severe mental illnesses had the highest rates of substance abuse and dependence—people with schizophrenia had over four times the risk of having a substance use disorder as others, and people with bipolar disorder had over six times the risk (Regier et al., 1990). Similarly, people with substance abuse or dependence were more likely to have co-occurring psychiatric disorders (see ■ Figure 21–2).

Characteristics of Clients with Coexisting Disorders

The same demographic factors that are associated with substance use disorders in the general population affect people with mental illness (see Chapter 13). Being male, unmarried, young adult, and poor are associated with higher risk of substance abuse.

CLINICAL EXAMPLE

Ramon is a 25-year-old man who was diagnosed with schizophrenia 6 years ago, when he was a student at a local junior college. After becoming ill, Ramon lost most of his friends because he was preoccupied with a delusional relationship with a radio talk-show host and spent most of his time alone in his room. He dropped out of college because his mental disorganization and frequent psychiatric hospitalizations interfered with his ability to attend classes. He has tried several times to work, but has not been able to keep a job.

After Ramon's most recent hospitalization, he moved into a psychiatric halfway house and began receiving weekly injections of a long-acting neuroleptic medication. He became much less delusional and started making friends. Several months ago, Ramon and two of his male friends from the halfway house moved into an apartment in a neighborhood known for its high incidence of crack cocaine use.

Ramon's case manager believes Ramon is using crack. He has lost weight, become aggressive and paranoid, and has been threatened with eviction for failing to pay his rent. Ramon was brought to psychiatric emergency services by the police after becoming agitated and threatening in a convenience store. In psychiatric emergency services, Ramon's urine toxicology screening was positive for cocaine.

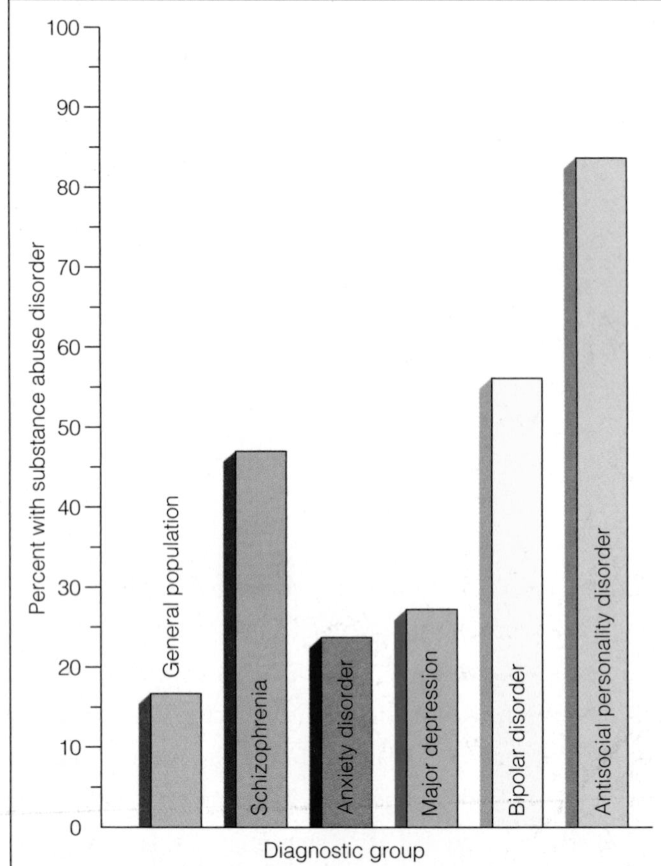

FIGURE 21–1 ■ *Lifetime prevalence rates for substance abuse disorder.*

Source: Based on data from *Epidemiologic Catchment Area Study*, Regier et al., 1990.

People with coexisting disorders display a wide range of clinical characteristics and service needs, depending on the nature and severity of their psychiatric and substance-related problems. Ries and colleagues (1997) proposed a classification scheme that categorizes individuals on two axes: severity of mental illness and severity of substance use disorder (see ■ Figure 21–3). Clients with high psychiatric severity have disabling conditions such as schizophrenia, bipolar disorder, or severe personality disorders that are made more difficult to manage when substance abuse or dependence is a complicating factor. Clients with low psychiatric severity (disorders such as dysthymia and anxiety disorders) would experience little disability if their symptoms were not aggravated by a substance use disorder and if they received adequate treatment.

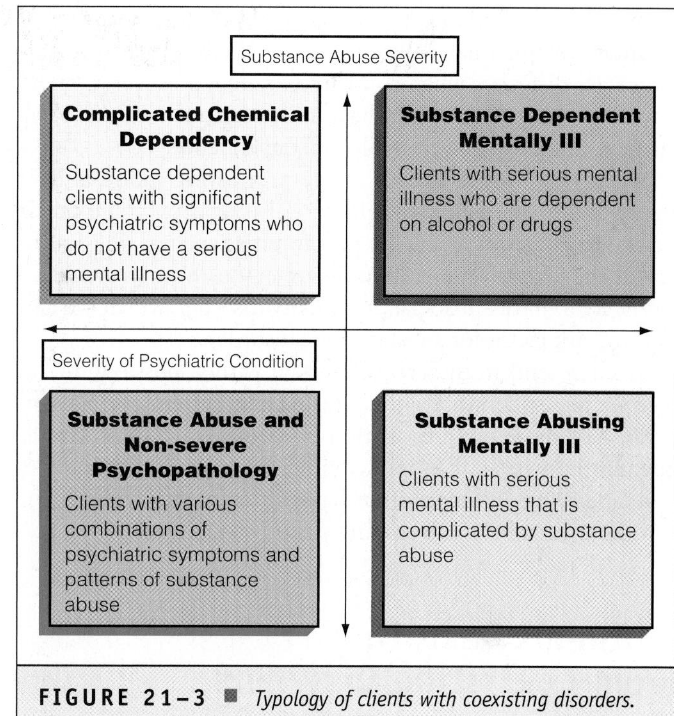

FIGURE 21–3 ■ *Typology of clients with coexisting disorders.*

RACIAL AND ETHNIC DIFFERENCES

There is limited information available on racial and ethnic differences in substance use disorders among people with coexisting mental illness. However, the available evidence suggests that people with psychiatric disorders are likely to abuse the same substances that are used, abused, and available to them in their families and communities. Since alcohol is socially acceptable, inexpensive, and widely available in the United States, it is the substance that has the highest rate of abuse in the general population (across ethnic groups and gender), as well as among those with co-occurring psychiatric disorders.

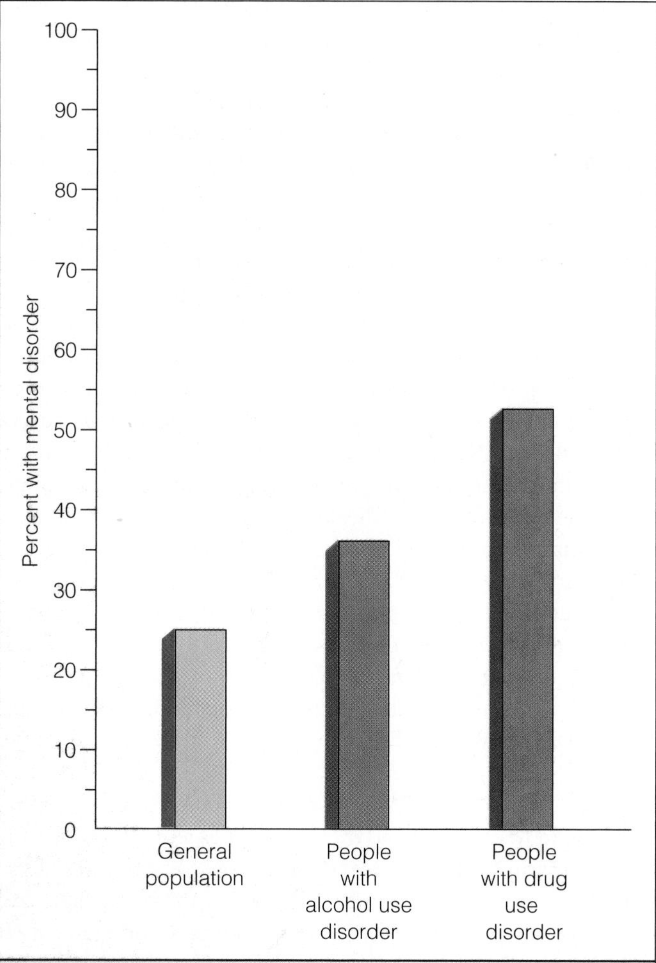

FIGURE 21–2 ■ *Lifetime prevalence rates for non–substance abuse mental disorder.*

Source: Based on data from *Epidemiologic Catchment Area Study,* Regier et al., 1990.

When racial and ethnic groups are looked at in the aggregate, differences in rates of substance use disorder are not striking. Native Americans tend to have higher rates of alcohol and drug disorders than others, and substance use disorder rates for Asian-Americans and Pacific Islanders tend to be lower (Center for Substance Abuse Treatment, 1999).

There is considerable variation in substance use patterns within ethnic groups based on such factors as socioeconomic status, geographic location, and degree of acculturation. Socioeconomic factors such as low income, poor education, and never having been married are all significant risk factors for substance abuse across ethnic, race, and gender groups for both alcohol and drug dependence.

Race and ethnicity may influence the frequency of complications associated with substance abuse. Compared to white men, African-American men suffer more consequences from problem drinking, such as higher mortality from liver cirrhosis and increased frequency of delirium tremens. Literature on Native Americans also suggests an increased risk for alcohol-related health and social problems (Center for Substance Abuse Treatment, 1999).

GENDER DIFFERENCES

Since men and women have different rates of substance use disorders and of some psychiatric disorders, there are gender differences in the range of coexisting psychiatric and substance use disorders. Women have a lower prevalence of all types of substance use disorders when compared to men; however, women, across ethnic groups, often have more serious and disabling medical complications from alcohol dependence.

Women are more likely to have preexisting mood and/or anxiety disorders than men. They are also reported to link their substance abuse with specific past traumas such as physical or sexual abuse much more often than men do. Women are much less likely to have antisocial personality disorder, which is a significant risk factor for substance use disorders.

Women tend to undergo treatment earlier, possibly due to their increased comfort with accessing help systems, or perhaps because of more rapid escalation of medical and social consequences known as the "telescoping" phenomenon (Brady & Randall, 1999). Women often have different motivations for entering treatment, such as child custody concerns.

Problems Resulting From Coexisting Disorders

MediaLink Case Study: PTSD and Substance Abuse

People with psychiatric illnesses are at high risk for problems caused by use of drugs and alcohol. Homelessness, involvement with the criminal justice system, problems in relationships with family and friends, and health problems such as infection with HIV and hepatitis C are common in people with coexisting psychiatric and substance use disorders.

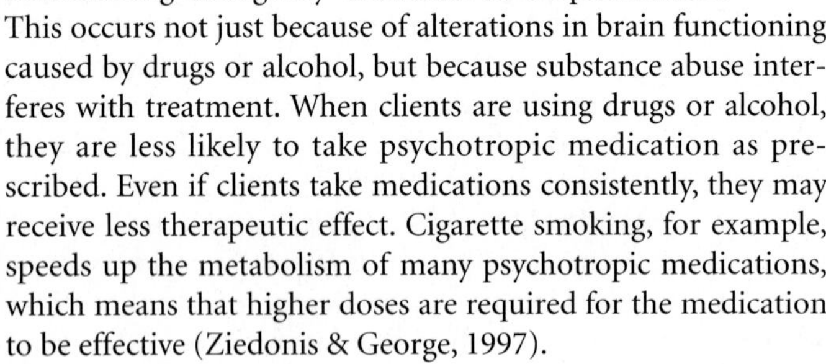

In addition, symptoms of mental illness may worsen when alcohol or drugs are used, leading to suicidal, assaultive, or disorganized behavior and necessitating emergency treatment or hospitalization. This occurs not just because of alterations in brain functioning caused by drugs or alcohol, but because substance abuse interferes with treatment. When clients are using drugs or alcohol, they are less likely to take psychotropic medication as prescribed. Even if clients take medications consistently, they may receive less therapeutic effect. Cigarette smoking, for example, speeds up the metabolism of many psychotropic medications, which means that higher doses are required for the medication to be effective (Ziedonis & George, 1997).

Biopsychosocial Theories

A number of different factors—genetic predisposition, family and social background, the effects of **psychoactive** drugs (drugs that alter the functions of the central nervous system) on brain chemistry, among others—have been suggested as contributing to the high rate of psychiatric/substance abuse **comorbidity** (having two or more disorders at the same time). Four general theories may help to explain this phenomenon:

1. Mental illness leads to substance abuse.
2. Substance abuse leads to mental illness.
3. A common factor causes both disorders.
4. Disorders develop independently.

MENTAL ILLNESS LEADS TO SUBSTANCE ABUSE

This theory proposes that mental illness increases vulnerability to substance use disorders. This supposition is supported by research indicating that the onset of a severe mental illness commonly precedes the development of problems with substance use (Hambrecht & Hafner, 1996). It is also true that symptoms associated with mental illness may be risk factors for substance use disorders.

Self-Medication

One theory is that mentally ill clients self-medicate with drugs or alcohol. Both psychological and biologic perspectives contribute to the understanding of **self-medication** (using drugs or alcohol to reduce symptoms).

Psychological Aspects. Khantzian (1985) is the person most commonly associated with the psychodynamic viewpoint on self-medication. Based on his clinical observations and interventions with addicts, Khantzian concluded that deficits in ego functioning lead to an inability to modulate painful feelings. The addict's **drug of choice** (preferred substance of abuse) is selected for its ability to pharmacologically compensate for difficulties in regulating feeling states.

Compton (1989) reformulated Khantzian's ego/self theory of substance dependence to fit Orem's nursing model for self-care. Orem's conceptualization of self-care includes all the actions that people take to maintain health and well-being (Lacey, 1993). Using Orem's self-care deficit theory, Compton defines lack of self-protective behavior and difficulty in handling painful feelings as self-care deficits that require nursing intervention.

Khantzian's theory helped clarify the adaptive function of substance use, making the behavior more comprehensible to health care providers. However, this psychodynamic theory has some significant limitations when applied to clients with severe mental illness. Khantzian's focus on drug use to regulate unpleasant feelings does not include other symptoms that mentally ill people may self-medicate, such as abnormal perceptions (hallucinations) and the physical discomforts associated with medication side effects. Also, the idea that, after a period of experimentation, people will settle on just one "drug of choice" is contradicted by research showing that **polysubstance abuse** (simultaneous abuse of more than one intoxicating substance) is the norm among people with serious mental illness (Meuser, Essock, Drake, Wolfe, & Frisman, 2001).

Biologic Aspects. Biologic, as well as psychological, factors are thought to contribute to the use of drugs and alcohol to self-medicate symptoms of mental illness. Some substances of abuse may stimulate neurotransmitter systems in the brain that have been altered both by the disease and by some of the agents used to treat schizophrenia. Animal studies indicate that addictive agents increase activity in brain systems dependent on dopamine (DA), a neurotransmitter whose functioning is altered in schizophrenia. The use of stimulants by people with schizophrenia may be seen as an attempt to "normalize" certain brain functions that have been impaired by the disease. In addition, nicotine relieves problems with sensory processing caused by schizophrenia and counteracts side effects of psychotropic medication, which may help to explain the extremely high frequency of smoking in this group (Ziedonis & George, 1997).

Although substance use may produce symptom relief, it is often true that this decrease in symptoms is short lived and likely to be followed by an exacerbation of symptoms. It is also true that the same substance may relieve some psychiatric symptoms and worsen others—for example, stimulants may briefly elevate depressed mood and increase energy, but exacerbate anxiety and psychotic symptoms.

Effects of Social Disadvantage Related to Mental Illness

The life circumstances associated with severe mental illness may increase the risk of substance abuse. Estroff's (1981) classic ethnographic study of people with chronic mental illness paints a vivid picture of the employment difficulties, poverty, and social isolation too often still experienced by such clients. Joblessness is a significant risk factor for misuse of alcohol and drugs, because it leads to poverty and because unemployed people have lots of time on their hands. Large amounts of unstructured time and few affordable recreational activities may make substance use an attractive way to kill time.

Poverty caused by living on disability income often limits mentally ill people to poor neighborhoods in which drugs such as crack cocaine are widely available. Being exposed to heavy substance use is most likely to influence mental health consumers who are socially isolated because of stigma and impaired social skills. People with psychiatric illnesses are likely to use drugs or alcohol because they feel it makes it easier to socialize with peers.

CLINICAL EXAMPLE

Daisy is a 38-year-old woman who was diagnosed with schizophrenia in her mid-20s and has been unable to work since she became ill. She spends most of her time alone in her room in a single-room-occupancy hotel. She began drinking heavily when she was married to a man who was an alcoholic, and continues to binge on alcohol when she receives her disability check. She prefers to drink at a bar near her hotel because "it's the only place I feel comfortable talking to guys."

SUBSTANCE ABUSE LEADS TO MENTAL ILLNESS

This model suggests that some cases of mental illness develop as a consequence of substance abuse. Acute effects of intoxication and withdrawal from drugs, such as psychoses produced by amphetamines and rebound depression following a cocaine binge, resemble psychiatric disorders. However, these symptoms usually resolve as the client detoxifies. The evidence is still inconclusive as to whether substance use can actually cause persistent mental illness in the absence of other predisposing factors.

Research does suggest that significant substance use may lead to an earlier onset and more severe course of psychotic illness (Kovaszny et al., 1997). In addition, recent research indicates that, even when other risk factors are taken into account, cigarette smoking leads to increased risk of developing depression and anxiety disorders (Johnson et al., 2000).

COMMON FACTOR CAUSES BOTH DISORDERS

This theory proposes that both substance use disorders and mental illness have a common underlying factor. Genetic vulnerability has been suggested as one such common factor, given the familial links between alcoholism and some psychiatric disorders.

Trauma is another factor that may predispose individuals to both psychiatric and substance use disorders. Childhood sexual abuse trauma is thought to be a predisposing factor for a number of psychiatric disorders, including depression, dissociative disorders, borderline personality disorder, and post-traumatic stress disorder, as well as substance use disorders. Combat trauma has also been linked with increased rates of both psychiatric and substance use disorders.

DISORDERS DEVELOP INDEPENDENTLY

In this theory, disorders arise independently of each other, but each influences the course of the other. For example, if a teenage boy with a family history of schizophrenia is involved with a drug-using peer group and started using drugs regularly, it could precipitate an earlier onset of schizophrenic symptoms. If the psychotic symptoms were severe enough to interfere with finishing high school and finding a job, the young man could find himself with unstructured time to spend using drugs.

MediaLink Care Plan: Emergency Treatment

NURSING PROCESS

Clients with Coexisting Disorders in Emergency Settings

Clients with coexisting disorders are likely to be a large part of the population served by nurses working in psychiatric emergency settings. Intoxication often leads to acute decompensations:

- Alcohol intoxication may lead to impulsive suicide attempts.
- Chronic cocaine use may produce intense paranoia.
- Stimulant or hallucinogenic drugs may produce or aggravate psychotic symptoms, such as hallucinations and delusions.
- The "crash" that follows a cocaine or speed binge may cause severe depression and acute suicidality.

Assessment

Given the high rate of substance abuse in individuals with mental illness, you should always include a comprehensive evaluation for substance use in any emergency assessment. Substance-related diagnoses are often missed for several reasons:

- Drug effects may mimic symptoms of mental illness.
- The client is too disorganized to provide accurate information about substance use.
- Psychiatric clinicians often receive inadequate training in assessing and treating substance-related disorders.

SUBJECTIVE DATA

Gathering useful subjective data from clients who are intoxicated may be difficult because of their mental disorganization. If possible, ask clients if they have used any drugs or alcohol, and if so, how recently. "Have you had any kind of alcohol to drink in the last 24 hours? How many have you consumed?" As well as including alcohol and street drugs such as marijuana, speed, phencyclidine (PCP), and cocaine, ask about over-the-counter drugs and inhalants, such as airplane glue or gasoline additives. The Assessment box below provides a concise format for collecting the information necessary to an emergency evaluation. Also ask anyone who accompanies the client about what substances were consumed, and the time and amount.

Even if clients are coherent enough to answer questions, the accuracy of their answers may be suspect. Clients may fear legal consequences if they admit to using illegal substances, may fear being stigmatized as a "junkie" or a "drunk," or may simply be unaware of what was in the street drugs they consumed.

Other subjective data that may indicate substance use are the client's reported symptoms. Although auditory hallucinations are common in people with psychotic disorders, visual or tactile hallucinations are uncommon and may indicate substance use.

You should also ask about use of prescribed medication—"Which medications do you take? Do you sometimes take more of your medications than prescribed?" Clients may overuse anticholinergic medications to get a "buzz," and narcotics and antianxiety agents may be taken in greater than the prescribed amounts for their euphoric effects. Besides taking prescribed medicines for their pleasurable effects, clients may have misunderstood how their medications should be taken, or be too disorganized to take them correctly. Information about psychoactive medications is very important when clients have consumed drugs or alcohol because these drugs can interact and cause serious complications, such as overdose or seizures.

In addition to asking about drugs that may be producing intoxication, it is important to evaluate withdrawal risk. Find out which substances have been used regularly, and in what amounts. Also ask if the client has ever experienced withdrawal, and if so, what the symptoms were like. People who have experienced severe withdrawal symptoms are at greater current risk of withdrawal.

OBJECTIVE DATA

Much information can be obtained from appearance, behavior, and vital signs, even when clients are disorganized or uncooperative.

Appearance Observe the client for signs of substance use and intoxication:

- Alcohol on the breath
- "Tracks" (needle marks) on the skin
- Slurred speech
- Ataxia

ASSESSMENT **Quick Substance Use Check Sheet**

Check all that apply.

1. What substances do you use?
   Alcohol { }
   Cocaine { } Crack { }
   Heroin { }
   Marijuana (*Pot*) { }
   Prescription drugs (*Vicodin, Demerol, codeine cough medicine, morphine sulfate, other pain meds, Valium, Ativan, etc.*){ }
   Over-the-counter meds (*Nyquil, antihistamines*){ }
   Designer drugs (*Ecstasy*) { }
   Inhalants (huffing) { }
   Tobacco { }
   Caffeine (coffee) { }
   Other drugs that you do that are important for your health care provider to know about to give you good care { }
   Please name____________________.
2. When did you last use the drugs you have checked? Be specific by hour and day______________.
3. How much do you use each day of the substances you have checked? Be specific.
4. When you stop using whatever substances you have taken, what withdrawal symptoms do you suffer?
   Anxiety and "shakes" [ ]
   Confusion [ ]
   Memory loss [ ]
   Nausea and vomiting [ ]
   Diarrhea [ ]
   Itching and numbness [ ]
   Sweating [ ]
   Paranoia and fear [ ]
   Hallucinations (auditory, and/or visual) [ ]
   Headache [ ]
   Seizures [ ]
   Others [ ]
   Please describe:____________________

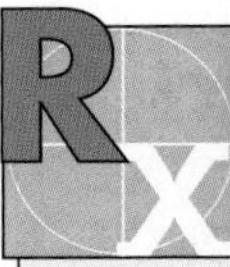

COMMUNICATION

Client Using Illicit Drugs

CLIENT: "What's the matter—you think I'm a speed freak or something? You probably think I belong in jail instead of here."

NURSE RESPONSE 1: "I'm not making any judgments about you, but we see clients from all walks of life who use amphetamines. Since some of your symptoms could be caused by stimulant use, we need to know if you've been using any of those drugs so we'll know how to provide the best treatment."

RATIONALE: Clients are likely to be more straightforward if they feel you are not judging them and if they understand that information about their drug use will be used to help them.

NURSE RESPONSE 2: "If you're concerned that any information you give me about drug use may get passed along to the police, I want to let you know that won't happen. Because our job is to provide treatment, we're not required to inform the police of patients' drug use."

RATIONALE: Clients who are using illegal substances have legitimate fear of the possible legal consequences. They are likely to provide more accurate information about drug use if they know that disclosure will not result in arrest.

Vital Signs Vital signs are important indicators of substance-related problems.

- Elevated heart rate and blood pressure may indicate stimulant overdose or alcohol withdrawal.
- Depressed vital signs may indicate sedative overdose.

Although the cause of altered vital signs may not be immediately apparent and may be due to physical problems other than substance abuse, any abnormality in vital signs indicates a need for closer monitoring and more extensive physical examination.

Neurologic Signs Similarly, abnormal neurologic findings indicate a need for more extensive medical evaluation.

- Changes in levels of consciousness, such as delirium or stuporousness, are not caused by psychiatric illness and indicate an organic cause.
- Observe the client's pupils: pinpoint pupils can be caused by opiate use, marijuana and amphetamines dilate the pupils, and PCP use can cause nystagmus.
- Abnormal motor behavior, such as ataxia, should be reported and further evaluated.

Mental Status Abnormal mental status findings are seen in substance-induced disorders but are not specific to them.

- Confusion, disorientation, and agitation are often seen in intoxicated individuals, but can also indicate other problems, such as dementia, head injury, or metabolic abnormalities.
- Paranoia is common in stimulant abuse but can also indicate paranoid schizophrenia.
- Hallucinations can be caused by hallucinogens, withdrawal from alcohol, or psychotic illnesses.
- Signs of impaired thinking, such as loose associations, are unlikely to be caused by substance use and are more likely to be due to schizophrenia.

Toxicology Toxicologic screening of the blood or urine is helpful in clarifying the contribution of substance use to the client's presentation.

- Clients who deny drug use may nevertheless show evidence of drugs in their urine.
- Obtain toxicology specimens as early as possible when the role of substance use is in question.
- Toxicology may fail to detect covert drug use. Most toxicologic screenings do not identify inhalants, and other drugs may be missed unless the screening is done at the earliest possible time.
- Clients in withdrawal will often test negative for substance use.

HISTORY

The client's history may offer some insight into his or her current presentation.

- Has the client been previously diagnosed with a mental illness? If so, were the presenting symptoms similar to those you are seeing now?
- Symptoms that are unusual for the client, or are more severe than usual, may indicate substance use.
- If the client has no known history of psychiatric illness, note current symptoms so they can be reevaluated when drug or alcohol effects have worn off.

Although just dealing with the combination of mental illness and substance abuse is a significant challenge to your assessment skills (as demonstrated in the Rx Communication feature), clients with coexisting psychiatric and substance use disorders are at increased risk for other medical and psychosocial problems that can make the diagnostic picture even more complicated. For instance, HIV infection caused by injection drug use can cause many psychiatric syndromes, including mood disorder, dementia, and psychosis. Malnutrition in a homeless, alcoholic client can contribute to Wernicke's encephalopathy. Although the effects of all these interlocking disorders may be too complicated to sort out during an emergency visit, you should perform as thorough an assessment as possible of physical, psychological, and social factors that led to the crisis admission (see the Assessment box on page 514).

ASSESSMENT **Obtaining a Substance Use History for Clients with Coexisting Mental Illness**

The topics below should be included in a comprehensive assessment of substance use patterns in clients with a coexisting psychiatric disorder.

1. **Psychoactive substances currently used.** Ask about all the categories listed below. If possible, describe these with terms commonly used in the client's peer group—see Chapter 13 for common terms for these substances.
   - Alcohol: beer, wine, and distilled spirits
   - Marijuana, other cannabinoids
   - Sedative/hypnotic drugs
   - Opiates (heroin)
   - Tranquilizers
   - Hallucinogens
   - PCP
   - Tobacco
   - Cocaine
   - Amphetamines and other stimulants
   - Inhalants
   - Prescription medications
   - Over-the-counter drugs
2. **Recent use of each substance.**
3. **Route of administration/safety issues.** The way the drug enters the body may cause additional health risks. For example, sharing needles to inject drugs increases the risk of blood-borne diseases like HIV. See Chapter 24.
4. **Age at first use.** Clients who began using substances in early adolescence or before are likely to have more entrenched habits. Drinking or using drugs at younger ages interferes with developmental tasks, so these clients may need additional help to learn coping skills.
5. **Family history of substance abuse.** Have the client's parents or siblings had problems with drugs or alcohol? Did they ever receive treatment? What were their experiences with recovery like?
6. **Effect on mental illness.** How does substance use affect the client's psychiatric symptoms, both immediately and after they are no longer intoxicated? Has use of alcohol or drugs caused a need for psychiatric emergency services or hospitalization?
7. **Negative consequences of substance use/abuse.** Ask about problems with physical and mental health, housing status, finances, school or work performance, relationships, spiritual well-being, and involvement with the criminal justice system.
8. **Understanding of the role of substance use in current difficulties.** Does the client see a connection between alcohol and drug use and problems identified above?
9. **Evidence of physical dependence (tolerance or withdrawal).**
10. **Past attempts at treatment/controlling use/harm reduction.** What motivated previous attempts at treatment or self-management? How successful have these attempts been? What factors helped or hindered?
11. **Stage of readiness for change (precontemplation, contemplation, determination, action, maintenance, relapse).** Does the client acknowledge any need for changing substance use habits? Does the client express ambivalence about changing? Is the client willing to take action to change?

Ways to Increase the Validity of Substance Use Assessment

- Assess when psychiatrically stable.
- Assess when not intoxicated or in withdrawal.
- Use self-report in conjunction with other sources of information (lab tests, collateral information).
- Assure that responses will remain confidential when possible.
- Evaluate if client has reasons for distorting report of substance use (legal, housing loss).
- Conduct substance use assessment after assessing other areas of functioning to build rapport.
- Use nonjudgmental interviewing techniques.
- Demonstrate knowledge of substance use patterns.
- Use simple, direct questions and clearly defined time frames (past month).
- Use open-ended questions.
- Normalize substance use.
- Repeat assessments over time.
- Integrate multiple sources of information.

Nursing Diagnosis: NANDA

The primary nursing diagnoses to be addressed in an emergency admission include risk of injury; risk of violence directed at self or others; and knowledge deficits.

RISK OF INJURY

Intoxicated clients often have impaired motor control and may injure themselves by falling. Impulsive acts such as punching walls can cause injury. Clients may incur injuries as a result of withdrawal complications, such as seizures.

RISK OF SELF-DIRECTED VIOLENCE

Suicidal behavior is a concern with clients who are intoxicated, due to lability and impaired impulse control. Those who are acutely depressed from "crashing" after a cocaine or amphetamine binge are also at increased risk for self-harm.

RISK OF VIOLENCE DIRECTED AT OTHERS

Intoxicated individuals are likely to be emotionally labile and impulsive. PCP users, in particular, may behave unpredictably, changing rapidly from being calm to being highly agitated. Such behavioral disinhibition increases the likelihood that clients may strike out at others.

KNOWLEDGE DEFICIT ABOUT DRUG AND ALCOHOL EFFECTS

Although clients are well aware of the euphoric effects of intoxicating substances, they may lack accurate information about long-term consequences of substance use. Clients typically lack knowledge about the impact of drug or alcohol use on mental illness.

Nursing Outcome Identification: NOC

Risk for injury will be decreased as evidenced by risk control. Specific outcomes related to maintaining client safety include aggression control, impulse control, and suicide self-restraint. If clients are stable enough to benefit from education as part of crisis intervention, improved knowledge of substance use control may be achieved.

Planning and Implementation: NIC

Stabilizing the client's physical and mental condition and preventing harm to the client and others are nursing care priorities for clients with coexisting disorders in an emergency setting.

RISK IDENTIFICATION

You should monitor vital signs and neurologic status closely to detect impending medical emergencies, such as seizures or delirium tremens. Serious complications such as these may require the client to be transferred to a medical emergency setting. Clients may require care for physical problems resulting from intoxication. Trauma may result from falls, fights, or self-inflicted injury.

RISK CONTROL

Clients who are highly agitated, threatening, or unpredictable may require seclusion and/or restraints to prevent them from becoming assaultive. Benzodiazepines, such as lorazepam (Ativan), may be helpful in controlling agitation. To avoid harmful drug interactions, administer medications with caution if in doubt about what substances the client has consumed. Encourage clients who are dehydrated or are withdrawing from alcohol to drink ample amounts of fluid.

SUICIDE SELF-RESTRAINT

Institute suicide precautions for clients whose admission was precipitated by a suicide attempt, if they acknowledge suicidal intent, or if they appear acutely depressed. As the client's mental status stabilizes, help the client identify ways to deal with suicidal feelings that do not involve self-harm.

KNOWLEDGE OF SUBSTANCE USE CONTROL

In some emergency settings, client education is a component of crisis intervention. The current crisis can provide dramatic evidence of the need for changing substance use habits. Peer counselors, former clients who have been trained in counseling, can share their experiences of recovering from coexisting disorders.

Evaluation

As clients stabilize, you should see improved control of aggressive and impulsive behavior so that the client is no longer dangerous to self or others. Stable vital signs and neurologic status indicate decreased risk of injury from withdrawal complications. Clients whose mental status has stabilized should be able to identify the role of substance misuse in their current crisis.

NURSING PROCESS

Clients with Coexisting Disorders in Inpatient Settings

During an inpatient stay, a client may be able to completely detoxify from the effects of chronic substance use. This provides an opportunity for further assessment, client and family education, and linkage with community resources. Resources such as Double Trouble (www.doubletroubleinrecovery.org), Dual Recovery Anonymous (www.draonline.org), the Dual Diagnosis Recovery Network (www.dualdiagnosis.org) and others can be found on the Companion Website for this book.

MediaLink Dual Diagnosis Resources

Assessment

Inpatient hospitalization presents an excellent opportunity for a more comprehensive nursing assessment of the client with coexisting disorders. Mental status may have cleared enough to make it possible for the client to cooperate, and additional sources of information can be consulted.

When performing assessments on clients with coexisting disorders, you may find it helpful to use a standardized substance use questionnaire to guide your interview. See the Assessment box on page 514 for areas to be covered in a substance use history. Ask specifically about every drug, giving several examples of drugs in each category.

A matter-of-fact, nonjudgmental approach is most likely to elicit useful information. Also, make it clear to the client why you need the information. Clients will usually provide more accurate information about recent drug or alcohol consumption if they know you are concerned about issues such as preventing withdrawal symptoms or avoiding inappropriate use of psychotropic medications. Eliciting information about the client's motivations for substance use may reveal symptoms, such as anxiety, that could be more effectively treated with prescribed medication.

Nursing Diagnosis: NANDA

Risk for injury continues to be a concern for clients who may be withdrawing from alcohol or sedative/hypnotic drugs. You will also need to focus on denial and knowledge deficits about the impact of drugs or alcohol on the course of the client's mental illness.

Nursing Outcome Identification: NOC

Desired nursing outcomes include control of aggression and impulsive behavior, and increased knowledge and understanding of substance use control. Teaching and motivational strategies should also lead to improved adherence to the regimen for treating both disorders.

Planning and Implementation: NIC

Although stabilization of the client's physical and mental status continues to be a concern on the inpatient service, hospitalization can also be an opportunity to educate and motivate the client to reduce substance use.

MONITORING FOR SIGNS OF WITHDRAWAL

When you know or suspect clients have been drinking heavily or using high doses of sedative/hypnotic drugs, continue to monitor vital signs and mental status for signs of withdrawal. Symptoms such as irritability or psychosis can be due to a psychiatric disorder, but confusion, disorientation, visual hallucinations, and fluctuating level of consciousness may indicate a drug withdrawal delirium. Your ability to recognize withdrawal signs and promptly institute an appropriate protocol for treating withdrawal can prevent serious complications such as seizures and aspiration. The most serious symptoms of withdrawal should resolve in a few days, although symptoms of anxiety, depression, and cognitive impairment may require several weeks to clear completely.

EDUCATING CLIENTS AND FAMILY

Hospitalization provides an opportunity to educate clients about addiction, and about the effects of substance use on people with mental illness (see the Client/Family Teaching feature below). A group format can be especially effective to provide this education. The model of Addiction Education Groups described by Pollack and Steubben (1998) is an example of a group psychoeducation program implemented in an inpatient setting. This model uses a monthly curriculum of topics such as denial and relapse, and utilizes didactic presentations, role-playing, and group discussions.

ENCOURAGING REFLECTION

In addition to providing structured education about drug and alcohol use (refer to the Case Study and Nursing Care Plan on pages 520–521), encourage clients to reflect on the consequences of their own substance use (see the Rx Communication feature: Bipolar Illness and Alcohol Abuse). Although denial or cognitive impairments resulting from mental illness often interfere with a client's ability to make cause-and-effect connections between drug and alcohol use and subsequent problems, a crisis-like hospitalization can make it clear to clients that drug or alcohol use has made their illness impossible to manage. Skillful questioning can help clients understand the role of substance use in their current psychiatric decompensation.

CLINICAL EXAMPLE

Tom Jones, an unemployed 28-year-old man with bipolar mood disorder, was admitted to an inpatient psychiatric unit after attempt-

CLIENT / FAMILY TEACHING

Facts on Substance Abuse and Mental Illness

- **People who are diagnosed with mental illness are at higher risk for substance abuse than others in the population.** You are not alone, and support and treatment is available.
- **Drugs or alcohol are often used in an attempt to help control the unpleasant symptoms of mental illness or side effects of psychiatric medications.** Usually the relief provided is only temporary, and will eventually lead to symptoms getting worse.
- People who abuse alcohol or drugs are more likely to engage in risky behavior, such as having unsafe sex, sharing needles, fighting, or attempting to kill or hurt themselves.
- **Treatment for mental illness is *less* effective when drugs or alcohol are being used.** When people are drinking or using drugs, they may not take their medications as directed, either forgetting to take them or taking extras to counter the effects of the drugs or alcohol. However, taking medication and participating in treatment are still extremely important to keep mental illness from getting worse. Drinking or "using" is not a good reason to avoid receiving mental health treatment.

Interactions Between Drugs and Mental Illness

- *Stimulants* such as caffeine (commonly found in coffee, tea, or soda), methampetamine ("speed"), and cocaine or crack can reduce the effects of antipsychotic and antianxiety medications. Strong stimulants such as speed can cause or worsen paranoia and hallucinations and increase the risk of seizures. They can also cause nervousness and restlessness. Withdrawal from these substances can cause a variety of symptoms such as headache, anxiety, and depression.
- *Depressants* such as alcohol or heroin can cause or prolong depression, and reduce the effects of antidepressant medications. They can lead to overdose when combined with some antidepressant or antianxiety medications. Alcohol withdrawal can include stomach and bowel problems, anxiety, seizures, and visual and tactile hallucinations. Withdrawal from heroin includes stomach and bowel problems as well as anxiety and severe bone and muscle pain.
- *Marijuana* and *hallucinogens* can cause distorted perceptions even in people who do not have a mental illness. They can also decrease the effects of antipsychotic medications. Marijuana may cause apathy, fatigue, and weight gain, which can add to the side effects of some antipsychotic medications.
- *Cigarettes* or other forms of tobacco can cause psychiatric medications to be processed too quickly by the body. This means you have to take more to get the same benefit, which increases the risk of side effects. Also, tobacco has been proven to cause cancer, lung disease, and heart disease, as well as several other serious health problems.

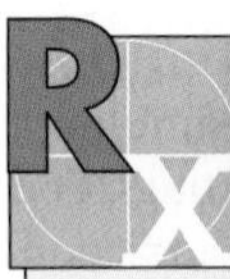

COMMUNICATION

Client with Bipolar Illness and Alcohol Abuse

CLIENT: "I got real sick even though I was taking my lithium. Beer is the only thing that helped when my voices got bad."

NURSE RESPONSE 1: "It sounds like the hallucinations quieted down when you were drinking, but what happened with the voices after the effects of the alcohol wore off?"

RATIONALE: Clients who drink or use drugs in response to bothersome psychiatric symptoms may find that symptoms briefly improve. However, symptoms usually get worse after the substance wears off. Clients may need help to see the pattern of short-term symptom relief followed by rebound exacerbation.

NURSE RESPONSE 2: "When you drink beer, you urinate more. How do you think that might affect your lithium level?"

RATIONALE: As well as drawing the client's attention to the direct effects of substance use on their mental illness, clients need to be aware of how drinking or using drugs can interfere with the effectiveness of treatment.

ing suicide. He described a period of depression and sleep difficulties that began a month before admission and became increasingly severe. He was bothered by auditory hallucinations telling him that nothing was going to get any better and that he should kill himself. Although Tom had been taking the lithium he had been prescribed, he claimed, "It just wasn't working for me anymore." Tom's blood lithium level on admission was 0.05.

Tom had begun drinking beer in increasing quantities during the few weeks before admission. At first, he drank only at bedtime "to help me get to sleep," but later began drinking during the day because he claimed, "it fuzzed the voices out so I could ignore them."

TREATMENT OF CONCURRENT MEDICAL PROBLEMS

Medications with euphoric effects, such as narcotic pain medications, must sometimes be used to treat injuries or infections related to substance use. Abuse-related phenomena such as tolerance or liver damage can affect the efficacy of these medications, and their use may raise emotional issues for clients and staff (see the Rx Communication feature: Post-Operative Client with Borderline Personality Disorder and Heroin Dependence feature).

EVALUATION

Freedom from symptoms of drug or alcohol withdrawal and improved knowledge and understanding of the need for substance use reduction and adherence to treatment are desired goals. Clients should be able to identify ways in which substance abuse interferes with management of their psychiatric disorder.

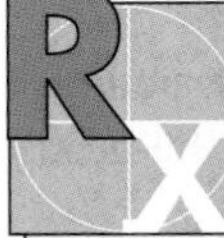

COMMUNICATION

Postoperative Client with Borderline Personality Disorder and Heroin Dependence

CLIENT: "I need something that will work for this pain! I had surgery yesterday and I can't even move. You nurses must think that because I shoot dope I'm just taking these pain shots to get high! If you don't give me some decent pain medication, I'm just going to wheel myself out of here and go shoot up!"

NURSE RESPONSE 1: "I'm sorry that you're in so much pain, and I'll do what I can to help you get better pain relief. The medication will work better if you get it as often as it can be given, instead of waiting until you're already in a lot of pain. We can also try some techniques to relax you and get your attention off the pain, like deep breathing, listening to a relaxation tape, or watching TV."

RATIONALE: Clients with borderline personality disorder often respond with rage when they feel that others are dismissing their concerns. This response may lead to impulsive behavior that is harmful to the client. Escalation of self-harming behavior can be avoided by empathic acknowledgment of the client's concerns, and a willingness to work with the client to satisfy her needs.

NURSE RESPONSE 2: "I'm sorry that your pain medication isn't working as well as it needs to. The pain medication you're taking is chemically similar to heroin. Since your body has developed a tolerance to heroin, you also won't get as much effect from the pain medication. I'll talk to your doctor and to our nurse expert on pain control about adjusting your medication dosage so you'll be more comfortable."

RATIONALE: Clients with heroin dependence develop physiologic tolerance to opiate drugs over time. When they require narcotic medications for pain, they may require a higher dose to obtain adequate pain relief.

They should also identify alternatives to substance use for managing symptoms of mental illness or undesirable treatment side effects.

Case Management

Since the services available to clients with coexisting disorders are often inadequate and unwelcoming, advocacy for your clients to receive services is a particularly important function as a nurse case manager. Substance abuse settings may exclude clients with coexisting mental illness because of bizarre or disruptive behavior, or because psychiatric symptoms such as depression or the negative symptoms of schizophrenia are interpreted as "lack of motivation." Mental health providers may feel that clients with coexisting disorders cannot benefit from treatment if they are still drinking or using drugs. Thus, clients may fail to receive treatment unless they are in crisis, leading to a "revolving door" pattern of emergency service use.

MODELS OF TREATMENT

Services for mental illness and substance abuse are often fragmented, so coordination of care is another important case management role. Three models of care are commonly used for treating clients with coexisting disorders: sequential, parallel, and integrated.

Sequential Treatment

In the sequential model, a client is treated first by the mental health system, then by the substance abuse treatment system, or vice versa. The decision about where the client is treated first may be made based on which disorder is most severe at the time, or on which disorder emerged first. For instance, a client who binges on alcohol when he becomes manic may first be hospitalized to treat the mania, then referred to an alcoholism treatment program when he is psychiatrically stable.

Parallel Treatment

Parallel treatment occurs when clients are treated simultaneously in both substance abuse and mental health settings. For example, a client with depression and crack cocaine addiction may participate in a residential program for crack-addicted women and their children while receiving antidepressant medication and group therapy at a mental health center. Coordination of care between the two settings can range from extensive to nonexistent.

Problems with Sequential and Parallel Treatment

These two models can work well for selected clients. They may provide suboptimal treatment, however, if the providers working with the client in either setting lack the training to understand how the two types of disorder may interact, or if the treatment methods and philosophies of the agencies are contradictory. These are some examples of the problems that can arise from sequential or parallel treatment:

- Behavior that is related to mental illness may be erroneously attributed to substance use, or vice versa, leading to misdiagnosis and inappropriate treatment.
- Treatment for one disorder may exacerbate the other. For instance, addiction treatment that is highly confrontational may be so emotionally intense that it causes decompensation in a schizophrenic client. Similarly, substance abuse relapse may result if benzodiazepine treatment for anxiety is not carefully monitored (see Box 21–1).
- Clients may receive contradictory advice from different settings. Mental health professionals may see adherence with psychotropic medications as essential to the management of a psychiatric disorder, but use of these medications might be regarded as "just another addiction" in a substance abuse setting.

In such circumstances, your role as coordinator of care is essential. You can help clients sort out conflicting instructions, as well as help to educate other care providers about the needs of clients with coexisting disorders.

BOX 21–1 Guidelines for the Use of Psychotropic Medication with Clients with Coexisting Disorders

- When it is not clear if psychiatric symptoms are due to mental illness or are caused primarily by substance use, medications should be used with caution. However, if psychiatric symptoms are severe, treatment should be instituted promptly even if the diagnosis is still unclear.
- Reevaluate the need for medication after a period of abstinence, or after acute symptoms clear.
- Be aware of potential interactions between substances of abuse and prescribed medication, but do not withhold needed medication just because the client is continuing to use alcohol or drugs.
- Consider other alternatives before medications with the potential for abuse (i.e., benzodiazepines or narcotic pain medications) are prescribed. If these medications are the most effective agents for treating a client's condition, monitor their use carefully.
- If clients are using alcohol or drugs to alleviate medication side effects, consider changing to a medication with less troublesome side effects.
- Atypical antipsychotic agents are associated with less drug craving (intense preoccupation with and desire for a drug) than older antipsychotic medications. These may be a better choice for substance-abusing clients with psychotic disorders.

Sources: Sowers, W., & Golden, S. (1999). Psychotropic medication management in persons with co-occurring psychiatric and substance use disorders. *Journal of Psychoactive Drugs, 31*(1), 59–70; and Wilkins, J. N. (1997). *Pharmacotherapy* of schizophrenia patients with comorbid substance abuse. *Schizophrenia Bulletin, 23*(2), 247–253.

Integrated Treatment

Integrated treatment for clients with severe mental illness and substance use disorders has become more widely available in the past decade. In this model, clients participate in one program that provides treatment for both disorders. Clinicians are trained in psychopathology, assessment, and treatment of both disorders, and offer substance abuse treatments that are specifically tailored for clients with coexisting mental illness (see the Intervention box below).

Recent studies of integrated treatment indicate that comprehensive integrated outpatient treatment for coexisting disorders can effectively engage clients in treatment and help them reduce substance use and attain remission of psychiatric illness. Program features that seem to produce the best outcomes include assertive outreach; motivational interventions; case management; a long-term, staged approach to recovery; and cultural competence (Drake et al., 2001). Research suggests that integrated treatment programs will become even more effective as this model continues to evolve (Ho et al., 1999).

In addition to the need for coordinated treatment for mental illness and substance abuse, clients with coexisting disorders may need your help to obtain the necessities of life. Decent, stable housing is one of the factors most important for clients with coexisting disorders to achieve and maintain sobriety (Alverson, Alverson, & Drake, 2000).

INTERVENTION

Guidelines for the Client with Coexisting Disorders

- Use matter of fact, nonjudgmental language when discussing substance use with clients. Try to understand the client's perception of his/her substance use.
- Help clients identify cause–effect relationships between their use of drugs or alcohol and the resulting consequences. Remember that the client's ability to understand these relationships may be impaired due to mental illness.
- Be straightforward in sharing your concerns about the consequences of a client's continued misuse of alcohol or drugs, but don't preach or nag.
- Collaborate with clients in setting short- and long-term treatment goals. Although you may recommend abstinence, be flexible in supporting interim goals that help clients reduce use and its associated harms.
- Support clients to identify and work toward goals that are important to them. Help clients understand how continued substance abuse may interfere with achievement of these goals.
- Be aware that both substance disorders and serious mental illnesses are chronic conditions in which progress may be slow and relapse is common. Take a long-term perspective, and appreciate and praise small steps forward.
- Relapse is part of the cycle of change. Help clients reframe lapses and relapses as learning opportunities to improve their recovery plan.
- Acceptance of the client as a person does not mean tolerating disruptive or abusive behavior from intoxicated clients.
- Encourage and support clients to get involved in self-help groups such as Alcoholics Anonymous if they are interested, but don't insist that they participate. Special self-help groups for people with co-existing disorders may be more acceptable to the client.

Community-Based Care

Working in a community setting allows you to learn much about the role of drug and alcohol use in your clients' lives, and to intervene in a variety of ways to decrease substance use and the negative consequences that may result. The frequency of contact and long-term nature of your relationships with clients allows for trust to develop, so clients feel able to talk about their drug use. In addition, knowledge about the client's social milieu and daily activities provides valuable information about which substances may be available and under what circumstances they are used.

As you develop an awareness of how substance abuse is affecting a client's course of illness and daily functioning, you can help the client see cause-and-effect relationships between substance misuse and adverse consequences. Clients with coexisting disorders may have a hard time making these connections. Denial is a common feature of addictive disorders, and logical thinking is impaired by thought disorder resulting from mental illness and cognitive deficits produced by the toxic effects of various drugs and alcohol.

Carey (1996) has described a model for working with clients with coexisting disorders in outpatient settings. This model incorporates key treatment principles articulated by experts in working with this population, such as integration, use of motivational approaches, harm reduction (see Chapter 13), and stagewise treatment. See Box 21–2 on page 520 for a description of the stages involved and their associated therapeutic tasks.

MediaLink Alcoholics Anonymous

GROUP TREATMENT

In addition to individual counseling, groups may be an extremely effective treatment modality for clients with coexisting disorders. In a group setting, clients feel less alone in struggling with mental illness and substance abuse, and can share experiences and coping strategies. Models of group treatment that address coexisting disorders include:

- 12-step models that incorporate the principles of groups such as Alcoholics Anonymous (www.alcoholics-anonymous.org).
- Professionally assisted groups to help prepare mental health clients for AA participation.
- Educational/supportive models that educate clients about both disorders and provide interpersonal support for **sobriety** (abstinence from use of intoxicating substances).
- Social skills training groups that teach clients skills necessary for sobriety, such as drink/drug refusal and obtaining a support person.
- Persuasion groups that develop awareness of the costs associated with substance use for clients who are not motivated to quit or reduce their use of drugs or alcohol.

Persuasion groups typically allow clients to attend group sessions even if they are under the influence of drugs or alcohol, as long as their behavior is not disruptive. You may have to exclude

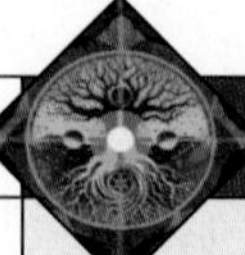

Case Study

Client with Coexisting Psychiatric and Substance Use Disorders

Bonnie Lewis is a 36-year-old woman who lives in a women's shelter. As a child, she was physically and sexually abused by her stepfather. She has required treatment for numerous suicide attempts over the years. Psychiatric diagnoses include major depression and borderline personality disorder. Bonnie also has a long history of alcohol and stimulant use. After completing a substance abuse program, she became an active participant in Alcoholics Anonymous, and has remained clean and sober for 8 months.

Bonnie appeared depressed the last time you saw her. She told you, "My mom died this time last year, and I get really sad when I think about it."

Today, Bonnie is malodorous and disheveled. She tells you that she "got stinking drunk" when she went to an appointment yesterday and ran into an old boyfriend, who invited her to join him in a few beers. Bonnie yielded to his persuasion and drank five or six beers "because I felt like it didn't matter anyway." After getting in an argument with her friend, Bonnie returned to the shelter. She is now very discouraged and says: "Once a drunk, always a drunk. I guess I'll never get clean and sober."

clients, however, who are abusive or threatening from group sessions. You should make clear to these clients that it is their disruptive behavior and not their substance use per se that is objectionable, and that they are welcome back when they can maintain appropriate behavior.

As you discuss with clients both the consequences and the desired effects of substance use, you may gain insight into how drugs or alcohol may be used to cope with symptoms of mental illness. Alternative coping strategies can then be taught. For instance, clients who use alcohol to relieve anxiety can learn relaxation exercises (Chapter 32) or cognitive strategies (Chapter 30) to reduce anxiety. The use of prescribed antianxiety medications may relieve anxiety as effectively as alcohol, but with fewer deleterious side effects.

SUBSTANCE ABUSE TREATMENT SETTINGS

Nurses in substance abuse treatment settings are also likely to work with clients with coexisting disorders and face difficulties determining whether psychiatric symptoms result exclusively from substance abuse, or whether an underlying psychiatric disorder is present. Accurate history about the onset of symptoms and their relationship to substance use can be difficult to obtain. If it can be determined that such symptoms as depression, paranoia, or hallucinations were present before substance use began, or during past periods of prolonged abstinence, you can assume the client has a mental disorder. Further consultation about managing the mental illness while in substance abuse treatment should be sought (see the Using Research Evidence feature on page 522). Similarly, if symptoms present during periods of substance use or withdrawal persist after more than a few weeks of abstinence, refer the client for a more complete psychiatric assessment.

When abstinence is well established, previous psychiatric diagnoses may need to be reviewed. For instance, clients thought to have bipolar disorder may have been diagnosed without knowledge of the role played by cocaine use in producing their severe mood swings. In contrast, substance abuse may mask the presence of other psychiatric disorders. The antipsychotic effects of opiates such as heroin may suppress the psychotic symptoms of schizophrenia.

BOX 21–2 Therapeutic Tasks Associated with Stages of Community Treatment for Clients with Coexisting Disorders

1. Establishing a working alliance.
   - Assist client to obtain food, clothing, shelter, and medications if necessary.
   - Communicate a sincere acceptance of the person, if not their substance use.
2. Evaluating costs and benefits of continued substance use.
   - Educate clients about effects of drugs and alcohol and their effects on psychiatric symptoms.
   - Identify and discuss client's life goals.
   - Clarify client's motivations for using drugs or alcohol.
   - Help client assess costs of substance use.
3. Individualizing goals for change.
   - Negotiate harm-reduction goals with client (may include reduced use or abstinence).
   - Discuss client's fears about recovery and provide reassurance.
   - Praise client for small successes.
4. Building an environment and lifestyle supportive of abstinence.
   - Provide structure to client (day treatment, frequent clinic appointments).
   - Help client identify people in social network who support sobriety.
   - Encourage client to attend meetings of self-help groups.
   - Engage client in enjoyable activities (recreation, education).
5. Coping with crises
   - Teach relapse prevention strategies.
   - Monitor for early signs of either psychiatric or substance abuse relapse.
   - Frame lapses as learning opportunities and assist client to resume sobriety.

Source: Adapted from Carey, K. B. (1996). Substance use reduction in the context of outpatient psychiatric treatment: A collaborative, motivational, harm reduction approach. *Community Mental Health Journal, 32*(3), 291–306. Reprinted with permission from Kluwer Academic/Plenum Publishers.

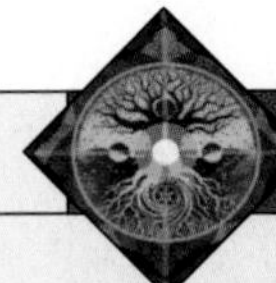

Nursing Care Plan

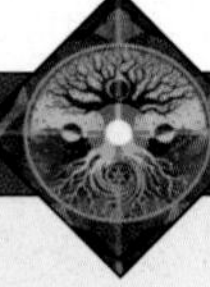

Nursing Diagnosis: Knowledge deficit related to substance abuse relapse.

Nursing Outcome: Knowledge, substance use control.

Short-Term Goals

- Client will describe potential for relapse in efforts to control substance use.
- Client will describe actions to prevent and manage relapses in substance abuse.

Interventions

- Educate client about relapse as a part of the process of changing addictive behavior (See Figure 13–3, Transtheoretical Model of Behavior Change).
- Teach client the difference between a **lapse** (brief incident of substance use) from a **relapse** (longer-term resumption of previous pattern of substance use).
- Praise client for seeking help to prevent her lapse from becoming a relapse.
- Educate client about common risk factors for substance abuse relapse. Help client identify personal risk factors or **triggers** (persons, places, or things that produce a desire to use an intoxicating substance).
- Assist client in analyzing lapse by identifying the risk factors present in recent situation.
- Ask client to recall other situations in which triggers were present and lapse did not occur. Help client identify successful coping mechanisms for dealing with **high-risk situations** (situations in which there is a high probability of a lapse or relapse), and suggest other possible successful responses.
- Rehearse/role-play situations in which client will be faced with her personal triggers for relapse.
- Use information gained from these discussions to help client prepare an "emergency card" that she can carry with her at all times. This should include phone numbers to call in emergencies or when she needs support to avoid drinking; the reasons why she wants to remain clean and sober; high-risk situations; and coping skills she can use to avoid relapse.
- Reinforce client's success in staying clean and sober in past months.

Rationale

- Normalizing lapses and relapses as a part of the change process decreases guilt and hopelessness.
- Identifying risk factors such as depressed mood and unresolved grief alerts client to the need to seek prompt assistance in coping with these problems.
- Rehearsing high-risk situations and having a written relapse prevention plan can help the client react quickly to avoid relapse when triggers are present.
- Identifying situations in which the client has successfully avoided relapse and reminding her of past success reinforces her sense of self-efficacy and hope.

Home Care

Psychiatric home care nurses are in an ideal situation to identify factors in the home that could either support or inhibit recovery for the client with coexisting disorders. The presence of household members who are drinking heavily or using drugs may make it difficult for a client to abstain. However, a loving relationship with someone sober who accepts the client's mental illness is an important "quality of life" factor that helps people become and stay sober (Alverson, Alverson, & Drake, 2000).

Families of clients with coexisting disorders may experience significant caregiving burden related to the client's disability and erratic behavior. Educating family members about how

USING RESEARCH EVIDENCE

Jeff B. is a 35-year-old man attending an outpatient day treatment program. He was diagnosed with schizophrenia at age 19 and has been hospitalized several times since then. He has been treated with a variety of typical antipsychotic medications, which he has taken "off and on" for years. He complains that when he takes his medications regularly "the discomfort is unbearable" and he feels "constant physical and emotional pain and pressure."

Your assessment of his current symptoms reveals that he is bothered by auditory hallucinations, delusions, paranoia, insomnia, restlessness, and muscle rigidity. Your substance use assessment reveals that Jeff became dependent on caffeine while hospitalized one year ago and is now drinking 5 to 6 cups of coffee per day. Six months ago, Jeff began drinking 5 to 6 beers per night in an attempt to improve his sleep. As his psychiatric nurse case manager, you formulate a nursing care plan that addresses the following considerations:

1. Jeff is suffering from psychiatric symptoms that are related to his illness, his medication side effects, and his use of substances.
2. Jeff is unaware of how abusing caffeine and alcohol affects his mood, psychiatric symptoms, and medication effects. You can help him make the connection between substance use and the relief, onset, and/or worsening of his symptoms.
3. Jeff is on a medication regimen that is ineffective and causing side effects. You can assist him in finding a medication regimen that gives him the best symptom control with the fewest unpleasant side effects.
4. Jeff can be educated about interactions between substances of abuse and medications.
5. If Jeff's symptoms continue in spite of changes in his medication regimen, improvement in his psychiatric symptoms, and a reduction in or abstinence from substances of abuse, he should be reevaluated for comorbid psychiatric conditions, such as depression.

The nursing care plan for Jeff is based on the following research:

Kasten, B. P. (1999). Self-medication with alcohol and drugs by persons with severe mental illness. *Journal of the American Psychiatric Nurses Association, 5*(3), 80–87.

mental illness and substance abuse interact (see the Client/Family Teaching feature on page 516) and supporting them to set limits on unreasonable behavior are ways you can be helpful to clients' families.

Maintaining a Positive and Hopeful Attitude

Working with clients with coexisting disorders can be difficult. Sometimes the sheer magnitude and complexity of their problems seems overwhelming, especially when few resources are available. It is easy to be frustrated when the best-laid treatment plan is undermined by a client's impulsiveness or poor judgment. It can also be painful to see clients suffer and become discouraged as they experience the losses and setbacks that are a common result of coexisting disorders.

Your ability to maintain hope in the face of adversity and envision a better future for your clients makes a crucial difference in your work—optimism is a key treatment principle when working with clients with coexisting disorders. See the Nursing Self-Awareness feature below for suggestions to help you provide compassionate care and avoid burnout.

Nursing SELF-AWARENESS — Maintaining Therapeutic Optimism

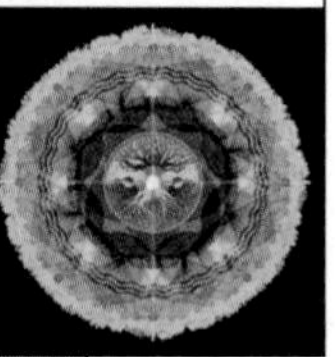

- **Realize that both mental illness and substance disorders are chronic, relapsing conditions.** Understand that progress may be slow and setbacks inevitable despite your best efforts and those of the client. Appreciate small steps forward and reframe setbacks as learning opportunities.
- **Understand that even if a client is not currently making much effort toward better management of his or her disorders, the development of a trusting relationship with you is helping to set the stage for movement toward recovery in the future.** "A positive, valued relationship with a mental health professional" is one of the factors that prompt mental health clients to move toward sobriety (Alverson et al., 2000).
- **Talk to people with coexisting disorders who are in recovery.** Hearing about how these individuals overcame challenges to become happier and more stable will give you more confidence that clients who are currently struggling with similar obstacles can also overcome them.
- **Don't be afraid to talk to clients about spirituality.** Mental health providers often underestimate how important spiritual concerns are in the lives of clients with coexisting disorders. Ask clients about their spiritual beliefs and practices, and be flexible in helping clients find support for their spirituality. Access to these inner resources is especially important when clients lack external support.
- **Find mentors who are successful in working with clients with coexisting disorders.** Seek their help in dealing with situations you find difficult or frustrating.
- **Take good care of your own physical, mental, and spiritual health.** You can role model healthy behavior for clients (never underestimate the power of a good example!), and renewing your own energy means you have more to give in your relationships with clients.

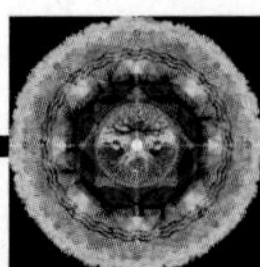

EXPLORE MediaLink

NCLEX review, case studies, and other interactive resources for this chapter can be found on the Companion Website at http://www.prenhall.com/kneisl. Click on Chapter 21 to select the activities for this chapter.

For animations, video tutorials, more NCLEX review questions, and an audio glossary, access the accompanying CD-ROM in this textbook.

BIBLIOGRAPHY

Alverson, H., Alverson, M., & Drake, R. E. (2000). An ethnographic study of the longitudinal course of substance abuse among people with severe mental illness. *Community Mental Health Journal, 36*(6), 557–569.

Brady, K., & Randall, C. (1999). Gender differences in substance use disorders. *Addictive Disorders, 22*(2), 241–251.

Carey, K. B. (1996). Substance use reduction in the context of outpatient psychiatric treatment: A collaborative, motivational, harm reduction approach. *Community Mental Health Journal, 32*(3), 291–306.

Center for Substance Abuse Treatment. (1999). *Cultural issues in substance abuse treatment* (DHHS Publication No. SMA 99-3278). Rockville, MD: Department of Health and Human Services.

Compton, P. (1989). Drug abuse: A self-care deficit. *Journal of Psychosocial Nursing, 27*(3), 22–26.

Drake, R. E., Essock, S. M., Shaner, A., Carey, K. B., Minkoff, K., Kola, L., et al. (2001). Implementing dual diagnosis services for clients with severe mental illness. *Psychiatric Services, 52*(4), 469–476.

Estroff, S. E. (1981). *Making it crazy*. Berkeley, CA: University of California Press.

Hambrecht, M., & Hafner, H. (1996). Substance abuse and the onset of schizophrenia. *Biological Psychiatry, 40*(11), 1155–1163.

Ho, A. P., Tsuang, J. W., Liberman, R. P., Wang, R., Wilkins, J. N., Eckman, T. A., et al. (1999). Achieving effective treatment of patients with chronic psychotic illness and comorbid substance dependence. *American Journal of Psychiatry, 156*(11), 1765–1770.

Johnson, J. G., Cohen, P., Pine, D. S., Klein, D. F., Kasen, S., & Brook, J. S. (2000). Association between cigarette smoking and anxiety disorders during adolescence and early adulthood. *Journal of the American Medical Association, 284*(18), 2348–2351.

Kasten, B. P. (1999). Self-medication with alcohol and drugs by persons with severe mental illness. *Journal of the American Psychiatric Nurses Association, 5*(3), 80–87.

Khantzian, E. J. (1985). The self-medication hypothesis of addictive disorders: Focus on heroin and cocaine dependence. *American Journal of Psychiatry, 142*(11), 1259–1264.

Kovaszny, B., Fleischer, J., Tanenberg-Karant, M., Jandorf, L., Miller, A. D., & Bromet, E. (1997). Substance use disorder and early course of illness in schizophrenia and affective psychosis. *Schizophrenia Bulletin, 23*(2), 195–201.

Lacey, D. (1993). Using Orem's model in psychiatric nursing. *Nursing Standard, 7*(29), 28–30.

Mueser, K. T., Essock, S. M., Drake, R. E., Wolfe, R. S., & Frisman, L. (2001). Rural and urban differences in patients with a dual diagnosis. *Schizophrenia Research, 48*, 93–107.

Pollack, L. E., & Steubben, G. (1998). Addiction Education Groups for inpatients with dual diagnoses. *Journal of the American Psychiatric Nurses Association, 4*(4), 121–127.

Regier, D. A., Farmer, M. E., Rae, D. S., Locke, B. Z., Keith, S. J., Judd, L. L., et al. (1990). Comorbidity of mental disorders with alcohol and other drug abuse: Results from the Epidemiologic Catchment Area (ECA) Study. *Journal of the American Medical Association, 264*(19), 2511–2518.

Ries, R. K., Sloan, K. L., & Miller, N. S. (1997). *Dual diagnosis: Concept, diagnosis, and treatment*. Unpublished manuscript.

Sowers, W., & Golden, S. (1999). Psychotropic medication management in persons with co-occurring psychiatric and substance use disorders. *Journal of Psychoactive Drugs, 31*(1), 59–70.

Wilkins, J. N. (1997). Pharmacotherapy of schizophrenia patients with comorbid substance abuse. *Schizophrenia Bulletin, 23*(2), 215–228.

Ziedonis, D. M., & George, T. P. (1997). Schizophrenia and nicotine use. *Schizophrenia Bulletin, 23*(2), 247–253.

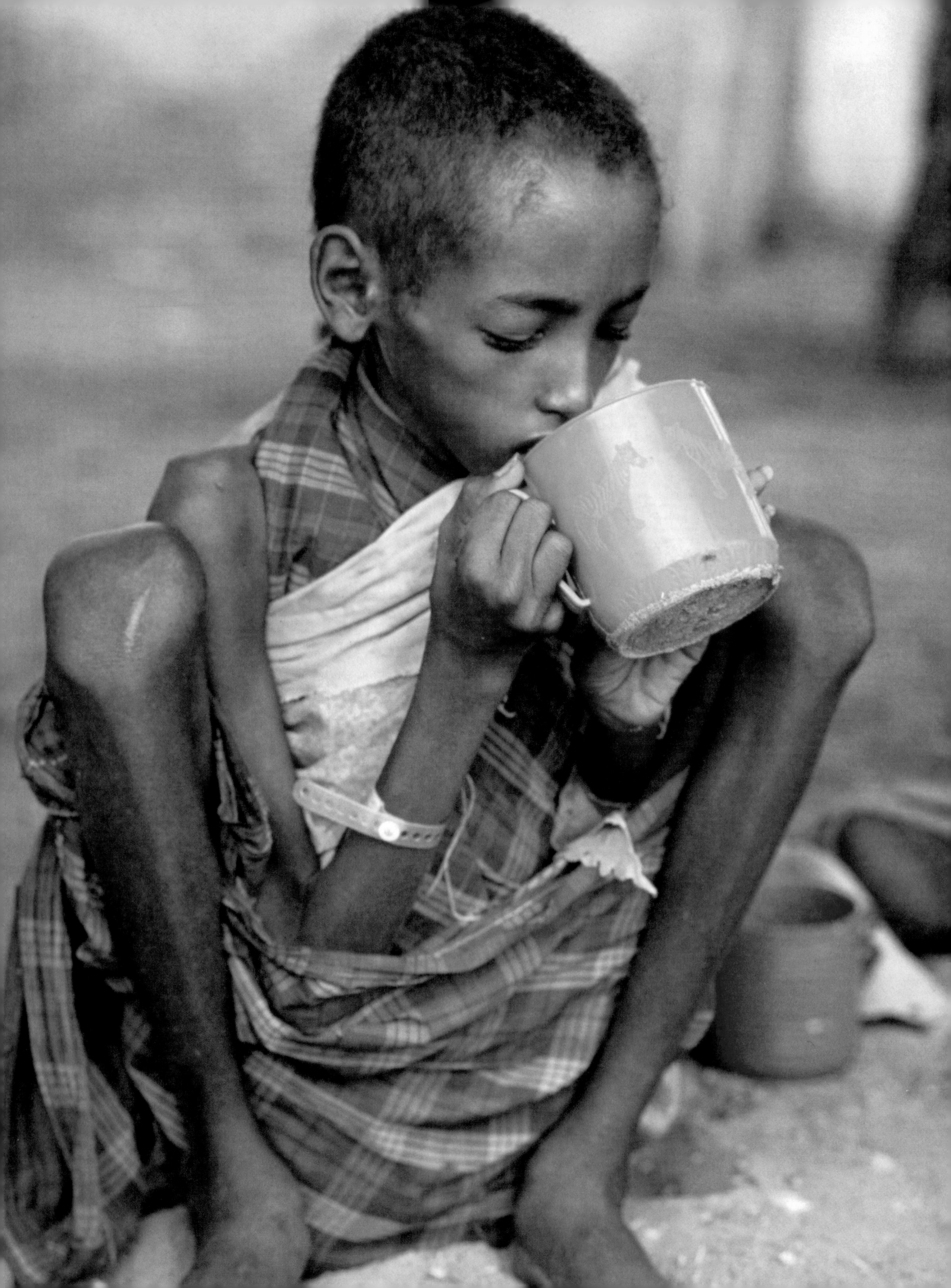

UNIT Four

Vulnerable Populations

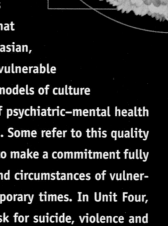

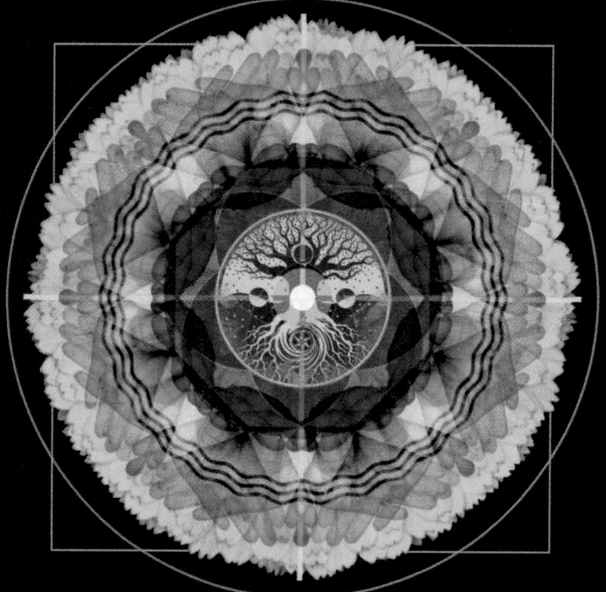

Abdi is a starving child squatting on the sand at a feeding center in Kismaayo, Somalia, in Africa. Learning of his life experience emphasizes the fact that to a large extent, people's health status may depend on the group or subgroup to which they belong. Furthermore, in the case of Abdi, his failing physical health can hold disastrous consequences for his ability to learn, to remember, and to carry out daily tasks of mental survival. A critical task for us as psychiatric–mental health nurses is to be aware of the disparities in mental health status among the diverse populations of the world. It follows, then, that we advocate for research that expands the focus from Caucasian, middle-class, heterosexual, able-bodied people to include vulnerable populations. We must gain a deeper understanding of current models of culture and the way culture shapes our thinking about and practice of psychiatric–mental health care. And we must develop a responsible or moral imagination. Some refer to this quality as a *common fire*, a shared vision of core values that allows us to make a commitment fully respectful of the common good in the shifting complexities and circumstances of vulnerable populations and in the face of the unknowns of contemporary times. In Unit Four, you will learn about some of these populations—people at risk for suicide, violence and abuse, HIV/AIDS, children, adolescents, and elders—and how you can serve as an advocate who works in a knowledgeable, compassionate, and forgiving way.

←

Source: Schiller/The Image Works

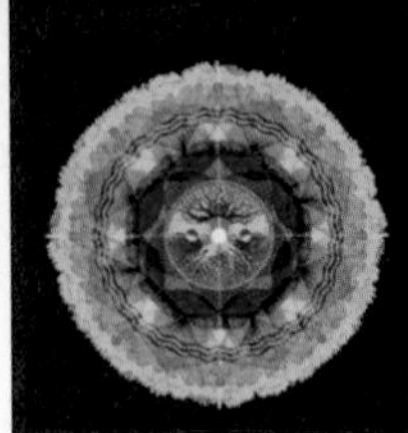

22

Chapter TWENTY-TWO

Clients at Risk for Suicide and Self-Destructive Behavior

CAROL REN KNEISL
ELIZABETH A. RILEY

KEY TERMS

cluster suicide
chronic self-destructive behavior
lethality assessment
psychological autopsy
self-destructive behavior
self-mutilation
suicide
suicide attempt
suicide precautions
suicide threat

FOCUS QUESTIONS

- Why might you feel anxious when working with suicidal or other self-destructive clients?
- What social, demographic, and clinical variables influence suicidal or self-destructive behavior?
- How would you carry out a lethality assessment?
- What are the crucial components of basic suicide precautions? Maximum suicide precautions?
- What strategies for intervention are helpful to survivors of suicide?

MediaLink 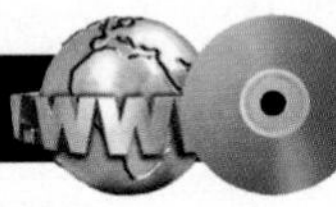 www.prenhall.com/kneisl

Additional resources for this chapter can be found on the Student CD-ROM accompanying this textbook, and on the Companion Website at www.prenhall.com/kneisl. Click on Chapter 22 to select the activities for this chapter.

CD-ROM
- Audio Glossary
- NCLEX Review

Companion Website
- Additional NCLEX Review
- Care Plan: Suicide Watch
- Case Study: Assessing Lethality

CHAPTER OUTLINE

CROSS REFERENCES

Other topics relevant to this content are: Behavioral contracts, Chapter 30; Crisis intervention, Chapter 33; Critical incident staff debriefing, Chapter 33; Ethical reasoning, Chapter 10; Medications for depression, Chapter 31; Neurotransmitter hypothesis of depression, Chapters 4 and 15; Right to treatment in the least restrictive setting, Chapter 11; Stress, anxiety, and coping, Chapter 5; Suicide risk in children, adolescents, and elders, Chapters 25, 26, and 27; Suicide risk in substance abuse, depression, and HIV, Chapters 13, 15, and 24.

CRITICAL THINKING CHALLENGE

Despite your attempts to convince Maureen that her family would not be better off without her, Maureen insists that she is determined to commit suicide. Maureen plans to run from the inpatient unit and jump in front of a moving car. In considering how best to help her, a staff member suggests that taking her shoes away would prevent Maureen from running away. How do you feel about taking belongings away from someone who is suicidal? Do you agree with this practice? How can you best help to maintain Maureen's safety? ■

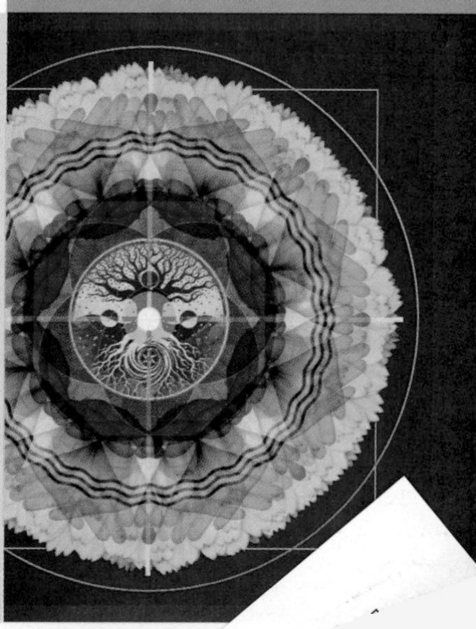

Self-destructive behavior has been a part of the human experience since time began. **Self-destructive behaviors** are maladaptive measures a person uses to restore inner equilibrium when overwhelmed or unable to cope with stressful life events. Distressed and unable to see that they have other options, people consider or attempt to harm themselves thinking that they can take away unbearable emotional pain.

Did you know that many people who commit **suicide,** the willful act of ending one's own life, have seen a nurse, physician, or other health care professional the same month they commit suicide? Over 90% of people who commit suicide have a psychiatric illness, and over 50% are under active psychiatric or mental health care (Fawcett, 2001).

Stigma and ignorance about mental illness, depression, and suicide may embarrass, shame, and silence individuals who really want to speak with others of their pain. Clients may believe that others, including nurses and other health care providers, will label them "crazy" if they speak of suicide. In fact, discussions of suicide do arouse intense and complicated emotions in others.

Suicide is a major public health problem in North America and in many countries around the globe. ■ Figure 22–1 is a visual of U.S. suicide rates by age, gender, and race. Box 22–1 demonstrates that suicide affects all age groups, both genders, and all cultures, religions, and socioeconomic classes as in the clinical examples that follow.

CLINICAL EXAMPLE

Sarah, age 17, is a petite brunette cheerleader. She comes to the school nurse stating that she just found out she has been rejected by the college of her choice.

Frank, a retired financial counselor, is a 68-year-old African-American man. His wife died last year and his children live two states away. He comes to the family nurse practitioner stating he just "feels sick."

Natalie is a 36-year-old divorced mother of two receiving Aid to Families with Dependent Children assistance. She comes into the outpatient clinic stating she has taken 32 diazepam (Valium), 10-mg tablets.

Tom is 24 years old. He is in the emergency room of the hospital and is comatose. His landlord found him in his room in a boarding house with bottles and pills all around him.

Be aware that any client in a health care, occupational, or community setting may, under certain circumstances, contemplate suicide.

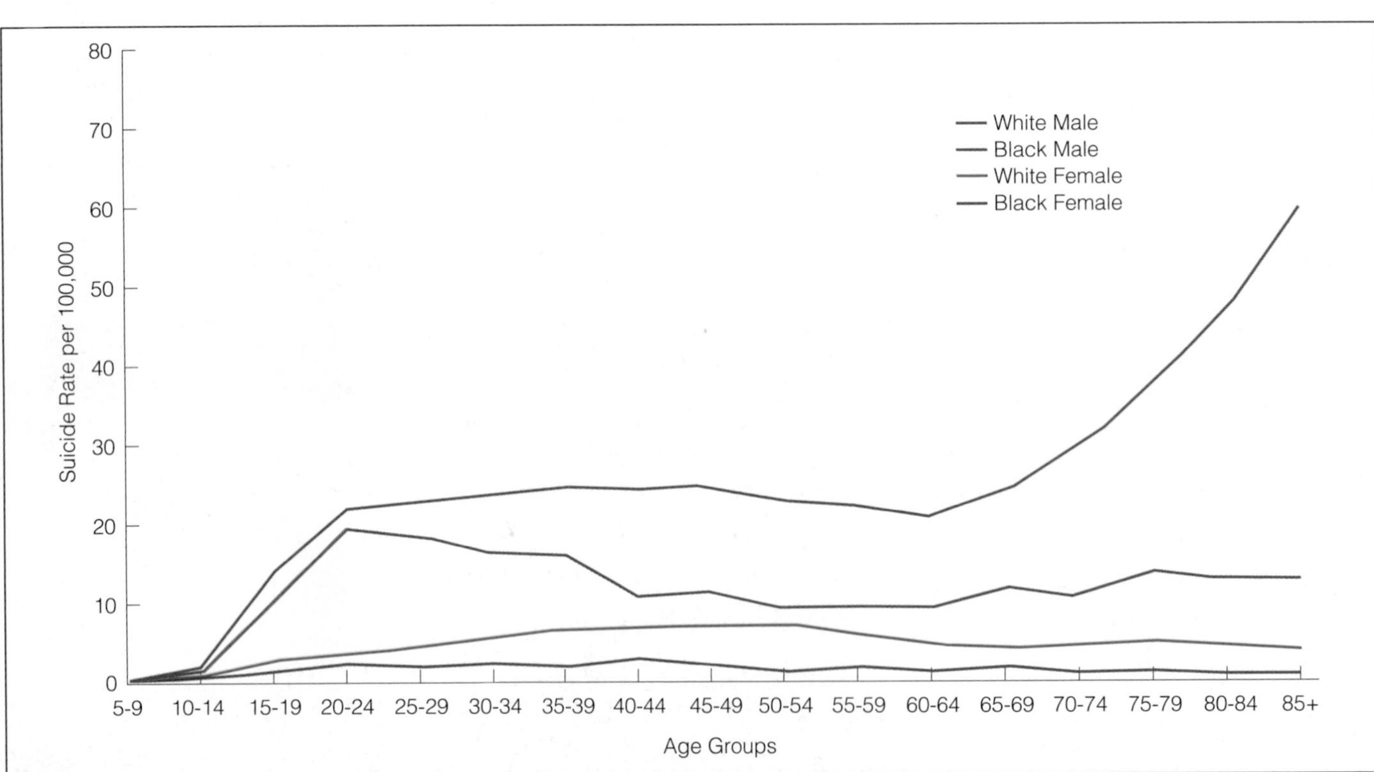

FIGURE 22–1 ■ *U.S. suicide rates by age, gender, and racial group.*
Source: National Institute of Mental Health, 1999.

BOX 22–1 Suicide Facts

- Suicide is the **third** leading cause of death among young people 15 to 24 years of age.
- Suicide is now the **eleventh** leading cause of death in the United States across all age groups.
- More people kill themselves each year than are murdered; for every **two people who are murdered**, there are **three persons who take their own lives.**
- There are more than **30,000** deaths from suicide each year.
- Over **700,000** people visit emergency departments for self-inflicted injury each year.
- There are **twice** as many suicides than deaths due to HIV/AIDS.
- In the month prior to their suicide, **75%** of older suicide victims had visited a primary care provider—many had a depressive illness that was not detected.
- More men than women die by suicide; the gender ratio is **four males to every one female**; however, **women attempt suicide three times more often** than men.
- The strongest risk factors for attempted suicide in adults are **depression, alcohol abuse, cocaine use, and separation or divorce.**
- The strongest risk factors for attempted suicide in youth are **depression, alcohol or other drug use disorder, and aggressive or disruptive behaviors.**

Source: National Institute of Mental Health, 2002.

Direct and Indirect Self-Destructive Behavior

In addition to suicide, other typical self-destructive behaviors include, but are not limited to, nail biting, hair pulling, scratching or cutting one's wrist or another part of the body, smoking cigarettes, driving recklessly, drinking alcohol, and using drugs. In general, these behaviors range from relatively innocuous acts at one end of the continuum, such as overeating and gambling, to more lethal ones at the other, such as driving recklessly in a blinding snowstorm. A completed suicide is the most violent self-destructive behavior.

People who are self-destructive may manifest several of the behaviors listed in Box 22–2. Those who are chronically self-destructive in indirect ways may also make suicide attempts or carry suicide to completion.

When the primary conscious goal of the behavior is self-injury, the term *direct self-destructive behavior* is accurate. Suicide is its most extreme form. In *indirect self-destructive behavior*, self-injury is an undesired effect rather than the primary conscious goal. It is important to understand that not all self-destructive individuals (in fact, only about 10% of those who purposefully injure themselves) go on to kill themselves.

MALADAPTIVE MEASURES

People who have experienced early childhood neglect, abuse, or trauma frequently have difficulty understanding how to process feelings verbally and how to intervene in situations in a productive fashion—that is, to avoid problems. Many of these individuals use **self-mutilation**—such as cutting themselves, burning themselves with cigarettes, burning themselves on a stove, pulling out their hair, biting their fingernails into the cuticles—to deal with anxiety and distress. Self-mutilation is likely to be related to early childhood abuse or neglect and trauma.

Self-destructive individuals do not see the behaviors as particularly problematic until the behaviors are out of control. These clients feel that the experience of the painful behavior helps change or improve their mood and their level of awareness, thereby enabling them to reconnect with themselves. Individuals such as those described in the clinical examples below perceive their painful behavior as being adaptive and helpful to them in dealing with their anxiety and distress.

BOX 22–2 Levels of Self-Destructive Behavior

- **Chronic self-destructive behavior:** Behavior that harms the self, is habitual, and generally poses a low level of lethality. Behaviors may include smoking, gambling, using drugs, self-mutilation.
- **Suicide attempt:** A desperate call for help involving different levels of risk. The attempt may be planned to avoid serious injury, or it may be one in which the outcome depends on the circumstances and is not under the individual's control. For example, someone who takes a heavy overdose of sleeping pills may or may not be discovered in time.
- **Suicide threat:** A threat that is more serious than a casual statement of suicidal intent and that is accompanied by other behavior changes. These may include mood swings, temper outbursts, a decline in school or work performance, personality changes, sudden or gradual withdrawal from friends, and other significant changes in attitude.

CLINICAL EXAMPLE

Katy, 29 years old, has had trouble adjusting and being a part of things since "as far back as she remembers." She has no idea how to effectively manage her life problems and her increasing stress. She often cuts her abdomen or her arms. Katy is quick to point out that this is in no way a plan to kill herself. Rather, she finds that it helps relieve tension and changes her perspective.

Josie, age 33, is a compulsive overeater and manages anxiety by literally eating nonstop. Since she has been trying to lose weight, she now pulls out her hair (a different type of self-destructive behavior) to manage internal feelings of increasing stress and discomfort. Her hair is starting to fall out more readily, and she has required several haircuts to keep her hair looking appropriate for her job.

Indirect self-destructive behavior can injure one's health and hasten one's own sometimes premature death.

The exact reason for indirect self-destructive behavior is unknown, although there is much speculation about it. Several interpretations are possible. For example, indirect self-destructive behavior may help people cope with a crisis, or deny mental pain or cope with it, thus avoiding depression. Indirect self-destructive behavior may also result from impulsivity in people who are unable or unwilling to consider the long-term effects of their behavior. Another possibility is that indirect self-destructive behavior is a coping mechanism that raises low self-esteem by denying helplessness. A self-punishing act tends to relieve unconscious guilt.

ETHICS AND SUICIDE

Do people have the right to commit suicide, and can or should nurses intervene when people try to kill themselves? The traditional belief is that mental health care professionals should do everything possible to prevent suicide. Nurses should know that, ethical concerns aside, they may be prosecuted under state laws, making it a crime to aid or abet a suicide, under any circumstance, even when a terminally ill person decides to end his or her life. Questions about a client's right to suicide and society's right to control suicide have not been answered. Engaging in the process of ethical reasoning presented in Chapter 10 will help you in your search for a personal position.

MEANING AND MOTIVATION IN SUICIDE

Suicide is never a random act. Whether committed impulsively or after painstaking consideration, the act has both a message and a purpose. In general, the purpose or reason for suicide is to escape or to end an intolerable situation, crisis, or relationship, such as:

- Escaping a terminal (especially painful) illness.
- Avoiding being a burden to others.
- Resolving an untenable family situation.
- Resolving an untenable individual situation.
- Avoiding punishment or exposure of socially or personally unacceptable behavior.

CLINICAL EXAMPLE

Helen's lung cancer has metastasized to her bones; any exertion causes spontaneous fractures and she is in constant pain. She has asked friends, family, and health care workers to help her escape her illness by ending her life.

Joan, a widow, fell three times last year and is now in a nursing home. She decided on suicide so that she would no longer be a burden to her family. Joan has not eaten in 7 days.

Matt, age 7, attempted to run into the path of a car. He had heard his mother say many times, "If it weren't for you, your Daddy and I would never have broken up." Matt believed that if he were dead, his parents would reunite, thus solving what he believes to be an untenable family situation.

Serena, age 33, had been admitted for the third time to a psychiatric unit because of thoughts of suicide. Jorge, her husband, has broken the last two family therapy appointments and went on vacation when she came into the hospital this time. Serena recognizes that Jorge will not be available to her, and can't tolerate the idea of divorce or looking for another mate. She believes that she is unlovable and will attempt to leave the hospital tonight to finally stop the pain.

Fletcher, 34, was a successful businessman. Last night, he was charged with drunken driving and vehicular homicide. Horrified that his unacceptable behavior would be exposed, he committed suicide after learning that his picture and the story would be in the morning newspaper.

Cognitive Style

Suicidologists have speculated about the cognitive style (method of thought processing) of clients who commit or attempt suicide. Although there is no single suicidal logic, some cognitive styles predispose to suicidal behavior.

Dichotomous thinking (the belief that there is only an either/or choice) is commonly seen in the suicidal person. The person falls into an imminently suicidal state when death seems the only escape. The thought processing of suicidal clients is generally constricted; that is, people who are suicidal have great difficulty (if they can do it at all) in considering alternatives to their current dilemma. *Constriction in thought* generally results in the belief that there are only two choices: a magical solution or death. Clients whose prior suicide attempts were highly lethal performed significantly worse than other groups on tests of executive functioning (logical reasoning, verbal learning, integrating old and new information). These differences could not be explained by prior education, occupation, or intellectual capacity (Keilp et al., 2001).

Ambivalence

People who are considering suicide are divided within themselves. They have two conflicting desires at the same time: to live and to die. Understanding the thinking of someone who is acutely suicidal requires an understanding of the concept of ambivalence. Ambivalence accounts for the fact that a suicidal person often takes lethal or near-lethal action but leaves open the possibility for rescue, allowing for the possibility of intervention (Aguilera, 1998). Failing to intervene and provide life choices increases the person's desperation, and death becomes the more focused choice.

Communication

Many people who are self-destructive have lifelong difficulties communicating their needs to others. Some people cannot express their needs or feelings; or, when they do, they do not obtain the results they hoped for. For them, self-mutilation or suicide becomes a clear and direct, if violent, form of communication. See the Rx Communication feature below for an example of communicating with a client who self-mutilates.

The message inherent in suicide is often aimed at a specific person, usually the significant other. The significant other's ability to recognize this message is the key to understanding and resolving the suicidal person's unmet need. Interrupting a suicide plan or suicidal thoughts requires hearing, understanding, and responding appropriately to messages of pain, loneliness, and hopelessness.

Intended Effect on Significant Others

According to the classic work of Schneidman (1985), suicide is more accurately described as a dyadic event between two unhappy people, motivated by real or perceived rejection, abandonment, guilt, revenge, or pity. Suicide can be better understood if viewed in the context of the relationship between two people: the suicidal person and the significant other. Broadly defined, the significant other can be a spouse, child, boss, landlord, friend, nurse, or other health care worker.

Suicidal people almost always communicate their intent to significant others before the fact or attempt, although the meaning of the message may not be clear until after the attempt or death. Schneidman (1985) found a clear communication of intent in 80% of cases studied. A suicide threat or suicide attempt can arouse feelings of sympathy, anger, hostility, anxiety, or desire for connectedness on the part of a significant other, thus altering the current relationship to meet the need of the suicidal person.

Nurses' Self-Awareness

As psychiatric–mental health nurses, we frequently find ourselves face to face with suicidal or self-destructive people. Few clients elicit such intense feelings of anxiety and helplessness. Suicidal individuals will cause you to question your abilities to help others and preserve life. Thus, it is critically important to be prepared for all of the emotional reactions—fear, anxiety, anger, and so on—that a suicidal client may evoke in you. Unless you understand them, these reactions may interfere with your ability to establish rapport.

Our attitudes toward suicidal clients have many sources. In addition to direct experience with suicidal clients, societal and ethical issues, as well as historical antecedents, influence what we think and how we feel about suicide and self-destructive behavior, euthanasia, abortion rights, the right to commit suicide, and the responsibility to prevent suicide. We can get caught up in the dilemma of how much responsibility to take for the self-destructive person and for how long.

All nurses must be competent to assess and intervene effectively with a suicidal client. This is not easy. Suicidal and self-destructive people seemingly defeat our best efforts by choosing death over life, or by being self-destructive. Although it is our responsibility to promote and maintain life, we cannot force the client to do so. Instead, we encourage clients to examine and understand how it is that they have reached this point.

Nurses working with self-destructive or suicidal clients may have a variety of feelings—frustration and anger among them. Before working with someone who is suicidal or self-destructive, it is critically important to assess personal feelings, experiences, conflicts, and memories that may either impede or facilitate your effectiveness. The inventory in the Nursing Self-Awareness feature on page 532 will help you to explore your own attitudes.

Biopsychosocial Theories

Suicide and self-destructive behavior are still not well understood by the public or by the scientific community. In fact, many peoples' understanding of suicide has been influenced by misconceptions. These myths, and the corresponding explanatory facts that negate them, are discussed in Box 22–3.

Suicide is a complex phenomenon, and there is no single explanation for its complicated process; however, sociocultural and biologic theories seem to contribute the most to our understanding of suicide. In addition to the section that follows, careful study of Chapters 15 and 20 will help you to understand the behaviors discussed in this chapter.

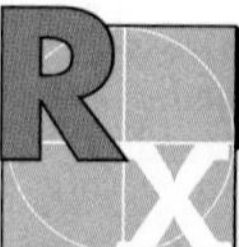

COMMUNICATION

Communicating with a Client Who Self-Mutilates

CLIENT: I just had to cut myself. There is no other way to be able to feel anything.

NURSE RESPONSE 1: I'm wondering how you felt when you cut yourself.

RATIONALE: Gathering more data will help you to understand the client better. You can help the client consider triggers and behaviors if you first encourage the client to identify and describe feelings and emotions around the event.

NURSE RESPONSE 2: Let's talk about what led up to your cutting yourself.

RATIONALE: While this response validates the behavior as real, it also asks the client to begin examining cause and effect.

Nursing SELF-AWARENESS — An Attitude Inventory for Working with Suicidal Clients

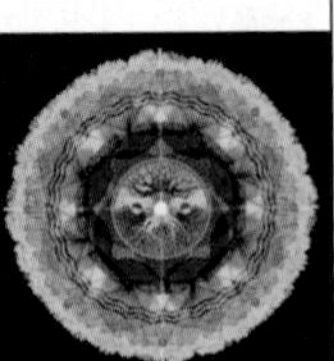

To increase self-awareness about managing your own anxiety in working with clients who are suicidal, ask yourself the following questions:

- What kinds of things frighten me?
- How do I feel about asking for someone else's help with a client if I'm unsure of myself or uncomfortable?
- Are suicidal clients asking me to take responsibility for their behavior?
- Are suicidal clients able to assume responsibility for their own behavior?

To increase self-awareness of your own feelings about self-destructive people, ask yourself the following questions:

- How do I feel about people who deliberately harm themselves?
- How do I understand self-destructive behavior?
- Do I believe that clients are capable of change?
- Do I believe that people ultimately have the responsibility for their own lives?
- Can a person who is mentally ill choose suicide as a reasonable course?

To increase self-awareness about your own anger, ask yourself the following questions:

- What kinds of things make me angry?
- How do I deal with my own anger? Do I tend to ignore it or hide it?
- How do I react to others when they are angry?
- How do I feel about people who don't change immediately?
- How do I deal with people who appear to do illogical things?
- How do I feel when people don't change their behavior when I've asked them to or when I talk to them about it?

To increase self-awareness about your own feeling of control, ask yourself the following questions:

- In what areas of my life and my work do I feel the need to take control?
- How do I feel when interventions do not go the way I would like them to?
- How do I handle control issues with clients?
- How do I feel about control issues with clients?
- How do I feel about my lack of control over others?

SOCIOCULTURAL THEORIES

Sociocultural theories about suicide propose that the social and cultural contexts in which the individual lives influence the expression of suicidality. The notion that suicide is an expression of interpersonal and societal, as well as intrapsychic, conflict is perhaps the most significant contribution sociologists have made to our understanding of suicide. The clinical examples on the facing page describe some social and cultural contexts for suicide:

- Having no close relationships with others.
- Experiencing a precipitous deterioration in one's relationship with society (such as the loss of a job or a close friend).

BOX 22-3 Suicide Myths Versus Suicide Facts

Myth: A suicide threat is just a bid for attention and should not be taken seriously.

Fact: All suicidal behavior should be taken seriously; a bid for attention may be a cry for help.

Myth: It is harmful for a person to talk about suicidal thoughts. The person's attention should be diverted when this occurs.

Fact: Of prime importance in helping a suicidal person is talking with that person in order to assess the lethality of the person's suicide plan.

Myth: Only psychotic people commit suicide.

Fact: The majority of completed suicides are committed by people who are not psychotic.

Myth: People who talk about suicide won't do it.

Fact: Most people do talk about their suicide intention before making a suicide attempt.

Myth: A nice home, good job, or an intact family prevents suicide.

Fact: People of all social and economic backgrounds commit suicide.

Myth: A failed suicide attempt should be treated as manipulative behavior.

Fact: Failed attempts are more likely evidence of a person's ambivalence toward suicide.

Myth: People who commit suicide are always depressed.

Fact: People who commit suicide are not always depressed, although depression is common. People can also be psychotic, agitated, organically impaired, or have personality disorders.

Myth: There is no connection between alcohol or drug use and suicide.

Fact: Alcohol, drugs, and suicide are often closely connected. A person who commits suicide may have become depressed, impulsive, and suicidal after using alcohol or other drugs.

Myth: Once suicidal, always suicidal.

Fact: Suicide attempts are often made during particularly stressful times in people's lives. If the suicide attempt is managed properly, people can and do go on with their lives without recurrent thoughts of suicide.

Myth: Suicidal people rarely seek medical help.

Fact: According to studies, 50% to 60% of suicidal people sought help within the 6 months that preceded the suicide.

- Having no personal freedoms and no hope of getting them.
- Considering self-inflicted death as honorable.

CLINICAL EXAMPLE

Gerald had decided that life was not worth living after retiring from his job with the federal government. He realized that no one would even know or care if he succeeded in killing himself. Without family or friends, Gerald has had no significant relationship since the death of his mother about 20 years ago.

Danielle thought that suicide was the best way to solve her problems after she lost her job at a local factory, and her boyfriend of 10 years precipitously broke off their engagement, left the area, and married someone else.

Jamie, who is a battered woman, believes that it doesn't make any sense to go on living. She has no close friends or relatives. Her husband will not allow her to drive, go shopping, go to work, and so on. She is unable to see an alternative and decides that a life regulated to this extent is not worth living.

In the Gaza Strip, a suicide bomber on a revenge mission detonated explosives strapped to his body as he rode his bicycle into an Israeli checkpoint, killing himself and three soldiers and wounding several bystanders. Those who claimed responsibility for the attack indicated their belief that the suicide bomber's death was an honorable one.

Similarities and differences exist in suicide rates among various ethnic and racial groups. When gender is considered, males in each group (Native Americans, white non-Hispanics, African-Americans, Hispanics, and Asian/Pacific Islanders) have higher suicide rates than females. When age is considered, Native Americans and African-Americans have the highest suicide rates during the adolescent and young adult years, while the highest suicide rates in those over 65 years of age occur in European-American non-Hispanics, Hispanics, and Asian/Pacific Islanders (Center for Mental Health Services, 2002). The percentage of suicide attempts was significantly higher among Hispanic Latina girls (19.3%) than in African-American or Caucasian groups (Rew, Thomas, Horner, Resnick, & Beuhring, 2001). Another study compared the relationship between suicide and major depression among whites, Puerto Ricans, Mexican-Americans, and Cuban-Americans. According to Oquendo et al. (2001), the rate of depression was significantly higher for Puerto Ricans (6.9%) and significantly lower in Mexican-Americans (2.8%) and Cuban-Americans (2.6%) compared to the 1-year prevalence rate for major depression for whites (3.6%). This study also found that annual suicide rates were higher for males than for females, and Mexican-American and Puerto Rican males had lower suicide rates than white males. The researchers raised the possibilities that depression differs in form or severity in these groups, or that unidentified factors protect against suicide in different subgroups.

BIOLOGIC THEORIES

The neurotransmitter receptor hypothesis of depression (see Chapters 4 and 15) holds that errors in the receptors for the specific neurotransmitter, serotonin, are critical in the development of depression and suicide. The research indicates that serotogenic hypofunction is associated with suicide and serious suicide attempts (Kamali, Oquendo, & Mann, 2001). There is considerable evidence that the serotonergic system is partly under genetic control and that as yet unknown genetic factors influence the risk for suicidal behavior. These genetic factors are thought to be independent of the factors responsible for the heritability of major psychiatric conditions associated with suicide (Mann, Brent, & Arango, 2001).

Normally, serotonin is released from one nerve cell, received by the next nerve cell, and then reabsorbed back into the first nerve cell. Many factors influence how much serotonin is passed from the first cell to the second cell, and how much is reabsorbed back into the first cell. Transmission can be influenced by:

1. The number of receptors.
2. The ability of the receptors to function properly.
3. Whether the body produces monoamine oxidase, which catabolizes serotonin (as well as norepinephrine and dopamine).

Positron emission tomography (PET) has helped researchers examine how serotonin affects the brain after the person has ingested the serotonin-releasing compound fenfluramine. Mann (2000) found that serotonin-induced brain metabolic activity was reduced throughout the frontal cortex. This finding is consistent with explanations for the physiologic basis of selective serotonin reuptake inhibitor (SSRI) antidepressant therapy. When the same study was repeated on persons who had attempted suicide (Mann, Brent, & Arango, 2001), serotonin activity was reduced in a small, specific area of the frontal cortex, immediately above the eyes. This area of the brain has been thought to be associated with the control of impulsive behaviors. Whatever the exact mechanism is when serotonin and serotonin metabolic activity is reduced, more violent lethal suicides and attempted suicides occur in these circumstances.

While there may be more effective medications available to treat depression, the suicide rate has not declined. Isometsa (2001) indicates that **psychological autopsies** (a review of the circumstances and events that preceded an individual's completed suicide) of suicide victims reveal that more than 90% have a comorbid mental disorder (most of them mood disorders and/or substance use disorders) and, furthermore, that they were undertreated, despite contact with psychiatric or other health care services.

NURSING PROCESS

Suicide and Self-Destructive Behavior

Working effectively with self-destructive clients requires understanding the meaning the self-destructive behavior has for the client, performing a lethality assessment, and helping the client enlarge his or her repertoire of adaptive coping behaviors. An example of how this can be done in clinical practice is in the Using Research Evidence feature.

Review these other chapters for information on suicide in specific populations: children, Chapter 25; adolescents, Chapter 26; elderly, Chapter 27; substance abusers, Chapter 13; people with HIV disease, Chapter 24.

Assessment

A thorough assessment always includes a self-assessment by the nurse, the identification of clues or cries for help, and an accurate lethality assessment.

SELF-ASSESSMENT

When assessing a suicidal client, be aware of and monitor your own reactions to this potentially life-threatening situation, because your reactions may interfere with your ability to accurately assess the situation. (Refer back to the Nursing Self-Awareness feature on page 532.) The suicidal client presents a unique challenge and will call on all your resources. You must be able to ask the right questions, as well as manage your own fears and anxieties. Helping a person who not only may not want your assistance, but who wants to deliberately harm or kill himself, is a very complicated process.

To assess the suicidal client, you must be compassionate enough to be able to form an effective link. The goal is to encourage the client to see you as an ally, yet you also need to maintain enough detachment to avoid being overwhelmed by the client's pain. The client will also bring many feelings into the interaction. Whether the feeling is anger, fear, anxiety, irritability, or hostility, remember that all emotions need to be tolerated, worked through, and evaluated.

CLUES OR CRIES FOR HELP

People intent on suicide almost always give either verbal or nonverbal clues of their plans or ideas. Up to 80% of all individuals who commit suicide may signal their need for help by making contact with the health care system 1 to 2 months before the suicide because of various physical complaints (Mann, 2000). Unfortunately, the cry for help is not always clear until after the event. Because people do want help, it is important that you ask questions about depression and suicide. Always be alert to patterns that may at first seem coincidental, as in the clinical example below.

CLINICAL EXAMPLE

Yusef, a 21-year-old man, was referred to a therapist by his physician. Although he described chronic "aches and pains" and "not feeling well," a physical exam revealed no physical problems. He did talk about how life was just not worth living, and he had a recent history of driving recklessly. After further discussion, he said that he had recently broken up with his girlfriend and admitted that his reckless driving had a suicidal intent.

The cry for help may be indirect or subtle. Examples of what a person might say are: "I just can't take it anymore," "There's no reason to go on," "Sometimes I think I'd be better off dead," "I won't be seeing you anymore," "Take care of my dog and cat," "Too bad I won't get to see my little brother grow up," and "Will you be sorry when I'm gone?" Sometimes the behavior of people intent on suicide provides the clue. They may:

USING RESEARCH EVIDENCE

Carolyn D., a 23-year-old college student, has been admitted to the inpatient unit after attempting suicide. Carolyn has just broken off her engagement with her fiancé. Within the 3 months prior to this admission, she experienced a major injury to her knee. The injury was severe enough to prevent her from achieving her life plan—being a dancer. Her family reports that she became increasingly despondent and said that she had nothing left to live for.

While on the unit, she has been unwilling to attend therapy group or any other scheduled programs. Carolyn tells you that she "can't talk right," that her "head isn't working," and that she feels she "can't talk in front of others." Her DSM-IV-TR diagnosis is Major Depression, and she has begun taking appropriate medications.

As her psychiatric–mental health nurse, you formulate a nursing care plan that addresses the following considerations:

1. Carolyn is depressed and is working through multiple losses. In order to be able to find alternatives to suicide, she will need to think and process her feelings in a less rigid fashion.
2. Providing a less demanding but secure environment will allow time to demonstrate to her that she has flexibility to develop new coping skills and behaviors in response to her losses.
3. Helping her to express feelings and perceptions will increase her self-awareness and her ability to plan methods for meeting her needs in the future. Validating Carolyn's perceptions provides reassurance and can decrease anxiety.

The interventions for Carolyn are based on the following research:

Keilp, J. G., Sackheim, H. A., Brodsky, B. S., Oquendo, M. A., Malone, K. M., & Mann, J. J. (2001). Neuropsychological dysfunction in depressed suicide attempters. *American Journal of Psychiatry, 158*(5), 735–741.

- Give away prized possessions.
- Make out or change a will.
- Take out, or add to, an insurance policy.
- Cancel all social engagements.
- Be despondent or behave in unusual ways.
- Be unable to sleep.
- Feel hopeless.
- Have trouble concentrating at school or on the job.
- Suddenly lose interest in friends, organizations, and activities.
- Have a sudden, unexplained recovery from a depression.
- Plan their funeral.
- Cry for no apparent reason.

An assessment for suicide should *always* be done whenever you suspect suicidal thought or intent.

Be alert to both clear and veiled communications about suicide. Once clues have been identified, the next step is to perform an accurate lethality assessment.

LETHALITY ASSESSMENT

A **lethality assessment** is an attempt to predict the likelihood of suicide. An accurate lethality assessment is essential in formulating a plan for helping a suicidal person. Assessment of risk factors is essential in order to determine the client's need for hospitalization (Hirschfeld, 2001). Carrying out a lethality assessment requires direct communication with the client about the client's intent. The Assessment box below presents a lethality assessment scale.

Another component of assessing lethality is a consideration of the lethality of the proposed suicide method. Box 22–4 compares the lethality of various suicide methods. There are some gender differences in suicide methods. Women tend to use less violent methods—drugs and carbon monoxide poisoning—while men tend to use more violent methods—firearms and hanging (Denning, Conwell, King, & Cox, 2000).

BOX 22–4 Lethality of Suicide Methods

Less Lethal Methods

- Wrist cutting
- House gas
- Nonprescription drugs (excluding aspirin and acetaminophen [Tylenol])
- Tranquilizers

Highly Lethal Methods

- Gun
- Jumping
- Hanging
- Drowning
- Carbon monoxide poisoning
- Barbiturates and prescribed sleeping pills
- High doses of aspirin and acetaminophen (Tylenol)
- Car crash
- Exposure to extreme cold
- Antidepressants

It is critical that you evaluate the client's ability and intent to act on an idea or plan. Beyond inquiring into the existence of a plan for suicidal action, ask questions and pay particular attention to whether or not steps have already been taken to implement such a plan. For example, has the person already stockpiled medication; written a suicide note; obtained (or have access to) knives or guns; spoken to others about purchasing a gun, writing a will, or giving away valued objects; recently purchased insurance? Also obtain information about prior suicide attempts as well as the client's history of violence and impulsiveness, alcohol and drug use, and family history of suicide or violence.

Assessment of suicide risk is not easily accomplished. One barrier is the nurse's fear of asking inappropriate questions.

ASSESSMENT Lethality Assessment Scale

Key to Scale	Danger to Self	Typical Indicators
1	No predictable risk of immediate suicide.	No notion of suicide or history of attempts; satisfactory social support network; in close contact with significant others.
2	Low risk of immediate suicide.	Has considered suicide with less lethal method; no history of attempts or recent serious loss; satisfactory support network; no alcohol problems; basically wants to live.
3	Moderate risk of immediate suicide.	Has considered suicide with highly lethal method but has no specific plan or threats; or has plan with less lethal method, history of less lethal attempts, tumultuous family history, reliance on drugs or medications for stress relief; weighing the odds between life and death.
4	High risk of imminent suicide.	Current highly lethal plan with obtainable means; history of previous attempts; unable to communicate with close friend; drinking problem; feels depressed and wants to die.
5	Very high risk of imminent suicide.	Current highly lethal plan with obtainable means; history of highly lethal attempts; cut off from resources; depressed and uses alcohol to excess; threatened with a serious loss (unemployment, divorce, failure in school).

Source: Adapted from Hoff, L. A. (1995). *People in crisis: Understanding and helping* (4th ed.). Menlo Park, CA: Addison-Wesley. This material is used by permission of John Wiley & Sons, Inc.

It is not possible to "cause" a person's suicide by assessing feelings and thoughts. Inquiring about suicidal thoughts may alleviate a person's anxiety about considering suicide, not "give them the idea."

These are some suggestions for questions that you might ask:

- "How bad are things for you?"
- "How down do you get?"
- "Are you worried about yourself?"
- "Do you ever think of harming yourself when you're down?"

Then proceed with questioning the client gently, but directly asking:

- "Have you ever thought of taking your own life?"
- "Have you ever been so sad that you wanted to end it all, maybe by dying?"
- "How long have you been feeling that way?"
- "How are you thinking of hurting/harming yourself?"

Do not use euphemisms—be direct and clear in your communication.

The client who asks you to promise not to tell anyone about a suicide plan poses a serious assessment problem. Never promise to keep clinical information a secret, and explain to the client that information is shared with the treatment team. You will probably need to discuss the issue of confidentiality further and explore the dynamics of the nurse–client relationship.

A comprehensive assessment, including a lethality assessment, will help you decide which interventions are indicated for the client. For example, a complete assessment of level of lethality can prevent unnecessary hospitalizations. Hospitalizations in and of themselves can create a crisis. However, when the suicide plan is lethal and there are inadequate supports to maintain the client in the community, hospitalization is the optimal option (Hirschfeld, 2001).

MediaLink Case Study: Assessing Lethality

Nursing Diagnosis: NANDA

Core nursing diagnoses apply to most suicidal clients:

- Risk for Self-Harm
- Risk for Self-Abuse
- Risk for Self-Mutilation
- Ineffective Individual Coping
- Low Self-Esteem

Several other nursing diagnoses (Anxiety, Impaired Verbal Communication, and Spiritual Distress) may be appropriate, depending on the situation.

Outcome Identification: NOC

Outcome criteria for the self-destructive client are:

- Acknowledge self-harm thoughts.
- Admit to use of self-harm behavior if it occurs.
- Be able to identify personal triggers.
- Learn to properly identify and tolerate uncomfortable feelings.
- Choose alternatives that are not harmful.
- Admit to the use of self-harm behavior if it occurs.
- Attempt to identify stressors.
- Cooperate with interventions designed to reduce suicidal thoughts and control behavior.

Planning and Implementation: NIC

The nursing interventions discussed below are based on the traditional belief that mental health care professionals should do everything possible to prevent suicide.

GENERAL GUIDELINES FOR ANY SETTING

The priority task is to work with the client to stop the constricted processing of suicidal thinking, long enough to enable the client and family members to consider alternatives to suicide.

The nature of the nursing interventions is in large part determined by the setting in which you encounter the suicidal client. The following list of interventions and suggestions offers general guidelines that are applicable in most settings:

- Take any threat seriously. Evaluate the threat before dismissing it.
- Talk about suicide openly and directly. Remember, asking about it will not put the notion into the client's head.
- Implement suicide precautions/restrictive status (discussed in greater detail later in this chapter)
- Search the client's room, especially if suicidal thoughts or a suicide attempt occur after admission.
- Decide (usually along with other members of the team) if a no self-harm/no-suicide contract will be used (a sample contract is in the Intervention box on page 537).
- House the client in areas that are accessible for easy observation.
- Select a room that is near the nurses' station. A two-person room is best.
- Be careful not to encourage staff behaviors that give clients or staff members a false sense of security.
- Organize a plan of care with the client. Discuss all important problems, prioritize them, and list several approaches to each problem. Write down this plan, noting who is responsible for which actions.
- Do not make unrealistic promises such as, "Don't worry, I won't let you kill yourself." Remain honest but hopeful. Making unrealistic promises diminishes your credibility with the client.
- Encourage the client to continue daily activities and self-care as much as possible. Assign tasks for the client that are distracting but not taxing.
- Decide with the client which family members and friends are to be contacted and by whom.
- Be prepared to deal with family members who may be confused, angry, or uninterested. Strive to remain neutral, and do not make assumptions about the family's behavior.
- Expect that the client will be experiencing shame, and work to help the client toward self-acceptance.

INTERVENTION

How to Develop No Self-Harm/ No Suicide Contracts

No self-harm/no suicide contracts are effective in many situations, and they work well with certain clients. They can be used in hospital or outpatient settings as a means of providing additional support to people who are likely to harm themselves.

Do

- Do fully assess the client to determine if a contract will be helpful.
- Do establish a relationship with the client prior to initiating the contract.
- Do use the contract as a way of connecting with and staying connected to the client.
- Do specify in the contract the intervals for reevaluation. In outpatient settings, the interval may be 1 week; the inpatient interval may range from every shift to every 1 to 3 days.
- Do have both nurse and client sign the contract and date it.
- Do have the client write out the contract if at all possible. Be creative if a client is unable or unwilling to write it out (the contract could be audiotaped, or the client and the nurse might each write half).

Don't

- Don't use a no suicide contract before performing a thorough assessment.
- Don't place more trust in a contract or more emphasis on a contract than you would on clinical judgment. A contract is a helpful therapeutic tool, but it does not replace good clinical judgment and is not a guarantee against legal liability (Range et al., 2002).

Clients who are acutely suicidal may agree to the contract even though they have no intention of adhering to it.

Sample No Self-Harm/No Suicide Contract

I, Cathy Smith, will not harm myself in any way. If I feel as if I am going to lose control, I will tell the staff (inform my nurse, call the crisis unit, call my therapist, etc.).

I will not bring, nor will I ask others to bring, harmful articles or substances onto the unit.

This contract lasts until 2/1/2003 and is renewable at that time.

Signed
Cathy Smith 1/26/2003
Nancy Jones, RN 1/26/2003

- Remove the client from immediate danger by confiscating pills or other harmful objects in the client's possession, or by moving the client to a physically safe environment.
- Relieve the client's obvious immediate distress. Does the client need a bath, clean clothing, food, sleep?
- Find out what, in the client's view, the most pressing need is. This may be to see a friend or family member, or to arrange for someone to pick up the children after school.
- Assume a nonjudgmental, caring attitude that does not engender self-pity in the client.
- Ask why the client chose to attempt suicide at this particular moment. The client's answer will shed light on the meaning suicide has for the client and may provide information that can lead to other helpful interventions.
- Provide for the client's safety through close observation and careful monitoring (see the section on client safety).
- Review the safety of the environment (see the section on safety in the therapeutic environment).
- Evaluate the client's need for medication.
- Evaluate the plan developed in collaboration with the client, and arrange for appropriate follow-up.
- Monitor your personal feelings about the client, and decide how they may be influencing your clinical work.
- Work with other team members to evaluate the issues fully. You don't always have all the pieces of the puzzle.
- Perform a physical examination. One woman had cut herself severely prior to coming to the hospital, but this injury was not discovered until the physical examination was performed.
- Recognize that people can and have hung or strangled themselves with shoelaces, brassiere straps, pantyhose, robe belts, craft materials, and so on. Remain alert: Razor blades may be found in pages of books; matches are relatively easy to hide; pills may be hidden in plastic wrap in a cake box or stuffed animals; light bulbs can be broken and used to cut oneself, as can wire from spiral notebooks. Clients are also able to drown in a bathtub, throw themselves through a plate-glass window, set themselves on fire, or drink bleach from the cleaning person's cart.

GENERAL GUIDELINES FOR THE EMERGENCY DEPARTMENT

Suicidal behavior is prevalent in the psychiatric emergency department. As many as 38% of psychiatric emergency department clients are thought to be at increased risk for suicide (Dhossche, 2000).

In the emergency department, whether in a psychiatric hospital or a general hospital medical center, the main goal of treatment is to save the person's life. Although the emergency staff may be excellent at technical interventions, they may voice or feel contempt for the client who is a "repeater," especially if the attempt is not a serious one. The client needs a professional, nonpunitive approach and a smooth transition to other caregivers or agencies. Leaving the person alone or with access to harmful objects is obviously a hazard to be avoided in a busy emergency department.

SUICIDE PRECAUTIONS/RESTRICTIVE STATUS

Maintain the client's safety in the least restrictive manner possible (client right of treatment in the least restrictive setting is discussed in Chapter 10). The length of time on restrictive status is of concern to the client as well as the staff. Remember that restrictions meet the safety needs of the client, but they do not constitute treatment. On an inpatient unit, times of highest risk for suicide are evenings, nights, and weekends. Two factors account for this. During these periods, clients' time is less structured, and fewer staff members are available.

MediaLink Care Plan: Suicide Watch

Suicide Protocols. Most psychiatric inpatient units have developed a set of protocols or guidelines for observing and monitoring client behavior, often referred to as **suicide precautions.** Systems of observation may have 3 to 6 levels. Restrictions may require a physician's order but can and should be implemented on an emergency basis by nurses or other clinical staff. These protocols are often labeled to reflect the rationale for their use. In addition to suicide precautions, they may be known by such names as *special awareness*, *observation*, *constant observation*, and *constant visual observation.* For sample protocols, see the Intervention box at right.

It is of critical importance that all staff members be familiar with the system being used and understand the rationale for its use. Maintaining and observing clients on these protocols is an important nursing responsibility.

Restrictive status should be reserved for the safety management of suicidal clients. Restrictions can confound therapeutic management, and their use simply to restrict the free movement of clients diminishes their effectiveness. In general, privileges and other components of unit restriction are better dealt with by other measures such as privilege systems. If there is doubt about the appropriate safety status, the client should remain on a more restrictive status until the team decides what measures are appropriate. If there is doubt or concern about moving a client to a different status, it is best to retain the more restrictive status until the clinical direction of treatment is clarified.

INTERVENTION

Sample Protocols for Suicide Precautions

Basic Suicide Precautions

Basic suicide precautions may be started without a physician's order, but a psychiatric consultation must be obtained as soon as possible.

- The client is to remain in the room with the door open unless accompanied by a staff or family member. The client may use the bathroom alone.
- Check the client's whereabouts and safety every 15 minutes. Place a check-off sheet on the client's door to document safety checks.
- Stay with the client while all medications are taken.
- Look through the client's belongings for potentially harmful objects. Make the search in the client's presence, and ask for the client's assistance while doing so.
- Check all articles brought in by visitors.
- Allow the client to have a regular food tray, but be sure to check whether the glass or any utensils are missing when collecting the tray.
- Allow visitors and telephone calls unless the client wishes otherwise.
- Check that visitors do not leave potentially dangerous objects in the client's room.
- Maintain the protocol until it is canceled by a psychiatrist.
- Inform the client of reasons for and details of precautionary measures. This explanation must be made by the nurse and by the physician and documented in the chart.

Maximum Suicide Precautions

Maximum suicide precautions can be instituted without a physician's order under emergency conditions, but a psychiatric consultation must be obtained as soon as possible.

- Provide one-to-one nursing supervision. The nurse must be in the room within arm's reach of the client at *all* times. When the client uses the bathroom, the bathroom door must remain open. A staff member should sit next to the client's bed at night.
- Do not allow the client to leave the unit for tests or procedures.
- Allow visitors and telephone calls unless the client wishes otherwise. Maintain one-to-one supervision during visits.
- Look through the client's belongings in the client's presence, and remove any potentially harmful objects, such as pills, matches, belts, shoelaces, pantyhose, brassieres, razors, tweezers, mirrors or other glass objects (such as light bulbs), wire, and craft materials.
- If suicide precautions are initiated after the client has been on the unit for any length of time, make a complete search of the room.
- Check that visitors do not leave potentially harmful objects in the client's room.
- Serve the client's meals in an isolation meal tray that contains no glass or metal silverware.
- Prior to instituting these measures, explain to the client what you will be doing and why. A physician must also explain this to the client. Document the explanation in the chart.
- Do not discontinue these measures without an order from a psychiatrist.

Signs of Clinical Improvement. Once a client has been recognized as a suicide risk and a safety plan has been implemented, the therapeutic work of addressing depression, psychosis, and precipitating factors must begin. The treatment focus shifts as the client begins to show signs of clinical improvement.

The following signs usually indicate clinical improvement and signal the need to review or change treatment plans, grant privileges, or plan discharges:

- Verbalizing a range of options other than suicide.
- Making long-term plans or discussing future events.
- Verbalizing hope.
- Responding to antidepressant and/or antipsychotic medications.
- Wanting to reconnect or moving toward reconnecting with family or significant others.
- Showing more energy.
- Sleeping better.
- Feeling less hopeless.
- Demonstrating a wider range of affective responses to situations that occur on the unit.

Removing Suicide Precautions/Restrictive Status. Restrictions should be changed gradually, rather than all at once. A realistic plan is to change one or, at the most, two variables at a time while observing, monitoring, and documenting client responses.

As the team begins to move the client off special status, it is important for all team members to keep communicating openly about the client. As the client begins to improve, the risk of suicide increases temporarily (especially if the client has increased energy and ability finally to act on the suicidal ideation). The following times are critical and call for careful evaluation:

- *When the decision is made to move the client off suicide precaution status.* Clients, especially those who have come to depend on the around-the-clock safety, comfort, and nurturance provided by a staff member, may experience the discontinuing of suicide precaution status as a loss. Gradual removal from suicide precaution status and careful monitoring of its impact on clients is indicated in these cases.
- *When the decision is made to increase access to "sharps"* (dangerous objects). This increased access may make it possible for a client to act on a suicidal impulse. Assess the client carefully before granting this access.
- *During the second or third week of antidepressant drug therapy.* At this time, clients have increased energy but their depression has not been resolved.
- *When the decision is made to grant a pass.* Decisions to grant pass privileges should be evaluated carefully. Where is the client going, and with whom? What time frame is being considered, and why? Perform a careful assessment both before and after the client goes on a pass. Additional searches may be needed at these times.
- *Prior to discharge and while formulating the discharge plan.* Remember that while clients are inpatients, they have staff available to them at a moment's notice. This is not the case once the client is discharged. It is crucial to evaluate the "holding environment" in the community. Refer the client to resources in the community, and schedule a follow-up appointment at the time of discharge. Family and significant others should participate in discharge planning. It is generally not a good idea to discharge a client (especially one who lacks immediate family support and must rely on agencies or clinics) on a Friday, over a long weekend, or when the mental health care provider will be on vacation or otherwise unavailable.

MONITORING SAFETY OF THE THERAPEUTIC ENVIRONMENT

The safety of the therapeutic environment should be evaluated periodically. Does it meet the needs of the current client population, and is the level of restrictions consistent with the milieu philosophy? Here are specific questions to consider:

- Are areas free of glass or sharps?
- Are hazardous objects and areas kept locked?
- Are closet or shower rods of the breakaway type?
- Are craft items safe?
- How many clients are there? What is the client population like now? Do they have character disorders? Serious depression?
- If the therapeutic environment is temporarily deemed to be unsafe—that is, if there are objects (such as liquor, razors, drugs) on the unit that can harm others—is there also a need to conduct a thorough "health-and-welfare search," in order to completely examine all areas of the unit for further contraband or other potential hazards?

It is also very important to educate the client's family and visitors about safety measures and their rationale. Taking this step helps ensure that family members and other visitors do not bring unsafe objects on the unit. Visitors must understand visit limits and unit policies in relation to passes. It is also necessary to explain the need for searches. Families and friends who repeatedly violate safety measures of the unit may require additional attention, and their visiting privileges may have to be restricted.

DOCUMENTING CLIENT BEHAVIOR AND TREATMENT

Documentation is essential for those working with suicidal clients on an inpatient unit. Documentation helps all staff members understand the rationale for changes and comply with ethical and legal requirements. In general, follow agency rules about documentation. Also be sure to document:

- All team reviews of client status and the names of the team members involved.
- Any decision to remove the client from a more restrictive status to a less restrictive one.
- The rationale for any changes in the treatment approach, especially changes in the level of restriction.
- Statements from clients about self-harm or denial of self-harm.
- Client responses to changes, passes, family, visitors.
- All telephone calls or interactions with family members.
- All searches carried out and the reason for them.

WORKING WITH FAMILIES

Including family members in the plan of care for the client is extremely important. Hospitalizations for suicidal ideation or a suicide attempt may be brief and may be terminated before antidepressant medication has had a chance to work. There are two important strategies that families need to know:

1. How to prevent suicide.
2. How to help their loved one avoid acting on suicidal thoughts when those thoughts occur.

Guidelines for families in preventing suicide are given in the Client/Family Teaching feature on page 540. You can also suggest some helpful Web sites to family members such as: American Association of Suicidology (www.suicidology.org), American Foundation for Suicide Prevention (www.afsp.org), and Suicide Prevention Advocacy Network (www.spanusa.org). Direct links to these resources can be found on the Companion Website for this book.

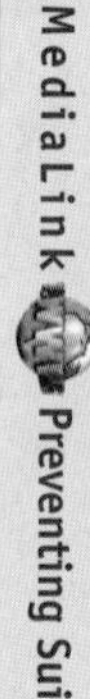

Evaluation

Suicide, like all crisis situations, calls for ongoing evaluation of the plan made by the nurse and client. Because events often occur rapidly, initial care plans may need to be changed almost daily. In addition to evaluating individual care plans, staff members who work with suicidal clients need to evaluate their overall approach and philosophy periodically.

CLIENT / FAMILY **TEACHING**

Helping Families Prevent Suicide

If you strongly believe that someone is close to a suicidal act, or the person has indicated that he or she is close to acting on a suicidal impulse, taking these steps can help you to prevent suicide.

- **Take the person seriously.** Stay calm, listen, but don't underreact. Express concern.
- **Listen attentively.** Maintain eye contact. Use body language to show concern, such as moving close to the person or holding his or her hand, if appropriate.
- **Do not promise secrecy.** You may need to speak to the person's health care professional in order to protect the person from him- or herself. Don't make promises that would endanger your loved one's life.
- **Ask direct questions.** Find out whether the person has a specific plan for suicide. If you can, determine what method of suicide is being considered.
- **Offer reassurance.** Stress that suicide is a permanent solution to a temporary problem. Remind the person that help is available and that things will get better.
- **Involve other people.** Don't try to handle the crisis alone or jeopardize your own health or safety. Call 911 if necessary. Contact the suicidal person's mental health professional, a crisis intervention team, a suicide hot line, a hospital emergency room, or others who are trained to help.
- **If possible, do not leave the person alone.** Make sure that arrangements are made for your loved one to be in professional hands.

Case Management, Community-Based Care, and Home Care

The treatment team needs to have a realistic approach when planning the care of a suicidal client. It may not be possible to meet all therapeutic goals in an inpatient setting. Even clients who are suicidal are often discharged well before antidepressant medication is at full therapeutic response (see Chapter 31 for a discussion of antidepressant medications). These clients will need intensive monitoring at home.

Case managers can ensure that planned therapeutic linkages occur once the client has been discharged. Linkages might be established with public health or home health nurses, community mental health nurses, or psychiatric–mental health nurse practitioners. Discharged suicidal clients should also be linked with a mobile crisis unit. Case managers can also find other appropriate resources in the community to meet an individual client's needs. Make sure that discharged clients and their families have all the telephone numbers they need—suicide/crisis hot line, mobile crisis unit, therapists, community resources. Clients should also have the time and date of their follow-up appointment. Case managers can assure that clients in the community have a suicide crisis plan in place that will help clients to avoid acting on suicidal impulses. Suggestions for a suicide crisis plan are in the Client/Family Teaching feature below.

Survivors of Suicide

The act of suicide has long-lasting ramifications for the survivors. Nurses who are working with the families or staff who have worked with the deceased must be alert to the potential aftereffects of the death. (Staff reactions are described later in the chapter.)

Farberow (1992), a suicidologist who studied the effects of suicide on survivors, identified these emotional experiences of survivors of suicide:

- Strong feelings of loss accompanied by sorrow and mourning.

CLIENT / FAMILY **TEACHING**

Helping an Individual Develop a Family Suicide Crisis Plan

For most people, thinking about committing suicide is temporary. It is important that when suicidal ideas occur to you that you have a crisis plan in place. This plan will help you avoid acting on suicidal thoughts when those thoughts occur. Your plan should contain the following elements:

- **Tell those you trust about your condition.** It is important for the people close to you to be totally familiar with your condition before it becomes a crisis. Discuss your plan with family and friends so that they can respond quickly and effectively if you need their help.
- **Recognize the earliest warning signs of a suicidal episode.** Learn to be sensitive to subtle warnings of illness. This is a time to take care of yourself with the utmost care. *Do not become angry or disgusted with yourself.*
- **Avoid drugs and alcohol.** Most deaths by suicide are the result of sudden, uncontrolled impulses. Since drugs and alcohol contribute to such impulses, it is essential to avoid them. Drugs and alcohol also interfere with the effectiveness of medications prescribed for depression.
- **Don't despair if your suicidal thinking recurs.** Suicidal thinking is the signal of a neurochemical imbalance. Call for help.
- **Contact your mental health provider, primary care provider, or clinic.** Have these phone numbers with you along with a back-up number such as a psychiatric emergency room or a suicide crisis line.
- **Predial your telephone with emergency numbers.** Having these numbers available will get you help sooner if you are feeling desperate.

- Anger at being made to feel responsible for the behavior of the suicidal person.
- Feelings of separation because their help was refused.
- Anxiety, guilt, shame, or embarrassment because the person committed suicide.
- Relief that the nagging, insistent demands of the suicidal person have ceased.
- Feeling as if one has been deserted.
- The arousal of impulses toward suicide.
- Anger caused by the belief that the suicide represents a rejection of social and moral responsibilities.

Families and other survivors of suicide may not receive the same degree of support as bereaved people whose loved ones died because of illness or accident. People in the support network (including other family members) may be uncomfortable and embarrassed and may stay away rather than help. If there is shame associated with suicide, that shame may be directed toward the survivors of suicide. A recent study by Jordan (2001) compared subjects' feelings about survivors whose loved ones died by suicide with their feelings about survivors whose loved ones died by accident or natural causes. This study found that survivors of suicide were viewed as more psychologically disturbed and ashamed. The respondents also believed that the suicide survivor could have done more to prevent the death.

Very often, suicide is denied or concealed by family members who wish to avoid feelings of shame or avoid being blamed for the death. This secrecy further impedes grief work, because survivors cannot resolve the loss unless they discuss it openly. Suicide exacerbates dysfunctional family dynamics, such as scapegoating or blaming other family members.

Besides making the usual preparations after death, which are stressful enough in themselves, families must deal with police investigations, the media, and insurance companies. This can precipitate extreme stress, especially if only limited support is available.

Survivors rarely seek assistance from mental health care professionals. They may be angry and believe that mental health care professionals "should have prevented this." Those who work with survivors, including nurses, must be prepared for this reaction. Families and all significant others who survive a suicide need nursing intervention, but it is especially warranted for the following:

- Families who lack support from usual sources.
- Dysfunctional families who react by blaming, scapegoating, or covering up the death as an accident.
- Children whose parent has committed suicide.
- Adolescents exposed to the suicide of a friend.

Plan outreach services for these groups. A typical plan might include telephoning the family immediately after the suicide and periodically until the first anniversary of the death, and providing for staff or a staff representative to attend services, if appropriate. Consider involving the family in a bereavement support group. Participants in bereavement groups were found to experience a significant reduction in overall depression, psychological distress, and grief (Constantino, Sekula, & Rubinstein, 2001). Psychoeducational services and family network intervention has also been found to be helpful (Jordan, 2001). Support from family and friends has been found to be the strongest protective factor (Callahan, 2000).

CHILD SURVIVORS

Children who experience a loss as the result of a parental suicide require urgent intervention to deal with the trauma. Be particularly sensitive with children who have lost a parent to suicide—they often have problems with grieving. A child who loses a parent is also at greater risk for suicide and depression (Pfeffer, Karus, Siegel, & Jiang, 2000).

ADOLESCENT SURVIVORS

Adolescents who are exposed to the suicide of a friend are at high risk for development of major depression and should be carefully screened, observed, and treated for depressive symptoms. A close relationship with the victim, visual exposure to the victim at the scene of death, having a conversation with the victim the day of the suicide, and both a personal and a family history of depression are all predictive of the development of depression subsequent to the suicide.

Cluster Suicide

Cluster suicide—an excessive number of suicides occurring in close temporal or geographic proximity to each other—is a phenomenon of great concern to those who work with adolescents. Clustering is most prevalent in the age group of 14 to 24, where it is two to four times more frequent than in older age groups.

Because of the influence of and close connections with their peer group, adolescents are at risk for cluster suicide. At highest risk are hospitalized or institutionalized adolescents. Clustering has been estimated to account for about 5% of teenage suicides in the United States. While that may seem at first glance to be a small number, it is an important one and a particular public health concern.

STAFF SURVIVORS OF CLIENT SUICIDE

Staff members are also survivors of a client's suicide. Client suicide during a course of treatment has sometimes been referred to as an "occupational hazard," and yet there seems to have been a general reluctance to examine and define the kinds of support needed for staff members after a suicide. Valente (1994) postulates that this may be related to a cultural influence that denies death and/or the hope or belief that if you are "a good enough nurse or therapist," you will be able to effectively prevent all suicides.

The reactions of staff members can be as varied as the roles they perform with clients. For example, the exact memories and reactions will vary with a nurse who finds a client hanging and administers first aid, a therapist who saw a client for his or her last session, and a psychiatrist who was the last person to evaluate the client. All are likely to experience the suicide as a traumatic event.

Support for staff members is critical after client suicide. Typical reactions to the suicide of a client may include sadness, anger, denial, and shame. Staff members may lack confidence and be unable to function. This would be a good time for nurses to review their reasons for becoming nurses in the first place. Thoughts of reconsidering what they do or where they work are common. The range of other common reactions among nurses, therapists, and physicians range from refusing to admit suicidal clients to their caseloads or their units to recognizing what the particular problems were and how they might manage them better in the future.

Outside therapists or crisis workers can be helpful for counseling and implementing critical incident stress debriefing (CISD). CISD is a seven-stage structured group in which those who have been affected by a traumatic event are given the opportunity to discuss their thoughts and feelings. See Chapter 33 for a complete discussion of CISD.

Staff members with little medical training or experience suffer more than those who have previously encountered illness and death. These workers need extra attention.

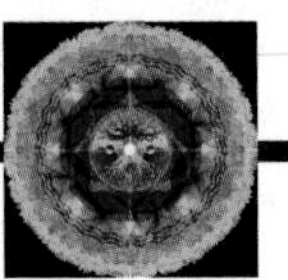

EXPLORE MediaLink

NCLEX review, case studies, and other interactive resources for this chapter can be found on the Companion Website at http://www.prenhall.com/kneisl. Click on Chapter 22 to select the activities for this chapter.

For animations, video tutorials, more NCLEX review questions, and an audio glossary, access the accompanying CD-ROM in this textbook.

BIBLIOGRAPHY

Aguilera, D. C. (1998). *Crisis intervention: Theory and methodology*. St. Louis, MO: Mosby.

Callahan, J. (2000). Predictors and correlates of bereavement in suicide support group participants. *Suicide and Life Threatening Behavior, 30*(2), 104–124.

Center for Mental Health Services. (2002). *At a glance—Suicide among diverse populations*. Retrieved June 30, 2002, from the World Wide Web, www.mentalhealth.org/suicideprevention/diverse.asp.

Constantino, R. E., Sekula, L. K., & Rubinstein, E. N. (2001). Group intervention for widowed survivors of suicide. *Suicide and Life Threatening Behavior, 31*(4), 428–441.

Denning, S. G., Conwell, Y., King, D., & Cox, C. (2000). Method choice, intent, and gender in completed suicide. *Suicide and Life Threatening Behavior, 30*(3), 282–288.

Dhossche, D. M. (2000). Suicidal behavior in psychiatric emergency room patients. *Southern Medical Journal, 93*(3), 310–314.

Farberow, N. L. (1992). The Los Angeles survivors—after suicide program: An evaluation. *Crisis, 13*, 23–24.

Fawcett, J. (2001). Treating impulsivity and anxiety in the suicidal patient. *Annals of the New York Academy of Science, 932*, 94–102.

Hawton, K., & Van Keeringen, K. (2000). *The international handbook of suicide and attempted suicide*. New York: John Wiley & Sons.

Hirschfeld, R. M. (2001). When to hospitalize patients at risk for suicide. *Annals of the New York Academy of Science, 932*, 188–196.

Isometsa, E. T. (2001). Psychological autopsy studies—A review. *European Psychiatry, 16*(7), 379–385.

Jordan, J. R. (2001). Is suicide bereavement different? A reassessment of the literature. *Suicide and Life Threatening Behavior, 31*(1), 91–102.

Kamali, M., Oquendo, M. A., & Mann, J. J. (2001). Understanding the neurobiology of suicidal behavior. *Depression & Anxiety, 14*(3), 164–176.

Keilp, J. G., Sackheim, H. A., Brodsky, B. S., Oquendo, M. A., Malone, K. M., & Mann, J. J. (2001). Neuropsychological dysfunction in depressed suicide attempters. *American Journal of Psychiatry, 158*(5), 735–741.

Lester, D. (2001). *Suicide prevention: Resources for the millennium*. New York: Guilford.

Mann, J. J. (2000). Serotonin activity in suicidal patients different from depressed patients. *Psychiatric News*. Retrieved from the World Wide Web, www.psych.org/pnews/00-04-07/serotonin.html.

Mann, J. J., Brent, D. A., & Arango, V. (2001). The neurobiology and genetics of suicide and attempted suicide: A focus on the serotonergic system. *Neuropsychopharmacology, 24*(5), 467–477.

Maris, R.W., Berman, A. L., & Silverman, M. M. (2000). *Comprehensive textbook of suicidology*. New York: Guilford.

Oquendo, M. A., Ellis, S. P., Greenwald, S., Malone, K. M., Weissman, M. M., & Mann, J. J. (2001). Ethnic and sex differences in suicide rates relative to major depression in the United States. *American Journal of Psychiatry, 158*(10), 1652–1658.

Pfeffer, C. R., Karus, D., Siegel, K., & Jiang, H. (2000). Child survivors of parental death from cancer or suicide: Depressive and behavioral outcomes. *Psychooncology, 9*(1), 1–10.

Range, L. M., Campbell, C., Kovac, S. H., Marion-Jones, M., Aldridge, H., Kogos, S., et al. (2002). No-suicide contracts: An overview and recommendations. *Death Studies, 26*(1), 51–74.

Rew, L., Thomas, N., Horner, S. D., Resnick, M. D., & Beuhring, T. (2001). Correlates of recent suicide attempts in a triethnic group of adolescents. *Journal of Nursing Scholarship, 33*(4), 361–367.

Schneidman, E. S. (1985). *Definition of suicide*. New York: John Wiley & Sons.

Valente, S. M. (1994). Psychotherapist reactions to the suicide of a patient. *Journal of American Orthopsychiatric Association, 64*, 614–621.

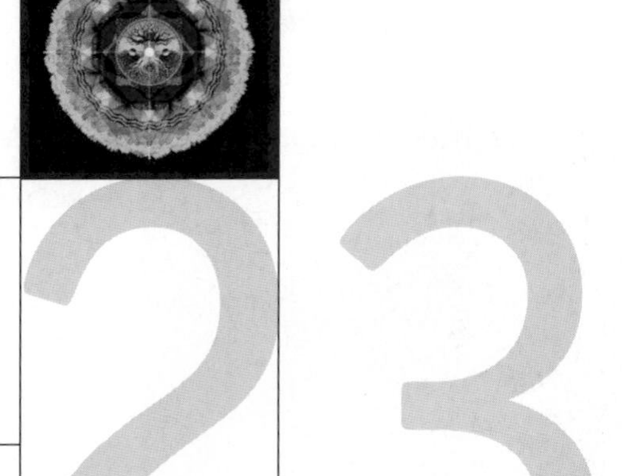

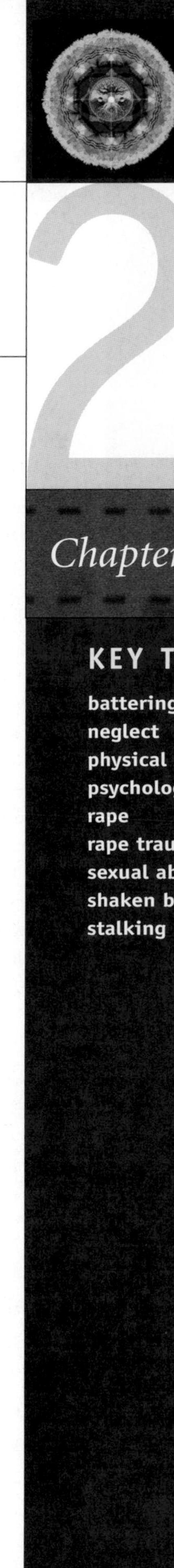

Persons at Risk for Abuse or Violence

KAREN LEE FONTAINE

Chapter TWENTY-THREE

FOCUS QUESTIONS

- **How would you describe the biopsychosocial causes of rape and intrafamily violence?**
- **Which principles are common to most treatment plans for victims of violence?**
- **What are your personal values regarding perpetrators of physical and sexual abuse?**
- **What are the long-term effects on victims of rape and intrafamily violence?**
- **What societal changes need to occur to decrease incidents of violence?**

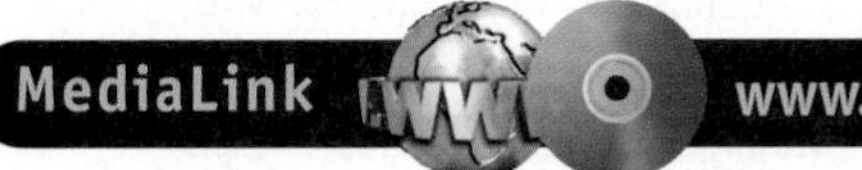

www.prenhall.com/kneisl

Additional resources for this chapter can be found on the Student CD-ROM accompanying this textbook, and on the Companion Website at www.prenhall.com/kneisl. Click on Chapter 23 to select the activities for this chapter.

CD-ROM
- Audio Glossary
- NCLEX Review

Companion Website
- Additional NCLEX Review
- Care Plan: Battering During Pregnancy
- Case Study: Child Sexual Abuse
- Learning from Clients: Sexual Abuse Video

KEY TERMS

battering
neglect
physical abuse
psychological abuse
rape
rape trauma syndrome
sexual abuse
shaken baby syndrome
stalking

CHAPTER OUTLINE

CROSS REFERENCES

Other topics relevant to this content are: Family dynamics and family therapy, Chapter 29; Repressed and recovered memory, Chapter 5; Stress management techniques, Chapter 32.

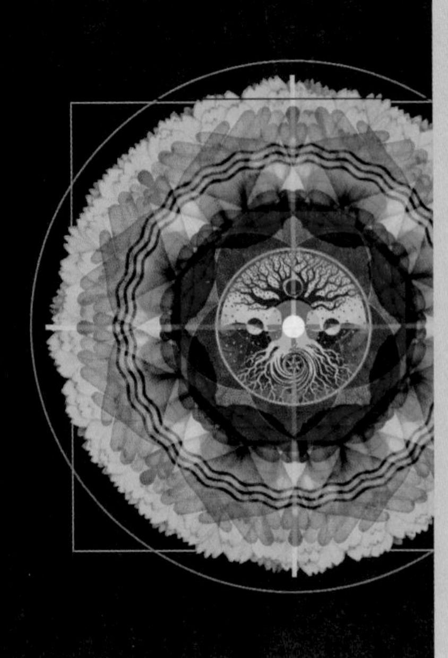

CRITICAL THINKING CHALLENGE

Beth is a 40-year-old professional woman in a long-term abusive relationship with Pat. Each time Pat beats Beth, he screams at her that she made him so angry that he had no other choice but to hit her. Even though she is a competent professional, Beth has difficulty seeing that she is not responsible for Pat's loss of control.

Much of the current sociocultural climate encourages beliefs and practices about abuse that can subtly, or overtly, support abuse. Do you believe that men would not be abusive if women did not make them angry? Do you believe that a wife should be below her husband in status by never making more money than he does? Do you believe that a man has a right to hit a woman if she nags or yells at him incessantly? Do you believe that violence against children, women, and the elderly flourishes due to tolerance for violence within American institutions such as the prison system? What do you think about the studies that show that the men who rape or commit incest are within the range of what is considered "normal" for men in our society? ■

Violence that is demonstrated as rape, or that occurs as physical or sexual abuse within the family, is a national health problem that confronts not only psychiatric–mental health nurses but also nurses in many different clinical settings. Victims are seen in the community, in pediatric units, in intensive care units, in medical–surgical units, in maternal care settings, in ambulatory care facilities, in geriatric units, and in psychiatric settings.

Nurses must assess and provide appropriate intervention for the emotional consequences, as well as the physical trauma, of violence and abuse including rape. Nurses may be called on to give legal evidence in the prosecution of a rapist. Within the community, nurses can establish, or refer victims to, support groups. They can also become active in increasing public awareness of rape through formal and informal teaching activities. Because of their unique position, nurses can be active in the prevention of rape and the treatment of rape survivors.

Nurses also need to be involved in the prevention, detection, and treatment of intrafamily violence. You need to develop a knowledge base and be able to identify factors that contribute to domestic violence in order to assume a preventive role. Part of this role is providing public education and becoming active in changes in public policy. This knowledge, along with increased awareness of the extent of the problem, helps nurses arrive at earlier, more accurate detection of intrafamily violence. Nurses must comply with state laws on the reporting of violence and referral for treatment. Some nurses with advanced education in family therapy are part of the therapy teams that intervene with violent families.

Rape

Rape is a crime of violence. It is second only to homicide in its violation of a person. The issue is not one of sex but one of force, domination, and humiliation. If you think rape is about sex, you have confused the weapon with the motivation. **Rape** refers to any forced sexual activity; the key factor is the absence of consent. Forcible rape by juveniles in both the United States and the United Kingdom has been on the increase, and teens now account for 18% to 20% of rapes (Murphy & Page, 1999).

There is no typical rape victim. Of reported rapes, however, 93% of the victims are female and 90% of the perpetrators are male. To communicate about rape issues, a rape victim will be referred to as a female throughout this chapter. One can be a victim of rape at any age, from childhood through old age. Police records indicate that a woman is raped every 6 minutes in the United States. And experts believe that 70% of rapes are unreported. It is believed that 1 out of every 3 women will be raped or sexually assaulted at least once in her lifetime; 60% to 80% of victims are raped by a spouse, partner, relative, or friend (Draucker & Madsen, 1999; McLeer & Rose, 1999; Smith & Kelly, 2001).

Of all women raped on college campuses, 50% are date rapes. In surveys of college men, 10% to 15% admitted that they had committed date rape on at least one occasion, and another 22% admitted they had used verbal coercion and deception to pressure a date into having sex. Women very rarely report rapes when they know their attackers, especially if they were in a dating relationship. The victim is often blamed, by herself and others, for being naive or provocative. A cultural value, slow to die, is: If a woman accepts a date and allows the man to pay all the expenses, she somehow "owes" him sexual access and has no right to refuse (Shaw, 1999). The U.S. Department of Justice has a Web site of interest (www.ojp.usdoj.gov/vawo/) in the Office of Justice Programs dealing with aspects of violence against women.

MediaLink Violence Against Women

Traditionally, husbands have not been charged when they raped their wives. It was not until 1974 in the United States and 1991 in Great Britain that the first cases of marital rape were prosecuted. Marital rape is often accompanied by extreme violence and is the most underreported type of rape. The attacks range from assaults that are relatively quick to those that involve sadistic, torturous episodes that last for hours. In some instances, women are forced to have sex with other people while their husbands/lovers watch (Draucker & Stern, 2001).

The myth of male rape has been that it occurs only where heterosexual contact is not possible, such as in prisons or in isolated living conditions. As more male rape victims report the crime, however, this myth is being shattered. Male rape is not a homosexual attack. Just as in female rape, the issue is one of violence and domination rather than one of sex. Some perpetrators are gay males who coerce partners or dates into sexual activity by use of threats or intimidation, as in date rape. Other perpetrators are heterosexual males who rape other males as a way of punishing and degrading them; this can occur among prison inmates or as part of gay bashing. Inmates who are sexually assaulted are often viewed by the public as deserving of their fate because of the crimes they have committed against society. Similarly, many people believe that gay men deserve to be raped as punishment for their "perverse" lifestyle (Hodge & Canter, 1998; Lips, 2001).

RAPE TRAUMA SYNDROME

Rape is a violent act against an innocent person. It changes lives forever because once people become victims, they never again feel completely safe. The victim's response to this act of violence is referred to as **rape trauma syndrome.** Some rape survivors do not develop major symptoms in response to the trauma, while as many as 25% continue to have signs of impairment a year after the assault. A variety of factors contribute to the response, including age or developmental state, a history of prior victimization, the relationship to the offender, precrisis coping abilities, and the ability to use support resources. Response factors related to the rape itself include the severity of the rape, the duration, the frequency, the number of offenders, and the degree of violence. Environmental factors contributing to a rape victim's response are the quality and continuity of social supports and community attitudes and values.

During the actual rape, some victims use the defense mechanism of depersonalization or dissociation to cope with the attack. By perceiving the attack as "not really happening to me," a victim protects her sense of integrity. Other victims rely on denial to block out the traumatic experience. The use of these defense mechanisms may continue through initial treatment and should be supported until the person is able to face the reality of the attack.

Some rape victims respond immediately with agitated and nonpurposeful behavior. They appear in the emergency department emotionally distraught and unable to respond to questions about what has occurred. Their level of anxiety may be so high that they may not be able to follow simple directions. After a period of shock and disbelief, many experience episodes of fear.

CLINICAL EXAMPLE

Doreen, a graduate student at the local university, was brought to the hospital by the police, who found her running down the street half-clothed. In the hospital she was able to tell the staff that she had been raped by her date, Mike, another graduate student. She exhibited outward calmness but kept repeating "This cannot have happened to me. My friends introduced us and he seemed so nice." She was unable to decide who to call to take her back to the dorm or what to tell her friends about what happened.

Fears may arise in response to any stimulus that brings back the rape memories. There are also fears of rape consequences such as pregnancy; sexually transmitted infections, especially HIV; talking to the police; and testifying in court. In addition, there are fears related to potential future attack, which underlie fears of getting close to men, of being alone, and of being in a strange place.

Rape usually results in a number of physical injuries. The victim may be beaten, stabbed, or shot. Profuse bleeding and trauma to vital organs may be critical problems. Most likely, the vagina or rectum will be sore or swollen. There may be tearing of the vaginal or rectal wall from forceful insertion of the penis or a foreign object. The throat may be traumatized from forced oral sex.

Rape trauma syndrome may have long-term consequences. Depression frequently develops within a few weeks of the assault. This post-trauma depression usually lasts about 3 months, and it is not unusual for the survivor to experience suicidal ideation. For some, the depression will develop into a major depressive disorder requiring medical intervention (Symes, 2000). Some survivors develop obsessional thoughts about the rape, which may be severe enough to interfere with daily functioning. Some experience flashbacks, some have violent dreams, and others may be preoccupied with thoughts of future danger.

Rape profoundly affects beliefs about the environment. If the assault occurred in the home, the normal feeling of safety within the home will most likely be destroyed. Belief in an inability to protect oneself in the future may lead to social withdrawal or phobic avoidance. A woman who is a survivor of marital rape suffers additional problems. Often, she must continue to interact with her rapist because she is dependent on him. She may be forced to pretend, to herself and to family members and friends, that the rape never occurred.

Sexual problems are one of the longest-lasting effects of rape. Nearly all adult rape survivors feel the need to withdraw from sexual activity for a period of time. For some, a period of celibacy is necessary to reestablish control and autonomy. Others may choose abstinence because they feel unclean or contaminated. Both the survivor and the sex partner must understand that the need for closeness and nondemanding physical contact continues. Expressing caring and affection through nonsexual touching minimizes the partner's feelings of rejection and reduces the rape survivor's feelings of self-blame and uncleanliness. Box 23–1 describes the phases of response to rape.

Biopsychosocial Theories

Theorists in many disciplines have studied the crime of rape in an effort to understand the causes and develop preventive measures. Most agree that rape is a crime of violence generated by issues of power and anger rather than by sex drive.

BOX 23–1 Phases of Response to Rape

Anticipatory Phase

Begins when the victim realizes the situation is potentially dangerous.
The victim may think about how to get away, may reason or argue with the offender, and recall advice people have given about rape.
Use of dissociation, suppression, or rationalization to preserve the illusion of invulnerability.
Possible physical action.

Impact Phase

The period of actual assault and immediate aftermath.
Intense fear of death or serious injury.
Expressive styles:

- Open expression of feelings—crying, sobbing, pacing.
- Controlled style—numbness, shock, disbelief.
- Compound reaction—reactivated symptoms of previous conditions, such as psychotic behavior, depression, suicidal behavior, substance abuse.

Somatic reactions—tension headache, fatigue, increased startle reaction, nausea, gagging.

Reconstitution Phase

Outward appearance of adjustment with an attempt to restore equilibrium.
Life activities are renewed, but superficially and mechanically.
Periods of anxiety, fear, nightmares, depression, guilt, shame, vulnerability, helplessness, isolation, sexual dysfunctions.

Resolution Phase

Anger at the assailant, at society, and at the judicial system.
The need to talk to resolve feelings.
The survivor seeks family and professional support.

INTRAPERSONAL THEORY

The intrapersonal perspective views rapists as emotionally immature individuals who feel powerless and unsure of themselves. They are incapable of managing the normal stresses of everyday life. The causes of rape are many, but the dynamics of the act are that perpetrators abuse their own and others' sexuality as a method of discharging anger and frustration. From this perspective, there are five types of rape:

1. Anger rape
2. Power rape
3. Sadistic rape
4. Gang rape
5. Date or acquaintance rape (Holmes, 1991)

An *anger rape* is distinguished by physical violence and cruelty to the victim. Believing that he is the victim of an unjust society, the rapist takes revenge on others by raping. He uses extreme force and viciousness to demean and humiliate the victim. The ability to injure, traumatize, and shame the victim provides an outlet for his rage and temporary relief from his turmoil. Rapes occur episodically as the rage builds up and he strikes out at others to relieve his pain.

In a *power rape*, the intent of the rapist is not to injure someone but to command and master another person sexually. The rapist has an insecure self-image, with feelings of incompetence and inadequacy. The rape becomes the vehicle for expressing power and strength. Seeing his victim as a conquest, the rapist temporarily has the feeling of omnipotence.

A *sadistic rape* involves brutality, bondage, and torture as stimulants for the rapist's own sexual excitement. For the rapist, the assault is an erotic experience. He plans very carefully, and the process of rape may be ritualized. Victims are often murdered after being raped.

A *gang rape* involves a number of perpetrators and may be part of a group ritual that confirms masculinity, power, and authority. The perpetrators may range in age from 10 to 30, but they are most typically adolescents. Victims are usually the same age as the gang members.

A *date rape*, or *acquaintance rape*, is forced sexual activity by a perpetrator who is known to the victim. Typically, there is less physical violence and more coercion and deception involved. Even during the high school years, it is estimated that 30% of female students are sexually or physically abused in their dating relationships.

Not all rapists are alike. Their motives and expectations vary. Most convicted sex offenders do not suffer from major mental disorders. Many meet the criteria for sociopathic, schizoid, paranoid, and narcissistic personality disorders. Rapists are typically young; 80% are under the age of 30, and 75% are under age 25. The majority report having been sexually and physically abused as children or adolescents (Burton & Rasmussen, 1998; Koss & Boeschen, 2000).

INTERPERSONAL THEORY

Most rapists do not have normal interpersonal involvements. Preoccupied with their own fantasies, they want to control and dominate others rather than engage in mutually satisfying relationships. With this model in mind, a rapist sees no need for consent to sexual activity, particularly from his wife. The husband may view the rape as merely a disagreement over sexual behavior. If the wife has said she does not want to engage in sex and the husband uses force, her control and autonomy have been violated. When sex occurs without consent, it is, in fact, rape.

SOCIAL LEARNING THEORY

The acceptance of interpersonal violence in a culture contributes to a higher incidence of rape. Society's approval of the use of intimidation, coercion, and force to achieve a goal promotes an excessive level of violence. Violent behavior is an expression of power and strength, and individual rights are disregarded.

Aggression is learned through three primary sources: family and peers, culture/subculture, and the mass media. The modeling effect occurs when potential offenders see rape scenes and other acts of violence against women in real life or in the media, through slasher and horror films, and in violent pornography. The media contribute to the process of desensitization; with repeated exposure, viewers become numb to the pain, fear, and humiliation of sexual aggression (Shaw, 1999).

FEMINIST THEORY

From the feminist perspective, rape is the result of long and deeply rooted socioeconomic traditions. Men dominate most political and economic activities, and women are viewed as subservient and relatively powerless. At the farthest extreme, women are viewed as property. Sexual gratification is not the prime motive in rape; rather, it is used to establish or maintain control of one person by another. When women are considered inferior to men, tacit approval is given for coercion and force. These stereotypes support the false beliefs that at times women deserve to be raped, that they may want or need to be raped, and that rape does not cause them much physical or emotional damage.

Sexist values affect people of all ages, both female and male. When schoolchildren were asked questions regarding rape, many believed it was acceptable for a man to force a woman to have sex if they are in a dating relationship. Some college students believe forced sex is acceptable if:

- A woman agrees and then changes her mind.
- The couple is engaged in heavy petting.
- Both partners willingly have their clothes off (Koss & Boeschen, 2000).

NURSING PROCESS

The Client Who Has Been Raped

Before the assessment process, clients must be informed of their rights, which include the following:

- A rape crisis advocate is present in the emergency department.
- The client's personal physician is notified.
- The client has privacy during the assessment and treatment process.
- Family, friends, or an advocate can be present during the questioning and examination.
- Confidentiality is maintained by all members of the staff.
- The client receives gentle and sensitive treatment.
- The client receives detailed explanations of, and gives consent for, all tests and procedures, including photographs.
- The client is given referrals for follow-up treatment and counseling.

As a nurse, you must respect the victim's autonomy and give the victim as much control as possible through every step of the assessment and treatment process. If this is not done, clients are susceptible to revictimization by members of the health care team.

Assessment

Rape victims must be assessed physiologically from head to toe for any serious or critical injuries that may have resulted from the assault. Before any further medical intervention occurs, clients must be informed of their right to have a rape crisis advocate with them during the assessment process. With the victim's permission, a vaginal or rectal examination is performed to determine necessary treatment and to provide evidence for legal action. With permission, photographs of the injuries may be taken for legal documentation. The physiologic assessment process must be carefully documented in writing to assist with possible prosecution of the perpetrator. Guidelines for physical assessment are given in the box below.

Victims who respond to rape in a controlled manner may be able to answer assessment questions, but those in a state of emotional shock and disbelief may find it difficult to engage actively in the assessment process. The method by which you complete the assessment depends on the person's response to the trauma. Documentation of assessment should be in subjective terms and objective quotes. Clear and concise depicting of the client is necessary for possible court proceedings. Guidelines for assessing the victim's mental status are given in the box on page 549.

Nursing Diagnosis: NANDA

The health care team must quickly establish physical and mental status priorities. Attention must then be given to long-range physical, emotional, social, and legal concerns of the survivor.

The nursing diagnosis for clients who have been raped is Rape Trauma Syndrome. If clients suffer from reactivated symptoms of a previous physical illness or mental disorder, or if they rely on alcohol or drugs to manage their trauma, they are given the more specific nursing diagnosis of Rape Trauma Syndrome: Compound Reaction. The nursing diagnosis of Rape Trauma Syndrome: Silent Reaction is applied when the client experiences high levels of anxiety, an inability to discuss the trauma, abrupt changes in relationships with men and/or changes in sexual behavior, and the onset of phobic reactions.

There is no corresponding DSM-IV-TR diagnosis for Rape Trauma Syndrome. Rape is, however, mentioned specifically as the type of trauma that may result in posttraumatic stress disorder. Rape victims may also experience one of the anxiety disorders, mood disorders, or sexual dysfunctions discussed in the DSM-IV-TR.

ASSESSMENT — Physical Assessment of the Rape Victim

Complete a head-to-toe physical assessment with particular attention to the following:

Head

- Evidence of trauma
- Facial bruises
- Facial fractures
- Eyes: swollen, bruised, hemorrhages

Skin

- Bruises
- Genital trauma
- Rectal trauma

Musculoskeletal

- Fractures of the ribs
- Fractures of arms/legs
- Dislocated joints
- Impaired mobility

Abdomen

- Bruises or wounds
- Evidence of internal injuries

Other

- Have physical injuries such as scratches, bruises, and cuts been recorded and photographed?
- Have fingernail scrapings been taken and preserved?
- Has blood typing been done?
- Have smears for sexually transmitted infections been taken of the mouth, throat, vagina, and rectum?
- Have combings of the pubic hair been made and preserved?
- Has genital trauma been recorded and photographed?
- Has rectal trauma been recorded and photographed?
- Have semen specimens been preserved?
- When was the client's last menstrual period?
- Has the clothing been inspected for rips, blood, and stains?
- Has the clothing been preserved?

ASSESSMENT **Nursing History Tool for Assessment of the Rape Victim**

Behavioral Assessment

Is the client able to respond verbally to questions?

Is the client able to follow simple directions?

Has the client bathed, douched, changed clothes, or done any self-treatment before coming to the hospital?

Affective Assessment

Which of the following emotions is the client experiencing? Describe with objective and subjective data.

Disbelief	Anxiety
Shame	Fear
Embarrassment	Guilt
Humiliation	Anger
Hopelessness	Depression
Vulnerability	Alienation from others

Cognitive Assessment

Is there evidence of defense mechanisms?

Is the client confused?

Has the client been informed of her rights?

Describe the client's attention span.

Is the client able to describe what occurred?

Is the client able to make decisions?

Who has the client informed about the rape? Family? Friends? Police?

Does the client need assistance in telling others?

Is the client blaming self for the attack?

Is the client experiencing flashbacks to the attack?

What does this event represent to the client?

Sociocultural Assessment

Who and where are the available support systems for the client? Family? Friends? Advocate? Clergy?

Is the client in need of temporary shelter?

Does the client know about available counseling?

Outcome Identification: NOC

The long-term goal of intervention is to help survivors of rape return to their precrisis level, or achieve a higher level of functioning. The following outcome behaviors demonstrate that the crisis has been resolved in an adaptive fashion:

- Control over remembering—can elect to recall or not recall the rape; decreased flashbacks and nightmares.
- Affect tolerance—feelings can be felt, named, and endured without overwhelming arousal or numbing.
- Symptom mastery—anxiety, fear, depression, and sexual problems have decreased and are more tolerable.
- Reconnection—increased ability to trust and attach to others.
- Meaning—has discovered some tolerable meaning to the trauma and to self as a trauma survivor; feels empowered.

Planning and Implementation: NIC

It is important to support defense mechanisms until clients are able to cope with the reality of the assault. Give them ample time to respond to simple questions; anxiety will decrease their ability to perceive input, thereby slowing down their response time. If clients are unable to express feelings, acknowledge the difficulty by saying, "I understand that it's difficult for you to describe your feelings right now. That's okay. You may be able to talk about them later." Communicate your knowledge and understanding of the usual emotional responses to rape. Statements such as "People usually experience a number of feelings, like anxiety, fear, embarrassment, guilt, and anger" will reassure clients that their feelings are a normal reaction to rape. Use the Nursing Self-Awareness feature below to help you in understanding your own feelings and attitudes.

ENCOURAGING COPING

Encourage the client to talk about the rape. Many clients will have a compulsive need to recount the assault. The emotional arousal of the trauma contributes to this intense pressure to talk. Listen patiently and supportively, understanding that compulsive retelling is a natural way by which the victim is gradually desensitized to the trauma.

***Nursing* SELF-AWARENESS**

Working with Rape Victims

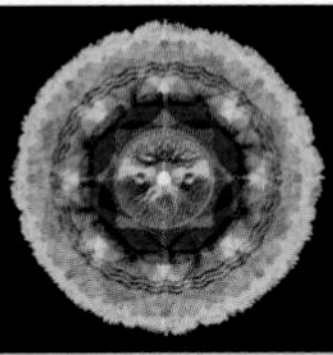

Take some time to think about and consider your reactions to the following questions:

- Are people being conditioned by their families, movies, and television into accepting rape as something allowable?
- Have you ever been in a situation in which genital or oral sex occurred without your complete consent or your partner's complete consent? How did you feel after it was over?
- Is acquaintance rape more emotionally destructive than stranger rape?
- Is it rape if the victim is under the influence of alcohol or drugs?
- Can a person who is mentally retarded, or suffering from a mental disorder, give consent to sexual activity?
- Is our society too tolerant of rapists?

Identify specific coping behaviors clients used during the rape such as screaming, fighting, talking, blacking out, and/or remaining passive. Initially, clients may experience distortions related to self-blame or guilt. Recognizing that their behavior was an adaptive mechanism for survival will raise their self-esteem and decrease their feelings of guilt. Repeatedly tell clients it was not their fault. Emphasize that survival is the most important outcome. Reassure them that their responses were all that was possible under the degree of fear that rape induces. A helpful statement might be, "I know you handled the situation right because you are alive."

IDENTIFYING AND PRIORITIZING CONCERNS

Help clients identify immediate concerns and prioritize them. Focusing on immediate problems lessens the client's confusion and the feeling of being overwhelmed. Next, help the client use the problem-solving process. Clients need to be empowered to make their own decisions and act on their own behalf. Restoring personal choice is a primary antidote to rape trauma. Informed choices help clients regain control and autonomy, both of which were violated during the rape.

PROVIDING ANTICIPATORY GUIDANCE

Help clients identify who to tell about the rape. Rape is both a personal and a family crisis. Victims often fear how family and friends will respond to the situation. Anticipatory guidance on your part will help them take advantage of available support systems. When significant others are involved, prepare them before they join the victim because they may not know how to best support their loved one. See the Client/Family Teaching feature below as a guide to family education.

Discuss beliefs about postcoital contraception and abortion if appropriate. Pregnancy may result from the rape, and clients must have information about available options. The most common medical intervention is a course of hormonal treatment. Elevated doses of oral contraceptive or DES (diethylstilbestrol) may be administered if the woman chooses to prevent conception. Mifepristone (RU-486) is a chemical that greatly diminishes the chances that a fertilized ovum will be implanted or that a placenta will develop. Inform clients about the need for follow-up medical evaluation and treatment for sexually transmitted infections, including a test for HIV/AIDS.

CONNECTING CLIENTS WITH HELPFUL RESOURCES

Provide a written list of referrals of community resources before clients are discharged from the emergency department. Crisis intervention counseling can help minimize the long-term emotional impact of rape. Every effort should be made to connect clients with aftercare services while they are still in the emergency department. Links to these resources can be found on the Companion Website for this book.

Group therapy provides an opportunity for victims to meet with other survivors of rape in a safe, supportive, and egalitarian setting. In this therapeutic environment, clients have their feelings validated as normal reactions to the assault and receive confirmation of their survival behaviors. The long-term goal of group therapy is to help survivors understand their distress and take charge

MediaLink Rape Victims: Community Resources

CLIENT / FAMILY TEACHING

Rape Myths Versus Rape Facts

Myth: Sexual assault is caused by uncontrollable sex drives.

Fact: Sexual assault is an act of physical and emotional violence, not of sexual gratification. Men assault to dominate, humiliate, control, degrade, terrify, and violate. Studies show that power and anger are the primary motivating factors.

Myth: Women provoke sexual assault, and sex appeal is of prime importance in selecting targets.

Fact: Women who have been sexually assaulted range in age from infants to the elderly. Appearance and attractiveness are not relevant. A man assaults someone who is accessible and appears vulnerable.

Myth: Women are usually sexually assaulted by strangers.

Fact: Studies show that the majority of those sexually assaulted are acquainted with their assailants.

Myth: Most sexual assaults are interracial.

Fact: As a national average, more that 90% of all sexual assaults occur between people of the same race, although attacks by men of color against white women are given more publicity. There is evidence of racial bias in our legal system: Although men of color are estimated to constitute a small proportion of sexual assailants, they are 48% of those convicted and 80% of those jailed for assault.

Myth: Sexual assault is unplanned and spontaneous.

Fact: Studies show that a majority of sexual assaults are planned in advance.

Myth: Women make false reports of sexual assault.

Fact: Statistics show that 2% of reports of alleged rape are unfounded; this is the same proportion as for all other crimes.

Myth: Men do not have to be concerned about sexual assault because it affects women.

Fact: Men, both straight and gay, are sexually assaulted. In addition, men have wives, friends, mothers, and daughters who may someday need help coping with the aftereffects of sexual assault. Rape will not cease until men stop raping.

Source: Lenehan, G. (1991). Sexual assault nurse examiners: a SANE way to care for rape victims. *Journal of Emergency Nursing, 17*(1):1–2. Reprinted with permission of Elsevier Science.

of their own recovery. Recovery is accomplished by counteracting self-blame, sharing grief, and by affirming the self and life.

Evaluation

As a nurse, you must challenge cultural values and beliefs that promote and condone sexual violence. Myths that support rape in any way must be confronted, and a new understanding of rape and rape victims must be developed. Changing the stereotypes of gender roles and the inequality of power inherent in heterosexual relationships can decrease the prevalence of sexual violence. It is only through this process that long-term changes will occur.

Community-Based Care and Home Care

In the 1990s Sexual Assault Nurse Examiner (SANE) programs were established to improve community response to sexual assault victims. The retraumatization of victims in the medical setting in the past included long waits in busy public areas; not being allowed to eat, drink, or urinate to avoid destroying evidence; and health care professionals untrained in forensic evidence collection procedures.

A SANE is a registered nurse who has advanced education and clinical preparation in forensic examination of sexual assault victims. SANEs provide respectful and prompt emergency medical–legal treatment. They offer victims compassionate care of both physical and psychological traumas. SANEs know what forensic evidence to collect and how to document injuries and other legal evidence. SANE programs provide improved medical and legal response to sexual assault victims (U.S. Department of Justice, 2001).

Intrafamily Violence: Physical Abuse

Domestic violence—violence within the family—occurs at all levels of society. The myth is that violence occurs only among the poor and undereducated, but the reality is that violence occurs also among the middle and upper classes and professional elite. In the past, these problems among wealthy or prominent people were kept hidden from the general public. With an increase in national concern, however, more publicity is being given to cases of domestic violence at all socioeconomic levels.

In this text, the word *family* refers to any one of these three categories of those people who are:

- Related by birth, adoption, or marriage.
- In an intimate relationship.
- In a domestic relationship, that is, sharing the same household.

Although the image of the American family is one of happiness and harmony, this ideal is often in conflict with the underlying reality of domestic violence. The home is the most frequent place for violence of all types. Women and children are more likely to be assaulted, raped, and killed by people who claim to love them. Perpetrators of violence do to intimates in their homes what they would not dare do anyplace else. The culture does not condone violence in schools, at work, or on the streets, but the culture continues to "allow" it within the privacy of the family. It almost seems as if family members believe they have a license to hit. **Battering**, a pattern of repeated physical assault, can be considered an epidemic in North America.

The incidence of domestic violence can only be estimated. Studies often include only those people who are willing to respond to surveys. Typically underrepresented in such studies are those who do not speak English, the very poor, the homeless, and those who are hospitalized or incarcerated at the time of the survey. The actual rates of domestic violence are probably much higher than reported. This domestic violence Web site has abundant information (www.nlm.nih.gov/medlineplus/domesticviolence.html).

MediaLink Domestic Violence

In all 50 states of the United States, nurses are required by law to report suspected incidents of child abuse, and in every state there is a penalty—civil, criminal, or both—for failure to report child abuse. In addition, not reporting child abuse is considered to be nursing malpractice. State laws vary for reporting the abuse of adults and the elderly. Domestic violence is a violent crime against which the victim has the right to be protected and for which the perpetrator can be arrested and prosecuted.

SIBLING ABUSE

The form of domestic violence most unrecognized occurs between siblings. Many people assume it is natural and even appropriate for children to use physical force with one another. Parents say things like "It's a good chance for him to learn how to defend himself," "She had a right to hit him; he was teasing her," and "Kids will be kids." With these attitudes, children learn that physical force is an appropriate method of resolving conflict among themselves. Children who are hit by their parents have more than double the rate of violence against siblings than children whose parents did not hit them. Hitting children increases the probability that they will be violent. Parents should not be complacent about sibling aggression; siblings cause 3% of all child homicides in the United States. Even though violence decreases with age, studies indicate that 63% to 68% of adolescent siblings use physical violence to resolve conflict (Bloom & Reichert, 1998).

CHILD ABUSE

Each year, approximately 2.8 million American children experience at least one act of physical violence, and 1.4 million are otherwise abused or neglected. Children who live in a home in which a parent is being abused are 1,500 times more likely to be abused than the national average. Younger parents are more likely to **physically abuse** children than older parents, and the abuse is often disguised as discipline. For many, hitting begins when they are infants and does not end until they leave home. Younger children are spanked, punched, grabbed, slapped, kicked, bitten, and hit with fists or objects. Adolescents are more likely to be beaten up and have a knife or gun used against them. Both men and women are equally likely to abuse young children. During adolescence, however, the abuser is more likely to be male (Hansen, Sedlar, & Warner-Rogers, 1999).

Acts of violence against children range from a light slap to a severe beating to homicide. Hitting or spanking children is condoned and even approved of as being necessary and good for the child. Many parents, however, do not realize the underlying messages they are giving the child by hitting (Straus, 1994):

- If you are small and weak, you deserve to be hit.
- People who love you hit you.
- It is appropriate to hit people you love.
- Violence is appropriate if the end result is good.
- Violence is an appropriate method of resolving conflict.

Shaken Baby Syndrome

Shaken baby syndrome is one of the most serious, yet frequently overlooked, forms of child abuse. It involves vigorous shaking of babies who are being held by the extremities or shoulders that causes whiplash-induced intracranial and intraocular bleeding. It is estimated that one-third have significant and permanent brain damage and one-third of the victims die. Not recognizing the danger, many parents shake rather than hit the child, mistakenly believing it is less violent (Ewing, 1997).

Child Neglect

Neglect is the most frequently reported type of child maltreatment. It differs from abuse in that it is an act of omission that results in harm. Neglect includes lack of adequate physical care, nutrition, and shelter. It also includes unsanitary conditions that often contribute to health and developmental problems. Lack of human contact and nurturance is considered to be emotional neglect (Gershater-Molko & Lutzker, 1999).

Homicide of Child

In the United States, homicide is one of the five leading causes of death before the age of 18. Sixty percent of children who are killed by their parents/caretakers are under the age of four, and 40% are less than one year old. Most of these deaths are from battering in response to colic in the infant and toilet training difficulties in the toddler. A small percentage of children are killed because they are unwanted, as the result of mercy killings, at the hands of a mentally ill parent, or in retaliation when one parent kills the child to inflict hurt on the other parent (Bloom & Reichert, 1998; Busby & Smith, 2000).

Homicide of Parent

Although it is a rare event, each year more than 300 parents are killed by their children in the United States. This accounts for 1.5% to 2.5% of all homicides. Both victims and perpetrators tend to be European-Americans, with 30% of the perpetrators being under age 18. The most frequent situation—90% of the cases—is one in which the teen has been severely abused and/or the mother is a victim of abuse. The adolescent's attempts to get help have failed, and the family situation becomes increasingly intolerable prior to the murder. A critical factor is the easy availability of guns in the home. The other 10% of cases involve either a severely mentally ill child who experiences hallucinations and delusions or the dangerously antisocial child who has extreme conduct problems (Ewing, 1997).

PARTNER ABUSE—HETEROSEXUAL

Although no socioeconomic class, ethnic group, religion, or age group is immune from domestic violence, most victims are women. And if the abused are mothers of dependent children, their children are likely to be victims also. Female partner abuse in heterosexual relationships is the most widespread form of family violence in North America. It is thought that 1 woman in 6 is physically abused by her partner, and that 3 to 4 million women are severely assaulted every year. If verbal and emotional assaults were included, the numbers would be much higher. Violence is the single largest cause of injury to women in the United States, with 20% of emergency department visits resulting from physical abuse. Three to four battered women are killed every day in the United States (Bloom & Reichert, 1998; Torres & Han, 2000).

Half the women who are abused suffer beatings several times a year. The other half may be beaten as often as once a week. The intensity and frequency of attacks tend to escalate over time. Compared to nonabused women, abused women are 5 times more likely to attempt suicide, 15 times more likely to abuse alcohol, and 9 times more likely to abuse drugs (Torres & Han, 2000).

Overwhelmingly, the first acts of partner violence occur in dating relationships. Physical abuse occurs among as many as 30% to 40% of adolescent and college students who are dating. Sadly, more than 25% of victims and 30% of offenders interpret violence as a sign of love (Centers for Disease Control and Prevention [CDC], 2000; O'Keefe, 1998).

You need to be aware of the numbers in relation to males being abused by females. It is estimated that there are between 100,000 and 150,000 heterosexual male partners who are abused by women who initiate the violence. They are generally not recognized as "real" victims, and when they do tell others, they are criticized for not standing up for themselves or for not fighting back.

PARTNER ABUSE—HOMOSEXUAL

Until very recently, there has been a public minimization or denial of physical abuse in lesbian and gay relationships. This denial has been supported by the myths that women are not violent people and that men can defend themselves. In reality, violence does occur in some gay and lesbian families, for the same reasons as in heterosexual families: to demonstrate, achieve, and maintain power and control over one's partner. In addition to physical or emotional abuse, the violent partner may use homophobic control—the threat of telling ("outing") family, friends, neighbors, or employers about the victim's sexual orientation.

In the United States, domestic violence is the third largest health problem for gay men, following substance abuse and AIDS. It is estimated that 20% to 25% of coupled gay men are victims. Men rarely talk about being victims for fear of being considered feminine if they admit that their partners are hurting them. Looking at violence in same-sex relationships demonstrates clearly that violence is not a gender issue but rather a power issue.

Homophobia and hatred of homosexuals in the United States contributes to the difficulties of battered lesbians and gays. They are cut off from the usual support systems available to heterosexual victims such as specialized counseling services and shelters. Most state laws regarding domestic violence exclude gays and lesbians with the use of terms such as *spouse* and *battered wife*. Gays and lesbians of color and those who live in rural areas are even more isolated than their counterparts. Since same-sex partnerships are not recognized as "legitimate," victims have no access to the legal system. Often, being victimized by one's lover is less frightening than being victimized by the legal system. Fear of being identified as gay or losing custody of children adds to the silence about the violence. Members of lesbian and gay communities are currently making an attempt to intervene with and support victims (Levy & Lobel, 1998; West, 1998).

ELDER ABUSE

One and a half million elderly people are mistreated each year nationwide. Elder abuse is any deliberate action or negligence that harms elderly people. Physical abuse is the nonaccidental use of physical force that results in bodily injury, pain, or impairment. Some older adults may have their basic physical needs neglected and suffer from dehydration, malnutrition, and oversedation. They may be deprived of necessities such as glasses, hearing aids, and walkers. Emotional neglect can mean leaving a person for long periods of time or failing to provide social contact. Some older people are **psychologically abused** by verbal assaults, threats, humiliation, and/or harassment. Remarks such as "One of these days I am going to poison your food and you won't know when" are considered psychological abuse. Families may violate an older person's rights by refusing appropriate medical treatment, forcing isolation or unreasonable confinement, denying privacy, providing an unsafe environment, or demanding involuntary servitude. Some are financially exploited by their relatives through theft or misuse of property or funds. Others are beaten and even sexually abused or raped by family members.

Perpetrators of elder abuse may be a spouse, child, grandchild, niece, nephew, some other relative, or a non-related caretaker. The abuse is most likely to be inflicted by a person with whom the victim lives. A number of factors contribute to the abuse of older adults. Perpetrators may have personal problems such as lack of support in caring for the older family member, alcohol or drug addiction, and a family history of violence. Family factors include unresolved previous conflicts and power struggles. The perpetrator may be retaliating for previous abuse suffered at the hands of the older person. Elderly people are often resistant to intervention because they fear that losing a caregiver will mean they will have to be put in an institution (Adelman, Lachs, & Breckman, 1999).

EMOTIONAL ABUSE

Although the focus of violence in this chapter is on physical abuse, it must be remembered that emotional abuse is often equally as damaging. Words can hit as hard as a fist, and the damage to self-esteem can last a lifetime. Emotional abuse involves one person's shaming, embarrassing, ridiculing, or insulting another either in private or in public. It may include destruction of personal property or the killing of pets in an effort to frighten or control the victim. Such statements as "You can't do anything right," "You're ugly and stupid—no one else would want you," and "I wish you had never been born" are devastating to one's self-esteem.

ABUSE OF PREGNANT WOMEN

Pregnancy is a time of increased risk for abuse. There are more incidents of violence during pregnancy than of hypertension, gestational diabetes, or placenta previa, all of which are screened for regularly. Indeed, 16% to 25% of women report abuse during pregnancy. A past history of abuse is one of the strongest predictors of abuse during pregnancy. Nonpregnant women are usually beaten in the face and chest. But pregnant women tend to be beaten in the abdomen, which can lead to miscarriage, placenta abruptio, fetal loss, premature labor, fetal fractures, pelvic fractures, rupture of the uterus, and hemorrhage. Battering during pregnancy is associated with severity of abuse. The man who beats his pregnant partner is an extremely violent and dangerous man. Battering during pregnancy is also a risk factor for eventual homicide of the female partner (Bloom & Reichert, 1998).

The first prenatal visit is often related to abuse status. Abused women are twice as likely to delay prenatal care until the third trimester. Many abused women report that the abuser forced them to avoid prenatal care by denying them access to transportation.

Physical abuse during pregnancy may be related to ambivalent feelings about the pregnancy, competition for attention with the developing fetus, increased vulnerability of the woman, increased economic pressures, and decreased sexual availability. Unfortunately, the abuse of pregnant women is often overlooked by health care professionals even when the victim appears in the emergency department with bruises, cuts, broken bones, and abdominal injuries.

MediaLink Care Plan: Battering During Pregnancy

STALKING

The term *stalking* has become not only a part of the American vocabulary but also a new classification of crime, and all 50 states have passed stalking laws. **Stalking** is the act of following, viewing, communicating with, or moving threateningly toward another person. Property damage and assault may accompany stalking. Victims often feel trapped in an environment filled with anxiety, stress, and fear that often results in their having to make drastic changes in how they live their lives.

Domestic stalking occurs when a former partner, spouse, or family member threatens or harasses a person. The stalker often makes it clear that the victim is his "property." The stalker is usually motivated by a desire to continue the relationship, which can evolve into an attitude of "If I can't have her/him, no one can." In some cases the stalker is angry and retaliating against the victim, whom he perceives as rejecting him. Frequently, there is a history of domestic violence, and the stalking often ends in a violent attack on or killing of the victim (Mullen et al., 1999).

CYCLE OF VIOLENCE

Domestic violence is the deliberate and systematic pattern of abuse used to gain control over the victim. The behavior is always intentional. Perpetrators choose to be violent and give themselves permission to be violent. Perpetrators are not out of control, as is commonly assumed. They may be enraged or cool and calculating, but in either case they have made a choice. The victim cannot "make them do it." Generally, perpetrators of domestic violence are law abiding and are dangerous only to their loved ones.

To the victim, domestic violence often happens without warning and without a buildup of tension. A pattern of violence usually develops. The first incident may be precipitated by frustration or stress. If the victim immediately refuses to accept the violence and seeks outside help, there are often no further episodes. If the victim submits to the violence, then physical force, without the stimulus of frustration or stress, becomes a way of relating, and the pattern becomes resistant to change. A typical cycle occurs when conflict escalates into a violent episode, after which the perpetrator begs for the victim's forgiveness. The victim stays in the system because of promises to reform. With the next episode of conflict, the cycle of violence begins again and becomes part of the family dynamics.

Violent people are often extremely jealous and possessive. They view other family members in terms of property and ownership. Abusers use violence in an attempt to prove to themselves and others that they are superior and in control. Their use of physical force temporarily obliterates their sense of inadequacy and compensates for a lack of internal resources.

The abuser is the most powerful person in the life of the abused. The abuser's purpose is to enslave the victim, while simultaneously demanding respect, gratitude, and love. Control over the victim is established by repetitive emotional abuse that instills terror and helplessness. Threats of serious harm or threats against other family members keep the victim in a constant state of fear. In order to have complete domination, the abuser isolates the victim. She often is forced to give up work, friends, and family. He may stalk her, eavesdrop, and intercept letters and phone calls. Control and scrutiny of the victim's body and bodily functions further destroy her sense of autonomy. She is shamed and demoralized when told what to eat, when to sleep, what to wear, when to go to the bathroom, and so on. For a victim who has been deprived long enough, the hope of a meal, a bath, or a kind word can be a powerful reward. All this abusive behavior alternates with unpredictable outbursts of physical violence. Such domestic captivity of women, along with traumatic bonding to the abuser, often goes unrecognized.

Victims can be further immobilized by feelings of anxiety and depression. Feelings of self-blame may be expressed in such statements as "If I hadn't talked back to my mother, she wouldn't have hit me," and "If I were a better wife, he wouldn't beat me." Guilt can contribute to depression, which further immobilizes victims and keeps them from leaving or seeking help for the family system.

Fear contributes to women's inability to leave abusive relationships. Often threatened with death at the idea of leaving, they live in fear of physical reprisal. Fearing loneliness, some women may believe being in a bad relationship is better than being alone. And leaving the relationship would not necessarily ensure the end of the abuse. The abuser is often most dangerous when threatened or faced with separation.

CLINICAL EXAMPLE

Sandy, age 20, met Brad at work. In the beginning of their dating relationship, Brad bought her small gifts and said sweet things to her. He told Sandy he'd never loved anyone else as much. Sandy believed him, quickly fell in love, and moved in with Brad. Several months later she called her parents from work and begged them to come and get her. Sandy told them that she didn't like the relationship with Brad but she didn't know how to get out of it. Brad had taken over Sandy's life, even controlling the use of the car her parents had helped her buy. He followed her everywhere and rarely let her out of his sight. Sandy insisted on returning to the apartment that night to get her car, telling her parents that Brad was not a violent person. However, Brad brutally beat her for having called her parents. Sandy moved back home and began trying to put her life back together. Even so, Brad continued to make harassing phone calls to Sandy. Because she had moved out so quickly, there were still financial matters she and Brad needed to clear up, so Sandy agreed to meet with him one evening. But instead of allowing her to end their 16-month relationship, Brad pulled out a gun and shot Sandy once in the back of the head.

For a partial list of reasons people remain in abusive relationships, see Box 23–2.

Fear also contributes to the inability to leave a partner in an abusive gay or lesbian relationship. Because many couples share close friends within the same community, victims may fear shaming their partners. They may also fear that friends will either deny the problem or take the abuser's side. Homophobia contributes to the victim's reluctance to seek help. Calling the police may result in ridicule or hostile responses from the officers. Victims may not seek help from family members to avoid reinforcing negative stereotypes about homosexuality, which might exacerbate the family's homophobia (West, 1998).

Biopsychosocial Theories

Domestic violence is easy to describe but difficult to explain. There is no single cause of this type of violence. It results from an interaction of neurobiologic, personality, situational, and societal factors that have an impact on families.

BOX 23–2 Why Do They Stay? Why Do They Go Back?

Fear Of physical reprisal if they resist, of being found and beaten again, of their children being hurt; *those who attempt to leave risk suffering worse violence and even death.*

Learned Helplessness They believe they have no choices and no control; have come to believe that violence is an accepted way of life.

Traumatic Bonding Results from alternating good and bad treatment; they have no sense of autonomy.

Emotional Dependence They are convinced that they are weak, inferior, and do not deserve better treatment; insecure over potential autonomy.

Financial Dependence They may not have a source of income; if the abuser is arrested, he may lose his job and the family will have no income; have been taught that they have to be submissive in exchange for financial support.

Guilt and/or Shame They have been convinced that they provoked the abuse; guilt over failure of the relationship; family/religious/cultural values against divorce or separation; shamed about remaining in the abuse relationship.

Isolation They have few, if any, friends; little support from family; no phone, no mail, no car.

Children They may believe two parents are better than one; they may be threatened with loss of custody; the abuser may threaten to harm or kidnap the children.

Hope They hope that if they change in the way the abuser wants them to, the abuse will stop; hope that the abuser will keep promises and stop the assaults.

NEUROBIOLOGIC THEORY

Neurobiologic theorists propose that genes and neurotransmitters may contribute to causing violent behavior. Although a genetic predisposition may make certain behaviors more likely, it does not make them inevitable. Two genetic mutations have been added to a growing body of evidence that supports a genetic–environmental link to violence. One defect appears to decrease serotonin (5-HT) levels, and the other raises norepinephrine (NE) levels in susceptible people exposed to certain environmental stresses such as violence and substance abuse. Low levels of 5-HT and high levels of NE are implicated in a lack of control, loss of temper, and explosive rage. These two neurotransmitters may work separately or together in different abnormal combinations to produce a strong tendency toward a variety of violent behaviors (Ratey, 2001).

INTRAPERSONAL THEORY

Intrapersonal theory suggests that the cause of violence lies in the personality of the abuser. It is thought that people who are violent are unable to control their impulsive expressions of anger and hostility. As many as 80% of male abusers grew up in homes in which they were abused or observed their mothers being abused. With these family dynamics, the child sees the father as frightening and intimidating and sees the mother as helpless and nonprotective. This early emotional deprivation contributes to an adult who is very needy of nurturance and support. He comes to adult relationships with unrealistic demands for time and attention. As the relationship develops, he discourages his partner's relationships with other people because of his low self-esteem and fear of abandonment (Sudermann & Jaffe, 1999).

SOCIAL LEARNING THEORY

Social learning theory proposes that violence is a learned behavior and people are conditioned to respond aggressively and violently. Children learn about violence from having observed it, from being a victim, and/or from behaving violently themselves. If the use of violence is rewarded by a gain in power, the behavior is reinforced. If there is immediate negative reinforcement within the family, a decrease in violent behavior will result. Learning to abuse is the first step in the battering process, but it does not necessarily lead vulnerable individuals to abuse. The social environment impacts how the potentially abusive person behaves. In other words, the person must have the *opportunity to abuse* without suffering negative consequences. There is the perception that he can "get away with it." Although learning may have occurred and opportunity is present, the potentially abusive person makes a *conscious choice* to abuse. The batterer is solely responsible for the violence.

In addition to family models, the media provide many models of violence to which children are exposed. Some movies and television shows demonstrate that "good" people use force to achieve "good" ends. Many of the stories make no attempt to justify the use of force for "good" ends; they simply present endless, senseless acts of cruelty by one human being upon another—violence without consequences. With these types of family and media examples, children develop values that tolerate, and even accept as normal, everyday violence between people.

FEMINIST THEORY

Feminist theory describes the sexist structure of the family and society as an important factor in domestic violence. The cultural value is that men have a right to keep women subordinate through power and privilege. Domestic violence is both a gender issue and a power issue. Victims are sometimes labeled as codependent in the abusive relationship, but such labeling is just another way of blaming the victim for the abuse.

The sexist economic system helps entrap women, who are often forced to choose between poverty and abuse. It is often difficult for women to find advocates and solutions within the male-dominated legal, religious, mental health, and medical systems. Society sanctions male violence by neglecting female victims. What remains unacknowledged is that women are being murdered on a regular basis, not by strangers, but by husbands and lovers (Gamache, 1998).

NURSING PROCESS

Intrafamily Physical Abuse

Addressing abuse that occurs within the family system requires an approach that is sensitive and effective.

Assessment

Nurses in all clinical settings must routinely assess clients for evidence of intrafamily violence. Considering the extensiveness of the problem, ask one or two introductory questions of every client. In assessing a child, say, for example, "Moms and dads try to help their children learn how to behave well. What happens to you when you do something wrong?" Or ask, "What is the worst punishment you ever received?" In assessing adults, you may begin with this approach: "One of the sources of stress in our lives is family disagreement. Could you describe how disagreements affect you? What happens when you disagree?" If the responses to these questions are indicative of violence, conduct a more in-depth nursing assessment. Guidelines for assessment are given in the box below.

Nursing Diagnosis: NANDA

The most important outcome of nursing assessment is identifying the existence of domestic violence. Priority must be given to critical and serious physical injuries. The severity and potential fatality of the situation must be considered, as well as the needs of dependent children and legal issues surrounding the case. Consider the following nursing diagnoses when analyzing your assessment data:

- Ineffective Family Coping, Disabling, related to an inability to manage conflict without violence.
- Ineffective Individual Coping related to being a victim of violence.
- Altered Parenting related to the physical abuse of children.
- Powerlessness related to feelings of being dependent on the abuser.
- Self-Esteem Disturbance related to feeling guilty and responsible for being a victim.
- Social Isolation related to shame about family violence.
- Risk for Violence, Directed at Others, related to a history of the use of physical force within the family.

ASSESSMENT **Nursing History Tool for Assessing Victims of Family Violence**

Behavioral Assessment

Tell me about how people communicate within your family.

What types of things cause conflict within your family?

How is conflict managed or resolved?

Who in your family loses control of themselves when angry?

Have you received verbal threats of harm?

Have you ever been threatened with a knife or gun?

In which ways have you been at the receiving end of a family member's violent outbursts? Slapped? Hit? Punched? Thrown? Shoved? Kicked? Burned? Beaten up?

Who in your family has needed emergency medical treatment?

In what ways have you attempted to stop the violence?

Have you attempted to leave the situation in the past?

What occurred when you attempted to leave?

Describe the use of alcohol in your family.

Describe the use of drugs in your family.

Affective Assessment

Who do you think is responsible for the use of physical force within your family?

In what way is this person(s) responsible?

How much guilt are you experiencing at this time?

Tell me about your fears. Lack of security? Financial problems? Child care problems? Living apart from spouse? Further physical injury?

What kinds of factors contribute to your feeling of helplessness to leave or stop the abuse?

How hopeless do you feel about your situation?

How would you describe your level of depression?

Cognitive Assessment

Describe your strengths and abilities as a person.

If you were describing yourself to a stranger, what would you say?

What are your beliefs about keeping your family together?

Tell me about your reasons for remaining in this situation. Promises of reform? Material rewards?

Do you believe/hope the violence will not recur?

What are your expectations of how children should behave?

What rights do parents have with their children?

What rights do spouses have with each other?

What are the rules about physical force within your family?

Sociocultural Assessment

How did your parents relate to each other?

Who enforced discipline when you were a child?

What type of discipline was used when you were a child?

What was/is your relationship like with your mother?

What was/is your relationship like with your father?

How did you get along with your siblings?

In your present family, who is the head of the household?

How are decisions made in your family?

How are household jobs assigned in your family?

Describe the recent and current stresses on your family. Unemployment? Financial problems? Illness? New family members? Deaths or separations? Child-rearing problems? Change in job status? Increase in conflict? Change in residence?

Who can you turn to for support in times of stress?

Describe your social life.

What types of contact have you had with the legal system? Phoned police? Peace bonds? Obtained a lawyer? Court cases? Protective services?

Outcome Identification: NOC

Achievement of the following outcome criteria is evidence that the plan of intervention was successful. The victims have:

- Recognized that they are not to blame for the violence of others.
- Ended the denial and minimization of domestic violence.
- Demonstrated an awareness of strengths, skills, and competence.
- Reestablished a sense of power over their own lives.
- Verbalized their right to express their own needs and to satisfy them.
- Established social networks to decrease isolation and secrecy.

Nursing SELF-AWARENESS

Working with Victims of Domestic Violence

Take some time to think about and consider your reactions to the following questions:

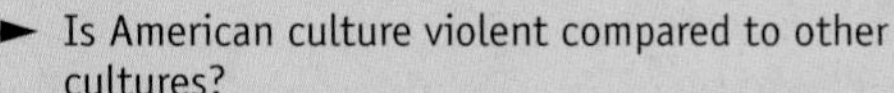

- Is American culture violent compared to other cultures?
- The United States was founded by violence. How has this influenced the values and behavior of present-day Americans?
- What is the difference between spanking a child and beating a child?
- Do you think the stalking laws are decreasing the level of violence in the United States?
- Are you for or against gun control?
- Would it be more difficult for a person to stab a family member than to shoot that person?

Planning and Implementation: NIC

Most victims of domestic violence would like it to end, but they may not know how to seek the help they need. It is extremely important that you be nonjudgmental in your interactions with all family members. Initially, clients may be unwilling to trust you because of family shame and fears of being accused for remaining in the violent situation. It is vital that you not impose your own values by offering quick and easy solutions to the very complicated problem of domestic violence. The Client/Family Teaching feature below will help you to debunk myths about family violence. Use the Nursing Self-Awareness feature above to help you in understanding your own feelings and attitudes.

The treatment of families experiencing violence requires a multidisciplinary approach, with a broad range of interventions. Nurses, social workers, physicians, family therapists, vocational trainers, police, protective services personnel, and lawyers must coordinate to intervene effectively in a situation of intrafamily violence.

In the initial contact with family members, assure their physical safety as much as possible. It is critical to assess the level of danger for the victim; homicide may be a real possibility if previous threats have been made. Also assess the level of danger for the abuser. The severity and duration of the violence are the factors that contribute most directly to victims killing their abusers in self-defense. If the level of danger is high, contact protective services or the police for emergency custody placement or removal to a shelter.

PROVIDING PSYCHOEDUCATION

Provide interventions to improve communication. Families experiencing violence often have poor communication skills.

CLIENT / FAMILY TEACHING

Myths and Facts About Domestic Violence

Myth: Family violence is rare.

Fact: Every year, 10 million Americans are abused by a family member.

Myth: Family violence is confined to mentally disturbed or sick people.

Fact: Fewer than 10% of all cases involved an abuser who is mentally ill. The vast majority seem totally normal and are often charming, persuasive, and rational.

Myth: Violence is trivial—a joking matter.

Fact: A woman is beaten every 15 seconds in the United States, and 2,000 to 4,000 women are murdered by their husbands or boyfriends every year. Every year, 2.5 million children are abused, and 1,200 die from the abuse. There are 1 million cases of elderly abuse annually.

Myth: Family violence is confined to the lower classes.

Fact: Social factors are not relevant. There are doctors, ministers, psychologists, and nurses who beat their family members. Violence occurs at least once in two-thirds of all marriages.

Myth: All members of the family participate in the family dynamics, therefore, all must change in order for the violence to stop.

Fact: Only the perpetrator has the ability to stop the violence. A change in the victim's behavior will not cause the abuser to become nonviolent.

Myth: Family violence is usually a one-time event, an isolated incident.

Fact: Violence is a pattern, a reign of force and terror. It becomes more frequent and severe over time.

Myth: Abused women like being hit; otherwise, they would leave.

Fact: Abused women are forced to stay in the relationship for many reasons. The perpetrator dramatically escalates the violence when a woman tries to leave.

Teach active listening with feedback, clear and direct communication, and communication that does not attack the personhood of others.

Identify the normality of conflict within all families by discussing how disagreements are inevitable. From there, discuss the use of the democratic process in conflict resolution and decision making. It is best to practice with minor, unemotional family problems at first.

Help family members identify methods to manage anger appropriately. All family members must assume responsibility for their own behavior. They can learn and practice talking out anger as it occurs. Make suggestions for appropriate expression, such as relaxation; physical exercise; and striking safe, inanimate objects (a pillow, a couch, or a punching bag). Guide the family in establishing limits and defining consequences if violence recurs. Emphasize that violence within the family will not be tolerated.

Help parents who are physically abusive develop and improve their parenting skills. Begin by recognizing their current positive parenting skills to increase their self-worth and help them engage in the learning process. Share your understanding that the use of violence is a desperate attempt to cope with their children. Confirming that they care about their children will increase the likelihood of their active participation in the treatment process.

Because domestic violence is often transgenerational, discuss with the parents how they were punished as children. Teach them about the normal growth and development of children. Unrealistic demands for children to comply beyond their developmental ability often result in violence. The first step in the problem-solving process is helping parents identify specific problems they experience with raising children. They can then go on to identify solutions, other than physical force, that are age appropriate for their children. They need support in implementing, practicing, and evaluating these new skills.

EMPOWERING VICTIMS

Practice feminist-sensitive therapy. This might also be called a survivor-centered approach—not specific techniques, but rather a perspective or way of seeing and understanding the context in which women and children live, recognizing the cultural values that underlie domestic violence. Using this approach, speak up and say that violence is wrong and will not be tolerated.

One of the primary goals of feminist-sensitive therapy is the empowerment of victims. The process of violence removes all power and control from a person, resulting in low self-esteem, anxiety, depression, and somatic problems. The following principles are basic to the empowerment of victims:

- A commitment to the belief that women and men are inherently equal.
- An egalitarian approach to the nurse–client relationship. The client is viewed as an equal partner rather than a helpless recipient of nursing interventions.
- Interventions that focus on the enhancement of the victim's power.
- An emphasis on the victim's strengths and abilities.
- Respect for the victim's ability to understand his or her own experiences.
- Family interventions that change destructive roles and expectations within the family system.
- A willingness to state clear value positions about domestic violence.

Through this approach, clients can become aware that they have choices in, and control over, their lives. Avoid trying to convince adult victims to leave their abuser. As difficult as it may be, you must be willing to support clients in their pain, rather than telling them what to do about their problems. For the most positive adaptive outcome, adult victims must be their own rescuers and take charge of their own safety and protection plan. If they need help with this process, teach them to ask for that help directly. This is not meant to imply in any way that you would abandon clients; rather, you stand by, support, and affirm the positive choices and decisions they make.

Help adult clients begin identifying ways in which they are dependent on their abusers. High levels of dependence make it difficult for victims to leave abusers without intense support. You can help them identify intrapersonal and interpersonal strengths to decrease their feelings of powerlessness. From there, clients can move on to identifying aspects of life that are under their control. Offer assertiveness training to help them develop new skills for relating to others in the future. But caution them, if they are still in the abusive relationship, because assertive behavior may escalate the violence.

TREATING THE ABUSER

Most abusers do not seek treatment unless it is court ordered or there are custody issues involved. It is frustrating to intervene with abusers who deny the reality of or the responsibility for the violence. Group therapy for abusers is sometimes helpful. The group setting is more effective than individual therapy because interactions with a number of people more successfully address the anger and control problems. The responsibility for aggression is always placed on the aggressor. Issues regarding the patriarchal and power views of relationships are discussed in great depth. Participants are asked to specify their abusive behaviors, identify the intentions behind those behaviors, and examine the effects of the abuse on their victims. Abusers learn that anger can be controlled and that violence is always a *choice.*

Evaluation

Nurses in acute care settings may not have the opportunity for long-term evaluation of the family system. Short-term evaluation focuses on:

1. The identification of domestic violence.
2. The family's ability to recognize that a problem exists.

3. The willingness of the family to accept assistance by following through with referrals.
4. The removal of the victim from a volatile situation.

Nurses in long-term settings or within the community have an opportunity to evaluate the effectiveness of the multidisciplinary treatment plan over an extended period of time. When violence no longer exists within the family system, the plan has succeeded. Sharing in the process of family growth and adaptation can be a tremendous source of professional satisfaction.

All nurses should evaluate their professional obligations and practice in counteracting those aspects of society that foster domestic violence. Domestic violence is a mental health problem of national and international importance, and nurses should be leaders in helping prevent it in future generations. Primary prevention includes the nursing interventions of parent education, family life education in schools, referral for appropriate child or elder care, establishment of support groups, and education of fellow nurses about the problem of domestic violence. It also includes community education about the pervasive effects of media violence on individuals and society. An example of a cultural perspective on domestic violence can be found at the Web site for the Institute for Domestic Violence in the African American Community (www.dvinstitute.org/).

Secondary prevention of domestic violence includes working with children who are victims or who have seen their mothers beaten, and making referrals for multidisciplinary intervention. Nurses must be community advocates in supporting hot lines, crisis centers, and shelters for victims of domestic violence. On the political level, nurses must make their voices heard in regard to policies and laws affecting children, women, and older people. Questions to guide the evaluation of nursing practice include:

- Have I, as a nurse, assessed each client for possible abuse?
- What action have I taken to decrease violence in the media?
- Have I been an advocate for gun control?
- Have I confronted the use of physical punishment within families?
- Have I volunteered to teach parenting classes at grade schools and high schools?
- Have I written to legislators to protest funding cuts in programs designed to help children, women, and older people?
- Have I spoken out on the need to increase the number of bilingual/bicultural counselors, lawyers, nurses, and physicians to attend to the needs of ethnic families?

Case Management

Case managers coordinate care for victims of domestic violence. The goal is to focus on the immediate problems. Intervention is directed toward developing rapport with the victim, clarifying the presenting problems, and enhancing the victim's existing problem-solving ability. Safety of the victim(s) is of primary importance. Once safety is assured, case management interventions include (McCloskey & Bulechek, 1996):

- Identification of effective and ineffective coping skills.
- Emphasis on victim's strengths and abilities.
- Development of problem-solving skills and new coping behaviors.
- Identification of available support systems.
- Group therapy with other victims and survivors of domestic violence.
- Evaluation of the effectiveness of new coping strategies.

MediaLink Domestic Violence: Cultural Perspective

Community-Based Care

Prevention of child abuse is a community function that involves the identification of risk factors and crisis intervention. Risk factors include:

- Parents who were abused as children.
- Adult relationship dysfunction.
- Poor self-esteem.
- Social isolation.
- Unrealistic expectations of children's abilities.
- Having a child with special needs.

Interventions are geared toward improving adult–adult relationships as well as adult–child relationships. Helping families connect with other families will decrease the sense of isolation. Parenting classes help families develop realistic expectations of their children according to developmental levels. It is very important that families of special needs children be referred to appropriate support groups.

Prevention of elder abuse involves supporting elderly individuals and caretakers in identifying and expanding social support networks. These community resources may be able to help with activities of daily living (ADLs), transportation, financial advice, and assistance with personal problems. Assist the caretakers in exploring their feelings about the older person in their care. Help them identify factors that are disturbing to them and that may contribute to neglect or abuse. Determine the caretakers' ability to meet their loved one's needs, and provide appropriate teaching. Provide community resource information, including addresses and phone numbers of agencies that offer senior service assistance.

The federal Gun Control Act of 1968 prohibits anyone who has been convicted of a felony from owning or possessing a firearm or ammunition. The 1996 amendment to the Act prohibits anyone who has been convicted of a misdemeanor involving domestic violence from owning or possessing a firearm or ammunition. There are no exceptions to this law including police or military personnel. Violation of this Act results in 10 years in prison and a fine of $250,000. Victims of domestic violence should be able to turn to the police and have their perpetrator arrested. This law, however, has been difficult to enforce and is being challenged by the National Rifle Association.

Home Care

Nurses involved in home care help women develop a "safe plan" or an "escape plan" to use when their safety is threatened. They should plan a quick, safe exit from their home along with having a safe place to go once they do leave. The plan needs to be easy and complete and it must be taught to their children. As part of the plan, you may suggest that they have all important documents (such as birth certificates and orders of protection), some money, a list of important phone numbers, and a couple of days' clothing gathered in one secure location. They should have a second set of car keys so they can leave quickly if they need to.

Intrafamily Violence: Sexual Abuse

Childhood sexual abuse is a major health problem in the United States. The majority of cases are probably unreported. Health care professionals, as well as families, have used denial to cope with ambiguous evidence of the cultural taboos of incest and sex with children. Use the Nursing Self-Awareness feature below to help you in understanding your own feelings and attitudes. In order to respond appropriately to cues that signal sexual abuse, you must understand the characteristics and dynamics of families involved. A note of caution must be added, however. With the recent increased publicity, there is a real danger of a witch-hunt developing; any hint or accusation of sexual abuse may be interpreted as absolute proof of guilt. Rumors and false accusations have destroyed individuals and families. You must assess carefully and maintain a balance between the extremes of denial and automatic belief of guilt.

Sexually abused children and adult survivors of childhood sexual abuse (hereafter referred to as adult survivors) are crying out for help. A few cry out loudly in protest, but most cry inwardly in silence. It is thought that as many as 1 in 3 girls and 1 in 7 boys are sexually abused before the age of 18. Many of these are single incidents. Boys are more frequently molested outside the family system than are girls. The period of abuse tends to begin and end at a younger age in boys (Morrell, Mendel, & Fisher, 2001; Shaw, 1999).

Sexual abuse occurs in all ethnic, religious, economic, and cultural subgroups. Affinity systems—immediate family, relatives, friends, neighbors, clergy, scout leaders—account for 75% to 80% of the abusers. Male perpetrators account for 90 percent of the reported cases. Although father–daughter incest is most reported, it is believed that sibling incest is the most widespread. Some siblings turn to each other for emotional nurturance and acceptance. In other instances a sibling uses coercion or violence to perpetrate the abuse. (National Center for Victims of Crime, 2001; Sholevar & Schwoeri, 1999).

Sexual abuse is defined as inappropriate sexual behavior, instigated by a perpetrator, for purposes of the perpetrator's sexual pleasure or for economic gain through child prostitution or pornography. Behavior ranges from exhibitionism, peeping, explicit sexual talk, touching, caressing, masturbation, oral sex, vaginal sex, and anal sex, to forcing children to engage in sex with one another or with animals.

> **Nursing SELF-AWARENESS**
>
> **Working with Victims of Child Sexual Abuse**
>
> Take some time to think about and consider your reactions to the following questions:
>
> - Do you think the rate of child sexual abuse is increasing, or is there just better reporting?
> - Do you think sex education can decrease the rate of sexual abuse?
> - Which situation do you think is more devastating—when force is used or when no force is used?
> - Does the fact that most perpetrators were sexually abused as children excuse their behavior? What if the perpetrator is only 11 years old?
> - Many fewer women than men are accused of sexually abusing their children. How do you explain this?
> - What needs to be done to decrease the incidence of child sexual abuse?

TYPES OF OFFENDERS

Some offenders prefer girls, others prefer boys, and some abuse both, as long as the victim is a child. Some are interested in adolescents or preteens, some in toddlers, and some in infants. Some offenders do not abuse until they are adults, but more than half start in their teens.

Juvenile Offenders

Many, if not most, of these cases are unreported. Family members often want to protect and shield the young offender. At other times, the behavior is rationalized as adolescent male experimentation. Fifty to sixty percent of juvenile offenders were sexually abused as children; they gradually develop offending behaviors as they reach adolescence. The other 40% to 50% show fairly high rates of other delinquent behaviors, and most are diagnosed with conduct disorder. Those offenders who were child victims tend to have an earlier age at onset of abusing, to have more victims, and to have male victims when compared with nonabused teen sex offenders. Juvenile offenders may seek victims within or outside the family system. The type of sexual offense often parallels their own experiences of abuse. The most frequent offense is sexual touching, which often escalates to rape and other sex crimes (Murphy & Page, 1999; Ryan, 2000).

Male Offenders

One research project that studied fathers who abused their daughters established five types of incestuous fathers (Schetky, 1999). *Sexually preoccupied abusers* (26% of the fathers) have a conscious and often obsessive sexual interest in their daughters. Many of them regard their daughters as sex objects, in some cases as early as birth. *Adolescent regressors* (33% of the fathers) become sexually interested in their daughters when they begin puberty. These men sound and act like adolescents around their daughters. *Self-gratifiers* (20% of the fathers) are not sexually attracted to their daughters per se, and during the abuse, they fantasize about someone else. In effect, they are simply using their daughters' bodies. *Emotional dependents* (10% of the fathers) see themselves as failures and feel very lonely and depressed. They see their daughters as romantic figures in their lives. *Angry retaliators* (10% of the fathers) abuse out of anger, either at the daughter or at the mother. This type of offender is most likely to have a criminal history of assault and rape.

Female Offenders

Female perpetrators have been largely overlooked but commit between 3% and 13% of sexual abuse cases. The most common types of sexual abuse by women are fondling, oral sex, and group sex.

Female offenders fall into four major types:

1. Teacher-lovers are older women who teach children about lovemaking.
2. Experimenter-exploiters are often girls who have had no sex education growing up. Baby-sitting is often an opportunity to explore younger children. Many of the girls in this group do not even realize what they are doing or that it is inappropriate.
3. Predisposers usually come from a family with a long history of physical and sexual abuse. These families have been dysfunctional over many generations.
4. Women coerced by males are those who abuse children because men have forced them to abuse. Usually, they have been victims as children and are easily manipulated and intimidated (Green, 1999).

ABUSIVE BEHAVIOR PATTERNS

Typically, adult perpetrators initiate sexual behavior in a manipulative or coercive manner. Often, the adult misrepresents the abuse as a game or "fun" activity. The behavior usually follows a progression of sexual activity, from exposure and fondling to oral, vaginal, and/or anal sex. Secrecy is imposed on the child by persuasion or threat. The abuser may say such things as "If you tell, you'll be sent away," "If you tell, I won't love you anymore," "If you tell, I will kill you," or "If you tell, I'll do the same thing to your baby brother."

Secrecy and silence are used by abusers to escape accountability. When secrecy fails and the child victims or adult survivors begin to talk to others about the abuse, perpetrators usually attack the credibility of the victims and try to make sure no one will listen. Perpetrators make such statements as "It never happened, she's lying," "He's exaggerating some innocent touching," and "Even if it did happen, it's time to forget the past and move on." Other perpetrators acknowledge the abuse but minimize the impact with such statements as "Better for her to learn about sex from her father than from some horny teenager" and "She didn't really mind; in fact, we have a very close relationship." Others use the defense mechanism of projection and blame the child for the abuse, as evidenced by such statements as "She's a very provocative child, and she seduced me," and "If he hadn't enjoyed it so much, I wouldn't have continued."

CHILD VICTIMS

Children know adults have absolute power over them, so they obey. When they have been threatened with abandonment or harm, they frequently choose to protect others. When asked, "Why didn't you tell sooner?" the answers are, "I didn't know who to tell," "I was scared," and/or "I did tell and no one believed me."

Children often feel responsible for the adult's behavior and ashamed that they have not been able to stop the abuse. Secrecy and guilt keep these children isolated, causing them to feel alienated from their peers. They may act out sexually by initiating oral or genital sex with other children or adults. The feeling of powerlessness is extremely potent because what the victim says and does makes no difference. When the repressed rage comes to the surface, it may be directed against the self in self-defeating and self-destructive ways, such as self-mutilation and suicide (Johnson, 1999).

Adolescent victims may run away from home to escape an intolerable situation. Because they have learned, at home, that sexual behavior is rewarded by affection, love, and attention, some turn to prostitution. Others are forced into prostitution as a way to support themselves while living on the streets.

Some child victims use denial to cope with the trauma. Acknowledging the abuse would mean acknowledging that the world is dangerous and that those who are supposed to protect and nurture failed and caused harm. Other victims minimize the impact, saying things like "It's not so bad; it only happens once a month" and "It's all right because it stopped when I was 11 years old."

Frequently, dissociation is the victim's major defense. The mind is "separated" from the body so the victim is not emotionally present during the sexual attack. Dissociation is evidenced by such statements as "I put myself in the wall, where he couldn't reach all of me" and "When he would come into my room, I would close my eyes and go to my favorite place. Only my body stayed on the bed; the rest of me wasn't there." When sexual abuse is severe and sadistic, the victim may develop dissociative identity disorder (DID).

ADULT SURVIVORS

Many adult survivors continue to believe that they were to blame for the abuse and should have been able to resist the adult. This self-blame often contributes to depression, anxiety, panic attacks, and low self-esteem. They feel worthless and different from other people. For some, anger is the only emotion experienced and expressed, all other feelings being repressed. Many adult survivors continue to hate their perpetrators, as well as nonabusing significant adults, for not protecting them (Sholevar & Schwoeri, 1999).

MediaLink Case Study: Child Sexual Abuse

CLINICAL EXAMPLE

Sonja describes her current sexual life as one of promiscuity and relates this to being sexually molested by her grandfather when she was between the ages of 4 and 7. This is her description of the abuse:

"Whenever I was alone with him in the car, he would fondle me and expose his penis to me. He would tell me I could touch it, it would be alright. So much of the time I tried to block everything out—it's hard for me to recall exactly what happened. Some of the things I remember clearly. I remember Grandpa's easy chair. When we were alone he would make me sit on his lap in that chair, and he would stick his fingers in me. This happened many times. One time he parked in an isolated area and played with me and made me touch him and kiss his penis. He tried to coax me to have intercourse. He told me it wouldn't hurt. But I cried and he masturbated into his handkerchief instead. Like most abuse victims, I was sworn to secrecy. He always bought me things or gave me money. I remember the day he died. I came home from school and when my mom told me, I cried. But deep down I was glad. I was really safe from him now. And I hated him for hurting me and making me tell lies all the time."

Adult survivors may believe they are only sex objects, to be used and abused by others. Some have a very strong aversion to sex and are filled with terror in sexual situations. Some are sexually inhibited and experience discomfort with sexual thoughts, feelings, and behaviors. Some engage in compulsive sexual behavior, perhaps as an unconscious way to validate their shame and guilt, or as a way to feel powerful. Many adult survivors go through a period of celibacy as they try to manage fear, anger, and distrust.

Confusion about sexuality is very common among male survivors. Sexual victimization of a male, by a male, carries a hidden implication that the victim is less than a man. Heterosexual survivors fear that the abuse has made, or will make, them homosexual. Intense homophobia and/or hypermasculine behavior may be an effort to disprove their fears. Gay survivors worry that their sexual preference may have caused the abuse. It must be remembered that childhood sexual abuse is not related to adult sexual orientation.

Some adult survivors engage in *self-mutilation*, as in cutting, slashing, or burning themselves. It is important to understand the meaning of such behavior. For some, the pain of self-mutilation proves their existence and reassures them that they are alive and real. Self-mutilation may be a plea for nurturance, as they come to the emergency department seeking care. Others nurture themselves by cleaning up the wounds after self-mutilation. For those who dissociate, self-mutilation may be a way to stop the dissociation with physical pain. Others self-mutilate as a form of self-punishment and a way to decrease guilt feelings. And finally, some self-mutilate as a way to reduce emotional pain through the feeling of physical pain. It is important to understand the function of the behavior in order to replace it with healthier behaviors that satisfy the same need.

MediaLink Learning from Clients: Sexual Abuse

Memory of Sexual Abuse

Research shows that many memories of past events are not reports but reconstructions. It is the difference between remembering facts and remembering events. What is remembered is the overall impression rather than the specific details. The details we add when we reconstruct our experience depend on our personality traits and cognitive styles. We may also create pseudomemories of events that never actually occurred, especially after being told of such "events" by trusted individuals. That is the reason that reports of remembered child abuse in adults should ideally be corroborated by other people (Chu et al., 1999; Paris, 1999). See the Caring for the Spirit feature on page 95 in Chapter 5.

Biopsychosocial Theories

There is no single cause of childhood sexual abuse. Rather, the abuse results from a combination of personality and family factors.

INTRAPERSONAL THEORY

There are many types of perpetrators of sexual abuse of children. Some traits are contradictory, and there is no agreement on a composite personality. Certain characteristics apply to many people, not just abusers. The descriptions are guidelines for assessment, not proof that the person actually committed sexual abuse.

Perpetrators usually have low self-esteem and feel more secure in interactions with children than with adults. Some were emotionally deprived as children and thus have a great need for constant, unconditional love, which is more easily obtained from children than from adults. Some perpetrators are described as lacking impulse control and the ability to experience feelings of guilt. Others are described as rigid and overcontrolled, while others are dominant and aggressive.

If perpetrators were sexually abused themselves as children, they may have learned to associate all feelings of love with sexual behavior. Most people who were sexually abused as children do not go on to sexually abuse others. Some victimized children, however, develop offending behavior in late childhood, adolescence, or adulthood. Most likely, there are a number of factors involved in why some abuse and others do not. The world of abuse is comprised only of victims (powerless) and perpetrators (powerful). Victims become perpetrators in an unconscious attempt to master the trauma of their own experiences and take over the power. The move from victim to offender may also result when anger and hostility concerning the past are externalized and projected onto new victims (Sholevar & Schwoeri, 1999).

FAMILY SYSTEMS THEORY

Intrafamily sexual abuse most typically occurs in families who have difficulty with cohesion, adaptability, and communication. Families who are enmeshed, that is, the members are immersed in and absorbed by one another, may be at risk for sexual abuse. In addition, incestuous families tend to be either rigid or chaotic in their adaptability. Rigid family systems have strict rules and stereotyped gender-role expectations, with minimal emotional interaction.

Children have no power and authority, even over their own bodies. They are not allowed to question or protest inappropriate sexual behavior. In contrast, chaotic family systems have either no rules or constantly changing rules. Within the chaotic system, there may be no assigned roles or no rules regarding appropriate sexual behavior, which may contribute to the incidence of sexual abuse (Burton & Rasmussen, 1998).

Communication patterns within the family system may contribute to the occurrence of sexual abuse. Incest depends on keeping the secret within the family. In family systems that avoid conflict, accusations of sexual abuse are not tolerated. Peace, and therefore silence, must be kept at all costs. (See Chapter 29 for a complete discussion of family dynamics.)

NURSING PROCESS

Intrafamily Sexual Abuse

A case study and nursing care plan for an adult survivor of childhood sexual abuse accompanies this section.

Assessment

It is vitally important that you acknowledge the reality of childhood sexual abuse. Nurses who deny the existence of the problem will miss the cues and fail to complete a detailed assessment. If you are knowledgeable about the incidence and the characteristics of the problem, you will be alert for cues that demand nursing assessment. Guidelines for assessment are given in the boxes on pages 564 and 565.

When assessing children, remember that some will exhibit most of the characteristics presented in this chapter, others will exhibit only some, and still others will exhibit none of the characteristics. Also remember that these same behavioral, affective, and cognitive characteristics may be symptoms of other emotional problems. Once it has been discovered that one child in a family is a victim of sexual abuse, suspect the abuse of siblings, both boys and girls, as well. Sometimes entire families are sexually abused before someone "tells."

You must appreciate the power of secrecy and how difficult it is for adult survivors to disclose such information, especially for men, who, in our society, are expected to be anything other than victimized. Routine questions on nursing histories may provide an opportunity for survivors to share their pain and obtain treatment as adults.

As a nurse, you are responsible for initiating the topic. Shame and confusion may keep the adult survivor from doing so. If you avoid the topic, you will be contributing to pathology by supporting the client's denial of reality. Failure to initiate a discussion of sexual abuse sends a message to clients that such abuse does not occur or does not matter. Now that childhood sexual abuse has been identified as a major health problem, nurses in every clinical setting must be alert for cues from both individuals and families.

When working with adult survivors, you must continuously assess the client's comfort level with the physical setting. Closed doors will increase anxiety in some clients, while others will request that doors never remain open. Some will be uncomfortable in a room with a couch or a bed rather than chairs. How close you sit can be an issue for some clients. Even normally appropriate physical contact, such as a handshake, may increase anxiety. Always ask permission before touching a client.

Nursing Diagnosis: NANDA

Based on assessment data, nursing diagnoses are formulated for the individual child victim, the family members, and/or the adult survivor. Possible diagnoses for the child victim include:

- Ineffective Individual Coping related to being a victim of sexual abuse.
- Powerlessness related to being a victim of sexual abuse.
- Post-Trauma Response related to being a victim of sexual abuse.
- Social Isolation related to keeping the family secret of sexual abuse.

For families experiencing sexual abuse, some possible diagnoses are:

- Ineffective Family Coping, Disabling, related to a child being sexually abused.
- Ineffective Family Coping, Disabling, related to an enmeshed family system that is either rigid or chaotic.
- Altered Parenting related to being a perpetrator of sexual abuse.
- Altered Family Process related to disruption of the family unit when abuse is discovered.

For adult survivors of childhood sexual abuse, some possible diagnoses are:

- Post-Trauma Response related to being an adult survivor.
- Spiritual Distress related to asking questions about fairness and justice in life or not being protected by a supreme being.
- Chronic Low Self Esteem related to self-blame for the abuse.
- Ineffective Denial related to amnesia for childhood events.
- Social Isolation related to difficulty in forming intimate relationships, mistrust of others.
- Sexual Dysfunction related to the trauma of abuse.
- Risk for Injury related to being revictimized as an adult.

Outcome Identification: NOC

Once you have established outcomes, you, the client, and the family mutually identify goals for change. Goals are specific behavioral measures by which you, clients, and significant others determine progress toward healing. The following are examples of some of the goals appropriate to people who have experienced childhood sexual abuse:

- Remains safe and free from harm.
- Utilizes a variety of therapies to express feelings about the sexual abuse.

ASSESSMENT

Nursing History Tool for Assessment of Individuals and Families for Intrafamily Sexual Abuse

Behavioral Assessment

Individual Child

Have there been any signs of regressive behavior in the child?

Is the child having sleeping problems?

Is the child exhibiting clinging behavior to the parents or others?

Does the child have friendships with other children?

Has there been any sexual acting-out on the part of the child?

Has the child ever run away or threatened to run away?

Has the child ever attempted suicide?

Perpetrator

Describe how discipline is handled in the family.

Do you see yourself as the dominant person in the family?

At what age do you believe parents should give up control of their children?

How many adult friends do you have?

Describe your relationships with these friends.

Describe your relationship with your spouse.

What kinds of sexual difficulties are you and your spouse experiencing?

When you were young, who was the closest family member with whom you had any sexual activity?

Family System

Describe who has responsibility (mother, father, both parents, or children) in the following areas of home management:

- Caring for the younger children
- Cooking
- Cleaning
- Paying bills
- Shopping
- Outside home maintenance
- Budget planning
- Decisions about leisure time
- Supervising children's homework
- Taking children to activities
- Putting children to bed

Who are the best communicators in the family?

Who talks to whom the most?

Who is unable to talk to whom very much?

How are secrets kept from one another within the family?

How are secrets prevented from leaking outside the family?

Affective Assessment

Individual Child

How helpless does the child feel about changing any of the family's problems?

In what way is the child responsible for family problems?

Does the child get enough love within the family?

Is the child more loved than the other children in the family?

Ask about the fears the child may have if any family secrets are told:

- Fears of not being believed
- Fears of being blamed for the problems
- Fears that your parents will not love you
- Fears that you will be moved to a foster home
- Fears that your parents will be taken away
- Fears of physical abuse

Perpetrator

Who loves you most within the family?

Who is able to give you unconditional support and affection?

Do you see yourself responsible for family problems?

How does fear of failure affect your life?

Family System

Describe the emotional relationships among family members.

Does everybody know each family member's business?

How is privacy protected within the family?

Do you have any fears of the family unit disintegrating?

What will happen if the family is separated?

Cognitive Assessment

Individual Child

Tell me about your nightmares.

How would you describe the family's problems?

What effect do these problems have on you?

What effect do these problems have on the rest of the family?

Who do you believe is responsible for these problems?

Perpetrator

Describe what kind of a person you are.

What are your personal strengths?

What are your personal limitations?

Describe how you handle new situations.

Do you enjoy changing situations?

Family System

Who sets the family rules?

Tell me about the most important family rules.

How do rules get changed within the family?

What are the expectations of the males in the family?

What are the expectations of the females in the family?

Sociocultural Assessment

What significant events have occurred for your family in the past year?

What support systems do you have outside the family?

How often do you visit with friends?

Who are the problem drinkers in the family?

How is the issue of drugs managed within the family?

ASSESSMENT

Physical Assessment of the Sexual Abuse Victim

Complete a head-to-toe physical assessment with emphasis on the following:

- Weight and nutritional status
- Throat irritation
- Gag reflex
- Episodes of vomiting
- Abdominal pain near diaphragm
- Smears of the mouth, throat, vagina, and rectum for sexually transmitted infections
- Genital irritation or trauma
- Rectal irritation or trauma
- Chronic vaginal infections
- Chronic urinary tract infections
- Pregnancy

- ► Verbalizes improved self-esteem.
- ► Manages negative emotions in an appropriate manner.
- ► Verbalizes a feeling of connectedness to significant others.
- ► Verbalizes improvement in sexual functioning.
- ► Utilizes community resources.

Planning and Implementation: NIC

The first priority of care with child victims is to ensure the safety of the child. Nurses are mandated by law to report any suspected child sexual abuse. See the Case Management section for details on a plan.

When families are enmeshed and either rigid or chaotic, help family members move to a moderate position between the extremes. With a rigid family, problem-solve ways in which the members can increase their flexibility of roles and rules. With a chaotic family, problem-solve ways to organize appropriate roles and formulate consistent rules. Throughout this approach, teach the family the problem-solving process.

WORKING WITH CHILDREN

Facilitate the child's ability to talk and to think about the abuse with decreasing anxiety. Create a safe and predictable environment in which the child feels supported. Make it clear to the child that you understand that talking about the abuse is difficult.

Plan interventions that will encourage affective release in a supportive environment. Child victims must be able to experience a range of emotions. Play therapy helps these children play out traumatic themes, fears, and distorted beliefs. It is a nonthreatening way to process thoughts and feelings associated with the abuse, both symbolically and directly. Art therapy provides an opportunity to express feelings for which there are no words. Therapeutic stories present the traumatic issues of abuse, link victims' feelings and behavior, and describe new coping methods. Journal writing can help children over age 10 cope with intrusive thoughts and feelings. They often choose to bring their journal into the one-to-one sessions with their therapist.

EMPOWERING SURVIVORS

Practice feminist-sensitive therapy. Because the process of sexual abuse is disempowering, it is important to empower survivors. The focus on traumatic stress therapy treats the trauma while acknowledging the process and result of victimization. Developmental therapy focuses on the "gaps" in the personality that occurred during the abusive process such as trust issues, identity issues, and relationship issues. Loss therapy focuses on helping the survivors identify and grieve over the things that they have lost during their childhood sexual abuse such as innocence, trust, nurturing, and memories.

In working with adult survivors, remember that they have been robbed of a sense of power and feel detached from others. Recovery includes restoring power and control. Be sure to avoid becoming a "rescuer," as that might send the message that clients are not capable of acting for themselves. Also be careful not to set yourself up as a powerful authority because that might recreate the type of relationship in which the abuse occurred. The most helpful approach is being ally, collaborator, and supporter as clients struggle through the healing process. Point out ways they have taken control of their lives, and help them identify situations in which they are able to make self-respecting choices.

SUPPORTING SPIRITUAL RECOVERY

Support the client's spiritual recovery. Betrayal by abusing adults is a spiritual issue. As nurses, we sometimes ignore a client's need for spiritual healing. Victims and survivors are consumed with spiritual questions like "Why did it happen to me?", "What's wrong with me?", and "Am I some evil person?" When people are sexually abused, they must struggle with questions of a God who either overlooked their pain and did not respond or did not even see their pain at all. Questions arise, such as "What's wrong with God?" and "Why didn't God stop it?" It is not unusual for survivors to be angry with God and hold God responsible for the abuse. This anger may in turn trigger fear and guilt for hating someone so powerful.

To recover from sexual abuse, survivors must place responsibility for the abuse where it belongs—100% with the offender. If they fail to do this, they will continue to be paralyzed by self-blame and guilt. The adult self needs to reach out and care for the hurt inner child by breaking down the walls that have isolated that child. Fully experiencing the rage and grief enables the survivor to move on to self-forgiveness and more complete healing. Spirituality includes a sense of connectedness to others. Survivors must begin the long journey of developing trusting relationships. They need to experience human contact and the warmth of the nurse–client relationship. When requested, refer clients to religious counselors who understand the emotional issues surrounding sexual abuse and who are sensitive to the need of survivors to work slowly through their spiritual struggles. See the Case Study and Nursing Care Plan for an adult survivor of childhood sexual abuse on pages 566–567.

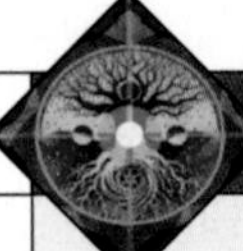

Case Study

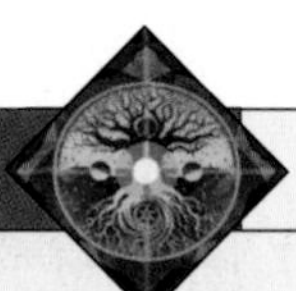

An Adult Survivor of Childhood Sexual Abuse

Identifying Information

Jill is a 35-year-old woman who is a full-time homemaker. Her husband, John, is president of an advertising firm. Jill and John have been married for 15 years and have three children, ages 14, 12, and 7.

Jill was sexually abused by her grandfather from a very young age until about 11 or 12 years of age. At times, the grandfather would involve Jill's brother, who is three years older, by forcing Jill and her brother to have sex for the grandfather's enjoyment. She states that she told her mother about the abuse when she was 9 or 10 but that her mother just ignored it. Her mother now denies that Jill told her about the abuse when it was occurring. Jill has tried to ignore her abuse history until several months ago when she saw a television program about incest. She has periods when she is filled with rage at her parents and grandfather.

History

No prior psychiatric history.

Jill was born and raised in Ohio and is the third child of five in an intact family. Jill describes her mother as "strict . . . she would threaten by saying 'wait until your dad comes home.' " When asked about her father, Jill states "He wasn't around . . . he was working . . . he was always distant." She describes the family communication as "dysfunctional; only certain people talk to certain other people. For example, none of us kids could talk directly to our father. We always had to go through our mother."

Jill describes herself as a "homebody." In the past, she attended social functions with her husband as necessitated by his employment position. These functions were not a great source of pleasure for her, however. Lately, she has had no desire to participate in any activities outside the home. She states that she has never had close friends. Her only friend is her husband, and she feels somewhat intimidated by him. She has a very close relationship with her children.

Jill has no current or past medical problems. She states she is in good health except for feeling "terrible at times."

Current Mental Status

Jill is oriented to person, place, and time. Her affect appears dysphoric, irritable, and constricted in range. At times she is filled with rage, saying "I am mad . . . mad at the world in general and at having to deal with all of this." She states that during her entire life she has spent much of her energy in "not thinking," "not imagining," and "not remembering" the abuse. She has attempted to keep a sense of distance and alienation from her inner emotional life. After viewing a televised program on incest, she now experiences "painful, bitter, brooding thoughts about the abuse." Jill is an anxious and angry woman with extremely low self-esteem and intense feelings of inadequacy. On one hand she views herself as unable to function in an autonomous, self-directed, and self-reliant fashion. Yet she sees the world as untrustworthy, betraying, and often cruel. Unable to rely on her own resources or depend on the support of others, Jill feels a sense of bitter futility and resignation. She identifies herself as a victim who is inevitably betrayed and disappointed. Many of her dynamics are consistent with adult survivors of sexual abuse. There is an intense rage at her parents for being unsupportive, unprotective, and unable to provide Jill with an inner sense of safety and security in herself and the world around her. This contributes to Jill's fear of autonomy and her conflict between her need to depend on others and her intense mistrust of the sincerity and commitment that others can offer. There is no evidence of psychotic illness or of a manifest thought disturbance.

Other Subjective or Objective Clinical Data

Jill states that she needs more emotional support from her husband. Her husband states that he cannot give it to her lately because he is often irritated because the house is messy and dirty. She thinks he is being perfectionistic. He has offered to hire someone to help, but Jill sees that as another failure on her part.

INCREASING SELF-ESTEEM

Design interventions to increase self-esteem. Adult survivors have a continuous internal monologue of negative statements like "You're weak, stupid, incompetent, unlovable, and unattractive." Negative statements become self-administered abuse and keep the survivor weak and powerless. Help clients become aware of the frequency and intensity of these negative thoughts. Teach them to consciously replace negative thoughts with positive ones. Often difficult at first, it becomes easier with practice.

REDUCING ANXIETY

Because adult survivors are often anxious, interventions to reduce anxiety are also necessary. Clients who learn progressive relaxation and controlled breathing are often able to avoid full-blown panic attacks. Teach the process, and talk clients through the stages of relaxation until they are able to reduce anxiety by themselves. When they are relaxed, instruct them to imagine a scene in which they feel safe and comfortable. Any time they need to, they can return to this safe scene where they are in total control. Daily practice facilitates the usefulness of these techniques. (See Chapter 32).

FACILITATING HEALING

Art therapy helps adults in the healing process. Making group murals to express both individual progress and a sense of unity among clients can be very effective. Music therapy, combined with movement or dance, may be a way for clients to experience very early memories. Journal writing is used more than any other expressive therapy and can be expanded to include poetry, songs, and plays.

Group therapy allows survivors to share their feelings and experiences with others who believe their stories. The group setting fosters mutual understanding and decreases the sense of isolation. Many adult survivors find self-help groups to be very supportive in the process of healing. (See Chapter 29).

Evaluation

Nurses in acute care settings may not have the opportunity for long-term evaluation. Short-term evaluation focuses mainly on

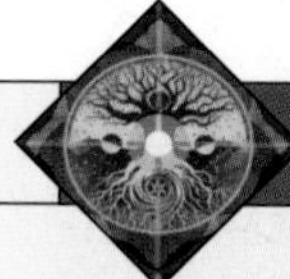

Nursing Care Plan

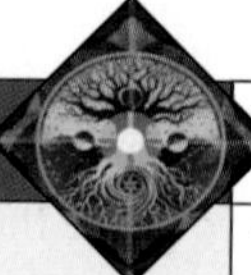

Nursing Diagnosis: Post-Trauma Response related to being an adult survivor of incest.

Expected Outcome: Client will resolve associated anger and anxiety.

Short-Term Goals	*Interventions*	*Rationale*
Jill discharges the energy of her anger appropriately. Jill uses relaxation exercises.	• Discuss feelings of guilt. Repeat often that children are never responsible for the incest but rather her grandfather is totally responsible. • Discuss her feelings of anger toward the grandfather and her parents for not protecting her as a child. • Connect feelings of low self-esteem to feelings of guilt and anger. • Assign journal keeping for recording feelings, thoughts, and memories. • Help Jill identify and grieve over things lost in childhood, such as innocence and trust. • Teach anxiety-reducing techniques such as muscle relaxation, deep breathing, and physical exercise.	Jill needs to place the responsibility for this abuse where it belongs. Survivors of abuse frequently take blame for the incest. Jill's current interactions with others is based on what she learned from these experiences as a child. Learning to relax and take care of herself was not taught to her as a child by the adults who raised her.

Nursing Diagnosis: Social Isolation related to withdrawal and decreased desire to interact with others.

Expected Outcome: Client will increase interactions with people outside her family.

Short-Term Goals	*Interventions*	*Rationale*
Jill will be able to initiate relationships outside the family. Jill will receive support and help from a self-help group.	• Help Jill identify the benefits of social interactions. • Help Jill identify a variety of available supportive people. • Give Jill positive feedback when she expresses an interest in or engages in interactions with others. • Provide assertiveness training. • Provide information on self-help groups for adult survivors where Jill can share with others and establish trusting relationships.	Jill may not know that she could feel better when she is regularly in contact with other people. Direct Jill's discovery of others by answering where and how and when questions on social interactions. Jill's ability to say "No," comfortably through assertiveness training will increase her comfort to be in relationships with others.

identifying child victims and adult survivors and referring them to appropriate community resources.

Nurses in long-term or community settings can evaluate the effectiveness of the treatment plan over an extended period. Questions to guide the evaluation of the child victim and family include the following:

- Has the child remained safe from further harm?
- Has the child returned to functioning at an appropriate developmental level?
- Is the child able to express feelings either verbally or through play or art therapy?
- Is the child verbalizing decreasing feelings of guilt and/or responsibility?
- Is the child developing peer friendships?
- Has the family structure become more flexible?
- Is communication more open within the family?

As a nurse, you have the opportunity to influence the care of adult survivors of childhood sexual abuse. Explain to others that the survivors' behavior is a posttrauma response that makes sense as an adaptation to trauma and perhaps a dysfunctional family. Intervene if staff members recreate the dynamics of the abusive relationship by assuming a position of power and control. It is very rewarding to share the growth of clients toward making self-respecting choices in their lives. Questions to guide the evaluation of adult survivors include:

- Has the person remained safe from further harm in adult relationships?
- Is the client able to talk about the childhood trauma? If not, is art therapy, music therapy, movement therapy, or journal writing effective in facilitating expression?
- Is the client able to identify situations in which he or she has been able, or hopes to be able, to make self-respecting choices?
- Is the client verbalizing increased spiritual comfort regarding the trauma?
- Is the client verbalizing less self-blame?
- Is the client verbalizing improved self-image?
- Is there evidence that the client is able to develop trusting and respectful relationships with adults?

Although, as a culture, we say that we protect our children, we do not in reality live out this value. We do not invest many of our energies—time, caring, and money—in the prevention of childhood sexual abuse. Our present approaches to treatment and to the social control of sexual abuse are not yet effective enough that we can be assured of the long-term safety of children. As nurses, we must all become active in the battle to stop childhood sexual abuse.

Case Management

As mentioned above, the first priority of care with child victims is to ensure the safety of the child. Nurses are mandated by law to report any suspected child sexual abuse. Protective services will implement one of four plans if the abuse is occurring within the family system:

1. The most frequent option is when the abuser is removed from the family. The nonabusing parent must protect the child from any contact with the abuser.
2. When the nonabusing parent is unable to protect the child, both the child and the abuser are removed from the home. This option maximizes the child's safety and decreases the child's feelings of responsibility.
3. In a few cases in which families have not used physical violence, where there is no substance abuse, and there is someone who can ensure the child's safety, the family may be allowed to remain intact while participating in intensive therapy.
4. In a few instances, the child may be removed from the family when that is the safest option. Unfortunately, this decision may place additional guilt on the child.

Community-Based Care and Home Care

Sexual harassment of women in the workplace and in schools has always existed as a hidden crime. Only recently has it been recognized for what it is—discrimination against and violation of the victim. It is on one end of the continuum of sexual violence, with the other end being childhood sexual abuse and rape. Girls and boys and women and men must be taught that they do not have to tolerate harassing behaviors. These behaviors include:

- Sexual teasing, jokes, remarks, or demeaning comments.
- Making sexually stereotypical comments.
- Showing offensive pictures.
- Invasive questions regarding personal life.
- Persistent pressure for dates.
- Letters, telephone calls, or e-mail of a sexual nature.
- Sexual gestures.
- Deliberate touching, cornering, or pinching.
- Invasive watching.
- Pressure for sexual favors.
- Actual or attempted rape.

Sexual harassment can lead to severe stress in the victims. Many experience depression, isolation, feelings of powerlessness, helplessness, fear, restlessness, inability to concentrate, somatic complaints, sexual problems, and loss of self-esteem. At

USING RESEARCH EVIDENCE

In your role as a community health nurse, you have been conducting health classes for girls and young women at a local school. During your class discussions, every one of the female students spoke about their fears regarding emotional, physical, and sexual abuse and assault. Upon further exploration, not only did the girls report many disturbing instances of harassing behaviors, but there was also a perception that there were no consequences for the perpetrators even when such behaviors were reported to adults.

Your reading of the literature supports this empirical experience and points to how sexual harassment has become one of the most insidious forms of violence affecting all females, children included. It is not hard to imagine how violence can become "normalized" in the lives of girls and young women. Listening to the reactions of girls to their numerous experiences matches current research being conducted by groups such as the Canadian Alliance of Five Research Centres on Violence.

As a nurse, you are in an ideal position to develop health education programs that incorporate strategies for coping under these circumstances. Strategies are needed to empower girls to deal with sexual harassment with healthy resistance. Acts of healthy resistance include speaking out, avoiding substance use, and learning how to manage conflict.

These interventions are based on data in the following study:

Berman, H., McKenna, K., Arnold, C. T., Taylor, G., & MacQuarrie, B. (2000). Sexual harassment: Everyday violence in the lives of girls and women. *Advances in Nursing Science, 22*(4), 32–46.

its most severe, harassment resembles the other sexual traumas of rape and child sexual abuse and may result in posttraumatic stress disorder.

The U.S. Equal Employment Opportunity Commission (EEOC) is the government agency that interprets and enforces employment laws. In 1980, the EEOC issued a position statement clearly stating that sexual harassment is considered a form of sexual discrimination and, therefore, an unlawful employment act. The intent of the law is to give people the opportunity to work in an environment that is free from sex-based discrimination, taunts, jeers, and insults.

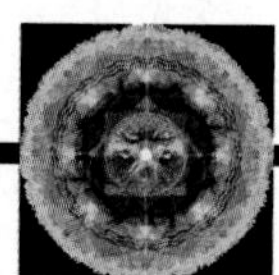

EXPLORE MediaLink

NCLEX review, case studies, and other interactive resources for this chapter can be found on the Companion Website at http://www.prenhall.com/kneisl. Click on Chapter 23 to select the activities for this chapter.

For animations, video tutorials, more NCLEX review questions, and an audio glossary, access the accompanying CD-ROM in this textbook.

BIBLIOGRAPHY

Adelman, R. D., Lachs, M. S., & Breckman, R. (1999). Elder abuse and neglect. In R. T. Ammerman & M. Hersen (Eds.), *Assessment of family violence: A clinical and legal sourcebook* (2nd ed.) (pp. 271–286). New York: John Wiley & Sons.

Alexander, C. J. (1997). *Growth and intimacy for gay men*. New York: Harrington Park Press.

Bloom, S. L., & Reichert, M. (1998). *Bearing witness: Violence and collective responsibility*. New York: Haworth Press.

Burton, J. E. & Rasmussen, L. A. (1998). *Treating children with sexually abusive behavior problems*. New York: Haworth Press.

Busby, D. M., & Smith, G. L. (2000). Family therapy with children who are victims of domestic violence. In C. E. Bailey (Ed.), *Children in therapy* (pp. 164–191). New York: W. W. Norton.

Centers for Disease Control and Prevention. (2000). National Center for Injury Prevention and Control. Dating violence. Retrieved from the World Wide Web, www.cdc.gov/ncipc/factsheets/datviol/htm. Oct. 1, 2002

Chu, J. A., Frey, L. M., Ganzel, B. L., & Matthews, J. A. (1999). Memories of childhood abuse: Dissociation, amnesia, and corroboration. *Am J Psychiatry, 156*(5), 749–755.

Draucker, C. B., & Stern, P. N. (2001). Women's responses to sexual violence by male intimates. *Western Journal of Nursing, 22*(4), 385–397.

Draucker, C. B., & Madsen, C. (1999). Women dwelling with violence. *IMAGE, 31*(4), 327–332.

Draucker, C. B., & Petrovic, K. (1996). Healing of adult male survivors of childhood sexual abuse. *IMAGE, 28*(4), 325–330.

Ewing, C. P. (1997). *Fatal families*. Thousand Oaks, CA: Sage.

Gamache, D. (1998). Domination and control: The social context of dating violence. In B. Levy (Ed.), *Dating violence* (pp. 203–208). Seattle, WA: Seal Press.

Gershater-Molko, R. M. & Lutzker, J. R. (1999). Child Neglect. In R. T. Ammerman & M. Hersen (Eds.), *Assessment of family violence: A clinical and legal sourcebook* (2nd ed.) (pp. 157–183). New York: John Wiley & Sons.

Green, A. H. (1999). Female sex offenders. In J.A. Shaw (Ed.), *Sexual aggression* (pp. 195–210). Washington DC: American Psychiatric Press.

Hansen, D. J., Sedlar, G., & Warner-Rogers, J. E. (1999). Child physical abuse. In R. T. Ammerman & M. Hersen (Eds.), *Assessment of family violence: A clinical and legal sourcebook* (2nd ed.) (pp. 127–156). New York: John Wiley & Sons.

Hodge, S., & Canter, D. (1998). Victims and perpetrators of male sexual assault. *Journal of Interpersonal Violence, 13*(2), 222–239.

Holmes, R. M. (1991). *Sex crimes*. Newbury Park, CA: Sage.

Johnson, T. C. (1999). Development of sexual behavior problems in childhood. In J. A. Shaw (Ed.), *Sexual aggression* (pp. 41–74). Washington, DC: American Psychiatric Press.

Koss, M. P., & Boeschen, L. (2000). Rape. In A. E. Kazdin (Ed.), *Encyclopedia of psychology*, Vol. 7 (pp. 1–6). Oxford, UK: Oxford University Press.

Levy, B., & Lobel, K. (1998). Lesbian teens in abusive relationships. In B. Levy (Ed.), *Dating violence* (pp. 203–208). Seattle, WA: Seal Press.

Lips, H. M. (2001). *Sex and gender* (4th ed.). Mountain View, CA: Mayfield.

McCloskey, J., & Bulechek, G. M. (1996). *Nursing interventions classification (NIC)* (2nd ed.). St. Louis, MO: Mosby.

McLeer, S. V., & Rose, M. (1999). Extrafamilial child sexual abuse. In J. A. Shaw (Ed.), *Sexual aggression* (pp. 210–242). Washington DC: American Psychiatric Press.

Morrell, B., Mendel, M. P. & Fisher, L. (2001). Object relations disturbances in sexually abused males. *Journal of Interpersonal Violence, 16* (9), 851–864.

Mullen, P. E., Pathe, M., Purcell, R., & Stuart, G. W. (1999). Study of stalkers. *American Journal of Psychiatry, 156*(8), 1244–1249.

Murphy, W. D., & Page, I. J. (1999). Adolescent perpetrators of sexual abuse. In J. A. Shaw (Ed.), *Sexual aggression* (pp. 367–389). Washington DC: American Psychiatric Press.

National Center for Victims of Crime. (2001). Retrieved October 1, 2002, from the World Wide Web, www.ncvc.org.

O'Keefe, M. (1998). Factors mediating the link between witnessing interparental violence and dating violence. *Journal of Family Violence, 13*(1), 39–57.

Paris, J. (1999). *Nature and nurture in psychiatry*. Washington, DC: American Psychiatric Press.

Ratey, J. J. (2001). *A user's guide to the brain*, New York: Pantheon Books.

Riggs, D. S., & Caulfield, M. B. (1997). Expected consequences of male violence against their female dating partners. *Journal of Interpersonal Violence, 12*(2), 229–240.

Ryan, G. (2000). Perpetration prevention. *SIECUS Report, 29*(1), 28–34.

Schetky, K. H. (1999). Sexual victimization of children. In J. A. Shaw (Ed.), *Sexual aggression* (pp. 107–128). Washington, DC: American Psychiatric Press.

Shaw, J. A. (1999). Sexually aggressive behavior. In J. A. Shaw (Ed.), *Sexual Aggression* (pp. 3–40). Washington DC: American Psychiatric Press.

Shirar, L. (1996). *Dissociative children*. New York: Norton.

Sholevar, G. P., & Schwoeri, L. D. (1999). Sexual aggression within the family. In J. A. Shaw (Ed.), *Sexual aggression* (pp. 75–105). Washington, DC: American Psychiatric Press.

Smith, M. E., & Kelly, L. M. (2001). The journey of recovery after a rape experience. *Issues in Mental Health Nursing, 22*, 337–352.

Stark, E., & Flitcraft, A. (1996). *Women at risk*. Newbury Park, CA: Sage.

Straus, M. A. (1994). *Beating the devil out of them: Corporal punishment in American families*. Lexington, MA: Lexington Books.

Sudermann, M., & Jaffe, P. G. (1999). Child witnesses of domestic violence. In R. T. Ammerman & M. Hersen (Eds.), *Assessment of family violence: A clinical and legal sourcebook* (2nd ed.) (pp. 343–366). New York: John Wiley & Sons.

Symes, L. (2000). Arriving at readiness to recover emotionally after sexual assault. *Archives of Psychiatric Nursing, 14*(1), 30–38.

Torres, S., & Han, H. R. (2000). Psychological distress in non-Hispanic white and Hispanic abused women. *Archives of Psychiatric Nursing, 14*(1), 19–29.

U.S. Department of Justice. (2001). Sexual assault nurse examiner (SANE) programs: Improving the community response to sexual assault victims. Retrieved October 1, 2002 from the World Wide Web, www.ojp.usdoj.gov/ovc/publications/bulletins/sane_4_2001/welcome.html.

Volavka, J. (1995). *Neurobiology of violence*. Washington, DC: American Psychiatric Press.

West, C. M. (1998). Leaving a second closet: Outing partner violence in same-sex couples. In J. L. Jasinski & L. M. Williams (Eds.), *Partner violence* (pp. 163–183). Newbury Park, CA: Sage.

Wiehe, V. R., & Richards, A. L. (1995). *Intimate betrayal*. Newbury Park, CA: Sage.

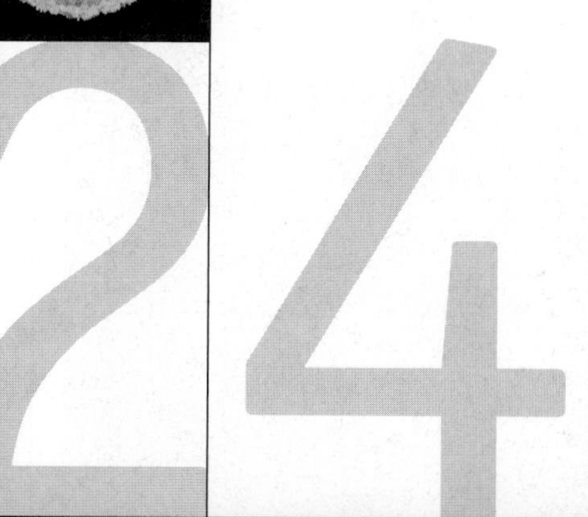

Chapter TWENTY-FOUR

Psychiatric–Mental Health Clients with HIV/AIDS

CAROL REN KNEISL

FOCUS QUESTIONS

- Why are certain psychiatric populations at risk for acquired immune deficiency syndrome (AIDS)?
- What are the neuropsychiatric impacts of human immunodeficiency virus (HIV) infection?
- How do you feel about caring for a mentally disordered person with HIV/AIDS?
- What modifications would you make in providing direct nursing care to people with HIV disease in psychiatric settings?
- What HIV risk-reduction education and counseling strategies regarding sexual behavior and substance abuse would be helpful in working with psychiatric–mental health clients and people in the community?
- How can psychiatric–mental health nurses support caregivers of people with HIV and AIDS and individuals experiencing AIDS-related bereavements?

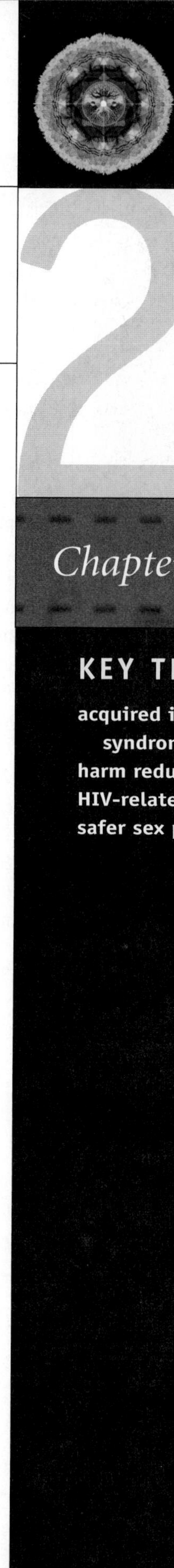

KEY TERMS

acquired immune deficiency syndrome (AIDS)
harm reduction
HIV-related dementia
safer sex practices

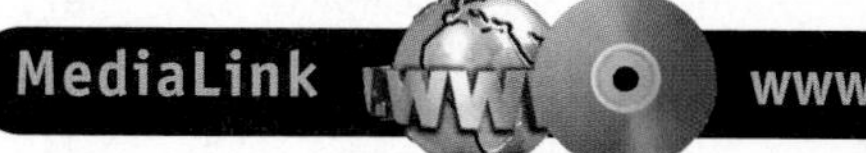

Additional resources for this chapter can be found on the Student CD-ROM accompanying this textbook, and on the Companion Website at www.prenhall.com/kneisl. Click on Chapter 24 to select the activities for this chapter.

CD-ROM

- T-cell Destruction by HIV Animation
- Audio Glossary
- NCLEX Review

Companion Website

- Additional NCLEX Review
- Care Plan: Coping with HIV Symptoms
- Case Study: HIV Dementia

CHAPTER OUTLINE

CROSS REFERENCES

Other topics relevant to this content are: Caring for clients with dementia and delirium, Chapter 12; Caring for depressed clients, Chapter 15; Caring for substance-abusing clients, Chapter 13; Enhancing compliance with pharmacologic treatment, Box 14–5 in Chapter 14, and Chapter 31; Visualization, therapeutic touch, and stress-management techniques, Chapter 32.

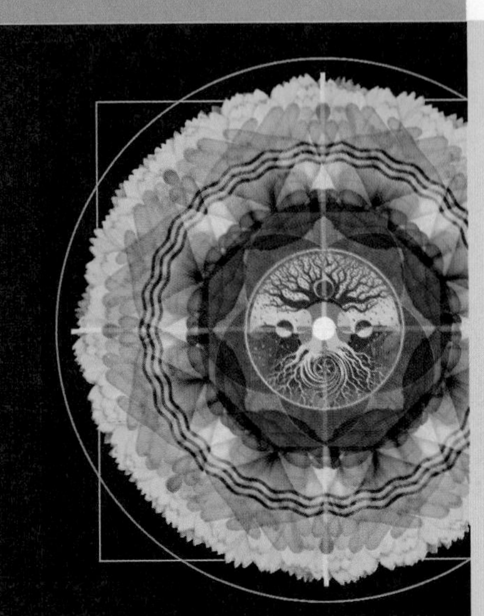

CRITICAL THINKING CHALLENGE

The community in which you live is against a needle and syringe prescription program for injection drug users (IDUs), but is considering establishing a needle and syringe exchange program as an HIV/AIDS prevention strategy. At the town meeting, several people voice their concern that a needle and syringe exchange program would not only facilitate, but also encourage, illicit drug injection. Because you are a psychiatric–mental health nurse, you are asked to comment. What would you say? ■

A chronic, potentially life-threatening illness, **acquired immune deficiency syndrome (AIDS)** is of clinical concern to all nurses, but especially to psychiatric–mental health nurses, who, by nature of their commitment and responsibility, become involved in human experiences. Clients with the human immunodeficiency virus (HIV), the virus that causes AIDS, require care that promotes quality of life and personal growth now that HIV is a chronic disease with the prospect of long-term survival (Sherbourne et al., 2000). Fully 61.4% of adults under care for HIV used mental health or substance abuse services (Burnam, et al., 2001).

Promoting quality of life and personal growth can be achieved only when psychiatric–mental health nurses are knowledgeable about the disease itself and are sensitive to the issues common to the communities hardest hit by this chronic illness:

- Men who have sex with men, their partners, friends, children, and families of origin.
- Male and female injection drug users (IDUs), their partners, friends, children, and families of origin, disproportionately represented in the African-American and Latino communities.
- The fastest growing group of persons newly infected with HIV—heterosexual women.

Be aware that the global face of HIV is changing. Health experts at the Joint United Nations (U.N.) Programme on AIDS (2001) indicate that:

- HIV/AIDS is now the fourth largest global killer and is rampant in sub-Saharan Africa.
- Other countries such as China, India, and the countries of the Russian Federation are poised for a similar epidemic.
- In Papua, New Guinea, more than one-third of the working-age population could die from AIDS by 2020.
- The rate for women in Canada went from 8.5% in 1995 to 24% in 2000.
- In 2000, 82% of those infected in the United States were African-American and Hispanic.

A more recent report is even more pessimistic by 15 to 20 million cases than the projections by the U.N. Joint Programme on HIV/AIDS. This report estimates that, by 2010, the five countries thought of as next-wave countries (Nigeria, Ethiopia, Russia, India, and China) will reach a total of 50 million to 75 million HIV/AIDS cases, swelling the global case toll to more than 80 million (National Intelligence Council, 2002). Russia is expected to suffer the fastest decline because its public health macrostructure is at its lowest point since World War II.

The focus of this chapter is on the understanding and skills essential to providing HIV/AIDS care to vulnerable psychiatric populations. This chapter is written with the assumption that, from earlier courses, you have basic knowledge of HIV disease, its cause, incidence and distribution, and modes of transmission; that you understand the basics of instituting universal precautions to protect yourself and others; and that you know how to provide physical care to people with HIV disease. It is not meant to be an all-inclusive chapter.

The HIV Mental Health Spectrum

Knox, Davis, and Friedrich (1994) identified a broad spectrum of people in the population with growing mental health care needs that are related to HIV. Their model of the HIV mental health spectrum remains relevant today and is illustrated in ■ Figure 24–1 on page 574.

THE GENERAL WORRIED POPULATION

The general worried population makes up the majority of people in this country. Although worried about transmission of HIV, they perceive themselves to be personally unaffected—that is, they are not infected, are not close to someone who is infected, and believe, perhaps naively, that they do not practice behaviors that put them at high risk. Identifying and reducing fears, promoting knowledge and reducing social naivete, and encouraging behavioral change are crucial roles of mental health care providers with this population.

HEALTH CARE PROVIDERS

Irrational fears, prejudice, and stress can lead to burnout and reduce the quality of health care. Although it is crucial that mental health care workers help set the tone and example for others in the community for appropriate attitudes and practices regarding HIV infection, some are reluctant to work with HIV-infected individuals. They cite fear of contagion (as the result of an accidental needlestick or being cut with a sharp instrument) as a primary concern. However, studies of health care workers that documented parenteral or mucous membrane exposure to the blood or body fluids of HIV-infected people indicate that the incidence is extremely low. Additional concerns are discomfort in working with the terminally ill, and discomfort with IDUs and men who have sex with men (Sherman & Ouellette, 1999). Worries about how best to protect themselves and their families are also common concerns. Providing empathic, supportive care requires confronting your own and your family's fear of infection as well as your own values and prejudices. (See also the section on ethical concerns and the Nursing Self-Awareness feature.)

SIGNIFICANT OTHERS AND FAMILY MEMBERS

Significant others and family members face many emotional challenges. Many families are facing the emotional challenge of multiple HIV diagnoses and injection drug use within the family. Family secrets about sexual or drug use behavior may be publicly disclosed along with an HIV diagnosis. At the same time they cope with these problems, significant others and family members are often the mainstay of emotional support for the person with HIV. They assume the burden of providing emotional support while coping with their own fears, providing physical care, and anticipating, then grieving, their loss. The issue of bereavement associated with HIV and AIDS is addressed later in the chapter. Family burden is discussed in Chapter 29.

INDIVIDUALS AT RISK

Individuals at risk are those who are most likely to have or to contract HIV, due to past or current participation in high-risk

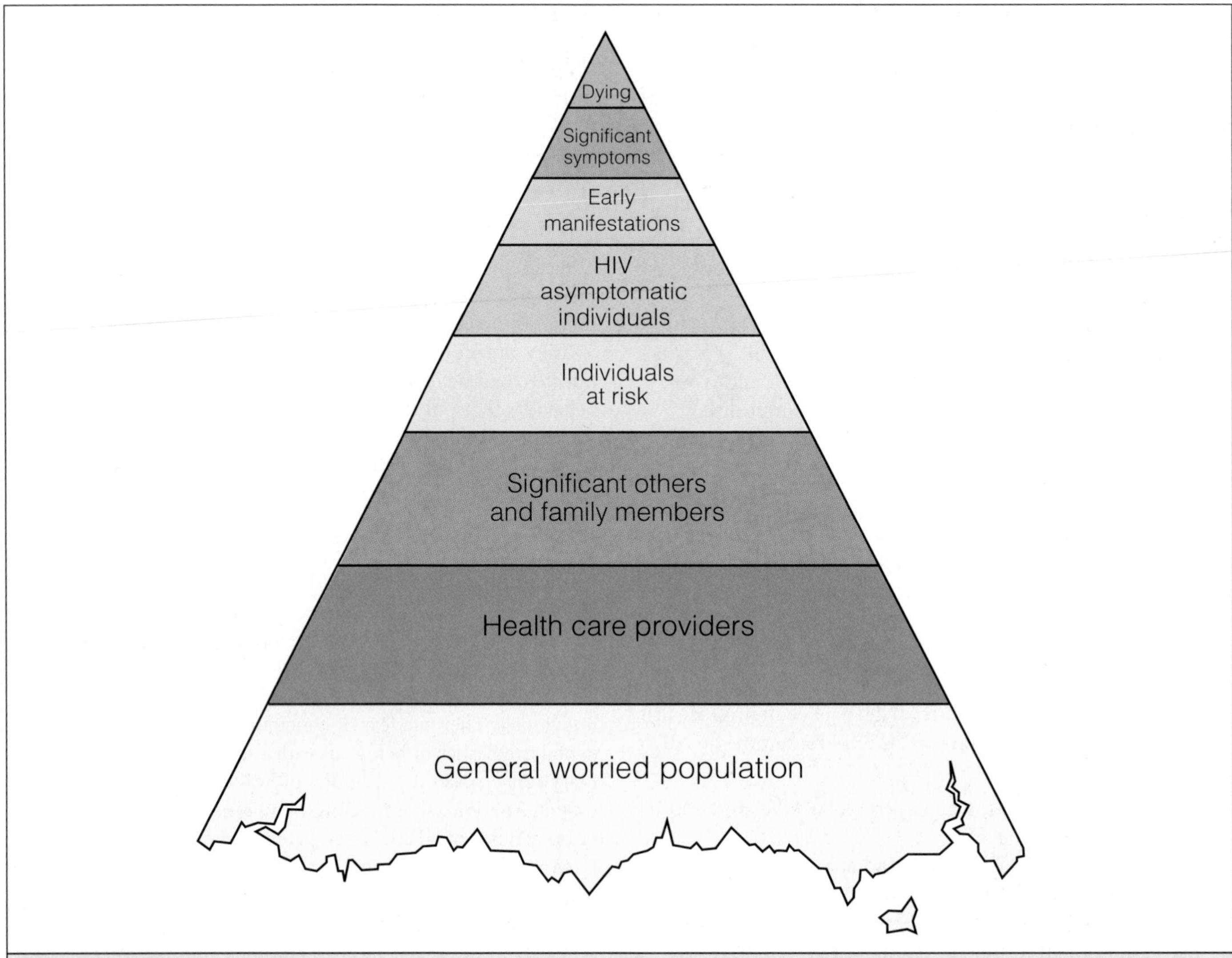

FIGURE 24–1 ■ *The HIV-mental health spectrum. This model shows populations requiring mental health care services related to HIV. Cross-sectional size represents population size and diversity. Distance from the base represents increasingly direct emotional effects of HIV infection and the increasing need for mental health intervention.*

Source: Adapted from Knox, M. D., Davis, M., & Friedrich, M. A. (1994). The HIV mental health spectrum. *Community Mental Health Journal, 30*(1), 77. Reprinted with permission from Kluwer Academic/Plenum Publishers.

activities. This specific group includes people who have not been tested for HIV and those who have received negative HIV antibody test results but are still considered at risk. Maladaptive human responses in individuals at risk could result in self-destructive and irresponsible behaviors such as unsafe sexual practices.

HIV ASYMPTOMATIC INDIVIDUALS

This category of individuals affected by HIV is referred to in the Centers for Disease Control and Prevention (CDC) classification system as HIV-seropositive (asymptomatic). This group consists of people whose HIV antibody tests confirm the presence of the virus but as yet exhibit no symptoms associated with immune system suppression.

People who are HIV-seropositive (asymptomatic) may experience many of the same responses as individuals at risk, in addition to problems of impaired adjustment and the development of a sense of powerlessness. This may be manifested in a variety of ways, including chronic depression and decreasing motivation. As asymptomatic people begin to deal with the reality of their condition, you may be able to help them engage in health-seeking behaviors. Wellness activities not only promote physical health but also empower the individual, thus promoting mental health.

INDIVIDUALS WITH HIV-RELATED CONDITIONS

This category on the HIV mental health spectrum includes individuals with HIV-related conditions (HRCs). These people are referred to in the CDC classification system as HIV-seropositive (symptomatic).

Individuals with HRC have begun to experience the physical effects of immune system deterioration. In addition to having physical manifestations, they may experience complex psychosocial responses as well as the other human responses previously discussed. These may include altered role performance and self-concept disturbance related to losses, and changes in their perceptions and abilities secondary to the development of physical symptoms and limitations.

PEOPLE WITH AIDS

People with significant symptoms are those with a formal diagnosis of AIDS, as defined by CDC guidelines. These are characterized by the development of potentially life-threatening complications because of extensive immune system suppression.

People with AIDS (PWAs) may experience any of the human responses of individuals throughout the HIV mental health spectrum. In addition, PWAs may experience a sense of hopelessness, social isolation, impaired social interactions, or spiritual distress associated with the effects of a chronic life-threatening illness.

LONG-TERM SURVIVORS

Although not listed in the HIV mental health spectrum, there is one other group of people of clinical concern to psychiatric–mental health nurses. People who have outlived the generally expected life span for people with HIV and AIDS are called long-term survivors. As more individuals with HIV infection are identified and new treatments are discovered to slow or halt HIV progression in a predictable fashion, the number of long-term survivors will continue to increase. This has obvious implications for mental health care professionals working with people affected by HIV infection. As the number of long-term survivors who have benefited from highly active antiretroviral therapy (HAART) increases, psychiatric–mental health nurses should expect to see increasing numbers of people struggling with issues related to HIV infection.

HIV Transmission Risks in Psychiatric Populations

The research overwhelmingly indicates that the major modes of transmission of the virus are:

- Intimate (oral sex, vaginally insertive heterosexual intercourse, anally receptive sex) unprotected sexual contact with an HIV-seropositive person.
- Parenteral injection of blood or blood products infected with HIV.
- Transfer of the virus from an HIV-infected mother to a fetus or newborn infant in utero, during labor or delivery, or in the early newborn period during breast-feeding.

Because of the nature of these major modes of transmission and the epidemiology of the epidemic in the United States, the following psychiatric–mental health populations are at high risk for contracting HIV:

- Intravenous drug users (because intravenous transmission is a major mode of transmission of the virus).
- The seriously mentally ill (because their judgment and problem-solving ability are compromised and they are likely to engage in unprotected sex).
- The homeless mentally ill (because they often trade sex for drugs or money).
- Clients whose mental disorder causes them to act recklessly (because they are likely to engage in unprotected sex or inject drugs).

A cross-sectional study by Stoskopf, Kim, and Glover (2001) found that persons with a mental illness are 1.44 times more likely to have HIV/AIDS, especially if they are substance abusers, diagnosed with a depressive disorder, or female.

INJECTION DRUG USERS

The second largest transmission category for HIV in North America and Europe is injection drug use through the transfer of small amounts of blood in shared needles or syringes. Active IDUs who are also hazardous alcohol users are thought to be at particularly high risk (Stein, Anderson, Charuvastra, Maksad, & Friedmann, 2002). Injection drug users also constitute a bridge to others—their fetuses, newborns, and sex partners—putting them at increased risk. Unfortunately, 60.4% of IDUs minimize their HIV risk, appraising their risk of infection as nil or small (Brown, Outlaw & Simpson, 2000).

Fully one-third of people with AIDS in the United States are IDUs or the sexual partners of IDUs (Centers for Disease Control and Prevention [CDC], 2002a). Of heterosexuals whose only known exposure was through sex with a person at risk, approximately two-thirds are female partners of male IDUs. As much as 47% of all women diagnosed with AIDS have been infected through injection drug use (Moser, Sowell, & Phillips, 2001). ■ Figure 24–2 illustrates the distribution of IDU-associated AIDS cases by exposure category.

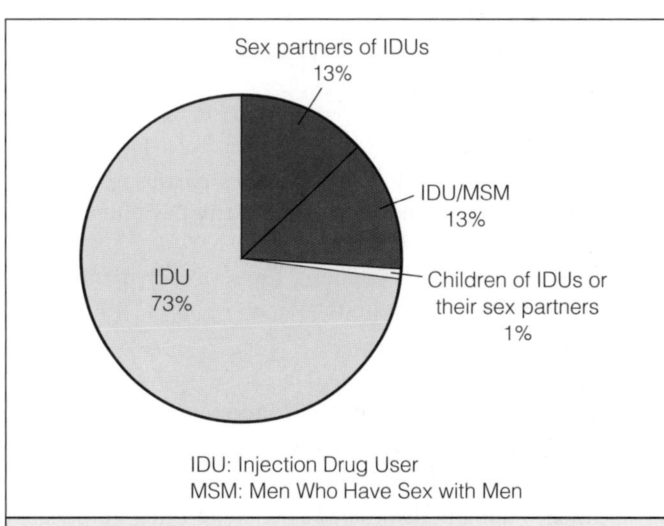

FIGURE 24–2 ■ *Proportion of IDU-associated AIDS cases, by exposure category, reported in 2000, United States.*

Source: Data from Centers for Disease Control. (2002b). *HIV/AIDS surveillance report, 13*(1).

THE SERIOUSLY MENTALLY ILL

Seroprevalence rates among the seriously mentally ill have been estimated to range between 4% and 23% (Lyon, 2001). It is for this reason that the Office on AIDS Research of the National Institutes for Health has identified the prevention and treatment of HIV in persons with serious mental illness as one of its highest priority research initiatives.

People with serious mental illness often engage in behaviors that put them at high risk for HIV infection. For example, a survey in which 79% of the sample had a primary diagnosis of schizophrenia found that 20% of mentally ill men and 51% of mentally ill women had been sexually active in the 12 months preceding the survey (Davidson et al., 2001). They were also eight times more likely to have injected illicit drugs and shared needles 7.4% of the time.

According to Brown and Jemmott (2000), seriously and mentally ill persons are thought to be especially susceptible to HIV risk-related behaviors for the following reasons:

1. Poor judgment
2. Limited impulse control
3. Deficits in problem-solving skills
4. Suicidal intent
5. Self-destructive tendencies

MediaLink T-cell Destruction by HIV Animation

CLINICAL EXAMPLE

On her last admission to the inpatient unit for treatment of a manic episode, Sadie had a persistent vaginal fungal infection that resisted treatment. HIV testing came back positive for the presence of HIV. Prior to this last admission, Sadie had not taken her lithium for 2 months. As Sadie's mania increased, so did her risk behavior. When elated, Sadie was game to try anything, from alcohol to crack cocaine, to unprotected sex with men she met at one of several bars she frequented. Sadie felt invulnerable.

Many of our mentally ill clients meet sex partners in bars or mental health clinics, and their sexual activities often involve the exchange of money or drugs for sex.

In most studies of HIV among the seriously mentally ill, there are several consistent findings:

- Having multiple sex partners
- Having sex partners who are IDUs
- Absence of, or inconsistency in, condom use
- Frequent use of alcohol and drugs in conjunction with sex
- A history of sexually transmitted infections

In addition, mentally disordered clients are often ambivalent about abstinence and the need to reduce the risk of infection with a sex partner. They may see themselves as more helpless than others in the general population when it comes to reducing risk, or, on the contrary, they may view themselves as invincible.

THE HOMELESS MENTALLY ILL

The homeless mentally ill who live in urban areas, particularly those who live in municipal shelters, are at particular risk for HIV, hepatitis C, and tuberculosis (TB). The high incidence of injection drug use in this population, along with exchanging sex for drugs or money, makes this group extremely vulnerable. The homeless mentally ill are likely to experience several barriers to beginning, maintaining, and completing treatment. Several practical matters—establishing a medication routine, having access to health care providers, and being supported by friends and family—are the usual barriers faced by homeless people. The specific cognitive barriers that result from mental illness and HIV infection add to the difficulty of obtaining prophylactic or early treatment.

The Biopsychosocial Impact of HIV/AIDS

HIV affects the biologic, psychologic, neurologic, developmental, sociocultural, economic, and ethical spheres of human life.

NEUROPSYCHIATRIC MANIFESTATIONS

Significant numbers of people with HIV experience neuropsychiatric manifestations (NPMs) for two major reasons:

1. Because the virus is capable of invading central nervous system (CNS) tissue, several of the opportunistic infections and neoplasms associated with AIDS also affect the CNS (see ■ Figure 24–3).
2. Prescribed pharmacologic treatment may have neuropsychiatric side effects.

Symptoms can range from anxiety and depressive symptoms to delirium, dementia, and coma. Neuropsychiatric side effects of medications used to treat HIV/AIDS are listed in ■ Table 24–1 on page 578.

Psychological

HIV disease threatens psychological integrity as well as physiologic integrity. The concept of loss is central to an understanding of the psychological impact of HIV and the depression, anxiety, and suicidal ideation that often accompany it. HIV disease is frequently linked with several different loss experiences for people with HIV and their families, friends, and caregivers. These include loss of the following:

- Energy, appetite, strength, and physical stamina
- Control of body functions such as elimination, mobility, speech, sight, hearing, and tactile sensations
- Control of body appearance due to dramatic weight loss, oozing wounds, skin breakdown, hair loss, skin lesions, or side effects of antiviral medications (e.g., persistent lipodystrophy syndrome)
- Self-worth and personal competence
- Mental clarity and cognitive ability

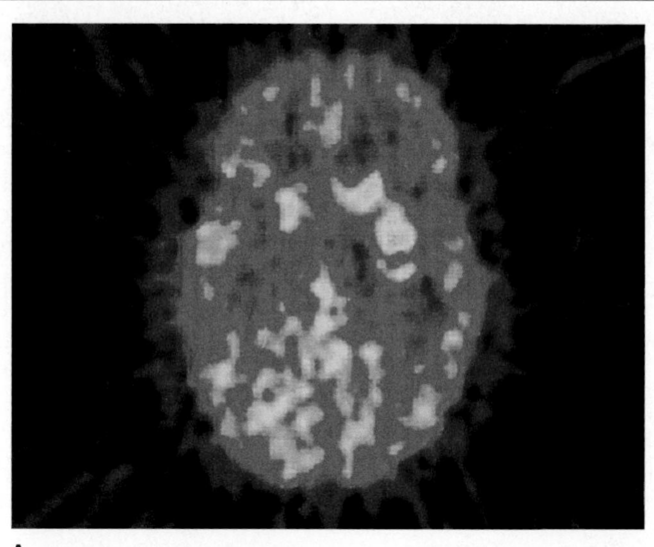
A

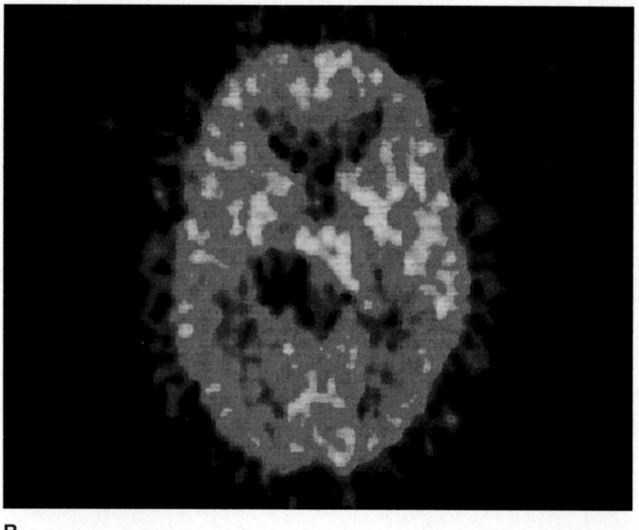
B

FIGURE 24–3 ■ *Opportunistic HIV Diseases of the Brain. PET scans facilitate a neurologic diagnosis by distinguishing between hot lymphomas and metabolically cold toxoplasmosis. (A) PET scan of an HIV-related lymphoma, the metabolically hot tumor on the right side of the scan. (B) In contrast, this scan shows HIV-related toxoplasmosis, indicated by the dramatic "hole" of a metabolically cold area.*

Source: Courtesy of Dr. Giovanni DiChiro and Dr. Ramesh Raman of the Neuroimaging Branch, National Institute of Neurological Disorders and Stroke, National Institute of Health.

- Privacy
- Self-sufficiency and self-determination
- Employment, health insurance, salary
- Physical intimacy, including sexual expression
- Friends and lovers to earlier deaths from AIDS
- Social support
- Hope
- Peace of mind and spirit
- Life itself

Psychological syndromes associated with HIV infection are generally related to the initial diagnosis of HIV, crisis points along the HIV mental health spectrum, or adjustment to the experience of chronic illness. Anxiety and depression are high (Morrison et al., 2002; Zinkernagel et al., 2001). Increased suicide risk can result from depression related to stress from the HIV diagnosis, treatment, and side effects of medications. The inherent lack of predictability and control, the fear of rejection and abandonment, hopelessness, and problems such as memory deficit and confusion also play a role. These factors, especially anxiety and depression, not only affect the client's quality of life but may also determine how closely the client adheres to the treatment plan (Holzemer, 2002).

Neurologic/Neurocognitive

Studies suggest that physiologically based clinical neuropsychiatric manifestations or disorders are common among PWAs. A neurologic syndrome or neurocognitive impairment may be the first clinical manifestation of HIV disease. Neurocognitive impairment is thought to be associated with high levels of HIV activity and severe immunosuppression (Ungvarski & Trzcianowska, 2000).

Focal Brain Processes. The most common focal brain processes are toxoplasmosis (a parasitic opportunistic infection), cryptococcal meningitis (a fungal opportunistic infection), cytomegalovirus (CMV) encephalitis (a viral opportunistic infection), progressive multifocal leukoencephalopathy (PML; a viral opportunistic infection), and CNS lymphoma (a neoplastic process). Signs and symptoms associated with these processes include focal deficits, altered level of consciousness, confusion, memory disturbances, headaches, and seizures.

HIV-Related Dementia. A syndrome caused by direct HIV infection of the CNS, **HIV-related dementia** is characterized as a progressive dementia that involves a progressive slowing and loss of precision in both cognitive and motor functions, with accompanying behavioral disturbances. Its cause is not fully known.

MediaLink Case Study: HIV Dementia

The signs and symptoms of HIV-related dementia include the following:

- Cognitive dysfunction: forgetfulness, loss of concentration, confusion, and slowness of thought.
- Declining motor performance: loss of balance, muscle weakness, and deterioration in fine motor skills such as handwriting.
- Behavioral changes: apathy, withdrawal, dysphoric mood, and regressed behavior.
- In addition, people with HIV-related dementia may experience other symptoms such as headaches or seizures.

HIV-related dementia is often initially confused with psychiatric depression but generally progresses in a period of months to the point at which the affected individual is bedridden.

TABLE 24–1 Neuropsychiatric Side Effects of Some HIV/AIDS Medications

Medication	Side Effect
Acyclovir	Agitation, anxiety, confusion, depersonalization, hyperacusia, hyperesthesia, insomnia, tearfulness, thought insertion, visual hallucinations
Amphotericin B	Anorexia, delirium, diplopia, peripheral neuropathy, sleep disturbance
Cotrimoxazole	Apathy, depression, headache, insomnia, loss of appetite
Didanosine (ddI)	Anxiety, confusion, insomnia, mania, peripheral neuropathy
Foscarnet	Confusion, headache, irritability, paresthesias, seizures
Ganciclovir	Agitation, delirium, irritability, mania, psychosis
Interferon	Anxiety, confusion, depression, sleep disturbance, weakness
Isoniazid	Agitation, anxiety, depression, hallucinations, impaired memory, paranoia, sleep disturbance
Methotrexate	Encephalopathy
Pentamidine	Anxiety, confusion, hallucinations
Procarbazine	Confusion, insomnia, loss of appetite, malaise, mania, nightmares
Stavudine (d4T)	Anxiety, confusion, depression, early morning awakening, insomnia, mania, sleep disturbance
Steroids	Depression, euphoria, mania, psychosis, sleep disturbance
Thiabendazole	Hallucinations, olfactory disturbances
Vinblastine	Anorexia, depression, headache
Vincristine	Agitation, ataxia, depression, hallucinations, headache, sensory loss
Zidovudine (AZT)	Agitation, anxiety, auditory hallucinations, confusion, depression, headache, insomnia, irritability, malaise, mania, restlessness, unusually vivid dreams

Source: New York State Department of Health AIDS Institute. (2001). *Mental health care for people with HIV infection: HIV clinical guidelines for the primary care practitioner*. New York: Author; Schulte, J. (2000). HIV infection: The quintessential biopsychosocial disease. In Kay, J., & Tasman, A. *Psychiatry: Behavioral science and clinical essentials*. Philadelphia: Saunders.

Individuals with HIV-related dementia may quickly succumb to opportunistic infections because they are unable to take care of themselves. HIV-related dementia has declined since the introduction of HAART. It has been reported that antiviral medications have a direct neuroprotective effect, in addition to their antiviral effects, of delaying or reducing the symptoms associated with HIV-related dementia (Herning, Better, Tate, & Cadet, 2002). Therefore, it is important to encourage clients to follow their medication regimen precisely.

Psychoneuroimmunology

There has been increasing emphasis in the scientific literature on the study of psychoneuroimmunology (PNI), introduced in Chapter 4. A growing body of evidence has demonstrated the interrelatedness of the body–mind–spirit connection and the immune system. Nurses need to be more aware of the psychological and neurologic effects on immune system disorders. There is widespread support for the use of holistic nursing practices and treatment approaches to boost the immune system, in accordance with the findings in the growing field of psychoneuroimmunology (see the accompanying Caring for the Spirit feature).

DEVELOPMENTAL EFFECTS

Most people with HIV disease are young adults or adults in their middle years. The period known as young adulthood is normally the healthiest and is characterized by peaks in muscular strength. Cognitive development should be completed and cognitive abilities should be refined at this stage. Recall that the psychosocial task of identity consolidation is the major developmental task of young adulthood. HIV disease may disrupt the person's ability to negotiate this challenge successfully.

Typically, the middle years are very productive in the arenas of work and family. During this period, adults consolidate relationships and occupational status and goals. HIV disease may interfere with the individual's ability to accept the responsibilities inherent in such roles as parent, worker, mate or partner, and so on. Questions of dependence and independence, thought to have been resolved previously, are reawakened as illness forces a return to earlier developmental phases.

Children and adolescents with HIV infection face delays or changes in skills on all developmental fronts—physical, cognitive, and psychosocial—as they confront acute life-threatening illness and chronic disability. Failure to thrive is a striking feature of this illness in children.

CARING FOR THE SPIRIT

Long-Term Survivors of HIV

Wars wage within our bodies every minute of every day. Most of the time we are unaware of the battles that go on within us. We have evolved legions of defenders—specialized cells that silently rout the unseen enemy. Their victories go unheralded. When our defenses are penetrated, our defenders are caught unprepared, or our defenders are routed and we've lost the battle. Then we develop a cold, the flu, or something worse. Why did I catch a cold from the sick toddler on the airplane when the woman next to me did not? Why didn't you come down with the flu when your roommate was sick? Why do only some of the people exposed to HIV develop the disease? Why do some people with HIV die within a year or two while others have survived, or even thrived, for 10, 20, or more years? We don't, as yet, have all the answers to these questions.

One particularly exciting field of research that has contributed toward answering these questions is *psychoneuroimmunology (PNI)*, the study of the communication between the mind, the brain, the endocrine system, and the immune system. Belief in the interconnectedness of mind, body, and spirit has long been a tradition of nursing. Recent scientific advances in PNI are important to nurses because they support the mind–body–spirit connection.

Perhaps the most common characteristics of people with AIDS who live long past the time predicted for them is their refusal to accept the diagnosis of HIV disease as a death sentence. They do not deny the diagnosis, but *they do defy the fatal outcome* that is supposed to be connected to it. Long-term survivors are extremely goal oriented and social. They treat their symptoms as if they were minor impediments in their lives; they are determined to prevail. Their immune systems seem to function better. They have higher T-cell counts and, in many cases, other immune system cells compensate for the ravaged T cells. Emotional distress, on the other hand, has been found to accompany negative immune function factors in HIV-infected individuals.

The highest incidence of illness and death occurs in people who experience stress after infection with HIV. This suggests that HIV-seropositive people should reduce their exposure to stressful events. Assertive coping, less stress, more self-nurturing, regular exercise, and a spiritual outlook have been associated with better immune status, suggesting that stress-reduction behaviors may be helpful in slowing the progression of HIV disease.

While we cannot promote the idea that clients are in total control of the disease process and the state of their health, or that the mind or the spirit can cure AIDS, we can and should teach clients the self-care and self-nurturing behaviors that long-term survivors are using to maintain their health. Assess the level of stress, quality of social support, and mood factors that influence the quality of life of people with HIV disease. Nursing interventions to help clients enhance neurologic, immunologic, and cognitive functioning should focus on improved nutrition, adequate sleep–wake patterns, hygiene, stress reduction, and social and spiritual support.

SOCIOCULTURAL AND ECONOMIC EFFECTS

Although HIV/AIDS continues to be a leading public health issue in the United States, public focus on the epidemic as a significant social and political issue appears to be waning. Webber (2000) believes that this waning of interest is taking place because HIV increasingly affects low-income people of color in urban areas, as well as women. Stigma and economic factors, including homelessness, combine to cause inequality in access to HIV care. In general, the poor have limited access to health services (Burnam et al., 2001).

Stigma

The sociocultural environment of people affected by HIV can be hostile to them. Most people with HIV are in one of two risk categories—men who have sex with men and injection drug users—that engender fear, anger, and prejudice. Persons in both risk categories experience stigma during hospitalization. There is some evidence to suggest that stigmatization of clients with HIV by nurses is stratified based on the means by which HIV had been contracted, with IDUs expressing the greatest feeling of stigma from nurses (Surlis & Hyde, 2001).

On the other hand, children with HIV disease or individuals who have contracted HIV from the transfusion of blood or a blood product are usually perceived as "innocents." However, they too may be feared and subject to discrimination.

Economic Factors

Days lost from work because of illness may cost people with HIV infection or AIDS their jobs and insurance benefits. Some insurers are avoiding or reducing claims by isolating high-risk applicants with HIV antibody tests, denying new policies to those at risk, and aggressively fighting existing policyholders' claims in court. Family and friends may be unable or unwilling to assist financially. Young adults find themselves having to seek public assistance such as Medicaid or rely on the generosity of pharmaceutical companies for help in meeting the costs associated with HIV disease.

AIDS services organizations (ASOs) provide a social and economic lifeline for people with AIDS. They provide emotional support counselors and pastoral counselors to the dying and their families; send out workers to clean, cook, shop, and provide transportation; run low-cost residences; and shuttle PWAs back and forth to hospital and clinic appointments. Programs such as these have helped lessen the financial impact. Unquestionably, HIV/AIDS presents an economic problem of severe proportions.

Homelessness

An increasingly critical problem is the lack of decent, appropriate housing for the growing number of people with HIV disease. HIV disease is disproportionately prevalent among individuals already at the economic edge and those who are targets of discrimination in housing and medical care: people of color, homosexuals, injection drug users, and homeless and runaway youths. In many communities around the country, available housing and services fall short of the need for appropriate residential care for thousands of people who have been made homeless by HIV-related illnesses, or whose struggle to survive on the streets has been worsened by the disease (National Resource Center on Homelessness and Mental Illness, 2002). Fatigue, repeated hospitalization, and recurring illnesses all require time off from work, resulting first in the loss of employment, then in the loss of housing. The lack of effective risk-reduction education programs among the homeless has led to predictable and dramatic increases in HIV-seropositivity among them. Studies estimate the predicted number of homeless with HIV to be between 3% and 20% (National Coalition for the Homeless, 2002).

Although most people with an impaired immune system can live independently, they require a safe environment that helps them avoid exposure to infectious disease, get adequate rest, meet their special nutritional needs, and have access to support services and home help when necessary.

ETHICAL CONCERNS

The ethical issues surrounding HIV/AIDS prompt many emotional responses. Review the ethical questions in the Nursing Self-Awareness feature below while being conscious of your own emotional responses.

NURSING SELF-AWARENESS

Ethical Issues Surrounding HIV/AIDS

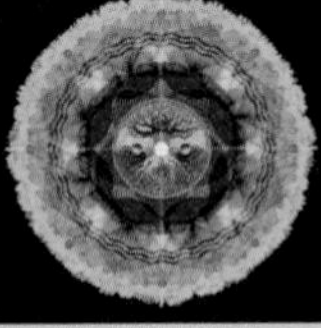

Engage in the process of ethical reflection discussed in Chapter 10 to analyze these and other issues to avoid further stigmatizing people with HIV disease.

- Should HIV antibody testing be made mandatory? If so, who should be tested: gay men, IDUs, pregnant women, people admitted to hospitals, prisoners, couples applying for marriage licenses, food handlers, health care workers, child care workers, people applying for health and life insurance—everyone?
- Is it in the public interest to identify, report, and make public the names of HIV-infected individuals or those at risk for HIV?
- Should people with HIV/AIDS be placed in quarantine for the public good?
- Can or should employers suspend, terminate, or refuse to hire people with HIV/AIDS? If they are teachers? Food handlers? Health care workers?
- Can or should insurance companies deny HIV-related medical insurance claims and life insurance policy claims?
- Should people who have had sexual contact with people with HIV or received infected blood products be traced and informed by public health authorities?
- Should people infected with HIV be tattooed to protect potential sex partners from infection?
- Do health care workers have a duty to inform those at risk when a person with HIV does not modify high-risk behavior?
- Can, or should, nurses or other health care professionals refuse to provide care to people with HIV disease?

Be aware that HIV-infected people are doubly stigmatized. They have an HIV diagnosis, and most of them are already members of other stigmatized groups.

Several state nurses' associations and national nursing organizations have published statements relative to nursing practice that clarify the professional nurse's responsibility in relation to the care of HIV-infected people. These statements and the Code of Ethics for Nurses of the American Nurses Association (ANA) (2001) address the need to provide appropriate care (both direct and indirect), health teaching, and advocacy regardless of the nature of the client's illness because of moral obligation. Be sure to familiarize yourself with your state nurses' association's statement on the care of HIV-infected people. The advocacy role of nursing organizations in the United States, Canada, Australia, and New Zealand is discussed later in this chapter.

Roles for Psychiatric–Mental Health Nurses

Psychiatric–mental health nurses will work with clients all along the continuum of HIV infection and disability. You may be involved in working with people with HIV disease in inpatient settings in psychiatric hospitals, psychiatric units in general hospitals, mental health clinics, community health agencies, HIV day treatment programs, hospices or homes, private practice, industry, or schools, as a citizen and neighbor, or even as an AIDS prevention street nurse as in one creative program in Vancouver, Canada (Hilton, Thompson, Moore-Dempsey, & Hutchinson, 2001). In addition, you will have an active role with healthy people, the family and friends of people with HIV, and bereaved survivors.

PROVIDING A THERAPEUTIC MILIEU

Proactive preparation and programming is critical in allaying the anxiety of staff members and clients when incorporating people with HIV disease into a psychiatric–mental health setting. Both staff members and clients may have concerns about disease transmission, inadequate knowledge regarding HIV and AIDS, and lack of understanding of the needs and behavior of people with HIV disease.

Protecting Privacy

Be concerned with protecting clients' privacy. Clients experience breaches in confidentiality because of institutional policies that make their disease conspicuous and from nurses' nonchalance in handling information about their disease (Surlis & Hyde, 2001). Clients also consider the sharing of stigmatizing medical information among nurses and other medical personnel, without their prior consent, as a breach of confidentiality (Whetten-Goldstein, Mguyen, & Sugarman, 2001) and make decisions on where to seek care based on the degree of professionalism of the staff. Obviously, clients who do not trust that you will respect their privacy are likely not to be forthcoming.

Modifying Agency Policies and Procedures

Special arrangements may need to be made about the scheduling of activities, visiting policies in an inpatient setting, and the provision of physical treatments, depending on the physical and neuropsychiatric manifestations of the disease and the extent of HIV disease progression. Staff will need to make individual decisions on a case-by-case basis. Clear communication with staff members and other clients is necessary for promoting consistency and preventing disruption of the milieu as a result of perceived inequities.

Clients with NPMs may present a special challenge to the staff and to the therapeutic environment. Their behavior may be erratic, frightening, and unlike that of the usual psychiatric client. This may require modification of usual unit procedure or activities. It may become necessary to exclude some clients, such as those with HIV dementia, from certain activities or to bend the rules to keep clients involved. To prevent other clients from perceiving that the client with HIV disease is receiving special treatment, openly discuss these issues with the other clients while continuing to ensure individual client confidentiality, as appropriate.

Not all clients react favorably to the presence of PWAs. Clients with paranoid disorders tend to have the greatest difficulty in accepting clients with HIV. They may become hostile, incorporate AIDS into paranoid delusions, insist on being transferred to another unit, or insist that PWAs be transferred to another unit.

You can help other clients by providing education, offering support, allowing the other clients to vent their fears and express their concerns, and emphasizing that the care of HIV clients is an important and normal part of the unit routine.

Implementing Infection Control Precautions

The use of standard infection control precautions in a psychiatric–mental health setting can also help minimize staff and client anxiety. Not all people with HIV (both staff and clients) are aware of their status or feel comfortable disclosing the information even if they are aware. Standard precautions, as prescribed by the CDC, will protect all staff members and clients against the transmission of HIV. This approach promotes confidentiality because appropriate precautions are taken in the care of all clients.

GIVING DIRECT CARE

Psychiatric hospitalization may be needed because the client is depressed, suicidal, or psychotic or has an AIDS-related behavior disturbance, probably because of a focal brain disorder or HIV-related dementia. Nursing care for clients with depression, suicidal ideation, psychosis, dementia, and delirium has been discussed in earlier chapters in this text (see Chapters 15, 22, 14, and 12). Incorporate these principles into your care of clients with HIV as appropriate.

Psychiatric–mental health nurses caring for clients with HIV or AIDS on inpatient units encounter a number of issues that are uncommon in psychiatric settings:

- The client may have a multitude of physical problems.
- The client has a condition that calls for infection control precautions.
- The quality of the nurse–client relationship is intensified through the additional contact required in giving physical care.
- The common problems of adherence to prescribed psychotropic medication become more complex because clients need also to be faithful to antiretroviral and other AIDS-related pharmacologic regimens (see Chapter 31 and Box 14–5 in Chapter 14 for guidelines to enhance adherence) and must contend with unwelcome side effects from antiretrovirals and antipsychotics.
- Physical problems can be mistaken as psychiatric problems, and vice versa. For example, it is important not to mistake delirium for depression (see Table 12–1 on page 239).
- Psychiatric–mental health nurses, who very seldom work with dying clients, find it necessary to confront the issue of caring for clients with life-threatening illnesses.

A necessary modification in the care of clients with HIV/AIDS has to do with the use of touch. The physical care needs of AIDS clients require modifying the usual psychiatric injunction of limiting physical contact with clients. Because AIDS is such an isolating and stigmatizing condition, giving a massage or holding the client's hand has therapeutic value. A variety of complementary and alternative therapies may be appropriate (Standish, Calabrese, & Galantino, 2001). For example, you might incorporate some of the complementary and alternative therapies, such as relaxation techniques, visualization, imagery, or massage, that are discussed in Chapter 32. Caring for clients with a dual diagnosis that includes HIV disease requires creative modification.

It may be beneficial to set up a separate support group for people with HIV disease, where they can discuss issues specific to HIV/AIDS in a supportive setting. If there aren't enough HIV clients for a group, then an ASO might provide support group services.

CLINICAL EXAMPLE

Jorge, an outpatient client at a mental health clinic based in a medium-size northeastern city, has both bipolar disorder and HIV disease. Jorge and Bill, his life partner, had recently returned to the city of their birth after an absence of 15 years. Although Jorge came from a large family, he has very limited contact with his family. Most of his family members are having trouble accepting Jorge's homosexuality. Bill and his family have taken on the caregiving responsibility for Jorge; however, Bill is becoming concerned about the extent of the emotional and physical care he needs to provide for Jorge since Bill is trying to manage his own alcohol abuse. The psychiatric–mental health nurse at the mental health clinic made a phone call to a local ASO, AIDS Family Services, and referred Jorge and Bill. The ASO offers several services—a support group for family members, friends, and partners; and a 12-step spirituality group—that Jorge and Bill could both benefit from.

An ASO can also be an important resource for HIV clients after discharge. The range of services available depends on the structure of the ASO but frequently includes counseling, support groups, buddy programs, educational programs, pastoral care, spirituality programs, financial assistance, housing referral, legal aid, and client advocacy.

Clients with NPMs such as HIV dementia, may offer the greatest challenge to the inpatient unit staff. Three important but frequently ignored nursing diagnoses that apply to clients with NPMs are:

1. Impaired Communication.
2. Spiritual Distress.
3. Impaired Home Maintenance Management.

Clients with NPMs of HIV disease often have special discharge planning needs or experience placement problems. Intervention strategies appropriate to these three selected nursing diagnoses are discussed in the following sections.

Intervening in Impaired Communication

Evidence exists that clients with both HIV infection and psychiatric disorders may not receive optimal care because their psychiatric disorders are a barrier to communication with health care workers (Treisman, Angelino, & Hutton, 2001). Incorporate the facilitative communication principles discussed in Chapter 8 in your work with these clients.

Dementia and other cognitive problems are also barriers to communication. Because a client's symptoms are generally progressive, interventions do not reverse the dementia but may enhance the quality of life for both the client and the primary caregiver. Here are several strategies:

- Convey unconditional positive regard, maintain a relationship, and maintain a sense of normality in interactions.
- Make verbal communication clear, concise, and unhurried; be sure to have the person's attention before starting; encourage the person to communicate; be comfortable with periods of silence; be aware of tone and volume of voice (this may prevent misperceptions).
- Use brief, direct statements: "Bill, eat this pudding" rather than "Why don't you and I have some pudding for dessert?"
- Ask questions that require only simple yes or no answers, and make only one request at a time.
- Be sensitive to the need to restate statements or questions at intervals.
- The client may have memory loss; therefore, reintroduce yourself as often as necessary.
- Remember that nonverbal communication and touch are important; nonverbal communication may eventually become the primary communication mode between the client and the nurse or the client and the primary caregiver.
- Remember who the person was in the past, because reminiscence and validation are important; provide familiar stimuli.
- Be sure not to equate aphasia or flat affect with the absence of feelings; use empathy and interpretation of behaviors/statements to understand what is happening (for example, when a person who is at home says, "I want to go home"); support the person's feelings.
- Provide an environment of sheltered freedom, that is, the least restrictive level that is safe (unhurried, consistent, structured, with decreased external stimulation).
- Avoid mechanical or chemical restraints as much as possible.
- Avoid infantilizing the person, but remember that you may need to set firm limits.
- Be flexible, try different approaches, and share information.

MediaLink Care Plan: Coping with HIV Symptoms

Intervening in Spiritual Distress

Spiritual distress is usually evidenced by guilt, recriminations and self-blame, hyperreligiosity, rejection of significant others, and expressions of despair. Guidelines for working with clients experiencing spiritual distress include:

- Give the person permission to experience personal feelings, no matter what they are, and encourage appropriate expression of these feelings.
- Accept the fact that primary caregivers may not be able to listen to the client's feelings. If the primary caregiver delegates this job, recognize the distress it may cause both the client and the primary caregiver.
- Recognize the stages of grieving, and allow people to progress at their own rate; don't push the client into a stage that you think is necessary.
- Share spiritual resources as appropriate; encourage the person to find comforting spiritual outlets (poetry or other literature may be used to encourage reflection).

Having a spiritual connection was found to be a positive factor for long-term survivors. In a study designed to measure both spirituality and religiousness, Ironson et al. (2002) found that long-term survivors scored higher than an HIV-positive comparison group on four factors—sense of peace, faith in God, religious behavior, and compassionate view of others. Long-term survival was also correlated positively to frequency of prayer and negatively to judgmental attitude.

Enhancing Home Maintenance Management

The following list gives guidelines for enhancing care in the home and community:

- If the client is in an inpatient setting, begin planning for discharge as soon as the client is admitted to the facility.
- Assess the client's abilities to function in the home, the family's or primary caregiver's abilities to function in the home, and the housing or home environment itself.
- Make referrals to home care professionals and other community agencies.

- Help the primary caregiver determine the appropriate level of care and realistically assess his or her own ability to provide home care; explore all role responsibilities and related factors; assist in redefining and prioritizing roles and functions.
- Determine the primary caregiver's learning needs, and facilitate the development of skills by identifying specific symptoms (such as memory loss) and developing strategies to address those symptoms.
- Provide respite care for primary caregivers.
- Provide emotional support to clients and primary caregivers, and refer them to additional support systems.

You can also refer clients and their families to the United States Department of Health and Human Services guide for home care of persons with HIV at www.hivatis.org/caring/ (CDC, 2001), which is available through a resource link on the Companion Website for this book.

RISK REDUCTION EDUCATION AND COUNSELING

Taking a leading role in risk reduction education and counseling is a crucial responsibility of all nurses. Teaching risk reduction can best be accomplished by listening, informing, and supporting clients in making choices that reduce their risk. Risk reduction education is directed toward three broad goals:

1. Educating clients, the public, other professionals, colleagues, friends, and neighbors in strategies to reduce the risk of contracting or spreading HIV.
2. Counteracting the myths, stereotypes, and hysteria that surround HIV and AIDS.
3. Correcting misinformation.
4. Before implementing risk reduction and prevention programs for people at risk for contracting HIV, consult current CDC guidelines at www.cdc.gov, which is available through a resource link on the Companion Website for this book.

Sexual Behavior

Some experts fear that educating people about **safer sex practices** (sexual practices that avoid the risk of HIV infection by preventing the transmission of body fluids during sexual activity) generates a false sense of security. These experts say the only safe sex is no sex. Realistically, however, abstinence is not a lifelong change that will be maintained by many. Counseling about high-risk sexual behaviors, low-risk sexual behaviors, and risk-free sexual behaviors makes more sense, especially in terms of the principles outlined in the list above. High-risk sexual behaviors are those in which there is an exchange of blood or body fluids. Receptive anal intercourse is thought to be of highest risk because of the trauma caused to the mucous membranes of the rectum. Any sexual activities that involve tissue trauma or exchange of blood or body fluids that may transmit HIV are high risk. This includes sharing of sex toys; and wet kissing (French kissing), fellatio (oral–penile contact), and cunnilingus (oral–vaginal contact) when there are breaks in the mucous membrane of the mouth.

MediaLink HIV/AIDS Home Care

The use of condoms (a barrier protection placed on the penis to prevent the transmission of body fluids during sexual activity) is important in minimizing risk, but they must be used correctly in order to be effective. The Client/Family Teaching feature below will provide you with information to share with clients and their significant others.

Since HIV is most commonly transmitted through sex, being sexually active without taking proper precautions is definitely high-risk behavior. It is crucial to understand that a person does not simply go to bed with one other person. When one calculates the possible length of the HIV latency period, a person goes to bed with everyone in the other person's entire sex history for approximately the past 10 years. ■ Figure 24–4 on page 584 is a sobering illustration of one person's hypothetical sex history.

MediaLink CDC Guidelines: HIV

CLIENT / FAMILY TEACHING

Effective Condom Use

Remember to include the following information about condoms in any risk-reduction program. Remind clients to use a new condom for each act of vaginal, anal, or oral sex.

- Latex condoms are safer to use than natural or lambskin condoms. *HIV may be small enough to pass through the pores in natural condoms.*
- Condoms with reservoir tips are safer than those without. *A reservoir tip provides space for the semen and helps prevent breakage.*
- Do not open condom packages until use. Open packages carefully. *This helps to prevent damage from rough handling or jagged fingernails.*
- Store condoms in a dark, cool, dry place. *Excessive heat or cold, sunlight, and moisture can damage the latex. Therefore, a wallet is not a good place to store a condom.*
- Apply the condom before any genital contact. Use the condom throughout sex from start to finish. *Semen and seminal fluid may be discharged in advance of ejaculation.*
- Place the condom at the tip of the erect penis and gently press the air out of the condom tip. *Air bubbles can cause condoms to break.*
- Hold the condom at the tip, roll it down, and smooth it over the entire erect penis. Uncircumcised men should pull back the foreskin before applying the condom. *This provides a more effective seal.*
- Use a water-based product for lubrication. *Insufficient lubrication can cause condoms to tear or pull off. Oil-based lubricants such as petroleum jelly, baby oil, vegetable oil, mineral oil, cold cream, or hand lotion may cause the latex to disintegrate.*
- After ejaculating, but before losing the erection, the man should hold the base of the condom firmly while gently withdrawing the penis. *This prevents the escape of semen from the condom.*
- Safely discard, and never reuse a condom.

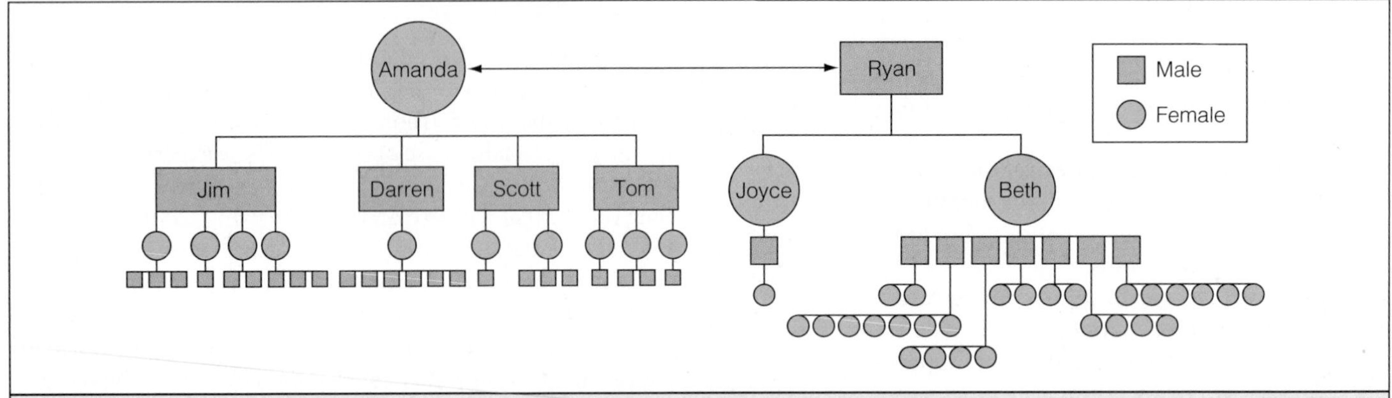

FIGURE 24–4 ■ *A Hypothetical Sex History. Amanda and Ryan think that they are only having sex with one another. However, they are hypothetically having sex with each others' sex partners for approximately the past 10 years (the HIV latency period). Imagine tracing the sex history of the last row of sex partners, represented by the dots. The explosive geometric progression could not be contained on one page.*

Substance Use

Prevention of risk to sex partners is important because IDUs serve as a bridge for transmitting HIV to their sex partners or to fetuses and newborns. The transmission of HIV and injection drug use is linked in the following ways:

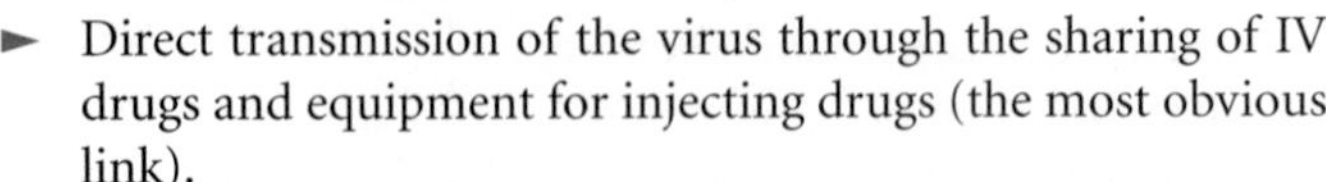

- Direct transmission of the virus through the sharing of IV drugs and equipment for injecting drugs (the most obvious link).
- Sexual transmission by infected IDUs to their sex partners.
- Neonatal transmission by infected women who are themselves IDUs or the sex partners of IDUs.

While these modes of transmission address injection drug users, there are other less well-known links to noninjection substance use and HIV. The use of poppers (volatile amyl and butyl nitrates in breakable glass capsules inhaled to enhance sexual pleasure) may be a cofactor in the susceptibility to HIV and in the development of AIDS because they are thought to lead to a generalized suppression of the immune system. Alcohol, as well as drugs such as amphetamines, cocaine, and marijuana, are also thought to damage the immune system. Another factor is lessened inhibition; that is, with loss of inhibition, a person under the influence of alcohol or drugs is more likely to engage in high-risk activities.

Harm Reduction. Realistic approaches to HIV risk-reduction education for IDUs consist of more than information about, and encouragement to obtain treatment for, substance abuse. According to the harm reduction approach, those who are not ready for treatment must be counseled on how to reduce the risk to themselves and to others. As a concept, harm reduction respects work on any positive change as a person defines it for himself or herself (Bigg, 2001) and focuses on minimizing the personal and social harms and costs associated with the spread of HIV through drug use. The major goal is to see to it that IDUs protect themselves against HIV (Hilton, Thompson, Moore-Dempsey, & Janzen, 2001) and other life-threatening diseases such as hepatitis C. Because harm reduction does not seek to eliminate drug use, it is considered controversial in several quarters.

Clients' risks to themselves derive from the practice of sharing drug use equipment with others. Teach clients to never share injectable drugs, needles, syringes, or other drug paraphernalia with others. As an HIV prevention strategy, increasing numbers of communities are providing needle and syringe exchange programs or writing laws to allow health care providers to prescribe needles and syringes, and pharmacists to dispense them. The best way of preventing transmission through injection drug use is for clients to use new, sterile needles and syringes, from a reliable source, each time they inject drugs. The ANA has supported needle and syringe exchange programs since 1993 (ANA, 1997).

If a new needle and syringe are not available, and the client will inject drugs anyway, the next best thing is for clients to clean their "works" (syringe and needle). Remind clients to clean needles immediately after use to reduce sterilization problems caused by clotted blood. Then, flush with bleach (held for 30 seconds) and then with water, three separate times. You should, however, inform clients that *cleaning used "works" with bleach is not reliable and should be used only when there is no safer alternative.*

Studies report that needle and syringe exchange programs have played a significant role in lowering the rates of needle sharing in the Netherlands, Australia, the United Kingdom, and the United States. Studies also report that needle and syringe exchange programs have served as sources of referrals into drug treatment programs. Additionally, needle and syringe exchange programs recapture used and potentially infectious syringes for safe disposal. The Using Research Evidence feature on page 585 provides an example of the nursing role in risk prevention and harm reduction.

A general counseling plan for clients with a dual diagnosis of HIV disease and substance use is given in the Intervention Box on page 585.

SUPPORT FOR CAREGIVERS

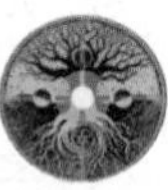

You can be a vital support link for the wide spectrum of people who are caregivers of persons with HIV disease.

USING RESEARCH EVIDENCE

Donald is a 35-year-old client on the inpatient unit in which you work. He is ready for discharge after his second admission for schizophrenia. Donald is also an IDU. He has injected drugs for 8 years and been in several substance abuse programs over this period of time. Each time, Donald has returned to using heroin.

During this admission, Donald consented to testing for the presence of HIV. The test came back positive. Donald is being treated with several medications to control the symptoms of his schizophrenia and to treat the HIV. In a conversation with Donald, you discover that he has been sharing needles with others. When you express concern, Donald tells you not to worry; he rinses his syringes and needles with water when he uses them, and sometimes with bleach.

You immediately institute risk prevention and harm reduction teaching. You tell Donald that HIV is often transmitted through shared injection equipment, that cleansing with water will not wash away HIV, and that bleach is not a safe alternative. Using sterile, never-used needles and syringes is the best answer. You plan to meet with Donald later in the afternoon after you've had an opportunity to investigate needle and syringe exchange programs in your community and the availability of physician prescription and/or pharmacist dispensing programs for IDUs. You will also contact the mental health outreach team that services Donald's neighborhood and the buddy program of AIDS Family Services to link Donald with a support group and a medication maintenance program.

These suggestions stem from the following research:

Contoreggi, C., Jones, S., Simpson, P., Lange, W. R., & Meyer III, W. A. (2000). Effects of varying concentrations of bleach on in vitro HIV-1 replication and the relevance to injection drug use. *Intervirology, 43*(1), 1–5; and Hilton, B. A., Thompson, R., Moore-Dempsey, L., & Janzen, R. G. (2001). Harm reduction theories and strategies for control of human immunodeficiency virus: A review of the literature. *Journal of Advanced Nursing, 33*(3), 357–370.

This spectrum includes nurses and other health care professionals; the family members, friends, and same sex partners of people with HIV; firefighters, police officers, and correction officers; and community volunteers. Nurses are now and will continue to be the health care professionals who are the front-line workers in providing health care to increasing numbers of people with HIV/AIDS.

Caring for people with HIV requires participation as a client advocate, effective multidisciplinary collaboration, and the ability to make appropriate referrals. To address the needs of this group adequately, one needs the ability to empathize with the individual with HIV and with primary caregivers and to act on the basis of that empathy. A primary caregiver is a person who is generally responsible for providing or coordinating daily care for a PWA who cannot perform self-care activities. Usually, a primary caregiver is a nonprofessional who is a significant other (life partner, spouse, family member, or close friend) of the person with AIDS.

Special emotional stamina is needed to care for PWAs. Not only must nurses and other caregivers care for and comfort those who face great suffering and death, they also care for and comfort those infected with the virus who have not developed the disease. At the same time they provide help, nurses must cope with their fears for their own and their family's health (especially if the nurses themselves are members of a risk group) and their own pain in caring for people who do not get well or whose future is uncertain.

Specifically, our skills and knowledge make us able to:

- Facilitate caregivers' expression of fears and concerns.
- Help caregivers acknowledge their susceptibility to increased stress and burnout in AIDS work.
- Instruct caregivers in complementary and alternative therapies (see Chapter 32).
- Identify what needs to be reorganized and renegotiated in the work environment to maintain the health of caregivers and clients such as: staff support groups, networking with AIDS providers in other agencies and communities, respite time for staff, time off to attend funerals or memorial services, rearranging staff assignments to avoid overloading or overburdening particular staff members, or creating get-away space for staff in the work setting.
- Provide help to caregivers unaccustomed to dealing with delirium and dementia, who may have unrealistic expectations about the client's ability to adhere to procedures and treatment as mental capacities diminish (see Chapter 12).

INTERVENTION

Counseling Plan for Clients with a Dual Diagnosis of HIV and Substance Use

In addition to the general counseling and risk-prevention teaching for anyone with HIV, incorporate the following steps into an intervention plan for a substance-using client with HIV.

- Confront denial or lack of commitment to minimize risk behavior.
- Check the need for, and the depth of, motivation for referral to chemical dependence or alcohol treatment programs.
- Encourage joining or continuing a commitment to the recovery process in treatment for chemical dependence or alcoholism.
- Help the client verbalize feelings of anger, grief, and loss generated by the diagnosis; the need for change in sexual and drug use behavior; possible delay in childbearing; or the fear of having exposed others to HIV or doing so through continued risk behavior.
- Stress the need to use tools learned in recovery from chemical dependence and alcoholism in coping with this life crisis.
- Continue to confront the drug abuse as you would with clients not diagnosed with HIV.
- Involve the client in a harm reduction program.

BEREAVEMENT SUPPORT

Millions of people will experience AIDS-related bereavements. There are several groups of people to whom the psychiatric–mental health nurse can provide bereavement support. The most obvious is the person with AIDS who grieves over a potentially fatal diagnosis, the loss of other friends or family to the disease, or any of the several other losses discussed in the section on the biopsychosocial impact of HIV/AIDS. In particular, clients who have sustained multiple and repetitive losses are at risk for depression (Sikkema et al., 2000). The bereavement coping challenges they face can be especially difficult and pronounced.

Bereavement support to family, friends, same sex partners, and caregivers should continue after death has occurred. Home visits to friends, lovers, and family members demonstrate your continuing interest and concern for the survivor's well-being.

CLINICAL EXAMPLE

When his client Antoine died of complications of AIDS, Jim, his nurse, made a home visit to Antoine's family. Jim helped Antoine's wife, children, mother, and three brothers plan remembrance rituals for a memorial service for Antoine.

Bereavement support groups and individual and family counseling can all be helpful, depending on individual situations and the availability of volunteers and professionals.

To provide adequate bereavement support to the survivors of people with AIDS (SOPWAs), it is important to consider a number of factors. SOPWAs represent a diverse segment of society:

1. Sex partners of PWAs
2. Children of PWAs
3. Parents and siblings of PWAs
4. Friends of PWAs
5. Health care providers of PWAs

Some SOPWAs may be in high-risk groups or may have HIV disease themselves, while some may have been unaware of the significant other's sexuality or lifestyle until diagnosis or death. Some survivors may have been responsible for the transmission of HIV, and many are members of minority groups and have few resources.

SOPWAs are often characterized by several factors that place them at high risk for complicated grief reaction. These factors are identified in the Assessment box below. It is important to assess survivors for the presence of these factors, which can interfere with adaptive grieving. The potential for dysfunctional grieving exists because multiple high-risk bereavement factors are characteristic of SOPWAs. Individual or group bereavement interventions can help survivors engage in the grief process in an adaptive fashion.

SELF-HELP

Self-help is one way in which persons with HIV disease can move to reestablish a sense of self-control and reduce feelings of helplessness and powerlessness. Self-help can occur on several levels, depending on the client's physical and mental abilities and motivation. Clients should participate as much as possible in their own care and in decision making that affects them. Encourage clients to join peer support groups and engage in HIV/AIDS advocacy activities in their communities. Some of the many resources available to you and your clients include:

ASSESSMENT High-Risk Bereavement Factors for SOPWAs

Stigma

Sources

- Discomfort with illness, death, and grief.
- Sexuality and drug use often associated with HIV/AIDS.
- Confusion and hysteria associated with HIV/AIDS.

Results for SOPWAs

- May need to mask the cause of death to self and others.
- Community may not recognize the significance of the loss.
- Support from others in mourning the loss or expressing feelings associated with bereavement may be absent.

Ambivalence

Sources

- Strained relationship with PWA

Results for SOPWAs

- May feel guilt.
- Progress in the grief process may be blocked.

Untimely Nature of Death

Sources

- Facing issues of mortality.
- Generally young age of PWAs.

Results for SOPWAs

- Anxiety, despair
- Unprepared to accept the death.

Concurrent Life Crises

Sources

- Fear of the possibility of having been exposed to a fatal illness.
- Guilt if the survivor feels he or she may have transmitted HIV.
- Experiencing the deaths of many other PWAs.

Results for SOPWAs

- Anger associated with being a SOPWA.
- Helplessness associated with being a SOPWA.
- Reoccurring need to grieve for many other PWAs.

- For general information on prevention, see: www.cdcnpin.org (CDC National Prevention Information Network)
- For general information and lists of AIDS organizations and support groups, see: www.aegis.com (AIDS Education Global Information System)
- For general information on treatment and clinical trials see: www.amfar.org (American Foundation for AIDS Research; amfAR)
- For information on research on AIDS and mental health, see: www.nih.gov/oa/ (NIH Center for Mental Health Research on AIDS)

Direct links to all of these resources can be found on the Companion Web site for this book.

Clients may benefit from such activities as nutritional counseling and psychological counseling. Boosting the immune system also helps keep people healthy. Stress-management techniques and visualization and imagery for self-healing and pain and symptom control (such as those discussed in Chapter 32) are believed to boost the immune system by reducing stress.

RESEARCH

Psychiatric–mental health nurses have a direct role in research and an indirect role in supporting ongoing research and encouraging the undertaking and funding of new research. Being knowledgeable about the current research and incorporating it into clinical practice enables the psychiatric–mental health nurse to act on the basis of what is currently known or supposed. For example, there is a growing body of knowledge about quality of life and how it affects the physical, psychological, and social well-being of people affected by HIV.

ADVOCACY AND POLITICAL ACTIVISM

Persons with HIV disease and their loved ones need advocates. Psychiatric–mental health nurses can be effective advocates by speaking out against dehumanizing measures that threaten well-being.

CLINICAL EXAMPLE

A proposition was introduced in California that could have forced public health officials to establish camps to quarantine people with AIDS, as well as anyone infected by HIV, whether healthy or unhealthy. This measure would also have flatly banned HIV-seropositive people from attending or teaching in public schools or holding jobs that involve food handling. The California Nurses Association was among the groups that actively spoke against the proposition and contributed to its failure.

As a citizen and an advocate, you need to be politically aware of pending legislation and move to influence it in a positive direction.

Earlier in this chapter, brief mention was made of nurses' associations with published statements about the care of people with AIDS and the role of nurses. National specialty groups such as the Association for Nurses in AIDS Care (ANAC) are also active in mobilizing the professional and political resources of the nursing community in the United States. You can reach ANAC at www.anacnet.org. Canadian nurses can contact the Canadian Association of Nurses in AIDS Care (CANAC) at www.canac.org. Nurses in Australia and New Zealand have the Australia/New Zealand Association of Nurses in AIDS Care at http://home.vicnet.net.au/anzanac. These resources can also be found on the Companion Website for this book.

It is every nurse's responsibility to find out what nursing groups are accomplishing or not accomplishing on local, state, and national levels. Beginning at the local level by becoming involved in community AIDS councils, self-help groups, and nursing organizations is a good way to start. Local involvement is a bridge to state and national involvement. You can also be part of a nationwide effort to lobby for adequate public and private funding for research, education, prevention, treatment, a vaccine, and a cure for HIV/AIDS.

MediaLink Self-Help for HIV/AIDS

MediaLink HIV/AIDS Nursing Organizations

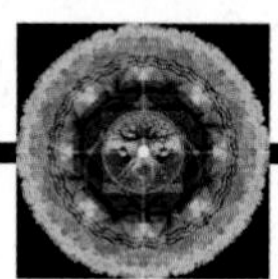

EXPLORE MediaLink

NCLEX review, case studies, and other interactive resources for this chapter can be found on the Companion Website at http://www.prenhall.com/kneisl. Click on Chapter 24 to select the activities for this chapter.

For animations, video tutorials, more NCLEX review questions, and an audio glossary, access the accompanying CD-ROM in this textbook.

BIBLIOGRAPHY

American Nurses Association. (2001). *Code of ethics for nurses*. Washington, DC: Author.

American Nurses Association. (1997). *Position statement: Needle exchange and HIV*. Washington, DC: Author.

Bigg, D. (2001). Substance use management: A harm reduction-principled approach to assisting the relief of drug-related problems. *Journal of Psychoactive Drugs 33*(1), 33–38.

Brown, E. J., & Jemmott, L. S. (2000). HIV among people with mental illness: Contributing factors, prevention needs, barriers, and strategies. *Journal of Psychosocial Nursing, 38*(4), 14–19.

Brown, E. J., Outlaw, F. H., Simpson, E. M. (2000). Theoretical antecedents to HIV risk perception. *Journal of American Psychiatric Nurses Association, 6*(6), 177–182.

Burnam, M. A., Bing, E. G., Morton, S. C., Sherbourne, C., Fleishman, J. A., London, A. S., et al. (2001). Use of mental health and substance abuse treatment services among adults with HIV in the United States. *Archives of General Psychiatry, 58*(8), 729–736.

Centers for Disease Control and Prevention. (2001). *Bright ideas 2002: Innovative or promising practices in HIV prevention and HIV community planning* (2nd ed.). Washington, DC: Author.

Centers for Disease Control and Prevention. (2002a). *Drug-associated HIV transmission continues in the United States*. Retrieved April 2, 2002, from the World Wide Web, www.cdc.gov/hiv/pubs/facts/idu.htm.

Centers for Disease Control and Prevention. (2002b). *HIV/AIDS surveillance report, 13*(1).

Contoreggi, C., Jones, S., Simpson, P., Lange, W. R., & Meyer IIII, W. A. (2000). Effects of varying concentrations of bleach on in vitro HIV-1 replication and the relevance to injection drug use. *Intervirology, 43*(1), 1–5.

Davidson, S., Judd, F., Jolley, D., Hocking, B., Thompson, S., & Hyland, B. (2001). Risk factors for HIV/AIDS and hepatitis C among the chronic mentally ill. *Australian and New Zealand Journal of Psychiatry, 35*(2), 203–209.

Herning, R. I., Better, W. E., Tate, K., & Cadet, J. L. (2001). Antiviral medications improve cerebrovascular perfusion in HIV+ non-drug users and HIV+ cocaine abusers. *Annals of the New York Academy of Science, 939*, 405–412.

Hilton, B. A., Thompson, R., Moore-Dempsey, L., & Hutchinson, K. (2001). Urban outpost nursing: The nature of the nurse's work in the AIDS prevention street nurse program. *Public Health Nursing, 18*(4), 273–280.

Hilton, B. A., Thompson, R., Moore-Dempsey, L., & Janzen, R. G. (2001). Harm reduction theories and strategies for control of human immunodeficiency virus: A review of the literature. *Journal of Advanced Nursing, 33*(3), 357–370.

Holzemer, W. L. (2002). HIV and AIDS: The symptom experience. *American Journal of Nursing, 102*(4), 48–52.

Ironson, G., Solomon, G. F., Balbin, E. G., O'Cleirigh, C., George, A., Kumar, M., et al. (2002). The Ironson-Woods spirituality/religiousness index is associated with long survival, health behaviors, less distress, and low cortisol in people with HIV/AIDS. *Annals of Behavioral Medicine, 24*(1), 34–48.

Joint United Nations Programme on AIDS. (2001). *AIDS epidemic update: December 2001*. Geneva, Switzerland: United Nations.

Knox, M. D., Davis, M., & Friedrich, M. A. (1994). The HIV mental health spectrum. *Community Mental Health Journal, 30*(1), 75–89.

Lyon, D. (2001). Human immunodeficiency virus (HIV) disease in persons with severe mental illness. *Issues in Mental Health Nursing, 22*(1), 109–119.

Morrison, M. F., Petitto, J. M., Ten Have, T., Gettes, D. R., Chiappini, M. S., Weber, A. L., et al. (2002). Depressive and anxiety disorders in women with HIV Infection. *American Journal of Psychiatry, 159*(5), 789–796.

Moser, K. M., Sowell, R. L., Phillips, K. D. (2001). Issues of women dually diagnosed with HIV infection and substance use problems in the Carolinas. *Issues in Mental Health Nursing, 22*(1), 23–49.

National Coalition for the Homeless. (2002). *HIV/AIDS and homelessness*. Washington, DC: Author.

National Intelligence Council. (2002). *The next wave of HIV/AIDS: Nigeria, Ethiopia, Russia, India and China*. Washington, DC: Author.

National Resource Center on Homelessness and Mental Illness. (2002). *How many people are homeless? Why?* Delmar, NY: Author.

Sherbourne, C., Haus, R. D., Fleishman, J. A., Vitiello, B., Magruder, K. M., Bing, E. G., et al. (2000). Impact of psychiatric conditions on health-related quality of life in persons with HIV infection. *American Journal of Psychiatry, 157*, 248.

Sherman, D. S., & Ouellette, S. (1999). Moving beyond fear: Lessons learned through a longitudinal review of the literature regarding health care providers and the care of people with HIV/AIDS. *Nursing Clinics of North America, 34*(1), 1–48.

Sikkema, K. J., Kalichman, S. C., Hoffmann, R., Koob, J. J., Kelly, J. A., & Heckman, T. G. (2000). Coping strategies and emotional wellbeing among HIV-infected men and women experiencing AIDS-related bereavement. *AIDS Care, 12*(5), 613–624.

Stein, M. D., Anderson, B., Charuvastra, A., Maksad, J., & Friedmann, P. D. (2002). A brief intervention for hazardous drinkers in a needle exchange program. *Journal of Substance Abuse Treatment, 22*(1), 23–31.

Standish, L. J., Calabrese, C., & Galantino, M. L. (2001). *AIDS and complementary and alternative medicine: Current science and practice*. London: Churchill Livingstone.

Stoskopf, C. H., Kim, Y. K., & Glover, S. H. (2001). Dual diagnosis: HIV and mental illness, a population-based study. *Community Mental Health Journal, 37*(6), 469–479.

Surlis, S., & Hyde, A. (2001). HIV-positive patients' experiences of stigma during hospitalization. *Journal of the Association of Nurses in AIDS Care, 12*(6), 68–77.

Triesman, G. J., Angelino, A. F., & Hutton, H. E. (2001). Psychiatric issues in the management of patients with HIV infection. *Journal of the American Medical Association, 286*(22), 2857–2864.

Ungvarski, P. J., & Trzcianowska, H. (2000). Neurocognitive disorders seen in HIV disease. *Issues in Mental Health Nursing, 21*(1), 51–70.

United States Department of Health and Human Services (2002). *Caring for someone with AIDS at home: A guide*. Retrieved June 25, 2002, from the World Wide Web, www.hivatis.org/caring/.

Webber, D. W. (2000). HIV/AIDS legal issues in the United States. *Canadian HIV AIDS Policy Law Review, 5*(4), 38–41.

Whetten-Goldstein, K., Nguyen, T. Q., & Sugarman, J. (2001). So much for keeping secrets: The importance of considering patients' perspectives on maintaining confidentiality. *AIDS Care, 13*(4), 457–465.

Zinkernagel, C., Taffe, P., Rickenback, M., Amiet, R., Ledergerber, B., Volkart, A.C., et al. (2001). Importance of mental health assessment in HIV-infected outpatients. *Journal of Acquired Immune Deficiency Syndrome, 28*(3), 240–249.

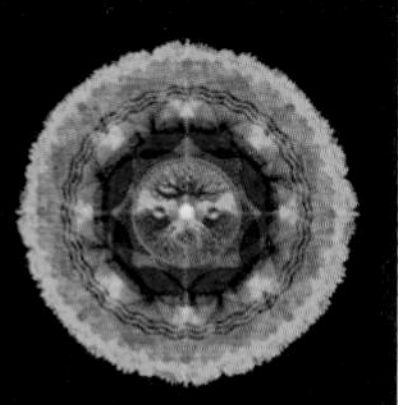

25

Chapter TWENTY-FIVE

Children

SANDRA WEISS

FOCUS QUESTIONS

- What are the similarities and differences between generalist and specialist roles in child psychiatric nursing?
- What are the key ideas in the major theories underlying the development of childhood psychiatric disorders?
- What symptoms are associated with each of the common psychiatric disorders of children?
- How would you conduct an assessment of a child with a mental health problem?
- What various approaches are available to child psychiatric–mental health nurses when diagnosing and treating children?
- How might your own attitudes toward children affect therapeutic outcomes of your work with them?

KEY TERMS

attention deficit hyperactivity disorder (ADHD)
autistic disorder
conduct disorder (CD)
developmental disorders
disruptive behavior disorders
elimination disorders
feeding and eating disorders
mental retardation
oppositional defiant disorder (ODD)
reactive attachment disorder
selective mutism
separation anxiety disorder
tic disorders
Tourette's disorder

MediaLink 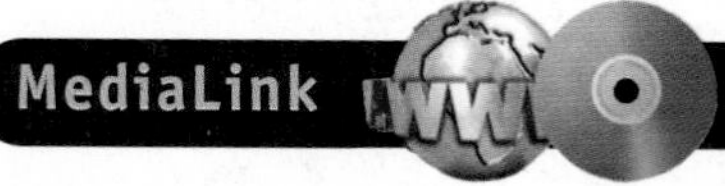 www.prenhall.com/kneisl

Additional resources for this chapter can be found on the Student CD-ROM accompanying this textbook, and on the Companion Website at www.prenhall.com/kneisl. Click on Chapter 25 to select the activities for this chapter.

CD-ROM
- Audio Glossary
- NCLEX Review

Companion Website
- Additional NCLEX Review
- Care Plan: Conduct Disorder
- Case Study: Child with ADHD
- Learning from Clients: Autism Video

CROSS REFERENCES

Other topics relevant to this content are: ANA Standards of Psychiatric–Mental Health Nursing, Chapter 1; Developmental theories, Chapter 2; Drug abuse, Chapter 13; Depression, Chapter 15; Eating disorders, Chapter 18; Family assessment and therapy, Chapter 29; Intrafamily physical and sexual abuse of children, Chapter 23; Suicide, Chapter 22.

CHAPTER OUTLINE

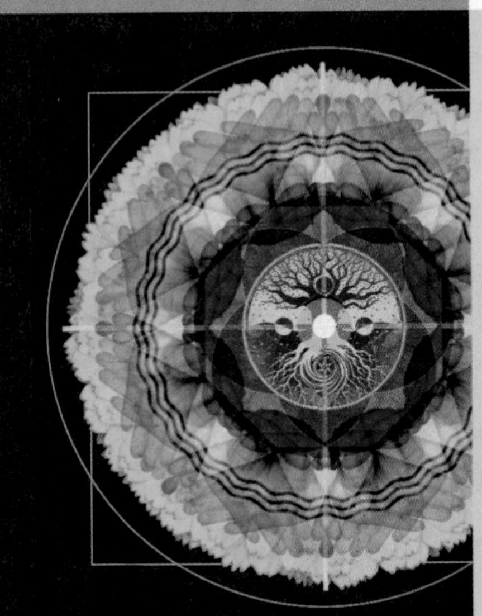

CRITICAL THINKING CHALLENGE

You are checking the charts of the children who will be your clients on the shift you have just begun. A nurse who is finishing her shift says to you as she is leaving: "So you'll be working with Kevin tonight, the little red haired guy with autism. I warn you . . . his mother is a real pain. . . . She is constantly asking questions and telling the staff what to do. I don't think they should even let her visit. If you ask me, she is the reason for all of the kid's problems."

What are your feelings about the nurse's comments regarding Kevin's mother? How might her attitude influence the care that Kevin and his family receive? How would you respond to the nurse and why? What do you know about autistic disorder and its causes? ■

There are more children in need of psychiatric care than ever before. About 1 in 10 children in the United States suffers from mental illness (National Institute of Mental Health [NIMH], 2000) but fewer than one in five of these children receive treatment. Available resources for prevention and treatment of mental illness are minimal and the number of mental health professionals prepared to work with children has dwindled.

The Office of the U.S. Surgeon General recently produced a report indicating that the unmet mental health needs of children and their families is a public health crisis (Department of Health and Human Services [DHHS], 2001). The report calls for a national action agenda to promote mental health in children and treat more effectively their mental disorders. Among the many important goals in this national agenda are plans to:

- Improve assessment and recognition of children's mental health needs.
- Eliminate racial/ethnic and socioeconomic disparities in access to care.
- Educate mental health providers as well as front-line, primary care providers to better recognize and manage children's mental health issues.

Nurses are in a key position to advance these goals. Growing recognition of the psychobiologic underpinnings of mental illness has resulted in a greater interest in using nurses for a variety of roles that demand knowledge of both mental and physical health. For example, nurses in child psychiatry must assess psychologic and physical symptoms, explain laboratory tests to children, administer medications that require strict and systematic monitoring, and work with children having a dual medical and psychiatric diagnosis (such as diabetes and conduct disorder). Child psychiatric–mental health nurses have the knowledge to perform these diverse clinical functions at a reasonable cost to society.

As a specialty, child psychiatric–mental health nursing had its inception in the early 1950s, when graduate programs opened and training funds became available through the National Institute of Mental Health (NIMH). The early child mental health teams did not include the nurse. In some residential programs, the majority of milieu staff were from other disciplines, and only one nurse was included for each shift, primarily to attend to the physical needs of the children and administer medications. As the community mental health movement developed, programs specifically for children began to offer appropriate roles for the child psychiatric–mental health nurse, including treatment, consultation, education, and medication supervision. Today, advanced practice nurses are often the primary caregivers for children with mental health problems, providing direct counseling, working with the family, and managing the child's medications. This comprehensive role is especially common in rural or inner city areas. Child psychiatric–mental health nurses also are the mainstay of hospital treatment programs where they are responsible for daily treatment plans, ongoing one-on-one or group counseling, and management of the child's medication regime. A growing role for child psychiatric–mental health nurses involves promotion of infant mental health in high-risk families where the infants have medical complications or the parents have a history of mental illness or substance abuse. They also function as liaisons to pediatric inpatient and outpatient settings, providing psychiatric consultation to the pediatric staff. In most cases, the nurse functions as part of an interdisciplinary team, along with child psychiatrists, social workers, psychologists, occupational therapists, recreational therapists, special educators, pediatricians, and child care workers. For more information, refer to the Association of Child and Adolescent Psychiatric Nurses at www.ispn-psych.org. Other specialists are used for consultations as indicated, particularly child neurologists, speech and language specialists, child abuse teams, clergy, and physical therapists.

A number of mental health problems typically appear in childhood, although they may continue into adulthood, or lead to other psychiatric disorders in later life. Each type of disorder has a particular constellation of symptoms or descriptive features that sets it apart from others. Remember that the disorders described in this chapter are not the only ones found in childhood.

MediaLink Specialty Certification

Developmental Disorders

All **developmental disorders** involve a lack of expected development or a regression after normal development. These impairments are sometimes in single areas or can involve a spectrum of deficits.

MENTAL RETARDATION

The major feature of **mental retardation** is significantly subaverage intellectual functioning (an IQ below 70 in children, or, in infants, clinical judgment based on cognitive tests). The degree of severity of intellectual impairment is described as mild (IQ 50/55–70), moderate (IQ 35/40–50/55), severe (IQ 20/25–35/40), or profound (IQ below 20/25). The child must also show deficits or impairments in adaptive functioning in at least two areas of life; for example, communication, social/interpersonal skills, or safety. The onset of this disorder occurs before the age of 18.

Mental retardation is found in approximately 1% of the population. The major risk factor for retardation is the early alteration of embryonic development as a result of exposure to toxins in utero (maternal drug use, for example) or chromosomal changes (such as Down syndrome). Other predisposing factors include inherited errors of metabolism (such as fragile X syndrome), pregnancy and perinatal problems such as prematurity or trauma, medical conditions acquired in infancy or childhood, and early environmental influences such as deprivation of nurturance or other stimulation.

SPECIFIC DEVELOPMENTAL DISORDERS

Three categories of developmental disorders involve specific cognitive impairments that are presumed to result from dysfunctions in the cortex of the brain: learning disorders, motor skills disorder, and communication disorders. These dysfunctions have been associated with genetic vulnerabilities, organic damage, and delayed maturation. Children from disadvantaged socioeconomic circumstances tend to receive these diagnoses more frequently, particularly boys.

Learning Disorders

A learning disorder may be diagnosed when a child's achievement on standardized tests in reading, mathematics, or written expression is substantially below what is expected for his or her age, schooling, or intelligence level. The problems are so major as to significantly interfere with the child's activities of daily living or academic progress.

Learning disorders affect 2–10% of the population, with about 5% of all public school students identified as having a learning disorder. Reading is the major learning problem.

Motor Skills Disorder

A motor skills disorder, marked impairment in the development of motor coordination, occurs in approximately 6% of all children. You may first notice this problem in a child's delay in achieving motor milestones such as walking or crawling, in "clumsiness," and in poor handwriting or sports performance. To be considered a psychiatric disorder, the impairment must significantly interfere with the child's academic achievement or activities of daily living and not be the result of a physical health problem such as cerebral palsy.

Communication Disorders

Communication disorders can be one of four different problems: impairments in language expression, in the understanding of language, in phonology, or stuttering. These impairments must be severe enough to interfere with academic achievement or social communication. Problems in language expression may include a markedly limited vocabulary, errors in tense, or difficulty recalling words or producing sentences with developmentally appropriate length or complexity. Problems in understanding language include difficulty understanding words, sentences, or specific types of words. The symptom of a phonological disorder is the failure to use developmentally expected speech sounds appropriate for a child's age and dialect. For example, the child may substitute one sound for another ("t" for "k") or omit sounds in words. Stuttering is a disturbance in the normal timing and fluency of speech; for instance, frequent repetitions, prolonged sounds, or pauses in the middle of a word. Word substitution is often used by a child to avoid problematic words.

While stuttering occurs in about 1% of prepubertal children, the prevalence of the other communication disorders is somewhat greater: about 3% to 5% of all children. However, under the age of 3, language delays occur in 10% to 15% of all children. Remember to evaluate any communication problems within the cultural and language context of a child, especially if the child is bilingual. The only known predisposing factor for the development of a communication disorder is a family history of the disorder. For stuttering, especially, family and twin studies provide strong evidence of a genetic factor in its etiology.

PERVASIVE DEVELOPMENTAL DISORDERS

The pervasive developmental disorders include autistic disorder, Rett's disorder, childhood disintegrative disorder, and Asperger's disorder. Each of these psychiatric conditions usually arises in the first years of life and is characterized by severe developmental impairment in several areas.

Autistic, disintegrative, and Asperger's disorders are much more common in boys, with autism having rates four to five times higher for boys. Rett's disorder has been found only to occur in girls. The reasons for these gender differences are not yet understood.

All of these disorders are rare, with autistic disorder having the highest incidence. It occurs in 2–5 children per 10,000. Regardless of the small percentage of children affected by pervasive developmental disorders, their impact on children and families is enormous. They also represent a substantial segment of the families to whom child psychiatric–mental health nurses provide care, because the problems these families encounter are severe and require much professional support (see The Rx Communication feature below).

Autistic Disorder

Sometimes referred to as autism, **autistic disorder** involves difficulties in both the quality of a child's social interaction and

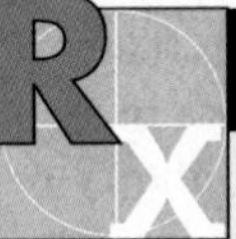

COMMUNICATION

The Parent of a Child with Autism

PARENT: I've had it. I just can't take this anymore. Kaetlin screams and flaps her arms every time I touch her. I can't even give her a bath without a huge scene. It's exhausting.

NURSE RESPONSE 1: I hear how frustrated and exhausted you are. Let's talk about *your* needs for a bit and figure out ways to get you some support and relief.

RATIONALE: This response shows the parent that the nurse empathizes with the parent's situation. It also provides an opportunity (a) for the parent to discuss her feelings in more detail, and (b) for the nurse to make concrete suggestions for decreasing the burden the parent is experiencing.

NURSE RESPONSE 2: Yes, it can be very exhausting. Other families I work with have these same experiences. Let's talk about some approaches that you might use to help Kaetlin handle her bath and other types of contact without getting so upset.

RATIONALE: First, this response provides comfort to the parent that the problem is not unique to her family but is shared by others. The nurse then offers her the opportunity to learn some specific strategies to better manage the child's behavior.

communication. In social interaction, the child may have problems making eye contact, fail to develop appropriate peer relationships, fail to spontaneously seek out shared enjoyment with other people, or show no social or emotional reciprocity. In communication, the child may have a delay in developing language or a total absence of speech; use language in a stereotyped, repetitive, or idiosyncratic fashion; show deficits in spontaneous, imaginative play; or have a restricted, repetitive repertoire of interests or behaviors (as in folding a facial tissue repeatedly or flapping his or her hands up and down).

There is also a diagnosis of mental retardation in about 75% of children with autism, usually in the moderate range. Autism appears prior to age 3. Parents may tell you that their baby does not want to cuddle, has an indifference to touch and affection, does not make eye contact, or is not facially responsive. Children may also have many associated behavioral problems such as hyperactivity, aggressiveness, self-injurious behaviors like head banging, temper tantrums, and unusual sensitivities to sensory stimuli (such as an oversensitivity to touch or a high threshold for pain). You may notice abnormal mood or affect as well; for example, a child may overreact or not react at all to the environment.

Rett's Disorder

Rett's disorder is the accumulation of multiple developmental deficits by a child after there has been a period of normal development during the first 5 months of life. Within the first or second year of life, the baby begins to show deceleration in head growth, loss of previously acquired hand skills and eventual stereotyped hand movements, loss of social engagement, poorly coordinated gait or trunk movements, and severely impaired language development with psychomotor retardation. The disorder is lifelong, with persistent and progressive loss of skills. Only modest developmental gains have been noted in a few children later in their childhood or adolescence.

Childhood Disintegrative Disorder

Childhood disintegrative disorder (CDD) is quite similar to Rett's disorder except that its period of normal development is much longer, with symptoms not appearing until ages 2 through 10. In addition, there is no head growth deceleration or loss of hand skills. Instead, the losses involve skills in expressive or receptive language, social skills, play, and bowel or bladder control. Some of the abnormalities of functioning that develop are similar to those in autistic disorder, such as impairments in social interaction, communication, and repetitive, restricted, stereotyped behavior. However, in autistic disorder, the abnormalities are usually noticed within the first year of life and do not reflect the pattern of developmental regression found in CDD.

Asperger's Disorder

Asperger's disorder has some but not all of the features of autism. Children with this disorder show the same problems with social interaction and restricted, repetitive behavior as in autism. However, there is no delay in language, in cognitive development, in age appropriate self-help and adaptive skills, or in curiosity about the environment. The onset of the disorder is also later than autism, most commonly in the preschool period. In contrast to CDD, there is no loss of previously acquired skills in Asperger's disorder.

MediaLink Learning from Clients: Autism Video

Attention Deficit and Disruptive Behavior Disorders

This category of child psychiatric problems includes attention deficit hyperactivity disorder and two **disruptive behavior disorders** (a group of mental illnesses including conduct disorder, oppositional defiant disorder and other related behavior problems that cause significant impairment in social, academic or occupational functioning): conduct disorder and oppositional defiant disorder. The symptoms common to all of these disorders involve behavior that is externally manifested or directed, often called *externalizing disorders.*

ATTENTION DEFICIT HYPERACTIVITY DISORDER

The most distinctive features of **attention deficit hyperactivity disorder (ADHD)** are the child's inattention to the surrounding environment, and hyperactivity and/or impulsiveness. Both of these symptoms must persist for at least 6 months, be apparent in two or more settings, be inconsistent with the child's developmental level, and cause clinically significant impairment in functioning. In addition, some of these symptoms must have been present prior to age 7. To determine whether inattention exists, look for behaviors such as making careless mistakes in schoolwork, not listening when spoken to, disliking tasks that require sustained mental effort, and being easily distracted. You will see hyperactivity in fidgeting or squirming, running around when the child is asked to stay seated, or talking excessively. Signs of impulsiveness are a child's difficulty waiting for his or her turn in activities, or interrupting others. Most children with this disorder have a combination of symptoms indicating both inattention and hyperactivity–impulsiveness, but some children have predominantly one or the other.

MediaLink Case Study: Child with ADHD

ADHD is most commonly diagnosed in early school years, when demands for sustained attention increase. By late childhood and adolescence, excesses in gross motor activity become less apparent, and symptoms may reflect primarily fidgetiness or even inner feelings of restlessness without any observable signs. A clinical example that includes ADHD is in the next section on conduct disorder.

Controversy has grown during the last 10 years about the number of children being diagnosed with ADHD. Community surveys have found the disorder in 17% of boys and 8% of girls of elementary school age. Girls are more likely to have symptoms only of inattention. Children with the disorder represent 40% to 70% of child psychiatric inpatients and 30% to 50% of child psychiatric outpatients (Dulcan & Martini, 1999). In light of these numbers, concerns have developed regarding possible overdiagnosis and overtreatment of ADHD. Some mental health professionals question whether the growing trend toward assessment and management of the disorder by pediatricians and internists is a problem because they may not be as skilled in differential diagnosis or treatment of psychiatric disorders. Another concern relates to the pressures by school personnel to control children's behavior, pressures that may influence parents and/or family practitioners to prescribe medication for ADHD when psychosocial management of the behavioral problems would be better. In response to these public and professional concerns, the American Medical Association commissioned a study which found that, in most instances, ADHD diagnosis and treatment seemed to be appropriate. Their analysis noted that ADHD has one of the strongest foundations of research of any problem confronted by medicine, including evidence that stimulants are a highly effective treatment, with typically mild and short-lived side effects (Goldman, Genel, Bezman, & Slanetz, 1998).

CONDUCT DISORDER

MediaLink Care Plan: Conduct Disorder

Conduct disorder (CD) is also one of the most frequently diagnosed problems for children. Boys show an incidence 3 to 5 times greater than girls. Its prevalence is up to 10% in inner city, urban areas (DHHS, 2001). The central feature of CD is repetitive and persistent behavior in which the basic rights of others or major age-appropriate societal norms or rules are violated. Look for behaviors that show aggression toward people and animals, destruction of property, deceitfulness or theft, or serious violation of parental or school rules. These symptoms may appear as early as 5–6 years of age, but occur more typically in later childhood or early adolescence. There are two subtypes of this disorder: childhood onset and adolescent onset. Childhood onset must show at least one symptom prior to 10 years of age. In the majority of cases, the disorder remits by adulthood, but those individuals with childhood onset are more likely to develop adult antisocial personality disorder (APD; see Chapter 20) than are those with onset in adolescence. The diagnosis of CD is made only when the behavior is symptomatic of a problem within the child and not a reaction to a social context of war, poverty, high crime, or fear for one's well-being.

Boys with the disorder are more likely to fight, steal, vandalize, or have school problems, whereas girls are more likely to run away, be truant, use drugs or become involved in prostitution. Girls usually do not show confrontational behavior, although we are seeing more of this over the last few years. While almost all cases of CD in childhood are boys, there is a more even gender balance in adolescent onset. Children with the disorder may have little empathy toward others, and in ambiguous situations, they often misinterpret the intentions of others as hostile and threatening, responding with aggressive behavior which they view as reasonable and justified (see the Rx Communication feature below). Self-esteem is commonly low but covered up by a facade of toughness.

CLINICAL EXAMPLE

Rob, a 9-year-old boy, was recently diagnosed with conduct disorder in addition to an earlier diagnosis of attention deficit hyperactivity disorder. Rob has been in numerous fights at school for the past 2 months. His grades have dropped substantially, and he was caught vandalizing school property. At home, he refuses to talk to his parents and hit his mother when she was yelling at him for stealing money from her purse.

Rob's long history of behavioral problems began with temper tantrums at 6 months of age. At the age of 3, he cut up the family sofa. His parents took him out of preschool because the teachers couldn't handle his behavior, especially his shoving other children and running around. During his early school years he had difficulty in concentrating and focusing on an activity for a sustained period of time, and interrupted ongoing activities. He has almost no friends in school.

Rob views his problems as the result of others' hostility and threats toward him. He expresses much anger toward the "school bullies" and all authority figures in his life.

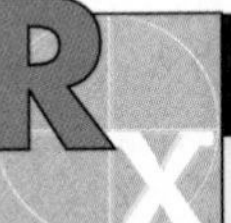

COMMUNICATION

A Child with Conduct Disorder

CHILD: I'm going to beat the crap out of that kid!

NURSE RESPONSE 1: You sound very angry at him. What is it that has made you feel so angry?

RATIONALE: This response reflects back to the child the feelings underlying the aggressive behavior and helps to facilitate the child's awareness of his anger. The follow-up question encourages the child to develop some insight regarding his anger and is general enough to allow issues to surface that may actually be unrelated to the other child.

NURSE RESPONSE 2: You know, Rob, that you will not be allowed to hurt anyone on the unit. If you're angry about something, I'll help you find ways to deal with your anger.

RATIONALE: This response clearly establishes limits on the child's behavior, reinforcing what is appropriate versus inappropriate behavior. The nurse also makes it clear that there are constructive ways to handle anger and that she will be there to help the child learn how to manage his feelings more effectively.

OPPOSITIONAL DEFIANT DISORDER

All of the features of oppositional defiant disorder (ODD) are usually present in conduct disorder, so it is not diagnosed if it meets the criteria for CD. ODD is a recurrent and hostile pattern of behavior toward authority figures. However, it does not involve the physical aggression, destructive behavior, deceitfulness, theft, or serious violation of rules shown in CD. ODD has a prevalence rate of 2% to 16%. It is more common in children from families in which the child experiences many different caregivers; families in which harsh, inconsistent, or neglectful child-rearing practices are used; where mothers are depressed; or where serious marital discord exists. The disorder is associated with problematic preschool temperaments and a high degree of motor activity by the child. ODD usually becomes apparent before age 8, with symptoms first appearing in the home and then later within other settings. The child may show low self-esteem, minimal frustration tolerance, swearing, mood lability, and precocious use of tobacco, alcohol, or illegal drugs.

Other Important Disorders of Infancy or Childhood

There are a number of other disorders that are typically diagnosed in childhood. With the exception of tic disorders, most of them rarely continue past childhood. They may, however, predict subsequent adult disorders of another type.

FEEDING AND EATING DISORDERS

Three disorders in this category are specific to childhood: pica, rumination disorder, and feeding disorder of infancy or early childhood. Anorexia nervosa and bulimia nervosa may also occur during later childhood, but these disorders are discussed in Chapter 18 because they are not unique to childhood, nor do they necessarily first appear in childhood.

Pica

Pica is a disorder in which the child persistently eats nonnutritive substances (such as paint, plaster, string, hair, cloth, animal droppings, insects, or leaves). To be considered a disorder, the behavior must be inappropriate for the developmental level of the child and not part of a culturally sanctioned practice. This disorder is most frequently seen in preschool children and in individuals who are retarded. Lack of adequate supervision, neglect, and poverty increase the possibility of the problem. Usually, the disorder lasts only for a few months, but it can continue into adolescence or adulthood.

Rumination Disorder

Rumination disorder is the repeated regurgitation and rechewing of food. It appears after a period of normal eating behavior in an infant or child. The child brings up partially digested food into the mouth, without any evidence of nausea or retching, and then chews and reswallows it. Sometimes the food is spit out. These symptoms are not associated with any medical condition or with any other eating disorder. Rumination disorder is most common in male infants between 3 and 12 months of age. You will see a characteristic straining and arching of the back in these babies, and they make sucking movements with the tongue, appearing to enjoy the process very much. However, between the times of regurgitation, babies are often irritable and hungry, and they eat a lot when fed. Because they regurgitate immediately after eating, there is common weight loss or failure to gain expected weight. Certain factors place an infant at risk for the disorder, including lack of stimulation, neglect, and problems in the parent–child relationship. In turn, the unsuccessful nature of the feeding experience and the aversive nature of the regurgitation may result in a parent's difficulty in providing responsive or loving care.

Feeding Disorder of Infancy or Early Childhood

In feeding and eating disorders, there is a persistent failure to eat adequately, accompanied by either a failure to gain weight or significant weight loss. Resulting malnutrition can threaten the baby's life. As with other disorders in this category, there is no medical condition causing the behavior. Babies with this problem are particularly irritable and difficult to console during feeding. At other times, they may appear apathetic or withdrawn. Infants who have preexisting developmental impairments or problems with regulation of the nervous system (for example, sleep–wake irregularities) may be less responsive to the parent, creating difficulties in the feeding process. In addition, parent behavior can make the feeding problem worse. For example, a parent may force the food into a baby's mouth too roughly or at too rapid a pace. There is a high incidence of parental psychopathology as well as child abuse or neglect associated with the condition. Although the disorder is most common in infancy (about 1% to 5% of all pediatric hospital admissions are for failure to thrive), it may have its onset as late as age 2 to 3. Most children eventually achieve improved growth patterns.

CLINICAL EXAMPLE

Chang, an 8-month-old Chinese boy, was referred to the child psychiatric clinic by pediatrics for an assessment. Chang's mother was dependent on alcohol and had several bouts of drinking during her pregnancy with Chang. As a result, he had low birth weight and many neurobehavioral problems at birth. Chang continued to have tremors and an increased startle response throughout his first 6 months of life. He was also highly irritable and difficult for his mother to console, especially during feeding. He had been followed by a nurse practitioner, Dawn, since the time he was 3 months of age. Dawn reported that he had not eaten well from the time he was born, was quite undernourished and failed to gain weight. Chang's failure to thrive became such a concern that Dawn hospitalized him for treatment of a number of resulting medical problems. During his hospitalization, an extensive diagnostic workup produced no clear reasons for his failure to eat and develop normally. The pediatric nurses, however, had noted his mother's frustration with Chang's lack of interest in eating. Her frustration would often lead to impatience and cause her to simply stop trying to get Chang to eat. They also charted some concern about her current alcohol use. They could smell alcohol on her when she came to the unit and there were times when she was verbally abusive to the staff.

The child psychiatric–mental health nurse noted that, most of the time, Chang's mother related to him with very little emotion. His mother commented to the nurse that "Chang has always been a difficult and stubborn baby, never happy with anything. I've given up trying to please him. He has a personality just like his father." The nurse also noticed that Chang's facial expression was solemn and he rarely made eye contact with anyone. He seemed listless and lethargic much of the time. When attempts were made to feed him, Chang would become very distressed, crying and trying to bang his head against the wall or floor. His mother commented that, because of such behavior, she rarely tried to pick him up anymore and would prop the bottle during his feeding.

REACTIVE ATTACHMENT DISORDER OF INFANCY OR EARLY CHILDHOOD

Reactive attachment disorder of infancy or early childhood is a markedly disturbed and developmentally inappropriate way of relating that is presumed to be the result of gross pathologic care. This pathologic care may be any of the following:

- Persistent disregard of the child's basic emotional needs for comfort, stimulation, or affection.
- Persistent disregard of the child's basic physical needs.
- Repeated changes of caregivers that prevent the formation of stable attachments.

However, not all children who experience gross pathologic care will develop the disorder.

Two types of this disorder are distinctly opposite in their symptoms. The *inhibited type* involves a failure to initiate and respond to most social interactions in a developmentally appropriate way. Children show excessively inhibited, hypervigilant, or ambivalent responses. Examples are a look of frozen watchfulness, resistance to comfort, and a mixture of approach and avoidance. In contrast, the *disinhibited type* involves an indiscriminate sociability or lack of selectivity in the choice of attachment figures. The child may be excessively familiar with strangers in demonstrating affection or seeking comfort and affection from a variety of adults who are not well known to the child. The severity and duration of the disorder depend on the degree of psychosocial deprivation and the nature of any intervention. If a supportive environment is provided, improvement does occur. Children with this disorder commonly have a feeding and eating disorder as well (see the Using Research Evidence feature below).

SEPARATION ANXIETY DISORDER

Separation anxiety disorder involves a developmentally inappropriate and excessive anxiety over separation from home or from attachment figures. Symptoms may include fear and worry about possible harm befalling attachment figures or about being separated from them. There is usually a reluctance or refusal to go to school, be without attachment figures, or go to sleep without them nearby. It is also common for the child to have somatic complaints when separation occurs or is anticipated. Children with this disorder frequently come from close-knit families and are often described as demanding, intrusive, or in need of constant attention. They may also be unusually compliant, conscientious, or eager to please. Depressed mood is typical and may increase over time.

USING RESEARCH EVIDENCE

Maria Vasquez was being seen at the family mental health clinic for PTSD and depression. She was a recent refugee who had experienced many traumatic events, most notably, seeing her own parents shot and killed. She was also the victim of domestic violence, being frequently beaten by her partner. The child psychiatric nurse practitioner at the clinic noticed that Ms. Vasquez regularly brought her 2-year-old son Mario with her to her treatment sessions. He would sit in the hallway while his mother met with her therapist. The NP was concerned that Mario showed very little facial expression, seemed uninterested in his toys, and was distant toward his mother. The nurse had recently read some clinical research which found that stress experienced by immigrants, as well as conflict and violence between adult partners, are strong predictors of mental health problems for preschool children. In light of these research findings and her observations of Mario, she approached the mother's therapist and proposed that Mario have a clinical assessment. With the mother's agreement, the nurse did a mental status exam with Mario and interviewed the mother about his behavior. The assessment indicated that Mario had symptoms of major depression as well as indications of reactive attachment disorder. Based on her assessment, the nurse then developed a care plan that included both play therapy and infant–parent psychotherapy.

These suggestions stem from the following research:

Weiss, S., Goebel, P., Page, A. & Warda, M. (1999). The impact of cultural and familial context on behavioral and emotional problems of preschool Latino children. *Child Psychiatry and Human Development, 29*(4), 287–301; and Zeanah, C., Danis, B., Hirshberg, L., Miller, D., & Heller, S. (1999). Disorganized attachment associated with partner violence. *Infant Mental Health Journal, 20*, 77–86.

The disorder occurs in about 4% of children and may appear after a stressful life event such as the death of a pet, a family illness, or immigration. There are periods of exacerbation and remission over the course of the disorder that persist for many years, including into adulthood.

ELIMINATION DISORDERS

The **elimination disorders** are encopresis and enuresis. In order to be classified as a mental disorder, these problems must not be due to any medical condition or to the physiologic effects of a laxative, diuretic, or other substance.

Encopresis

Encopresis is the repeated passing of feces by the child into inappropriate places such as clothing or a corner of the room. This is usually involuntary behavior, but it may be intentional in some situations. There are two subtypes of the disorder. The first involves constipation and continuous leakage of feces during the day and during sleep. Incontinence stops once the constipation is treated. The constipation may develop for psychological reasons, often related to a general pattern of anxious or oppositional behavior that leads the child to avoid defecation. Health problems causing dehydration, or the side effects of medication, may also initially create the constipation, but once it has developed, a child may retain stool because of painful defecation or anal fissure. The second subtype does not involve constipation or incontinence. Feces are normal and soiling is intermittent, with feces usually found in an obvious place. Children with this subtype often have a dual diagnosis of ODD or CD. With either subtype, smearing the feces may result from attempts to clean or hide the feces, or it may be a deliberate effort to make a mess.

Enuresis

Enuresis is the repeated voiding of urine into the bed or clothes, either during the day or at night. The *nocturnal type* is most common and typically occurs during the first part of the night. The *diurnal type* (during waking hours) happens most typically in the early afternoon of school days. This type may be related to social anxiety and a resulting reluctance to use the toilet, or it may be because the child becomes preoccupied with play or other activities. Some children show a combination of both day and night enuresis.

For both encopresis and enuresis, there is a primary and secondary type. With the *primary type*, the child has never been toilet trained. In the *secondary type*, the disturbance develops after a period of using the toilet appropriately. Of course, the problem is not diagnosed as a mental disorder unless the child has reached a chronological age at which elimination problems should not be apparent (at least age 4 for encopresis and age 5 for enuresis).

Predisposing factors for both disorders include inconsistent or lax toilet training, or psychosocial stressors such as entry to school or a sibling birth. In contrast to encopresis, about 75% of all children with enuresis have a parent or sibling who has had the disorder.

Both disorders are more common in boys, with prevalence rates for enuresis being higher (5% to 10% of 5-year-olds) than for encopresis (1% of all 5-year-olds). Neither disorder is typically chronic. Most children become continent by adolescence. The degree of immediate and long-term impairment depends to a great extent on the amount of resulting peer rejection, punishment and rejection by the caregiver, and a child's overall self-esteem.

SELECTIVE MUTISM

Selective mutism is the persistent failure to speak in specific social situations, even though the child can speak in other situations. Of course, the failure to speak must not be the result of a lack of normal language skills or knowledge of a certain language. The child can be excessively shy, fearful of embarrassment, withdrawn, clinging, and negative; or you may see temper tantrums or oppositional behavior, especially at home. Mutism is rare, but slightly more common in girls. Usually, the disturbance lasts for only a few months, but it can continue for several years.

STEREOTYPIC MOVEMENT DISORDER

Stereotypic movement disorder is a pattern of motor behavior that is repetitive and nonfunctional and one that the child appears driven to do. Examples of such movements are rocking, twirling objects, head banging, self-biting, picking at skin or body orifices, or hitting parts of one's own body. The specific behaviors may change over time from one type of behavior to another. The disorder can result in tissue damage or be life threatening, and it is frequently associated with mental retardation. Sometimes children try to restrain themselves from the behavior, for example, by putting their hands in their pockets; but if the restraint is interfered with, the behaviors resume. Onset of the disorder may follow a stressful event.

TIC DISORDERS

There are three disorders classified as tics: Tourette's disorder, chronic motor or vocal tics disorder, and transient tic disorder. In each of these conditions, there is a rapid, recurring, nonrhythmic, stereotyped movement or vocalization that occurs suddenly and involuntarily. Tics are worse during stress but occur less frequently when the child is focused intently on an activity such as reading.

Most **tic disorders** appear to be transmitted through a genetic or constitutional factor, which gives the child a vulnerability to developing the disorder. However, about 10% of children with the disorder have a "nongenetic" form; these children frequently have a dual diagnosis with another mental disorder or a medical condition such as epilepsy. Regardless of type, boys are more likely to develop tic disorders than girls.

Tourette's Disorder

Tourette's disorder involves multiple motor tics and one or more vocal tics, which can occur simultaneously or at different periods during the illness. The diagnosis requires that there is never a tic-free period for more than 3 months. Vocal tics are words or sounds such as yelps, barks, snorts, or coughs. *Coprolalia* is a specific type of vocal tic in which obscenities are uttered. *Motor tics* include such behavior as eye blinking, protruding the tongue, sniffing, retracing steps, or twirling when walking. The disorder may begin as early as age 2, but more often it starts during childhood or early adolescence. Tourette's disorder normally lasts for a life-time with periods of remission, but in most cases the symptoms decrease during adolescence and adulthood.

Chronic Versus Transient Tic Disorders

Chronic motor or vocal tic disorder differs from Tourette's disorder in that it involves *either* motor tics or vocal tics, but not both, as is required for a diagnosis of Tourette's disorder. Transient tic disorder differs from all of the above in its duration. While the others require that the problems have occurred for at least a year, transient tic disorder does not last longer than 12 months.

PEDIATRIC AUTOIMMUNE NEUROPSYCHIATRIC DISORDERS ASSOCIATED WITH STREPTOCOCCAL INFECTIONS (PANDAS)

The symptoms of children who have tic disorders or other disorders such as obsessive–compulsive disorder may get worse following streptococcal infections (e.g., strep throat). The mental health problems resulting from such an exacerbation of symptoms are referred to as PANDAS. (See Chapter 16 for more detailed discussion.)

Adult Disorders That May Begin in Childhood

A few disorders that are diagnosed more frequently in adulthood may begin in childhood. These include anxiety disorders, mood disorders and schizophrenia.

ANXIETY DISORDERS

In addition to separation anxiety, which was described earlier, children can have many other anxiety disorders. Panic disorder and agoraphobia are rare in children. Specific phobias, however, may be seen in children even before age 5 and are considered one of the most common childhood anxiety disorders. Children develop fears, especially of animals and blood-related events. Severe social phobia is also found in children and may lead to school avoidance. The onset of obsessive–compulsive disorder (OCD) is common for children aged 9 to 11. Because children may not have developed "insight" yet, the requirement for OCD that they recognize the excessive nature of their behavior is waived for children. Generalized anxiety disorder (GAD) and posttraumatic stress disorder (PTSD) are also found in children. Children with GAD are often shy and may act more mature and serious than expected for their age. They often are perfectionistic and highly compliant to demands of authority figures. PTSD in children is often associated with child abuse. In contrast to the adult experience of "flashbacks" of the traumatic event, children typically reexperience traumatic events as nightmares or through repetitive reenactment during play. Remember that memories of events that cannot be described verbally can still be brought forth in play or dreams by children who are as young as 2 or 3 years of age. Early treatment of all types of anxiety disorders in children is very important because they can lead to many social problems, including rejection or neglect by peers, academic failure, and inadequate development into an autonomous, secure adult. These anxiety disorders are discussed in detail in Chapter 16. In general, their symptoms are similar in children and adults.

MOOD DISORDERS

Mood disorders are discussed fully in Chapter 15, so they will not be covered in detail here. However, a few issues related to mood disorders in children are important to note. One class of mood disorders, bipolar disorders, is very rare in childhood. In contrast, another class, depressive disorders, is quite common in children, with depressive symptoms occurring even in the first year of life. Diagnoses are usually not made during infancy, because developmentally, children often do not have the ability to reflect on their feelings even if the feelings are strongly affecting them. Also remember that children may not be able to accurately report symptoms even if they are experiencing them.

The two types of depressive disorders are major depression and dysthymia. Major depression involves a definite change in behavior from the child's normal functioning. The child begins to show a depressed or sad mood or a lack of pleasure (anhedonia) in almost all activities at least 50% of the time. There are some important differences in how children and adults may manifest these symptoms. Children may describe things as bad, gloomy, blue, or empty when they are depressed. You may see a bland, frozen look on their faces or only fleeting smiles, as if they are smiling because it is socially expected rather than because they feel like smiling. On the other hand, you may see no evidence of sadness in children but rather a persistent irritability around even small matters. Pervasive boredom is a common sign of anhedonia in children. Another sign is social withdrawal, especially when a child avoids or rejects opportunities to play. Other symptoms of depression in children include unexplained somatic complaints, poor school performance, sleep and appetite changes, and/or psychomotor agitation and increased risk taking. The most common type of depression in children is called *reactive depression*, meaning that it occurs in response to a particular situation, such as the trauma of hospitalization or an extended separation from a parent.

Dysthymia is a chronic disorder in which there are periods of depressed affect interspersed with normal mood. Symptoms of later adult dysthymia often begin in childhood, even if not diagnosed until later. Because of this early and chronic quality, the person is often described as a "depressive personality." Although the symptoms of dysthymia are the same for children and adults, children are likely to show greater evidence of irritability, not simply depressed affect, and may react negatively or shyly to praise. They may respond to positive relationships with testing, anger, or avoidance. Other symptoms of dysthymia are similar to those described for major depression, except that the child may show more evidence of low energy and low self-esteem. A key predisposing factor for childhood dysthymia is the presence of an inadequate, rejecting, or chaotic home environment.

There is strong evidence of a familial pattern for both major depression and dysthymia, with clear support for a genetic, biochemical etiology. Although there is a greater incidence of depressive disorders for women in adulthood, the prepubertal incidence is the same for boys and girls (about 2% of all children).

Schizophrenia

Occuring as early as age 5 or 6, childhood-onset schizophrenia is rare. Its incidence is about 1 in every 1,000 children, mostly boys. The features of schizophrenia (delusions, hallucinations, disorganized speech and behavior, and negative symptoms) are the same in children as adults. Be aware, however, that failure to reach expected levels of speech and behavior may be seen in children rather than a deterioration into disorganization. (Schizophrenia is discussed fully in Chapter 14.)

CLINICAL EXAMPLE

Shauna, an 11-year-old, described hearing the voice of her mother calling her name and yelling at her, although her mother was not present. At times, she heard her own voice telling her to do things such as chores for her mother. She experienced her mother's voice as coming from outside her head and her own voice as coming from inside her head. She reported seeing a woman who looked like her mother and she thought was her mother. She also believed that her mother was watching her. Shauna described going to the bathroom in the morning and "daydreaming" that objects were weapons (e.g., cotton swabs were sticks to stab people, and washcloths were used to smother people). All these experiences seemed real to Doris as they happened. Shauna also believed that the world was coming to an end. She described hearing on the news that a hole was breaking apart pieces of the earth, and she thought this was going to happen. She also expressed concern that a heat wave might result in there not being enough air to breathe.

It is difficult to make the diagnosis in children, however, because delusions and hallucinations are less detailed and more accepted developmentally as normal fantasy or imaginary playmates. Visual hallucinations are more common in children than in adults but are almost always accompanied by auditory hallucinations. Disorganized speech (such as in communication disorders) or disorganized behavior (as in ADHD or autistic disorder) may result in other diagnoses when they are actually symptoms of schizophrenia.

Biopsychosocial Theories

Five major theories guide existing views regarding the etiology of childhood psychopathology and the therapeutic approaches underlying its prevention and treatment. These are psychodynamic theory, object-relations theory, attachment theory, cognitive–behavioral theory, and biologic diathesis theory. Although many specific schools of thought fall within these perspectives, only the central features of these overarching theories will be discussed here.

PSYCHODYNAMIC THEORY

Psychodynamic theory originated with Sigmund Freud in his conceptualization of psychoanalysis but has evolved substantially since its original formulation. Much of Freud's speculation regarding psychosexual stages of development has been rejected, but many components of his personality theory continue to serve as a foundation for assessment and treatment in child psychiatry (Gabbard, 1994).

A central component of this theory is the concept of *psychic determinism*, which proposes that the child's initial perceptions of the world are defined substantially during the first 5 to 6 years of life and will influence the child's later views and behavior in a causal way. While this stance seems almost a given in today's world, the concept was unheard of when Freud first proposed it. Psychodynamic theory also holds that the child is born with instincts or drives for the gratification of needs to ensure survival. *Libido* is described as the psychic energy that makes the child try to meet these needs. If the needs are not satisfied during development, the child may become so fixated on meeting the needs that they influence much of his or her behavior.

Because the ego and superego prevent the id from getting all needs met, Freud proposed that children attempt to cope with the anxiety associated with need deprivation through the unconscious mental processes known as defense mechanisms (see Chapter 5). Defense mechanisms commonly employed by children are repression, reaction formation, and projection. The child comes to deal with the world through these distorted views in an attempt to defend against painful unconscious issues. However, the unconscious content continues to influence the behavior and conscious thoughts of the child, often in ways which severely impair his or her ability to function in life. Defense mechanisms are, therefore, considered to be symptoms of mental health problems. The focus of treatment is attempting to bring repressed conflicts and issues into awareness so that they can be addressed and resolved. A primary way in which this occurs is through *transference*, a process whereby the child unconsciously directs feelings and desires from other relationships in life onto the therapist. So the relationship between therapist and child is used as a focus for interpretation and change in working with the child.

OBJECT-RELATIONS THEORY

Object-relations theory is built upon the foundation of psychodynamic theory and is based in the work of Fairbairn, Winnicott, Klein, Mahler, Stern, and others (Dilts, 2001). In this theory, an *object* is defined as a person or thing in the child's environment that has psychological significance to the child.

A major assumption of this theory is that rather than being driven simply by physical needs or instincts that enhance survival, infants have an innate biologic need for relationships. These relationships increase in quality and complexity as a child develops. Initially infants are undifferentiated from the object they seek (the primary caregiver) and are in a state of diffuse, unorganized experiences. The child is totally dependent on the mother to organize the child's different experiences into an understandable whole. As the young child begins to differentiate—that is, separate and develop a sense of his or her own self as an individual—the relationships with interpersonal "objects" in the world of the child are internalized and become the internal mental representations that form the self.

The differentiated self forms the basis for the child's future views of his or her own worth and the availability and responsiveness of others. Ultimately, it determines whether or not the child becomes healthy, strong, and creative. Development of the self is considered to depend primarily on the relationship between parent and child, and how effectively a parent responds to the baby's needs and assists in organizing experience. Object-relations theorists maintain that an individual will repeat in relationships throughout life what is learned about self and others from the individual's initial experience with the primary caregiver.

ATTACHMENT THEORY

Attachment theory builds on the psychodynamic concepts of psychic determinism and the impact of unconscious processes. As in object-relations theory, relationships are viewed as the organizing principle for the development of psychologic well-being in the child. However, the concept of *security* within the relationship is the main focus of attachment theory. Attachment theory was originally described by Bowlby and later extended by Ainsworth and others (Cassidy & Shaver, 1999).

Attachment refers to the socioemotional bond of the child to another person (the attachment figure) who is perceived as strong or powerful and who can be turned to for protection and support in situations of perceived danger or adversity. Infants are viewed as coming into the world with an innate neurobiologic structure called the attachment behavioral system. This evolutionary-based adaptive system monitors and processes information regarding uncertainty, stress, or potential danger as well as the accessibility of the attachment figure during these situations. The infant appraises both the environmental conditions and his or her emotional state to determine how much proximity or contact is needed in order to feel secure. The child then uses attachment behaviors (proximity or contact-promoting behaviors such as calling, approaching, or clinging) to acquire a sense of security.

The ways the attachment figure responds to the child's attachment behaviors are considered critical to the foundation of the child's internal working models (Weinfield, Sroufe, Egeland, & Carlson, 1999). These models are ways of viewing relationships that will come to guide the child's evaluation of his or her own capacity to handle stress, as well as the responses he or she expects of others in times of need. Four major patterns of attachment have been identified as resulting from the initial experiences with the primary attachment figure:

1. Secure
2. Insecure-avoidant
3. Insecure-resistant
4. Disorganized

While the first three patterns reflect different internal working models, the last pattern is viewed as a lack of any integrated or consolidated model to guide attachment behavior during situations where comfort or felt security is needed.

Secure working models involve a view of the attachment figure as available and responsive, and they encourage the child to seek security through proximity and contact. *Insecure-avoidant* children appear indifferent to stress and uncertainty, although their physiologic responses suggest otherwise. They actively avoid their attachment figure during stressful times and focus on other things, such as play. Research suggests that this pattern results from an insensitivity of the caregiver to the child's needs for comforting and an active rebuffing of the child's attempts to be comforted during distress.

Children with *insecure-resistant* patterns of attachment tend to resist interaction and contact with the caregiver when it is available, yet show proximity-seeking behavior when it is not available. They shift between excessively seeking comfort, and being difficult to settle or soothe when contact is acquired. Primary caregivers of these children tend to be unpredictable in their accessibility, less adaptable, hesitant, and occupied with caregiving routines rather than providing tender, sensitive care.

Infants with a *disorganized* attachment pattern show unexplainable or disoriented behaviors toward the attachment figure during distress, such as frightened expressions and freezing while greeting the parent with raised arms, smiling while forcefully striking the parent's face, or extended rocking or ear pulling. Some parents of these children behave in frightening or threatening ways toward the infant or else reverse roles with the infant, acting timid or deferential to the child even when he or she is very small.

These various patterns can be seen in children by 12 months of age and eventually stabilize into cognitive frameworks that influence all of their intimate relationships in adulthood. While the primary attachment relationship is seen as central to the development of these life patterns, other significant relationships and the child's own degree of resilience or temperamental vulnerability are recognized as important mediators in developing secure or insecure attachment patterns.

COGNITIVE–BEHAVIORAL THEORY

The origins of cognitive–behavioral theory stem from Skinner's behavioral learning school of thought. However, current views integrate more recent cognitive theory and social learning theory traditions (Dilts, 2001). The basis of this theory is the importance of the environment in the child's psychologic development. The environment encompasses everything to which the child is exposed, including the immediate caregiving environment (the family, school, and neighborhood), as well as the larger sociocultural milieu within which values and expectations are developed. Infants are viewed as coming into the world with a relatively "blank slate," and they develop personality by being conditioned to respond in certain ways by others in the environment. Bandura emphasized the importance of modeling as well, whereby children learn by watching others and what happens to those people as a result of their behavior.

The original views of behavioral theory were that positive and negative reinforcement alone could condition a child's behavior. These approaches do show success in a variety of disorders (Bosch & Ringdahl, 2001; Eikeseth, Smith, Jahr, & Eldevik, 2002; Green, Brennan, & Fein, 2002). Bandura expanded this conceptualization to emphasize the child's ability to deliberate consciously on what occurs and make certain choices about behaviors that are used. He describes this as "reciprocal determinism." In this view, the environment provides information that influences the child in choosing how to behave, but *interpretation* of the environment is the determinant of the child's behavior, not the environment itself. However, without the environment, the child has no stimulus toward growth or development.

Cognitive theorists emphasize that psychopathology results from particular mental sets or cognitive schemata which involve distortions of reality. Children's experiences with the environment create these schemata, or ways of viewing the world, which then influence what is perceived and how it is processed and understood in all future interactions. Biased or inaccurate ways of thinking or processing information can take a number of forms; for instance, interpreting things as worse than they are, overgeneralization, selective perception, disqualifying the positive, jumping to conclusions, or personalizing events that are not actually related to the child. These distortions are brought about by the irrational beliefs stemming from the child's schemata. External events and relationships set off particular schemata that have been established early in life and that can create major problems in the child's ability to function appropriately, or that are adaptive for the child. Treatment is thus focused on a reeducation or relearning process aimed at the child's irrational beliefs and their related behaviors. This process can occur individually or in a group situation (Heyne, King, Tonge, & Cooper, 2001; Schortt, Barrett, & Fox, 2001).

BIOLOGIC THEORY

A *biologic diathesis* is some constitutional predisposition to the development of a disease. There is no single view regarding how a diathesis for mental illness is acquired. Rather, there are many hypotheses regarding the particular biologic characteristics that may make children vulnerable to developing certain psychiatric disorders (Nelson & Bosquet, 2000; Schore, 2001).

For example, there is considerable evidence for the role of neurobiologic factors in the development of disorders such as autistic disorder and childhood-onset schizophrenia. Children with these disorders have more physical anomalies, neurologic soft signs, and brain abnormalities on electroencephalograms (EEGs) and in computed tomagraphy (CT) and magnetic resonance imaging (MRI) scans. These problems are considered potential causes of the mental disorder (Charney, Nestler & Bunney, 1999).

There is growing support for the existence of certain abnormalities in neurotransmitter secretion. Serotonin (5-HT) has been of major interest in a number of disorders. For instance, studies suggest that 5-HT levels may be elevated in autism but depleted in childhood depression. However, it is unclear whether the dysfunction in neurotransmitter levels causes the disorder, or whether the disorder may create nervous system changes that cause the neurotransmitter abnormality.

Studies also indicate that problems with nervous system responsiveness may be related to certain psychiatric disorders. For example, children with schizophrenia have unusually high autonomic system reactivity when in baseline or resting states, and children with ADHD appear to have a lowered excitability in the reticular activating system of the brain, requiring more stimulation in order to feel optimally aroused.

While the exact relationship between these biological factors and mental illness is not yet understood, there are three likely sources of these abnormalities: a genetic predisposition, perinatal complications resulting in CNS injury, and early childhood trauma. Twin and adoption studies continue to provide evidence in support of genetic etiology for many disorders, including pervasive developmental disorders, schizophrenia, and depression. Adopted children and their biologic parents show a much stronger likelihood of both having these disorders than adoptive parents and children. In addition, when one twin has a disorder, the other is much more likely to have the disorder than might be another sibling, parent, or other relative.

Perinatal complications, including perinatal asphyxia, congenital anomalies, and intrauterine exposure to drugs and alcohol have also been found to be associated with psychiatric disorders. Similarly, lead poisoning, central nervous system (CNS) trauma, and infections in childhood have all been implicated as possible causative factors.

Finally, there is a growing body of research that suggests that early psychological trauma from severe neglect or abuse may create deficits or abnormalities in brain structure and function (Perry, 1999). It was previously thought that a child's biologic makeup could influence his or her psychosocial outcomes but not the reverse. Evidence now indicates that psychological trauma in the first few years of life can create changes in the size of the brain, the number of neuronal pathways affecting certain brain functions (such as emotion) and the amount and function of neurotransmitters in the brain (Paris, 1999).

MULTICAUSAL MODEL

While each of the perspectives just described is often considered in isolation, there is growing acceptance of a multicausal, multidimensional nature in any etiology of mental illness. Box 25–1 on page 602 lists potential risk factors that have been identified for childhood mental illness.

Although various schools of thought may emphasize specific risk factors, as nurses, we need to view mental health in an inte-

BOX 25–1 Risk Factors for Developing Mental Health Problems in Childhood

- Inherited metabolic deficiencies or nervous system abnormalities.
- Injury, or toxic exposure or physical complications in utero or during the perinatal period.
- Medical conditions of infancy or childhood (such as epilepsy, low birth weight).
- Early deprivation of nurturance or stimulation (parental absence or loss, neglect or rejection, large family size, foster placement).
- Family history of a psychiatric disorder.
- A chaotic home environment (family violence or severe marital discord).
- Disadvantaged socioeconomic status (poverty, violence, hopelessness).

grative, interactive way. In this view, the child's genetically determined attributes or vulnerabilities are seen to interact with life experience to influence mental health outcomes (see ■ Figure 25–1). Many children show tremendous hardiness and resilience in the face of horrible life experiences, while other, more vulnerable children may be severely affected by even a minimally stressful or adverse experience. Not only do the child's characteristics affect how the child will respond to and internalize what is experienced, but he or she can influence what the environment provides as a result of a genetically given temperament or biomedical status.

It is important to remember that children both:

- Actively elicit and seek out certain responses and experiences.
- Perceive what is given by the environment through the looking glass of their unique genotype.

These factors interact with what is actually available in the environment to determine the degree to which a child achieves mental health or develops a mental illness. In a multicausal model, there is no certain etiology, no predictable set of risk factors, and no specific therapeutic approach having a standard effectiveness. The unique fit between a particular child and a particular set of life experiences must be considered to understand the child's mental health problems and develop an appropriate intervention.

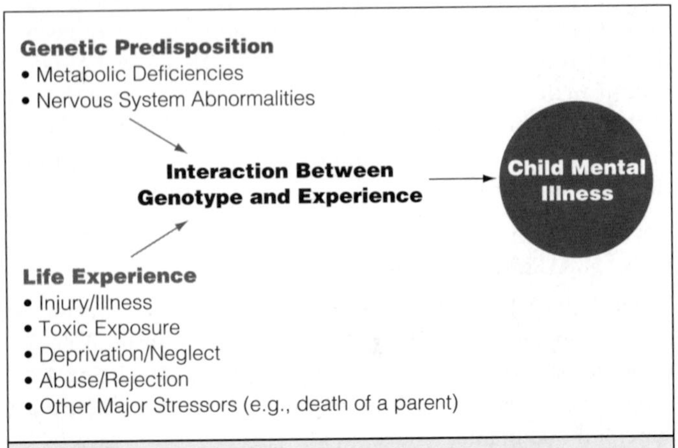

FIGURE 25–1 ■ *Interactive model of child mental illness.*

NURSING PROCESS

Children

The assessment, diagnosis, planning, implementation, and evaluation activities undertaken by the child psychiatric nurse are always in collaboration with the child, the family, and professional colleagues who are part of the child's care. The degree to which these individuals are active partners in the nursing process will influence the resulting quality and efficacy of your nursing care.

Assessment

Your ability to perform a valid assessment depends on your knowledge of developmental norms and your cultural sensitivity, including gathering pertinent cultural information within which to consider a particular child's behavior.

CULTURAL AND DEVELOPMENTAL CONTEXT

Your nursing assessment must occur within the context of a child's cultural background and developmental stage. What can be defined as "normal or functional" versus "dysfunctional or abnormal" is relative to the meaning certain behaviors have within a culture and the child's developmental capabilities. For instance, temper tantrums can be viewed very differently within different cultures. It has been noted that Hispanic families often see tantrums as the result of a nervous temperament or a fragile personality. In contrast, African-American families frequently think tantrums are the child's "acting up" (Kohlenberg, Joseph, Prudent, & Richardson, 1995). These different perceptions bring about different responses by the parent, which may, in turn, affect the child's behavior over time.

Asking families what they believe about the cause of their child's problems is a good way to assess their culture-specific beliefs. You can also find out what their parents and grandparents have said about the problems as well as traditional resource people within their communities (such as spiritual advisors or healers). Also be sure to ask whether they have used any traditional remedies or cultural practices to deal with the child's problems. It is important to show respect for a family's unique views of mental illness and to build a mutually acceptable approach to your assessment.

Regarding developmental norms, you must determine whether a behavior (such as temper tantrums or separation anxiety) is understandable or appropriate based on the child's age. Stage of development affects the symptoms you will see, a child's expected responses to life stress, and the child's ability to understand and communicate with you about certain problems. Be sure to allow adequate time for full responses to open-ended questions, active listening, and careful observation of patterns of behavior. Assessment should be an ongoing process rather than a one-time session. Do not assume that observations can be generalized to other times and settings.

The most basic assessment includes a history-taking interview and a clinical assessment of the child.

THE HISTORY-TAKING INTERVIEW WITH PARENTS

For history taking, include the child as well as the parents in this discussion. Parents are a better source for facts such as onset, developmental milestones, or context surrounding the symptoms, but including the child is helpful in a number of ways. First, it decreases the child's feelings of being left out, talked about, or powerless in the situation. You will find it very useful to hear an older child's response to the parents on certain issues or how the child's view may differ. In addition, you can learn much by paying attention not only to what the parents say, but to the nonverbal communication among family members. The way in which they interact will give important clues regarding the family's functioning in areas such as closeness, conflict, decision making, and flexibility. Because there may be certain information that parents are not comfortable discussing in front of their child, be sure to give them some time with you alone in addition to this total family approach. See Chapter 29 for specific suggestions on assessing family process.

There are four important aspects of history to be acquired. First, discuss the history of the child's current problem, including major concerns or complaints, how long it has been since the problem first began, the specific symptoms, and their previous and current efforts to address the problem.

Next, talk with the family about their own history and family process. This aspect of the assessment can include a genogram or family time line, discussion of child-rearing beliefs and behaviors, supports and stressors for the family, the history of any separations between parents and the child, and any psychiatric or other illness in the family.

CLINICAL EXAMPLE

The maternal grandmother of a suicidal child who was scheduled for admission to an inpatient unit tried to block the admission. She insisted that the child was possessed by a demon and wanted the child to stay with her so she could pray over her and give her healing herbs. The child psychiatrist and the child psychiatric nurse spent time with the parents discussing the pressure they experienced from the child's grandmother. They mentioned to the parents that psychiatric services are unfamiliar to the grandmother's generation and cultural beliefs. They also reviewed the basis for the recommendation of hospitalization. The parents were encouraged to make their own decision based on their experience with their child and their concerns for her safety. Ways to involve the grandmother and her traditional medicines were suggested, and the professionals offered to be available to discuss the grandmother's questions and concerns.

The child's medical history is a third area for the interview. Find out about any childhood illnesses, allergies, medications, and so on. And finally, have the parents describe the child's developmental history. Starting with pregnancy or birth complications, progress through the child's development to identify any lags or events in achieving developmental milestones. Find out both the parents' and the child's view of the child's temperament, interests, and skills.

During this aspect of the interview, you can also identify the nature of the child's sociocultural environment (home, neighborhood, school) and how it may support or inhibit the achievement of developmental tasks. Be sure to find out about the nature of the child's friends as well.

CLINICAL ASSESSMENT OF THE CHILD

The clinical assessment of the child involves a mental status exam by the nurse and referral of the child for a complete physical and neuropsychologic evaluation. These latter evaluations are important in order to rule out any medical conditions and identify any neurologic or cognitive problems that may be associated with the child's psychiatric symptoms.

A mental status exam consists of both a semistructured interview and an unstructured play session with the child. If the child is nearing adolescence or is ambivalent about unstructured play, try games instead, as a medium through which you can observe the child's way of relating and approaching various situations. For both aspects of the exam, a relaxed, conversational approach is the most effective, where the child has the opportunity to tell you his story about problems he may be having and his relationships with family, peers, and teachers. Research has shown that children are the best source regarding the nature and extent of their symptoms (better than parents). Frame questions in ways that are developmentally appropriate for the child. Even 3- to 6-year-olds can give excellent feedback about their symptoms if questions are developmentally appropriate. Asking simple, informal questions like what kind of animal they would like to be, what they would want if they could have three wishes, or what was the saddest thing that ever happened to them, can provide a great deal of information regarding speech, modes of thinking and perception, and feeling states. Having children draw and discuss pictures of themselves and their family can be very useful for understanding their view of the world. The drawing in ■ Figure 25–2 on page 604 by a six-year-old girl named Emma is an excellent example.

Observing a child play with puppets, clay, or a sand tray can also provide invaluable information about motor behavior, thought content, affect and impulse control. In addition, there are many children's books using stories about abuse, depression, divorce, or hospitalization as themes. These stories portray children and animals with problems that relate to a variety of mental health challenges faced by children. They can serve as a stimulus for questions such as "How do you think that puppy might feel?" or "What would you do if you were that little girl?". These stories offer children opportunities to project their own thoughts and feelings onto the characters in the stories and

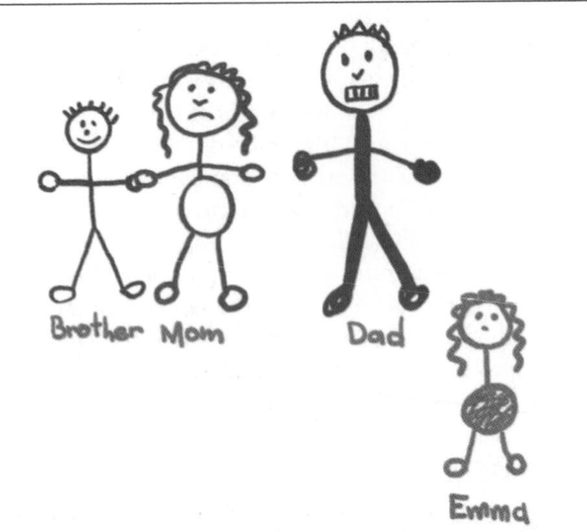

FIGURE 25–2 ■ *Family drawing by Emma, a 6-year-old girl. Emma's drawing has a number of distinctive features. She has placed herself at a distance from the rest of the family, suggesting feelings of isolation, rejection, or perhaps fear. The heavy lines around her father's body may indicate that he is seen as aggressive or angry. This interpretation is supported by the father's mouth, which appears to be open as if yelling or showing his teeth. Her brother looks happy, and her mother's downturned mouth looks a bit sad. Emma's drawing of herself is quite small, in contrast to others in the family (especially her brother, who is actually younger and smaller than Emma). Her smallness could indicate some insecurity, low self esteem, or perhaps a desire to withdraw from the world and not be noticed. The center of Emma's body is shaded, suggesting some anxiety about that part of her body. She is also missing her mouth and hands. This could imply a sense of inadequacy or powerlessness to act or speak.*

share them with you. Areas for assessment during the mental status exam are shown in the Assessment box at right.

ASSESSING POSSIBLE MALTREATMENT

You should always be alert for possible signs of maltreatment during your assessment. Take special notice if a parent seems evasive, unconcerned, or resistant to your questions or any follow-up procedures. Some of the most important signs of maltreatment in a child are detailed in Box 25–2. Maltreatment can involve child neglect or outright abuse. In neglect, parents fail to recognize when a problem exists or to meet their child's normal emotional and physical needs. Abuse can take many forms. It may be physical, involving severe disciplinary practices (e.g., beatings) or unexplained injury to the child (e.g., burns or bruises). Before age 12, boys are at greater risk of physical abuse but girls are more at risk as teenagers. Abuse can also be emotional, such as a child's being verbally demeaned or rejected. And, of course, sexual abuse is possible. Sexual abuse can include exposure from exhibitionism, molestation or fondling, nonassaultive intercourse, or rape. Girls are more likely than boys to be victims of sexual abuse by a 10-to-1 ratio. Chapter 23 has more information on child abuse.

ASSESSMENT

Guidelines for Children

Areas to Assess During the Mental Status Exam

General Appearance and Demeanor

- Grooming, alertness, eye contact, and overall attitude toward clinician

Motor Behavior and Coordination

- Activity level, gross motor and fine motor control, nature of movements, posture

Mood and Affect

- Overall mood state, manner of expressing feelings, range and intensity of emotions, evidence of dysphoric state (anger, anxiety, sadness)

Speech and Language

- Clarity and articulation, rhythm and organization, appropriateness of word choice

Thought Process

- Ability to understand and express meaning in an age-appropriate way, evidence of any loss of connectedness between ideas (loose associations), repeated behaviors or mannerisms (perseveration), or tangentiality of child's response to your questions

Thought Content

- Themes in play and talk, fears, evidence of beliefs that have no basis in reality

Perceptual Disturbances

- Threshold and tolerance for sensory input, evidence of hallucinations or illusions

Cognitive Function

- Orientation to person, time, and place; ability to follow through on requests; attention and concentration; distractability

Impulse Control

- Ability to manage behavior appropriately in response to needs and desires

ASSESSING SUICIDE RISK

Suicide by children has increased threefold over the last two decades. NIMH notes that there are over 300 suicides a year among children aged 1 to 14 (NIMH, 1999), and the numbers continue to rise despite increasing awareness by parents and professionals. These statistics probably underestimate the scope of the problem, because professionals and families tend to label suicidal acts as accidents. Depending on age, children may not conceptualize death as an irreversible state, and to that degree, suicide may be accidental.

Some people cannot believe that children can be depressed or would want to end their lives. Suicide attempts by children belie the myth of the "happy child" in our culture. The follow-

BOX 25–2 Signs of Maltreatment

- Unexplained or unusual history of physical injuries for the child
- Fearful and withdrawn or hyperalert and placating behavior by the child
- Unexplained developmental delays in child's language or motor behavior
- Malnutrition and dehydration
- Medical problems such as vaginal bleeding or recurrent urinary tract infections

ing clinical example illustrates denial and lack of information on the part of parents of a suicidal child:

CLINICAL EXAMPLE

A 7-year-old boy set up a rope over a door to hang himself. His attempt was stopped by his parents. The door, a second entrance to the room, was nailed shut and painted, but the subject of suicide was not discussed. His parents failed to recognize the same symptoms in the child 2 years later. At this time, however, severe behavioral problems in school, and pressure by school personnel, forced the parents to seek a psychiatric evaluation.

Although suicide in children under 12 occurs infrequently, suicidal ideation or suicide threats by a child always deserve attention and merit careful study. Even the most obvious gesture can prove fatal, especially in a child whose assessment of physical danger is immature and unrealistic. Children commit suicide by simple but lethal methods such as poisoning, shooting themselves with firearms (Miller, Azrael, & Hemenway, 2002), hanging, or darting into the path of moving cars.

It is unclear what drives a child to suicide. However, there are characteristic presuicidal symptoms and life circumstances of the suicidal child. The symptoms are known as depressive equivalents; that is, the symptoms may indicate a masked depression. The symptoms of masked depression are:

- Boredom or restlessness.
- Irritability or lethargy.
- Difficulty concentrating.
- Apparently purposeful misbehavior.
- Somatic preoccupation.
- Excessive dependence on or isolation from others, notably adults.

Children at higher risk for suicide are those who have experienced significant losses, family discord, abuse, and neglect or have other psychiatric problems, such as depression or other mood disorders (Lyon & Morgan-Judge, 2000).

A careful assessment of suicide risk should be done whenever a child expresses ideas about suicide or makes an attempt. The assessment interview should consider the degree of risk while exploring the family situation and the external events that preceded the thoughts or the attempt.

The meaning behind the attempt must be explored. Young children are less able to verbalize, and thus require more structure and planned activities in order to make an appropriate assessment. For example, there are books to help children talk about suicide. Be sure to carry out the following:

- Obtain a promise from the child, in the form of a contract, not to cause self-harm for a specified period of time (see the discussion of no suicide/no self-harm contracts in Chapter 22).
- Secure the support of the family in creating a safe environment for their child by making sure that all potentially lethal objects and medications are secured and out of sight.

If the family appears to be unable or unwilling to agree to the contract or to create a safe home environment, it may become necessary to hospitalize the child.

An outpatient treatment plan is outlined carefully with parents prior to initiating the plan. Adherence to the treatment plan will be enhanced if you ensure the following:

- Appointment dates and times.
- Contact with the family and the child between sessions.
- Family psychoeducation.
- The purpose and the goals of treatment are understood by the family.

Also see Chapter 22 for a discussion of child survivors of the death by suicide of a parent.

Nursing Diagnosis: NANDA

Your nursing assessment will provide information for both a psychiatric diagnosis using DSM-IV-TR criteria and nursing diagnoses.

Nursing diagnoses are the critical foundation underlying all planning, implementation, and evaluation activities with a child. Once you identify a child's problems, determine which of the NANDA diagnoses best match the problems. Then, prioritize the diagnoses based on their urgency or their need for attention before other problems can be addressed. There are some diagnoses specific to children in the NANDA classification system, such as Disorganized Infant Behavior, Altered Growth and Development, and Risk for Altered Parent–Child Attachment. Many other general diagnoses are relevant to children, such as Impaired Communication, Anxiety, or Sensory/Perceptual Alterations. Many family and parent-related diagnoses are also quite relevant.

Outcome Identification: NOC

After determining your nursing diagnoses, identify outcomes that are important for the child and/or family to achieve specific to each diagnosis. These outcomes are behaviors or skills that are necessary in order to bring about positive mental health changes.

Planning and Implementation: NIC

Each nursing diagnosis provides the basis for planning and implementation of nursing care. The care plan involves identification of specific outcomes that you want to achieve for each nursing diagnosis, along with your nursing interventions for each expected outcome. The most widely used treatment approaches are shown in the Intervention box below, along with a rationale for when they are likely to be useful. There are, however, many other innovative approaches that can also be used (Brue & Oakland, 2002; Montgomery, 2001; Muratori, Picchi, Casella et al, 2002; Schaefer, 1999; Webster-Stratton, Reid, & Hammond, 2001).

INFANT–PARENT PSYCHOTHERAPY

Infant–parent psychotherapy is effective for early intervention with infants who are at risk for later mental health problems either as a result of their own perinatal risk/medical complications or their caregiver's mental illness. Infant–parent psychotherapy is also a great resource in treatment of pervasive developmental disorders, feeding disorders, and reactive attachment disorder. In this treatment approach, the child psychiatric–mental health nurse works closely with both the primary caregiver (usually the mother) and the infant. The nurse focuses on three components: the infant's behavior, the parent's attitudes and feelings about the child, and the interaction between parent and infant.

Infant Behavior. Individual work with the infant aims to identify specific difficulties in the child's temperament and to help manage these difficulties more effectively. *Temperament* is the constitutional makeup of the infant at birth, specifically the child's behavioral and psychophysiologic attributes. For instance, infants who have been drug exposed in utero may be very sensitive to stimulation from lights, sounds, or touch; may cry frequently and be difficult to console; and have trouble developing regular patterns of sleep. The nurse may need to help an infant with such a temperament develop better regulation of his sleep patterns and responses to distress through a variety of activities that reduce stimulation and help calm and soothe the infant. In this way, the child may feel less distressed and begin to feel more secure with people. The nurse may also work to improve the baby's interpersonal skills or capacity to respond through interventions that help the child learn how to be a more active social partner. These skills are important to the infant's ability to engage the parents and respond in ways that reward their caregiving. In addition, parents who watch the nurse work with the infant develop a better understanding of the child's unique temperament and needs.

Parental Attitudes and Feelings. Focusing on the parent's attitudes and feelings toward the child is essential, especially for caregivers whose feelings about the baby or attitudes about parenting are distorted in some way. For example, distortions can occur as a result of a parent's own maltreatment as a child or current mental illness. Interventions with the parent may include exploration of feelings about the parent's own history and family relations and how they are affecting the care of the child. They may also help to minimize the caregiver's psychological distress through empathy and support so that she can rework the model she holds in her mind of her relationship with the infant. The goal of these interventions is to increase the capacity to nurture the child and to find satisfaction in the role as a caregiver.

Interaction Between Parent and Infant. Infant–parent psychotherapy provides interaction guidance in order to sensitize the parents to appropriate caregiving practices. The nurse does this by modeling specific ways of interacting with the infant, suggesting approaches for the parents to try, supporting and praising the use of positive interactions, and speaking for the infant so the parents become more aware of the baby's potential experience during caregiving (e.g., "Oh, I feel so safe and loved when you snuggle me close like this . . .").

Each of the components of parent–infant psychotherapy attempt to enhance the *goodness-of-fit* between parent and infant in order to increase their mutual enjoyment in one another and provide the infant with a more supportive foundation for optimal mental health (Lieberman, Silverman, & Pawl, 2000). This therapeutic approach can change the way the child behaves toward the parent, the way the parent interprets the child's behavior and defines the parent role, and the way the parent behaves toward the child (Sameroff & Fiese, 1999). Parent–infant psychotherapy clearly reflects an interactive model of mental illness and integrates every one of the theories described earlier.

INTERVENTION

Guidelines for Various Treatment Approaches Used with Children

Approach	Rationale
• Infant–parent psychotherapy	Parent's attitudes and caregiving style are the focus for intervention.
• Play therapy	The child's emotions and previous experience are the focus for intervention.
• Cognitive–behavioral therapy	The child's attitudes, beliefs, and behaviors are the focus for intervention.
• Family therapy	The dynamics of family interaction are the focus for intervention.
• Medication	A neurobiologic deficit or abnormality is the focus for intervention.

PLAY THERAPY

Play therapy builds on the foundation of the psychodynamic, object-relations, and attachment theories described earlier (Chethik, 2000). Although play therapy is used as part of most assessment protocols and to treat a variety of mental health problems, you may find it quite helpful for nursing diagnoses associated with attention deficit disorders, disruptive behavior disorders, mood disorders, and reactive attachment disorder.

Types of Play. There are four major types of play, which are also related to stages of play development in children. During the first year of life, *sensorimotor play* is the child's focus. This play involves attempts to assimilate sensory information and gain control over objects in the environment, by mouthing toys or pulling them around, for instance. During the second year of life, *construction or combinatorial play* becomes the child's focus, as in putting together shapes or stacking blocks. From ages 2 to 6, *symbolic or pretend play* emerges. At this age, the capacity to fantasize and put the self cognitively into other situations or other people's shoes enables play therapy to become a central vehicle for treatment of the child. The themes of the child's play are now motivated by inner psychologic dynamics. At age 5 or 6, children develop the capacity for and interest in *game play*. In games with rules, children are required to assume the perspective of others, remain attentive, and control their impulses. The ways in which children interact with others around the rules and activities provide another base of information regarding their inner world and how they view others.

Nondirective play is normally viewed as the best way to begin play therapy. The symbols and themes that emerge in play provide a core of information for assessment and subsequent treatment. They give us the same type of information that we gather through verbal communication with adults. Remember that symbols (such as aggressive behavior toward a father doll) can have several meanings and should never be interpreted in a standardized fashion. Always consider the way a symbol is used in the play as it may relate to the particular context of the child's life before interpreting a symbol's subjective meaning to a child. Your impressions must be verified or refuted based on a variety of different types of information collected over time.

CLINICAL EXAMPLE

Twelve year old Laura had been sexually molested by her father as a preschooler. Her father was sent to prison for the sexual molestation of another preschooler. During Laura's therapy session, she asked the nurse therapist to go to the playroom. She built a fortress of large multicolored blocks. She put a chair inside the structure and sat down, stating, "This is a dungeon. A rainbow dungeon." As the nurse used gentle questions to help Laura talk about what the dungeon meant to her, she began to speak hesitantly of her father and the ambivalence she had about his sexual abuse. Although the dungeon symbolized how trapped and tormented she felt during the times she was molested, they also were the only times she felt loved and cared for by her father. This was the feeling symbolized by the rainbow dungeon.

There is a general belief that toys with ambiguous meaning and diverse uses foster symbolic play more effectively because they allow the child to project his or her own identity and function onto the toy. However, there may be times when you want to move the child more directly into specific play themes through structured play. In these situations, toys with an obvious identity or function may be selected for a play session (as in addressing themes of parental separation or abuse). Structured play is rarely used until nondirective play has enabled a full assessment of relevant themes and issues, and the child's trust around anxiety-laden issues has been developed.

Purposes of Play Therapy. Play therapy can serve many purposes. A major use is for *catharsis*, the release of strong emotions in order to provide relief from the inner tension they may be causing the child. It is also believed that expressing the themes, even though they may not be conscious for the child, provides some kind of cognitive relief. Catharsis can be facilitated through many forms of play, including drawings, doll play, clay modeling, or the acting-out of certain feelings through pounding toys or punching dolls or bags. Another purpose of play therapy is *abreaction*, the reliving through play of past events and their related feelings. Through abreaction, the child gradually can assimilate previous experiences that have been traumatic or painful. Assimilation occurs through the release of related emotions, as well as through integrating what happened into the child's ongoing view of himself and the world. The basis of this integration is the opportunity, through play, to gain mastery over an experience in which the child most likely had no control. Mastery comes from reenacting the event in the child's own way, working through the feelings that were part of the experience, and modifying, over time, how it happened and what the outcome may have been.

Another frequent use of play therapy is to help the child try out other ways of relating to the world or responding to situations. At about 3 years of age, children have the capacity for role-play. In taking on certain roles, children can learn how others may feel or think (by putting themselves in somebody else's shoes). Role-play can occur through the child's taking on a character himself, or projecting that character onto a puppet or doll.

Therapeutic Interventions. Regardless of the specific purpose of play therapy, your interventions should involve a combination of reflection and interpretation to help the child gain greater awareness of the unconscious issues becoming apparent. *Reflection* involves simple commenting on what is happening in the child's play—for example, "The boy doll is hitting the father doll again." Such a statement includes no interpretation but has the potential to help the child become more aware of what is happening in the play. Reflection is the major intervention used by more inexperienced clinicians, including the generalist nurse.

It is also the mainstay for clinical specialists during their initial work with the child. However, there should be a few sessions of play observation without any reflective comment, to allow the child to gain comfort in the play, before eliciting any anxiety that may arise as a result of reflection.

The use of *interpretation* begins after rapport and trust have been established, and it can range from subtle to very direct. Subtle interpretations are more removed from the child and speak to the potential meaning behind the toy's behavior—for instance, "The boy doll is hitting the father doll because he's very angry at him." More direct interpretations are used over time as the nurse develops greater confidence in the validity of the interpretations for the child—for example, "I wonder if you feel like the boy doll. You seem angry at your dad for leaving." Obviously, these more direct interpretations must integrate anything observed in the play with your total assessment of the child's issues and problems in the real world.

COGNITIVE–BEHAVIORAL THERAPY

The approaches used in cognitive-behavioral therapy stem from cognitive-behavioral theory, described earlier. Two major differences exist between this modality and play therapy. First, cognitive-behavioral approaches focus on the child's conscious rather than unconscious issues. Second, emphasis is placed on more effective coping in the present rather than on mastery over unresolved feelings associated with the child's past experiences. Cognitive–behavioral approaches have been particularly successful in treating problems associated with depression, conduct disorder, ADHD, and anxiety in children 9 and older (Ellis, 1997). Behavioral techniques, without the cognitive component, are also widely used to address therapeutic goals for children with mental retardation, learning and communication disorders, pervasive developmental disorders, tic disorders, and elimination disorders (Mash & Barkley, 1998).

Cognitive Restructuring. Cognitive–behavioral treatment is a reeducation and relearning process involving the development of new ways of thinking about life and new behaviors that are more adaptive and more functional for the child. The cognitive aspects of therapy attempt to modify inaccurate or biased ways of processing information that result in distortions of what is actually occurring in the child's world. This process of cognitive restructuring involves strategies such as finding out what the child means by statements he makes, teaching him to question the "evidence" he's using to maintain any irrational beliefs, helping him identify other options for what a situation might mean, listing advantages and disadvantages of a particular belief, and teaching the child to use self-talk or directives to himself to help change or reframe a situation—for example, "Stop and wait; don't get angry until you find out more." You can coach the child to think differently about problems, thereby helping him more effectively make sense of the world. In this way, the child begins to modify his perceptions of interactions with others and his expectations for the future.

Behavioral Approaches. The behavioral aspects of therapy are based to a great extent on classical and operant conditioning techniques. The major classical conditioning technique is systematic desensitization, which involves the pairing of a negative stimulus (such as a feared situation or animal) with a positive stimulus (such as candy or relaxation exercises). The pairing is done in a progressive way, so the child begins to handle situations that are increasingly fearful or aversive. For example, a child may initially look at pictures of a dog that scares him while having a favorite snack, and progress through a series of more frightening situations. Eventually, the child is asked to touch a dog in the context of many positive rewards, which counteract the negative impact.

Examples of operant conditioning techniques are contingency contracting, the use of tokens, modeling, and behavioral role-play groups. *Contracting* involves setting goals with a child, with specific consequences (positive and negative) clearly identified for achieving or not achieving the goals. *Tokens* can also be used in contracting, whereby points are accumulated or lost depending on the child's following through with agreed-upon behavior. These tokens can then be exchanged for various rewards that are important to the child. When a *modeling* intervention is used, children with specific problems are exposed to real or filmed examples of other children who model effective responses to difficult situations. *Behavioral role-play* takes modeling a step further to help the child try out new behaviors before applying them in the real world.

Milieu Therapy. Cognitive–behavioral approaches, such as the ones just described, serve as the basis for most milieu therapy in child psychiatric inpatient settings. These settings are for children with more severe mental health problems, who may require around-the-clock assessment to determine the exact diagnosis, or intensive, consistent care for life-threatening or violent conditions. The use of behavioral interventions on inpatient units allows nursing staff to give continuous feedback to the children about the appropriateness of their behavior. The children receive rewards such as verbal praise, a sticker, or points for appropriate behavior. For example, children who have a problem hitting others all the time may receive a sticker and verbal praise for no hits hourly, until they associate their behavior with the reward. At that time, the need for feedback may decrease to a less-frequent schedule, and later to the need for only verbal reminders of the desired behavior.

At the same time staff members are trying to reward children for positive behavior, children also need to know that certain hostile or aggressive behaviors cannot be tolerated. When children cannot behave in acceptable ways, you can have them take a time-out from the activity by sitting in chairs until they are able to pull themselves together. If that does not work, the time-out may be taken in a quiet room free of objects and stimulation. If isolation is also too difficult, you may need to use a restraining hold to help them calm down. As children are able to calm down, help them see why they needed a time-out and what they could do differently next time. The goal is to have children learn what precedes episodes during which they get out of control, and learn ways to avoid the negative consequences of out-of-control behavior such as fights with other children. It is through effective limit setting that we can help children separate their feelings from their behavior and learn more adaptive ways of expressing themselves.

CLINICAL EXAMPLE

Jervis was a strong, very large 8-year-old boy with mild retardation. He was on a child psychiatric unit for evaluation after he severely injured another child during a fight. When the other children on the unit would make fun of him or make faces at him, Jervis would strike out at them, often punching and knocking them to the floor. The child psychiatric clinical nurse specialist, Rita, brought the unit staff together to develop a behavioral program for Jervis. Rita also met with Jervis to discuss a behavioral contract with him. Part of this discussion was to identify the things Jervis liked most and least on the unit because these would be used as part of his rewards or sanctions for meeting his part of the contract. For instance, he loved his television time, making cookies with the staff, and playing ball outside in the courtyard. But he disliked helping with clean up after meals and sitting in the corner for a "time-out" from games or other activities. The contract with Jervis was to help him learn better control of his anger when other children teased him. If he ignored the children or came to one of the staff to express his frustration or get their help in resolving the problem, he got a red star. If he struck out at the children, he got a blue dot. These were kept on a bulletin board in his room. For each red star, he could negotiate with staff for an extra something on his list of "likes." For each blue dot, he would either lose a chance to participate in one of his favorite activities or he would have to do something on his list of "dislikes."

Family Involvement. Family involvement in cognitive-behavioral approaches with children is also very common. For instance, you can help parents implement contracting and other behavioral approaches within the home. Involving parents as active members of their child's hospital treatment team has a profound impact on the degree to which the inpatient treatment is carried over into the real world of the child and the family. In both inpatient and outpatient settings, you can work closely with parents to help them understand the use of cognitive-behavioral strategies in their parenting practices. For example, they can learn to apply reward systems and time-outs, as well as help their children use self-talk to better understand situations before they do something impulsively. Remember also to give written and verbal information to parents so that they become truly informed partners in their child's care. The Client/Family Teaching feature below is an example of some useful information for families at various stages in the child's treatment.

FAMILY THERAPY

Family therapy goes beyond family involvement in the child's treatment to focus on treatment of the entire family (Hanna & Brown, 1999). This method is selected when interactions among family members need attention in order to address specific problems exhibited by the child. The goal is to increase the likelihood that improvements in the child's mental health will occur and will be supported in the home with consistent and sustained family patterns (Ziegler & Bush, 1999).

CLINICAL EXAMPLE

The staff on an inpatient unit found they needed to help the parents of Nathan, a 12-year-old boy with conduct disorder, plan his weekend day passes. Nathan reported that he barely saw his parents while home on pass. Both parents worked most of the time, and when they were home, they argued a lot. So Nathan hung out at the local mall with his friends and got into trouble. This situation was interfering with Nathan's recovery and his transition back into the home. The family therapist and primary nurse brought the family together to talk about the issues related to Nathan's use of time on his weekend passes. The overt goal of the first meeting was to help the family better structure Nathan's time and their availability to him. But it became clear that there was a great deal of conflict between the parents as well as much hostility directed at Nathan during the family discussions. Because the family conflict had implications for the success of Nathan's treatment, the entire family was scheduled for a number of therapy sessions.

CLIENT / FAMILY TEACHING

Important Types of Information to Discuss with Families

- The symptoms their child may have as a result of the disorder
- Theories about the causes of their child's problems
- Options for treating the symptoms and the rationale for the recommended treatment
- Potential side effects of any medications used in treatment and how to manage the side effects
- What they can do to help reduce the likelihood of the symptoms occurring
- Specific suggestions for how they can manage various symptoms if they do occur
- Who they should contact regarding concerns they may have about symptoms or medications
- Strategies for coping with their own stress related to the child's problems
- Informational resources and support groups available to assist them

Family therapy approaches are described fully in Chapter 29, but there are a few issues specific to family therapy when children are included.

If children under age 7 are involved in family therapy, the nurse may choose to alternate having the child present and seeing the parents or other family members only. The child's presence provides information for clinical assessment, allows for direct comment on and discussion of the dynamics that occur among parents and children, and provides opportunities for the nurse to model effective interaction with the child, as well as teach the family about normal development and positive parenting. However, there may be issues for discussion that are beyond the child's capacity to understand and/or inappropriate for discussion in front of the child. Meeting with the parents alone enables these issues to be more openly addressed in a setting with fewer distractions.

Family play therapy is another option with young children that enables their full participation. Usually, the first half of the family session involves either directive or nondirective play. In the second half, the parents talk with the therapist about family issues that arose during the play, while the child continues to play or engages in discussion as desired or when invited.

Older children can be involved with more typical family therapy approaches. The developmental status of the child's capabilities and the nature of the child's problems should guide the nurse's decisions with the family regarding the specific strategies to use.

MediaLink Psychiatric Medications: Children

PSYCHOPHARMACOLOGY

The nature of drug therapy is detailed in Chapter 31. However, there are important considerations in using medications with children. First, one can never assume that the actions and side effects of any drug will be the same for children as for adults. Determining the dosage of a drug by body weight is thus not appropriate. Only recently have studies been undertaken to carefully examine the impact of medications on children at various developmental stages. Not only do children at various stages have different medication needs in terms of rates of absorption, excretion, sites of action, and toxicity, but these may change for the same child as he or she develops. Children must, therefore, be carefully monitored, with ongoing titration, if they are kept on a drug over extended periods of time.

Second, the developmental impact of a drug on a child must be weighed alongside the potential benefits it has for a specific mental health problem. Some research has shown that the developing neurotransmitter systems of young children can be very sensitive to medications and it is unclear how this fact may impact their brain development (NIMH, 2000). Medications are often used with children to address a behavioral problem that may be disturbing to their family or teachers, yet their use may interfere with the developmental capacity of the child. For instance, antipsychotic medications such as chlorpromazine (Thorazine) cause cognitive dulling and may interfere with learning. They also cause tardive dyskinesia, movement disorders that occur after chronic use (Conner, Fletcher, & Wood, 2001; Stigler, Potenza, & McDougle, 2001). Stimulants may increase learning potential for children with ADHD, but they can affect the physical growth potential of the child. Such risks have significant implications for children who are developing and who may experience cumulative effects of medications over many years. All the benefits and risks must be balanced against one another in a full and open discussion with the child's family.

Three classes of drugs are most commonly used with children: stimulants, antidepressants, and low-dose antipsychotics. Mood stabilizers and antianxiety agents however, are also prescribed. ■ Table 25–1 outlines these major classes of drugs, their uses and common side effects. Refer to Chapter 31 for a detailed discussion of psychopharmacology. You can refer families to the American Academy of Child and Adolescent Psychiatry Web site for information on children and psychiatric medications (www.aacap.org).

Stimulants. The stimulants most frequently used with children are methylphenidate (Ritalin), pemoline (Cylert), and dextroamphetamine sulfate (Dexedrine), primarily for the treatment of ADHD. Some stimulants have been approved only for children over 6 years of age while others may be used for ages 3 and up. Methylphenidate (Ritalin) appears to have fewer side effects, though dextroamphetamine sulfate (Dexedrine) has a longer duration of action and is less expensive. It is very important to monitor for vital sign changes or signs of depression. An increase in symptoms (rebound effect) may occur as each dose wears off every 3 to 4 hours, so maintaining a consistent schedule for taking the drug is important for the parent or for you as the nurse who manages a child's medication. There has been a fair amount of controversy regarding the long-term effects of stimulants on the growth of children. Some studies have found deficits in weight and height for children treated with these drugs. But other research suggests that growth catches up once the stimulant is discontinued. No studies however, have looked at growth effects in children treated continually from childhood through adolescence. Until then, we won't know whether growth deficits are persistent and whether they are the result of stimulant use versus some maturational delays related to ADHD itself.

Antidepressants. Of the three types of antidepressants, tricyclic antidepressants (TCAs) have been the most widely used with children, especially imipramine (Tofranil). But they can create cardiac rate and rhythm changes (a greater risk for children than adults) and can be highly toxic if overdosed accidentally by a child. Because of these issues, adults must closely supervise their administration and keep the medication in a safe place. The selective serotonin reuptake inhibitors (SSRIs) such as sertraline (Zoloft) and fluvoxamine (Luvox) are being carefully evaluated for use with children and appear to be working well. Because of their fewer side effects, it is highly likely that the SSRIs will become the drugs of choice for treating depression and obsessive–compulsive behavior in children. Monoamine oxidase inhibitors (MAOIs) are rarely used for children because they require careful dietary control to prevent untoward interactions. Such control is very difficult for children.

Antipsychotics. Antipsychotics (also called neuroleptics) are less effective in reducing psychotic symptoms for children

TABLE 25–1 Classes of Drugs Used With Children

Drug Class	Disorders Treated	Side Effects
Stimulants	ADHD	Anorexia and weight loss
	Conduct disorder	Abdominal pain
	Mental retardation	Headache
	PDD	Sadness or mood lability, irritability
Antidepressants	Depression	Fatigue, drowsiness
	OCD	Nausea, upset stomach
	Enuresis	Dry mouth
	Separation anxiety	Constipation
	ADHD	Anorexia
	Tourette's disorder	Restlessness, agitation, headaches, dizziness, insomnia
Antipsychotics	Schizophrenia	Sedation, lethargy
	Tourette's disorder	Cognitive dulling
	PDD	Tardive dyskinesia
	Severe conduct disorder	Weight gain, tremor, rigidity, drooling
Mood stabilizers	Bipolar disorder	Tremor
	Mental retardation	Weight gain
	PDD	Enuresis, hypothyroidism
Antianxiety agents	Anxiety disorders	Fatigue, drowsiness
	Sleep disorders	Addiction

than they are for adults. In addition, children don't respond as well to the medication used to control the acute extrapyramidal side effects (e.g., tremor or drooling) of the more traditional antipsychotic drugs. Last, tardive dyskinesia (involuntary problems with movement) and cognitive blunting can have major implications for a child's academic potential and ability to function effectively later in life. The newer antipsychotics such as clozapine (Clozaril) have fewer of these side effects than the typical antipsychotics like haloperidol (Haldol) or thioridiazine (Mellaril) and also appear more effective in reducing psychotic symptoms for children. Only haloperidol (Haldol) and thioridiazine (Mellaril), however, have FDA approval for young children between 3 and 18. It's important for you to be aware of the sometimes inappropriate use of antipsychotics to reduce agitated behavior or sedate children with mental retardation or pervasive developmental disorders (PDD). Although drugs like haloperidol (Haldol) may be appropriate for some children who could injure themselves or others, drugs should not be used as a substitute for careful supervision or behavioral interventions that could modify and control problem behaviors.

Mood Stabilizers. Lithium carbonate (Lithane) is the mood stabilizer used with children. Its primary use, however, is for aggression and agitation across a variety of disorders (e.g., mental retardation or PDD) rather than for managing mania; evidence of mania is rare before adolescence. In general, children have a poorer response to lithium than do adults. In addition, children under 7 are more prone to side effects of lithium than are older youth or adults, so its use must be cautiously considered. The potential hypothyroidism that may result from the use of lithium has especially negative consequences for a child because of the impact of thyroid disease on so many facets of development.

Anxiolytics. Benzodiazepines such as diazepam (Valium) and chlordiazepoxide (Librium) are only infrequently used with children. Most clinicians believe that symptoms of anxiety or sleep disturbances should be treated first with psychosocial interventions or perhaps antidepressants unless these methods have proved unsuccessful and the symptoms are causing severe impairment or distress for the child. Remember that benzodiazepines can become addictive if used over a period of time so they are normally discontinued after a few weeks.

Nursing Interventions. Nurses play an important role in monitoring the child on medication and educating the child and parents about the medication.

- Monitor side effects daily in inpatient settings and weekly in outpatient settings.
- If the child is being treated in an outpatient setting, work closely with parents and teachers to record the child's behavior.
- Assess the concerns the child has about side effects and stigmatization by peers related to the medication.
- Take time to assess the parents' beliefs and fears about the medications. Parents are often concerned about the potential for the child to become dependent on medication, as well as its side effects. Give parents an opportunity to discuss their worries and questions and become informed about the medication.

- Prepare the child and the parents for a potential increase in symptoms when a medication is removed or decreased. Plan other interventions to help the child and family at this time.

Evaluation

The purpose of evaluation is to determine whether interventions are effective and how you should modify your care if necessary. The focus of evaluation should be on the nursing outcomes you have identified in your work with a particular child. But it's important to choose concrete and observable aspects of the child's behavior. Tangible changes or improvements are more readily assessed than vague statements that cannot be measured or observed in some way. For example, assessing an increase in the child's self-esteem is very difficult, but evaluating specific behaviors indicating esteem (such as positive statements about self or improved grooming) will make your evaluation easier and more useful.

SITUATIONAL AND DEVELOPMENTAL CONTEXT

Acquiring input from as many sources as possible is also essential to effective evaluation of children. Have you obtained information from the child, parents, other nursing staff, or school personnel? Depending on the situation, it may or may not be possible to conduct a comprehensive evaluation, but it should be your goal whenever possible. Finally, outcome criteria for evaluation must be congruent with appropriate developmental and sociocultural expectations. Frustration tolerance, for example, is far different in the 4-year-old than the 14-year-old. For this reason, an accurate evaluation must consider the norms for age-appropriateness. Similarly, expectations should take into consideration the child's sociocultural norms. For instance, a child who exhibits aggressiveness or informality with adults may have had such behaviors encouraged at home, yet they are viewed by the larger society as disrespectful toward authority. Children need to fit in with their own communities and social context as well as society as a whole, so these factors must be weighed as various outcomes are identified for your interventions.

SELF-EVALUATION

In addition to the outcome criteria you establish to assess the effectiveness of your interventions, another critical feature of evaluation is the ongoing review and evaluation of your own process as a child psychiatric nurse.

CLINICAL EXAMPLE

Eleven-year-old Luisa had a history of living with extended family and several hospitalizations. Luisa's mother was ambivalent toward her, often openly rejecting her (such as limited visitations and missed family sessions). Luisa's predicament stimulated a lot of feeling among the staff about bad mothers and good mothers, and the staff was protective of the child and angry at the mother. The staff was encouraged to examine the mother's own deprivation by an abusive mother and the difficulties in raising this very troubled child.

Are you aware of your attitudes and behaviors in working with specific children? How are these affecting your interventions with each child? For some key areas to consider in evaluating your potential impact, see the accompanying Nursing Self-Awareness feature.

Working with children, particularly children with emotional problems, may activate feelings about your own unresolved issues with your family of origin or current family. You may then react as if the child is feeling or acting in ways that you might have felt or acted, and project your own issues onto the child, rather than responding to their actual therapeutic needs. Nurses may also respond to children or parents with certain stereotyped attitudes or beliefs, rather than being open to each child and parent as individuals. Self-awareness and ongoing self-monitoring are essential skills for child psychiatric nurses to acquire. Without this capacity, we can have little assurance that we will be truly therapeutic in providing nursing care.

Case Management, Community-Based Care, and Home Care

All of the content within this chapter applies to care of children within both inpatient and outpatient settings. It is important, however, to note that advanced practice nurses who are specialists in child psychiatry are now assuming growing responsibilities as primary care providers, case managers, counselors, and

***Nursing* SELF-AWARENESS**

Promoting Aware Child Psychiatric Nursing

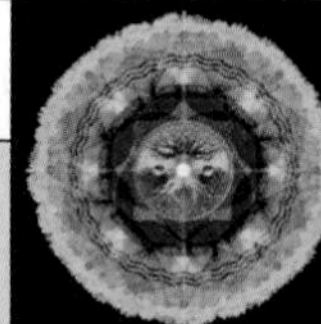

To assist you in your own self-growth and in examining your attitudes and behavior toward child psychiatric clients, answer the following:

Attitudes

- What do I like about this child?
- What don't I like about this child?
- Is there anything about this child's personality or problems that reminds me of myself or my own childhood?
- What feelings arise in me when I'm working with this child? What is it about the child or me that might cause these feelings?

Behavior

- How are my views/feelings about this child affecting the way I relate to the child? How are they helping my therapeutic work? How are they hindering my therapeutic work?
- How is the child responding to my interventions?

Self-Growth

- What am I learning about myself as I work with this child?
- Am I fully exploring these issues with my supervisor so that I can improve both my working relationship with this child and my insight as a child psychiatric nurse?

crisis team members in community mental health agencies. Because mental health work with children entails close relationships with parents and school systems, the nurse's role in the community typically involves visits to the home and school as well as contacts with the juvenile justice system, family shelters, foster care placements, and social services. The community-based child psychiatric–mental health nurse has multiple responsibilities including risk assessment, medication monitoring, symptom management, supportive counseling, teaching, and coordination of overall care.

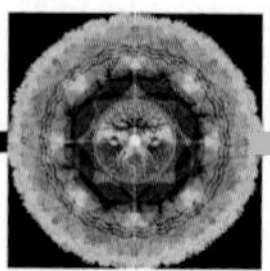

EXPLORE MediaLink

NCLEX review, case studies, and other interactive resources for this chapter can be found on the Companion Website at http://www.prenhall.com/kneisl. Click on Chapter 25 to select the activities for this chapter.

For animations, video tutorials, more NCLEX review questions, and an audio glossary, access the accompanying CD-ROM in this textbook.

BIBLIOGRAPHY

American Psychiatric Association (2000). *Diagnostic and statistical manual of mental disorders* (4th ed., Text Revision) (DSM-IV-TR). Washington, DC: Author.

Boris, N., Wheeler, E., Heller, S., & Zeanah, C. (2000). Attachment and developmental psychopathology. *Psychiatry, 63*(1), 75–84.

Bosch, J., & Ringdahl, J. (2001). Functional analysis of problem behavior in children with mental retardation. *American Journal of Maternal Child Nursing, 26*(6), 307–311.

Brue, A., & Oakland, T. (2002). Alternative treatments for attention-deficit/hyperactivity disorder: Does evidence support their use? *Alternative Therapies in Health and Medicine, 8*(1), 68–70.

Cassidy, J., & Shaver, P. (1999). *Handbook of attachment*. New York: Guilford Press.

Charney, D., Nestler, E., & Bunney, B. (1999). *The neurobiology of mental illness*. New York: Oxford University Press.

Chethik, M. (2000). *Techniques of child therapy: Psychodynamic strategies*. New York: Guilford Press.

Conner, D., Fletcher, K., & Wood, J. (2001). Neuroleptic-related dyskinesias in children and adolescents. *Journal of Clinical Psychiatry, 62*(12), 967–974.

Department of Health and Human Services (2001). *Surgeon General's report on child mental health*. Rockville, Maryland: Public Health Service.

Dilts, S. (2001). *Models of the mind: A framework for biopsychosocial psychiatry*. Philadelphia: Brunner-Routledge.

Dulcan, M., & Martini, D. (1999). *A concise guide to child and adolescent psychiatry*. Washington, DC: American Psychiatric Press.

Eikeseth, S., Smith, T., Jahr, E., & Eldevik, S. (2002). Intensive behavioral treatment at school for 4- to 7-year-old children with autism. *Behavior Modification, 26*(1), 49–68.

Ellis, A. (1997). *The practice of rational emotive therapy*. New York: Springer.

Gabbard, G. (1994). *Psychodynamic psychotherapy in clinical practice*. New York: American Psychiatric Association.

Goldman, L., Genel, M., Bezman, R., & Slanetz, R. (1998). Diagnosis and treatment of attention-deficit/hyperactivity disorder in children and adolescents. *Journal of the American Medical Association, 279*, 1100–1107.

Green, G., Brennan, L., & Fein, D. (2002). Intensive behavioral treatment for a toddler at risk for autism. *Behavioral Modification, 26*(1), 69–102.

Hanna, S., & Brown, J. (1999). *The practice of family therapy: Key elements across models*. Belmont, CA: Brooks/Cole.

Heyne, D., King, N., Tonge, B., & Cooper, H. (2001). School refusal: Epidemiology and management. *Pediatric Drugs, 3*(10), 719–732.

Kohlenberg, T., Joseph, H., Prudent, N., & Richardson, V. (1995). Cultural responses to behavioral problems. In S. Parker & B. Zuckerman (Eds.), *Behavioral and developmental pediatrics* (pp. 353–358). Boston: Little, Brown.

Lieberman, A., Silverman, R., & Pawl, J. (2000). Infant-parent psychotherapy: Core concepts and current approaches. In C. Zeanah (Ed.), *Handbook of infant mental health* (pp. 472–484). New York: Guilford Press.

Lieberman, J., & Tasman, A. (2000). *Psychiatric drugs*. Philadelphia: Saunders.

Lyon, D. E., & Morgan-Judge, T. (2000). Childhood depressive disorders. *Journal of Nursing Scholarship, 16*(3), 26–31.

Mash, E., & Barkley, R. (1998). *Treatment of childhood disorders*. New York: Guilford Press.

Masters, K., Bellonci, C., Bernet, W., Arnold, V., Beitchman, J., Stevens, P., et al. (2002). Practice parameter for the prevention and management of aggressive behavior in child and adolescent psychiatric institutions, with special reference to seclusion and restraint. *Journal of the American Academy of Child and Adolescent Psychiatry, 42*(2), 4S–25S.

Miller, M., Azrael, D., & Hemenway, D. (2002). Firearm availability and unintentional firearm deaths, suicide, and homicide among 5–14 year olds. *Journal of Trauma, 52*(2), 267–275.

Montgomery, P. (2001). Media-based behavioral treatments for behavioral disorders in children. *Cochrane Database System Review, 1*, CD002206.

Muratori, F., Picchi, L., Casella, C., Tancredi, R., Milone, A., & Patarnello, M. (2002). Efficacy of brief dynamic psychotherapy for children with emotional disorders. *Psychotherapy and Psychosomatics, 71*(1), 28–38.

National Institute of Mental Health (2000). *Treatment of children with mental disorders*. Rockville, Maryland: Department of Health and Human Services, Public Health Service. NIH Publication # 00-4702.

Nelson, C., & Bosquet, M. (2000). Neurobiology of fetal and infant development: Implications for infant mental health. In C. Zeanah (Ed.), *Handbook of infant mental health* (pp. 337–359). New York: Guilford Press.

Paris, J. (1999). *Nature and nurture in psychiatry: A predisposition-stress model of mental disorders*. Washington, DC: American Psychiatric Press.

Perry, B. (1999). Effects of traumatic events on children. *In maltreated children: Experience, brain development and the next generation* (pp. 2–23). New York: Norton.

Sameroff, A. & Fiese, B. (1999). Transactional regulation: The developmental ecology of early intervention. In S. J. Meisels & J. Shonkoff (Eds.), *Early intervention: A handbook of theory, practice and analysis*. New York: Cambridge University Press.

Schaefer, C. (1999). *Innovative psychotherapy techniques in child and adolescent therapy*. New York: John Wiley & Sons.

Schore, A. (2001). Contributions from the "decade of the brain" to infant mental health. *Infant Mental Health Journal, 22*(1–2), 1–69.

Schortt, A., Barrett, P., & Fox, T. (2001). Evaluating the FRIENDS program: A cognitive–behavioral group treatment for anxious children and their parents. *Journal of Clinical Child Psychology, 30*(4), 525–535.

Stigler, K., Potenza, M., & McDougle, C. (2001). Tolerability profile of atypical antipsychotics in children and adolescents. *Pediatric Drugs, 3*(12), 927–942.

Webster-Stratton, C., Reid, J., & Hammond, M. (2001). Social skills and problem-solving training for children with early-onset conduct problems: Who benefits? *Journal of Child Psychology and Psychiatry, 42*(7), 943–952.

Weinfield, N., Sroufe, L., Egeland, B., & Carlson, E. (1999). The nature of individual differences in infant–caregiver attachment (pp. 68–88). In J. Cassidy & P. Shaver (Eds.), *Handbook of attachment*. New York: Guilford Press.

Weiss, S., Goebel, P., Page, A., Wilson, P., & Warda, M. (1999). The impact of cultural and familial context on behavioral and emotional problems of preschool Latino children. *Child Psychiatry and Human Development, 29*(4), 287–301.

Wilens, T., Spencer, T., & Biederman, J. (2000). Pharmacotherapy of attention-deficit/hyperactivity disorder. In T. Brown (Ed.), *Attention-deficit disorders and comorbidities in children, adolescents and adults* (pp. 509–535). Washington, DC: American Psychiatric Press.

Zeanah, C. Danis, B., Hirshberg, L, Benoit, D., Miller, D. & Heller, S. (1999). Disorganized attachment associated with partner violence. *Infant Mental Health Journal, 20*, 77–86.

Zeigler, R., & Bush, A. (1999). *Sharing care: The integration of family approaches with child treatment*. Philadelphia, PA: Brunner/Mazel.

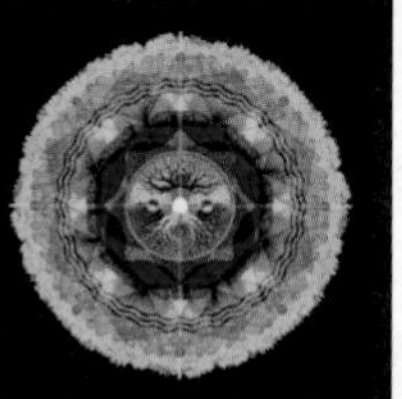

Adolescents

CAROL BRADLEY-CORPUEL

26

Chapter TWENTY-SIX

FOCUS QUESTIONS

- **What is the relevance of biologic and developmental data in the assessment of adolescents?**
- **Why is a humanistic interactionist perspective important in a comprehensive assessment of adolescent problems?**
- **Can you give an example of an adolescent acting out a "life script"?**
- **How would you construct a client contract for use with an adolescent in treatment?**
- **Why is a keen self-awareness of your own adolescence and unresolved issues important when working with adolescents?**

KEY TERMS

acting-out
ecstasy (MDMA)
life script
scapegoating

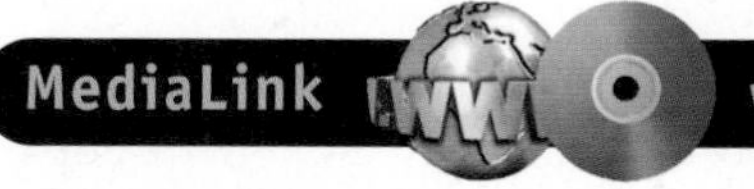

www.prenhall.com/kneisl

Additional resources for this chapter can be found on the Student CD-ROM accompanying this textbook, and on the Companion Website at www.prenhall.com/kneisl. Click on Chapter 26 to select the activities for this chapter.

CD-ROM
- Audio Glossary
- NCLEX Review

Companion Website
- Additional NCLEX Review
- Care Plan: Acting Out Teenager
- Case Study: Psychoeducation in the School

CHAPTER OUTLINE

CROSS REFERENCES

Other topics relevant to this content are: ANA Standards of Psychiatric–Mental Health Nursing, Chapter 1; Behavioral contracts, Chapter 30; Cultural competence, Chapter 6; Depression, Chapter 15; Developmental theories, Chapter 2; Drug abuse, Chapter 13; Eating disorders, Chapter 18; Family assessment and interventions, Chapter 29; Milieu therapy, Chapter 11; Psychobiology, Chapter 4; Suicide, Chapter 22; Therapeutic communication, Chapter 8; Violence in the psychiatric setting, Chapter 34.

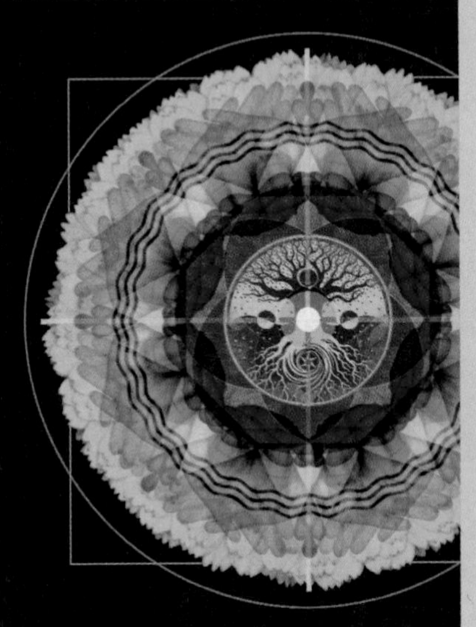

CRITICAL THINKING CHALLENGE

Your 15-year-old patient, Angela Cook, informs you that her mother has sent her to your community clinic for contraception and information on “safe sex.” Your own personal beliefs advocate sexual abstinence before marriage for religious as well as preventive health reasons. Moreover, you feel compelled to be a “better parent” to this young girl and feel inclined to dissuade her from sexual intercourse at this early age.

How do you reconcile your own personal convictions with the client’s need for preventive health care and education? ■

What is adolescence? Some sources define it simply as the time of physical and psychosocial development between the ages of 12 and 20. Others describe it as a period of "normal psychosis." Still others see it as an attempt by a tyrannical subculture to overtake adult America. It is not necessary to accept the latter two definitions verbatim to understand their implications. Most people recognize the immense stress that occurs during adolescence and the importance that managing the stress has for an adolescent's future.

Whether a generalist or clinical specialist, the nurse in today's health care setting integrates professional capabilities, skills, and roles to intervene with adolescents to achieve optimal social, emotional, cognitive, and physical development. Using expertise in identifying relevant deviations in the developmental process, the nurse works closely with the systems (family, school, community, and institution) on which adolescents are emotionally and economically dependent.

Trying to understand adolescents is a challenge to anyone. For the nurse who chooses to work with adolescents, the challenge offers considerable rewards. Nurses who can recollect their own experiences and reactions during this tumultuous time will better appreciate the dilemma of adolescent clients.

Biopsychosocial Theories

A sound theoretic knowledge base helps you differentiate between the "normal" and "abnormal," or the usual and unusual, behaviors of adolescents. In particular, you can do a comprehensive assessment by focusing on the psychologic development of the individual and the evolution of the adolescent as a biopsychosocial being. You can accomplish the first task with an understanding of developmental theory and the second with an appreciation of biologic and humanistic interactionist theories.

BIOLOGIC THEORY

Psychiatric–mental health nursing in the twenty-first century requires that you integrate a biologic focus into your practice, to accommodate both changing client needs and an expanding biologic knowledge base. An appreciation of hormonal changes, growth spurts, stress and immune function, chronic illness, depression, and other mental disorders can help you evaluate adolescents from a more effective and comprehensive perspective.

Findings of Neuroimaging

More specifically, in recent years clinician researchers have begun the use of neuroimaging in children and adolescents. For example, magnetic resonance imaging (MRI) and spectroscopy are being used to better delineate the anatomic, functional, and biochemical defects of mood disorders in children and adolescents. Findings such as reduced prefrontal cortex volumes in depressed subjects, reduced metabolite levels with lithium treatment in manic patients, and increased neurochemical compounds in the temporal and frontal lobes of adolescents with bipolar disorder seem to be contributing to the increasing evidence that bipolar disorder in children and adolescents is similar to that in adults (Botteron, 1999; Davanzo, 1999; Moore, 1999). Such biologic findings in the brain may help make the case that these youth have a "medical" disorder, allowing them to obtain medical coverage for their debilitating illness from third-party payers. Equally profound is the correlation that neuroscientists have established between aggressivity and brain levels of corresponding neurotransmitters. Study results of limbic deficits and uncontrolled aggression in monkeys reared in isolation now have human correlates. Specifically, studies of physically and emotionally neglected children reveal distinct neurophysiologic deficits, such as diminished neurons and corresponding neurochemical changes. These findings contribute more objective data to the importance of the more subjective experience of parental–child bonding (Lewis, Amini, & Lannon, 2000).

Effects of Chronic Illness

Of equal importance in the literature has become the effect of chronic illness on the adolescent's mental health. Asthma, head injury, diabetes, epilepsy, and many of the less common chronic physical diseases can result in depression. Equally at risk for depression are adolescents with various learning disabilities or specific neuropsychiatric illnesses, such as attention deficit/hyperactivity disorders (ADD/ADHD); disruptive behavior disorders; tic disorders; eating disorders; anxiety disorders, including obsessive–compulsive disorder (OCD) and post-traumatic stress disorder (PTSD); and schizophrenia and related conditions (American Psychiatric Association [APA], 2000).

Effects of Psychotropic Medications

There is increasing impetus to study the clinically significant effects that various psychotropic medications may have on the brain when administered during the developing phase that spans from birth through adolescence. The National Institute of Mental Health (NIMH), the National Institute of Child Health and Human Development (NICHD), and the National Institute on Drug Abuse (NIDA) have requested research grant applications to study the clinical use of psychotherapeutic medications in children and adolescents. In particular, this program incentive, entitled "Developmental Psychopharmacology," is related to Mental Health and Mental Disorders and Biology of Brain Disorders, one of the priority areas of the *Healthy People 2010* initiative. The U.S. Public Health Service is committed to achieving the health promotion and disease prevention objectives of this comprehensive, nationwide agenda. *Healthy People 2010* contains 467 objectives organized into 28 focus areas, each reflecting the identified major health concerns in the United States at the beginning of the twenty-first century. A limited set of the objectives, known as the Leading Health Indicators, are:

1. Physical Activity
2. Overweight and Obesity
3. Tobacco Use
4. Substance Abuse
5. Responsible Sexual Behavior

6. Mental Health
7. Injury and Violence
8. Environmental Quality
9. Immunization
10. Access to Health Care (U.S. Department of Health and Human Services [DHHS], 1999a)

DEVELOPMENTAL THEORY

An understanding of developmental theory helps you identify deviations in adolescent growth and development processes and intervene appropriately. The theories of Freud, Erikson, and Sullivan provide considerable insight into the adolescent's struggle to attain adulthood.

The development of an adolescent's sense of identity entails a preoccupation with self-image. It also entails a connection between future role and past experiences. In the search for a new sense of sameness and continuity, many adolescents must repeat the crisis resolutions of earlier years to integrate these past elements and establish the lasting ideals of a final identity. According to Erikson, these crisis periods or stages are reviews of the adolescent's sense of trust, autonomy, initiative, and industry, in that order. Equally important for an adolescent's development is cognition. Piaget's research revealed three stages of cognitive development. The third stage, called formal operations, develops between ages 12 and 14 and results in the adolescent's ability to conceptualize on an adult level. The adolescent has the capacity to think abstractly, to be self-reflective, and to adopt a multidimensional perspective on problems. (For a discussion of developmental theories as they relate to adolescent growth and development, see Chapter 2.)

HUMANISTIC INTERACTIONIST THEORY

As a nurse, you not only need knowledge about developmental theories and psychobiology, you must also integrate humanistic interactionist principles into assessment and interventions to develop a trusting, caring interpersonal relationship with adolescent clients. The adolescent developmental period is a time in the individual's life when identity, values, and goals are in a state of flux. You should take into account not only the immediate situation but also the impact of the developmental stage; the social, ethnic, and cultural factors; family influences; and psychodynamic conflicts on the adolescent's behavior.

In order to accomplish this, you must explore the meaning of the identified problem or behavior. The list of questions in Box 26–1 can help guide this exploration.

It is insufficient to base the nursing response to the adolescent's needs and dilemmas solely on behaviors without a more comprehensive evaluation of these other factors. This approach can lead to ineffective treatment, a temporary ceasing of the initial behaviors with an upheaval of symptoms in another area, and possibly a sterile treatment environment without any meaningful therapeutic alliance. Only by considering all aspects of the adolescent client as a biopsychosocial being can you truly understand the meanings of such behaviors to the client and intervene effectively in the situation.

BOX 26–1 Exploring the Meaning of an Adolescent's Identified Problem or Behavior

- What meaning does this behavior or problem hold for the adolescent?
- What message is he or she conveying through this behavior?
- What impact does this problem have on the client in this developmental stage? Is this a usual or unusual problem or behavior for the adolescent's peer group?
- How have resulting changes, if any, affected the adolescent and his or her relationships with others?
- What goals does the client have for the immediate and distant future?
- What personal strengths does the adolescent have to help deal with this problem?
- What considerations have you and the client given to other developmental, familial, biologic, or sociocultural factors involved?

The Role of the Nurse

The nurse can assume numerous roles within a variety of treatment modalities to help maintain the health and well-being of adolescent clients and identify abnormal or problem-causing behavior during this difficult period of development. Studies suggest that 15% to 25% of children and adolescents suffer from some type of mental health disorder and that 50% to 80% of this population do not receive adequate mental health care (Post, Carr, & Weigand, 1998).

IN THE OUTPATIENT SETTING

In the changing world of health care the outpatient arena for services to adolescents yields many diverse roles for the psychiatric–mental health nurse.

As a Community Health Nurse

In the school, clinic, or community health agency, you have excellent opportunities to observe adolescents engaging in the normal activities of daily living. You have frequent occasions to counsel adolescents in the problems that confront them daily and to advise school or clinic staff members in their encounters with adolescents. The nurse who knows how to deal with normal adolescent problems will also be adept in identifying obstacles to effective resolution of emotional problems and suggesting further treatment.

Within the School. School is the most influential experience in an adolescent's life outside the home. Adolescents spend more waking time in school activities than in any other activity, and most of their successes, problems, and conflicts are demonstrated in the school setting. Even adolescents who are supposedly truant from school are often on the school grounds, perhaps meeting their friends at lunch-time, playing cards in the library, or "hanging out" on the school steps. Such an "absent" student may suddenly appear at the school nurse's door because of "boredom" or a physical complaint.

Unfortunately, the school nurse's role in the early recognition and treatment of predelinquent individuals has been minimized or has gone unrecognized. There are several reasons for this. One reason is that school administrators and teachers tend to view the school nurse as a person who deals only with physical sickness and medical emergencies. They may not be aware that because of the intimate quality of a nurse–client relationship or the comprehensive and holistic nature of nursing assessments, the nurse may be helpful in exploring an area of conflict in an adolescent's life or intervening with a disruptive student. Such early intervention could prevent more serious problems in later years. Many studies have indicated a direct correlation between the problems of early school life and family dysfunction and the incidence of subsequent juvenile delinquency, depression, and suicidal behavior. (American Medical Association [AMA], 2000; APA, 2000; Berenson, 1998; Lewinsohn, Rohde, Seeley, Klein, & Gotlib, 2000; Muscari, 1999; Post et al., 1998). See Box 26–2 for a list of problems demonstrated by adolescents in the school setting that call for early intervention.

Another reason is that administrators tend to limit the nurse's activities to the school itself. They may see no need for the nurse to make home visits to meet with a sick student's family or view problems first-hand. Many school districts lack the time and money to provide for counseling families or individuals in a formal setting. As the role of the independent nursing practitioner expands, and as legislation for third-party reimbursement for independent practice becomes a reality in more states, nurses will be better able to assume more autonomy and responsibility in meeting student needs more comprehensively and effectively.

Within Community-Based Care. The nurse who is employed in the community agency can seize every opportunity to provide an active school health program and to educate school administrators and faculty members about the importance of preventive care. For example, the nurse in a viable school health program can provide preventive counseling not only to troubled adolescents in school but also to their preschool siblings during routine home visits. Nurses can establish productive relationships with teachers, help other faculty members encourage parent-teacher conferences, take an active part in developing the curriculum, and help adolescents on probation or parole return to school.

Within Social Programs. The many problems encountered by today's youth—substance abuse, teenage pregnancy, family violence, street crime, and school failure—are increasingly being recognized in professional, community, and social arenas. The American Academy of Child and Adolescent Psychiatry (AACAP) has developed various tools to disseminate information. The AACAP Facts for Families and the Violence Fact Sheet are two such options to inform lay persons and professionals of the incidence of violent behavior among our youth. See Box 26–3 for a summary of the Violence Fact Sheet (AACAP, 1999). Reports of the Surgeon General are well established as landmark publications on selected topic areas. Recent examples directly impacting adolescents include the Surgeon General's Report on Mental Health and the Surgeon General's Report on Youth Violence (DHHS, 1999b, 1999d). Various committees and organizations are coordinating efforts to stem the tide of youth violence. In a recent news conference, the Commission for the Prevention of Youth Violence outlined a 65-page report emphasizing that nurses, physicians, and public health experts must work together to uphold the cornerstone of prevention in

MediaLink Case Study: Psychoeducation in the School

BOX 26–2 Problems Demonstrated by Adolescents in the School Setting That Call for Early Intervention

- Antisocial behaviors such as stealing, setting fires, bullying others
- Avoidant social behavior
- Chronic illness
- Depression
- Disruptive classroom behavior
- Substance abuse
- Excessive daydreaming
- Hypochondriasis
- Learning difficulties
- Poor school performance, or a dramatic shift in school performance
- Temper tantrums

BOX 26–3 Violence Fact Sheet: American Academy of Child and Adolescent Psychiatry

- In 1996, the National Center on Child Abuse and Neglect reported 969,018 cases of violent crimes committed against children.
- In 1996–1997, 10% of all public schools reported at least one serious violent crime to police or law enforcement (Bureau of Justice Statistics and Office of Juvenile Justice and Delinquency Prevention, U.S. Department of Justice, 1999).
- Gunshot wounds to children ages 16 and under have increased 300 percent in major urban areas since 1986.
- According to FBI reports 2,900 juveniles were arrested for murder in 1996.
- Estimates indicate that as many as 5,000 children die each year as a result of mistreatment and abuse from parents or guardians.
- Every day in America 16 children and youths are killed by firearms (Children's Defense Fund, 1998).
- Nearly a million U.S. students took guns to school during 1998 (Parents Resource Institute for Drug Education, 1999).
- Each year 123,400 children are arrested for violent crimes in the U.S. (Office of Juvenile Justice and Juvenile Delinquency Prevention, 1997).
- Persons under age 25 make up nearly 50 percent of all victims of a serious violent crime (The Institute for Youth Development, 1998).

Source: Reprinted with the permission of the American Academy of Child and Adolescent Psychiatry, copyright 2003.

dealing with youth violence (AMA, 2000). In stating that more school suspensions and more prisons "are not the answer," the commission outlined seven interrelated priorities for preventing youth violence:

1. Support the development of healthy families.
2. Promote healthy communities.
3. Enhance services for early identification and intervention for children, youth and families at risk for or involved in violence.
4. Increase access to health and mental health care services.
5. Reduce access to and risk from firearms for children and youth.
6. Reduce exposure to media violence.
7. Ensure national support and advocacy for solutions to violence through research, public policy, legislation, and funding.

The National Library of Medicine has compiled the Current Bibliography on Youth Violence Prevention Resources. This extensive listing can be found at www.nlm.nih.gov/pubs/cbm/youthviolence.html through a resource link provided on the Companion Website for this book.

MediaLink Youth Violence Prevention

Research has demonstrated that innovative social programs can be effective alternatives to hospitalization or incarceration. Recent data from the National Youth Survey (NYS), a long-term study of violent offenders, point compellingly to the influence of the adolescent offender's peer group. Many well-intended attempts to rehabilitate severely delinquent youths typically place them in settings with other delinquents such as "group homes." One alternative is the Therapeutic Foster Care program. Serious and chronic delinquents (i.e., with an average of 14 arrests, including 4 for felonies) are placed in the homes of carefully selected couples who are specially trained for working with these troubled youth. Evaluations of this program thus far indicate that it is more effective in reducing delinquency than the usual group home placement, is less expensive, and has fewer runaways and fewer program failures (National Institute of Mental Health [NIMH], 1999b). Another home-based model of therapy is Multisystemic Therapy (MST). MST therapists work in collaboration with the family, identifying and using family-identified strengths, goals and treatment strategies to change how the youth function in their natural settings at home, in school, and in their neighborhoods. MST therapists working in the home have small caseloads and are available 24 hours a day, 7 days a week. Treatment teams usually consist of professional counselors, crisis caseworkers, and psychiatrists or psychologists who provide the clinical supervision. In a series of randomized clinical trials in comparison with control groups, MST has proven effective in reducing long-term rates of criminal offenses (even 4 years posttreatment), in reducing long-term rates of rearrest by 25% to 70%, and in reducing the rates for out-of-home placements (NIMH, 1999a).

With the promise for change that these innovations bring, community health nurses are in a prime position to play a key role in the movement toward proactive partnerships among schools, families, and the community in enhancing the health and ensuring the future of our nation's youth.

As a Nurse Counselor/Therapist

Whether in the clinic, home, school, or community health setting, the psychiatric nurse has many opportunities to organize individual, group, or family counseling sessions. Nurses can function within a variety of treatment roles, according to their experience and capabilities.

As an Individual Therapist. The nurse's qualifications and role in the clinic, school, or community setting may allow for counseling adolescents on an individual basis. Sometimes the nurse can establish a trusting alliance and facilitate communication with the client. Sometimes, however, the adolescent is too threatened to talk openly with the nurse in this intimate setting. Some adolescents view the nurse as an authority figure and resist all efforts to communicate. You may make more headway with this mode of treatment when it is used in conjunction with group therapy. Unless certified to provide this service, you should counsel the adolescent only for the purposes of identifying the problem area and referring the client to a qualified professional for individual psychotherapy.

As a Group Therapist. It is usually more effective to work with adolescents in a group. Because the values, acceptance, and recognition of peers are so important during adolescence, the group can provide the support for dealing with problems and effecting change. In addition, involving the adolescent's peers helps dilute the conflict with adults that may exist in one-to-one work. In the school setting, health education groups can provide an acceptable forum for peer interaction and discussion of difficult topics. Otherwise, the nurse should practice as a group therapist only as a certified individual or with adequate supervision by a certified individual. Knowledge of group dynamics is crucial to be an effective group leader.

As a Family Therapist. Being a parent of a "normal" adolescent is difficult, at best. As the child grows into adulthood with all its perplexing questions and problems, parents normally worry about their child's safety and well-being. They may feel rejected because they are no longer needed in the same way. Because many parents of relatively normal adolescents share this plight, they can usually find receptive listeners who will give them comfort and support.

The problems of the parents of emotionally disturbed adolescents are more complicated. Many such parents have a strong sense of failure because their children did not turn out "right." Their feelings of guilt, frustration, and helplessness are likely to increase if their child is institutionalized. They probably felt confused and resentful when experts offered them smug and guilt-provoking advice. Unlike the parents of other adolescents, these parents may have no one in whom to confide, either because they lack the support and understanding of others, or because their own self-reproach prevents them from seeking out such confidants.

Meetings with family members may be indicated if the adolescent's role in the family seems to compound the problems presented in the school or agency setting. An important part of the problem-solving process is organizing initial interviews with parents and family members. Use the information gathered during these meetings to determine whether the problems stem from difficulties posed by the larger system (the family), and, if so, whether family therapy is indicated.

Show compassion and understanding for the parents' dilemma without blaming them or their offspring. Parents will be more receptive to family therapy and to exploring their part in the adolescent's problems if they sense that you will support them, too. Stress and psychologic symptoms evidenced by parents can serve as markers for emotional or behavioral problems in adolescents. As examples, depressive symptoms in the child or adolescent have been highly correlated with parental depression, parental neglect, unusual hostility between parent and child, and ineffective parenting. One recent long-term study of depressed adolescents identified the independent variable of family members with recurring major depression as predictive of recurrent major depressive disorder in young adulthood (Lewinsohn et al., 2000).

Any tendency to feel self-righteous or superior to the disturbed adolescent's parents is an obstacle to effective treatment. Such feelings are readily communicated to parents and can only validate their fear of blame and increase their reluctance to participate in therapy with their child. By the same token, resist any temptation to overidentify with the parents, thereby inadvertently perpetuating the family system's problems. The adolescent and the family need a neutral party who can play an objective, knowledgeable, and supportive role in helping them change. The adolescent's chances for resolving the underlying conflicts and maintaining a healthy life are virtually nonexistent if the family system remains unchanged.

Parents, school, and agency staff must understand the objectives and goals of treatment to appreciate the progress the client has made and avoid reinforcing the client's previously maladaptive behavior. The following incident illustrates the problems that arise when parents and school authorities, particularly those who must deal directly with behavior problems in the classroom, lack psychologic sophistication.

CLINICAL EXAMPLE

Jeremy, a 13-year-old boy, was referred to the school nurse because he was introverted and isolated. He made no contact with either his peers or his teachers and rarely spoke unless addressed directly. After he had spent 3 months in group and individual therapy sessions with the nurse, Jeremy began to come to the grade counselor's office of his own accord to talk about his depression and the problems he had been having in his family. Both the grade counselor and the boy's family believed this to be an indication that his difficulties had worsened, and they began to complain to the nurse about his illness! Not only were Jeremy's parents and counselor ignorant of the goals of treatment and the behaviors expected to come with change, but apparently they were also uncomfortable with the changes in Jeremy's behavior and with the implications of these changes for their relationships with him.

The client's siblings may experience many different feelings. Sometimes they share in the parents' guilt and shame. Sometimes, however, they are pleased and relieved when the "troublemaker" is out of the family and hospitalized. You should extend the same understanding to the siblings as to the parents, helping them see how each member of the family contributes to the problem. If the troubled adolescent is hospitalized, another member of the family, usually a sibling, may assume the role of the "bad" or "sick" person in the family because the identified "bad" person is no longer at home. Be aware of this tendency. If you are not skilled in assessing the need for family therapy or in providing this service, refer the family to a competent family therapist (see Chapter 29).

You may identify a need for all of the above therapies in dealing with a client's problems. In some cases, an informal discussion with you is all that is warranted. In other cases, you may identify problems that require considerable attention. Sometimes a period of unsuccessful treatment is necessary to determine that outpatient therapy is ineffective and that hospitalization is indicated. Before making such a recommendation, you need to establish a trusting relationship with the client and the client's parents. An excellent source, Facts for Families, has been developed by the AACAP to help you provide concise and current information on issues that affect children, adolescents, and their families. Translations into Spanish, French, and German languages are also available on the World Wide Web (www.aacap.org/publications/factsfam/index.htm), and through a resource link for the Companion Website of this book. Moreover, there are sources available to help you with specifically "how to say it," particularly regarding medications and neuroimagery (Wilens, 1999).

MediaLink Facts for Families

IN THE INPATIENT SETTING

Admission into a hospital or other residential treatment facility may be indicated under the following circumstances:

- If the adolescent is unable to control impulsivity.
- If the degree of destructive or antisocial behavior escalates beyond normal limits.
- If the adolescent cannot form meaningful, stable relationships within the everyday environment (as in the case of family dysfunction).

The existence of any of these conditions warrants counseling or professional treatment. A combination of two or more is likely to make treatment on an outpatient basis virtually ineffective, indicating the need for hospital or residential treatment.

Hospitalization of the disturbed adolescent has these possible advantages:

- It provides additional structure within which to handle the physically and psychologically destructive elements of the adolescent's behavior.

- It removes the individual from the stresses of a disturbed family environment.
- It offers opportunities for supporting existing ego strengths and for promoting whatever ability the client has for forming relationships.

Adolescents are sometimes institutionalized because their ideas are strange or threatening to their families, or because the responsible authorities seek to punish the adolescent's unacceptable behavior. The results can be disastrous. Therefore, it is important to make accurate assessments and to implement early treatment when indicated. You can play a crucial role in making such assessments, undertaking appropriate interventions, and educating parents, teachers, and school officials to recognize such needs.

As a Staff Nurse in a General Hospital Setting

Adolescents with emotional problems may have symptoms of physical illness and as a result may be admitted to a general hospital setting for evaluation and treatment. Clients with anorexia nervosa, in particular, may be referred for inpatient treatment on general adolescent medical units. As a staff nurse in such a setting, you can take the opportunity to reach out to adolescents in these programs.

As a Consultant in a General Hospital Setting

Staff nurses from a psychiatric inpatient unit of a general hospital may be consulted by other nursing staff about emotionally disturbed adolescents who have been admitted to their general medical or surgical units. Some general hospital settings have clinical nurse specialists in psychiatric liaison positions as consultants.

As a Staff Nurse or Clinical Specialist in a Psychiatric Setting

In inpatient psychiatric settings, the staff nurse or clinical nurse specialist may assume any of the previously mentioned roles. Nurses in inpatient settings also have numerous opportunities to observe and assess the family dynamics among the adolescent's family members and possibly to intervene. Nurses involved in family therapy sessions can perceive maladaptive ways of relating and take direct steps to work toward change. However, you need not work within the structured format of a therapy hour to have an impact on the family system. The Intervention box at right delineates specific parent behaviors and corresponding interventions by the nurse in the therapeutic environment. In addition, depending upon the focus for your treatment there are a variety of behavioral checklists and rating scales that might prove useful to you in your assessment of the adolescent's behavior (Barkley, Edwards, & Robin, 1999).

Because inpatient nursing entails around-the-clock care, the nurse has the responsibility to maintain the therapeutic envi-

INTERVENTION

Guidelines for Intervening with Specific Parent Behaviors

Parent Behavior

- Initiates loud verbal arguments during visits with adolescent.

Nursing Interventions

- Stop the immediate behavior, pointing out the disruptiveness to the unit.
- Refer adolescent and family to family therapist to resolve differences and learn more adaptive ways of relating in supportive atmosphere of family therapy.
- Suggest that family therapist contract with family for one or more of the following:
  - Staff will monitor visits.
  - Family will bring up potentially volatile topics only within the structure of family meetings and not on the unit during visits.
  - Staff will intervene if arguments ensue on unit.
  - Staff may limit visiting time on unit.

Parent Behavior

- Has history of physical violence against adolescent.

Nursing Interventions

- Upon admission, contract with adolescent and family for no acts of violence against people or property.
- Monitor visits with adolescent on unit.
- Limit or deny passes with parents until progress is demonstrated.
- Depending on abilities with impulse control, refuse visiting privileges with adolescent until progress is seen in family therapy.

Parent Behavior

- Is unable to set limits with adolescent during unit visits (is adversely influenced by manipulative attempts, tolerates verbal abuse, etc.)

Nursing Interventions

- Intervene if demands or behavior could lead to physical harm, unit rule breaking, or other negative results.
- Point out problem and refer adolescent and parents to family therapy.
- Role-model appropriate and effective limit setting with adolescent, if necessary.
- Offer to discuss situation with parents and adolescent if desirable in immediate situation.
- Offer emotional support to parent who needs to talk.

Parent Behavior

- Has limited interaction with adolescent during unit visits.

Nursing Interventions

- Initiate discussion among adolescent and family members related to visit and treatment goals.
- Refer problem and give observations to family therapist.
- Initiate discussion with parents to allow exploration of difficulty, if desired.
- Suggest that family members and adolescent discuss problem in family therapy.
- Plan outings or special-occasion celebrations to include family, if appropriate.

ronment. The role of the inpatient staff nurse includes the following:

- Maintaining physical and psychologic safety of the unit.
- Setting verbal and physical limits on client behavior.
- Establishing meaningful one-to-one relationships with clients.
- Identifying client strengths and promoting more adaptive coping skills.
- Role-modeling socially acceptable behaviors.
- Participating in group therapies and other structured activities.

As a Milieu Therapist

Many authors have described the importance of the therapeutic environment, indicating the strong influence of the treatment environment on the treatment outcome. (For a complete discussion, see Chapter 11.)

Because of adolescents' needs for peer acceptance, their overwhelming uncertainties and fears, and their everchanging behaviors and attitudes about identity, their chances for success in inpatient treatment are increased by a peer group setting. Much has been written about the value of the therapeutic environment in dealing with adolescent problems, including the problems of substance abuse and similar destructive activities. Without the social interaction and living-learning situations provided by the peer group, psychotherapy may be sterile and ineffectual.

The therapeutic environment provides valuable experiences for adolescents for the following reasons:

- Adolescents more readily hear and accept limits from peers than from adults.
- Adolescents more readily respond to feedback, both negative and positive, from peers than from adults.
- Shared goals and objectives facilitate group processes and the development of cohesion among adolescent group members.
- Group interaction allows for the expression of appropriate feelings and identification with peers with similar feelings.
- Group interaction provides opportunities for learning how to develop relationships with others.
- Group structure allows for the testing of new, more adaptive behaviors.
- Adolescents receive feedback from the peer group and have the opportunity to give feedback in a supportive environment.
- The group format provides an opportunity to work out specific issues of conflict with adult group leaders while receiving the support and understanding of peers.

NURSING PROCESS

Adolescents

Adolescents present behaviors and problems unique to their developmental stage. Without knowledge and understanding about potentially difficult areas, you may respond with confusion, anger, and even hostility, which will cause feelings of frustration and failure for both yourself and your adolescent clients. The following pages contain numerous examples of either typical behaviors expected of the "normal" adolescent or problem behaviors that may provide the impetus for referral to a treatment setting, or both. In many situations, you may simply need to focus on the difficult issues encountered in working with adolescents. That information is given in the Assessment section. Situations that represent an identified problem necessitating treatment are discussed under Planning and Implementation.

It will be important for you to keep in mind that over the course of normal development, children and adolescents experience symptoms of anxiety, dysphoria, oppositionality, or conduct disorder. On the other hand, there are factors that can contribute to missed or inaccurate diagnoses in the assessment of an adolescent:

- Symptom overlap, which can blur diagnostic boundaries.
- Effects of normal development on symptom presentation.
- High rates of comorbidity in youth with mental illness.
- Perception of informants (i.e., parents/guardians, teachers, or other family members).

Moreover, two other trends that can minimize the effectiveness and comprehensive nature of an adequate assessment in the adolescent are:

- The impact of managed care with emphasis on brevity in patient contact.
- The emphasis in clinical training on the rigid adherence to DSM-IV-TR criteria without the exploration of developmental and risk factors, current stressors, temperament, cultural and/or family dynamics (Berenson, 1998).

For nurses, the above dilemmas make the language of nursing diagnosis even more beneficial and user friendly. We can use nursing diagnoses as tools to adequately describe the client's behavior without rigidly adhering to a medically diagnostic label. We can communicate the adolescent's experience to family, lay personnel, and non–mental health professionals without having to resort to specialized terminology. For a more thorough discussion of the nursing process and the use of nursing diagnoses with psychiatric clients, see Chapter 7.

Assessment

Accurate and comprehensive assessments can be obtained only by viewing the adolescent as a biopsychosocial being. Only by integrating knowledge from biology, psychology, and humanistic interactionist theory can you understand what a particular behavior means to an adolescent. If you can remember your own adolescent experiences—the conflicts and uncertainty as well as the elation and the triumphs—you will better appreciate the adolescent's turmoil. It is equally important that you discover who the individual adolescent is. Meanings of behavior, values, and actions can vary from client to client and may not reflect meanings or values that you hold. For example, the client

MediaLink Care Plan: Acting Out Teenager

who has trouble with competitive feelings may be reluctant to accept an invitation to play a game of Trivial Pursuit. And because adolescents are developmentally between childhood and adulthood, they frequently have the feelings and choices of adulthood without an adult's abilities in verbal discourse and impulse control. As a result, adolescents may "act out" feelings and decisions nonverbally, in a childlike way. This is particularly true of the emotionally disturbed adolescent.

ACTING-OUT

The concept of acting-out is complex. The term has been used to describe a variety of behaviors, ranging from antisocial, destructive acts to unconscious impulses expressed in action rather than in symbolic words or symptoms. Acting-out may, and often does, include destructive actions and seemingly undefinable behaviors. The term describes a recreation of the client's life experiences, relationships with significant others, and resulting unresolved conflicts.

These are all components of what is commonly called the client's life script, which unfolds as the client relates, reacts, and behaves in accustomed ways. Through observation of and interaction with the client, you can uncover the meanings that various behaviors and actions hold for the individual. For example, the child who has assumed the "black sheep" role in the family seeks to recreate that familiar role with others outside the home, particularly in the inpatient setting. The following clinical example illustrates one girl's relationship with her parents as replayed with the staff on an inpatient unit.

CLINICAL EXAMPLE

Liza is 14 years old. She has been on the unit for 6 days. She is an attractive, engaging young person who has been friendly with both staff and clients. Liza has been on the periphery of several rule-breaking incidents but has not been directly involved. She has begun to establish close ties with Jim, a nurse, and engages in frequent lengthy discussions with him about her innermost feelings and fears. One evening she candidly talks to him about the callous way in which she was treated by one of the other nurses, a woman, in regard to a gynecologic problem. Liza says with undisguised fear and embarrassment that she is afraid the situation will repeat itself. She expresses great respect for Jim's knowledge and style and asks him to attend to any subsequent problems himself rather than report her dissatisfaction with Jane, the other nurse.

The implications for treatment are many. The most important factors for Jim to consider are what meaning Liza's behavior has for her and what would be the most therapeutically effective way to deal with the situation. The client's presenting problems and the expectation that the client will act out previous conflicts and life scripts have provided Jim adequate information on which to base an appropriate intervention. The client's attempt to seduce the nurse, and the need for nurses to examine their own behavior and motivations, are discussed in detail later in this chapter.

CLINICAL EXAMPLE

Jim recognizes the "pull" from Liza to feel that only he can adequately handle the situation. He remembers that Liza's home situation is chaotic. Liza's mother and father frequently fight over who is the better parent. Jim surmises that Liza also plays a part in these fights. The present situation seems to indicate that he is about to be played off against Jane, just as Liza perhaps plays one parent against the other. Jim responds by reiterating his concern for her dilemma and suggesting that Liza speak with Jane about the situation that is causing her concern.

In this example, it is clear that the client is attempting to recreate her home situation, using two of the nurses to reenact the roles of her parents. Had Jim been seduced into playing the father's role in the script, he would have re-created the family's conflict on the unit. The ideal solution is for staff to interrupt this pathologic process by substituting a healthier way of resolving the problem. Thus, Jim does not react with compliance or with anger to Liza's attempts. Instead, he recognizes the significance of her behavior and deals with the situation in a concerned yet healthy way, suggesting a resolution to the immediate problem that demonstrates respect for both Liza's and Jane's abilities to resolve the conflict.

Such situations are commonplace with adolescents. They require nursing staff to evaluate the client's psycho-dynamics and psychopathology as well as their own inner feelings and behavior. For these reasons, it is imperative to identify transference and countertransference issues and to discuss them with your clinical supervisor. Transference and countertransference are discussed in Chapter 28. But these situations are not limited to the inpatient setting. This fact alone obliges you to be alert in observing and assessing verbal and nonverbal communication and to understand your own feelings and behavior in order to make accurate assessments and appropriate interventions. In this way, you will be most effective when working with adolescents.

COMMUNICATION

Communication with adolescents is an art in itself. To become proficient in this area, you must accept and understand the following:

- Adolescents tend to act out feelings and conflicts rather than verbalize them.
- Adolescents have an unconventional language of their own.
- Adolescents, especially disturbed ones, may use profanity frequently.

- Many clues can be obtained simply by observing an adolescent's behavior, dress, or environment.

If you learn the skills of interviewing and the use of nonverbal cues and messages, you can use them comfortably and naturally in communicating with adolescents.

Nonverbal Cues. Adolescents give many nonverbal cues to their specific emotional struggles, underlying confusion, or transitory moods. A glance around their rooms or a brief study of their dress can tell you more than several direct questions would elicit. Sometimes adolescents give obvious cues. A client who wears a coat around the unit may be planning to run away. Other less obvious behaviors, which are often outside the client's conscious awareness or control, can also yield vital information. A sudden escalation of horseplay among the boys around bedtime is an example. You would probably be correct in identifying this behavior as an expression of anxiety related to sexual identity and fears of homosexual feelings. Interactionist theory holds that the adolescent boy's newfound sexual feelings and changing body image provide unfamiliar ways of relating to members of his own sex. As a result, he regresses to preadolescent behavior, which served him well in handling close feelings then but now proves inappropriate. In this instance, firm limit setting is in order. Avoid interpreting the behavior or paying undue attention to the specifics. (Testing and limit setting are discussed later in the chapter.)

Slang and Obscenities. Adolescents create a language all their own. This takes some understanding and acceptance. In seeking their identity, adolescents establish a form of communication unique to the group. To gain acceptance into the adolescent world, the adult must accept this need to use ambiguous (to the adult) yet specific (to the adolescent) terms to express themselves. In many cases, you must communicate with adolescents by using their slang.

This slang often includes obscene and profane words. This is particularly true of disturbed adolescents, who have an especially difficult time expressing anger and fear appropriately. The words they use often reveal the nature of the emotional conflict. For example, a young male adolescent grappling with his sexual identity and aggressive feelings may resort to sexually graphic words when he feels anxious or afraid. You may sometimes find it productive to use similar words to give explanations or to clarify communication. Understandably, some nurses have difficulty tolerating profane or sexually graphic language. However, you must evaluate your clients' underlying reasons for using such language, to help them understand their feelings. Only then can you encourage clients to use more appropriate means of expression. If clients sense that the reason you want them to speak more appropriately is only to make you, the nurse, feel more comfortable, the end result will not be satisfactory.

The adolescent psychiatric client often presents with symptoms of disturbed communication, which can affect all realms of daily living, particularly in relationships with peers, family members, and nonparental authority figures. Giving information is one way you can help decrease communication deficits and facilitate relationships with others. Other nursing behaviors are outlined in the Planning and Implementation section. (For the general principles of therapeutic communication, see Chapter 8.)

Confidentiality. An emerging body of research underscores the importance of discussing confidentiality with the adolescent. There will be health concerns, thoughts, and feelings that the adolescent client will want to keep private. Assurances of confidentiality will increase the likelihood that the adolescent will disclose sensitive personal information to you. Confidentiality, however, cannot be unconditional in that some information, such as sexual abuse, must be disclosed by law and other information, such as a suicidal plan, must be discussed with the parents and/or the rest of the treatment team. In discussing confidentiality with the adolescent, one way of clarifying this dilemma might be to simply state, "What you and I discuss is confidential. However, you need to know that *if it means harm to you or to someone else* [emphasize these words], it will be important for me to talk it over with your parents/other members of the team [whoever is most appropriate to the situation]. In that case, I will first discuss it with you to determine the best way in which to present our concerns to others."

ANGER AND HOSTILITY

Expressions of anger and hostility are common on an adolescent unit. Anger expressed verbally usually takes the form of profanity. How effectively we deal with expressions of anger and hostility depends on how effectively we handle our own angry or hostile feelings. You will compromise your effectiveness as a nurse if you are uncomfortable with expressions of anger or hostility, or view anger and hostility as negative or to be avoided at all costs.

Nurse's Self-Assessment. A subject that is rarely considered is anger felt and expressed by the nurse toward the client. The general focus on the client's need for understanding and good care seem to make it unacceptable to display negative feelings toward the client. In the nursing care of adolescents, however, a constant all-giving and all-accepting attitude by the nurse, particularly during times of testing, would be not only nontherapeutic but also illogical and dishonest. Testing behavior is at an all-time high, and adolescents need honest feedback. The adolescent sometimes escalates the provocative behavior to evoke an angry reaction. For you to pretend that you are not angry in such a situation is as undesirable for treatment as it would be to pretend that you are fond of the client. Being honest about your feelings is a prime prerequisite in establishing and maintaining meaningful and productive relationships with adolescent clients. This does not mean that you should give vent to all your thoughts or impulses. Be aware of your reactions, and use good judgment in handling them. The questions in the Nursing Self-Awareness feature on page 626 will help you assess your own ways of dealing with anger.

ANXIETY AND RESISTANCE

Normal adolescents frequently feel anxious as they experience change and inner turmoil in adapting to a new identity. The anxiety evidenced by disturbed adolescents in treatment can

Nursing SELF-AWARENESS — A Self-Awareness Inventory for Working with Adolescents

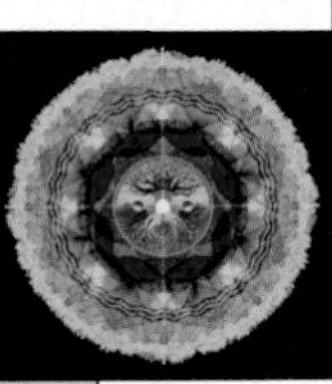

To increase self-awareness about your own way of dealing with anger:

- What kinds of things make me angry?
- How do I deal with my anger? Do I tend to ignore or hide it, or do I show that I am angry?
- Do I sometimes use profanity or act out my feelings in a physical way? How do I feel about others who do this?
- What do I think about how I handle anger?
- How do I feel about how I handle anger?
- How do I react to others when they are angry?

To increase self-awareness about your tendency to be seduced or manipulated:

- Is this client's friendliness compromising the professional role boundaries between us to "personalize" our relationship?
- Do I feel compelled to respond in a personal rather than a therapeutic way, possibly revealing information about my own life and lifestyle?
- Do I feel uncomfortable with the client's flattering comments or probing questions?
- Do I tend to forget that this person is a client?
- Is the client encouraging me to keep secrets from other staff or to "side" with client against other staff?

To increase self-awareness about your own sexual attitudes and feelings:

- How would I describe my adolescence as it related to my developing sexuality?
- What do I remember about the development and changes in my body?
- How did I feel about these changes?
- How would I describe my adolescent relationships with members of my sex?
- How would I describe my adolescent relationships with members of the opposite sex?
- What events stand out in my mind when I recall my sexual experiences during adolescence?
- How have these past relationships, events, and feelings influenced me today?

indicate many other things. The changes required are much more threatening to disturbed adolescents than to normal adolescents. If treatment is to be successful, clients must look at the meaning of their behavior and must change many of their earlier interactional patterns. This can be frightening. For example, it is more comfortable to play the role of the "bad seed" or "bad kid," with its known pitfalls and expectations, than to attempt a change that entails many uncertainties and unknowns.

Clients feel threatened and anxious when the nurse does not act according to their expectations, because they must then find other ways of handling the situation. They must also deal with the anxiety. Frequently this anxiety is channeled into a game of "cops and robbers," as the client once again assumes a familiar role and maintains the negative or unhealthy image. The anxiety caused by unfamiliar roles is dissipated by further testing and acting-out. Do not take this as an indication that therapy is not working. It may simply indicate that the client needs to move ahead more slowly with insightful discoveries and needs your support in doing so.

Keep in mind that to such adolescents, "opening up" in a trusting way does not hold the same positive promise that it might for you. Adolescents who have been rejected or have experienced loss following close relationships in the past will feel wary of your expressions of interest or concern and will be cautious about repeating such experiences. They may respond to you with testing behaviors, anger and mistrust, or outright rejection. Adolescents who expect rejection assume some control over the relationship if they reject others before being rejected themselves.

Nurse's Self-Assessment. Sometimes nurses find it difficult to allow adolescents to grapple with their anxieties and fears. At other times, you may not recognize the client's behavior as a symptom of anxiety or depression. The following clinical example demonstrates the value of a comprehensive assessment, of exploring all possible reasons for a client's resistance to your efforts before implementing action.

CLINICAL EXAMPLE

Kathy was the quietest and most aloof client on the unit. She had isolated herself from the other clients during the week that followed admission and avoided conversing with staff members outside meetings. One evening she seemed especially receptive to the new nurse, Ellie, who was able to interest her in a sewing project. Ellie, who was a new graduate, felt pleased that Kathy had responded warmly to her during their time together. The next day, Kathy did not speak to Ellie and seemed to avoid her at all costs. Later, Ellie noticed that the dress Kathy had been sewing was torn into shreds and stuffed into the wastepaper basket. Ellie interpreted this quite personally. She felt deeply hurt and rejected. In her discussion with her supervisor, Ellie showed her disappointment and anger. Her supervisor observed that, although the good time and feelings that Ellie and Kathy had shared the evening before were genuine, Kathy had not experienced many such times before with her parents or other adults. She suggested that Kathy was probably angry with Ellie for pointing up what she, Kathy, had missed. The supervisor suggested that Ellie be patient with Kathy. Perhaps later Ellie could reestablish the bond, and they would be able to talk about what had happened.

Fortunately, Ellie did not act on her angry feelings. Had she done so, she might have impulsively assessed Kathy's behavior as "hopeless," interpreting Kathy's anxiety and resistance as an inability to trust, or she may have begun to relate to the client in a vindictive way, withdrawing from Kathy in turn. Instead, she sought advice. Ellie's supervisor recognized that Ellie wanted badly to do well and needed positive feedback. She also realized that Ellie did not understand the nature of giving to emotionally disturbed adolescents. Had Ellie not sought advice, she might have acted on her angry feelings, further alienating Kathy and causing herself more anger and frustration. Without an understanding of Kathy's actions, Ellie would have continued to expect kindness in return for kindness and would have been keenly disappointed.

SEDUCTION AND MANIPULATION OF THE NURSE

In working with adolescents, there is always a risk of seduction of the nurse, or being manipulated into relating in a nontherapeutic way. These factors contribute to the problem:

- The intimate nature of the nurse's involvement with the adolescent client.
- The narcissism inherent in this age group.
- The nurse's all-accepting attitude in working with the adolescent client.

Narcissism in this age group is caused by the child's withdrawal from the parents and their value system. This withdrawal leads to a general self-centeredness, overevaluation of the self, heightened self-perception, decreased ability for reality testing, and extreme self-absorption. The result is that the people to whom adolescents turn become all-important and perfect in their eyes. Nurses may be strongly tempted to respond accordingly.

Nurse's Self-Assessment. The dangers inherent in this situation are not simply the two possible extremes: total submission to temptation, resulting in a sexual relationship with the client; or strong denial of temptation by maintaining a rigid, unapproachable stance that makes it impossible to establish a meaningful, trusting relationship. Neither of these extremes is unknown.

It is tempting to respond to the adolescent's idealized view, to be the "savior" who succeeded with this difficult person where everyone else has failed, to feel superior to the imperfect parents, the harassed school teacher, the skeptical juvenile judge, or other members of the staff on the unit. However, you should not give in to such temptations. Complications will most certainly develop that at best will temporarily compromise your effectiveness and at worst will render the treatment program completely ineffective. Liza's example of acting-out demonstrates this. Jim, the evening nurse, could have been seduced by Liza to collude with her against the day nurse, Jane, had he not been keenly aware of the possibility.

Nurses who work intensively with adolescents often face situations in which their own unresolved feelings are aroused. You must choose whether to act on these impulses or to explore their origin. Of course, one is not always conscious of these unresolved feelings. It would be unrealistic to expect you to be totally aware of the meaning of your behavior at any given moment. Nonetheless, the skilled clinician is usually acquainted with the issues or conflicts that have caused problems in the past. In doubtful cases, the knowledgeable nurse will seek consultation from such a clinician. The clinician can help you assess the situation and understand what part you may have played in initiating it. Nurses who wish to explore their personal conflicts further may then seek counseling or therapy. You can use the questions in the Nursing Self-Awareness box to assess the nature of such interactions with clients.

In addition, nursing staff would benefit from establishing one or more of the following to provide a consistent format for assessing and evaluating ongoing situations with adolescent clients:

- Each nurse's own ongoing supervision with preceptor or nurse supervisor.
- A regularly scheduled meeting (perhaps monthly) for all nursing staff to discuss difficult situations and conflicting feelings.
- Staff meetings (perhaps weekly) in which all disciplines identify interpersonal obstacles and plan interventions toward more optimal treatment.

SEXUAL BEHAVIOR OF THE ADOLESCENT

The biologic changes that occur in late childhood and early adolescence are rapid and pervasive. Do not underestimate the importance of the adolescent's experimentation and attitude in sexual matters. Likewise, evaluate your own attitudes and feelings about sexual issues as they relate to past experiences and current activities. Conflicts in such matters or resentments left over from the past will certainly affect your decisions or interaction with clients regarding sexual matters. Again, while it is not necessary for you to resolve all these issues, it is highly desirable to be aware of areas of conflict that might make it difficult to view a situation objectively or set rational limits. Refer again to the Nursing Self-Awareness feature to increase your self-awareness about sexual attitudes and feelings.

Until adolescents master their anxieties and fears about their sexual identity and gain control over sexual urges, they will exhibit a variety of behaviors and attitudes that may confuse or trouble you. In the past decade, rates of sexual activity among adolescents have stabilized and perhaps even begun to decrease as the use of condoms reportedly has increased. Perhaps these two observations provide some explanation for the sustained drop in adolescent pregnancy rates that has occurred since the mid-1990s. Although these trends are encouraging, 15- to 19-year-old adolescents have the highest rates of *Neisseria gonorrhoeae* and chlamydia infection of any other age group in the United States. It is estimated that one-fourth of the 12 million cases of sexually transmitted diseases diagnosed annually occur among adolescents (Joffe, 2000).

Heterosexual Behavior. Heterosexual activity is normal and desirable during adolescence. However, nurses working with either normal or disturbed adolescents will sometimes see them engage in sexual activities that do not seem healthy or growth producing. For example, the adolescent girl who seeks punishment rather than true pleasure in her sexual exploits will display them in an overt, exhibitionistic way in a place where a particularly moralistic person will discover her and give her the reprimands she desires. She may be testing a parent's values in an attempt to resolve her own inner conflicts. Adolescents in an inpatient treatment setting where sexual intercourse is forbidden may engage in sexual intercourse where you or another staff member will be sure to discover them. The experience may reinforce their image of sexual behavior as "bad" behavior. Or it may simply provide a means of acting out their defiance of the rules, thereby earning the familiar "bad kid" label. The incident involving the nurse Barbara and the clients Laurie and Bill in the Planning and Implementation section is an excellent example of this situation. There is an increasing body of research on dating violence including date rape. One study of 5,000 high school students cited more than 23% of girls and 9% of boys as victims of forced sex. The researchers found a correlation between severe dating violence and poor mental health (Jackson, Cram, & Seymour, 2000).

Homosexual Behavior. Preadolescents usually choose a member of the same sex with whom to experience intimate or loving feelings. This does not necessarily mean that a sexual relationship will ensue, although it often does. Homosexual activity may continue into the adolescent years.

Generally, however, adolescents begin to view homosexual feelings as a threat to the development of their identity. As a result, they may ward off such feelings by engaging in frantic sexual activity with a member of the opposite sex. This is particularly true for boys. It is normal for an adolescent boy to be afraid of his own passive wishes and to label them homosexual. He had probably been brought up to identify with physical displays of strength or aggressive displays of power. Thus, an incident in which he feels threatened or powerless would produce feelings of sexual impotence, a fear of castration, a feeling of dependence or weakness, and a greater fear of homosexuality. The adolescent boy in treatment may act out these feelings, or he may attempt to reaffirm his masculinity with inappropriate displays of aggression or destructive behavior.

At the other extreme are adolescents who engage in predominantly homosexual activities. Many of these individuals find relationships with the opposite sex threatening or unrewarding and continue to seek intimacy with people of the same sex. Some feel more comfortable with companions of the same sex and are satisfied with these relationships. Others use their homosexual affiliation to express and act out hostility directed against their parents and their parents' values.

Since nurses who work with adolescents may encounter any of these situations, they must attempt to understand the meaning that homosexual behavior has for the client. The clients may need to explore their feelings and anxieties openly. Open discussion with an understanding yet knowledgeable professional may help resolve many of the concerns and conflicts inherent in adolescent sexual behavior.

Clients who use homosexuality to express hostility toward their parents will undoubtedly act out with the staff as well. Remain objective and nonjudgmental with these clients, allowing them to deal with the feelings of anger or depression that may result from addressing the conflict.

Although homosexual behavior during adolescence does not predict adult sexual preference, some adolescents make a lasting identification as homosexuals during these years. Such adolescents will not experience conflicts about homosexual relationships or need to flaunt them or act out with the staff in an angry or hostile way. In such cases, however, you may have to deal with your own negative feelings about homosexuality, if any exist. It is important for you to consider what their relationships mean to clients and to respect them.

Pregnancy. Adolescent pregnancy may reflect social and family expectations and unconscious motivations. Some teenage girls are quite pleased to be pregnant and suffer no emotional consequences from motherhood. In general, however, a conscious, deliberate decision to become pregnant at this age is manipulative. The goal may be to escape a difficult family situation, to express hostility toward parents, or to act out a life script in which the daughter is seen as "bad." The adolescent girl who did not receive adequate nurturing as a child could be acting out dependence needs by giving her baby the love and caring she herself did not receive. In so doing, she feels loved and cared for in turn.

Be sensitive to motivational factors in dealing with emotionally deprived adolescents. Use existing educational tools and interpersonal relationships to help adolescent girls understand their needs and motivations in becoming pregnant. It is also important to educate teenagers of both sexes about sex and birth control. Many high schools are now recognizing this need and providing such information in birth control clinics or through health education classes. Too often parents and professionals alike deny the adolescent's sexual activity until an unwanted pregnancy occurs.

DIETARY PROBLEMS AND EATING DISORDERS

The eating habits and food preferences of disturbed adolescents can reveal a lot about the nature of their inner turmoil. A comparison between the client's diet and that of a normal, healthy adolescent may show little difference in variety but probably a great difference in quantity. Teenagers who have been deprived of early nurturing tend to eat more than others and probably place a higher value on mealtimes and on receiving their "share" of the food. You may notice that adolescents consume more milk than usual during periods of stress or anxiety. In general, girls want to follow food fads or unreasonable dietary regimens to become slim and attractive. This usually gives you an opportunity to engage in health teaching about nutrition and exercise, and to express a cooperative interest in their developing feminine identity. In the last decade, particular attention has been given to the athletes in our society. Although females often receive messages that "thin is in," female athletes also receive messages about body size and performance. As a nurse, you may be likely to uncover the female athlete "triad" of disorders, including eating disorders, amenorrhea, and osteoporosis

(Post et al., 1998). (Eating disorders are discussed in Chapter 18.)

DEPRESSION AND SUICIDE

Both depression and suicide are thought to be underreported among adolescents. It is reported that at least 5% of adolescents have a major depressive disorder, and nearly one-fourth of students in a national survey reported having seriously considered killing themselves in the last year. In this survey, 17.7% of students had a suicidal plan and 8.7% had attempted suicide, with 3% of them needing treatment from a physician or nurse for the injury (Joffe, 2000). The Surgeon General's Call to Action to Prevent Suicide introduces the AIM (Awareness, Intervention, and Methodology) approach for addressing suicide. The report recognizes the need to address the problems of undetected and undertreated mental and substance abuse disorders in conjunction with other public health approaches. Box 26–4 contains data from this report relevant to the young (DHHS, 1999c). In addition to the dramatic statistics provided by this report are the equally important data regarding implications for sexuality and ethnic considerations. (See Chapter 22 for a complete discussion of suicide, including assessment and nursing intervention.)

SUBSTANCE USE AND ABUSE

According to the Spring 2000 Monitoring the Future survey of approximately 45,200 students in 8th, 10th, and 12th grades, the use of several drugs has declined substantially in recent years. Inhalants, LSD, crystal methamphetamine, and Rohypnol are all down from the peak levels of the mid-90s. In addition, use of the drug ecstasy (MDMA), a synthetic compound with both stimulant and mildly hallucinogenic properties, has also declined. Marijuana remains the most widely used of the illicit drugs, with 16 percent of the 8th graders, 32 percent of the 10th graders, and 37 percent of the 12th graders indicating some use in the prior 12-month period. Although the rate of alcohol use is high by most standards, it has remained fairly stable over the past several years. Nearly a quarter (22%) of the 8th graders and half of the 12th graders report having taken an alcoholic beverage in the past 30 days. One in every twelve 8th graders (8.3%) reports being drunk at least once in the past 30 days, as do a third (32.3%) of the 12th graders (National Institute on Drug Abuse, 2001).

Vulnerable youth are at increased risk for HIV infection. Several case studies indicate substance abuse and mental illness as important comorbidities for HIV-infected adolescents, including a high prevalence of anxiety, depression, and bipolar illness, often predating the HIV diagnosis (Futterman, Chabon, & Hoffman, 2000).

Adolescents give many reasons for using drugs: to experiment, to get high, to "get inside my head," to have fun, to understand more about life. Adolescents may also use drugs to cope with feelings of worthlessness or loneliness, or to avoid uncomfortable feelings.

BOX 26–4 **At a Glance: Suicide Among the Young**

- For young people 15 to 24 years old, suicide is the third leading cause of death, behind unintentional injury and homicide. In 1996, more teenagers and young adults died of suicide than from cancer, heart disease, AIDS, birth defects, stroke, pneumonia and influenza, and chronic lung disease *combined*.
- Americans under the age of 25 accounted for 35% of the population, and 15% of all suicide deaths in 1996. The rate among children aged 10 to 14 was 1.6/100,000, the rate for children aged 15 to 19 was 9.7/100,000, and the rate for young people aged 20 to 24 was 14.5/100,000.
- Important risk factors for attempted suicide in youth are depression, alcohol or other drug use disorder, and aggressive or disruptive behaviors.
- Over the last several decades, the suicide rate in young people has increased dramatically. From 1952 to 1996, the incidence of suicide among adolescents and young adults nearly tripled, although there has been a general decline in youth suicides since 1994. From 1980 to 1996, the rate of suicide among persons aged 15 to 19 increased by 14% and among persons aged 10 to 14 years by 100%. For African-American males aged 15 to 19, the rate increased 105%.
- Among persons aged 15 to 19, firearm-related suicides accounted for 63% of the increase in the overall rate of suicide from 1980 to 1996.
- The risk for suicide among young people is greatest among young white males; however, from 1980 through 1996, suicide rates increased most rapidly among young black males.
- Males under the age of 25 are much more likely to commit suicide than their female counterparts. The 1996 gender ratio for people aged 15 to 19 was 5:1 (males to females), while among those aged 20 to 24 it was 7:1.
- Although suicide among young children is a rare event, the dramatic increase in the rate among 10- to 14-year-olds underscores the urgent need for intensifying efforts to prevent suicide among persons in this age group.
- It has been widely reported that gay and lesbian youth are two to three times more likely to commit suicide than other youth and that 30% of all attempted or completed youth suicides are related to issues of sexual identity. There are no empirical data on completed suicides to support such assertions, but there is growing concern about an association between suicide risk and bisexuality or homosexuality for youth, particularly males. Increased attention has been focused on the need for empirically based and culturally competent research on the topic of gay, lesbian, and bisexual suicide.
- In a survey of students in 151 high schools around the country, the 1997 Youth Risk Behavior Surveillance System found that Hispanic students (10.7%) were significantly more likely than white students (6.3%) to have reported a suicide attempt.
- Among Hispanic students, females (14.9%) were more than twice as likely as males (7.2%) to have reported a suicide attempt, but Hispanic male students (7.2%) were significantly more likely than white male students (3.2%) to report this behavior.

Source: U.S. Public Health Service. (1999). *The Surgeon General's call to action to prevent suicide*. Retrieved from the World Wide Web, December 28, 2000, www.surgeongeneral.gov/library/calltoaction/fact3.htm.

CLINICAL EXAMPLE

According to Cindy, a 15-year-old high school sophomore, her 3-year history of substance abuse has involved regular marijuana use 1 to 2 times a week, occasional use of Valium (which she sneaks from her mother's 5-mg tablet prescription bottle), Seconal ("street reds") on two occasions, and LSD on two occasions.

Cindy describes herself as a "loner" who has few friends and keeps to herself at home and at school. She leaves the house each morning for school before the others are awake "to avoid the hassles with my mother and sisters." She describes one female classmate to whom she feels close but states that their time together is usually brief and usually involves smoking marijuana in the morning just before school. Cindy has recently been suspended from school as a result of the school principal's discovery of Cindy and her friend smoking marijuana outside the cafeteria.

Cindy is lonely and depressed, and has extreme feelings of worthlessness. She characterizes herself as "bored," "bad," and "hopeless." Cindy says that when she uses drugs, her situation doesn't seem as bad.

ASSESSMENT

Behavioral Changes Associated with Teenage Drug Abuse

- Unexplained periods or reactions of moodiness, depression, anxiety, irritability, oversensitivity, or hostility.
- Strongly inappropriate overreaction to mild criticism or simple requests.
- Lessening in accustomed family warmth; avoids interaction and communication with parents, withdraws from family activities.
- Preoccupation with self, less concern for the feelings of others.
- Loss of interest in previously important hobbies, sports, activities.
- Loss of motivation and enthusiasm (amotivational syndrome).
- Lethargy, lack of energy and vitality.
- Loss of ability for self-discipline and assuming responsibility.
- Need for instant gratification.
- Change in values, ideals, beliefs.
- Changes in friends, unwillingness to introduce friends.
- Secretive phone calls; callers refuse to identify themselves or hang up when someone other than the adolescent answers.
- Unexplained absences from home.
- Disappearance of money or items of value from home; handling of money becomes secretive.
- Desire for increased sensory stimuli.

Although the general public may disagree about whether drugs are harmful, the fact remains that using drugs—or at least experimenting with them—is acceptable to many adolescents.

Assessing Drug Abuse. How can you determine when drug *use* becomes drug *abuse*? Generally, the adolescent who abuses drugs or alcohol exhibits at least one of these following characteristics:

- The adolescent's performance at school or work increasingly deteriorates.
- The adolescent is frequently caught high or in the act of getting high by parents or other authority figures.
- The adolescent increasingly resorts to alcohol or drugs in times of stress or boredom.
- The adolescent has seriously deficient interpersonal relationships and can relate only when under the influence of drugs or alcohol.
- The adolescent may lose interest in interpersonal relationships altogether, preferring to be high alone rather than to be with others.

A list of behavioral changes associated with teenage drug abuse can be found in the Assessment box at the top of the page.

Use of a mnemonic tool such as the CRAFFT questionnaire as discussed in the Assessment box to the right (Knight, Shrier, Bravender, et al., as cited in Joffe, 2000) may help you to keep your assessment of the adolescent's drug use focused on the health consequences rather than have you debate how much alcohol or drug is "too much."

Nurses are most effective when they can determine what the particular drug or high does for the client. A boy with a poor self-image and low-esteem may say that it makes him "feel like a man." A particularly shy or introverted girl may say that it makes her "outgoing and friendly." You may discover that being high helps rid disturbed adolescents of angry or depressed feelings. Indeed, in the treatment setting, the client frequently resorts to smoking marijuana or "popping" uppers or downers to escape uncomfortable feelings.

Nursing Diagnosis: NANDA

The use of nursing diagnoses with adolescent clients can lend meaning and substance to the clients' behavior that might be overlooked with a DSM-IV-TR diagnosis alone. For example, look back at Cindy, the 15-year-old with a 3-year history of substance abuse. Limiting your assessment to a DSM-IV-TR diagnosis alone might yield a substance use disorder, a cannabis use

ASSESSMENT

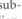

CRAFFT Screen for Adolescent Substance Abuse Assessment

C = Driving a *Car* after using drugs or alcohol or riding with a driver who has used drugs or alcohol
R = Using drugs or alcohol to *Relax*, to feel better about oneself, or to fit in
A = Using drugs or alcohol while *Alone*
F = *Forgetting* things because of drugs or alcohol
F = Having *Family* or *Friends* indicate that he or she needs to cut down on usage
T = Getting into *Trouble* because of drug or alcohol use

disorder, or a substance-induced mood disorder. While this tells you something about her drug history, it does not reveal any specifics such as current stressors; temperament; or cultural, social, or family dynamics that might contribute to or even underlie her drug abuse. Specifically, your assessments (and interventions) become more comprehensive and universally informative with an exploration of any or all of the following: Ineffective Individual Coping, Ineffective Family Coping, Chronic Low Self-Esteem, and/or Hopelessness. By using the various subsystems provided by nursing diagnoses, you can establish a more comprehensive picture of the client's difficulty and immediately become more goal-oriented in assessing and planning care. Moreover, in many treatment settings, mental health care professionals are reluctant to give adolescents a DSM-IV-TR diagnosis during these formative years to avoid having them be psychiatrically labeled (possibly erroneously). Such labeling may result in inadequate treatment, self-fulfilling prophecy, or both, in subsequent mental health care contacts.

Outcome Identification: NOC

Your choice of NOC expected outcomes and NIC interventions will depend primarily upon your individualized assessment and that adolescent's stated goals. Otherwise, your goals and your interventions for the client become one-sided, superficial, and ineffective.

With 15-year-old Cindy, for example, an expected outcome that she will no longer use drugs after discharge might be unrealistic. Expected outcomes that would yield more success yet demonstrate client improvement might be one or all of the following:

- Client will approach nurse and discuss temptation to use drugs when she is feeling angry or sad.
- Client will attend all family meetings.
- Client will discuss sad or angry feelings in therapy meetings.
- Client will be able to correlate drug usage with negative feelings or upsetting situations.

Likewise, correlating interventions to support the above expected outcomes might include one or all of the following:

- Establish a no-drug contract with client.
- Adopt neutral, matter-of-fact attitude when discussing drug usage.
- Encourage client to seek out nurse when feeling tempted to use drugs.
- Draw a parallel for client between drug usage and sad or angry feelings.
- Encourage client to talk about feelings in individual therapy, group meetings and family meetings.

Planning and Implementation: NIC

As nurses in numerous roles and diverse settings, we are in prime positions to recognize and intervene early with pathologic symptoms and behaviors.

PLANNING FOR PREVENTION

By preventing certain factors or circumstances in the early stages of life, health improvements are made possible at later stages. As one progresses along the chain from primary prevention and education/self-care, to secondary prevention with its risk factors and early problem recognition and treatment, to tertiary prevention with its more complicated and serious forms of illness and risky behaviors, it is obvious that services become increasingly more technological, expensive, and exclusive.

ESTABLISHING A CONTRACT WITH THE ADOLESCENT

Contracts can be particularly useful with adolescents because they can feel powerless in a treatment setting, especially when "referred" by parents or the legal system. Moreover, with this increased sense of control over their own behavior, adolescents become your collaborators in their treatment rather than objects of your treatment plan.

With most adolescents, a written contract is best, for these reasons:

- The goals and expectations are less easily forgotten.
- The process seems more formal and "serious."
- There is less room for misinterpretation and manipulation.

Contracts seem especially helpful in situations of substance abuse, eating disorders, suicidal behavior, and impulsive or manipulative behaviors. Whether verbal or written, the contract can be simply stated to promote clarity, consistency, and cooperation. Here is an example:

- I will not take drugs or bring drugs into the unit.
- I will not call or accept calls from my drug friends while in the treatment program.
- I will go directly to my outpatient therapy appointment and return immediately to the unit.
- I will not harm myself or others. If I feel like hurting myself, others, or property, I will tell the staff.

If written, the contract is signed by the client, dated, and cosigned by you. The contract is renegotiated at regular intervals (hourly, daily, or weekly), depending on the goals, the severity of the symptoms, and the degree of compliance with the agreement. The form of the contract is less important than the way you and the client jointly set the goals and expectations, carry out the contract, set limits and renegotiate changes, and evaluate the final outcome. Chapter 30 discusses contracting with clients in general, and Chapter 22 discusses no-suicide contracts.

INTERVENING INTO ANGER AND HOSTILITY

Depending on the degree to which the client is experiencing and expressing anger and hostility, you may choose any of a variety of interventions. These range from doing nothing other than observing the client's behavior, to physically restraining someone who is attempting destructive action (see Chapter 34). In some situations, a disturbed adolescent's ability to express anger directly to another person can be a sign of success in treatment. The choice of interventions also depends on your own experiences with such feelings, your knowledge and understanding of this client's life experiences with anger, and the external limits imposed by the mental health agency.

In choosing an appropriate nursing intervention, attempt to discover what meaning anger and hostility have for the client by asking the following questions:

- How has this person handled anger in the past?
- Does the client have a history of aggression toward objects or people?
- If so, what were the consequences of this behavior?
- How does the adolescent feel after such a reaction?
- What kinds of things make this client angry? Which of these would be most likely to occur on the unit or in our setting?

CLINICAL EXAMPLE

Steve had expressed great interest in building a model airplane. He had saved up his money and had taken a long time to choose "just the right one" at the hobby shop. After spending most of the afternoon constructing and painting it, he was interrupted by a phone call from his mother. She told him that she would not be able to attend the family meeting that week, giving a number of specious-sounding reasons. This was the third consecutive week that she had missed. Each time, she gave questionable reasons for being unable to attend. Steve was disappointed and angry. He slammed down the receiver, yelling obscenities in response to the nurse's questions, and ran into his room. There he began to destroy the plane by throwing it repeatedly against the floor.

In this example, Steve was not hurting himself or another. Although he did destroy property, the plane belonged to him, and he was free to do with it as he chose. The nurse resisted any impulse to stop Steve from damaging his plane. Since it was of significant value to him, he later regretted having taken out his anger on it. However, the situation provided Steve with an opportunity to explore his actions, and he later asked the nurse why he would destroy something that he valued so much after his mother had disappointed and angered him. The parallel between this situation and hurting himself with drugs right after he had argued with his mother was only too apparent.

Incidents in which the nurse bears the brunt of a client's anger or hostility do not offer such obvious solutions. Disturbed adolescents may not think twice about addressing a female nurse as "bitch" and coupling such a greeting with a request for a favor. Adolescents direct insults and hostile remarks at nurses for many reasons, most of which have little to do with the nurses as people but a lot to do with them as adults or authority figures.

There are as many suggestions for intervention as there are people who will be involved in such exchanges. In choosing interventions, consider the meaning behind the client's behavior, your own relationship with this client, your immediate feelings, and the result desired. For example, if the client calls you "bitch" the first time you meet, you may interpret this as a form of testing and may choose to respond immediately with a bewildered look at this unwarranted display of hostility. Later, you may approach the client, expressing a naive curiosity as to the origin of the hostile feelings: "Hey, I don't understand what happened between us a few minutes ago. We just met, and you're calling me a bitch. What's that all about?" This simple question conveys two messages. First, it indicates to the client that you are not accustomed to this kind of salutation. Second, it indicates that you are more interested in the motivation for the remark than in curtailing its use.

If the client resorts to name calling only when angry or under stress, you may decide to ignore the words and deal only with the feelings involved. For example, if a client has angrily left an ongoing family meeting and then calls you a bitch, you can probably assume that the anger is displaced. It is probably a result of overwhelming feelings experienced during the meeting. You may elect simply to say, "I know you're not angry at me right now. It seems like the meeting is pretty heavy, though. Do you want to talk about why you don't want to be in there now?" In neither situation is the name calling intended as a personal affront. However, the way you handle it determines both the outcome of the immediate situation and your chances of furthering your relationship with the client.

The adolescent's reaction to your intervention largely determines its effectiveness. For example, with Steve, the boy who destroyed his plane, the nurse's goal was to help Steve understand the impulsive reaction that destroyed something he loved and to encourage a more appropriate and direct expression of anger at his mother. He was able to do this as well as draw a parallel between anger at his mother and his drug abuse, which hurt himself. If the nurse's goal had been simply to stop the destruction of his property, Steve could have felt even greater anger and frustration, and he might have turned his aggression toward himself, the nurse, or the environment. Certainly if Steve had escalated his destructive behavior, turning his aggression toward himself or others, then direct limit setting, including physical restraints, would have been indicated.

In first-time encounters with any client new to the setting, do not be surprised or dismayed about less-than-optimal success with intervention. It may take some time and trial and error to assess the client's behaviors and choose the most effective interventions.

INTERVENING INTO TESTING AND LIMIT SETTING

As young adolescents attempt to adjust to the upheaval in their emotional lives and begin to emancipate themselves from parental figures, a good deal of testing is to be expected. This is normal. However, the meaning that testing holds for the disturbed adolescent is a more complicated matter.

Adolescents who lack early nurturing have difficulty with interpersonal relationships. In many cases, parents were emotionally unable to provide parenting. In other cases, they chose not to impose their values on their children. In either case, the children never developed the internalized values that reduce conflict and avert crisis during adolescence. This causes identity diffusion, which in turn results in emptiness, a lack of basic trust, and difficulties with intimacy on any level.

In the treatment setting, testing for these clients seems to consist of making limitless and absolute demands. Although these clients often react to imposed limits with cries of injustice, they often really seem to be asking for limits as an indication of caring.

CLINICAL EXAMPLE

Julie had been on the unit only 2 days. During that time she had seen several of the older clients run away from the unit, commonly known as going AWOL, and had witnessed the staff members' attempts to encourage those remaining on the ward to deal with whatever feelings they were experiencing. Toward the end of her second evening, Julie abruptly jumped up from a conversation with a nurse and ran toward the open door. The surprised nurse immediately followed, running down the stairs after her. A smiling Julie was waiting at the bottom step when the nurse arrived, quite breathless and thoroughly confused, and began her barrage of questions. Julie quickly answered, "I just wanted to see if you cared enough to come after me."

In this situation, no further action was necessary.

Sometimes the client may use annoying or destructive behavior to test you. At these times, firm limit setting without further interpretation or exploration may be indicated. In other instances, the client may be reacting to some real threat or uncomfortable situation.

CLINICAL EXAMPLE

Joanne was quietly playing pool by herself when she noticed her therapist talking to a new female client. Her volatile nature gave way to jealousy and rage, and she immediately began to hit the billiard balls off the table, making a lot of noise and startling everyone around her. The nurse who had been observing her witnessed the change in her behavior and understood the reaction. Without questioning Joanne's apparent anger, she stepped up to the table and challenged her to a game, which Joanne immediately accepted. Since Joanne prided herself on her pool-playing ability, she quickly channeled her energy and competitive feelings into the game and won. She then sought out her therapist and happily announced her victory.

Had the nurse not understood what had triggered Joanne's outburst, she might have become angry with her for making noise and set limits on her privilege to play pool. This would certainly have produced a helpless and even angrier Joanne, who probably would have escalated her behavior. Since the nurse was perceptive and adept in handling such situations, the results were more satisfying to both parties. Because of the nurse's action, Joanne was able to save face by winning at pool and was not forced into a situation where she would feel more helpless. What other interventions might have been equally effective with Joanne? In your relationships with adolescent clients, you might find yourself inclined to respond with a myriad of seemingly unrelated interventions. With a combination of increased clinical experience, a personalized assessment of the adolescent and the immediate situation, and knowledge of current practice studies, you will be most effective in your interventions. The Using Research Evidence feature on page 634 provides an illustration of basing a plan of interventions for an adolescent who is acting out.

INTERVENING INTO SCAPEGOATING

Scapegoating—a process by which an individual or group of individuals is identified as different from others and becomes the object of the group's fears, frustrations, or anger—is common in many groups, but particularly in adolescent groups. It occurs in three stages:

1. Frustration generates aggression.
2. Aggression is displaced on other people.
3. Through a process of blaming, projecting, and stereotyping, this displaced aggression is rationalized and finally justified, since the identified scapegoat is "different" in some real way.

The members of a group tend to attack the scapegoat because they are afraid to attack the person on whom their feelings are actually focused. Adolescents readily identify peers who are "different" and project on them their own fears and insecurities about their changing images. The client identified as the scapegoat is the object of much teasing and many hostile remarks. Refrain from attempting merely to rescue the scapegoat, as this may augment the other clients' anger and frustration and encourage an escalation of the hostility. Set limits on the behavior and then ask the group to focus on what is going on, to acknowledge the anxiety or other uncomfortable feeling that preceded the scapegoating incident. If possible, anticipate the occurrence of scapegoating in times of stress and try to circumvent the process before it gets out of control.

Also be aware that identified scapegoats share some responsibility for their predicament by presenting themselves to the other clients in a different or provocative stance. In some instances the scapegoat of choice has an inner need to be punished and meets the group's urgent need to punish as well. You can be valuable to these clients by helping them explore whatever function this role serves for them.

INTERVENING INTO SEXUAL BEHAVIORS

With a self-awareness and understanding of feelings and attitudes about sexual issues, you can more readily plan interventions with sexual behaviors of the adolescent client.

USING RESEARCH EVIDENCE

Brent is a large, muscular 13-year-old who is admitted to the crisis unit in your community after his parents called the police. He had been shouting obscenities at his mother, pushed his elderly father to the floor, and broke the windows of neighbors' cars parked along the street as he ran from his home. Within an hour of his arrival on the unit, he began breaking light fixtures in the hall and in other clients' rooms with a broom he found in a closet. Other clients were visibly distressed and frightened by his fury.

Your plan for intervention options is based on current research results. For example, in your review of studies of cognitive–behavioral therapy and anger management, you consider the possibility that Brent will more quickly and effectively gain self-control of his behavior if you work with him on specific techniques in private. Consequently, you set limits on his free activity on the unit and insist that he take a "time-out" in his room before you talk with him privately about the incident.

Your initial nursing assessment revealed that Brent's low self-esteem and guilt make it difficult for him to talk openly and freely with adults about his anger. Because of this finding and research literature on group work with adolescents, you also ask him to talk about the circumstances around his admission and the incident on the unit with his peers at the next morning's group session.

Finally, given the goal/task phase for Brent's family treatment, you decide to confront him with his behavior in the impending family therapy sessions scheduled before his discharge from the unit.

This set of multiple intervention strategies is based on the following research:

Diamond, G. M., Diamond, G. S., & Liddle, H. A. (2000). The therapist-parent alliance in family-based therapy for adolescents. *Journal of Clinical Psychology, 56*(8), 1037–1050.

Horner, S. D. (2000). Using focus group methods with middle school children. *Research in Nursing & Health, 23*(6), 510–517.

Mahon, N. E., Yarcheski, A., & Yarcheski, T. J. (2000). Positive and negative outcomes of anger in early adolescents. *Research in Nursing & Health, 23*(1), 17–24.

Miranda, A., & Presentacion, M. J. (2000). Efficacy of cognitive–behavioral therapy in the treatment of children with ADHD, with and without aggressiveness. *Psychology in the Schools, 37*(2), 169–182.

Masturbation. Masturbation is a normal sexual activity for people of all ages, from the beginning of sexual awareness to senescence. If you have a relatively healthy attitude toward masturbation, it is not likely to cause problems unless the client masturbates in inappropriate places or uses masturbation to express hostility. You may be confronted with an adolescent boy who fondles his genitals when he is anxious or feels threatened. Understanding his behavior as an indication of anxiety, you may elect to ignore the gesture and explore the nature of his anxiety with him. At other times, the boy may make a masturbatory gesture to convey contempt or hostility. In this case it would be ludicrous to feign indifference in response.

Your reaction depends on all the previously mentioned factors, such as the nurse–client relationship and the behavior that preceded the gesture. Generally, however, it is wise to comment on the client's gesture, for example, by mentioning it as an attempt to "make me uncomfortable," and then to allow the client the opportunity to express his feelings verbally. It is unlikely that this intervention will produce a tumultuous outpouring of feeling resulting in immediate resolution. However, it does allow you to acknowledge both the client's and your own feelings, perhaps paving the way for a more appropriate exchange in the future.

Heterosexual Behavior. The adolescent often uses sexual behavior as a means of acting out other conflicts and as a testing ground for the nursing staff's feelings and attitudes.

CLINICAL EXAMPLE

This is the third time Barbara, a nurse, had gone into Laurie's room to check on two clients, Laurie and Bill, who were an identified couple on the unit. Although there was a rule against clients having sexual intercourse with each other, Laurie and Bill had been discovered in the act each evening Barbara was on duty. Barbara found these discoveries disconcerting. She began to wonder whether she was the only staff member who checked on clients, since no one else had reported any sexual activity. She decided to bring the subject up in the next nursing care plan meeting to find a more effective way of dealing with the situation.

Imagine Barbara's surprise when the group agreed that Barbara was actually partly responsible for Laurie and Bill's acting-out. While they supported Barbara, they evaluated the problem and gave Barbara feedback regarding her non-verbal messages. It seemed that her frequent checking on clients conveyed her expectation that they were up to something. Barbara acknowledged that she expected that sort of behavior from them and was quite afraid of discovering them in the act of intercourse. The group helped Barbara see that her own expectations were being met. Laurie and Bill were doing exactly what she expected them to do—maybe even wanted them to do. Laurie and Bill were following their scripts of being "bad" and expressing their hostility to Barbara. When Barbara heard how other staff members spent time with the couple to encourage them in indirect ways to join the larger group activities and compared her own behavior to that of her peers, it became apparent to her how obvious her anxiety and unconscious messages actually were. She then began to question her own attitudes about sexual matters and to explore why she feared discovering the couple engaged in sexual intercourse.

In this example, the client couple used sexual behaviors to act out their own underlying feelings. Had Barbara's assessment been limited to the immediate situation, she would have focused only on their unacceptable behavior and would not have been open to the implications for her. By seeking out information and feedback from her peers, she made a discovery about herself and realized more effective ways of anticipating and possibly circumventing such client behaviors rather than having to intervene after the fact. Had Barbara not asked for feedback, the problem would have continued, with an increase in the sexual behaviors and in Barbara's frustration. The situation would have then demanded intervention by an astute supervisor or an empathic colleague.

Homosexual Behavior. In situations in which homosexual behavior is an expected developmental step or a lifestyle without expressions of anger or hostility toward parents or staff, little or no intervention may be indicated. However, when homosexual behavior is used to act out feelings of impotence, or aggressive behavior is used to counteract feelings of intimacy, limits must be imposed.

Try to anticipate such behavior and provide other ways for the adolescent client to demonstrate his masculinity, perhaps by organizing a game of football or tennis, if he is fairly proficient at these skills, or engaging him in some other activity in which he excels. The point is to reestablish the adolescent's feeling of competence and control. Without such intervention, his feelings of impotence will escalate to the point where he will most certainly act them out in a negative way. The client who uses homosexuality to express defiance against authority figures will most assuredly flaunt homosexual activities and consistently incur the anger, embarrassment, or both, of staff and clients alike.

INTERVENING WITH SUBSTANCE ABUSE

You will benefit from self-awareness and an appreciation for the feelings that working with substance abusers can evoke. For example, the nurse who feels angry and punitive with the client who abuses drugs or overidentifies with the client and finds adventure in the client's drug stories cannot establish a therapeutic relationship with the client. Feelings of disdain or envy can compromise nursing care and, indeed, may make the client's treatment ineffective. Only by viewing substance abuse as a symptom of a broader illness can you be effective in dealing with adolescents. Nurses who have contact with adolescents, especially in school or community settings, should familiarize themselves with the general effects of various drugs and the first aid treatment for each (see Chapter 13).

In the example of 15-year-old Cindy with the expected outcomes and interventions proposed earlier, you will know that your outcomes were met if:

- Client approaches nurse to discuss temptation to use drugs.
- Client attends and participates in family meetings.
- Client verbalizes negative feelings.
- Client correlates negative feelings with temptation to use drugs.
- Client demonstrates alternative ways of dealing with stressful situations, such as talking to others, becoming involved in peer group activities, or using "quiet time" in anticipation of family meetings.

Even with the "best" success with an adolescent, you may find that you can expect to be successful "only 80% of the time." The adolescent will take some time to "try out" new behaviors and coping mechanisms. Equally important is to acknowledge that the client may need to take two steps forward and one backward as progress is made. Moreover, as stressful situations arise, the adolescent will be inclined to resort to "old" patterns of behavior. With Cindy's situation, she may resist attending a difficult family meeting or may even bolt from the room when confronted with her behaviors or feelings. Either act alone does not mean that she is not showing progress or improvement.

Interventions are determined to be effective or ineffective by the use of subjective and objective behavioral criteria as described above. These criteria should reflect your individualized plan of care and the mutually agreed-upon goals between you and the client. Only then can you expect to see the merits of your professional interventions and reap the rewards that can come from working with this special population.

Evaluation

Evaluating nursing interventions with adolescent clients can be tricky for numerous reasons:

- The adolescent client may need to test the limit one more time following a nursing intervention to avoid appearing "too compliant" or to "save face" with the group.
- Although it is important to set limits, it is equally important to be flexible. To set a limit and immediately "draw the line" with the next infraction is to invite the client to step over that line to test its seriousness.
- Quick judgments should not be made if immediate results are not obtained. Persistence and consistency are the keys to success.
- The behaviors that brought the adolescent to psychiatric treatment will continue long after treatment and nursing interventions are begun. Despite a well-designed nursing care plan and client contract, the adolescent will resort to previous maladaptive ways, immature and impulsive acts, or destructive behaviors in the face of change, particularly if this change represents improvement or growth (such as an increase in privileges or an impending discharge). The nurse who thinks the nursing interventions are not effective may feel hopeless about progress and convey that hopelessness to the client and the rest of the treatment team.
- Use of a behavioral contract without understanding the underlying reasons or factors contributing to the adolescent's problems will result in a superficial approach with an equally superficial evaluation.

If the adolescent had the desire or the impulse control simply to "act right" after being given the rules and consequences, then the client would be doing so already, and psychiatric treatment would not have been necessary. The adolescent needs the structure and consistency of a nursing care plan and client contract without the rigidity that can be imposed by a "now or never" behavioral plan with absolute consequences.

You can make a more adequate evaluation if you attempt to be aware of the social context and meaning of the behavior to the adolescent. For example, you may be wrong in determining that an indicator of increased self-esteem for a female client would be to stop dyeing her hair purple. Dyeing one's hair an unusual color may have been an indication of low self-esteem during your adolescent years, but for the client in question, that may or may not be the case. For that adolescent client and her peer group, purple hair may be a well-defined status symbol.

Evaluation is determined to be effective or ineffective by the use of various subjective and objective behavioral criteria reflecting the client care goals.

Case Management, Community-Based Care, and Home Care

While many formal psychiatric disorders appear at first among young adults (see Chapters 14 and 15), psychiatric–mental health nurses will most likely encounter troubled adolescents in community-based settings such as schools, emergency rooms, jails and detention centers, detoxification programs, sexually transmitted disease (STD) clinics, and other outpatient settings that provide programs for angry, abused, neglected or otherwise troubled teenagers. Psychiatric–mental health nurses may also encounter adolescents who are experiencing a temporary crisis and are in need of support and counseling while in abortion clinics, group homes, homes for young mothers, and drunk drivers' schools. The section earlier in this chapter about psychiatric–mental health nursing roles in outpatient settings addresses in detail the skills you will need to address such client problems.

Of particular concern to psychiatric–mental health nurses who are committed to advocate for troubled and troublesome teens is the reauthorization of the U.S. Welfare System Reform that repealed the 1996 Aid to Families with Dependent Children program. As Stevens (2000) has aptly argued, under a banner of self-sufficiency and the righteousness of work, the new law called the Personal Responsibility and Work Reconciliation Act mandates payment to families only if the mother works full-time outside the home. Consequently, the teenagers of poor mothers live like Margarita, age 13, who describes her experience as living on the edge. She and her sisters have slept outside in a gas station, watched their mother be arrested for drugs, and have all spent months in a group home after Child Protective Services removed them from their mother's custody. Many of the teens like Margarita are alone most of the time with little parental guidance.

CLINICAL EXAMPLE

Nick's mother works two jobs as a night receptionist and a daytime maid at a local motel. Nick, age 15, has no one to talk to about the gangs and violence in his school or about the fact that he is falling so far behind in his schoolwork. Many of his friends have started drinking beer and sniffing glue before engaging in random violence and petty theft. His mother's long work hours leave him alone to feed his little brothers fast food and put them to bed. He then falls asleep on the couch with the TV flickering, having not done his homework yet again.

Psychiatric–mental health nurses who work with adolescents like Margarita and Nick need to pay particular attention to roles as case managers and clinicians who can practice in community and home-based settings. The skills required in these roles include:

- Assessing conflicted adolescents and problematic families wherever you encounter them.
- Educating faculty, school administrators, and parents about the importance of preventive attention and the resources available to help teens and their families.
- Preventing youth violence and drug abuse if possible.
- Advocating for home-based therapy models.
- Refining skills as an individual, group, and family therapist with adolescents and their families.
- Health teaching about sensitive topics like drug use, STDs, unwanted pregnancy, and the consequences of anger and violence.
- Working as a political advocate to avoid putting a sizable portion of our country's families at risk for the poverty that in turn puts teens at risk.

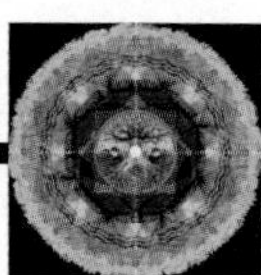

EXPLORE MediaLink

NCLEX review, case studies, and other interactive resources for this chapter can be found on the Companion Website at http://www.prenhall.com/kneisl. Click on Chapter 26 to select the activities for this chapter.

For animations, video tutorials, more NCLEX review questions, and an audio glossary, access the accompanying CD-ROM in this textbook.

BIBLIOGRAPHY

American Academy of Child and Adolescent Psychiatry. (1999). *Violence fact sheet*. Washington, DC: AACAP. Retrieved from the World Wide Web, October 11, 2002, www.aacap.org/web/aacap/info_families/NationalFacts/99ViolFctSh.html.

American Medical Association. (2000, December 13). AMA, youth violence commission emphasize prevention to stop youth violence [Announcement]. Washington, DC: AMA Member Communications. Retrieved from the World Wide Web, October 11, 2002, www.ama-assn.org/ama/pub/article/2403-3590.html.

American Psychiatric Association. (2000). *Diagnostic and statistical manual of mental disorders* (4th ed.), (Text Revision) (DSM-IV-TR). Washington, DC: Author.

Barkley, R. A., Edwards, G. H., & Robin, A. L. (1999). *Defiant teens: A clinician's manual for assessment and family intervention*. New York: Guilford Press.

Berenson, C. K. (1998). Diagnostic dilemmas, part II: Frequently missed diagnoses in adolescent psychiatry. *Psychiatric Clinics of North America, 21*(4), 917–926.

Botteron, K. N. (1999, October). *Prefrontal limbic neuromorphometry in early onset depression*. Paper presented at the meeting of the American Academy of Child and Adolescent Psychiatry 46th Annual Meeting, Chicago, IL.

Davanzo, P. A. (1999, October). *1HMR spectroscopy of juvenile onset bipolar disorder*. Paper presented at the meeting of the American Academy of Child and Adolescent Psychiatry 46th Annual Meeting, Chicago, IL.

Diamond, G. M., Diamond, G. S., & Liddle, H. A. (2000). The therapist-parent alliance in family-based therapy for adolescents. *Journal of Clinical Psychology, 56*(8), 1037–1050.

Futterman, D., Chabon, B., & Hoffman, J. D. (2000). HIV and AIDS in adolescents. *Pediatric Clinics of North America, 47*(1), 171–188.

Horner, S. D. (2000). Using focus group methods with middle school children. *Research in Nursing & Health, 23*(6), 510–517.

Jackson, S. M., Cram, F., & Seymour, F. W. (2000). Violence and sexual coercion in high school students' dating relationships. *Journal of Family Violence, 15*(1), 23–36.

Joffe, A. (2000). Why adolescent medicine? *Medical Clinics of North America, 84*(4), 769–785.

Lewinsohn, P. M., Rohde, P., Seeley, J. R., Klein, D. N., & Gotlib, I. H. (2000). Natural course of adolescent major depressive disorder in a community sample: Predictors of recurrence in young adults. *American Journal of Psychiatry, 157*, 1584–1591.

Lewis, T. B., Amini, F., & Lannon, R. A. (2000). *A general theory of love*. New York: Random House.

Mahon, N. E., Yarcheski, A., Yarcheski, T. J. (2000). Positive and negative outcomes of anger in early adolescents. *Research in Nursing & Health, 23*(1), 17–24.

Miranda, A., & Presentacion, M. J. (2000). Efficacy of cognitive-behavioral therapy in the treatment of children with ADHD, with and without aggressiveness. *Psychology in the Schools, 37*(2), 169–182.

Moore, G. J. (1999, October). *Proton MRS in bipolar disorder: A pilot study in adolescents*. Paper presented at the meeting of the American Academy of Child and Adolescent Psychiatry 46th Annual Meeting, Chicago, IL.

Muscari, M. E. (1999). Prevention: Are we really reaching today's teens? *American Journal of Maternal/Child Nursing, 24*(2), 87–91.

National Institute on Drug Abuse. (2000, December 14). *Monitoring the future national results on adolescent drug use: Overview of key findings, 2000* [News release]. Washington, DC: L. D. Johnston, P. M. O'Malley, & J. G. Bachman. Retrieved from the World Wide Web, October 11, 2002, http://monitoringthefuture.org/pubs/monographs/overview2001.pdf.

National Institute of Mental Health. (1999a). *Youth in a difficult world* (NIH Publication No. 99-4587). Washington, DC: U.S. Government Printing Office.

National Institute of Mental Health. (1999b). *Teens: The company they keep* (NIH Publication No. 99-4588). Washington, DC: U.S. Government Printing Office.

Post, D., Carr, C., & Weigand, J. (1998). Teenagers: Mental health and psychological issues. *Primary Care: Clinics in Office Practice, 25*(1), 181–193.

Stevens, P. (2000). A nursing critique of U.S. welfare system reform. *Advances in Nursing Science, 23*(2), 1–11.

U.S. Department of Health and Human Services. (1999a). *Healthy people 2010*. Rockville, MD: Office of Disease Prevention and Health Promotion. Retrieved from the World Wide Web, October 11, 2002, www.health.gov/healthypeople/LHI/lhiwhat.htm.

U.S. Department of Health and Human Services. (1999b). *Mental health: A report of the Surgeon General—executive summary*. Rockville, MD: U.S. Department of Health and Human Services, Substance Abuse and Mental Health Services Administration, Center for Mental Health Services, National Institutes of Health, National Institute of Mental Health. Retrieved from the World Wide Web, October 11, 2002, www.surgeongeneral.gov/library/mentalhealth/summary.html.

U.S. Department of Health and Human Services. (1999c). *Suicide among the young: The Surgeon General's call to action*. Washington, DC: U.S. Public Health Service. Retrieved from the World Wide Web, October 11, 2002, www.surgeongeneral.gov/library/calltoaction/fact3.htm.

U.S. Department of Health and Human Services. (1999d). *Youth violence: A report of the Surgeon General*. Rockville, MD: U.S. Department of Health and Human Services. Retrieved from the World Wide Web, October 11, 2002, www.mentalhealth.org/youthviolence/surgeongeneral/SG_Site/home.asp.

Wilens, T. E. (1999). *Straight talk about psychiatric medications for kids*. New York: Guilford Press.

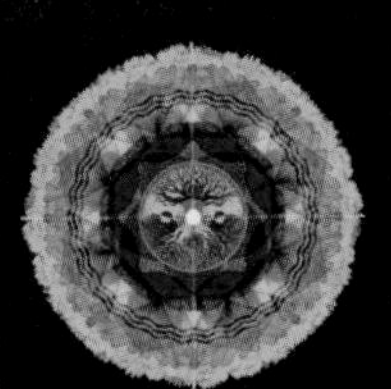

27

Chapter TWENTY-SEVEN

Elders

GLORIA KUHLMAN
HOLLY SKODOL WILSON

KEY TERMS

life review
palliative care
psychogerontology
reality orientation
reminiscence therapy
remotivation therapy
resocialization groups
restorative care

FOCUS QUESTIONS

- **What age-related demographic projections have implications for planning future mental health services for elders?**
- **What are the best known theories of aging and the major ideas associated with each one?**
- **What are the key components of a biopsychosocial assessment of an older client?**
- **Can you differentiate normal physical and psychosocial changes that accompany aging from mental disorders that afflict elders?**
- **How would you describe community support programs such as adult day care, restorative programs, and assisted living to elders and their families?**
- **What feelings do you experience when caring for elders who suffer from mental disorders?**

MediaLink 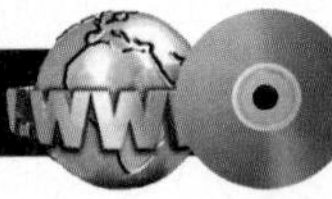 www.prenhall.com/kneisl

Additional resources for this chapter can be found on the Student CD-ROM accompanying this textbook, and on the Companion Website at www.prenhall.com/kneisl. Click on Chapter 27 to select the activities for this chapter.

CD-ROM
- Audio Glossary
- NCLEX Review

Companion Website
- Additional NCLEX Review
- Care Plan: Elder Feeling Like a Burden
- Case Study: Feeling Old

CHAPTER OUTLINE

CROSS REFERENCES

Other topics relevant to the content in this chapter are: Delirium and dementia, Chapter 12; Depression, Chapter 15; Elder abuse, Chapter 23; Polydrug use among elders, Chapter 13; Psychotropic medications, Chapter 31; Schizophrenia, Chapter 14; Sleep disorders, Chapter 19; Suicide lethality assessment, Chapter 22.

CRITICAL THINKING CHALLENGE

A recently retired 65-year-old man is brought to your clinic by his wife, who states that he "just sits around all day watching TV and won't do anything." She tells you that he used to be very active in his work and seemed to love it. He also played golf or spent time in his garden on the weekends. She reveals that he now seems unable to concentrate and has become bitter and difficult to live with. On interviewing the client, you find that he had been a successful owner of a small hardware store with his younger brother, who recently died of a heart attack while working at the store. Your client retired from the business soon thereafter at his family's insistence. He goes on to tell you that his memory is impaired, he has difficulty sleeping, and that he has lost his robust appetite. The other members of the clinic's treatment team want to perform a dementia workup but you are not convinced and would like to gather further data before beginning the dementia assessment. What areas would you assess? ■

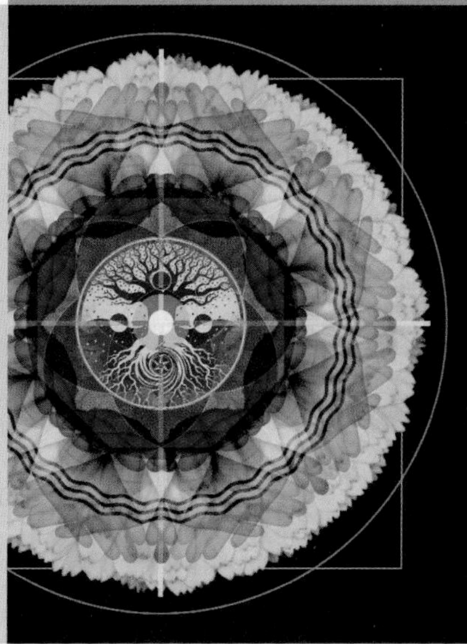

The population of American elders is growing faster than the nation as a whole. In 2000, the U.S. Bureau of Census reported that by the year 2050, 21% of the population will be age 65 and older. The over-65 population, which includes the middle-old (75 to 84) and the old-old (85+) reached 34.8 million or more than 12% of the U.S. population in 2000.

The rest of the world has experienced a similar population explosion in the over-65 age group. According to the Bureau of the Census (2000) estimate for the world population, by the year 2050 the numbers of old-old will continue to increase dramatically, especially in the United States, China, and India. As a consequence of improved pharmacologic and other treatments, the number of individuals afflicted with schizophrenia, dementia, and mood disorders once associated with decreased longevity will experience a relatively normal life span. An unprecedented growth in the number of elders with chronic mental illness will have a significant impact on the need for quality geropsychiatric care. Simultaneously, family caregivers who are aging themselves will also strain geropsychiatric care resources.

It is important to examine the age distribution of the over-65 population carefully. Grouping elders into an aggregate of all those over the age of 65 tends to blur important distinctions. The old-old group tends to have the greatest incidences of depression, delirium, dementia, and other chronic disabling conditions. Of this group, 49% have some limitations in their ability to perform activities of daily living (Eliopoulos, 2001). Therefore, the stereotypic frail elderly who consume many health care resources and maintenance services constitute only 5% of the over-65 population. A large proportion of healthy older people, particularly older women alone (who outnumber single elderly men by 2.5 to 1) will benefit most from supportive psychosocial services often provided by psychiatric–mental health care nurses.

The implications of a growing population of aging "baby boomers" with different mental health needs are important for planning programs and funding allocation. The data clearly underscore a need for more health professionals who are versed in the multiple requirements of older adults. Nursing's role in **psychogerontology** and in geriatrics is expanding as the needs and real numbers of elders increase (Eliopoulos, 2001). Psychogerontology refers to a subspecialty within gerontology focused on the psychosocial care of elders.

The aim of this chapter is to provide a comprehensive discussion of health promotion and advocacy for elders with mental health needs. It also discusses the DSM-IV-TR mental disorders commonly seen in later life and presents specific strategies for applying the nursing process with elders using North American Nursing Diagnosis Association (NANDA), Nursing Outcomes Classification (NOC), and Nursing Intervention Classification (NIC) terminology. Finally, contemporary issues including end-of-life care, restorative programs, and community-based support are also addressed.

Roadblocks to Mental Health Services for Elders

Elders are the most underserved population in need of supportive and tertiary mental health care. This discussion highlights four roadblocks to mental health care services—ageism, myths, stigma, and health care financing—and examines the demographic realities that compel us to break through these disabling roadblocks through self-awareness, health promotion, and client advocacy (see ■ Figure 27–1).

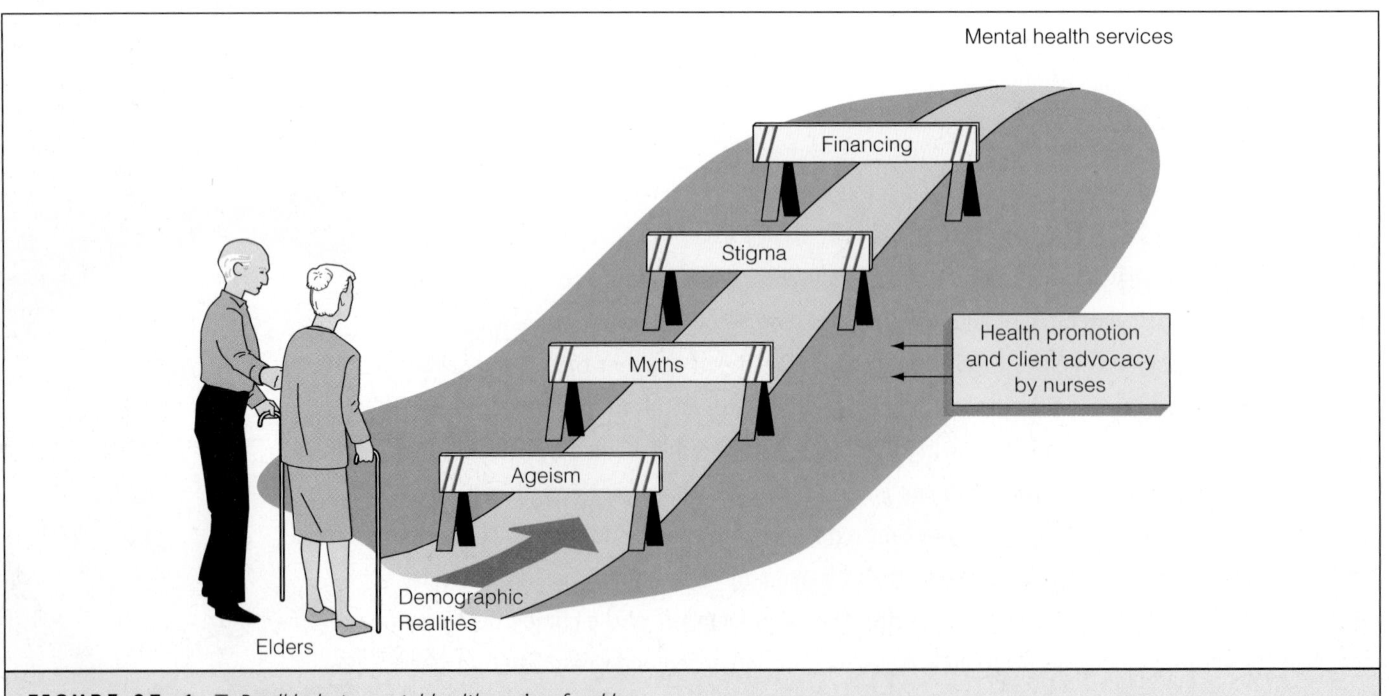

FIGURE 27–1 ■ *Roadblocks to mental health services for elders.*

AGEISM

A primary roadblock to adequate mental health services for elders is ageism—a prejudice against people because they are old. In many contemporary Western cultures, aging is often viewed with disdain and dislike. Elders are criticized for being unattractive, incompetent, socially irrelevant, and unhealthy. In the past, older adults were considered inappropriate candidates for mental health interventions and resources. According to Eliopoulos (2001), ageism stems from the belief that elders present a financial and emotional drain to the family and society. Other experts suggest that ageism results from our fears of facing our own aging process and mortality. Ageist attitudes can be internalized by elderly people, causing decreased self-worth and self-esteem, whatever the source.

When caring for elderly clients, be aware of their feelings and your own. Your personal biases can influence your clinical assessment and your decisions about interventions. You can provide invaluable support, insight, and feedback to colleagues who are working with older adults. Consider using the Nursing Self-Awareness feature below as a discussion point. We know that elders are as responsive to mental health services as are members of any other aging group. By modeling positive attitudes toward aging and by advocating quality of life and health care for elders in all settings and at all levels of function, you can help dispel ageist influences.

MYTHS

Mental health care professionals and elders themselves often equate growing old with growing sad, disengaged, inactive, socially isolated, and dependent. Such myths all too often inhibit people from seeking treatment for feelings and behaviors that they believe are a normal part of aging. Misled by these myths, health professionals can be less inclined to refer elders for mental health services. We now know that advancing age does not condemn an individual to senility, social isolation, loneliness, or dependence. Most elders live independently and contentedly well into late life unless they can no longer drive and live alone, or live in rural areas without transportation or even in urban areas where they are unable to access health care resources.

Psychiatric–mental health nurses can serve as elder advocates by educating the public, other health care professionals, and elders and their families about the differences between normal aging and changes associated with pathologic conditions. Recognizing that aging itself is not a problem increases the likelihood that problems that do arise will be assessed and treated.

STIGMA

Despite recent advances in mental health care, the stigma associated with mental illness remains very real to elderly people. Elders rarely seek mental health services and often hide their psychic pain for fear of being labeled "crazy" or losing control and being institutionalized.

Nurses have the opportunity to educate the public about mental disorders and state-of-the-art treatments that are available to all age groups. In so doing, we can help to decrease the stigma associated with psychiatric illness and treatment. The National Alliance for the Mentally Ill (NAMI) has made important advances in this direction by circulating information about the biological basis for many psychiatric disorders. You can refer elders who feel reluctant about acknowledging a psychiatric problem to the NAMI Web site at www.nami.org, which can be found through a resource link provided on the Companion Website for this text. As people learn more about research that confirms brain mechanisms associated with psychiatric disorders, traditional stigma associated with seeking mental health services is likely to decrease. At the present time, however, the primary care provider for many mentally ill elders is their family physician or adult nurse practitioner.

MediaLink NAMI

MediaLink Case Study: Feeling Old

HEALTH CARE FINANCING

Financial barriers, physical disability, and transportation problems are some factors that limit access to services, especially for mentally disordered elders. The financial barriers are particularly serious. Medicare, the major form of health care financing for elders, covers only a portion of the costs for its beneficiaries. Long-term care coverage and coverage for chronic conditions

Nursing SELF-AWARENESS — Attitudes Toward Aging

A bias against elders because of their age can result in discrimination against them even by mental health professionals. Ask yourself the following questions and discuss your responses with other students, faculty, or colleagues.

1. Am I uncomfortable around people who are old, infirm, or confused?
2. Do I have positive role models for aging with grace?
3. Do I dread growing old myself?
4. Should elders be encouraged to do as much as possible for themselves or be cared for by others?
5. How do I feel about old people who are sexually active and insist on trying to look and act young?
6. Do most elders become rigid and set in their ways once they age?
7. Am I well informed about the differences between mental disorder in elders and the normal aging process?
8. Do I equate advanced age with unattractiveness, incompetence, and senility?
9. Am I well informed about community resources and support systems available for elders and their family caregivers?
10. How do I feel when caring for an elderly person who is demanding and dependent?

Reflection on such questions can promote your beginning awareness of any attitudes that might interfere with quality care for elders.

MediaLink AARP

are sorely lacking. Community and home-based care is limited at best, and Medicare does not cover many mental health services at all. Expensive prescription medication plans and large copayments for services reimbursed through Medicare add to an older person's psychosocial stressors. These gaps and lack of coverage will reach crisis levels as baby boomers reach old age and require long-term care services. For the mentally ill elderly, the crisis is even more intense since many long-term care facilities do not admit identified geropsychiatric clients/patients. Nurses must become active voices in lobbying for policy change to improve financing for elder care that covers the range of acute and chronic illnesses. The American Association of Retired Persons (AARP) is an excellent information source related to these topics. The AARP Web site, www.aarp.org can be found through a resource link on the Companion Website for this text.

Biopsychosocial Theories of Aging

Distinguishing between normal aging changes and mental disorder in later life is a challenge. Many variables affect mental health as a person ages. Theories of normal aging are presented in the following section as biologic and psychosocial. Not all theories identified here have been fully confirmed through systematic research, and some, such as the disengagement theory, remain controversial.

BIOLOGIC THEORIES

Biologic theories of aging include genetic, wear-and-tear, immunology, nutritional, and environmental theories.

Genetic Theory

MediaLink Education and Genetics

Since the initiation of the Human Genome Project in 1990 by the Department of Energy and the National Institutes of Health, which aimed to map and sequence the human genome in its entirety, definitions of health and illness have been transformed by knowledge of genetics (Lea & Williams, 2002). According to genetic theories, aging is a process that operates over time to alter cellular structures. Harmful genes activate in late life to stop cell growth and division. This theory supports the idea that the life span is predetermined and people's aging experience is programmed by their genetic makeup. The National Coalition for Health Professional Education in Genetics, initiated by the American Medical Association, the American Nurses Association, and the National Human Genome Research Institute, can be contacted through this text's Companion Website at www.nchpeg.org.

Wear-and-Tear Theory

The wear-and-tear theory proposes that the accumulation of waste products from metabolism damages DNA synthesis, leading eventually to organ malfunction (Steen, 2001). In short, cells wear out. Even though the theory allows for individual rates of cell decline that can be accelerated from abuse and slowed by care, the emphasis is one of loss and decline in later life.

Immunology Theory

This theory explains age-related decline in people's immune systems. As a person ages, his or her ability to defend against foreign organisms declines with a corresponding increase in susceptibility to diseases, including cancer and serious infections. Theorists suggest that the changes that take place with aging allow the body to misidentify old, irregular cells as foreign bodies and the body then attacks these cells (Steen, 2001). Multiple neurochemical and viral theories are being developed as cellular research advances. For example, free radical theory posits that free radicals cause the damage to cell membranes as one ages.

Nutritional Theory

Nutritional theory focuses on the idea that the quality of one's diet is important to how one ages (Knoll, 2001). The quality of one's diet (amounts of fresh fruits and vegetables especially) is as important as the quantity because vitamin and nutrient deficiencies or excesses have an influence on disease processes.

Environmental Theory

A number of environmental factors are known to threaten health and may be associated with aging. The ingestion of lead, arsenic, pesticides, and other substances can seriously harm the body, as can smoking and air pollution. Environmental factors such as crowded living conditions and high levels of noise are known to be stressful and to drain a person's coping capacity. All can affect one's vulnerability or vigor while aging (Eliopoulos, 2001).

PSYCHOSOCIAL THEORIES

Psychosocial theories of aging include the disengagement and activity theories, which contrast sharply with each other.

Disengagement Theory

First proposed in the 1960s, the *disengagement theory* described what was considered to be an inevitable process in which elders willingly withdrew from social contacts and responsibilities, feeling relief about turning matters over to the younger generation (Bergstom & Holmes, 2000). This theory has become controversial because many older adults continue to be engaged and responsible well into later life unless limited by immobility that can lead to involuntary social isolation. Recent research emphasizes the need for continued mental activity in order to sustain health throughout the life span (Schroots, 1996). See the section on *restorative care* later in this chapter.

Activity Theory

Quite the opposite of disengagement theory is activity theory (Schroots, 1996). This theory proposes that the way to age successfully is to stay active and involved. Exercise and social interaction are believed to contribute to mental health and satisfaction in late life. Consequently, elders are encouraged to remain as active as possible for as long as possible.

Psychiatric Disorders in the Elderly

Ageist attitudes in our culture are responsible for many misconceptions about mental disorders among elders. Older people are believed to be more prone to mental illness than are young people. For several reasons, however, it is difficult to obtain exact incidence and prevalence rates for mental disorders in later life. Elders are often difficult to reach with community-wide surveys, they are reluctant to respond to personal questions that deal with emotional problems, and most either do not seek treatment for emotional problems or they consult primary care providers rather than psychiatric professionals.

Symptoms of mental illness in the elderly often differ from those of other age groups. While the DSM-IV-TR (American Psychiatric Association [APA], 2000) has enhanced our ability to make valid and reliable diagnoses of mental disorders, there are few age-specific categories. Thus, despite the DSM-IV-TR extensive, detailed descriptions of each problem category, clinicians and researchers continue to have difficulty applying the written descriptions of symptoms to elderly people.

Epidemiologic studies indicate that elders suffer no more than other groups from adjustment disorders, personality disorders, and grief reactions (Schwartz, Gunzelmann, Hinz, & Brahler, 2001). Older adults do have a disproportionately high incidence of depression and are somewhat more likely to become paranoid. They also frequently experience sleep disruptions that may or may not meet the diagnostic criteria for a formal sleep disorder. A growing body of information suggests that substance use disorders, particularly alcoholism and prescription medication abuse, are more serious problems among elders than had been thought in the past (Johnson, 2000).

MOOD DISORDERS

Mood disorders are primarily characterized by disturbed affect or emotional experience. When they occur in elders they may present as:

- Sustained elation and hyperactivity such as in a manic episode.
- Changes from elation to depression such as in bipolar disorder.
- Pervasive depressed mood not accompanied by mania such as in major depression.

Depression is the most preventable and most treatable mental disorder in later life (Eliopoulos, 2001).

Depression in the Elderly

Geriatric depression is widespread in general practice and even higher in hospitals and nursing homes. Depression robs the person of later life satisfaction, inhibits ego integrity, and may substantially decrease life expectancy. Elders have the highest rate of suicide of any age group and a range of physical disturbances intensified by depression (Salvatore, 2000).

Although the signs and symptoms of depression are relatively consistent throughout the life span, certain characteristics of depression are particular to elders. It is crucial for clinicians to remember that depression in older adults that responds well to treatment may appear with cognitive changes similar to those that accompany other organically based, irreversible disorders. Loss of executive function (often a diagnostic clue to dementia) includes disturbances in planning, sequencing, organizing, and abstracting. Such cognitive impairment can also be a sign of depression.

In addition to cognitive changes, another sign of depression in older adults is an excessive preoccupation with physical symptoms known as *somatization*. Expressing discomfort through the body may be more familiar and comfortable than recognizing and describing psychic pain. Such is the case in the following example.

CLINICAL EXAMPLE

Mr. Gambino, a 79-year old widower, came to his physician's office complaining of "not feeling well." After a physical examination, the doctor told Mr. Gambino that he had a weight loss of 10 pounds, mild chronic obstructive pulmonary disease (COPD), and slight hypertension, but was otherwise in good health for his age. Mr. Gambino responded angrily, "I know I am dying but it doesn't matter because I have nothing to live for now that my wife is dead. She's been gone for 6 months and everyone says I should be feeling better, but I feel worse! I can't eat, can't sleep, and I don't have enough energy to even wash my car!" Mr. Gambino says he is tired all day but cannot sleep at night. "I am up at 3:00 AM and can't go back to sleep." He says he tries to eat but does not cook well and "the food just doesn't taste right."

Clearly, Mr. Gambino presents with a number of physical complaints that may shift the focus away from distressing emotions to more acceptable medical conditions that are less stigmatizing. Other possible somatic signs of depression to watch for include:

- Chronic complaints of constipation.
- Muscular pain.
- Chest tightness.
- Headaches.
- Difficulty breathing.
- Chronic gastrointestinal upset.

Psychiatric–mental health nurses must be persistent and perceptive in looking for signs of depression. Depressed, apathetic elders may believe they are supposed to feel blue and "down in the dumps" as they age. We need to talk with them and their families about depression as a pathologic condition often caused by biochemical imbalances that can be corrected. Interventions for depression in the elderly should be instituted as aggressively and comprehensively as with any other age group.

Depressive symptoms may also result from social and economic circumstances such as social isolation and neglect. They may be the result of a medical condition such as a stroke, Parkinson's disease, or even a hip fracture. Consequently, it is imperative to include a comprehensive geriatric assessment of an elderly client before beginning a treatment regimen. An older person's response to traumatic events may be tied to functional disability and requires multiple areas of intervention.

Suicide Among Elders

Data from nearly all industrialized countries report that suicide rates rise progressively with age. The highest rates occur in men age 75 and older (Salvatore, 2000). Compared with the general population, suicide attempts are more lethal and approached with a greater degree of premeditation and planning when made by elders. Older adults who present a greater suicide risk include:

- Men.
- Widowed or divorced people.
- Caucasians.
- Those of lower socioeconomic status.
- Those with chronic pain and terminal illness.
- Alcoholics.
- Those with mental disorders.
- Those with neurologic deficits due to stroke and brain injury.

Suicidal elders have been known to seek help in the emergency room, often for a vague nonspecific physical problem prior to their self-destructive act. Accurate assessment of suicide potential requires active listening and direct questioning. A suicidal older client may present with any of the following:

- Verbal cues (I'm going to end it all; life is not worth living; I won't be around much longer).
- Behavioral cues (completing a will, making funeral plans, acting out, withdrawing, somatic complaints).
- Situational cues (a recent move, loss of a loved one, the diagnosis of a terminal illness).

For detailed information on suicide and the assessment of suicide potential including a lethality assessment, see Chapter 22.

SCHIZOPHRENIA

The number and proportion of older adults with schizophrenia will increase considerably with the movement of baby boomers into old age over the next 30 years. This generation of people with chronic mental illness has not spent years in institutions like the elderly mentally ill of past generations. There is little research on late-life schizophrenia and less on its treatment. This population of clients poses particularly critical issues when we realize the fact that 85% of older individuals with schizophrenia live in the community and will be approaching the age when long-term care becomes necessary at the same time nursing homes are severely restricting admission of psychiatric clients (Cohen & Talavera, 2000).

An individual with *late life schizophrenia* may be a psychotic person who has grown old or may be a person who did not experience psychotic symptoms until late in life. People with late-onset schizophrenia are often women with less severe negative symptoms, better premorbid functioning in early adulthood, and less impairment in the areas of learning, abstraction, and cognitive flexibility. They also require smaller doses of neuroleptic medication to manage their psychotic symptoms.

ADJUSTMENT DISORDERS

Elders often experience dramatic life changes because of losses due to death, relocation, dependence, loss of autonomy, retirement, illness, and financial stress. One or a combination of life changes and losses may contribute to the development of an *adjustment disorder*. The essential feature of adjustment disorders is a maladaptive reaction to an identifiable psychosocial stressor or stressors that occurs within 3 months after the onset of the stressor and has persisted for no longer than 6 months (APA, 2000). People experiencing adjustment disorders may have a variety of psychiatric symptoms, including:

- Anxious mood.
- Depressed mood.
- Mixed emotional features.
- Physical complaints.
- Withdrawal.

ANXIETY DISORDERS

Anxiety is common across age groups and increases in frequency with advancing age (Schwartz et al., 2001). Adjustments to physical, emotional, and socioeconomic changes as one ages add to the variety of causes for anxiety. Anxiety reactions in the elderly may manifest themselves as somatic complaints, rigid thinking and behavior, insomnia, fatigue, hostility, restlessness, confusion, and increased dependence. Physiologic indicators of anxiety include increased blood pressure, pulse, respirations, psychomotor restlessness, and increased voiding (Eliopoulos, 2001). Many of these manifestations of anxiety are noteworthy in the following example.

CLINICAL EXAMPLE

Mrs. Pyun, age 82, is rushed to the emergency room by her bridge group with what they think might be a heart attack. Mrs. Pyun is short of breath and sweating, her pulse is rapid, her hands are shaking, and she can't sit still during the assessment. She is tearful and cannot tell the advice nurse what is wrong. She says, "I don't know why I feel this way. I just know something bad is going to happen. I have to leave and get home. Why are you asking me all these questions? No, I don't have chest pain. I tried to tell them I was just nervous. I get this way sometimes."

Unfortunately, anxiety disorders and panic attacks are often overlooked in older clients because, as with depression, they present with a predominance of physical complaints that mask the underlying disorder. In addition, anxiety in elderly people often co-occurs with depression. The anxiety is treated but the depression persists, leading to a cycle of anxiety–depression and physical illness.

DELUSIONAL DISORDERS

Delusions in elders are considered to be a cognitive mechanism for maintaining a sense of power and control. The delusions may be comforting (belief that one is being guarded by an angel from God) or threatening ("The UPS driver has turned me into Homeland Security because he thinks I am a terrorist"), but whatever the content, they customarily form a structure for understanding a situation that otherwise seems unmanageable. Persecutory delusions involve the belief that one is under investigation, being harassed, or at the mercy of some powerful force. With somatic delusions, the predominant theme is an imagined physical disorder or abnormality of appearance. Somatic delusions in older people are frequently characterized by extremely morbid content ("My blood is leaking into my skin and will poison anyone who touches me").

Delusions in the elderly are often associated with delirium, depression, dementia, or anxiety disorders. Persecutory delusions may be a response to an older person's diminishing sense of self-mastery. Delusions involving suspiciousness and persecutory ideation are among the most unsettling for elders' caregivers and families. As older adults gradually give up important areas of function, such as financial management, driving, cooking, and shopping, they may begin to develop delusions that people are robbing them or poisoning their food. They respond to these delusions by "dismissing" or rejecting their caregivers in an effort to regain control over these areas of life. Delusions may also result from internalized ageist attitudes, sensory losses (particularly hearing impairment), and social isolation as is the case in the following example.

CLINICAL EXAMPLE

Ms. Colgán is an 88-year old woman living alone in a rural suburb of Calgary, Canada. Her cottage is somewhat isolated on a country road, and the long winters have kept her inside and isolated. A sister who has financial power of attorney pays her bills, and she primarily eats canned soups that she prepares for herself. Ms. Colgán rarely wears her hearing aids and spends most of her time watching TV with the sound turned up to the highest volume. Recently, she called her sister demanding to know what all these people are doing in her house. She believes that they are there to take her money and poison her food. After a careful assessment by the community mental health nurse, it became clear that Ms. Colgán was mistaking the actors on TV for people in her home.

As a psychiatric–mental health nurse, you must work to establish trust and consistency with delusional elders. It is important to assess the situation to validate that any persecutory and somatic content is not reality based. Clients need social interaction with caring people and consistent reality orientation. Relieving social isolation and correcting sensory losses may go far to solve the problem. Delusional processes associated with delirium often abate when the cause of the delirium is treated. Medication in small doses, geared toward relieving underlying anxiety or depressive disorder, may be helpful, although adherence is often a problem because of the client's suspiciousness.

SUBSTANCE-RELATED DISORDERS

The extent of alcoholism and drug and alcohol-related problems among older adults is not known. In the past, it was believed that the elderly constitute the age group with the lowest rates of alcohol and illegal drug use because of influences in early life such as prohibition and a historic disapproval of drinking by women. These beliefs are changing as baby boomers age. It is important to note that the elderly are more vulnerable than younger people to the effects of alcohol and other substances and that they are the largest consumers of over-the-counter (OTC) preparations and prescribed medications (Flodin, 1990). Alcohol abuse and drug dependence among elders are now recognized as serious problems (Johnson, 2000). Alcohol abuse can predispose elderly people to accidents, nutritional deficiencies, and disease that may lead to loss of autonomy. When older drinkers seek medical help for alcohol-related problems such as malnutrition, injuries from falls, and sleep problems, they rarely present alcoholism as their primary complaint. Unfortunately, the presenting problems may be treated and other symptoms mistakenly attributed to the aging process.

Clinical manifestations of alcohol abuse in the elderly include:

- Tolerance (requiring more of the substance for the same effect).
- Alcohol-related physical health problems such as gastritis, liver problems, and pancreatitis.
- Physiologic dependence on alcohol (the experience of withdrawal symptoms).
- Unexpected reaction to prescription medications.
- Multiple social complications (problems with family relationships and social isolation).
- Frequent behavioral problems such as aggression, memory gaps, and traffic accidents or DUIs.
- Self-care neglect such as incontinence, malnutrition, dehydration, and poor hygiene and home maintenance.

Many late-onset alcoholics are believed to have turned to drinking in response to stressful life events such as bereavement, illness, divorce, retirement, marital stress, or depression. Assessment for drug and alcohol abuse in elders, especially socially isolated elders who have suffered recent losses, should be approached with care. All clients must be educated about the risks of mixing medications with alcohol; approach elders in a nonjudgmental way when addressing this topic. Preventing drinking as a reaction to stress may be accomplished by providing social support and mental health services for elders at risk for social isolation and depression. Referral to resources such as Alcoholics Anonymous (www.alcoholics-anonymous.org) is a recommended intervention, especially when combined with other psychiatric supports (see Chapter 21 for information about treating people with the dual diagnosis of mentally ill chemical abuser).

DISORDERS OF AROUSAL AND SLEEP

MediaLink OTC Medication Use

The quantity and quality of sleep change with the aging process. Elders experience more frequent awakenings during the night, spend increased total time awake at night, and take longer to fall asleep. Changes in sleep patterns are believed to be related to changes in internal body rhythm, emotional stress, physical illness, and the effects of medications or drugs. Over one-third of people over 60 complain of sleep disturbances (Youngstedt, Kripke, Elliott, & Klauber, 2001). Elders nap more during the day and use a disproportionately high amount of OTC and prescription sleeping aids. Yet, the chronic use of sedatives and hypnotics by elders has not been shown to improve the quality of sleep and can lead to many undesirable and dangerous side effects. Elders excrete these drugs more slowly than the young and thus are prone to develop toxic effects, including delirium, daytime drowsiness, and loss of equilibrium. Respiration can be significantly disturbed with the use of sleeping medication.

Clinicians and clients alike must be cognizant of the risks associated with medications, especially when combined with alcohol or even herbal and other supplements. We should be more willing to try nonpharmacologic therapies if indicated. The National Council on Patient Information and Education and the Federal Drug Agency launched a campaign called "Be MedWise" to educate consumers on OTC medication use. For information go to www.bemedwise.org or use the Companion Website for this textbook.

MediaLink End of Life Care

Nonpharmacologic guidelines that are recommended for improving sleep for elders include:

- Steady daily physical activity.
- A cool, well-ventilated room.
- A light bedtime snack.
- Stress reduction to promote relaxation.
- Regular arousal time.
- Avoiding long naps during the day.
- Clean bed linen.
- Avoiding caffeine, tobacco, and alcohol.

Palliative and End-of-Life Issues with Mentally Ill Elders

Death and dying have been characterized as a crisis that is a natural part of life. Death itself has been called the ultimate loss, which is a uniquely personal experience that each of us faces alone. While more imminent for older adults, the need for improved care near the end of life is not unique to elders. Each death evokes different needs and behaviors and provides an opportunity for you as a nurse to address physical, psychological, social, and spiritual needs of clients and their families. The increased use of technology at the end of life, diminished inpatient care resources, and an aging population have all created a demand for palliative care.

PRECEPTS OF PALLIATIVE CARE

The World Health Organization (WHO) defines **palliative care** as the active total care of clients whose disease is not responsive to curative treatment. Not all palliative care occurs at the end of life, and much of it aims to help clients and their families to reach personal goals, reconcile conflicts, and derive meaning at the end of life (Ferrell & Coyle, 2002). Addressing such end-of-life issues is especially complicated when an elder client is exhibiting alteration in mental status due to delirium or dementia or associated with a preexisting psychiatric illness.

Palliative care requires attention to helping clients achieve comfort and a good quality of death and dying. While fears of pain, abandonment, and loss of control are among the most common symptoms for which nurses must provide relief, other end-of-life symptoms of particular concern to psychiatric–mental health nurses include:

- Delirium
- Agitation
- Anxiety
- Depression
- Loneliness
- Hopelessness
- Grief
- Social isolation
- Suffering
- Spiritual distress

In 1997, the American Association of Colleges of Nursing (AACN) hosted a panel of experts in order to develop guidelines concerning end-of-life care. These guidelines are considered to be the definitive statement on the knowledge and skills needed by nurses who are committed to improving palliative care. The statement entitled, *Peaceful Death: Recommended Competencies and Curricular Guidelines for End-of-Life Nursing Care* can be found at www.aacn.nche.edu/publications/deathfin/htm or through the Companion Website for this text. An additional Web-based resource can be found at the City of Hope Pain/Palliative Care Resource Center located at www.prc.coh.org.

An understanding of family dynamics as well as social, cultural, and religious beliefs may result in the need for additional supportive services of social workers, hospital chaplains, or other members of the interdisciplinary team. The entire team should be aware of the client's wishes and respond in an appropriate manner to his or her requests. An example of this is provided in the Using Research Evidence feature on page 647.

SPIRITUALITY AND END-OF-LIFE CARE

One of the precepts of palliative care is the notion of honoring the preferences, values, and culture of the client and family, especially with respect to suffering, whether it be physical, psychosocial, or spiritual. Spiritual assessment and care is a signifi-

USING RESEARCH EVIDENCE

Doris is 97 years of age and squarely among the percentage of elders who typically die in a nursing home. Her family is now challenged to decide whether she may die at home or must remain in a nursing home because of her increasing dementia. Unfortunately, Doris has lived long enough to lose her decisional capacity and her family is left with decisions about resuscitation, feeding tube placement, and use of antibiotics. Her grandchildren had been dealing with care decisions on a day-to-day basis and expressed considerable anguish, burden, and guilt when faced with decisions that required them to envision the dying trajectory.

Recognizing that Doris's family caregivers were experiencing a profound deficit in their ability to envision Doris's trajectory of dying, the mental health case manager engaged Doris's grandchildren in the advance care planning process. This provided a forum in which they could explore and discuss preferences and goals for end-of-life care. The case manager's care plan included translating medical information into an understanding of the trajectory of Doris's disease, the exploration of values and goals, and reduction of confusion, burden, and guilt. As a consistent counselor, the case manager was able to share her knowledge about palliative care options, was comfortable discussing death and dying, and exhibited sensitivity to the complexities of end-of-life decision making in a culture where multiethnic values, old age, and Western medicine may clash. This nursing care plan was based on the research evidence cited below.

Forbes, S., Bern-Klug, M., & Gessert, C. (2000). End-of-life decision making for nursing home residents with dementia. *Journal of Nursing Scholarship, 32*(3), 251–258.

cant component of end-of-life care. Spiritual integrity is a basic human power that gives meaning, purpose, and fulfillment to life and death. Literature has described the spiritual dimension as a striving for self-transcendence or search for a higher power and meaning that is greater than the self. Spirituality may or may not include formal religious participation. According to Joint Commission on Accreditation for Health Care Organizations (JCAHO) (2000) standards, certain clients require a comprehensive spiritual assessment. Among them are those receiving care at the end of their life, those who are being treated for emotional or behavioral disorders, and those in recovery from alcohol or drug dependence. Spiritual care according to hospice philosophy is nonjudgmental and all-inclusive and focuses on healing, forgiveness, and acceptance. Spiritual interventions can include any of the practices identified in the Caring for the Spirit feature on page 648.

Suffering is defined as a highly personal state of severe distress that transcends the physical, psychological, social, and spiritual dimensions and threatens the intactness of the person. According to Ferrell (1996), failure to respond to the spiritual needs of clients and their families coping with end-of-life issues may intensify the depth of suffering.

Historically, the role of the psychiatric–mental health nurse did not require expertise in palliative and end-of-life care. However, as the current population of psychiatric clients age and geropsychiatric care settings expand, addressing end-of-life care issues will become a major challenge and critical to management of a client's psychiatric illness. Effective communication with clients and their loved ones is essential. Communication strategies require that you accomplish the following:

- Be clear about the client's goals and expectations of care and treatment.
- Avoid euphemisms for words like *death* and *dying.*
- Be specific when using words such as *hope* and *better.*
- Listen to and honor the preferences, values, and cultural beliefs of clients and their loved ones (Norton & Talerico, 2000).

NURSING PROCESS

Elders

The following sections provide specific strategies for applying the nursing process when providing care to elders.

MediaLink Care Plan: Elder Feeling Like a Burden

Assessment

Assessment of the elder includes the assessment interview, a biologic assessment, consideration of cognitive status, an assessment of psychological/emotional status, an assessment of strengths and coping strategies, an assessment of sexuality, an attempt to determine social and financial status, and a focused effort to be astute to any indicators of elder abuse.

THE ASSESSMENT INTERVIEW

The variety of theories on aging and the complex interrelationship of physical, emotional, and environmental factors affecting mental health of elders require an individualized, comprehensive, and multidimensional approach. If feasible, a multidisciplinary team approach is most effective in providing validation of assessment impressions, accurate diagnoses, and appropriate intervention strategies.

The interview is the initial step in the assessment process and important to differentiating between psychiatric disorders and the normal aging process. Chapter 9 of this text offers a comprehensive overview of assessment procedures that should be adapted for elders. Guidelines for interviewing elders appear in the Assessment box on page 648.

Interviewing requires skill and heightened sensitivity and typically takes more time with older adults than with members of other age groups. Sensory loss, confusion, agitation, wandering, communication disorders, cultural influences, shame, and the fear of stigmatization may inhibit the expression of feelings in elders. They may be unaware of their behavior or expect neg-

CARING FOR THE SPIRIT

Supporting and Nurturing Spirituality of Elders in End-of-life Care

The word *spirituality* is rooted in the Greek language as a word for breath, breathing, and inspiration. Spirituality has evolved to mean something more than religiosity in nursing literature due to the influences of philosophies of holism and humanism as described in Chapter 2 of this text. Spirituality is recognized as a source of inner peace, hope, trust, faith, meaning and strength (Taylor, 2002). Attending to a client's spiritual quality of life and spiritual well-being has emerged as an important role for nurses. Spiritual needs, problems, concerns, distress, and pain all have been considered as nursing diagnoses, particularly among those receiving end-of-life care.

In addition to conducting and documenting a spiritual assessment and facilitating religious practices if the client wishes, a number of strategies are available to you as you attempt to provide care that supports and nurtures the spirituality of your clients. Consider learning more about each of them and adding them to your repertoire.

Engaging Spirituality Through Nature

Feelings of wonder, awe, and transcendence; a renewed sense of vigor; increased mindfulness; the sense of being present in the moment; an awareness of humility; and a better perspective all have been attributed to the benefits of experiencing nature. Finding ways to bring the influences of the natural environment into clients who are confined in nursing homes, hospice care, or hospitals can help clients draw strength and courage from things as simple as the image of a rainbow or the fragrance of pine needles.

Listening to Storytelling, Life Review, and Reminiscence

Encouraging a client to make an audiotape, dictate letters, create a photo album or scrapbook, or create other artistic expressions to depict the wholeness of his or her life can help the client establish a sense of satisfaction from a life well lived. Reminiscence and life review are identified as useful nursing interventions later in this chapter. Experts who teach about listening to clients' stories suggest guidelines for nurses using this approach. A major guideline is the idea of developing a list of questions that encourage awareness of positive aspects of a life story and reflection and enthusiasm on the part of the client telling the story. Questions might include: "How would you like the rest of your story to be?" "How has what has happened to you shaped who you are today?" "What do you think are the major themes in your life story?"

Assisting with Journal or Diary Writing

Keeping a journal offers a client a way in which to express inner thoughts. A journal can consist of narratives on topics such as "What do I stand for?", "What personal quality do I feel best about?", or "What makes me feel joy?" However, a journal can also take the form of sketches, song lyrics, descriptions of dreams, poetry, or prayers that can be original or collected from various sources.

Making and Appreciating Art as Spiritual Expression

According to Taylor (2002), creating art and sharing it with others allow clients to leave a legacy, build a sense of community and make sense of experiences. You can encourage clients to participate actively by drawing, painting, or sculpting or passively by collecting healing images such as mandalas, icons, or wilderness landscapes or photographs. Listening to music can help decrease anxiety, depression, agitation, and aggressive behavior as well as improve relaxation and peace of mind.

The strategies for supporting and nurturing spirituality described above represent only a sample of the possibilities. They all require self-disclosure on the part of clients who may feel vulnerable. Extreme sensitivity is required of the nurse who uses them in practice. Some clients will prefer to discuss these topics with a member of the clergy or a spiritual advisor. Their wishes must be respected.

---

ative changes as a normal part of aging. It is imperative to solicit interpretations from family and other staff members to help fill in aspects of the clinical picture and validate information provided by the client in the individual interview. See the Rx Communication feature on page 649 for an illustration of communicating with a confused elder.

ASSESSMENT

Guidelines for Interviewing Elders

1. Try to make the assessment interview as pleasant as possible by conveying a sense of respect and caring.
2. Be close to the client; use touch when appropriate.
3. Be clear in stating the purpose of the interview and the length of time it will take.
4. Attend to verbal, nonverbal, and environmental cues as well as to the cognitive and behavior status of the client.
5. Repeat the purpose and the time frame of the interview if the client forgets.

Assessment information about elders should include objective and subjective data regarding the client's physiologic status, psychological status, cognitive status, and social and financial status. A variety of self-report screening tools have been designed for use specifically with elderly clients. These require minimal special training to administer and help the nurse to obtain subjective assessment information. These tools may also be used as objective measures of the outcomes of interventions. Several of the most commonly used tools and scales are listed in the Assessment box on page 649.

The following section provides guidelines for obtaining subjective and objective assessment information about the client's physiologic, cognitive, emotional, and psychosocial status.

BIOLOGIC ASSESSMENT

Before a definitive psychiatric diagnosis can be made, all medically based illnesses that may present with psychiatric symp-

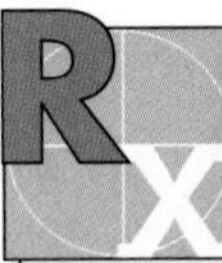

COMMUNICATION

Communicating with a Confused Elder

CLIENT: I don't know why I am here. My brother takes care of my finances. He doesn't think I take proper care of myself, but I am as I am and I want him to leave me A-LONE!

NURSE RESPONSE 1: Give me an example of something that your brother told you was your "not taking proper care of yourself."

RATIONALE: Response 1 focuses on collecting more information about the genuine safety risks faced by this 84-year-old woman who lives alone in a small New York City apartment. She has been referred to your clinic so that such an assessment can occur.

NURSE RESPONSE 2: What has your brother told you about why you are here at the clinic?

RATIONALE: This response requests concrete information from the client rather than any interpretations. It also has the potential to provide a picture of memory impairments she might be experiencing.

toms (depression, confusion, restlessness, and anxiety) must be ruled out. In addition, a complete medical and neurologic examination is necessary to differentiate irreversible conditions from treatable conditions such as pseudodementia. Many emergency room admissions for psychiatric problems in the elderly prove to have an underlying biologic etiology such as an infection or dehydration.

Objective assessment information includes lab results, a complete history, and physical exam, including weight, vital signs, and a description of the physical appearance of the client. Standard diagnostic laboratory analyses appear in ■ Figure 27–2 and should include complete blood chemistry, electrolytes, glucose tolerance, complete blood count (CBC), urinalysis, thyroid studies, blood urea nitrogen (BUN), creatinine, and liver function tests.

Other procedures important for ruling out infections, space-occupying lesions, drug toxicities, and cancers include chest radiography, drug toxicology screening, computed tomography (CT) scanning, positron-emission tomography (PET) scanning, electrocardiogram (ECG), electroencephalogram (EEG), and lumbar puncture. A dementia workup should include serologic tests for syphilis, folate, B_{12} levels, and trace minerals.

Subjective assessment information includes clients' perceptions of their physical health and a description of their chronic illnesses, symptoms, and self-care activities.

ASSESSMENT

Screening Instruments Frequently Used in Assessing Elders

- The *Iowa Self-Assessment Inventory*—Useful for obtaining a functional assessment of elders in a variety of settings.
- The *Geriatric Depression Scale*—Useful for collecting information about symptoms of depression.
- The *Short Portable Mental Status Questionnaire (SPMSQ)*—Useful for assessing mental status, including orientation, memory, and other cognitive functions.
- The *Mini Mental State Examination*—Also used to assess mental status of elders.

COGNITIVE STATUS

A thorough mental status examination is essential. Objective information includes the presence and extent of cognitive impairment. Include the family and other caregivers to determine the course of any mental changes. Ask: "Did the changes happen gradually (Alzheimer's disease [AD], drug toxicity, metabolic imbalances), suddenly (depression, cerebrovascular accident [CVA], drug toxicity) or in a graduated, stepwise fashion (multi-infarct dementia)?

The *Short Portable Mental Status Questionnaire* (SPMSQ) is a simple, reliable, and valid 10-item cognitive performance evaluation tool. It was designed to assess and monitor cognitive changes in an elderly client. Keep in mind, however, three important points when using standardized assessment tools with elders:

1. Older people are sensitive to fatigue, boredom, medications, and environmental influences that can affect results on a mental status measurement tool.
2. Tools like the SPMSQ cannot distinguish delirium from dementia.
3. Assessment instruments designed for use with other age groups may not be accurate or complete for use with elders.

Subjective information regarding cognitive status includes clients' own perceptions of their mental status. Questions to ask include:

- How has your thinking been lately?
- Is your memory as good as it used to be?
- Have you been able to keep track of your medications? The days of the week? Mealtimes?

PSYCHOLOGICAL/EMOTIONAL STATUS

Objective data about the client's psychological and emotional status require synthesis of impressions from both the content and process of the assessment interview and mental status examination. Avoid the overuse of psychiatric terminology but rather strive for descriptions accompanied by examples of the client's behavior and direct quotations. Be sure to include significant negative findings such as the absence of delusional thoughts, the absence of suicidal ideation, and the absence of hallucinations. Your assessment should include not only

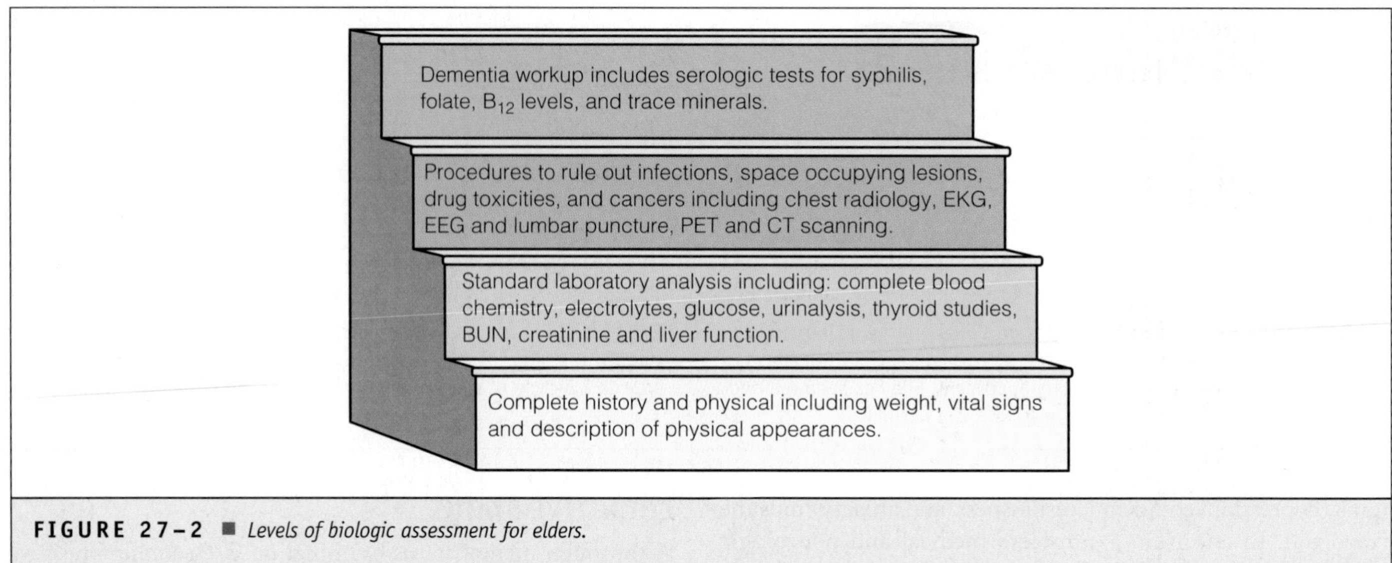

FIGURE 27–2 ■ *Levels of biologic assessment for elders.*

pathology and problems, but also health, adaptive strengths, and personal assets.

STRENGTHS AND COPING STRATEGIES

Aging is a process punctuated by positive and negative stress-producing events. Elders are people who have learned to cope with stress. Data about an elder's coping strategies and strengths are as important as information about his or her psychiatric symptoms. You can shift the conversation in this direction by making a statement like "You certainly have lived a long, full life. Would you share with me some of your survival secrets?".

The Assessment box below provides you with sample questions to gather data about an elder's strengths and coping strategies.

ASSESSMENT

Assessing Psychological Strengths

- What are some of the things you like about yourself?
- What are some of the upsetting, stressful, difficult times you can remember?
- What did you do to comfort yourself when your spouse/partner died?
- How did you make it through the death of your child (or friend)?
- What kinds of things do you do to cheer yourself up?
- What makes you happy or content?
- How do you nurture yourself?
- What do you do to have fun? To relax?
- What things do you think you can do to get through rough times?
- How have the passing years affected your sexuality?
- Are you happily married or partnered?
- What are you most concerned about right now?
- What kind of help do you feel you need?

Having gained an understanding of an elder client's strengths and coping strategies such as spiritual practices, love of music, or reaching out to help others, you can support and mobilize them through your plan of care.

Sexuality

Sexuality is an important area often overlooked when assessing elders. Remember that sexual activity can and does continue into later life and that sexuality includes a broad, multidimensional component of personal identity. Sexual expression includes body image, affection, love, flirtation, social roles, and interaction. Films like *Harold and Maude* and *Innocence* portray richly and with humor sexual expression among elders. Older people who do abstain from sexual expression often do so because they lack the opportunity or they perceive negative social pressure and norms regarding sexuality in people of their age.

Approach the topic of sexuality in a tactful, caring, and nonjudgmental manner. An elderly client who does not wish to discuss sexual issues most likely will make that clear by stating it directly, not answering the question, or changing the subject. An elder who was socialized in a different, more conservative era may not be comfortable discussing sex. Yet elders who matured in the 1960s may have entirely different attitudes toward their continuing sexuality.

SOCIAL AND FINANCIAL STATUS

The quality and quantity of social support (past and present) available to an elder must be assessed. Social support has been confirmed as important for optimal functioning even with psychiatric disturbances. Maintaining a meaningful social network suggests strong interpersonal skills that can be mobilized to help negotiate stresses and losses in later life. Formation of a new social network when others have dissolved is easier for an elder with social skills and the personal resources of assertiveness, friendliness, and warmth. Consider the following clinical example.

CLINICAL EXAMPLE

Irene is a 75-year-old widow who recently broke her hip while cross-country skiing. At first she felt depressed, embarrassed, and socially isolated by her injury and immobilization. She longed for her usual schedule of hiking, swimming, international travel, and attendance at plays and concerts. Because Irene had circles of friends, had regularly hosted holiday parties at her home, and was generous with her time and energy in interactions with her adult children and grandchildren, her social support network rallied to help her as soon as they learned of her condition.

Friends and family brought in the gourmet health food that she loved and stayed with her to keep her company while she ate it. Others sent clever, encouraging cards and notes. One friend telephoned her each day until she was able to be out and about. Because of her long-term positive relationships with her sons, she was able to ask one to mail her some of his favorite books and the other to set up Internet and e-mail connections for her computer. Irene made a rapid and full recovery both physically and psychologically. The stress of her unexpected injury and recovery process was met with her cheerful, resilient personal strengths. Instead of being derailed by her accident, she emerged even stronger from surviving it.

Elders who often manage on a low, fixed income may be plagued by financial problems that affect their mental and physical health. Some communities offer services for helping older people manage their finances. As a case manager for an elderly client, it is imperative that you learn about available financial aid and assistance programs. The removal of financial strain can dramatically improve the health of an aging person who is pressured by inadequate funds or inexperience with financial management. Sample questions for obtaining information about a client's social and financial status are listed in the Assessment box at right.

Elder Abuse

The mistreatment of elders is a serious, underreported, underdetected phenomenon. Elder mistreatment may take many forms, including physical abuse, neglect, exploitation, abandonment, and psychological abuse (see ■ Table 27–1 on page 652).

Elders who are at the greatest risk for abuse and neglect are those who are dependent on others for care. The degree of dependence may overwhelm the caregiver and the result may harm the elder. Stressors related to caregiving can overwhelm any caregiver, but the caregiver of a frail elder is often an adult child of the elder who has additional family and work role responsibilities or a spouse who is also aging. (See Chapter 29 for more information on family stress and burdens of caregiving.)

ASSESSMENT

Guidelines for Assessing Social and Financial Status

- How many phone calls and e-mails do you get in a week?
- How frequently do you have visitors?
- How frequently do you visit others?
- Are you happily married/partnered?
- How would you describe your relationship with your family members?
- Do you have someone you can trust and confide in?
- Do you find yourself feeling lonely?
- Do you have transportation to get to doctor/nurse appointments or to the hospital if needed?
- How is your financial situation? Do you worry about spending or running out of money?

An increasing number of states provide legal alternatives for the removal of an elder to a protective situation. Nursing home or respite care placement, discussed later in this chapter, may be necessary. However, most elders react negatively to such placement and want to return to the potentially harmful home situation. In-home assistance is becoming available in most areas, and such home health services can decrease the strain on caregivers. Home visits made by a case manager or community health nurse can provide an opportunity to assess the possibility of elder abuse in any of its forms and to plan for services to meet needs of elders and their family caregivers.

Nursing Diagnosis: NANDA

Once a comprehensive, multidimensional assessment is accomplished, nursing diagnoses are identified. The NANDA nursing diagnoses likely to be associated with DSM-IV-TR disorders in elders are covered in this section.

MAJOR DEPRESSION

NANDA diagnoses associated with the DSM-IV-TR disorder of major depression include the following.

Low Self-Esteem. Low self-esteem is a hallmark feature of depression. Not only do elders internalize social ageist biases, but also they are often plagued with irrational guilt in the form of intrusive, obsessional, self-deprecating thoughts.

Risk for Violence: Self-Directed. Feelings of hopelessness, low self-esteem, obsessive–compulsive symptoms, apathy, and powerlessness often contribute to suicidal ideation and attempts in depressed elders.

Activity Intolerance. Psychomotor agitation and or retardation are both symptoms of depression. Psychomotor agitation affects social interaction, self-care abilities, and the sleep–wake cycle. Psychomotor retardation is a common vegetative sign of depression in elders. People who suffer from psy-

TABLE 27–1 Forms of Mistreatment of Elders

Physical Abuse	Neglect	Exploitation	Abandonment	Psychological Abuse
• Direct beatings • Infliction of pain • Signs of coercion (abrasions, sprains, dislocation)	• Withholding food • Withholding fluids • Withholding medical attention	• Taking Social Security or pension checks • Taking possessions against person's will	• Dropping elder off at ER • Leaving incapacitated elder alone at home • Failure to provide for basic services	• Continuous degrading • Threatening • Using other scare tactics when the elder cannot provide for his or her own needs

chomotor agitation experience compromised self-care abilities and lack of physical exercise, and are at risk for developing complications of decreased mobility.

Self-Care Deficit: Feeding. Many depressed elders lose weight dramatically. A weight gain secondary to overeating and decreased activity occurs less frequently.

Altered Health Maintenance. Depressed elders are at risk for developing physical health complications secondary to poor self-care and poor health maintenance habits.

Sleep Pattern Disturbance. Often, older clients with depression experience sleep pattern disturbances, particularly early morning awakening. Occasionally, depressed elders report excessive sleeping.

Altered Thought Processes. Elders may present with cognitive changes such as short-term memory loss that accompanies depression. Concentration may be impaired and lack of motivation hinders the ability to learn new information and avoid social isolation. Chapter 12 in this textbook provides detailed information on memory impairment.

ADJUSTMENT DISORDER

NANDA diagnoses most likely to be found in elders with adjustment disorder are covered below.

Dysfunctional Grieving. Elders may become immobilized with stress associated with loss. Often, depression ensues, with an identified stressor as the only factor differentiating an adjustment disorder from major depression.

Self-Care Deficits. Individuals may lose interest in and motivation to perform self-care activities. Grooming, hygiene, and other activities of daily living are neglected. In some cases, elders are at risk for developing serious physical illnesses as a result of failing to adhere to medication regimens and refusing to eat or engage in other health care practices.

Altered Role Performance. The experience of losses often leads to changes in social interaction and role performance. Social withdrawal and loneliness as well as changes in mental status can occur due to lack of social stimulation.

Hopelessness. The experience of loss coupled with a pervasive dysphoria can place an older person as risk for developing dependence and loss of function as his or her self-concept and motivation wane.

ANXIETY DISORDERS

Elders suffering from anxiety disorders also suffer from the following NANDA diagnoses.

Ineffective Individual Coping. Anxiety symptoms often impair a person's ability to concentrate and think clearly. Consequently, judgment is affected and the client decreases activities in order to avoid stressful situations.

Activity Intolerance. Anxiety is often associated with psychomotor agitation and restlessness.

DELUSIONAL DISORDERS

NANDA diagnoses most likely to be found in elders with delusional disorder are covered below.

Altered Thought Processes. Elderly people with delusional disorders often become paranoid and suspect others of trying to rob them, cheat them, or harm them in some way. They may also have delusions about their body or bodily functions. Delusions may be accompanied by feelings of fear, paranoia, anger, and anxiety. Behavioral manifestations of these feelings include suspiciousness, aggression, lashing out, social isolation, and unusual eating behaviors.

Impaired Social Interaction. Delusions that are centered on family members and caregivers strain interpersonal relationships and may make them impossible to maintain.

Outcome Identification: NOC

Outcomes associated with NANDA diagnoses common among elders appear in the following section.

IMPROVEMENT IN ALTERED THOUGHT PROCESSES

Subjective indications of improvement in thought processes include client reports of thinking more clearly, improved concentration, and ability to remember recent and remote events. Individuals who presented with delusions and other signs of psychosis will note that they feel more like themselves and will be able to make more accurate, reality-based interpretations. Other NOC outcomes specific to this nursing diagnosis include:

- *Cognitive orientation:* Ability to identify person, place, and time.
- *Concentration:* Ability to focus on specific stimulus.
- *Decision making:* Ability to choose between two or more alternatives.
- *Information processing:* Ability to acquire, organize, and use information.
- *Memory:* Ability to cognitively retrieve and report previously stored information.
- *Consciousness:* Ability to arouse, orient, and attend to environment.

RENEWED HOPE AND SELF-ACCEPTANCE

Expressions of hope and self-acceptance, renewed involvement, and motivation in activities and planning for the future indicate improvement and replace dependence, apathy, and negative self-talk.

Other NOC outcomes relevant to this diagnosis in elders include:

- Expressions of faith, will to live, reasons to live, meaning in life, optimism, and belief in self and others.
- Ability to identify personal strengths.
- Ability to recognize behaviors that reduce feelings of hopelessness
- Demonstrating interest in social and personal relationships
- Interest in and satisfaction with life goals.

RESUMPTION OF SELF-CARE AND HEALTH MAINTENANCE

Clients will resume their prior level of self-care and health maintenance. Other NOC outcomes relevant to this nursing diagnosis with elders include:

- Ability to perform most basic physical tasks and personal care activities.
- Ability to dress self.
- Ability to maintain neat appearance.
- Ability to maintain own hygiene.

APPROPRIATELY PACED ACTIVITY, REST, AND PSYCHOMOTOR ACTIVITY

Vegetative signs will be replaced with more appropriately paced activities, movement, gait, speech, appetite, and sleep–wake cycle. Anxiety and fear will be replaced with subjective feelings of calm, restfulness, and well-being.

PLEASURE IN EATING AND NORMAL WEIGHT

Clients will report that their appetites are returning to premorbid level with increased pleasure associated with eating. Weight will return to normal range.

DECREASED PREOCCUPATION WITH DEATH AND DYING

Clients will report that suicidal ideation has markedly decreased if not resolved. Morbid preoccupation with death and dying will also decrease.

Planning and Implementation: NIC

The following section presents psychiatric–mental health interventions that are frequently effective when working with elders.

REMINISCENCE THERAPY AND LIFE REVIEW

Reminiscence therapy and **life review** are useful interventions for elders who are experiencing self-esteem disturbance, grief, hopelessness, powerlessness, altered role performance, and social isolation. Reminiscence therapy uses the recall of past events, feelings, and thoughts to facilitate pleasure, quality of life, or adaptation to present circumstances. Although it can be used throughout the life span, it is of special significance when working with elders.

Reminiscing can and should be encouraged for elders individually and in groups. Creative use of food, music, pets, and special events can facilitate the process and make it fun. Materials such as photo albums, journals, and video recorders provide ways for older people to establish a record of their lives, creating a legacy for those who follow.

REALITY ORIENTATION

Reality orientation is a structured program for elderly clients that emphasizes awareness of time, place, and person. The approach provides consistency and a constant reminder to clients of where they are, why they are there, and what is expected. The periodic use of reality orientation tests the elder's level of confusion and disorientation. The rationale for reality orientation is the need to use the part of the person's mind that remains intact.

SOCIALIZATION ENHANCEMENT

Socialization enhancement with elders usually takes place in **resocialization groups** conducted in senior centers, adult day care, and nursing homes. The goal of resocialization groups is to facilitate the elder's ability to interact with others and to renew interest in his or her surroundings. One form of resocialization group is that focused on **remotivation therapy**, in which the emphasis is on stimulating interest in the environment and relationships with others. Group discussion focuses on topics chosen by members of the group and may include world affairs, current local activities, and happy experiences. In the discussions, group members are encouraged to pool knowledge and develop stimulating discussions related to the topic at hand.

ANIMAL-ASSISTED THERAPY

Animal-assisted therapy or *pet therapy* involves the purposeful use of animals to provide affection, attention, diversion, and relaxation to clients. The animals, often obtained through community-based SPCA/Humane Society volunteer programs, are trained to respond to elders in a calm, nonthreatening manner. Small animals can be held in an older person's lap, while larger animals are trained to stand next to a wheelchair and allow the client to stroke or pet them without having to hold them.

EXERCISE PROMOTION AND THERAPY

Exercise and movement therapy can help induce relaxation, maintain flexibility, restore balance, and enhance joy in older clients. Such interventions may include stretching and reaching activities, complex exercises for those able to mirror the leader, or very simple and concrete movements such as handholding for those who are physically or cognitively incapacitated.

SUPPORT GROUPS

Social support and group interventions are useful when working with clients who experience altered family processes, knowledge deficits, ineffective coping, dysfunctional grieving, social isolation, and spiritual distress. They use a group situation or environment to provide emotional support and information for members.

Groups are the treatment of choice for many older clients, especially those in long-term care facilities because several people can benefit and transportation is not a problem.

MEDICATION ADMINISTRATION

Used judiciously, medications can be an effective adjunct to other interventions when working with clients who suffer mental disorders in later life. The high incidence of adverse drug reactions in older clients underscores the need for careful monitoring and conservative dosages. ■ Table 27–2 summarizes recommended dosages for categories of psychotropic drugs used with elders. (See also Chapter 31 of this text for in-depth information.)

It is important that you as a psychiatric–mental health care nurse recognize that elders are more prone to side effects of

TABLE 27–2 Dosage Ranges of Psychotropic Medications Used with Elders

Category	Dosage Range
Antipsychotics: Atypical	
Olanzapine (Zyprexa)	5–10 mg/day
Risperidone (Risperdal)	0.25–6 mg/day
Antipsychotics: Conventional	
Chlorpromazine (Thorazine)	10–800 mg/day
Fluphenazine (Prolixin)	PO: 0.25–20 mg/day, IM: 2.5–10 mg/d, Decanoate: 12.5–25 mg/1–4 wk
Haloperidol (Haldol)	PO: 0.25–15 mg/day, IM: 2–5 mg q4h prn, Decanoate: 50–100 mg/4 wk
Trifluoperazine (Stelazine)	PO: 0.5–40 mg/day, IM: 1–2 mg q4–6h Max 10 mg/d
Anxiolytic Agents	
Buspirone (BuSpar)	10–60 mg/day
Anxiolytic Agents (Benzodiazepines)	
Clonazepam (Klonopin)	1.5–20 mg/day
Lorazepam (Ativan)	0.5–2.0 mg/day
Oxazepam (Serax)	10–30 mg/day
Mood Stabilizers	
Carbamazepine (Tegretol)	400–1200 mg/day
Lithium	300 mg tid
Valproate (Depakote)	125 mg bid to max 60 mg/kg/d
Monoamine Oxidase Inhibitors (MAOIs)	
Isocarboxazid (Marplan)	10–30 mg/day
Phenelzine (Nardil)	15–90 mg/day
Tranylcypromine (Parnate)	30–60 mg/day
Sedative/Hypnotic Benzodiazepines	
Flurazepam (Dalmane)	15–30 mg/hs
Temazepam (Restoril)	7.5–15 mg/hs
Atypical Antidepressants	
Bupropion (Wellbutrin)	50–300 mg/day
Nefazodone (Serzone)	50–600 mg/day
Trazodone (Desyrel)	25–150 mg/day
Selective Serotonin Reuptake Inhibitors (SSRIs)	
Citalopram (Celexa)	20 mg/day
Fluoxetine (Prozac)	10–80 mg/day
Paroxetine (Paxil)	10–80 mg/day
Sertraline (Zoloft)	25–200 mg/day
Tricyclic Antidepressants	
Amitriptyline (Elavil)	10–150 mg/day
Desipramine (Norpramin)	75–150 mg/day
Imipramine (Tofranil)	PO: 75–300 mg/day
Nortriptyline (Pamelor)	10–150 mg/day

Source: Wilson, B. A., Shannon, M. T., & Stang, C. L (2003). *Nurse's drug guide 2003*. Upper Saddle River, NJ: Prentice Hall. Adapted by permission of Pearson Education, Inc., Upper Saddle River, NJ.

psychiatric medications and observe for their occurrence. Among them are:

- Extrapyramidal symptoms (dystonias, akathisia, tremor, pseudoparkinsonism).
- Constipation.
- Anticholinergic effects (urinary retention, blurred vision, dry mouth, sexual dysfunction).
- Cardiovascular effects (postural hypotension, arrhythmias).
- Drug interactions resulting in delirium, confusion, or disorientation.
- Sedation.

Medications within each psychotropic class vary widely with the intensity of the above listed side effects and ideally should be monitored by an especially prepared psychogerontologist who is knowledgeable about the appropriate doses and possible side effects of these drugs.

Evaluation

Identified outcomes and their measurement in both subjective and objective terms guide the evaluation step in the nursing process. When working with elderly mentally ill clients, realistic expectations must be formulated. Ultimately, clients' own values, culture, and preferences, particularly in the late stages of life, should be honored as the gold standard. Families and significant others should, whenever possible, be involved along with the client in the evaluation process.

Case Management, Community-Based Care, and Home Care

Care of mentally ill elders takes place in a variety of settings including at home, in day care programs, in geropsychiatric or dementia units of hospitals, in outpatient clinics, in assisted living programs, and in long-term care facilities such as nursing homes. Goals for care provided in the community emphasize:

- Maintaining optimal functional independence.
- Supporting clients and families across settings.
- Delaying institutionalization.
- Enhancing self-esteem and personal integrity.
- Educating clients and family caregivers about treatment strategies.
- Ensuring coordinated supportive daily activities that enhance the client's ability to cope and compensate for deficits.

RESTORATIVE CARE

According to Resnick and Fleishell (2002), **restorative care** is a planned, systematic program that focuses on restoration and maintenance of optimal function and assisting older adults to compensate for impairments. It also emphasizes prevention of deterioration whenever possible.

In order for it to be successful everyone working in the environment must adopt a philosophy of restorative care. This approach is particularly relevant to long-term care facilities such as nursing homes where functional impairment is often accepted as the normal consequence of old age.

COMMUNITY-BASED PROGRAMS

While the philosophy of restorative care is clearly applicable to care of elders who live in nursing homes or other long-term care facilities, it also guides many other community-based programs. Senior centers, adult day care, respite centers, and community support services such as Meals on Wheels and Whistle Stop Wheels that respectively bring prepared food and transportation to elders being cared for at home are all designed to promote the elder's optimal independent functioning and reduce the stress and burden on family caregivers.

Community-based programs offer alternatives to institutionalization. In the case of senior centers, the emphasis is on (1) health and wellness promotion and (2) social, educational, and recreational activities. Adult day care programs are another alternative to institutionalization. Adult day care programs represent a community resource for elders who need nursing, medical, and rehabilitative services beyond socialization and education. Many adult day care facilities and assisted living centers offer a *respite* option wherein elders can remain overnight in order to relieve family caregivers of their burden at least temporarily. Both of these community programs allow elders to continue living at home.

Assisted living communities are a relatively new option for elders who require support and can no longer remain in their own homes. Such communities take several forms but usually offer a range of assistance levels from independent apartment units through nursing home–like complete care. Unfortunately, this option is rarely available to elders who have sparse financial resources.

The next level of care for frail or mentally disordered elders is admission to a nursing home or other long-term care facility. Even when long-term care is an option, the decision to institutionalize a demented loved one is usually made only when family caregivers have reached the brink of their own tolerance levels, putting their own health at risk, the elder no longer recognizes them, or it becomes physically impossible to manage him or her due to violence or incapacity. As a nurse, especially when serving as case manager, you should be well informed about your community's resources for mentally ill elders and their family caregivers.

RESISTANCE TO CARE

Descriptions like *uncooperative*, *stubborn*, *noncompliant*, and *aggressive* have all been used when characterizing elders who are resistant to care. These behaviors are commonly noted as the biggest problems when caring for a mentally disordered elder in a community or home setting. Werner and colleagues' (2002) research on interventions used by nurses with psychogeriatric clients resisting care identified frequently mentioned reasons for disruptive behavior and resistance to care among elders. These included:

- Cognitive impairment.
- Fear.
- Excessive demands.
- Acute illness and pain.
- Environmental stress such as noise.

This team of nursing and health care researchers adopted the definition of *resistance to care* as client behaviors that prevent, oppose, or interfere with the caregiver's efforts to provide help. Resistance to care by mentally disordered elders can take the form of pushing, hitting, screaming, and cursing. Werner and associates' research, as well as research of others, suggest the following as potentially useful nursing interventions:

- Consult with the primary caregiver (family member or nursing staff member) who is in most frequent contact with the client about strategies that worked in the past.
- Talk and reason with the client.
- Allow the client to eat or dress independently.
- Distract the client by initiating social activity.
- Wait and return at a later time to resume the activity.
- Allow the client to refuse care such as dressing where there are few health consequences.

Dealing with mentally ill elders is challenging, particularly in the home or community. More nursing research is needed to determine strategies that work, especially with elders who are resistant to care.

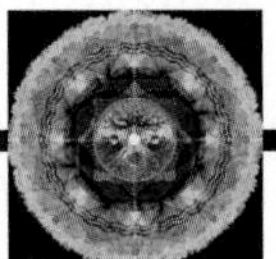

EXPLORE MediaLink

NCLEX review, case studies, and other interactive resources for this chapter can be found on the Companion Website at http://www.prenhall.com/kneisl. Click on Chapter 27 to select the activities for this chapter.

For animations, video tutorials, more NCLEX review questions, and an audio glossary, access the accompanying CD-ROM in this textbook.

BIBLIOGRAPHY

American Psychiatric Association (2000). *Diagnostic and statistical manual of mental disorders* (4th ed., Text Revision). Washington, DC: Author.

Bergstom, M. J., & Holmes, M. E. (2000). Lay theories of successful aging after the death of a spouse—review. *Health Communication, 12,* 377–406.

Bureau of the Census (2000). *Sixty-five plus in the United States*. Statistical brief. Washington, DC: U.S. Department of Commerce, Economic and Statistics Administration.

Cohen, C. I., & Talavera, N. (2000). Functional impairment in older schizophrenic persons. *American Journal of Geriatric Psychiatry, 8*(3), 237–244.

Eliopoulous, C. (2001). *Gerontological nursing* (5th ed.). Philadelphia: Lippincott.

Ferrell, B. R. (1996). *Suffering*. Sudbury, MA: Jones & Bartlett.

Ferrell, B. R., & Coyle, N. (2002). An overview of palliative nursing care. *American Journal of Nursing*, 102(5), 26–32.

Flodin, N. W. (1990). Micronutrient supplements: Toxicity and drug interactions. *Progress in Food & Nutrition Science, 14,* 277–331.

Forbes, S., Bern-Klug, M., & Gessert, C. (2000). End of life decision making for nursing home residents with dementia. *Journal of Nursing Scholarship, 32*(3), 251–258.

Johnson, I. (2000). Alcohol problems in old age: A review of recent epidemiologic research. *International Journal of Geriatric Psychiatry, 15,* 575–581.

Joint Commission on Accreditation for Health Care Organizations. (2000). *Hospital accreditation standards*. Oakbrook, IL: Author.

Knoll, J. (2001). Antiaging compounds—review. *CNS Drug Reviews, 7,* 317–345.

Lea, D. A., & Williams, J. K. (2002). Genetic testing and screening. *American Journal of Nursing, 102*(7), 36–43.

Norton, S. A., & Talerico, K. A. (2002). Facilitating end-of-life decision-making strategies for communicating and assessing. *Journal of Gerontological Nursing, 26*(9), 6–13.

Resnick, B. & Fleishell, A. (2002). Developing a restorative care program. *American Journal of Nursing, 102*(7), 91–95.

Salvatore, T. (2000). Elder suicide: a preventable tragedy. *Caring, 19,* 34–37.

Schroots, J. J. (1996). Theoretic developments in the psychology of aging—review. *Gerontologist, 36,* 742–748.

Schwartz, R., Gunzelmann,T., Hinz, A., & Brahler, E. (2001). Anxiety and depression in the general population over 60 years old. (German). *Deutsche Medizinische Wochenschrift, 126,* 611–615.

Steen, B. (2001). Biological aging—a mini review (Swedish). *Lakartidningen, 98,* 1924–1928.

Taylor, E. J. (2002). *Spiritual care: Nursing theory, research and practice.* Upper Saddle River, NJ: Prentice Hall.

Werner, P., Tabak, N., Albert, R., & Bergman, R. (2002). Interventions used by nursing staff members with psychogeriatric patients resisting care. *International Journal of Nursing Studies, 39*(4), 461–467.

Youngstedt, S. D., Kripke, D. F., Elliott, J. A., & Klauber, M. R. (2001). Circadian abnormalities in older adults. *Journal of Pineal Research, 32,* 264–272.

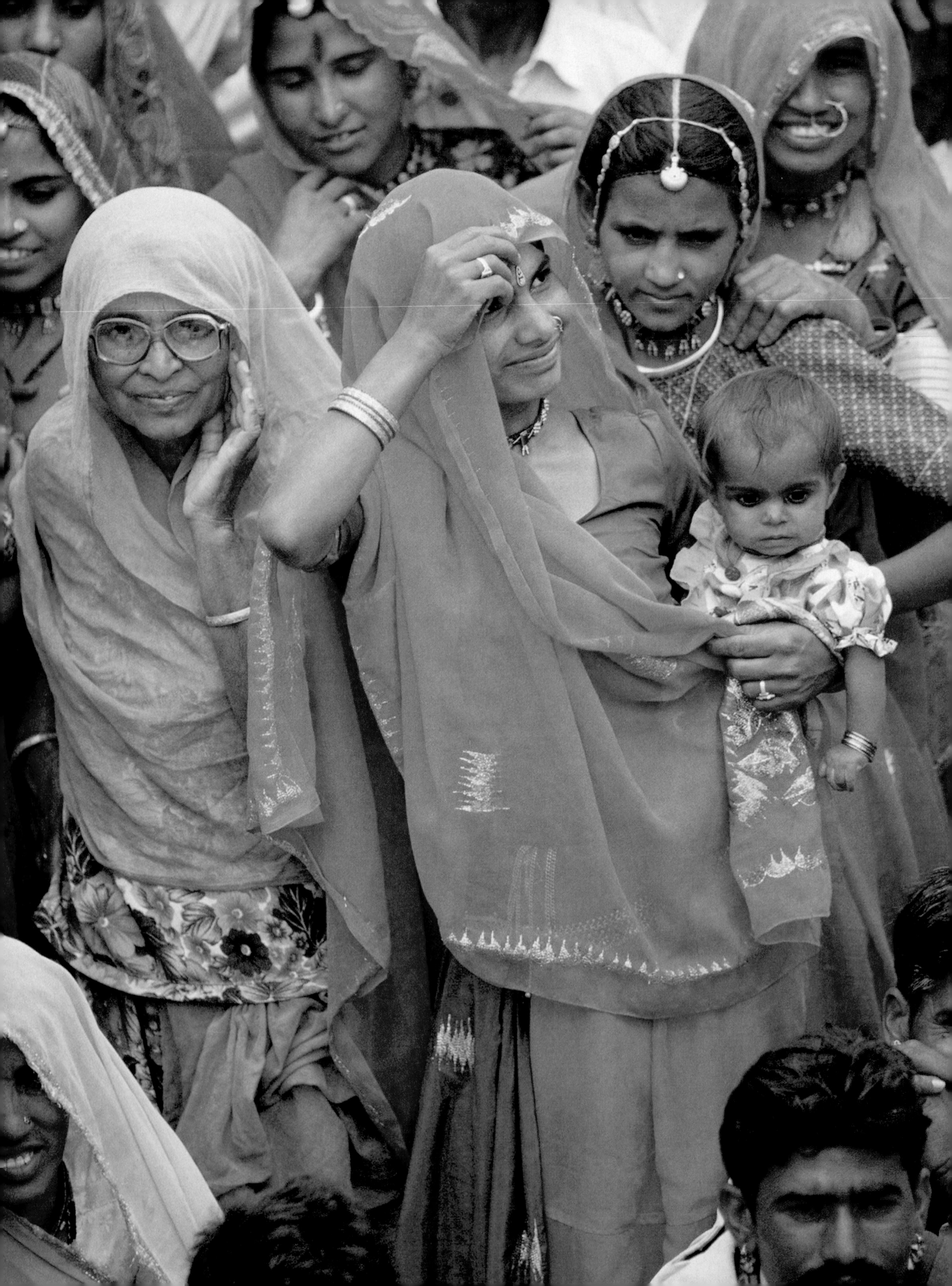

UNIT *Five*

Nursing Intervention Strategies and Outcomes

The Ramdas family joyfully celebrates at a traditional family festival in Rajasthan, India. The strength expressed in their family and community bond reflects how culture and groups build not only vulnerabilities but also strengths. When it comes to mental health, the most effective community-based prevention programs and treatment programs are outreach oriented. This mandates that we build partnerships with our clients' families and communities. Our interventions must reflect the habit of interpersonal perspective taking—seeing through the eyes and responding to the concerns of others. Our interventions must reflect the habit of critical thinking that allows us to identify coherent patterns and reflect evaluatively on them. Our interventions must reflect our capacity to resist becoming overwhelmed, discouraged, and bewildered so that we can respond creatively to the challenges we encounter and build a practice based on evidence, including evidence from clinical wisdom and cultural competence. In Unit Five, you will learn about a broad spectrum of psychiatric–mental health nursing intervention strategies including counseling individuals, groups, and families; cognitive, behavioral, pharmacologic, and alternative/complementary healing; as well as crisis intervention and forensic psychiatric nursing.

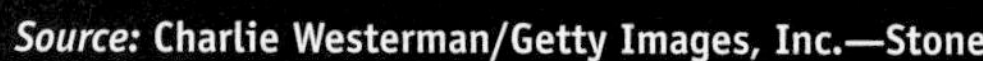

Source: Charlie Westerman/Getty Images, Inc.—Stone

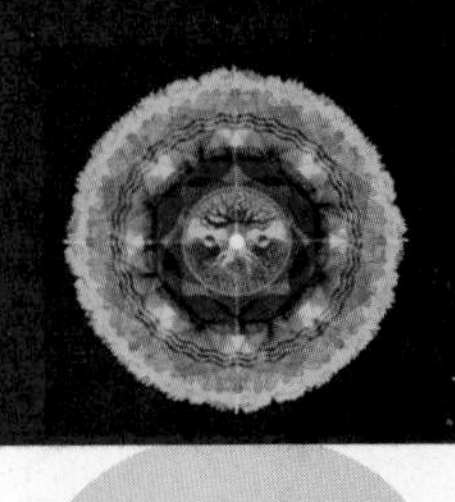

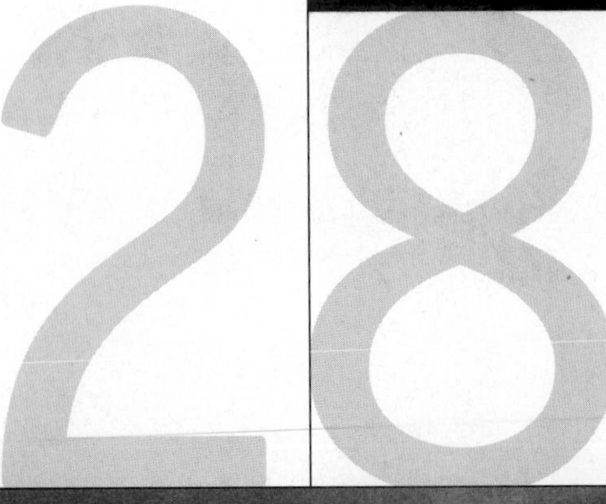

Counseling the Individual

BETH MOSCATO

Chapter TWENTY-EIGHT

KEY TERMS

acting-out
countertransference
resistance
therapeutic alliance
therapeutic nurse–client relationship
transference

FOCUS QUESTIONS

- **What are the common shared characteristics of one-to-one relationships?**
- **Which client abilities and behaviors are most often associated with growth-producing outcomes?**
- **If you were asked to analyze the following special concerns as they relate to psychiatric–mental health nurses—critical distance, self-disclosure, gift giving, the use of touch, and values—what aspects would you emphasize?**
- **How would you explain the three phases of the therapeutic nurse–client relationship and the main objectives and therapeutic tasks of each phase?**
- **What actions would you take in establishing and maintaining one-to-one relationships within the context of the client's cultural background?**

MediaLink 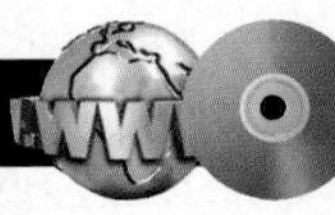 www.prenhall.com/kneisl

Additional resources for this chapter can be found on the Student CD-ROM accompanying this textbook, and on the Companion Website at www.prenhall.com/kneisl. Click on Chapter 28 to select the activities for this chapter.

CD-ROM
- Audio Glossary
- NCLEX Review

Companion Website
- Additional NCLEX Review
- Case Study: Resistive Client

CHAPTER OUTLINE

CROSS REFERENCES

Other topics relative to this content are: Assessment strategies and techniques, Chapter 9; Communication strategies, Chapter 8; Culturally competent care, Chapter 6; Facilitative personal characteristics of psychiatric–mental health nurses, Chapter 1.

CRITICAL THINKING CHALLENGE

You have just met with your first psychiatric client to develop a therapeutic nurse–client relationship. Despite your best efforts within the meeting, your client, Sammy, gave you "a hard time." There were long periods of silence broken by angry and explosive statements directed toward your abilities. You are uncertain whether Sammy will meet with you again. How do you feel about Sammy's behaviors and your performance as a nursing student? What steps can you take to deal with this first contact and the uncertainty of subsequent contacts with this client? ■

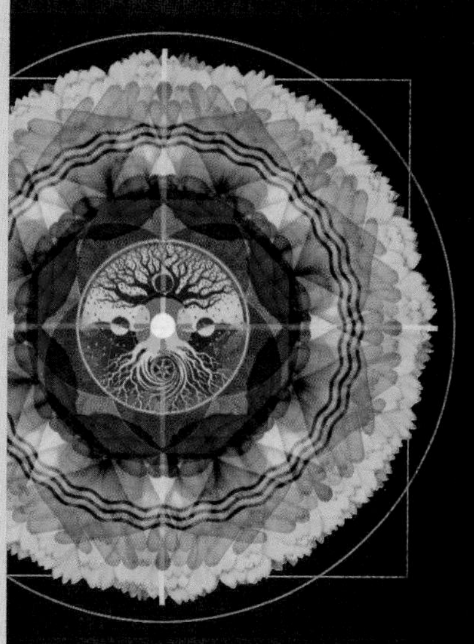

In the twenty-first century, psychiatric–mental health nursing continues to expand its neuropsychiatric focus. There has been an explosion of knowledge in our understanding of the neurobiologic basis of mental illness, in diagnostic technology, and in the discovery of newer and better psychopharmacologic approaches (see Chapters 4 and 31) that has moved us toward a neuropsychiatric paradigm of care. A neuropsychiatric paradigm is less stigmatizing and allows treatment to reach more people than a psychosocial view alone (Flaskerud & Wuerker, 1999). At the same time that clients may have their needs for safety, structure, and medication met, they may also express their longing for a deeper connection with mental health staff and more insight-oriented treatment (Thomas, Shattell, & Martin, 2002). The challenge for us is to integrate both biologic and psychosocial concepts while maintaining our nursing focus on caring. The therapeutic nurse–client relationship provides the opportunity to meet this challenge.

The **therapeutic nurse–client relationship,** also called the one-to-one relationship, is one in which the nurse uses theoretical understandings, personal attributes, and appropriate clinical techniques to provide the opportunity for a corrective emotional experience for clients. It has evolved as the cornerstone of psychiatric–mental health nursing theory and practice, largely based on almost 50 years of work by Hildegard Peplau. Memorial tributes to Peplau upon her death in 1999 by nurses around the world recognized her as the "mother of psychiatric nursing" (Barker, 1999; Haber, 1999). Her theory of interpersonal relations in nursing, including the stages of the nurse–client relationship, created the basis for psychotherapeutic nursing (Peplau, 1952, 1997).

We are challenged to creatively adapt the time-honored principles of Peplau's work under changing conditions such as the brevity of inpatient psychiatric treatment. The current health care economic climate with its focus on managed care has changed the face of the traditional therapeutic nurse–client relationship advocated by Peplau. Nevertheless, we incorporate the principles of the therapeutic nurse–client relationship in our everyday work—brief encounters as well as consistent long-term relationships.

The therapeutic nurse–client relationship may evolve in any nursing situation—between a nurse and a client with leukemia, between a nurse and an offender in a jail, between a nurse and a high-risk pregnant woman, or between a home care nurse and a client with emphysema. Of particular relevance, however, is the relationship that evolves between psychiatric–mental health nurse and client.

This chapter demystifies the characteristics, processes, phases, and problems of one-to-one relationships so that beginning psychiatric–mental health nurses can approach them with increased awareness of their own interpersonal effectiveness. Practical guidelines on how to facilitate interpersonal effectiveness with clients are included. The principles, processes, and phases discussed in this chapter also apply to family, group, and community interventions or therapies.

The One-to-One Relationship

The one-to-one relationship between psychiatric–mental health nurse and client is a mutually defined, collaborative, and goal-oriented professional relationship.

It may be viewed as a series of sequential nurse–client interactions with the following additional elements:

- The interactions occur over a designated period of time (daily, weekly, monthly).
- The interactions take place in a unique nurse–client structure, characterized by specific phases, processes, and problems.
- The interactions occur in a designated setting that tends to remain stable over time (home, private practice office, mental health clinic, inpatient psychiatric unit, medical unit).

A one-to-one relationship has three distinct phases:

1. The orientation (beginning) phase, characterized by the establishment of contact with the client.
2. The working (middle) phase, characterized by the maintenance and analysis of contact.
3. The termination (end) phase, characterized by the termination of contact with the client.

Each phase of a one-to-one relationship is distinguished by important goals and therapeutic tasks, discussed in detail in the nursing process sections of the chapter.

Shorter hospital stays for inpatient clients change the timing of, and expectations for, the inpatient one-to-one relationship. Although the components themselves do not change, the schedule will. Inform the inpatient client of the brevity of the length of the relationship between client and nurse. Announce the time frame during the beginning phase, and reinforce it throughout the other phases.

THERAPEUTIC ALLIANCE

The major task and overriding characteristic of the one-to-one relationship is the creation of a therapeutic alliance between nurse and client. The **therapeutic alliance** is a conscious relationship between a facilitative person and a client. It is fundamental to the therapeutic change process (Bjorklund, 2000). In this process, the nurse forms a mature alliance with the growth-facilitating aspects of the client. Each implicitly agrees to work together to help the client address personal problems and concerns. More specifically, the nurse identifies and provides feedback regarding the client's patterns of reaction, abilities, and potentials. The client can use these assets to handle unresolved problems constructively. The establishment of the therapeutic alliance enhances informal one-to-one relationships and is essential in formal one-to-one relationships (Krauss, 2000). Such a binding alliance between nurse and client allows the one-to-one relationship to continue, especially when the client experiences increased anxiety and resistance to change. The personal qualities of the nurse that enhance the ability to forge a therapeutic alliance are discussed in Chapter 1.

CULTURAL CONTEXT

Because cultural context influences nursing care, a sensitive and systematic consideration of the client's cultural and ethnic background is an essential part of the psychiatric nursing process in one-to-one relationship work. Cultural forces shape the expression of distress and the formation of symptoms (Flaskerud, 2000). Culture also influences the client's expectations of the nurse–client relationship and the client's interpretations of the events that take place in it. The nurse consistently evaluates the influence of culture within the one-to-one relationship as well as the effects of the therapeutic relationship on the client's values and life experiences. General considerations of cultural diversity are interwoven within this chapter and are further described in Chapter 6.

CHARACTERISTICS

In addition to having three distinct phases, the therapeutic nurse–client relationship has several common characteristics.

Professional

One-to-one relationships reflect a professional, rather than social, relationship. Psychiatric–mental health nurses use their personalities, interpersonal skills and techniques, and theoretic knowledge of psychiatric–mental health nursing practice in a purposeful, goal-directed manner to facilitate a useful change in their client's lives. This professional relationship differs from a social relationship in several significant ways. ■ Table 28–1 summarizes the major differences between professional and social relationships.

A professional one-to-one relationship can be either informal or formal. Spontaneous, informal nurse–client relationships are at one end of the continuum, and formal individual counseling or psychotherapy is at the other end.

Informal. Informal nurse–client relationships may be prearranged and planned, but more often they occur spontaneously. They consist of a set of interactions limited in time. There is minimum structure and a sense of immediacy. These relationships occur in numerous medical and nonmedical settings and are particularly common in psychiatric institutions and community mental health settings.

Formal. The more formal one-to-one relationship is used in crisis intervention, counseling, or individual psychotherapy. It requires more planning, structure, consistency, nursing expertise, and time. The formal one-to-one relationship occurs in various psychiatric settings, including psychiatric institutions, community mental health centers, and private practice.

The choice and effectiveness of informal or formal relationships depend on:

- The client's level of functioning.
- The psychiatric–mental health nurse's current abilities and skills.
- To some degree, the time that is available to both participants.

■ Table 28–2 highlights the similarities and differences of informal and formal relationship work. The differences are discussed throughout this chapter.

Mutually Defined

A one-to-one relationship is mutually defined by the two participants. Both psychiatric–mental health nurse and client voluntarily enter the relationship and specify the conditions under which it is to evolve. For example, the client may seek immediate alleviation of symptoms rather than long-term individual psychotherapy. Nurse and client identify together where and when they will meet and other conditions of their participation. This contractual aspect of the one-to-one relationship is explored further in the discussion of the beginning (orientation) phase of therapy later in the chapter. Once the one-to-one relationship is established, its maintenance depends on the commitment of both participants.

Collaborative

Both participants enter a relationship in which goals, strategies, and outcomes evolve within the context of the therapeutic work

TABLE 28–1 Differences Between Professional and Social Relationships

Characteristic	Professional Relationship	Social Relationship
Purpose	Systematic working-through of troublesome thoughts, feelings, and behaviors. Planned evaluation (through stages).	Companionship, pleasure, sharing of interests. Evolves spontaneously.
Role delineation	Roles for nurse and client with explicit use of psychiatric nursing skills and interventions.	Generally not present, except for broad social norms governing the particular type of relationship (friend versus lover).
Satisfaction of needs	Client is encouraged to identify, develop, and assess ways to meet own needs more effectively. Does not address personal needs of the nurse.	Mutual sharing and satisfaction of personal and interpersonal needs.
Time frame	Usually time-limited interactions with an expected termination.	Usually not time limited, in either duration or frequency of contact. No planned termination.

TABLE 28–2 Similarities and Differences of Informal and Formal One-to-One Relationships

Characteristic	Informal Relationship	Formal Relationship
Setting	Varied.	Generally psychiatric settings.
Frequency and duration of contact	Flexible, depending on client need or tolerance. Example: short, frequent intervals daily.	Structured. Example: once weekly, with possible crisis sessions. Duration usually set at 30 minutes or 1 hour.
Duration of relationship	May or may not involve time commitment. Generally a few days to a few weeks.	Involves time commitment: weeks to months, for short-term work; months to years, for long-term work.
Type of dysfunction	In general, more effective with severe dysfunction.	In severe dysfunction, may be useful after client is stabilized on medication.
Use of therapeutic contract	May involve simple therapeutic contract.	Utilizes therapeutic contract; the more specific, the better.
Fees	Usually not relevant.	May be relevant. May be part of therapeutic contract.
Degree of skill required	Nursing student or psychiatric nurse.	Advanced degree beneficial but not essential.
Degree of supervision	Some degree and type of supervision always necessary.	Consistent supervision or consultation usually necessary.
Degree of effectiveness	For both, depends on client's level of functioning, skills of the psychiatric–mental health nurse, and time allotment.	

together. Mutual collaboration implies that each participant brings personal abilities, capabilities, and power to the relationship. Thus, the psychiatric–mental health nurse does not assume responsibility for client behaviors but actively works with the client to assess the self-defeating and growth-promoting aspects of specific behaviors. Mutual collaboration also means that nurses assess and are accountable for their own behavior with clients. Ongoing supervision often helps the nurse meet these particular goals.

Goal-Directed

A therapeutic nurse–client relationship is always goal directed. The client is expected to identify and achieve specific physical, emotional, and social goals within the context of the relationship. Client goals vary widely in type and depth. For example, in informal relationship work, a client's goal may be to initiate one peer relationship within an inpatient psychiatric unit. Other examples include resolution of a divorce involving children and shared personal possessions, or coming to terms with the client's impending death. Often the client's initial goal is to solve an immediate problem, and this serves as a basis for establishing more extensive psychosocial goals. The psychiatric–mental health nurse also formulates therapeutic goals to enhance the growth-producing elements of the relationship. Inpatient clients with serious symptomatology may have difficulty connecting and modifying behaviors in the time allotted. Goals that can be worked on in the future and in various settings are the goals more likely to be achieved.

Open

The one-to-one relationship between nurse and client may be viewed as an experience in *shared dignity*. The psychiatric–mental health nurse adapts to allow clients to reveal their humanness freely and openly. Each aspect of the nurse's verbal and nonverbal behavior either encourages or inhibits clients from further revealing their humanness. The Using Research Evidence feature on page 665 shows how one nurse used several interventions to encourage a client to reveal her humanness.

Negotiated

In the one-to-one relationship, the client is an active decision maker and is personally accountable for the work. The atmosphere of give and take within the relationship emphasizes mutuality, reciprocity, and interpersonal fairness. Establishing a clearly defined, mutually agreed-on therapeutic contract represents a prime example of negotiation in one-to-one work. (The therapeutic contract is covered later in the chapter.)

Committed

Commitment is based on the therapeutic contract between nurse and client. The contract establishes the limits of the relationship as well as the time and energy allotted to it. At some point in the relationship, the nurse is confronted by the reality of the client's dysfunction. The beginning psychiatric–mental health nurse may respond by actively colluding with the client to deny or ignore the dysfunction and remain on a superficial, social level of communication. This collusion protects the

USING RESEARCH EVIDENCE

Sharon is a 15-year-old with a history of self-abusive behavior. She had been the victim of repeated incestuous experiences with her stepfather over several years, despite her mother's knowledge of such activity. On an inpatient adolescent evaluation unit, she met daily in an informal one-to-one relationship with a nursing student, of whom she seemed fond. One day Sharon received a message from the team leader stating that the student had the flu and was unable to meet with Sharon that day but planned to meet again the following day. When the team members asked about Sharon's reactions to this, Sharon refused to speak. She rushed out of the dayroom area, ran to her room, and pounded her fist into the cement wall numerous times, fracturing her right hand in two places.

The next day, the nursing student approached Sharon. Sharon offered no comment. The student's inquiry regarding the previous day's message also met with no comment. The student stated her concern for Sharon's welfare and her confusion regarding Sharon's injury. Sharon remained silent. The student stated her wish to sort things out together as they had done in the past and then sat quietly with Sharon. After a couple of minutes, Sharon began crying and talked about feeling alone.

The nursing student clarified communication (e.g., Was the previous day's message received? Understood?). She remained available without withdrawing despite Sharon's silence. She promoted trust by stating her concern for Sharon's welfare and injury as well as her willingness to work things out together. She accepted Sharon's initial silence and subsequent feeling of loneliness.

This nursing student effectively used several interventions based on her understanding of recent studies such as the one cited below.

Forchuk, C., Westwell, J., Martin, M., Bamber-Azzapardi, W., Kosterewa-Tolman, D., & Hux, M. (2000). The developing nurse–client relationship: Nurse's perspectives. *Journal of the American Psychiatric Nurses Association, 6*(1), 3–10.

nurse from having to address the client's helplessness, desperation, hostility, or raw grief. The nurse who does not let the client express these feelings is not sufficiently committed to the client.

The opposite is also nontherapeutic. The overcommitted psychiatric–mental health nurse may assume an omnipotent or rescuer role to "cure" the client. This role robs the client of active decision-making power and accountability. The client will test the nurse's commitment in some phase of the relationship. Both nurse and client need to deal with this test explicitly on verbal and nonverbal levels. A sense of positive connectedness with the client strengthens the sense of commitment.

Responsible

Personal responsibility for the one-to-one relationship is also based on the therapeutic contract between nurse and client, and it, too, will be tested by the client in some phase of the relationship. Beginning psychiatric–mental health nurses usually encounter responsibility problems as they begin to perceive unattractive, dysfunctional, or blatantly offending interpersonal behavioral patterns or habits in their clients. Both nurse and client must deal explicitly with "who is responsible for what." In addition, the nurse should avoid making any agreements with a client that the nurse may be unable to fulfill.

The personally responsible psychiatric–mental health nurse will insist on clinical supervision. Supervision provides novice, as well as experienced, nurses with the opportunity to learn therapeutic techniques and attitudes. It enables them to receive validation, insight, and support during the difficult times that may accompany therapeutic relationships (Laskowski, 2001) and enables them to analyze how they affect the one-to-one relationship and its outcome. In addition, clinical supervision helps one to examine the experience, expression, reporting, and evaluation of psychiatric disorders as influenced by cultural diversity. Supervision is further discussed later in this chapter.

Authentic

Spontaneity and authenticity are important in one-to-one relationships. Psychiatric–mental health nurses need to create an atmosphere that conveys permission to express pain and pleasure. Expressions of joy and assessments of client abilities, talents, and capabilities are an often neglected, yet essential, aspect of relationship work.

Meaningful

Psychiatric–mental health nurses work with clients in a search for meaning in their lives. It is essential that nurses establish their own personal meaning and integration of self (see Chapter 1), for these are key resources in treatment. For psychiatric–mental health nurses to be effective, they must already possess the personal skills to deal with the client's symptoms. They must have personally worked through any problems that resemble those of the client. For example, nurses who cannot cope with their own feelings of depression cannot be effective with severely depressed clients.

Phenomena Occurring in One-to-One Relationships

Sometimes you may initially sense confusion about what is happening in the nurse–client therapeutic relationship. This uneasiness may be difficult to identify, describe, and explore. Remember to keep the following phenomena in mind when you are attempting to "make sense" of a one-to-one relationship.

RESISTANCE

Resistance refers to all the phenomena that interfere with and disrupt the smooth flow of feelings, memories, and thoughts. It inevitably surfaces in the course of one-to-one work and most often occurs as the client begins to address self-defeating thoughts, feelings, and behaviors.

Resistance is often mistakenly seen as the client's struggle against the nurse. Instead, the client is struggling against the anxiety associated with change (Engle & Holiman, 2002), against self-awareness, and against responsibility for actions. Newman (2002) cautions us to be aware of the tendency to react adversely to client resistance. Although the client's behavior patterns may have self-defeating aspects, they have also provided some satisfaction or prevented some discomfort. The client may also resist giving up a defense that offered protection from the anxiety associated with unbearable thoughts and impulses. Thus, resistance in therapeutic one-to-one relationships is best understood as the client's struggle against change.

Manifestations

In general, you may suspect resistance when the client's behavior appears to block the progress of the relationship. Resistance is usually expressed in five different forms (Messer, 2002):

1. Resistance to the recognition of feelings, fantasies, and motives.
2. Resistance to revealing feelings toward the nurse or therapist.
3. Resistance as a way of demonstrating self-sufficiency.
4. Resistance as the clients' reluctance to change behavior outside of the nurse–client relationship.
5. Resistance as a result of the failure of empathy on the part of the nurse or therapist.

You must exercise caution in evaluating a client's behavior as resistive. The client's silence may indicate pensiveness, a pause before emotive expression, or a sense of completion. The client who is habitually late may have real difficulties adjusting a full personal schedule to accommodate the sessions. Resistance to specific topics or concerns may indicate that the client is not ready for investigative work. Likewise, the client may resist giving up a defense that is desperately needed to keep anxiety about a present situation at manageable levels.

Remember that the client has a right to resist one aspect of or the entire therapeutic process, as a matter of choice. However, the client's resistive behavior should be openly discussed, rather than ignored.

MediaLink Case Study: Resistive Client

Acting-Out

Acting-out is a particularly destructive form of resistance in which the client puts into action (that is, "acts out") a memory that has been forgotten or repressed. It is important to recognize that the client is externalizing an inner conflict to people in the immediate environment. Rather than verbalizing conflicts or feelings, the client displays inappropriate behaviors. Examples of acting-out include forcefully slamming a door, dressing provocatively, or slapping someone. In acting-out, the client acts toward a mate, friend, relative, or other person those feelings and attitudes that the client does not express toward the nurse. An example of acting-out is developing third-person relationships to absorb the emotions and fantasies that belong in the therapeutic relationship. Exaggerated feelings of intense hostility toward the nurse may lead to violence or physical harm to the client, nurse, or the third person. Intense feelings of love for the nurse or therapist may precipitate an affair or marriage with the third person.

Acting-out contains a vital seed for change. That is, it can form the basis for the client's understanding of, and eventual giving up of, destructive and inappropriate behaviors (Richarz & Romisch, 2002). Acting-out is difficult to deal with because the client does not talk about the feelings that precipitate the behavior and later tends to conceal or rationalize the behavior. Acting-out can abruptly break up treatment, unless it is identified and dealt with explicitly. Specific nursing interventions regarding acting-out include the following:

- Bring acting-out to the attention of the client.
- Encourage the client to *talk about* impulses rather than to act them out.
- Encourage identification of feelings *before* putting them into action.
- Increase frequency of contact.
- Look for evidence of transference phenomena toward the nurse.
- With repeated dangerous acting-out, consider withdrawing from the relationship unless the client sets limits on these behaviors.

Acting-out can be demonstrated by the nurse who manifests parental, erotic, sexual, or hostile nonverbal behaviors, such as:

- Placing hands on hips or pointing a finger while setting limits on a client's behavior (parental).
- Patting a client on the shoulder and offering reassurance (parental).
- Blushing and giggling when a client makes a sexual remark (sexual).

These behaviors by the nurse encourage gross acting-out by the client.

Parental or caretaker behaviors that express the need to nurture the client are the most common among beginning psychiatric–mental health nurses. These behaviors may indicate a countertransference problem (discussed later in this chapter) for the nurse and discount the client's ability to ensure his or her own well-being. Recognition of acting-out by the psychiatric–mental health nurse is essential and reinforces the need for formal supervision.

General Intervention Strategies

Several consecutive approaches are used as general nursing intervention strategies for resistance. They begin with the nurse's awareness of the resistance. Helpful intervention strategies include the following:

- Labeling the resistant behavior with the client. The nurse may allow the resistance to occur several times to demonstrate its presence to the client. It is as if the nurse were holding up a mirror for the client, reflecting and clarifying the specific resistant behavior.
- Exploring the accompanying emotion and history of its development.
- Exploring what function the resistance may serve, especially any self-defeating aspects.

- Facilitating working through the resistance by fully understanding and appreciating its implications in the client's life.

This sequence may occur repeatedly before a resistant behavior is resolved.

TRANSFERENCE

Transference is a normal phenomenon that may surface and inhibit effectiveness in any phase of one-to-one relationship work and in any setting, including nonpsychiatric settings (Pearson, 2001). **Transference** is the result of unresolved childhood experiences with significant others. Instead of remembering the past, the client "transfers" unresolved feelings, attitudes, and wishes into present significant relationships in an attempt to resolve them in a more satisfying manner. Thus, the client misunderstands the present according to the unresolved problems of the past. The client is unaware of the nature of this action.

It is important to understand that transference is a form of resistance. The client unknowingly resists any recollection of childhood conflicts. Instead, the client transfers these conflicts to present relationships, including the nurse–client relationship.

You may suspect that a client is in transference when the client repeatedly assigns meanings to the nurse–client relationship that belong to one or more of the client's past relationships. It is as if the client's ability to assess the nurse–client interactions becomes confused and thwarted by the unfinished conflicts belonging to past interactions with significant others. Thus, you may be viewed as parent, sibling, lover, or friend.

Explore the meaning of individual words, gestures, events, and situations in the current one-to-one relationship to determine how these reflect or replay distortions in past relationships. The therapeutic task is to separate feelings, thoughts, and behaviors that belong to the current one-to-one relationship from those that represent unresolved conflicts in past relationships.

Increasing awareness of the transference process often frees the client to work through past conflicts and explore the more creative, self-actualizing aspects of personal identity as they evolve in the current relationship. You must not behave like the client's parent or any other transference figure has behaved. Rather, help the client bring an unconscious event into consciousness, to examine its cause and meaning. The following example illustrates how transference may surface in a clinical setting:

CLINICAL EXAMPLE

Conrad Weber, hospitalized for depression, was assigned to a primary counselor, a male psychiatric–mental health nurse. Over the course of several meetings with his counselor, Conrad assumed a cowering, ingratiating manner. He seemed to resemble a little boy awaiting punishment from an intimidating, punitive father. This interpersonal orientation was observed by other male staff members who informally initiated interaction with Conrad on the unit.

The counselor chose not to explore Conrad's past relationships. The aim of short-term work was to focus on concrete ways to decrease depressed feelings in Conrad's present life situation. The counselor addressed ingratiating behaviors in the nurse–client relationship only when they had an adverse effect on their short-term work together.

In this example, the primary counselor chose to focus on present rather than past relationships in an effort to stabilize the hospitalized client. Transference may be dealt with in many ways, depending on the client's functioning, the counselor's theoretic orientation, and the type of therapy.

Positive Transference

Transference may be positive or negative. Positive transference—that is, positive feelings for the therapist—occurs when the client generally has had satisfying past relationships with significant others during childhood. The therapeutic relationship is usually able to progress in this instance.

Negative Transference

In negative transference, the client shows a number of reactions based on forms of hate (hostility, loathing, bitterness, contempt, annoyance). Although there are both positive and negative aspects to every transference, a predominantly negative transference is uncomfortable for client and nurse alike. The client does not like to be aware of and express this hate, and the nurse does not like to be the target of it. When negative transference appears unresolvable, it may be advisable to terminate relationship work rather than run the risk of further client dysfunction.

COUNTERTRANSFERENCE

While transference involves the client's reactions to the psychiatric nurse, **countertransference** involves the nurse's reactions to the client. The psychiatric–mental health nurse may develop powerful counterproductive fantasies, feelings, and attitudes in response to the client's transference or personality. Countertransference is now thought to be almost inevitable in psychotherapeutic situations (Gabbard, 2001; Ellis, 2001).

Countertransference is suspected when the nurse repeatedly assigns meaning to the nurse-client relationship that belongs to the nurse's other past relationships. In countertransference, the psychiatric–mental health nurse's ability to assess the nurse–client interactions becomes confused or thwarted by unresolved past conflicts. Thus, the nurse may unconsciously use behaviors (as parent, sibling, lover, or friend) that attempt to replay in the current situation some past identity with significant others. Countertransference indicates unresolved conflict in the nurse. This conflict may be expressed in acts of omission or commission and they may be covert or overt.

Look for the following signals that countertransference may be occurring:

- Irrational friendliness toward or irrational concern about the client.
- Reacting with annoyance or irrational hostility toward the client.
- Feeling uneasy during or after meeting with the client.
- Dreaming about the client.
- Preoccupation with the client during leisure time.

Be alert for what Kiesler (2001) calls *behavioral deviations from baseline,* the actions that a therapist takes with clients that are out of line with standard expectations for therapist behaviors.

Countertransference is a normal occurrence, requiring supervision or consultation to prevent degeneration of the one-to-one relationship. Supervision may enable the nurse to separate feelings, thoughts, and behaviors that belong to the current relationship from those that represent unfinished conflicts in past relationships.

It is reassuring that most countertransference problems can be resolved by self-assessment with professional supervision. Once the countertransference process is identified, the nurse can consciously develop therapeutic, goal-directed responses. Avoid self-disclosure of countertransference to clients. Sharing these feelings may overwhelm clients and burden them in a destructive way (Gabbard, 2001). In rare instances, however, referral to another nurse is appropriate when the first nurse cannot control the disturbed attitudes and emotions.

CONFLICT BETWEEN CARETAKER AND THERAPIST ROLES

Nurses may erect rigid defenses aimed at denying their personal feelings because of the emotional demands of nursing. For example, some procedures actually require the nurse to violate a client's emotional or physical state (injections, dressings). Defending against feelings becomes one way for the nurse to cope with inflicting pain on another person. You can deal effectively with the feelings of clients only to the extent that you explore your own personal feelings.

Continued assumption of the caretaker role also undermines your therapeutic effectiveness. The caretaker role tends to involve sympathy rather than empathy. The difference between these two responses is significant to therapeutic outcomes.

A one-to-one relationship requires that you help the client actively explore the meaning underlying the client's personal pain, distress, or discomfort. Avoid the caretaker role in which you alleviate pain. Rather, encourage clients to develop ways to do so for themselves. Similarly, the caretaker role requires nurses to make decisions for clients. It does not encourage clients to be accountable for their own decisions.

CRITICAL DISTANCE

It is important to observe how the client uses physical space. Hall (1966) asserts that people need to keep a critical distance between themselves and others to maintain their well-being. That specific distance depends on the relationship between the individuals. Nurses may allow physical distance between themselves and clients, especially early in a relationship. This distance promotes verbal communication and minimizes any existing anxiety and hostility. Moving rapidly toward closeness, especially in establishing the nurse–client relationship, may overwhelm the client and increase anxiety.

The physical distance between the psychiatric–mental health nurse and the client can be indicative of other therapeutic processes. For example, a client may sit in a chair at a great distance from you during initial meetings but move closer and closer as the working relationship is established. Assess the possible interpersonal implications of proximity (nearness) for each client. As the relationship progresses, assess whether physical distance or proximity reduces client anxiety. The client's need for critical distance during the therapeutic process usually increases as the client experiences panic or near-panic levels of anxiety. See Chapter 8 and Figure 8–3.

SELF-DISCLOSURE

Self-disclosure means being open to personal feelings and experiences, being "real" as opposed to hiding behind a professional facade.

How much should a nurse share with a client? Under what circumstances is it appropriate? The wisdom of disclosing personal information to clients has been the subject of much debate. Some argue that self-disclosure impedes therapeutic work; others argue just the opposite—that self-disclosure facilitates therapeutic work. A recent study by Barrett and Berman (2001) of clients at a university counseling center revealed that clients not only liked self-disclosing therapists more, but that they also reported lower levels of symptom distress. A study that examined how community mental health nurses promoted wellness with young adult clients who were experiencing an early episode of psychotic illness found that revealing oneself put both clients and nurses at ease and helped to dispel the perception of clients that they take part in a one-sided relationship (McCann & Baker, 2001). How much to share and under what circumstances remains an area for further research.

It may be helpful to view self-disclosure on a continuum. One end represents underdisclosure; the other, overdisclosure. When evaluating any self-disclosure at a given time, ask yourself the questions in the Nursing Self-Awareness feature on page 669.

Facilitative self-disclosure must be judiciously used within the context of the therapeutic relationship, where attention is given to its timing, appropriateness, and degree. For example, use self-disclosure cautiously with a severely dysfunctional client with poor ego boundaries. This client may not be able to separate thoughts and feelings that belong to the client from those that belong to the nurse. The client might misinterpret the nurse's self-disclosure or might not be able to make sense of the disclosure. The client may also fear engulfment; that is, the nurse's feelings might be perceived as so threatening that they overwhelm the client. Self-disclosure should foster the development of the therapeutic relationship rather than threatening its

Nursing SELF-AWARENESS

Self-Disclosure

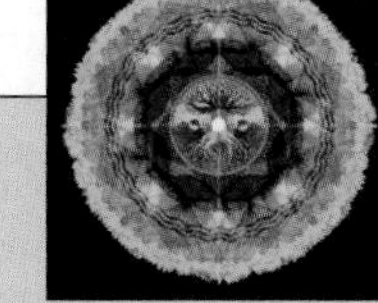

Determining whether or not to self-disclose will be made clearer by answering these questions:

- What is the purpose of the revelation; who is this self-disclosure for?
- Does this self-disclosure meet the client's therapeutic goals, or does it meet my needs?
- Will this self-disclosure take the focus away from the client?
- Does this self-disclosure foster the development of a more productive therapeutic relationship?

1. Will it encourage the client to disclose what the client has withheld or suppressed?
2. Will it encourage the client's cooperation?
3. Will it help the client to consider another point of view?
4. Will it support the client's positive movement in addressing life problems?
5. Will it encourage empathic understanding?

continuance. Beginning nurses should always discuss self-disclosure with an instructor/supervisor first.

When the nurse chooses to disclose personal information in a given instance, evaluation must follow. The client's reaction and subsequent exploration together can be a gauge for measuring how this client perceives and responds to self-disclosures by the nurse. As the nurse expresses feelings about the evolving relationship, the client may feel free to reciprocate. At times, the nurse may choose to role-model emotive expression.

When the nurse chooses to avoid self-disclosure in a given instance, several communication techniques may be helpful. For instance, a client might ask the nurse to disclose marital status, home address, religious affiliation, or a pressing personal problem. Auvil and Silver (1984) offer these ways to deflect a request for self-disclosure:

- *Use honesty.* "I don't want to share my home address with you."
- *Use benign curiosity.* "I wonder why you're asking me this today?"
- *Use refocusing.* "You were talking about how your father treats you. I wonder why you changed the topic? You were saying that . . ."
- *Use interpretation.* "I notice that every time you talk about your father, you change the subject and ask me a question." (pause)
- *Seek clarification.* "You keep asking me my home address. I wonder what concerns you might have about me today."
- *Respond with feedback and limit setting.* "I'm really uncomfortable when you ask me who pays my tuition. Talking about my finances isn't part of our agreement to work together." Adding "the last time we met, you were deciding if you were going to call your boss on the phone . . ." helps restructure the situation.

Use these communication techniques in the context of the therapeutic relationship, and assess and evaluate client responses in an ongoing manner. You can also refer to the facilitative communication techniques in Chapter 8.

GIFT GIVING

The giving of gifts may be a special concern in therapeutic relationships. Gift giving may take various forms: a fleeting social amenity (the purchase of a cup of coffee), a gesture (the loan of a favorite book), or the presentation of a valued object (the giving of an original painting). Like self-disclosure, gift giving in any instance must be met with ongoing assessment and evaluation to determine its form, intent, appropriateness, and meaning in the context of the therapeutic relationship (Shapiro & Ginzberg, 2002). No rule covers all instances of gift giving. Several broad guidelines can help you evaluate the particular situation.

During Orientation Phase

During the orientation phase of a therapeutic relationship, the client may overtly offer or ask for a gift. This gesture may be as incidental as offering you (or asking for) a cigarette. Examine this overture, keeping in mind several possible motivations:

- The client may seek to bribe or manipulate you, thereby seeking to control the direction of the therapeutic relationship. (Chapter 16 deals with manipulation.)
- The client may seek to "buy" your time and attention.
- The client may ask for small gifts to reinforce a helpless, "take-care-of-me" interpersonal stance.
- Of course, the client may have no covert intent and may simply need a cigarette.

In the orientation phase, it may be helpful not to accept or give any gift you feel uncomfortable about. Explore the client's intent. Often, this mutual exploration not only clarifies the client's intent but also helps define the parameters of the evolving relationship and models the exploratory process for the client.

During Working Phase

During the working phase, particularly after the client has shown positive growth, the client may offer a gift in the form of a craft or skill. As in the orientation phase, the intent of the gift needs to be made explicit. Encourage this exploration by asking questions such as, "How is it that you're sharing this gift with me?" or "What feelings might you want to share with this gift?"

A client might give a gift during the working phase for several reasons:

- The client may wish to acknowledge the mutual work that has taken place.
- The client may wish to show appreciation for being allowed to share concerns with another person.
- A gift may be a smoke screen to block further exploration of a major dynamic.
- A gift may outwardly cover up anger or frustration felt inwardly.
- Finally, a gift may indicate the client's perception that the therapeutic work is finished.

In every instance, assess the intent of the gift, as well as its timing and appropriateness, in the context of the therapeutic relationship.

During Termination Phase

Gifts are most often given during the termination phase of one-to-one relationships. In this phase, a gift may have several overt and covert meanings:

- The client may wish to give a token of appreciation for positive personal growth that has taken place.
- The client may desire to change the therapeutic relationship into a social one.
- The client may wish to prolong sessions to avoid the final goodbye.

Some nurses accept a small gift from a client at the time of termination if feelings regarding the gift have been explored and clarified. (The gift may be an appropriate remembrance of a mutual and positive growth experience.) Exploring the significance of a termination gift will ensure the maximum therapeutic benefit for the client (Shapiro & Ginzberg, 2002). You may find receiving a gift at times awkward and "artificial." Yet such a situation gives you the opportunity to help the client toward further self-expression and self-knowledge.

USE OF TOUCH

Physical contact is used cautiously in therapeutic work. It is best to avoid unplanned physical contact without therapeutic rationale. Clients with poor ego boundaries may become intensely threatened and feel overwhelmed by physical contact. For example, a client may lose the ability to distinguish self from the nurse during simple hand contact. Such contact may be perceived as a hostile or sexual gesture, although you do not intend it that way. In contrast, an acutely grief-stricken client, too distraught to focus on words, might receive needed support from being held.

When considering any use of touch, ask yourself:

1. Does touch meet the client's therapeutic goals, or does it meet my needs?
2. Does touch foster a more productive therapeutic relationship?

Evaluate the use of touch, like self-disclosure, in the context of the therapeutic relationship, paying attention to its timing, appropriateness, and type. For example, a client is thrilled to achieve an on-the-job goal that has taken much personal time and effort. You determine that a firm handshake and a statement of congratulations are facilitative in this instance and at this working phase of the relationship. If you are unsure of the effect of such a gesture, a frank inquiry may be in order: "How did you feel when I shook your hand a few moments ago?" Again, the client's reaction and subsequent exploration can be a gauge for measuring how the client perceives and responds to the use of touch.

VALUES

Address client values and beliefs that interfere with adaptive functioning. The following people hold cultural values and beliefs that may interfere with constructive change:

- The abusive spouse who believes the partner should be subservient, and, conversely, the partner who defers personal needs to preserve the relationship.
- The abusive parent who believes that to "spare the rod" is to "spoil the child."
- The child raised with the family injunction that family problems should not be discussed outside the home, who may view the nurse's actions as an invasion of privacy.

It is also possible that religious beliefs may interfere with change. For example, a client may believe that since God takes care of His people, there is no need to solve personal problems. Or, a client may believe that divorce or homosexuality is a sin, and therefore will never be forgiven (or forgive self).

Initially, you should become aware of the specific values and beliefs that influence the immediate relationship work. It is often useful to label the value or belief with the client, exploring its history, importance, cultural context, and impact. Nonjudgmental, alternative values may be discussed if the client initiates such an exploration. The humanistic nurse respects the client's values and beliefs, and the client's ultimate choices regarding personal value systems.

NURSING PROCESS

Orientation (Beginning) Phase

The primary goal of the orientation phase is to establish contact, to begin developing a working relationship with the client. Establishing contact includes the initial encounters between nurse and client—how they approach and interact with each other, both verbally and nonverbally. You and the client meet to discuss how you will work together toward a common goal. See the Rx Communication feature on page 671 for an example of an early dialogue related to goal setting. You are aware of having impact on the client and acknowledge the client's personal impact as a unique individual. A sensitive and systematic consideration of the client's cultural and ethnic background is important at each phase of the one-to-one relationship.

The time required for each phase ideally depends on the severity of client dysfunction, the number and types of problems surfacing during treatment, and the type of therapeutic contract. Although these phases are presented here in their entirety to develop a comprehensive theoretic framework, nurses rarely experience them in such detail and sequence. You are more likely to experience the development of several short-term goals and to experiment with several subsequent interventions in any phase of relationship work. Nevertheless, an exploration of each phase will increase your familiarity with the flow—that is, "what comes next"—and may also provide a framework in which you can see client and nurse behaviors as partial expressions of a specific phase.

In informal relationships, contact usually begins when the nurse seeks out the client. Establishment of contact may involve developing client awareness of your presence, followed by working to communicate with the client verbally. In formal relationships, contact may begin when the client inquires about services or when the psychiatric–mental health nurse contacts

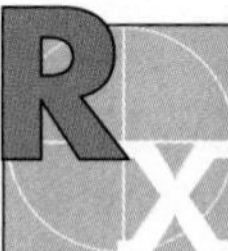

COMMUNICATION

The Initial Contract

CLIENT: What, exactly, are we supposed to be doing together?

NURSE RESPONSE 1: I'd like to meet with you every day while you're here. This will give you an opportunity to talk about yourself and the things that are of concern to you.

RATIONALE: In addition to providing structure about the sessions, the nurse lays the groundwork for the focus on the client.

NURSE RESPONSE 2: That's something that you and I can decide together tomorrow morning when we meet here at 9:30.

RATIONALE: The nurse reminds the client of the time for their meeting and sets the stage for mutual collaboration and negotiation.

the client following referral. In formal relationships, the sense of working together in a therapeutic alliance enables the client to endure anxiety and deal with resistance to change, which inevitably surface during the course of one-to-one relationships. This phase of the therapeutic relationship concludes with mutual agreement on a therapeutic contract, which may be verbal and quite simple. The contract spells out the client's goals for treatment and the nurse's professional responsibilities.

Assessment

Client assessment begins at the first moment of contact. Assessment continues throughout the therapeutic relationship but is particularly important during the orientation phase. Remember that shortcuts taken in assessment procedures almost always jeopardize the ultimate quality of care. Crucial areas of concern may go unaddressed or be treated superficially.

An important part of client assessment is to determine what the client is likely to accomplish in the time allotted. Consider the extent of the client's responsiveness to you during this early stage of relating, the severity of the client's symptoms, the client's level of resistance, and the priorities for the care of the client. Emphasize the treatment needed to reach the most important and obtainable goals. Together, you and the client take this opportunity to shape the nature of the client's care within the limits of the current health care environment.

SUBJECTIVE DATA

Observation, a process long regarded as essential to clinical nursing practice, is of particular importance in one-to-one relationship work. Note elements in the nurse-client interaction that are missing, distorted, or imbalanced. What the client avoids discussing is often more crucial than what is shared.

OBJECTIVE DATA

Objective data collection ideally includes the following: mental status examination, complete physical examination, nursing history, and psychologic testing, as needed. Which examinations are done and by whom are generally determined by the agency or institution in which the psychiatric–mental health nurse works, and by the psychiatric–mental health nurse's expertise in these specific areas.

INTERVIEW

Interviewing is a process that generally occurs in the orientation phase of one-to-one relationships. Although a psychiatric–mental health nurse may use the structured initial interview in formal one-to-one work, it is rarely used in informal relationships.

The initial interview has the following purposes:

- To initiate trust building.
- To establish rapport with the client.
- To obtain pertinent client data.
- To initiate client assessment.
- To make practical arrangements for treatment.

The initial interview is crucial because it sets the stage for subsequent therapeutic contact.

Amount of Structuring. Structure the initial interview to establish rapport, decrease anxiety, and convey willingness to address the client's suffering. Begin by introducing yourself, inviting the client to be seated, and making a statement about information thus far known about the client's seeking of services. An open-ended question, such as "How is it that you are here today?" provides an opportunity for the client to talk about concerns. Inform the client that the purpose of the initial interview is to obtain an overview of the client's current situation and then determine the availability of appropriate services.

Essential Data. One primary purpose of structuring the initial interview is to collect essential data (see Chapter 9). Address client resistance if it surfaces during the initial interview. This resistance may occur when the client has initiated services at someone else's request or insistence, has fears and misconceptions about therapy, or has had an unsatisfactory therapeutic experience in the past. Nursing intervention calls for explicit exploration of the specific resistance before further data collection.

Anxious clients may be confused about or misinterpret information given during the initial interview. Manifestations of anxiety must be differentiated from manifestations of resistance. You may need to repeat information several times or in subsequent meetings.

CLINICAL EXAMPLE

Selena, a 35-year-old woman, has been referred to the outpatient mental health clinic after several visits for minor medical problems. You note from the record a pattern of medication refills for antianxiety medication from her primary care provider. You also notice that she had been referred for mental health care on two other occasions, but failed to keep those appointments.

This information is valuable because it provides direction for appropriate nursing diagnoses related to both behavior and affect, the identification of appropriate outcomes, the setting of specific client-centered goals, and the implementation of appropriate interventions.

Nursing Diagnosis: NANDA

Following a comprehensive assessment, you will need to gather and organize all the data collected and formulate preliminary nursing diagnoses. The word *preliminary* is used to imply the ongoing potential for revision as client behaviors unfold during the course of the nurse-client relationship.

The goal in organizing the data is to understand the data as they reflect the client's unique, private world. Look for dominant themes or central issues in the client's responses. The dominant themes and central issues will be unique to each individual client. Select NANDA nursing diagnoses that derive from these themes and issues.

Outcome Identification: NOC

The major outcomes of the orientation phase are establishing contact and beginning to form a working relationship between client and nurse. The working relationship in this initial phase is the framework on which the client constructs behavioral change in the next phase. ■ Table 28–3 highlights common signs of a working relationship. Other individual outcomes will be determined by the specific dominant themes and central issues of the client.

Planning and Implementation: NIC

The interventions discussed below are common elements during the orientation phase. The development of additional interventions is based on assessment and nursing diagnoses for each individual client.

THERAPEUTIC CONTRACT

A plan for action actually forms the *therapeutic contract* negotiated in a one-to-one relationship. The therapeutic contract is a concrete, detailed, and mutually negotiated acknowledgment of the client's personal goals for treatment plus the nurse's professional responsibilities.

It may be modified over time but always serves as a tool for evaluating the benefit to the client and the effectiveness of the nurse. In an informal therapeutic relationship, the therapeutic contract may differ from the usual care plan often developed in outpatient and inpatient settings. For example, an initial contract may begin as a very simple agreement concerning the time and place of subsequent meetings together.

The client's personal goals for treatment may be long-term or short-term goals, but they always specify detailed, observable outcomes as in the following Clinical Example.

CLINICAL EXAMPLE

Nicole is a 30-year-old woman admitted to an inpatient psychiatric unit following an overdose of risperidone (Risperdal). During past hospitalizations, Nicole has been emotionally labile, has had trouble following her treatment schedule, and was easily frustrated by the limits and compromises of living in the hospital, demanded medication, and threatened suicide. Nicole's primary nurse proposed that they work together to identify goals and behaviors for improved personal and interpersonal functioning. Nicole identified problems of feeling empty, having poor relationships with others, and being angry; she chose to focus on the overall goal of improved social skills. Nicole agreed to the following expectations:

- *I will participate in a one-to-one relationship with my nurse and express my feelings verbally.*

TABLE 28–3 Signs of a Working Relationship

For Nurse	For Client
Sense of making contact with the client.	Nonverbal and verbal evidence of liking the nurse.
Sense that the client is responding well to the relationship.	Sense of relaxation with the nurse.
Sense that the nurse can facilitate client growth regardless of the severity of client dysfunction.	Sense of confidence in the nurse.
Sense of commitment to addressing the client's problems.	Nonsuperficial (in nature and depth) problems addressed.

- *I will identify uncomfortable situations involving other people and discuss the interactions with my nurse at appointed times.*
- *I will continue my routine treatment activities until the appropriate time to meet with my nurse.*

Strive for the most concise, detailed, and accurate description of client goals in the beginning phase. Clearly stated goals facilitate subsequent mutual evaluation during the middle and end phases of one-to-one work. Goals may focus on:

- Decreasing or eliminating troublesome behaviors.
- Increasing socialization.
- Increasing living skills.

Client goals most often contribute to the establishment of a working relationship when they are specific, address intrapersonal or interpersonal behavior patterns, and specifically delineate the degree of change necessary for client self-satisfaction.

At times, client goals may be long-term or even inappropriate. In this situation, help the client define initial steps toward the long-term goal. For example, a readmitted mentally ill client may pinpoint discharge as an important goal. You may then work with this client to identify the steps needed to achieve this goal. One step may be to maintain self-care in the area of bathing/hygiene. When severe dysfunction limits client input into planning, the nursing staff may supplement goals that are determined to be beneficial to the client.

In a formal therapeutic relationship, as in individual psychotherapy, the therapeutic contract is more detailed and generally includes three practical matters:

1. Determination of the place, duration, and time of the meetings.
2. Establishment of fees and payment intervals, if any.
3. Consideration of optional referral sources, should the client be unable to negotiate an agreement on the first two matters.

In formal therapeutic relationships, the therapeutic contract may not reflect client problems and strengths in their entirety. At that moment, the client may not determine that an area is, in fact, a problem. Thus, the therapeutic contract in formal relationship work reflects the *client's* definition of personal goals at one moment in time. The psychiatric–mental health nurse, in this instance, remains aware of other probable problem areas and assesses these areas with the client in an ongoing manner, as appropriate.

Regardless of the form that goal identification takes, the therapeutic contract serves the following purposes:

- To facilitate humanistic involvement with the client as an individual.
- To involve the client as a full partner in the therapeutic process.
- As a basis for communication in the therapeutic process.
- To provide continuity for the client and everyone involved with the client.

The initial goals of the therapeutic contract may be modified or deleted in subsequent phases of the one-to-one relationship as appropriate or necessary.

TRUST

Concerns about trust surface in this first phase of the relationship. Trust between nurse and client evolves over time as the client tests the emotional climate of sessions, risks self-disclosure, and observes the nurse's follow-through on responsibilities delineated in the therapeutic contract. You can promote trust by responding to all the client's feeling states without being judgmental or attempting to control emotive expression. The following interventions enhance initial trust:

- Listening attentively to client feelings.
- Responding to client feelings.
- Exhibiting consistency, especially regarding appointment times.
- Viewing situations from the client's perspective.

Consistency and listening were validated by Forchuk et al. (2000) as positive, helpful influences in encouraging trust.

Self-awareness of personal feeling states on the part of the nurse also enhances trust. It allows the client to disclose uncomfortable, even forbidden, feelings in safety. A common failing among those learning relationship skills is focusing on technique. This produces mechanical, unfeeling responses. It is also important to avoid giving premature reassurances about trust, which may inhibit exploration of this vital therapeutic issue and create distance between nurse and client.

CONFIDENTIALITY

Client concerns about the level of confidentiality also surface in this first phase of the therapeutic relationship. Keeping clients' confidentiality has been ranked by nurses as among the top ten caring behaviors (Brunton & Beaman, 2000). The issue of confidentiality must be explicitly addressed when the client makes even vague reference to it. Explicitly state which people will have access to client revelations (clinical instructor, case supervisor, consultant, colleague), and explore how the client feels in response to this information.

TUNING IN TO PROCESS

The beginning nurse often attends carefully to the *content* of the client sessions—what the client says—and only after considerable experience becomes actively attuned to *process.* Process here does not mean nursing process but rather a complex communication skill that enables the nurse to focus on several aspects of the nurse–client relationship at the same time. Process involves attention to all nonverbal and verbal client behaviors. It involves responding to client "themes," such as anger, hopelessness, and powerlessness. The challenge for the nurse is to become wise enough to learn what to ignore and sensitive enough to know what to emphasize (Guy & Brady, 2001). The experienced nurse is simultaneously aware of both content and process, interweaving both for maximum therapeutic effectiveness.

ADDRESSING THE CLIENT'S SUFFERING

Interventions during the orientation phase are valid and important, even if you do not reach the working phase with a particular client (because of time limitations or because the client is unable to agree on goals). The psychiatric–mental health nurse intervenes by directly addressing the client's suffering within the context of the client's cultural and ethnic background. This intervention allows clients to share how they perceive, experience, and manifest the problem. The following example illustrates how the nurse encourages a depressed client to "move outside himself."

CLINICAL EXAMPLE

Client: *This depression is like a big log weighing on my chest.*

Nurse: *How might I, or someone else, know that you are suffering in this way?*

Client: *Well . . . I sigh a lot . . . I don't move a lot, only when I have to . . . I wouldn't look at you, or bother to talk to you. I guess when I feel like this, I close people out. Yeah, I close everyone out, even my wife.*

Nurse: *So when you suffer in this way, you "close people out." And what is this like for you?*

Client: *I'm alone and lonely. Not a soul on earth cares for me.*

CLARIFYING PURPOSE, ROLES, AND RESPONSIBILITIES

An additional therapeutic task is to intervene directly in clarifying the purpose of the relationship work, the role of the nurse, and the responsibilities of the client. When this preliminary exploration of purpose, roles, and responsibilities is explicit and detailed, each participant better understands how to move within the relationship. It also decreases anxiety and the chance that a client may use the relationship to obtain special privileges. From the first meeting the nurse also intervenes to reinforce effective coping skills and increase client self-esteem. The Intervention box below summarizes the goals, tasks, and subsequent nursing interventions of the orientation phase of one-to-one relationships.

Evaluation

In the orientation phase, evaluation includes your initial comprehensive evaluation of client behaviors, any initial steps toward the development of client self-evaluation, and your ongoing self-evaluation. The more specific and goal-oriented the therapeutic contract, the easier it is for the client and nurse to evaluate the effectiveness of the therapeutic relationship.

In addition to evaluating the effectiveness of each therapeutic task, you must evaluate the important goal of the orientation phase: Has a working relationship evolved between the client and nurse, and, if so, to what degree? Table 28–3 lists the signs of a working relationships.

NURSING PROCESS

Working (Middle) Phase

Once contact is established, attention turns to maintenance and analysis of contact in the working phase. *Analysis of contact*

INTERVENTION

Goals, Tasks, and Interventions of the Orientation Phase

Goal: Establishing contact and beginning to form a working relationship with the client.

Therapeutic Tasks	Nursing Interventions
Clarify the purpose of relationship work, the role of the nurse, and responsibilities of the client.	Provide information regarding purpose, roles, and responsibilities in relationship work to alleviate initial client anxiety.
	Immediately and explicitly address any misconceptions, fantasies, and fears regarding relationship work and/or the nurse.
Address client suffering directly, offering to work with the client toward its alleviation.	Use facilitative characteristics, especially empathic understanding.
	Avoid premature reassurance (allow trust to evolve).
	Be explicit about who has access to client's revelations (degree of confidentiality).
Negotiate therapeutic contract (client's definition of personal goals for treatment and the nurse's professional responsibilities.)	Whenever possible, encourage delineation of goals that are specific, address intrapersonal and interpersonal behavioral patterns, and designate the degree of change necessary for client self-satisfaction.
	In informal relationship work, the contract generally includes a determination of time and place for working together to the extent that client ability permits.
	In formal relationship work, the contract generally includes place, duration, and time of therapy; fees and payment intervals, if any; and optional referral sources.

refers to an in-depth exploration of how the client relates to others as manifested in the nurse–client relationship. In this working phase, the client may address developmental and situational problems, as well as interpersonal problems. It is called the working phase because during this phase, the nurse and client actively and systematically identify, explore, link, modify, and evaluate specific behaviors, especially those determined to be dysfunctional for the client.

The client's clearly stated goals in the therapeutic contract are now explored. The nurse has the following two therapeutic goals:

- *Behavioral analysis.* The nurse and client determine the dynamics of the client's response patterns, especially those considered to be dysfunctional. Such analysis also addresses dysfunctional thought and emotive patterns, because these inevitably alter the client's behavior.
- *Constructive change in behavior.* This applies particularly to dysfunctional response patterns.

Thus, the psychiatric–mental health nurse and client work together to analyze behavior and institute behavioral change.

Assessment

Assessment is continued, detailed, and expanded upon. Your observations of nonverbal, verbal, and environmental responses continue to have vital importance as the client begins to address personal response patterns. In addition, you continue to assess emotive, cognitive, cultural, and behavioral aspects. Filling in gaps of information not obtained in the orientation phase, you may now acquire a detailed assessment about a subject the client was unable to share or ignored earlier. The following example illustrates that what was not said (that is, what was avoided, blocked, rejected) by the client may have more significance than what the client shared.

CLINICAL EXAMPLE

During initial sessions, 18-year-old Maureen avoided any inquiries about her parents, other than to say that she lived alone. After several sessions, the nurse again asked about the parents. Maureen replied softly with tears welling in her eyes. "They're dead. They died in a car crash 2 years ago." She slowly related how, since their deaths, she has spent so much energy trying to survive that she has barely felt much of anything. Subsequent sessions dealt with her apparent delayed grief reaction.

The new data caused the nurse to revise and update the tentative nursing diagnoses and make a marked change in the direction of the sessions. Such shifting is not uncommon in one-to-one relationships. When a change in direction occurs, assess if the sudden change indicates the need to avoid a certain topic, or indicates a move toward a deeper level of emotive expression.

In the working phase, you facilitate many aspects of assessment with the client. First, collaborate with the client in identifying important behavioral trends and patterns. Once a pattern is identified, explore it in elaborate detail to determine its origin, causes, operation, and effects on the client and the people in the client's world. Environmental factors (familial, political, economic, or cultural) are separated from intrapersonal factors (depression or anxiety) contributing to the pattern. The client figuratively holds the pattern to the light to examine and make sense of its every aspect. The elements of one pattern will inevitably link with others, so that the major life patterns gradually unfold. The first part of the Intervention box on page 676 summarizes the therapeutic tasks undertaken to achieve this objective and offers specific nursing approaches to helping the client.

There are two noteworthy considerations regarding therapeutic tasks of the first goal, behavioral analysis:

1. As clients begin to describe and reexperience conflict, they consciously or unconsciously use defenses to ward off the anxiety this awakens. The development of a good working relationship enables clients to tolerate increased anxiety in the working phase.
2. As clients become familiar with self-assessment, they may modify original personal goals, or develop additional goals, in keeping with what they have learned.

It is important during the working phase to encourage client self-assessment of growth-facilitating and growth-inhibiting behaviors. After assessing one specific response, the client is often able to transfer this skill to begin assessing other aspects of life as well. A realistic self-assessment process is perhaps the most valuable skill that the client can "take home." It is often thrilling to experience the client "taking over" and further applying realistic assessment skills developed in one-to-one work.

Nursing Diagnosis: NANDA

In the working phase, nursing diagnoses may be revised, expanded, or deleted to more accurately reflect a central pattern of concern in the evolving one-to-one relationship. As the working phase proceeds, the priority assigned to a nursing diagnosis may change, for example, when the client is able to implement positive change in some areas. Those nursing diagnoses designated as "potential problems" may move up or down on the priority list, depending on what interventions, if any, have been effective. A potential diagnosis may decrease in priority after preventive health education, if both the client and the nurse evaluate this intervention as beneficial.

Outcome Identification: NOC

The initial goal of behavioral analysis of the client's response patterns continues throughout the working phase. The major identified outcomes are:

INTERVENTION

Goals, Tasks, and Interventions of the Working Phase

Goal: Behavioral analysis (mutual determination of dynamics of response patterns identified by client, especially those considered dysfunctional).

Therapeutic Tasks	Nursing Interventions
Identify and explore important response patterns in detail.	Explore response pattern in depth, including origin, causes, operation, and effect of pattern (intrapersonally and interpersonally).
	Separate environmental factors (familial, political, economic, cultural) from intrapersonal factors.
	Link elements of one response pattern to other patterns as appropriate, for a gradual unfolding of central life patterns.
Analyze, with the client, client's mode of conflict resolution.	Encourage a detailed exploration of how the client reacts to reduce anxiety associated with conflict.
	Increase awareness of defenses employed to ward off anxiety awakened by such exploration.
Facilitate client self-assessment of growth-producing and growth-inhibiting response patterns.	Encourage client to evaluate each response pattern to determine which are self-defeating and/or thwart gratification of basic needs.

Goal: Constructive change in behavior, especially in dysfunctional response patterns identified by the client.

Therapeutic Tasks	Nursing Interventions
Address forces that inhibit desired change (troublesome thoughts, feelings, and behaviors).	Help the client challenge personal resistance to change.
	Use problem-solving strategies, active decision making, and personal accountability.
	Help the client learn and apply problem-solving strategies.
	Encourage the client to assert own needs when external environmental conditions (group, agency, institution) are an inhibiting force.
Create an atmosphere offering permission for active experimentation to test and assess the effectiveness of new behaviors.	Allow freedom to make and assess mistakes and blunders.
	Avoid parental judgment of any behavioral experimentation; encourage client self-assessment instead.
Facilitate the development of coping skills to deal with anxiety associated with constructive changes in behavior.	Address, rather than avoid, anxiety and its manifestations.
	Strengthen existing growth-promoting coping skills, especially regarding unalterable conditions (terminal illness, physical deformity, loss of significant other by death).
	Encourage the development of new coping skills and their application to actual life experiences.

- The client develops an awareness of current behavioral patterns.
- The client understands how and when those patterns manifest themselves.
- The client may gain insight into the potential causes of those patterns.
- The client assesses which behavioral patterns are ineffective and self-defeating.
- The client attempts to change ineffective behavioral patterns and develop new, more effective behaviors.

Planning and Implementation: NIC

In the working phase, planning is ideally done collaboratively between client and nurse. Such planning involves frequent consideration of the client's initial goals. When planning has been systematic and thorough, there is hardly a moment to worry about "what to do." The short-term and long-term treatment goals in the form of the therapeutic contract are a map indicating the direction, momentum, and the steps that are needed to reach a designated point.

There is, however, a potential danger in the implementation of the planning component: moving too quickly and incompletely through an exploration of the client's feelings and thoughts in an attempt to reach a designated goal. *Slowness* and *thoroughness* are all-important here. Change needs to take place in the client's feelings, thoughts, and behaviors. If change does not occur in all aspects, then it is destined to be short-lived and ineffectual in the long run and may contribute to client discouragement.

When the client is working on an issue that is unresolved at the end of a meeting, It is often helpful to summarize the unfinished work for the next meeting. This technique may help the client anticipate, plan, or prepare to tackle this area of concern again. Personal experiments, such as trying out new behaviors in real situations, may be encouraged between sessions. Some clients may be able to continue working through a problem on their own between meetings.

Active intervention is especially important to achieve the second goal of the working phase, constructive changes in behavior, particularly in self-defeating, growth-inhibiting behavior patterns. Behavioral change flows from the first goal of behavioral analysis. The objectives are interrelated and essential for successful therapeutic work. Understanding and insight need to be complemented by behavioral implementation. This statement deserves much attention, because particular clients may consistently generate and thrive on sophisticated insights while continuing to assume a powerless stance about implementing constructive change in their condition. The Intervention box on page 676 highlights therapeutic tasks and specific nursing interventions for the second goal in the working phase.

You can also use active experimentation to test the effect of new behaviors. The introverted male client who resolved to establish relationships with women may assume various postures (cavalier, paternal, seductive) with a female nurse to determine the appropriateness of these behaviors before displaying them outside of sessions. Permission to "try on" or role-play new behaviors must also include the freedom to make mistakes. Errors and blunders are rich sources of additional learning and occasional fun. Clients who can see humor in errors in a nondefeatist manner have acquired a new skill. Encourage them to apply this skill, and any other coping skills learned in relationship work, to normal maturational and situational crises encountered throughout life.

In inpatient settings, work with other staff members to make the whole team aware of the meaning of the client's behavior as positive actions that may be exaggerated at first. For example, some staff members may encourage a depressed client to verbalize anger and begin by shouting. If there is no staff collaboration, the client may receive negative feedback (room restrictions) for testing out new coping skills.

PROBLEM-SOLVING STRATEGIES

Problem-solving strategies, as a mode of intervention, are particularly important in the working phase. Problem-solving strategies are essential after the client has identified, explored, and assessed important behavioral patterns. Encourage clients to use the sequential problem-solving strategies discussed in the Intervention box at right. Reminding clients to be patient is supportive and reassuring. Problem-solving abilities improve with time and experience.

CHALLENGING THE CLIENT'S RESISTANCE TO CHANGE

Challenging the client's resistance to change is an appropriate intervention in the working phase. There are two major categories of forces that inhibit desired change:

1. Intrapersonal forces, which may arise from troublesome thoughts, feelings, or behaviors. Examples include thoughts that hamper the client's sense of worth, the client's inability to control and express emotion appropriately, or the client's inability to relate to others in a meaningful manner.
2. The client's personal resistance to change, which is the greatest inhibiting force. In fact, the client's challenge to this resistance constitutes the major work in one-to-one relationships.

Problems of resistance and general intervention strategies are discussed earlier in the chapter. Of equal significance is the previous discussion of transference and countertransference phenomena, since these phenomena may require careful, planned nursing interventions. Sometimes transference and countertransference are so intense that they become a problem for the beginning psychiatric–mental health nurse.

INTERVENTION

Problem-Solving Strategies

- **Observation.** Observation as a problem-solving strategy involves gathering and analyzing facts about a potential problem area. It eliminates opinions and impressions and emphasizes facts. (Observation as an aspect of assessment is discussed earlier in the chapter.)
- **Definition.** Definition is perhaps the most significant and far-reaching problem-solving strategy. It involves an initial specification of a problem, followed by a question. Starting a problem-solving exploration with the word "How" ("How is it?" "How does it manifest itself?" "How has this come about?") focuses on the process regarding a specific problem. It is generally more useful than asking "Why," which emphasizes rationale. (Questioning as a communication technique is explored in Chapter 8.)
- **Preparation.** Preparation involves collecting additional pertinent data related to the basic problem that may prove useful in later stages of problem-solving strategies. This enables the nurse and client to anticipate which data might be most useful.
- **Analysis.** As a problem-solving strategy, analysis involves breaking down the relevant material into subproblems so that each subproblem may be assessed separately.
- **Ideation.** Ideation involves accumulating alternative ideas on how to resolve the basic problem.
- **Incubation.** Incubation is used when the problem-solving process or one aspect of it is set aside for a period of time to allow for illumination.
- **Synthesis.** As a problem-solving strategy, synthesis involves putting together all elements of the basic problem, subproblems, and possible alternatives.
- **Evaluation.** Evaluation consists of making judgments about the ideas that result.
- **Development.** As a final problem-solving strategy, development involves planning the implementation of these ideas.

Evaluation

Several levels of evaluation occur simultaneously in the working phase. First, do an ongoing evaluation of the client's various levels of intrapersonal and interpersonal functioning. Feedback from family, community agencies, or the client's employer may enhance any current comprehensive evaluation. For example, does the client seem to be facing an impending crisis? If so, you may choose to switch from intrapersonal exploration to a crisis intervention strategy. Second, encourage client self-evaluation, as explored in previous discussion. Finally, constantly perform self-evaluation as a helping person growing in skill and experience. Nursing self-evaluation is done by informal discussions with staff and other mental health care personnel and by formal clinical supervision.

"On-the-spot" evaluations of relevant short-term and long-term goals can occur during any meeting with the client. For example, as the client talks about increasing socialization skills, the nurse may reflect: "Let's look at our contract together. You originally wanted to date a woman of your choice for two hours during an evening without leaving the situation. How do you think this compares with what you're now saying has happened?" Support any effort at evaluation on the part of the client and explore what else needs to happen for the client to achieve the short-term goal. An additional area of evaluation involves the client's "trying on" alternative behaviors to determine whether these new behaviors may work.

The client and nurse should mutually evaluate the appropriateness of goals in any one of the following areas in the light of the client's current functioning:

- Degree of the client's success in achieving specific goals.
- The client's growth-producing and growth-inhibiting behavior patterns.
- Unfinished business that must be resolved to achieve a desired goal.

The working phase may also involve ongoing evaluations of the status, characteristics, and depth of the nurse-client relationship. The client may view the nurse in different ways (parent, sibling, friend) at various times. It is only when the client makes these views explicit that the nurse may intervene to clarify roles and responsibilities in a facilitative manner.

The psychiatric–mental health nurse and the client have moved through the first two phases of therapeutic relationships when:

- They have established a working relationship.
- They have analyzed the dynamics of the client's behavioral patterns.
- The client has effectively instituted behavioral changes in keeping with the therapeutic contract.

In informal relationship work, the nurse may touch on only one or two aspects of the working phase. Even the advanced psychiatric–mental health nurse rarely addresses all therapeutic tasks in this phase of relationship work.

NURSING PROCESS

Termination (End) Phase

During the termination phase of one-to-one relationships, the psychiatric–mental health nurse and client discontinue contact. This phase is as important as the previous two phases, although both the nurse and the client frequently avoid it because of past difficulties with separation.

The goal of the end phase is termination of the one-to-one relationship in a mutually planned, satisfying manner. Remind the client that termination was first addressed in the orientation phase, when the duration of the relationship was discussed. Also emphasize the growth and positive aspects of the relationship, rather than focusing exclusively on separation.

A smooth and complete termination sometimes occurs in actual practice. In informal relationship work in inpatient settings, termination more often occurs with the client's abrupt departure or planned medical discharge. Even in formal relationship work in community settings, contact often ceases without explanation after a series of missed appointments, or with a phone call by the client to inform the therapist of the client's decision to terminate, or with the client abruptly leaving a session and failing to resume subsequent contact. In these instances, the nurse can call or write the client and suggest an additional session to deal with either the therapeutic good-bye or a willingness to continue the relationship work. Termination requires careful preparation, adequate time for the client to work through the feelings about ending, and an opportunity for the nurse to explore personal reactions with a clinical instructor, colleague, supervisor, or consultant.

Assessment

Assessment as a component of the nursing process in the resolution phase deals primarily with determining when the client may be ready to terminate, how the client deals with termination, and how the nurse deals with termination. Criteria that indicate a client's readiness for termination are presented in the Assessment box below.

ASSESSMENT

Termination Readiness

The following criteria may be useful to determine whether the client is ready to terminate:

- **Relief from the presenting problem.** Symptoms no longer interfere with the client's comfort.
- **Achievement of treatment goals.** These ideally are planned goals included in the therapeutic contract between the nurse and client.
- **Improvement in social functioning.** The client experiences increased satisfaction in interpersonal relationships.
- **Acquisition of adaptive coping strategies.** Ideally, these strategies include the client's use of effective problem-solving strategies on a daily basis.
- **Acquisition of more effective defense mechanisms.** A client who cannot achieve adaptive coping strategies should develop more effective defense mechanisms to ensure stabilization.
- **Attainment of identity.** The client experiences self-satisfaction and no longer needs to depend on the nurse for a sense of well-being.
- **Disruption due to a major impasse in the one-to-one relationship.** Stubborn resistances may surface and persist on the part of the client. Uncontrollable countertransference may develop on the part of the nurse.

Many factors influence how the client reacts to termination. These factors include:

- *Degree of client involvement.* The greater the degree of client involvement, the more intense the client's reaction to termination.
- *Length of treatment.* In general, the longer the nurse-client relationship lasts, the more time should be spent in exploring all aspects of termination.
- *Client's past history of significant losses.* A client who has lost significant others may reexperience past conflicts and emotional responses.
- *Ability to separate from others.* The reaction to termination is influenced by how well the client has mastered the early separation–individuation phase of development.
- *Degree of success achieved.* Reaction to termination depends on how successful and satisfying the relationship has been for the client.
- *Degree of transference in the relationship.* The greater the transference in the nurse–client relationship, the more intense the client's reaction to termination.

Be alert to client responses during termination. Any number of responses—repression, regression, anger, denial, sadness, withdrawal, avoidance, acceptance, joy—may surface, and it is not unusual for several to surface at once. When repressing, the client shows no emotional response. Regression on the part of the client is an extremely common response to termination. Regressive behavior may range from statements of abandonment and hopelessness to an inability to tend to personal hygiene. The central message conveyed is: "See? I can't make it without you!"

Nurses's Self-Awareness. Finally, assessment involves how you personally manage separation in the one-to-one relationship. Like the client, you can have any number of responses. Some common responses are:

- Regret that the client did not achieve more than the client actually did.
- Hesitation to give up the dependence elements of the relationship.
- Collusion with the client to prolong sessions to avoid the inevitability of separation.

Nursing Diagnosis: NANDA

Nursing diagnoses during termination should reflect the termination behaviors manifested by the client. A wide variety of nursing diagnoses may be relevant. Potential nursing diagnoses that stem from regression during the termination phase may be: self-care deficit, hopelessness, powerlessness, and ineffective individual coping. Nursing diagnoses should be modified as necessary, as the client moves through the termination experience.

Outcome Identification: NOC

The ideal outcome occurs when the nurse–client relationship terminates after achieving all identified and measurable personal behavioral changes. Such resolution seldom occurs in psychiatric practice, especially since brief hospital stays are now the rule rather than the exception. Often, the client achieves more limited behavioral changes and agrees to return for future work or referral as necessary. At other times, the client achieves symptom relief only.

Outcomes are compromised when the client is unable to make progress due to lack of insight or mental capacity. Chronic catastrophic life circumstances (such as severe medical illness, life-threatening poverty, prison, etc.) may interfere with growth-producing behaviors. On rare occasions, the client's condition deteriorates and the client is unable to benefit from the nurse–client relationship.

Planning and Implementation: NIC

Planning involves preparing for the final good-bye (the subject of this section) and mutual planning about where the client may seek future help if the need arises (the subject of the next section).

Intervention strategies vary according to the client's behaviors. You may respond to the client who is repressing the reality of termination by repeatedly observing that he or she is not addressing the issue of the impending separation. You may then attempt to explore this avoidance with the client. Useful interventions for clients who are regressing in response to termination include:

- Addressing the possible underlying fears of abandonment.
- Emphasizing the growth achieved by the client.
- Continuing to focus on the realities of separation.

The acting-out client may protest termination in numerous ways before the termination date, such as attempting suicide, psychiatric hospitalization, quitting a job, or rejecting the nurse. In general, the underlying feelings, fears, and fantasies need ventilation, exploration, and working through, as do reactions of anger, depression, and grief. An exception to this general guideline is the client who uses distraction maneuvers to prevent termination, such as introducing explosive new material in final sessions. In this situation, you may use limit setting rather than exploration because of time constraints. In other words, there may be "unfinished business" despite planning and effort.

The nurse has the final task of participating in an *explicit and therapeutic good-bye* with the client. Nursing responsibilities in this final phase include anticipating your own personal reaction to separation and, optionally, expressing this reaction in a manner that does not burden the client. In addition, you may share a special wish for the client, based on the client's particular assets within the therapeutic relationship.

A therapeutic good-bye gives the client a sense of freedom to move on to other relationships. The end phase may take from one meeting to several months of meetings, depending on the duration of the one-to-one relationship. In general, the longer the duration of the relationship, the longer the time needed to deal explicitly with the termination of contact. The Intervention box below summarizes the goal, therapeutic tasks, and specific nursing interventions of the termination phase.

Ideally, the client can completely work through feelings regarding separation so that there is no unfinished business between nurse and client. The nurse-client relationship has given the client the opportunity to depend on another in a realistic and mature manner. The direct, explicit good-bye is frequently the first such experience for the client. It is usually a moment of unique humanness for both the nurse and the client.

Evaluation

Evaluation is a vital component of the nursing process during the termination phase. You have the task of helping the client evaluate the therapeutic contract. The criteria for evaluation are the goals formulated in the orientation and working phases of the one-to-one relationship. Each goal is evaluated in terms of measurable, observable behavior. Were the goals appropriate, practical, and specific to the client? What are the therapeutic gains? What are the areas for possible further therapeutic work? How does the client evaluate motivation, effort, progress, and outcome? Has the client worked through most feelings about separation from the nurse?

You will also help the client evaluate the therapeutic experience in general, which may set the stage for future psychotherapeutic work. Would the client seek a similar experience in the future, if deemed necessary? You may also invite feedback from the client about your impact on the therapeutic relationship. Raingruber (2001) has found that the participants in a therapy session—clients and nurses—are the best evaluators of the effectiveness of therapeutic interventions.

The nurse's own personal, ongoing self-evaluation also warrants emphasis here. It is essential to continuously evaluate which of your own behaviors consciously or unconsciously promote, inhibit, or actively block growth-producing client abilities. Clinical supervision is essential if the one-to-one relationship is to be effective. Professional supervision helps you use transference effectively and recognize countertransference phenomena. The supportive function of supervision may be used to monitor your own needs, thereby minimizing the likelihood of severe clinical stress and burnout. There are various methods of evaluation: process recordings, videotapes, client evaluations, audiotapes, didactic instruction, and referral to specific clinical readings. There are several kinds of supervision available, such as intradisciplinary supervision with a psychiatric–mental health clinical nurse specialist, or interdisciplinary supervision by another mental health care professional (psychologist, psychiatrist, psychiatric social worker). An ethnic consultant can help to evaluate the influence of transcultural issues, including specific culture-bound syndromes. All of these people can be helpful, depending on their skills and availability. Supervision helps the psychiatric–mental health nurse effectively define, initiate, use, and evaluate client and self in any therapeutic relationship.

Case Management, Community-Based Care, and Home Care

The likely possibility that not all client goals have been achieved during a brief hospitalization makes case management and community-based care more important than ever. The Clinical Example on page 681 illustrates how a primary nurse in an inpatient setting can continue the therapeutic nurse–client relationship after discharge and can also function as a case manager.

INTERVENTION

Goals, Tasks, and Interventions of the Termination Phase

Goal: Termination of contact in a mutually planned, satisfying manner.

Therapeutic Tasks	Nursing Interventions
Help the client evaluate the therapeutic contract and the therapeutic experience in general.	Encourage the client's realistic appraisal of personal therapeutic goals (motivation, effort, progress, outcome) as these evolved in treatment.
	Provide appropriate feedback regarding the appraisal of goals.
	Review the client's assets and therapeutic gains.
	Review areas for further therapeutic work.
Encourage the transference of dependence to other support systems.	Encourage the client to develop reliance on others in client's immediate environment (spouse, relative, employer, neighbor, friend) for empathic, emotional support.
Participate in explicit therapeutic good-bye with the client.	Be alert to the surfacing of any behavior arising on termination (repression, regression, acting-out, anger, withdrawal, acceptance).
	Help the client work through feelings associated with these behaviors.
	Anticipate own reaction to separation and share in a manner that does not burden the client.
	Allow time and space for termination; the longer the duration of the one-to-one relationship, the more time is needed for the termination phase.

CLINICAL EXAMPLE

You have worked with Gustavo, a 65-year old male, during his brief 5-day stay on your unit. The treatment team's goal was to stabilize his mood and begin antidepressant medication. You have spent 45 minutes each day developing a therapeutic nurse–client relationship with Gustavo.

Following his discharge, you function as his case manager, connecting him with a job training program, a social club for mental health clients, and a medication psychoeducation group. You also meet with Gustavo in the outpatient clinic weekly for 4 weeks, then every 2 weeks for the next 2 months, and finally, monthly for the next 4 months.

When a referral is made to another psychiatric–mental health nurse or therapist, a home care nurse, a self-help group, a community agency, or a job training program, it is often wise to arrange for an initial contact with the referred person or agency before the nurse–client relationship terminates. This is a way to identify and deal with any initial misconceptions about what will take place after discharge and to ensure follow-up. The shift to dependence on other support systems (family, friends, referrals) is a therapeutic task that should be jointly managed, at least initially, by the nurse and the case manager.

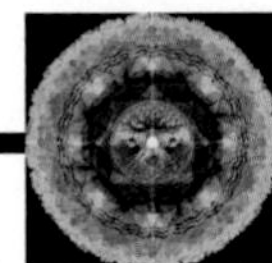

EXPLORE MediaLink

NCLEX review, case studies, and other interactive resources for this chapter can be found on the Companion Website at http://www.prenhall.com/kneisl. Click on Chapter 28 to select the activities for this chapter.

For animations, video tutorials, more NCLEX review questions, and an audio glossary, access the accompanying CD-ROM in this textbook.

BIBLIOGRAPHY

Auvil, C. A., & Silver, B. W. (1984). Therapist self-disclosure: When is it appropriate? *Perspectives in Psychiatric Care, 22*, 57–61.

Barker, P. (1999). Hildegard E. Peplau: The mother of psychiatric nursing. *Journal of Psychiatric and Mental Health Nursing, 6*(3), 175–176.

Barrett, M. S., & Berman, J. S. (2001). Is psychotherapy more effective when therapists disclose information about themselves? *Journal of Consulting Clinical Psychology, 69*(4), 597–603.

Bjorklund, P. (2000). Medusa appears: A case study of a narcissistic disturbance. *Perspectives in Psychiatric Care, 36*(3), 86–94.

Brunton, B., & Beaman, M. (2000). Nurse practitioners' perceptions of their caring behaviors. *Journal of the American Academy of Nurse Practitioners, 12*(11), 451–456.

Ellis, A. (2001). Rational and irrational aspects of countertransference. *Journal of Clinical Psychology, 57*(8), 999–1004.

Engle, D., & Holiman, M. (2002). A gestalt-experiential perspective on resistance. *Journal of Clinical Psychology, 58*(2), 175–183.

Flaskerud, J. H. (2000). Ethnicity, culture, and neuropsychiatry. *Issues in Mental Health Nursing, 21*(1), 5–29.

Flaskerud, J. H., & Wuerker, A. K. (1999). Mental health nursing in the 21st century. *Issues in Mental Health Nursing, 20*(1), 5–17.

Forchuk, C., Westwell, J., Martin, M., Azzapardi, W.B., Kosterawa-Tolman, D., & Hux, M. (1998). Factors influencing movement of chronic psychiatric patients from the orientation phase to the working phase of the nurse-client relationship on an in-patient unit. *Perspectives in Psychiatric Care, 34*(1), 36–44.

Forchuk, C., Westwell, J., Martin, M., Bamber-Azzapardi, W., Kosterewa-Tolman, D., & Hux, M. (2000). The developing nurse-client relationship: Nurses' perspectives. *Journal of the American Psychiatric Nurses Association, 6*(1), 3–10.

Gabbard, G. O. (2001). A contemporary psychoanalytic model of countertransference. *Journal of Clinical Psychology, 57*(8), 983–991.

Guy, J. D., & Brady, J. L. (2001). Identifying the faces in the mirror: Untangling transference and countertransference in self psychology. *Journal of Clinical Psychology, 57*(8), 993–997.

Haber, J. (1999). Hildegard Peplau. The mother of psychiatric nursing. *Nursing and Health Care Perspectives, 20*(4), 228.

Hall, E. (1966). *The hidden dimension*. New York: Doubleday Anchor Books.

Kiesler, D. J. (2001). Therapist countertransference: In search of common themes and empirical referents. *Journal of Clinical Psychology, 57*(8), 1053–1063.

Krauss, J. B. (2000). Protecting the legacy: The nurse-patient relationship and the therapeutic alliance. *Archives of Psychiatric Nursing, 14*(2), 49–50.

Laskowski, C. (2001). The mental health clinical nurse specialist and the "difficult" patient. *Issues in Mental Health Nursing, 22*(1), 5–22.

McCann, T. B., & Baker, H. (2001). Mutual relating: Developing interpersonal relationships in the community. *Journal of Advanced Nursing, 34*(4), 530–537.

Messer, S. B. (2002). A psychodynamic perspective on resistance in psychotherapy: Vive la resistance. *Journal of Clinical Psychology, 58*(2), 157–163.

Newman, C. F. (2002). A cognitive perspective on resistance in psychotherapy. *Journal of Clinical Psychology, 58*(2), 165–174.

Pearson, L. (2001). The clinician–patient experience: Understanding transference and countertransference. *Nurse Practitioner, 26*(6), 8, 11.

Peplau, H. E. (1952). *Interpersonal relations in nursing*. New York: Putnam.

Peplau, H. E. (1997). Peplau's theory of interpersonal relations. *Nursing Science Quarterly, 10*(4), 162–167.

Raingruber, B. J. (2001). Three perspectives regarding what works and does not work in therapy: A comparison of judgments of clients, nurse–therapists, and uninvolved evaluators. *Journal of the American Psychiatric Nurses Association, 7*(1), 13–21.

Richarz, B., & Romisch, S. (2002). Acting-out: Its functions within analytic group psychotherapy and its transformation into dreams. *International Journal of Group Psychotherapy, 52*(3), 337–353.

Shapiro, E. L., & Ginzberg, R. (2002). Parting gifts: Termination rituals in group therapy. *International Journal of Group Psychotherapy, 52*(3), 319–336.

Thomas, S. P., Shattell, M., & Martin, T. (2002). What's therapeutic about the therapeutic milieu? *Archives of Psychiatric Nursing, 16*(3), 99–107.

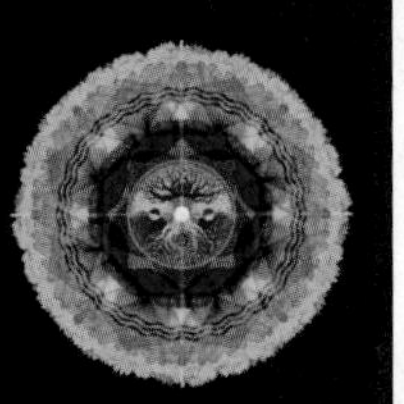

Group and Family Interventions

CAROL REN KNEISL

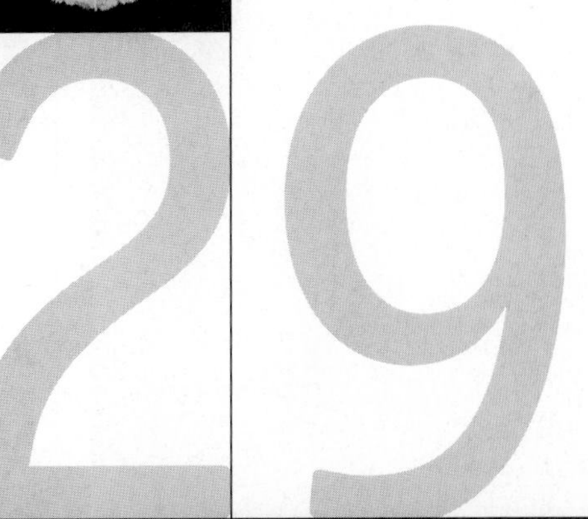

Chapter TWENTY-NINE

FOCUS QUESTIONS

- How would you create and maintain a therapeutic group?
- What purposes do therapeutic groups fulfill?
- What steps would you take to apply the process of here-and-now activation to a therapeutic group?
- If asked to describe families in terms of their relationships, associations, and connections, on which elements would you focus?
- What strategies would you use to assess and intervene with families?
- How does understanding group and family processes help you to promote and maintain an individual's mental health?

MediaLink 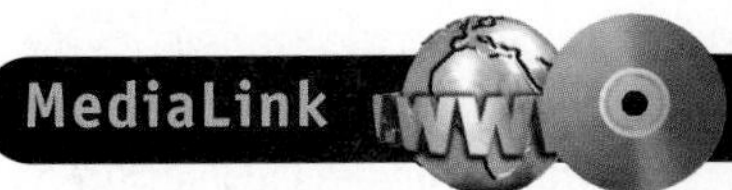 www.prenhall.com/kneisl

Additional resources for this chapter can be found on the Student CD-ROM accompanying this textbook, and on the Companion Website at www.prenhall.com/kneisl. Click on Chapter 29 to select the activities for this chapter.

CD-ROM
- Audio Glossary
- NCLEX Review

Companion Website
- Additional NCLEX Review
- Case Study: Orienting Client to Group Therapy

KEY TERMS

cohesion
family burden
family system
genogram
goblet issues
here-and-now activation
life script
self-fulfilling prophecy
self-reflective loop

CROSS REFERENCES

Other topics relevant to this content are: Client government groups and community meetings, Chapter 11; Cognitive and behavioral interventions for groups and families, Chapter 30; Intrafamily physical and sexual abuse, Chapter 23; Intervening with family members of clients with mental disorders, Chapters in Part II, Clients with Mental Disorders; Orienting families to inpatient admission procedures and policies, Chapter 11; Support groups, such as Alcoholics Anonymous, for substance abusers, Chapter 13.

CHAPTER OUTLINE

CRITICAL THINKING CHALLENGE

You are present at a multidisciplinary case conference presentation. Mark James, your 22-year-old client, is being discharged from his first hospital admission for schizophrenia to the home he shares with his father and his two sisters. Mark has been alienated from his mother since his parents' divorce when he was 17 years old. Mark's mother has failed to show up for the discharge conference. The mental health team has recommended family therapy to the James family. You perceive what you think is annoyance on Mr. James's face, and one of Mark's sisters appears embarrassed. Although you would not be the James family therapist because you are not a clinical specialist, you recognize how important Mark's family can be to his progress. What actions can you take to address the family's unspoken concerns and needs? ■

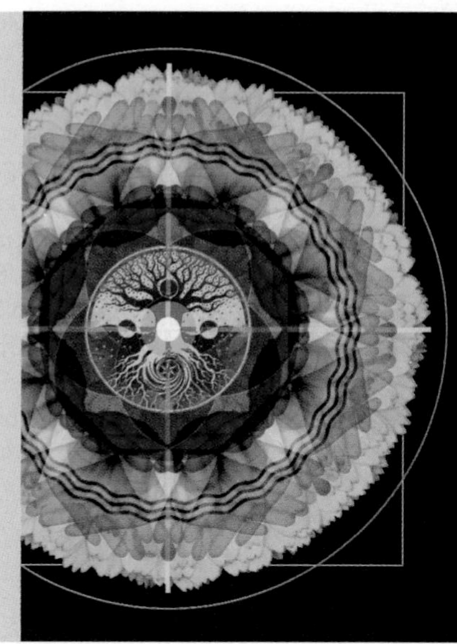

Why are groups and families important? Most people are born into a group—the family—and our survival from the moment of birth depends on relationships formed with other human beings. The sense of self, of being, of personal identity derives from the ways in which we are perceived and responded to by the other members of the groups to which we belong. We interact with others at all stages of our lives in various groups—family groups, peer groups, work groups, play groups, worship groups.

The family is the context in which most people, including nurses, develop their first relationships with other people. Their view of the larger social world outside their own unique family is molded by the events that happen within families and that influence the development of the individual. Nurses encounter families in many areas of their practice—in the emergency room, the intensive care unit, the school, the cancer hospital, the community health setting, and the mental health care setting. Preventive approaches to family mental health, assessment of families in trouble, and intervention on their behalf must be based on an understanding of how families grow and interact and how family coping patterns develop.

Many of the goals we set for ourselves cannot be achieved without membership in groups and families. Other people are important to each of us, just as we are important to others. Through cooperation and coordination we can achieve objectives and reach goals that we could not through individual effort alone. In this way, groups and families help us improve the quality of our lives.

Much of the nurse's professional life is spent in groups—groups of clients and groups of colleagues with whom the nurse plans and implements the delivery of health care services. Recent studies indicate that group interventions, relatives' groups, and multiple-family groups, will become increasingly more important in this economy as a result of the need to provide treatments that are also cost effective (Leff, 2000; Ormont, 2000; Taylor et al., 2001).

To use groups rationally and effectively and to effectively intervene with families, nurses must understand the forces that underlie small group interactional processes and family processes, and recognize their own patterns of participation. Group and family interventions are ways that psychiatric–mental health nurses can provide psychoeducation for their clients and their families, and the opportunity to seek validation, give and receive interpersonal feedback, and test new and different ways of being that may improve the quality of life. Mental health can be preserved, maintained, and restored through interaction with others in productive groups and families.

Nurses have long been involved in working with clients and their families in small groups brought together for health teaching, psychoeducation, or supportive purposes. All nurses, regardless of level of education, can lead therapeutic groups or psychoeducation groups, and all nurses can assist families, as long as they understand and apply group and family dynamics in their interventions. Informal groups exist on units in inpatient facilities and in community-based agencies as well. The disciplined application of group and family psychotherapeutic principles undergirds the nurse's therapeutic use of self in unplanned encounters in these settings. However, the role of the psychiatric–mental health nurse as group psychotherapist or family therapist is reserved for advanced practice clinical specialists prepared at the master's level and above (see Chapter 1, which discusses psychiatric–mental health nursing roles in relationship to education, preparation, and certification).

Small Group Dynamics

Several forces modify and shape groups, influencing their effectiveness. These forces are discussed in the sections that follow.

TRUST

Trust develops in relationships when people disclose more and more of their thoughts, perceptions, attitudes, and reactions to one another and find that their disclosures have been made in a safe environment among persons who respect their self-disclosures. The group member who makes a suggestion; discloses an attitude, feeling, experience, or perception; gives feedback; or confronts another member engages in trusting behavior and assumes the risks inherent in trusting. Trusting and being trusted are intimately linked to risk taking. The level of trust among the members of a group determines the extent of risk-taking behavior in the group. When trust exists, individual members will risk sharing more. Since trust takes some time to build, do not expect that trust will necessarily exist in short-term inpatient groups in which membership changes frequently in a brief period of time.

COHESION

Cohesion can be defined as a spirit of common purpose. In groups that cohere, the members have a desire for mutual association. Cohesion is the primary factor keeping a group in existence and working effectively.

A group is cohesive when its members are attracted to it. People are attracted to a therapeutic group for a wide variety of reasons. The group may meet their needs for affiliation, interpersonal security, self-knowledge, or therapy. It may have members who not only are available for human interaction but also have important shared attitudes, values, interests, and beliefs. An attractive group has explicit, mutual, and attainable group goals with clear paths to goal attainment.

What indicates that the spirit of cohesion exists in a given group? Attendance is high, the members arrive on time, and the members stay with the group. Its members engage in an interdependence that is cooperative rather than competitive. The activities the group undertakes are satisfying and successful, and there is a high degree of member participation. Communication networks are open, central, and flexible in a warm and friendly atmosphere, and "we" is frequently heard in discussions. The members like and trust one another. They enjoy interacting with one another and participation is high.

Cohesive groups are not born—they are developed. Cohesion does not become evident until the group has come together long enough to have shared experiences that provide the basis for attraction. An outpatient group has an existence lengthy enough to provide time for cohesion to develop. Inpatient groups are usually too brief to become cohesive.

How can a group's tendency to cohere be enhanced? Some methods are increasing the trusting and trustworthy behavior of members, the affection expressed among members, the expressions of inclusion and acceptance among members, and the influence that members have on one another. Another method for building cohesion is structuring cooperative relationships among the group members.

GROUP ROLES

Group roles center on the influence relationships that exist within the group. The primary influence relationship is leadership. Group dynamics theory tells us that leadership functions within a group can be fulfilled by the person designated as the leader, and by members who engage in leadership behavior. This approach to understanding leadership behavior is called the *distributed functions approach* and stems from the classic research of Benne & Sheats (1948).

The distributed functions approach to group leadership is based on two major beliefs:

1. Any member of a group may become a leader by taking actions that serve group purposes.
2. Different members may perform various roles in a group.

Each member may play more than one role during a meeting of the group and a wide range of roles in successive participations. Any member may play any or all of the roles. The various functional roles may be grouped in two categories:

1. *Task roles* are related to the task of the group. The job of people assuming these roles is to facilitate and coordinate group efforts in the selection, definition, and solution of a group problem.
2. *Maintenance roles* are oriented toward building group-centered attitudes among the members and maintaining and perpetuating group-centered behavior.

Sometimes members of a group satisfy individual needs that are irrelevant to the group task and may also be negatively oriented to group maintenance functions. These are called *self-serving roles.* If a group is to function effectively, it must perform a self-diagnosis to determine what the needs of the group are and how they can be met, so that the self-serving roles no longer present obstacles to effective functioning. Task, maintenance, and self-serving roles are described in Box 29–1 (see page 687).

Distributing leadership functions among group members is important because it teaches people the diagnostic skills and behaviors needed to accomplish the group's goals and maintain good interpersonal relationships. Of course, in psychotherapy groups, some functions or activities may be largely, or even solely, the province of the therapist.

POWER AND INFLUENCE

It is impossible to discuss group dynamics without discussing power because it is impossible to interact without influencing, and being influenced by, others. This process constantly occurs within groups, forcing members to adjust to one another and modify their behavior and, sometimes, their attitudes and beliefs. Power is defined as the ability to do or act, to have possession of command or control over others, to achieve the desired result. The terms *power* and *influence* are used interchangeably in this chapter.

Power and influence are not negative forces. Do not confuse the judicious use of power in building effective groups with the use of power to control, manage, and manipulate others. Become aware of how you can employ power and influence in the service of your clients and your profession.

A group in which certain members have much power and others have little power is likely to be in trouble. The unequal distribution of power affects both the task and the maintenance functions of a group. Members who believe they have little influence within the group are unlikely to feel committed to

BOX 29–1 Group Roles and Functions

Role	Function
Task Roles	
Information seeker	Asks for information that would clarify issues
Information giver	Offers facts, ideas, and own experiences
Elaborator	Fleshes out ideas and suggestions (arranging seating; distributing handouts)
Coordinator	Identifies the relationships among the group suggestions and ideas
Opinion seeker	Asks for beliefs that would clarify group values
Opinion giver	States beliefs about group function and group values
Maintenance Roles	
Encourager	Moves the group in a positive direction by encouraging and praising the contributions of others
Compromiser	Minimizes conflict by seeking alternatives
Standard setter	Reminds group of the standards to be achieved
Follower	Goes along with the group
Group observer	Keeps the groups records; interprets data
Harmonizer	Keeps the peace; smoothes over conflict
Self-Serving Roles	
Recognition seeker	Boasts, brags about accomplishments, calls attention to self
Blocker	Disagrees, opposes, and resists
Aggressor	Attacks groups members, ideas, or values
Dominator	Manipulates others, seeks control through excessive talking; interrupts others
Self-confessor	Expresses personal and self-oriented, rather than group-oriented insights and feelings
Playboy	Fails to become involved in group process

Source: Adapted from Benne, K. D., & Sheats, P. (1948). Functional roles of group members. *Journal of Social Issues, 4,* 41–49. Reprinted with permission from Blackwell Publishing.

group goals and to the implementation of group decisions. Their dissatisfaction with the group decreases its attractiveness and reduces its cohesion.

Group Development Theory

The interpersonal needs approach discussed in this section can be used to understand the development, dynamics, and functioning of small groups, from self-help groups to psychoeducation groups to psychotherapy groups. The interpersonal needs approach helps us to understand how groups develop and the factors that determine how effective they are.

The basic assumption of the interpersonal needs approach known as FIRO (Fundamental Interpersonal Relationship Orientation), a classic group dynamics theory, is that people need people. In addition, people need to establish some equilibrium between themselves and the others in their environment. This equilibrium is determined by the interaction of three basic interpersonal needs, and it appears to be synonymous with interpersonal compatibility (Schutz, 1958b).

THREE BASIC INTERPERSONAL NEEDS

An interpersonal need is one that can be satisfied only through relationships with people. Schutz reasoned that every individual has three interpersonal needs: inclusion, control, and affection.

Inclusion

The interpersonal need for *inclusion* is the need to establish and maintain relationships with others that offer interactions and associations satisfying to the individual. To put this another way, the inclusion need consists of the ability to take an interest in others to a satisfactory degree, and the ability to allow other people to take an interest in you to a satisfying degree to yourself. This need determines whether a person is outgoing or prefers privacy. Compare the inclusion needs illustrated in ■ Figure 29–1 (see page 688).

Control

The interpersonal need for *control* is the need to establish and maintain a satisfactory relationship between oneself and other people with regard to power and influence. Stated another way, the control need consists of the ability to take charge to a satisfactory degree, and the ability to establish and maintain a feeling of respect for the competence and responsibleness of others to a satisfying degree to yourself. Compare the control needs illustrated in ■ Figure 29–2 (see page 688).

Affection

The interpersonal need for *affection* is the need to establish and maintain a satisfactory relationship between the self and other people with regard to love and affection. Put another way, the affection need consists of being able to love other people or to be close and intimate to a satisfactory degree, and having others love you or be close and intimate with you to a satisfactory degree. Compare the affection needs illustrated in ■ Figure 29–3 (see page 688).

GROUP PHASES

According to this approach any group, given enough time, moves through three interpersonal phases—inclusion, control,

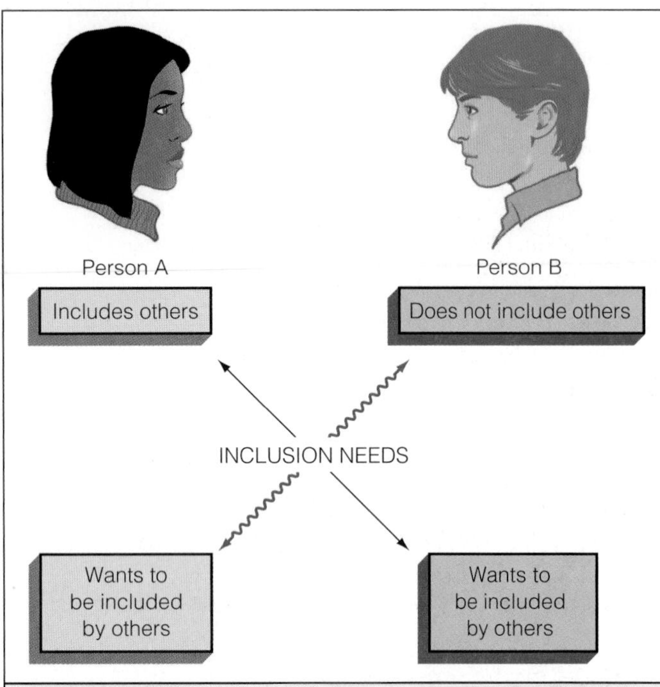

FIGURE 29–1 ■ *Inclusion needs. While both people want to be included by others, only one (Person A) includes others. Therefore, Person B's needs for inclusion are met. However, Person A will feel frustrated because her need to be included is not being met.*

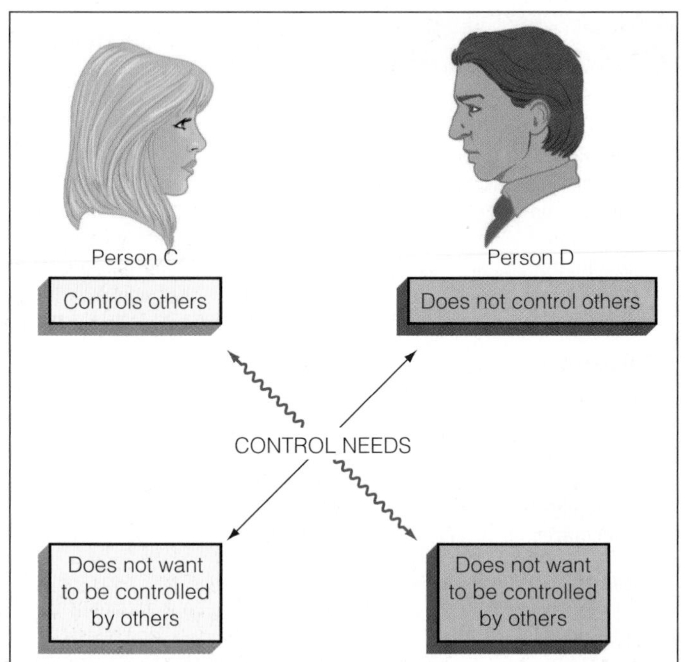

FIGURE 29–2 ■ *Control needs. This situation has the potential for great conflict. Person D, who is happiest in a lackadaisical atmosphere, will resent, and perhaps sabotage, Person C's efforts to control. Person C is likely to intensify her control efforts in response.*

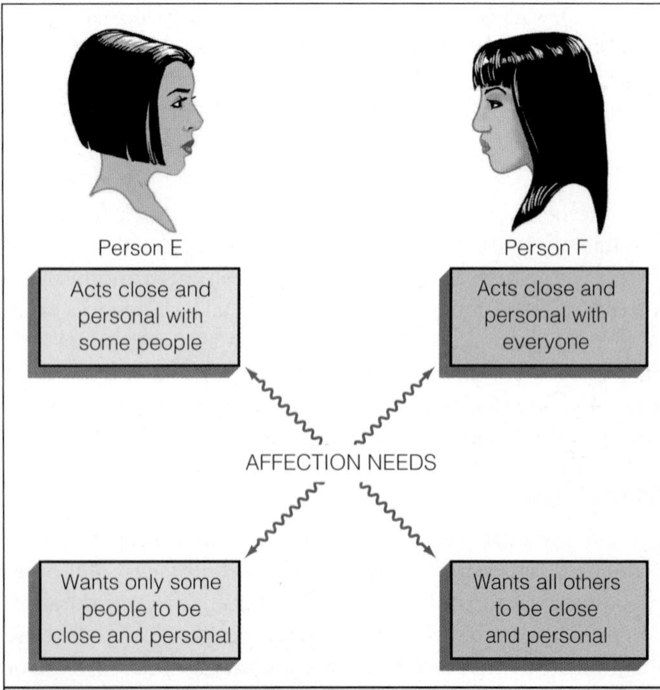

FIGURE 29–3 ■ *Affection needs. Both people in this situation are getting some of their affection needs met if Person F is one of the people with whom Person E wishes to be close and personal. If not, Person E could back away emotionally if she views Person F as intrusive. Backing away would likely cause frustration on Person F's part.*

and affection, in that order—that correspond to the three basic interpersonal needs.

Inclusion Phase

The first or inclusion phase is concerned with the problem of *in or out*. People attempt to find their place in the group and are concerned with learning whether they will be acknowledged as individuals or left behind and ignored. Because these concerns give rise to anxiety, this phase is dominated by behavior centered around the self. Overtalking, withdrawal, exhibitionism, and sharing other group experiences and biographies are some examples.

Frequently, what Schutz (1958a) calls **goblet issues** predominate. These are issues of minor importance to the group that help the members get to know one another better and to test out each other. Goblet issues are a vehicle for sizing people up. Goblet issues may revolve around the weather, sports, rules of procedure, and so on. If goblet issues continue to a significant extent beyond this initial phase of the group, they will impede group progress.

Control Phase

The second or control phase is concerned with the problem of *top or bottom*, which becomes central after problems of inclusion have been resolved. Concern about decision-making procedures predominates. The problems that emerge in this phase center around two concerns:

1. How responsibility is shared.
2. How power and influence are distributed.

There are struggles for leadership and about the structure, rules of procedure, and methods of decision making. Members are attempting to establish comfortable positions for themselves in terms of responsibility and influence.

Affection Phase

The third or affection phase is concerned with the problem of *near or far*, and it follows satisfactory resolution of the preceding two phases. Individual members are now faced with the problem of becoming emotionally involved with one another. Concerns about not being liked by, being too close to, or not being close enough to others, become relevant. The behavior in this phase is generally characterized by high emotion—positive feelings, jealousy, hostility, and pairing are some examples. Schutz (1958a) describes this phase as one in which, like porcupines, people attempt to get close enough to receive warmth, yet avoid the pain that sharp quills can inflict.

Interweaving of Phases

None of these phases is distinct, since all three problem areas are present at all times, even though only one predominates. Schutz (1958a) uses a tire-changing analogy, what he calls *tightening the bolts*, to describe the sequence of the phases. Changing a tire is best done by tightening the bolts just enough to hold the wheel in place. Then each bolt is tightened further until it is secured. The leader helps the group work on all three interpersonal need areas in similar fashion, returning to and working over each area to a more satisfactory level than was reached the last time. The interpersonal needs approach of Schutz is based on the belief that the way to attack problems within groups is by investigating what is going on among the individuals in the group and attempting to improve their interpersonal relations.

Group Therapy Theory

There is great diversity and flux in the field of group therapy. Many types of groups are found in mental health care settings or in communities at large. However, certain common principles seem to apply to all therapeutic groups, although specific methods and techniques may vary according to the purpose of the group or the skills and theoretic orientation of the therapist or group leader.

Irvin Yalom (1995) uses the term *interactional group therapy* to describe a process of group therapy in which member interaction plays a crucial role. The common principles that apply to interactional group therapy are discussed below.

The psychiatric–mental health nurse, even if not a clinical specialist or advanced practice nurse qualified as a group psychotherapist, can incorporate many of these principles of group therapy into the leadership role in therapeutic groups as well as in informal groups in the milieu. The principles will need to be modified for use in short-term groups, such as those in effect on most inpatient units. Modifications for short-term inpatient groups are discussed throughout this section. Essential differences between inpatient and outpatient groups are identified in ■ Table 29–1 (see page 690).

ADVANTAGES OF GROUP THERAPY

The advantages of group therapy stem from one major factor: the presence of many people, rather than a solitary therapist, who participate in the therapeutic experience. Specifically, group therapy provides the following:

- Stimuli from multiple sources, revealing distortions in interpersonal relationships so that they can be examined and resolved.
- Multiple sources of feedback.
- An interpersonal testing ground that allows members to try out old and new ways of being in an environment specifically structured for that purpose.

MediaLink Case Study: Orienting Client to Group Therapy

QUALIFICATIONS OF GROUP THERAPISTS

Mental health care professionals may believe, in error, that group therapy is less complex and therefore "easier" than one-to-one work, for example, because the presence of more people makes interactions between therapist and client less intense. Although it is true that the interactions between any one member and the therapist may be less intense because interactions are dispersed among others, it does not follow that anyone can be an effective group therapist. Rather, group processes are very complex because the interactions occur among many different personalities. To be effective, the group therapist should have the following special preparation:

- Education in small group dynamics.
- Education in group therapy theory.
- Clinical practice with groups.
- Expert supervision of the clinical practice (with ongoing supervision and/or consultation, depending on level of expertise).

The ANA Standards of Psychiatric–Mental Health Clinical Nursing Practice identify the group psychotherapist role as appropriate for clinical specialists prepared at the master's level (see Chapter 1). Experienced therapists report that it is also valuable to have been a member of a therapy or sensitivity training group, before becoming a group leader.

Psychiatric–mental health nurses at the generalist level are qualified, with appropriate preparation, to lead the therapeutic support groups described later in this chapter.

THE CURATIVE FACTORS

Yalom (1995) contends that 11 interdependent curative factors or mechanisms of change in group therapy help people. These factors constitute a rational basis for the therapist's choices of tactics and strategies. They are identified and defined in ■ Table 29–2 (see page 691).

TYPES OF GROUP LEADERSHIP

Groups can be led by a therapist working alone or by cotherapists working together in a variety of ways.

TABLE 29–1 Differences in Inpatient and Outpatient Groups

Inpatient Groups	Outpatient Groups
The composition of the group changes depending on who has been admitted and who has been discharged.	The composition of the group is stable, usually over its life.
Members may be selected because they happened to be clients on a particular unit or assigned to a particular therapist.	Selection criteria play a major role in designing the group.
Although clients may be assigned to one or another of available groups depending on appropriateness, selection interviews are not usually conducted.	Selection interviews are standard practice to prepare clients for the group experience and to establish and clarify the group contract.
Attendance is compulsory and clients are often wary of, or ambivalent about, attending the group.	Clients usually choose whether or not to join a group. Those who choose to join are motivated.
Membership length is determined by the length of hospitalization. When the client is discharged, membership in the group ends.	The group continues for a predetermined length of time identified in the group contract—often 1 year or more.
The goal is relief of symptoms and possibly some degree of self-awareness.	The goal is insight-oriented.
Sessions are usually 45–50 minutes long, daily, or several times a week.	Most outpatient groups are approximately 1½ hours in length, once a week.
Because of the continually changing membership, inpatient groups rarely become cohesive.	Group cohesion can be expected to develop over time.
Group members have 24-hour exposure to one another.	Members in outpatient groups are discouraged from having relationships with other members outside the meetings.
The inpatient therapist provides a greater degree of structure and takes on a more active role.	The outpatient therapist is less active and waits for the structure and the process to unfold.
Because the therapist has limited ability to select who will be in the group, the group tends to be heterogenous in terms of vulnerability or ego strength as well as personality characteristics.	Outpatient therapists usually design their groups to balance the behavior and characteristics the members bring to the group. The members are more likely to be homogenous in terms of their ego strength.

Single Therapist Approach

Groups led by a single therapist are common. They have an economic advantage in that only one therapist need be involved. A disadvantage is that the therapist cannot compare analyses of the group process with a cotherapist or get instant feedback or validation from a peer. Therapists working alone, however, do not have to direct their energies toward creating and maintaining a relationship with a colleague.

Cotherapy Approach

Groups led by two therapists, who share responsibility for leadership of the group to varying degrees, are gaining in popularity. The two models seen most often are the junior–senior and the egalitarian styles of cotherapy.

Junior–Senior Cotherapy. In the junior–senior approach, the therapists have unequal responsibilities toward the group. The senior member of the team is usually the more experienced or educated. Besides having major responsibility for the success of the group, the senior therapist is responsible for training the junior member of the team.

This approach is commonly used in agency settings, because it provides in-service training of new personnel and nonprofessionals under the guidance and watchful eye of an experienced group leader. However, relationship problems frequently surface when the roles of the leaders are not clear, or when one or both leaders are unable, or unwilling, to remain in the designated roles. The members of the group may also be unclear about the subordinate/superordinate roles and unsure of how to deal with and respond to leaders of unequal abilities and responsibilities.

Egalitarian Cotherapy. In the egalitarian approach to cotherapy, two therapists of relatively equal ability and status share equally in responsibility for the group. The method is also used for training, with both cotherapists working under clinical supervision.

Two nurses considering an egalitarian cotherapy relationship with each other need to engage in preliminary work to determine whether such a relationship is feasible for them. Exploration should include:

- Discussing each therapist's theoretic approaches, intervention styles, past experiences with groups, background, and personality characteristics.
- Considering and resolving such issues as how and when feedback is to be given, how disagreements between them

TABLE 29–2 Curative Factors of Group Therapy

Factor	Definition
Therapist	
Instilling hope	Imbuing the client with optimism for the success of the group therapy experience.
Universality	Confirming that the client is not alone or unique in misery or hurt.
Imparting information	Giving instruction, advice, or suggestions.
Altruism	Finding that the client can be of importance to others; having something of value to give.
Client	
Corrective recapitulation of the primary family group	Reviewing and correctively reliving early familial conflicts and growth-inhibiting relationships.
Development of socializing techniques	Acquiring sophisticated social skills, e.g., being attuned to process, resolving conflicts, and being facilitative toward others.
Imitative behavior	Trying out bits and pieces of the behavior of others and experimenting with those that fit well.
Interpersonal learning	Learning that one authors one's interpersonal world, and moving to alter it.
Group cohesiveness	Being attracted to the group and the other members with a sense of "we"-ness rather than "I"-ness.
Catharsis	Being able to express feelings.
Existential factors	Being able to "be" with others; to be a part of a group.

Source: Adapted from Yalom, I. D. (1995). *The theory and practice* of group *psychotherapy* (4th ed.). New York: Basic Books. Reprinted with permission of Basic Books, a member of Perseus Books, LLC.

are to be handled in the session, and the general conditions under which they will work together.

- Agreeing that decisions on client selection, length and number of sessions, time, and place are made together, and that decisions of an emergency nature made by one therapist in the absence of the other are based on mutually agreed-upon procedures for just such situations.

Obviously, egalitarian cotherapists must establish and maintain clear channels of communication. Not only must they expend a great deal of time and energy in preparation for the group experience, they must also plan for pre-session and post-session meetings, joint analysis of data, and joint supervision or consultation.

CREATING THE GROUP

The effectiveness of a group depends greatly on the conditions under which it is created. Much as architects design buildings, therapists design groups with certain functions and characteristics in mind.

Selecting Members

Selecting the members is one of the most important functions of group leaders or group therapists, since the quality of the interpersonal relationships among the members constitutes the core of successful group treatment. This is one of the major differences between group and individual therapy.

Clients may be admitted to an inpatient group on the basis of being hospitalized on a particular unit that mandates group therapy for all clients, or being assigned to a particular therapist. Group therapists or leaders of therapeutic groups in inpatient units may have little leeway about including specific individuals in the group. Therefore, inpatient groups tend to have a more heterogeneous composition; that is, the members may vary significantly in terms of their vulnerability or ego strength. They also tend to be more ambivalent about group therapy. You are encouraged to attempt to apply the principles below, regardless of the nature or location of the group.

It is more difficult to identify the characteristics of people who make good candidates for group therapy than those of people who do not make good candidates. We know that a person's motivation for therapy in general, and group therapy in particular, is of primary importance. Inclusion in a therapy group should also be at least partially determined by the effect a prospective member will have on the others, in terms of the prospective member's ability to bring the curative factors into play (Yalom, 1998).

Inclusion is also determined by the balance, in terms of behavior or characteristics, a prospective member will bring to the group. Will the person's subdued presentation prevent a member with similar behavior from being marginal and alone in the group? Does the person's age, occupation, or sex match another's so that the member will not feel singled out as different or deviant? The factor that appears to be most important, according to Yalom (1998), however, is that members are homogeneous in terms of their vulnerability or ego strength. Highly vulnerable members retard the progress of the less vulnerable, and vice versa. Yalom's research indicates that, if at all possible, avoid including in the group individuals who use denial to a significant extent, differ significantly from others in the group in relation to psychopathology, or have a pervasive dread of self-disclosure (Yalom, 1995).

Selection Interviews

Selection interviews are standard procedure for long-term outpatient groups. They are useful as well for short-term inpatient groups and groups in day hospitals to help determine the most appropriate type of group for each individual client.

The pregroup interview session has two major purposes: selecting the members and establishing the initial contract. Cotherapists should always interview potential members jointly, and both should make all decisions regarding membership. The interview session gives members and therapists the opportunity to be exposed to one another. The therapists should accomplish the following tasks in the selection interview:

- Determine the motivation of the potential member.
- Encourage the client to ask questions about the group.
- Correct erroneous prejudgments or misinformation the client has about group therapy.
- Inquire about any major pending life changes that may prevent the client's full and continued participation in the group.
- Inquire about what hurts—what the client sees as a need to work on.
- Establish and clarify the initial group contract.

During this period, therapists and members have a chance to decide whether they can work together in the specific group under consideration. Outpatient clients as well as therapists can choose whether they will participate or not. Because clients in outpatient groups have the choice of being a member of the group or not, they tend to be motivated to learn and to change.

Group Contract

The group contract identifies the shared rights and responsibilities of therapists and members. It is a negotiated set of rules or arrangements for the structure and functioning of the group. It may be written or verbal, and it should cover the elements discussed below.

Goals and Purposes. The purpose of the group must be clear to all involved. In interactive group psychotherapy, the purpose is to bring about enduring behavioral and character change. The interactive group psychotherapy experience takes place largely in the present, in the here-and-now.

Goals may be long term or short term and are both group oriented and individualized. Some goals may be identified as early as the selection interview, and others may be added as they emerge during the life of the group. Goals may be altered as appropriate.

Time, Length, and Frequency of Meetings. The time, length, and frequency of meetings should be determined by the therapists after consideration of the clients' needs. Most outpatient clients find one 80- to 90-minute session per week useful. Shorter periods may not allow adequate time for discussion. Longer periods generally tax the endurance and alertness of both members and therapists. Inpatient groups generally meet several times per week, or even daily for about 45 to 50 minutes, although they may be longer or shorter depending on the anxiety and tolerance levels of the particular clients.

Place of Meetings. The physical environment is important and influences the interaction among members. It is best to choose a pleasant room with comfortable chairs, preferably placed in a circle. The room should be private and free from external distractions.

Starting and Ending Dates. If the group has a predetermined life span and the inclusive dates are known, members should be told the dates. Groups without fixed termination dates usually plan termination individually as each member is ready to move away from the group. Starting and ending dates are determined in inpatient groups by the length of the client's hospitalization.

Addition of New Members. Open groups accept members after the first session; closed groups begin with a certain number of members and do not add new members. Open groups maintain their size by replacing members who leave the group. They may continue indefinitely or have a predetermined life span. Open groups are more common in short-term inpatient units where there is rapid turnover. Once the client leaves the inpatient setting, membership in the group ends. This means that since most hospitalizations are of 1 to 3 weeks' duration, there is little time for cohesion to develop. Cohesion develops in outpatient groups because of their length—1 or more years in duration, and 52 or more meetings.

Closed groups are more common in settings where the stability of membership is likely. Such settings include private practice settings, residential facilities of various types, and prisons. A major problem with the closed group is that it runs the risk of extinction as members leave the group for various reasons.

Attendance. It is important that members make a commitment to attend every session. Absences hinder the establishment of cohesion and have a demoralizing effect, especially when perceived as evidence that a member lacks interest or that the group is not attractive and valuable to its members. Stability of membership and high attendance have been demonstrated to be critical factors in the successful outcome of group therapy (Yalom, 1995).

Confidentiality. Some rules regarding confidentiality should be established, and clients' concerns about which people will have access to information concerning them should be explored. Many therapists like to use tape recorders so that their work can be evaluated afterward by supervisors. They must obtain client agreement to use of a tape recorder.

Rules about confidentiality and access may be determined by the therapists' employing agency. In some instances, therapists may be required to make regular notes concerning each member's participation. Therapists may also wish to establish with group members guidelines on confidentiality that allow the therapists to share content with professionals who provide clinical supervision to the therapist, or when clients are dangerous to themselves or others. A good rule of thumb is: *Promise only what you can safely deliver*. Members should also be held accountable for maintaining the confidentiality of the group.

Member Interaction Outside the Group. Members in outpatient groups are discouraged from having relationships with other members outside the meetings. This is impossible in inpatient groups because the members may have 24-hour exposure to one another on the hospital unit and may also interact with the group therapist while the therapist is functioning in other roles. In fact, interaction with one another is encouraged.

Participation of Members and Therapists. Therapists and clients should reach an understanding about the responsibilities of participants. Clients should be fully informed participants in the therapeutic process. Participants should share their expectations about the behavior and functions of clients and therapists and should clearly understand the modes of participation. Interaction patterns should form pathways among all members and the therapist as illustrated in ■ Figure 29–4 (left).

It is important for the inpatient group therapist to provide significantly more structure for the group and to take on a more active role than would be necessary in an outpatient group. Hospitalized inpatients are likely to be in crisis and to be more dysfunctional than outpatients. Passivity on the therapist's part would be destructive to the group and could increase a client's distress. Yalom (1998) suggests a protocol for structuring an inpatient group that is listed in the Intervention box at right.

Fees. Fees for outpatients should be determined in advance and arrangements for payment made. Most mental health care agencies have a sliding fee scale determined by the client's income and ability to pay. Clients should know whether fees will be charged for missed sessions. Fees for inpatients are included in the cost of hospitalization.

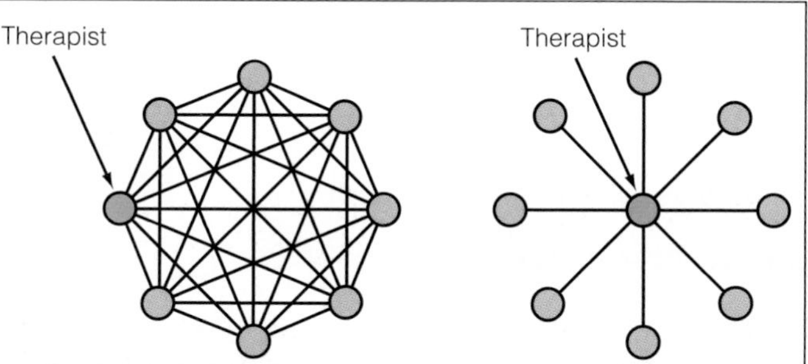

FIGURE 29–4 ■ *Comparison of positive and negative interaction patterns in group therapy. The desirable interaction pattern is on the left. The diagram on the right, in which communication is primarily to or through the therapist, is undesirable.*

INTERVENTION

Structuring an Inpatient Group

1. 3–5 minutes of orientation, warm-up, or preparation
2. 20–30 minutes for an agenda go-around in which each member may share personal concerns or problems
3. 20–30 minutes in which the therapist attempts to fit the members' agendas together by finding commonalities or threads to work on
4. 3–5 minutes to review the work of the group and to identify the issues or concerns that remain up in the air

Source: Adapted from Yalom, I. D. (1998). *The Yalom reader*. New York: Basic Books. Reprinted by permission of Basic Books, a member of Perseus Books, LLC.

STAGES IN THERAPY GROUP DEVELOPMENT

There is comfort in being able to predict, to some extent, the behavior of members at specific points in the group's life. Therapists organize predictions around stages or phases in the therapeutic experience, hoping to be prepared for expressions of behavior. You must bear in mind, however, that human experiences are dynamic and fluid and do not always progress as neatly as predicted.

The Schutz framework, presented earlier, gives clear indications of how group life develops in terms of meeting inclusion, affection, and control needs. This section focuses on the characteristics of member behavior and therapist interventions in the orientation phase (where inclusion needs are more salient), the working phase (where control needs are more salient), and the termination phase (where affection needs are more salient) of interactional group therapy. As members' problems in living are revealed, group life becomes richer and more complex. Therefore, there is no "cookbook" method that a therapist can follow to respond to every situation. The Intervention box on page 694 is simply a guide for identifying some common member behaviors and therapist interventions at various points in the life of the group.

HERE-AND-NOW EMPHASIS

The core of interactional group therapy is the here-and-now. According to Yalom (1995), the here-and-now work of the interactional group therapist occurs on two levels:

1. Focusing attention on each member's feelings toward other group members, the therapists, and the group.
2. Illuminating the process (the relationship implications of interpersonal transactions).

Thus, group members need to become aware of the here-and-now events—what happened—and then reflect back on them—why it happened. Yalom (1995) has called this the **self-reflective loop** (see ■ Figure 29–5, page 694).

INTERVENTION

Characteristic Member Behaviors and Nursing Interventions in Phases of Group Therapy

Member Behavior	Nursing Interventions
Beginning Phase	
Anxiety is high.	Move to reduce anxiety; avoid making demands until group anxiety has abated.
Members are unsure of what to do or say; need to be included.	Be active and provide some structure and direction; suggest members introduce themselves; work to sustain therapeutic rather than social role; include all members and encourage sharing but limit monopolizing.
Members are unclear about contract.	Clarify contract; give information to dispel confusion or misunderstandings.
Members test therapists and other members in terms of trustworthiness, value stances, etc., often through goblet issues.	Capitalize on opportunity to "pass" tests by proving trustworthy and by being open to and accepting the values of others.
Beginning attempts at self-disclosure and problem identification are made.	Focus on related themes; begin exploration; begin to focus on here-and-now experiences in session.
Members have sense of "I"-ness, little sense of "we"-ness.	Encourage involvement with others through curative factor of *universality*.
Middle Phase	
Sense of "I"-ness is replaced by "we"-ness.	Encourage cohesion; provide opportunity for expression of warm feelings.
Self-disclosure increases.	Encourage exploration and move to problem solving.
Members are more aware of interpersonal interactions in the here-and-now.	Encourage members to participate in observing and commenting on the here-and-now; make process comments.
Additions and losses of members evoke strong reactions.	Prepare members for additions and losses where possible; provide opportunity to talk about addition and loss experience.
Ability to maintain focus on one topic increases.	Encourage exploration of topic area in depth.
Termination Phase	
Feelings about separation may run the gamut (anger, sadness, indifference, joy, etc.).	Provide adequate time in as many sessions as necessary to work through affective responses; be sure members know the termination date in advance; help members leave with positive feelings by identifying positive changes that have occurred in individual members and in the group.
Members may feel lost and rudderless.	Explore support systems available to individual members; bridge the gap where possible (to another agency, another therapist, etc.); keep in focus the task of resolving the loss.

Steering the Group into the Here-and-Now

The first task of the therapist is to steer the group into the here-and-now. Yalom calls this process **here-and-now activation.** As the group progresses and becomes comfortable with awareness of the here-and-now, much of the work is taken on by the members. Initially, however, a primary task of the therapist is to actively steer the group discourse in an ahistoric direction. In other words, events in the session take precedence over those that occur outside or have occurred outside.

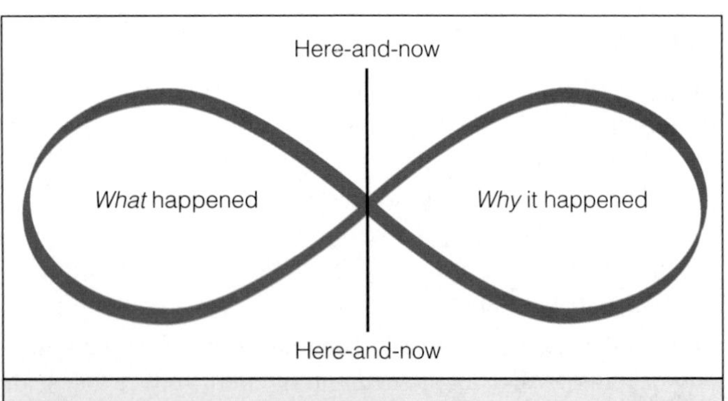

FIGURE 29–5 ■ *The self-reflective loop.*

Illuminating the Process

If the group is to engage in interpersonal learning, the therapist must illuminate the process. This is the second task of prime importance. The group must move beyond a focus on content toward a focus on process—the how and the why of an interaction. The process can be considered from any number of perspectives. The perspective chosen should be determined by the mood and needs of the group at that particular time. The group must recognize, examine, and understand the process. The task of illuminating it belongs mainly to the therapist, as in the Clinical Example below.

CLINICAL EXAMPLE

Every time Jim makes a comment in group, Al either sneers or smirks. As soon as Jim finishes speaking, Al contradicts whatever Jim has said. The group members focus on the content of the disagreements between Jim and Al. Margaret, the clinical nurse specialist who is the group therapist, steers the group in the direction of analyzing the dynamics of the relationship between these mem-

bers and the possible purposes their disagreements can serve for the group (e.g., controlling the direction of the group's efforts, meeting Al's control needs, or keeping the group anxiety down by keeping the focus away from other, more anxious members).

Process commentary is anxiety-producing for new or inexperienced therapists and group members because there are so many injunctions against it in social situations. For example, commenting on someone's nervousness at a party is generally taboo. It not only makes the nervous person uncomfortable, but also puts the process commentator in a high-risk situation. The comment may well be taken as criticism or viewed as inappropriate to the social context, and the commentator is vulnerable to retaliation from others. It is essential to educate members about this difference and to prepare them to hear, respond to, and eventually initiate process commentary.

The process of focusing on the here-and-now is akin to the process that is called *clearing the air* (making covert interpersonal difficulties overt) in Schutz's framework. Clearing the air is a major step in the interpersonal needs approach. Although this step is initially uncomfortable, the final result is rewarding. The following interpersonal difficulties can be made overt:

- Withdrawal or silence by members.
- Inactivity and unintegrated behavior by members.
- Overactivity and destructive behavior by members.
- Power struggles between members.
- Battles for attention among members.
- Dissatisfaction with the leader.
- Dissatisfaction with the amount of recognition a member receives for contributions.
- Dissatisfaction with the amount of affection and warmth demonstrated in the group.

In concert with Yalom's principles, the interpersonal needs approach of Schutz is based on the belief that the way to attack problems within groups is by investigating what is going on among the individuals in the group, and attempting to improve their interpersonal relations.

Focusing on the here-and-now experience differentiates interactive group psychotherapy from many other group therapies or therapeutic groups such as those discussed later in this chapter.

Therapeutic Groups

Nurses have long been involved in working with clients and their families in small groups brought together for health teaching, psychoeducation, or supportive purposes. This section discusses several different types of therapeutic groups in which nurses participate.

Developing and planning a therapeutic group should be a systematic process. ■ Figure 29–6 illustrates a step-by-step process that could be undertaken to determine the clinical need for the group and to develop and implement the group.

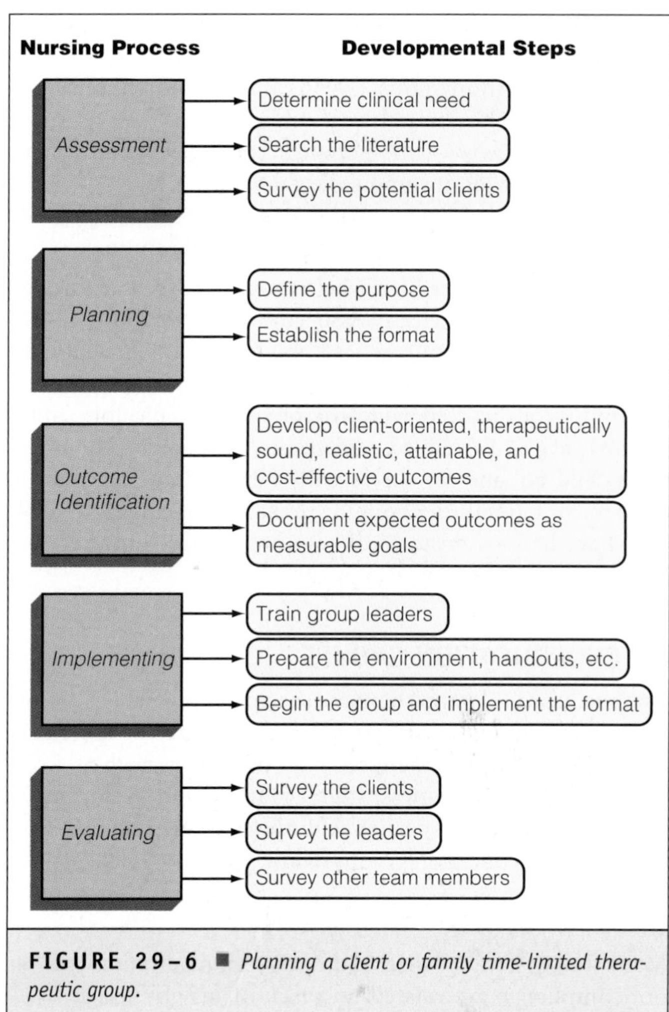

FIGURE 29–6 ■ *Planning a client or family time-limited therapeutic group.*

SELF-HELP GROUPS

The major operating principle in self-help groups is that the help given to members comes from the members themselves. A mental health professional is viewed as unnecessary. In fact, many of these groups developed because of the failure of programs planned and implemented by professionals.

The role of the nurse in self-help groups is that of a resource person. You need to be informed about such groups so that you can refer potential members to groups appropriate to their needs, or to provide consultation when invited to do so. In most self-help groups, leaders are former members. Alcoholics Anonymous is a well-known example of this principle.

There is a wide variety of self-help groups, for example:

- Recovery Incorporated (www.recovery-inc.com) and Schizophrenics Anonymous (www.sanonymous.org), concerned with mental disorder.
- Alcoholics Anonymous (www.alcoholics-anonymous.org) and Narcotics Anonymous (www.na.org), concerned with substance abuse.
- Al-Anon and Ala-Teen (www.al-anon-alateen.org), concerned with the families of alcoholics.
- Rational Recovery (www.rational.org), concerned with substance abuse.

- Overeaters Anonymous (www.overeatersanonymous.org), concerned with overeating.
- Gamblers Anonymous (www.gamblersanonymous.org), concerned with compulsive gambling.
- Gam Anon (www.gam-anon.org), concerned with the families and friends of compulsive gamblers.
- Child Abuse Listening and Mediation, Inc. (CALM) (www.calm4kids.org), concerned with child abuse.

In Canada, a directory of self-help groups is available through the Canadian Mental Health Association at (www.cmha.ca).

All of these resources can be accessed through the Companion Website for this book.

Groups for divorced, widowed, or single people, for parents of runaways and troubled adolescents, for parents who abuse their children, and for the recently bereaved are common in most major cities throughout the world. Client clubs for people who have had a colostomy, ileostomy, laryngectomy, mastectomy, or amputation are also popular.

PSYCHOEDUCATION GROUPS

Psychoeducation groups have the sharing of mental health care information as a primary goal. They also have the secondary benefit of facilitating the discussion of feelings such as isolation, helplessness, sadness, stigmatization, and/or anger and possible strategies for dealing with these feelings. Some examples of psychoeducation groups follow.

Medication Teaching Groups

Many studies have shown that the causes of medication noncompliance are related to a lack of insight and understanding by clients of their illness and of their drug treatment. In addition, drug side effects such as dry mouth, blurred vision, impotence, sedation, and akathisia can be difficult to tolerate. Medication teaching groups provide an opportunity for psychiatric–mental health nurses to educate clients about medications, their side effects, the nature and course of their mental disorder, the possibility of relapse without continued drug treatment, and the positive effect medications have on their lives.

Social Skills Training Groups

Social skills training can be accomplished effectively in groups. Small groups provide structure and support, while clients are coached in simple yet essential social interactions. It is best to form groups of clients who function at similar levels. Provide structure by clearly setting the time for group meetings, beginning and ending each session with a statement of goals, and recapping what the group has accomplished.

Social skills training has been found to decrease anxiety and psychopathology and increase self-control in clients with generalized social phobia (van Dam-Baggen & Kraaimaat, 2000), and to improve community life (recreational, residential, and vocational) for clients with schizophrenia by enhancing social competence (Roder, Zorn, Muller, & Brenner, 2001). Social skills training groups often focus on communication skills. For example, relationship risk factors for couples are reduced by teaching conflict resolution and communication skills (Freedman, Low, Markman, & Stanley, 2002). Social skills training groups for incarcerated adult offenders focus on role-plays with performance feedback, modeling, and anger reduction (Bourke & Van Hasselt, 2001).

Groups of Medically Ill Clients and Their Families

Groups composed of medically ill clients are increasingly common, as psychiatric–mental health nurses move into general health care settings offering liaison and consultation services to clients and staff. Group work is useful for chronically ill or disabled clients, preoperative and postoperative clients, clients with regulative medical problems (such as diabetes, cardiac disease, or kidney disease), dying clients, elderly clients, and clients with psychophysiologic disorders, among others.

Such groups generally focus on the stress associated with illness and have as their goal the reduction of stress. Groups may be composed of clients alone, family members alone, or a combination.

ACTIVITY THERAPY GROUPS

Activity therapies are manual, recreational, and creative techniques to facilitate personal experiences and increase social responses and self-esteem. Activity therapies are generally the province of health and recreation specialists.

Some activity therapies, such as the creative arts therapies, are organized and conducted in groups. Creative arts therapies provide many people with a comfortable opportunity for social exchange. Although there are specifically educated creative arts therapists, their numbers are small. Nurses may lead such groups or use their principles to reach beyond the ordinary realm of verbal communication with clients.

Poetry Therapy Groups

The goal of poetry therapy groups is to help members get in touch with feelings and emotions through the use of poetry. Poems that are read aloud provide the stimulus for understanding and catharsis. They are selected as the therapeutic medium because they are powerful but not explicit avenues of communication. It is not necessary to be able to write poetry to be a member or leader of a poetry therapy group, although some members or leaders may be stimulated to write poems of their own.

Art Therapy Groups

In art therapy groups, the art produced by each member gives the art therapist or group leader a personal insight into the artist's personality. The art is produced during the session and is used as the basis for discussion and for exploring members' feelings.

Music Therapy Groups

Music therapy consists of singing, rhythm, body movement, and listening. It is designed to increase group members' concentration, memory retention, conceptual development, rhythmic behavior, movement behavior, verbal and nonverbal retention, and auditory discrimination. It is also used to stimulate members' expression and discussion of affect.

Dance Therapy Groups

Dance therapy combines movement and verbal modes. In dance, members find it easier to express nonverbally the feelings and emotions that have been difficult to realize and communicate by other means. The person's inner sense is often reflected in body movements, and dance therapists work to help members integrate their experiences verbally as well as nonverbally.

Bibliotherapy Groups

In bibliotherapy groups, literature is the means for achieving a therapeutic goal. The purpose of a bibliotherapy group is to assimilate the psychological, sociologic, and aesthetic insights books give into human character, personality, and behavior. Literature provides a stimulus for group members to compare events and characters with their own interpersonal and intrapsychic experiences.

STORYTELLING GROUPS

Storytelling groups—a process by which group members create a story together—can stimulate interaction and imagination. Wenckus (1994) used an approach in which the group leader or the group members chose one person to be the main character in a story. The group leader can give direction to the story by having an opening question in mind that is likely to determine the direction of the story. Questions a group leader could ask include:

1. Where would you go if you were given a trip?
2. What would you do if you won the lottery?
3. What would you title your biography?
4. What would your epitaph say?
5. If your fairy godmother could grant your wish, what would it be?
6. What is your favorite room in the house you grew up in?

Storytelling can be very effective in helping clients talk about feelings they would otherwise have suppressed and to connect with one another. It can assist elders in reminiscence work. In addition, storytelling can be fun, generate laughter, and reduce stress, no matter the client's age.

COMMUNITY CLIENT GROUPS

Psychiatric–mental health nurses in community settings are involved with a variety of community groups. These settings include schools, youth centers, industries, neighborhood centers, churches, prisons, summer camps, single-room occupancy boarding houses, transitional facilities such as halfway houses, apartments for the elderly, and residential facilities for delinquent youths and runaways. Clients may also be people who have direct contact with these groups, such as teachers, youth counselors, prison guards, police officers, and camp counselors.

GROUPS WITH NURSE COLLEAGUES

Nurses who work together may form discussion and counseling groups to help reduce their job-related stress and to help them deal with problems of interpersonal relationships in more satisfying ways. Nurses in various intensive care and other high-pressure settings identify with increasing frequency the need for group work services that the psychiatric–mental health nurse can provide. The psychiatric–mental health nurse may also identify the need and offer this opportunity to colleagues.

Family Dynamics

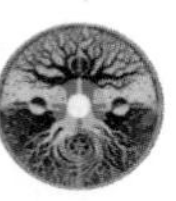

There are several dynamics that take place in families and influence both family and individual functioning. Some theories that help to explain family dynamics are discussed below.

FAMILY STRUCTURES

The traditional nuclear family is a two-parent, time-limited, two-generation family consisting of a married couple and their children by birth or adoption. In today's society, less than one in five children have grown up in the traditional nuclear family structure. Contemporary families look like any one of the following:

- A mother, a father, and 2.2 children (traditional nuclear family).
- A couple with eight children—three of hers, three of his, and two of theirs (blended family).
- A 32-year-old single electrical engineer and his three foster children.
- A divorced woman and her two teenagers.
- A widowed man, his child, and his parents.
- A grandmother raising her three grandchildren.
- Two lesbian mothers and their child.
- Three single women friends sharing an apartment neither could afford alone.
- Two gay men who live together in a committed relationship.

North American family forms continue to change. For that reason, sensitive psychiatric–mental health nurses reject a narrow definition of family and adapt their clinical practice to the wide variety of family constellations that exist in contemporary society.

FAMILY CHARACTERISTICS AND DYNAMICS

Whether they are functional or dysfunctional, families have certain characteristics and dynamics. In a family, each person's behavior is contingent on and affects the behavior of the others. This creates some interesting and complex turns in family relationships.

Family Roles

Members of a family must determine how to accomplish family developmental tasks. They do so by establishing roles, patterns of behavior sanctioned by the culture. Jackson (1968) believes that families set roles by operating as a rule-governed system, an ordered format designed so that members may be aware of their positions in relation to one another. Families decide which roles will exist within the system, socialize members into the roles, and then expend energy maintaining members within their roles.

When members are unable or unwilling to perform assigned roles, the family experiences stress. For the health of the **family system**—not only family members but also their relationships, their communication with one another, and their interactions with the environment—roles often must be negotiated in other than stereotyped ways. When the roles are not negotiated satisfactorily, family disequilibrium results.

Boundaries

Families have *boundaries* as well. Boundaries define who participates in the family, the amount or intensity of emotional investment in the family, the amount and kind of experiences available outside the family, and particular ways to evaluate experiences in terms of the family. Boundaries may be clear, rigid, diffuse, or conflicting.

Power Structure

Most families have a hierarchical power structure in which the adults wield the power. The power structure is often developed in this way because it creates a safe environment in which young children can grow and develop, and because it is easy to operate. However, stress develops when disagreements exist about who holds the power.

CLINICAL EXAMPLE

Tom, the 17-year-old son in the M family, always used the family car without permission. Although some serious arguments ensued between Tom and his father, no restrictions were placed on Tom's behavior, and the car keys continued to hang on a key rack in the front hall. Tom's paternal grandfather, who lived with the M family, took Tom's side in his arguments with his father. Grandfather M took the stance that "boys will be boys". One evening when the family car was in a repair shop for some minor work, Tom "borrowed" his grandfather's new car. Tom was involved in a collision about an hour later. Although no one was injured, Grandfather M's car was extensively damaged and had to be towed away. Later that night, the adults of the M family managed to come together to agree on a stance concerning Tom's use of the family car that they could mutually support.

Once the adults in the M family were able to acknowledge their internal power struggle and come to an agreement on what rules were to be set and by whom, the family system was subject to less stress.

When children mature and become capable of assuming greater responsibility for their own functioning, power is often diffused among all members of a family system in a more democratic fashion. Certain families, however, do not allow power to be redistributed, thus hindering the individual development of the members with less power. In some dysfunctional families, there is chronic discord about power.

Relationship Strains or Conflicts

Relationship strains or conflicts can occur in the family or among various parts of the family, or outside of it. A strain can exist between the individual members of a family—for instance, between two siblings with differing views on an issue. Conflict or strain can also occur between a member of the family and the rest of the family, or between a minority of family members and the other members. This commonly occurs when a previously and unanimously held family view is challenged by one or more members. Strain can also exist between a family and the community when a family view differs from that of the community at large.

RELATIONSHIP AND COMMUNICATION INTRICACIES IN FAMILIES

Some of the relationship complexities described below exist in all families, but dysfunctional families handle them differently than functional families do. Functional families allow for individuation and growth-producing experiences.

Self-Fulfilling Prophecy and Life Scripts

A **self-fulfilling prophecy** is an idea or expectation that is acted out, largely unconsciously, thus "proving" itself. In families, self-fulfilling prophecies are often seen in the guise of family life scripts. A **life script** is a plan decided not by the fates, but by experiences early in life. People with life scripts are following forced, premature, early childhood decisions. Most people live a scripted life, at least to some extent.

There is an endless variety among life scripts. The Miss America script is decided for the 5-year-old girl whose parents enroll her in the Little Miss New York State (or Alabama or Colorado) competition. There are "My Son the Doctor, Delinquent, Alcoholic, and Drug Addict" scripts. A person with a script, either "good" or "bad," is terribly disadvantaged in terms of autonomy or life potentials. According to self-fulfilling prophecy, unless people recognize what the script is and take steps to change it, they are prevented from living to their potential.

Family Myths and Themes

Family myths and themes help families maintain balance by permitting them to resist change. *Family myths* are well-integrated beliefs, shared by all family members, about each other and their positions in family life. The beliefs are unchallenged, even though family members may have to resort to distortions to maintain the myth. The family myth is related to the family's inner image—how the family appears to its members.

CLINICAL EXAMPLE

A myth in the Lundqvist family was that the father had the ability to make wise decisions. Individual members in this family participated to maintain the myth of the father as a wise man by gearing interactions with him in such a way that he appeared to make high-level family decisions single-handedly.

The *family theme* is the family's perception of its development and history. Family themes are important because they shape the fates of individual members and determine the pressures with which each person must contend.

CLINICAL EXAMPLE

The Weber family had a theme constructed around second-generation grandparents of Austrian descent, who were able to provide their oldest son with a law school education through their hard work. This family conceived of people on welfare as "lazy," thus reaffirming its view of the value of working hard and becoming educated.

Energy in the family is directed toward upholding particular images of the family—as the most hard-working, religious, popular, talented, financially successful, nonconformist, or whatever—in order to maintain the front the family strives to present to others.

Family Coalitions

Of all the forms of communicative exchange, dyadic communication is the most common. In fact, many families begin with a couple, a dyad. The presence of a third person always has an effect on an existing dyad. When the couple gives birth to or adopts a child, or a third person enters the family, the relationship becomes triadic. A triad is not a stable social situation, because it actually consists of a dyad plus one. Shifting alliances characterize triads or triangles in families. For example, adult partners may unite to discipline the child, mother and child may unite to argue for a family vacation, or father and child may join forces to go fishing together. Triangles are dysfunctional when issues are solved in families by shifting the intimacy among members, rather than by working the actual issue through or when interaction among family members is determined by fixed triangles. Fixed and rigid triangles are an effort to reduce stress and restore balance in a dysfunctional family. In actuality, fixed and rigid triangles perpetuate problems in families. Such coalitions always result in someone feeling "left out" (Bowen, 1988). A problematic family triangle is illustrated in ■ Figure 29–7.

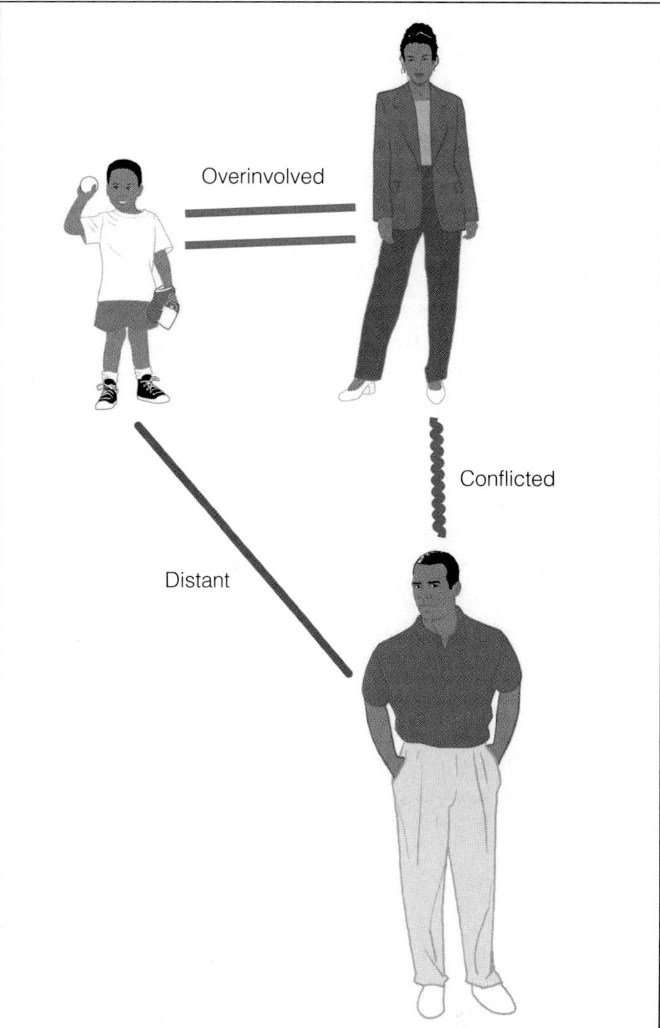

FIGURE 29–7 ■ *A family triangle. In this family, the relationship between husband and wife is conflicted. Mother and son are overinvolved. Father and son have a distant relationship.*

Coalitions arise basically to affect the distribution of power. By joining forces, two people can increase their influence over a third. Parents frequently pair up to discipline their child better. However, the child may also attempt to pair up with one parent to avoid discipline. In families with a number of children, typical coalitions involve children closest in age or children of the same sex.

Deviations in the Adult Partners' Coalition

In some families, problems develop from the couples' inability to form a satisfying coalition in terms of intimacy and control. Several common deviations within the family are examined in the sections that follow.

Schism. Families in which the children are forced to join one or the other camp of two warring spouses or adult caretakers are called *schismatic families.* The constant fighting in these families is most likely a defense against intimacy or closeness. In schismatic families, the adult partners devalue and undercut each other. This makes it difficult for the children to want to be like either of them.

Skew. Families in which one mate is severely dysfunctional are called *skewed families*. The other mate, who is usually aware of the dysfunction of the partner, assumes a passive, peacemaking, submissive stance to preserve the relationship. The passive partner is caught between effectively responding to the view of "reality" of the outside world and giving up this view within the home, accepting the dysfunctional mate's view. On the surface, a skewed couple may appear to be complementary. Their relationship is actually lopsided and unsuited to many basic family tasks, however.

Enmeshment. A fast tempo of interpersonal exchange is characteristic of *enmeshed families*. Interactions within the family are of high intensity and are directed more toward issues of power than toward issues of affection. In enmeshed families, one adult is often overcontrolling and becomes anxious over the possibility of losing control over the children.

Disengagement. Abandonment—to the other extreme from enmeshment, is characteristic of *disengaged families*. Family members seem oblivious to the effects of their actions on one another. They are unresponsive and unconnected to each other. Structure, order, or authority in the family may be weak or nonexistent. Assuming control and guidance increases the anxiety of the parent, who may feel overwhelmed and depressed. In these families, a child often assumes the parental role.

Pseudomutuality and Pseudohostility

A family in which *pseudomutuality* occurs functions as if it were a close, happy family. This pattern of relating has the following characteristics:

- Persistent sameness in the structuring of roles.
- Insistence on the desirability and appropriateness of the role structures within the family, despite evidence to the contrary.
- Intense concern over deviations from the role structure or emerging autonomy.
- Marked absence of spontaneity, enthusiasm, and humor in participating together.

In these families, the members do not form intimate bonds with one another as individuals. Instead, an inordinate amount of energy is expended in maintaining ritualized and stereotyped ways of behaving and relating. Such a family requires its members to give up their sense of personal identity.

Pseudohostility exists in families characterized by chronic conflict, alienation, tension, and inappropriate remoteness. As in pseudomutuality, family members deny the problems in an attempt to negate the hostility. Family members view their differences as only minor ones. Both pseudomutual and pseudohostile family environments are stifling milieus.

Family Assessment

Assessing and intervening with the families of your clients is an essential role. Unfortunately, some mental health care professionals still have a bias against family involvement. This bias is a remnant of now-discredited theories that poor parenting and dysfunctional family interaction patterns give rise to mental illness (Mohr, Lafuze, & Mohr, 2000). A related bias is the belief by some that if families "cause" schizophrenia, then the family's contact with the client should be limited for the client's sake. Besides violating family rights, this bias prevents social interaction with family members that might serve as a normalizing force by confronting clients with reality (Myin-Germeys, Nicolson, & Delespaul, 2001). Here is a question you can use to check if you have a bias against the family's rights: *Am I responding to this family any differently than I would to the family of a client with a medical condition?*

In addition, your experiences in your own family influence how you perceive and react to your client's family. Truthfully answering the self-assessment questions in the Nursing Self-Awareness feature below will help you to determine how your own family experiences might influence your behavior with your client's family.

The family who has cared for the client with a mental disorder has an in-depth understanding of the client's illness, history, and ability to function in the community. Include the family's insights in the assessment phase, and, if appropriate, use them in the planning of care, particularly care after discharge.

Family assessment involves gathering data in several different areas and can be done both formally and informally. Do not overlook natural opportunities to assess families and their needs. During visits, join the family for a few minutes to learn about their understanding of the treatment program, their con-

Nursing SELF-AWARENESS

The Influences of Your Own Family Experiences

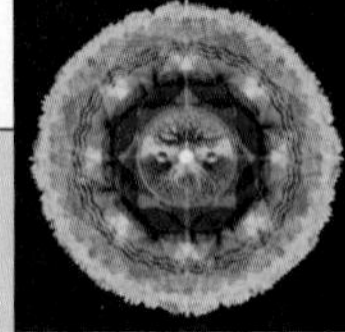

It is helpful when working with families to first come to an understanding of the experiences you bring with you from your own family. Filling in the blanks on the following statements will facilitate your self-understanding and recognition of the biases you bring with you to your work with families.

1. When someone in my family talks too much, I usually . . .
2. When one of my family members is silent, I usually . . .
3. When someone in my family cries, I usually . . .
4. When my family members are excessively polite and unwilling to confront each other, I usually . . .
5. When there is conflict in my family, I usually . . .
6. When one individual in my family is verbally attacked, I usually . . .
7. If there is physical violence in my family, I usually . . .
8. My typical intervention "rhythm" (fast/slow) is . . .
9. My style is characteristically more (nurturing/confronting) . . .
10. The things that make me most uncomfortable in my family are . . .

cerns, and their questions. More formal assessments using interview guides or strategies such as a family genealogy or time line (discussed later in this chapter) are also available. Whichever methods you use, remember that a trusting relationship with key members of the client's family is essential for establishing a flow of information and planning care. Remember, however, to secure clients' permission before information is released to their families, and encourage clients to involve their families in their treatment (Marshall & Solomon, 2000). Clients' rights in relation to sharing of information is discussed in Chapter 10.

DEMOGRAPHIC INFORMATION

Data pertaining to gender, age, occupation, religion, and ethnicity should be obtained. In addition to gathering discrete bits of information (the father is a 39-year-old Latino, physician's assistant, and a member of St. Ann's Roman Catholic parish), it is important to gather more detailed information that will give insight into family functioning:

- How actively does the family pursue religious/spiritual activities?
- What is the link of religion/spirituality to the family's value system, norms, and practices?
- What is the family's racial, cultural, and ethnic identification in relation to sense of identity and belonging?
- Who in the family is employed? What are their attitudes about employment?

MEDICAL AND MENTAL HEALTH HISTORY

Here, substantive information should also be gathered. You will want to know about past medical and mental health treatment; past and present illnesses; and pertinent health facts in the family of origin, the extended family, and in the family history.

Gather information about the developmental stage of the family.

- What were (are) the problems in transition from one developmental level to another?
- How has the family solved problems at earlier stages?
- What shifts in role responsibility have occurred over time?

FAMILY INTERACTIONAL DATA

This is probably the most complex data to obtain. For example, you will want to gather information about family rules.

- What family rules foster stability in the family?
- What rules foster maladaptation?
- How are rules modified?
- What happens when all members do not agree about the family rules?

You will also need to determine the roles of family members.

- What are the formal roles for each member?
- What are the informal roles (scapegoat, controller, decision maker, and so on)?
- Do the roles seem to have a good fit in the family?

Most important, gather information on how family members communicate.

- What are the channels of communication—who speaks to whom?
- Are the messages clear?
- What is the extent of unclear or ambiguous messages, mixed messages, or missed messages?
- Do members "hear" one another?

Assess levels of cohesion by noting who accompanies the client during admission.

- Is it the whole family or just one member?
- Does the client come in alone? (Visits from family are a rich source of information.)
- Who visits, how often, and for how long?
- How do family visitors behave with the client?
- Do the members spend time interacting and sharing activities, do they sit quietly together, or do they maintain physical and emotional distance from one another?

Document these patterns of family interactions, and monitor the effect of family visits on the client.

FAMILY BURDEN

In a report on the experience of stigma in families with mentally ill members, Muhlbauer (2002) noted that more than 4 million American families live with severely mentally ill members. Most families of mentally disordered individuals report that caring for the ill member is a very important, largely underappreciated, stigmatized, and frequently expensive, all-consuming, and lifelong task (Karp, 2000). **Family burden** is a term that refers to the difficulties and responsibilities of family members who assume a caretaking function for relatives with psychiatric disability.

Family burdens reported most often are financial strain, violence in the household, reductions in the physical and mental health of family caregivers, disruption in family routines, worry about the future, the impact of stigma, the mental health system itself as a stressor, and feeling overwhelmed or unable to cope. Families also report having these needs:

- Information about the disorder itself.
- Information about how to manage day-to-day problems due to the client's symptoms.
- Information and access to resources about medications and their side effects.
- Strategies for helping the seriously mentally ill family member accept treatment (Amador & Johanson, 2000).
- Support in their role as caregiver.

Gathering information about the family burden will help you to determine what kind of support would be most helpful to this family. A family support group? Referral to NAMI (discussed later in this chapter)? Respite care to give the family a break from their caregiving role? Family therapy?

FAMILY SYSTEM DATA

Determine how the family interacts with the outside world.

- How permeable or rigid are its boundaries?

- What is the extent to which the family fits into the larger culture of which it is a part?
- To what degree could the family be considered deviant from the larger culture?

Within the family, determine what are the family alliances.

- Who supports whom?
- Which members are in conflict with one another, or with the family as a whole?
- Are there extended family supports?
- What other social supports are available to the family?

NEEDS, GOALS, VALUES, AND ASPIRATIONS

Determine whether essential needs are met.

- Are physical needs met?
- At what level does the family meet the social and emotional needs of its members?
- What are the individual needs of family members, and how do they fit with the family needs?
- Is the family willing or able to meet the individual needs of its members?

Determine the extent to which individual family members' goals and values are articulated and understood by the other members.

- Are the goals and values shared by all?
- Do some members compromise?
- Do other members simply give up and give in?
- Does the family as a whole allow individual members to pursue individual goals and values?

FAMILY GENOGRAM

From the study of families in detail, it becomes apparent that patterns are spread over generations. The timeline, or **genogram,** is highly effective as a visual representation of family patterns from one generation to the next. By drawing it on a long, narrow piece of paper and taping it to the wall during the family's sessions, the therapist can use it repeatedly as therapy progresses. Colored lines can differentiate individual family members. Colored flags, pins, or stickers can identify and call attention to significant events in the family history. Births, deaths, marriages, and leave-takings should be noted. Any of several family tree or genealogic tracing formats for the family timeline can be used. One example is illustrated in ■ Figure 29–8. Other genograms can be developed to explore specific issues.

Cultural Family Genogram

A cultural family genogram is a useful tool for working with culturally diverse families (Congress, 2000). You can use a culturagram to become more aware of the cultural differences between yourself and the family and between the family and other families, assess a family's strengths, and point to areas where intervention may be useful. A cultural family genogram might include the following elements:

- What language is spoken at home and in the community?
- What significance does race, skin color, and hair play within the group?
- What role does religion and spirituality play within the everyday lives of the family members?
- What prejudices or stereotypes does this family have about themselves and other members of their cultural group?
- What prejudices or stereotypes does this family have about other cultural groups?
- What are the health beliefs in this family's culture?
- How does this culture view mental health professionals?
- What values does this family have about family, education, and work?
- What are the pride/shame issues of this cultural group? How are they manifested in this family?

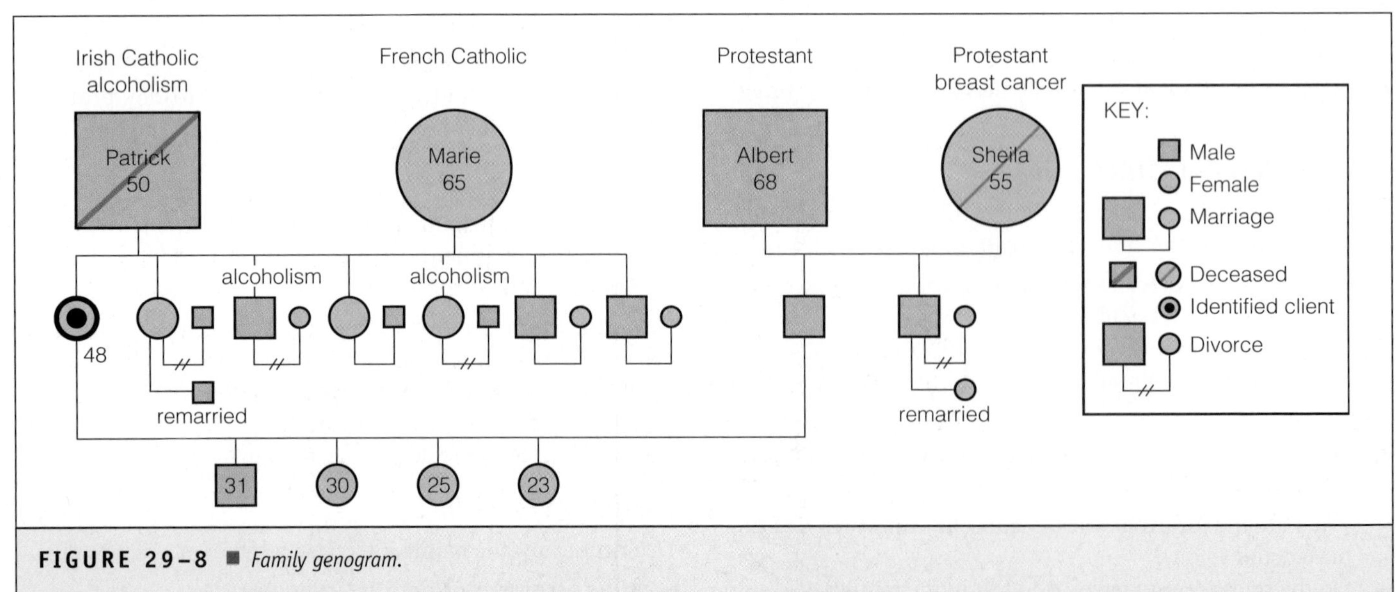

FIGURE 29–8 ■ *Family genogram.*

Spiritual Family Genogram

A spiritual genogram that is a multigenerational map of family members' religious and spiritual affiliations, events, and conflicts enables clients to make sense of their families' religious/spiritual heritage. It also helps them to explore the ways in which their experiences with spirituality affect couple or family issues (Frame, 2000).

Forensic Family Genogram

A forensic family genogram is a useful tool for forensic nurses for both assessment and intervention purposes. Kent-Wilkinson (1999) suggests a three-generational map to help offenders see the patterns in their lives as a way to begin to understand their personal circumstances. As part of the legal chart, it provides the courts with information about the events and factors in the individual lives of offenders in the form of a graphic database.

Family Interventions

Two main goals for involving family members in a client's treatment plan are:

1. Enlisting the family as an ally in promoting and bringing about therapeutic progress (Atwood, 2001).
2. Supporting family caregivers (Doornbos, 2002).

Three main forms of family intervention in current use are: family psychoeducation, referral to NAMI, and family therapy.

Advocating services for family caregivers is an important service that psychiatric–mental health nurses can provide. Services directed toward supporting the family caregivers of persons with serious and persistent mental illnesses may have the potential to improve outcomes for both the caregivers and the clients (Doornbos, 2002). Although there seems to be a consensus about the need for coordinated family-based services, they are not always implemented (Coffey, Olson, & Sessions, 2001). This is an area for active advocacy by the psychiatric–mental health nurse.

FAMILY PSYCHOEDUCATION

Family members can benefit from psychoeducation groups designed specifically to help them cope with their loved one's illness. Family psychoeducation has also been found to reduce psychotic relapse and rehospitalization (Bustillo, Lauriello, Horan, & Keith, 2001). Family education groups educate family members about the specific mental disorder including its signs and symptoms, the medications the client takes, the signs and stages of relapse, the treatment plan, and the fluctuating course of mental illness. They also learn about life events that cause stress for the client, how to prevent relapse, and how to manage behavior that is disturbing to others. Unfortunately, the use of family psychoeducation in routine clinical practice is limited. Family members are most likely to receive information about diagnosis and medications and least likely to receive information about the treatment plan (Marshall & Solomon, 2000). However, nurses can be influential in persuading their agencies to develop family psychoeducation programs, much like the one discussed in the Using Research Evidence feature below.

Family psychoeducation groups also serve a supportive function in an accepting environment. Family members are informed about local and national groups and organizations that provide educational and counseling services and respite care. A family psychoeducation program is a good bridge to referral to NAMI or to family therapy.

USING RESEARCH EVIDENCE

You are a member of the program development committee at the outreach clinic in which you work. The committee chair, Mrs. Brady, has suggested that the committee develop an online Internet support group for families of the clinic's clients. Her rationales are that in an era of diminishing health care resources, an online therapeutic support group makes good financial sense, would not require the provision of extra clinic space or other clinic resources, and makes it easier for families because they would not have to leave their homes.

You voted against this proposal. Your rationales are that despite the popularity of online support groups, little is known about their therapeutic effectiveness, member responses can be misinterpreted, there is no opportunity to check nonverbal against verbal communication, and families would not have the opportunity to interact on a personal face-to-face level.

Your argument was persuasive, and the other members of your committee also voted against the proposal. The committee chair gave you the task of coming up with an alternative by the next meeting.

You have decided to propose a family psychoeducation group based on evidence-based practice shown to reduce relapse rates and facilitate recovery. On the one hand, you know that in-service programs to persuade clinicians to adopt family psychoeducation techniques have a limited track record. Clinicians often cite intense work pressure and skepticism about the interventions as reasons for their lack of enthusiasm. Your proposal recommends organizational consultation with family psychoeducation experts, and differential rewards to those who implement family psychoeducation techniques. The differential rewards would be based on performance standards and evaluations, performance-based pay, positive feedback from clients and families, and public recognition for their efforts.

Your proposal is based on the results of the following studies:

Amenson, C. S., & Liberman, R. P. (2001). Dissemination of educational classes for families of adults with schizophrenia. *Psychiatric Services, 52*(5), 589–599; Cudney, S., & Weinert, C. (2000). Computer-based support groups: Nursing in cyberspace. *Computer Nurse, 18,* 1–6; Dixon, L., et al. (2001). Evidence-based practices for services to families of people with psychiatric disabilities. *Psychiatric Services, 52*(7), 903–910; and Finfgeld, D. L. (2000). Therapeutic groups online: the good, the bad, and the unknown. *Issues in Mental Health Nursing, 21*(3), 241–255.

REFERRAL TO NAMI

The National Alliance for the Mentally Ill (NAMI) is a grassroots, self-help, advocacy and support organization of families, consumers (a term used by NAMI to describe people diagnosed with and receiving treatment for severe mental illness), and friends of people with severe mental disorders. NAMI provides several services to families and consumers, including general information on mental disorders, psychiatric medications, mental health policy positions; referral to state and local affiliates and support groups throughout the country, and support from trained volunteers—consumers and family members—who know what it's like to have a mental disorder or to have a family member with a mental disorder. One program of special interest to families is the NAMI Family-to-Family Education Program. The special features of this course, prepared by families for families, has both a personal and a social focus and is outlined in Box 29–2.

NAMI also provides educational services to mental health care providers. The NAMI Provider Education Program for line staff at public agencies who work directly with people with severe and persistent mental illness is a 10-week course to educate providers on how to include families in the care of the client. The program is based on principles of competence (stressing empowerment and collaboration) and adaptation, rather than psychopathology, and shifts the emphasis from the causes to the effects of mental disorders (Marsh, 2000).

MediaLink NAMI Provider Education

You can refer consumers and families in need (as well as other health care providers) to the NAMI HelpLine at 1-800-950-NAMI (6264). You can also suggest the NAMI Web site at (www.nami.org), which can be accessed through a direct link on the Companion Website for this book.

FAMILY THERAPY

In general, family therapists believe that the emotional symptoms or problems of an individual are an expression of emotional symptoms or problems in a family. Therefore, family therapists view the family system as a unit of treatment. Their concerns are basically with the relationships between the family members, not with the intrapsychic functioning of individual family members.

Traditional family therapy has been criticized for its reliance on outdated theories and ineffective interventions, especially in relationship to the treatment of families with a member with a serious and persistent mental illness (discussed earlier in this chapter in the section on Family Assessment).

Forms of Family Therapy

There are two basic forms of family therapy: insight-oriented family therapy and behavioral-oriented family therapy (Snyder, Wills, & Grady-Fletcher, 1991) into which all schools of family therapy fit. Some examples of insight-oriented family therapy approaches are:

- Psychodynamic: problems are believed to arise because of developmental delays, or current interactions or stresses.
- Family of origin therapy: in which the goal is to foster differentiation among the members and decrease emotional reactivity and triangulation (Bowen, 1988).

Some examples of behavioral-oriented family therapy are:

- *Structural:* The focus is on systems, subsystems, boundaries, and schismatic, skewed, enmeshed, or disengaged families (Minuchin & Fishman, 1981; Navarre, 1998).
- *Strategic:* Problems arise because of inequality of power, flawed communication, and repetitive and maladaptive family interaction patterns (Haley, 1996; Satir, 1983).
- *Cognitive/behavioral:* The focus is on changing thinking and behavior, problem solving, and the development of skills (see Chapter 30 for a complete discussion of cognitive and behavioral strategies).

BOX 29–2 NAMI Family-to-Family Education Program

Emotional Understanding and Healing (Personal Realm)

- *Speaking Pain:* Guaranteeing a safe, protective place where family members can debrief the traumatic events and feelings they have experienced.
- *Normalizing:* Teaching the specific guideposts of the emotional process traumatized people go through in their process of adaptation and recovery.
- *Coming Out:* Creating a group-bonding process that will encourage candid self-disclosure.
- *Empathic Identification with the Victim:* Helping family members understand the subjective experience of their relative with a mental illness.
- *Modeling:* Providing teachers who have borne this personal trauma and have "come through."
- *Restoring One's Own Lifeline:* Showing the way to put living with trauma into a life perspective that fosters self-care and self-realization.

Power and Action (Social Realm)

- *Breaking the Silence:* Encouraging family members to recognize and express their anger at discrimination and stigma.
- *Consciousness Raising:* Providing a premeditated, detailed "informational overload" regarding the neurobiological aspects of brain disorders to disconfirm learned stereotypes about mental illness.
- *Empowerment:* Modeling peer mastery of basic biomedical knowledge.
- *Assertiveness and Skill Training:* Introducing and practicing new coping and communication techniques.
- *Liberation:* Releasing family members, through group support and mutual affirmation, from the gross misperception of their experience.
- *Solidarity:* Fostering self-respect and pride in families as examplars of courage, strength, and perseverance.
- *Activism:* Showing families a way to join the fight against social injustice by linking them with family advocacy groups on local and national levels.

Source: Adapted from Goals of NAMI's Brand of Family Education. Retrieved June 17, 2002, from the World Wide Web, www.nami.org. Reprinted with permission NAMI.

These lists are general, and not exhaustive. Discussion of these theories and their specific interventions are beyond the scope of this book.

Qualifications of Family Therapists

Being a family therapist requires a firm and clear understanding of all of the dynamics and forces that influence families. Family therapists should be specially educated in the practice of family therapy and strongly committed to a belief in the importance of the family. Nurse family therapists should be clinical specialists or advanced practitioners prepared in graduate programs that provide both theory and supervised clinical practice in this specialized area. Refer families to qualified nurse family therapists or other qualified family therapists. Families can also receive help in finding a therapist on the Web site of the American Association for Marital and Family Therapy (www.aamftmorg) or through the Companion Website for this book.

The Unit of Treatment

Most family therapists recommend that all people in the family constellation participate in the assessment phase of family therapy. Not all agree on which people make up the family constellation or the treatment unit. Some include all members of the nuclear family; others include members of the extended family; and still others, large numbers of people in the family's social network. Different coalitions may be seen together at different times to accomplish specific goals. For example, mates are often seen together for the first few sessions.

Children 4 years of age and younger are often not included in ongoing family therapy sessions. They may misinterpret, or be frightened by, the dialogue. In addition, small children tend to be disruptive. Some therapists, however, make it a point to bring all the children into some family therapy sessions to see how the family as a whole operates.

Contract or Goal Negotiation

The negotiation phase of family therapy is begun by identifying what each member would like changed in the family. When each family member and the therapist have identified important goals, they begin negotiating a set of attainable goals that everyone is willing to work on. Compromise is needed to achieve a working goal. At this time, the family therapist, along with the family, may also identify the means—tasks, strategies, and so on—that will be used to reach the negotiated goals.

INTERVENTION

The Role of the Family Therapist

- Creating a safe setting in which family members can risk looking at themselves and their actions
- Teaching family members how to share their observations with one another
- Asking for and giving information in a matter-of-fact, nonjudgmental, congruent way
- Responding as a role model whose meaning or intent can be checked on without fear
- Setting rules for interaction to ensure that all family members participate; interruptions, acting-out, or making it impossible to converse are not tolerated; no one speaks for anyone else
- Clarifying the content and relationship aspects of messages
- Pointing out significant discrepancies, incongruities, or double-level messages
- Helping everyone speak out clearly so that each can be heard
- Viewing the family as a system and not taking sides
- Showing that anger, pain, and the "forbidden" are safe to look at
- Reeducating family members to be accountable
- Delineating family roles and functions and teaching explicitly about role responses and role choices

MediaLink Marital/Family Therapy Resource

Intervention

Therapy for a family system involves understanding and use of the here-and-now, and of the basic processes that occur in the system. Guidelines for interventions employed by family therapists are listed in the Intervention box above.

Terminating Family Therapy

Family therapists use various criteria to determine when termination is appropriate. Family therapy is often terminated when family members can:

- See how they appear to others.
- Give feedback to others, telling them how they appear.
- Share their hopes, fears, and expectations with one another.
- Openly discuss problems with one another.
- Openly disagree with one another when appropriate.
- Give clear messages.
- Check meaning with one another.
- Ask for clarification.
- Support one another.
- Achieve the family's goals.

Termination in family therapy occurs in a flexible way, helping families achieve realistic goals, thus ending therapy with a feeling of accomplishment.

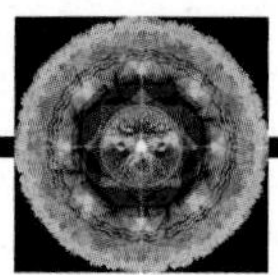

EXPLORE MediaLink

NCLEX review, case studies, and other interactive resources for this chapter can be found on the Companion Website at http://www.prenhall.com/kneisl. Click on Chapter 29 to select the activities for this chapter.

For animations, video tutorials, more NCLEX review questions, and an audio glossary, access the accompanying CD-ROM in this textbook.

BIBLIOGRAPHY

Amador, X., & Johanson, A-L. (2000). *I am not sick, I don't need help! Helping the seriously mentally ill accept treatment: A practical guide for families and therapists.* Peconic, NY: Vida Press.

Amenson, C. S., & Liberman, R. P. (2001). Dissemination of educational classes for families of adults with schizophrenia. *Psychiatric Services, 52*(5), 589–592.

Atwood, N. C. (2001). Combining individual and family treatment: Guidelines for the therapist. *New Direction in Mental Health Services, 91,* 31–46.

Benne, K. D., & Sheats, P. (1948). Functional roles of group members. *Journal of Social Issues, 4,* 41–49.

Bourke, M. L., & Van Hasselt, V. B. (2001). Social problem-solving skills training for incarcerated offenders: A treatment manual. *Behavior Modification, 25*(2), 163–188.

Bowen M. (1988). *Family therapy in clinical practice* (2nd ed.). Northvale, NJ: Jason Aronson.

Bustillo, J., Lauriello, J., Horan, W., & Keith, S. (2001). The psychosocial treatment of schizophrenia: An update. *American Journal of Psychiatry, 158*(2), 163–175.

Coffey, E. P., Olson, M. E., & Sessions, P. (2001). The heart of the matter: An essay about the effects of managed care on family therapy with children. *Family Process, 40*(4), 385–399.

Congress, E. P. (2000). Crisis intervention with culturally diverse families. In Roberts, A. R. *Crisis intervention handbook: Assessment, treatment, and research* (2nd ed.) (pp. 430–452). New York: Oxford University Press.

Dixon, L., McFarlane, W. R., Lefley, H., Lucksted, A., Cohen, M., Falloon, I., et al. (2001). Evidence-based practices for services to families of people with psychiatric disabilities. *Psychiatric Services, 52*(7), 903–910.

Doornbos, M. M. (2002). Family caregivers and the mental health care system: Reality and dreams. *Archives of Psychiatric Nursing, 16*(1), 39–46.

Frame, M. W. (2000). Spiritual ecomaps: A new diagrammatic tool for assessing marital and family spirituality. *Journal of Marital and Family Therapy, 26*(2):217–228.

Freedman, C. M., Low, S. M., Markman, H. J., & Stanley, S. M. (2002). Equipping couples with the tools to cope with predictable and unpredictable crisis events: The PREP program. *International Journal of Emergency Mental Health, 4*(1), 49–55.

Haley, J. (1996). *Learning and teaching therapy*. New York: Guilford Press.

Jackson, D. D. (1968). *Communication, family, and marriage*. Palo Alto, CA: Science and Behavior Books.

Karp, D. A. (2000). *The burden of sympathy: How families cope with mental illness*. London: Oxford University Press.

Kent-Wilkinson, A. (1999). Forensic family genogram: An assessment and intervention tool. *Journal of Psychosocial Nursing and Mental Health Services, 37*(9), 52–56.

Leff, J. (2000). Family work for schizophrenia: Practical application. *Acta Psychiatrica Scandanavia Supplement, 102*(407), 78–82.

Marsh, D. (2000). *Serious mental illness and the family: The practitioner's guide*. New York: John Wiley & Sons.

Marshall, T. B., & Solomon, P. (2000). Releasing information to families of persons with severe mental illness: A survey of NAMI members. *Psychiatric Services, 51*(8):1006–1011.

Minuchin, S., & Fishman, H. (1981). *Family therapy techniques.* Cambridge, MA: Harvard University Press.

Mohr, W. K., Lafuze, J. E., & Mohr, B. D. (2000). Opening caregiver minds: National Alliance for the Mentally Ill's (NAMI) provider education program. *Archives of Psychiatric Nursing, 14*(5), 1235–1243.

Muhlbauer, S. (2002). Experience of stigma by families with mentally ill members. *Journal of American Psychiatric Nurses Association, 8*(3), 76–83.

Myin-Germeys, I., Nicolson, N. A., & Delespaul, P. A. (2001). The context of delusional experiences in the daily life of patients with schizophrenia. *Psychological Medicine, 31*(3), 489–498.

Navarre, S. (1998). Salvador Minuchin's structural family therapy and its application to multicultural family systems. *Issues in Mental Health Nursing, 19,* 557–565.

Ormont, L. (2000). Where is group treatment going in the 21st century? *Group, 24,* 185–192.

Roder, V., Zorn, P., Muller, D., & Brenner, H. D. (2001). Improving recreational, residential, and vocational outcomes for patients with schizophrenia. *Psychiatric Services, 52*(11), 1439–1441.

Satir, V. (1983). *Conjoint family therapy.* Palo Alto, CA: Science and Behavior Books.

Schutz, W. C. (1958a). Interpersonal underworld. *Harvard Business Review, 36,* 123–135.

Schutz, W. C. (1958b). *The interpersonal underworld: FIRO.* Palo Alto, CA: Science and Behavior Books.

Snyder, D. K., Wills, R. M., & Grady-Fletcher, A. (1991). Long-term effectiveness of behavioral versus insight-oriented marital therapy: A 4-year follow-up study. *Journal of Consulting Clinical Psychologists, 59*(1), 138–141.

Taylor, N. T., Burlingame, G. M., Kristensen, K. B., Fuhrlman, A., Johansen, J., & Dahl, D. (2001). A survey of mental health care provider's and managed care organization attitudes toward, familiarity with, and use of group interventions. *International Journal of Group Psychotherapy, 51*(2), 243–263.

van Dam-Baggen, R., & Kraaimaat, F. (2000). Group social skills training of cognitive group therapy as the clinical treatment of choice for generalized social phobia? *Journal of Anxiety Disorders, 14*(5), 437–451.

Washington, O. G., & Moxley, D. P. (2001). A model of group treatment to facilitate recovery from chemical dependence. *Journal of Psychosocial Nursing and Mental Health Services, 39*(7), 30–41.

Wenckus, E. M. (1994). Storytelling: Using an ancient art to work with groups. *Journal of Psychosocial Nursing and Mental Health Services, 32,* 30–32.

Yalom, I. D. (1995). *The theory and practice of group psychotherapy* (4th ed.). New York: Basic Books.

Yalom, I. D. (1998). *The Yalom reader.* New York: Basic Books.

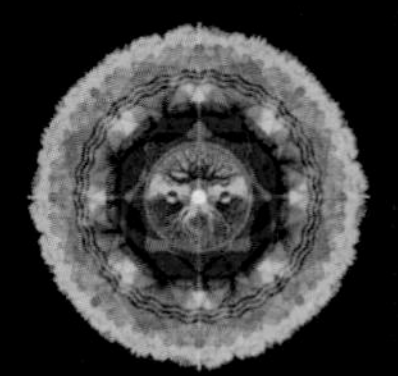

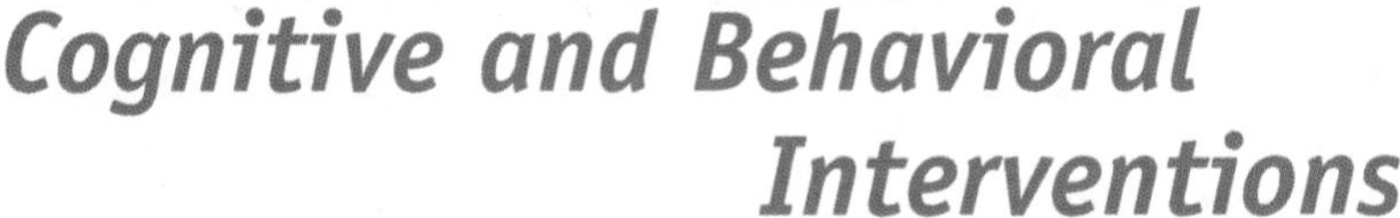

Cognitive and Behavioral Interventions

EILEEN TRIGOBOFF

30

Chapter THIRTY

FOCUS QUESTIONS

- **What are examples of humans expressing themselves in cognitive and behavioral ways?**
- **How are conditioning and association related to human learning?**
- **What therapeutic intervention would you use in a cognitive behavioral framework?**
- **Which diagnostic group would benefit from cognitive–behavioral-based case management?**
- **How would you design a behavioral contract to promote a change in health-related behaviors?**

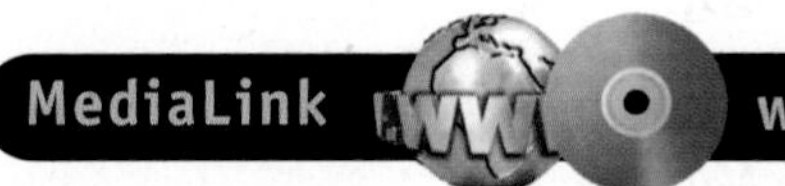

MediaLink www.prenhall.com/kneisl

Additional resources for this chapter can be found on the Student CD-ROM accompanying this textbook, and on the Companion Website at www.prenhall.com/kneisl. Click on Chapter 30 to select the activities for this chapter.

CD-ROM
- Audio Glossary
- NCLEX Review

Companion Website
- Additional NCLEX Review
- Case Study: Developing Behavioral Goals

KEY TERMS

behavior modification
mastery imagery
negative imagery
negative reinforcement
positive imagery
positive reinforcement
response prevention

CHAPTER OUTLINE

CROSS REFERENCES

Assessing clients, Chapter 9; Behavioral interventions with children, Chapter 25; Counseling options with individuals, Chapter 28; Cultural competence and psychiatric epidemiology, Chapter 6.

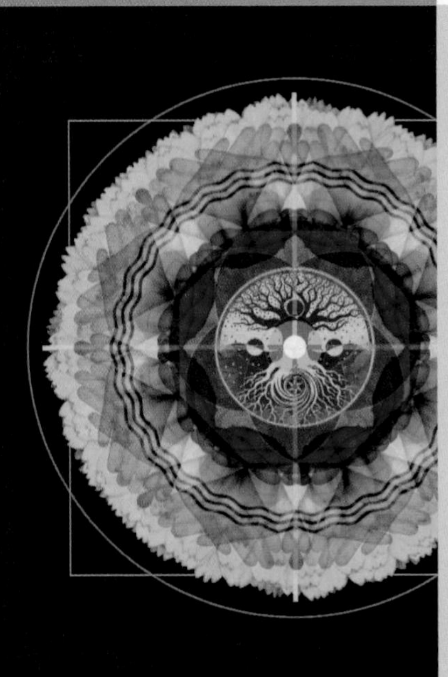

CRITICAL THINKING CHALLENGE

Steven Norah is a full-time college student who has been depressed for some time and has not made significant progress in a long-term therapy situation that specifically focused on his childhood and developmental issues. You discussed his treatment responses with other members of the treatment team during his recent hospitalization for an exacerbation of his depressive symptoms. Steven has expressed frustration at his inability to "get better and leave the depression behind." His depression and his routine ways of thinking and behaving continue in an unchanged, habitual manner.

The team believes a cognitive–behavioral approach would give Steven a better chance at recovery from depression. Changing his thoughts and his behaviors could change his feelings and diminish depressive thinking. Once changes occur, Steven has the opportunity to feel competent and successful; a distinct difference from his current view of himself. How would you introduce this change in therapeutic methods? What would you say to describe the differences that would occur? ■

Humans express themselves through thoughts and behaviors. We think and we act, then we have feelings about these thoughts and actions. Problems in certain areas of mental health can be linked to problems in the way a person thinks and behaves. Making specific changes in a maladaptive or problematic pattern of thinking and behavior could have a positive and healthy impact on an individual's mental health. This concept of human learning has led researchers into developing the *cognitive* (thought) and *behavioral* (action) therapies (Beck, 1976; Beck, Freeman, & Associates, 1990; Skinner, 1974, 1989). The National Science Foundation Behavioral and Cognitive Sciences site at www.nsf.gov/sbe/bcs/ can be accessed through the Companion Website of this text.

The design of cognitive therapy, behavioral therapy, and cognitive–behavioral therapy for certain psychiatric–mental health diagnoses focuses on how an individual can learn and make changes. An example of a cognitive change would be finding out what the routine thoughts are that a depressed individual has a habit of thinking, such as saying to oneself, "I'm no good at anything. I'm such a failure." You can imagine what the emotional impact of hearing that repeatedly would be like. Altering those sentences to something like "There are things I can do well and things I need to work on" offers that individual an opportunity to be more realistic and avoid chronically focusing on an unhealthy perspective. Over time, this change in thinking allows the client to spend time with neutral and positive thoughts about oneself, substituting for and displacing disturbing and negative thoughts. This is how a cognitive change can influence an emotional change for the better. This process is what forms the basis for cognitive therapy (Skinner, 1989).

Cognitive and behavioral interventions make use of the principles of cognitive functioning and behavior in Box 30–1. They are tailored to the client's needs and may be applied as single therapeutic entities and in combination. Each therapeutic mode is explored in this chapter.

BOX 30–1 Principles of Cognitive Functioning and Behavior

Principles of Cognitive Functioning

1. What people think affects how they feel.
2. What people think is often based on thinking habits.
3. If we change thinking, there can be a change in feelings.

Principles of Behavior

People do things:	When they are rewarded in a way that is meaningful for them. When something they don't like is removed.
People don't do things:	When they get punished. When something they like is taken away from them.

MediaLink Behavioral/Cognitive Sciences

Cognitive Therapy

Let's explore the idea of cognitions affecting feelings. Have you ever thought something about yourself, had an expectation that resulted in your feeling a particular way? For example, as a student, did you ever expect an excellent grade on a test because you studied hard and you thought you knew the material well? When the grade came back as a "B," you may have felt disappointed, betrayed, even demoralized because your efforts were not sufficiently rewarded. Your feelings about the grade you received would be different if your expectation of yourself was that you would study hard and do your best and the grade would reflect that effort, whatever that grade might be. The difference in those feelings is the difference between those cognitions. Thoughts can affect feelings.

ATTRIBUTIONS

Humans learn to think and act through cognitive behavioral learning processes. Initially, people make *attributions*; we label or assign a certain meaning to a circumstance or a set of circumstances (such as expecting to receive a grade of A). Then we attribute associated features or characteristics to that circumstance or set of circumstances (such as being a good student or knowing the material). Next, we expect a certain outcome from that circumstance and we behave consistently with that expectation. Finally, there are feelings we have that are congruent with the experience. The basic idea is that thoughts and behaviors lead to feelings.

MODELING AND SELF-EFFICACY

Other concepts in this process of human learning involve *modeling* and self-efficacy. Modeling involves imitating another (or others) in the expectation that one will receive the rewards others seem to be getting. See ■ Figure 30–1 on page 710 for an example of how people learn through modeling the behaviors of others. You may have experienced modeling throughout your education, especially once you selected nursing as your career. You would have had the opportunity to witness nurses who are competent and effective and you would strive for that level of skill in order to receive rewards.

Human learning also occurs through *self-efficacy*. Self-efficacy involves a feeling of effectiveness through one's own actions. People learn and adapt when put into circumstances demanding new or different skills. There is a tendency under those circumstances to acquire beliefs that life and problems can be coped with successfully through acquiring skills, practicing them, observing successful outcomes, and building confidence in a sense of self-efficacy.

Over time, consistent use of labeling, making attributions, modeling behavior, and experiencing self-efficacy feelings set a pattern of thinking in place for the person. The pattern explains events for that person while shaping expectations about interactions and other behaviors. The patterns can be shaped in adaptive or maladaptive ways, depending on the circumstances

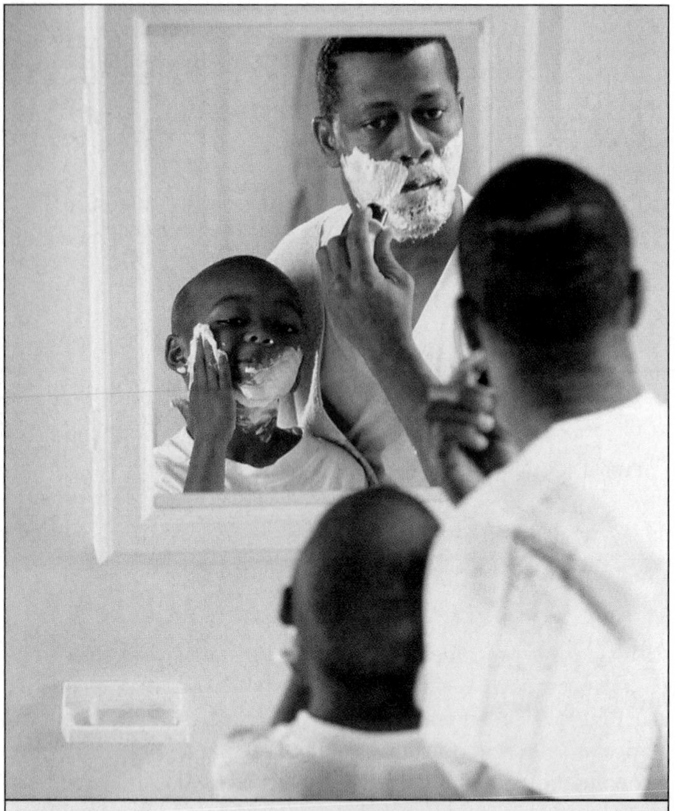

FIGURE 30–1 ■ *Modeling. Imitative learning is also a form of complex learning.*

Source: Andy Sacks/Tony Stone Images.

CLINICAL EXAMPLE

George is a 45-year-old male being treated for schizophrenia. His symptoms are coming under reasonable control with medications and therapy; however, he has been having difficulty lately with his mother. Whenever she cannot visit him, he becomes depressed and agitated. The nurse spoke with him about his current problems, and together they identified an irrational thought George had about his mother. He thought, and felt, that if she didn't visit him every 7 days because she had to work overtime, that meant she did not love him. George felt he would never be able to be "a man" without his mother's love. Once George realized he had that thought about her visiting, he was able to talk to her about her feelings for him. George had to concentrate and work to replace his automatic and irrational thoughts with statements to himself that his mother's love does not need to be renewed—it is always there. George recognized that their visiting schedule and their relationship were not connected. He prepared a number of neutral and positive statements to repeat to himself whenever the old irrational thoughts would appear. Eventually, George was able to tolerate changes in the frequency of his mother's visits.

and the multiple variables that come into play. Unrealistic thought patterns are maladaptive in that they make demands on the individual that cannot be met or cannot be resolved. For example, an elderly adopted woman may believe she has no worth because her birth mother gave her away. In her case, it is unrealistic to assume she might know the reason her mother had her adopted was a malevolent one and, as her birth mother is not likely to be discovered, the demand that she live with this negative perception taints her life.

COGNITIVE THERAPY TECHNIQUES

The purpose of cognitive therapy is to first identify thoughts and thinking that are unrealistic or otherwise problematic for the individual. Once the problematic thoughts are identified, they are examined for their impact on the individual. Nurses are instrumental in helping a client see how a particular set of thoughts can create a problem. Once the connection is made between the set of thoughts and the problem, those thoughts are then addressed. Substituting neutral or positive thoughts for the problematic thinking schema takes place over time. Correction of the automatic problematic thinking is a retraining experience. The individual must unlearn the maladaptive cognitive style then relearn adaptive cognitions.

Positive Imagery

Positive imagery consists of thinking in a positive way about how an event or experience will unfold. This tends to promote the likelihood that the individual will proceed with the activity as envisioned. Positive imagery can also be applied to past events. It is a reframing of the actions taken. For example, a woman is attacked at her parked car and blames herself for being weak, unprepared, and frightened. Positive imagery reframes the woman's actions as perfectly understandable under those circumstances and walks her through the events with this different perspective. It gives her permission to react to frightening events with fear. When directed toward an upcoming event, positive imagery can be a cognitive rehearsal. Thinking in advance about how a set of behaviors or an event will occur guides the individual. This positive attitude about actions helps the individual perform more competently in a variety of situations and with an array of skill sets.

Mastery Imagery

Mastery imagery shapes the individual's thoughts about being in control or having mastery over a particular situation. The point to this technique is to practice imagined successful behavior change. Imagining interacting competently and in an adult manner with someone who abused you in childhood is an example of mastery imagery.

CLINICAL EXAMPLE

Christine imagines and rehearses interacting with her usually overdemanding and agitated supervisor. She would typically respond in a similarly agitated and haphazard manner, resulting in mistakes and problems with her feeling of self-efficacy. Christine's mastery imagery establishes a new routine that consists of interacting with her supervisor in a consistently calm and thorough manner.

Negative Imagery

Another useful cognitive therapy tool to help change maladaptive behaviors is **negative imagery** or envisioning negative events and outcomes. Significant learning can occur by thinking about and thinking through a set of events and responses (Peden, Hall, Rayens, & Beebe, 2000). Thinking in a focused and different manner can help a client refrain from problematic behavior. The steps to this process include:

1. Identification of currently held imagery.
2. Recognition of the real impact of the behavior.
3. Substitution of a negative imagery for the currently held imagery.

The client is taught to identify the imagery invoked (the thoughts) when beginning a maladaptive behavior, such as substance use. It may be something like "Club drugs will be fun" or "I am so much more relaxed and able to interact better when I use this stuff." This is positive imagery. It will promote the use of the substance even though that substance use will interfere with and damage relationships important to the client. The real impact of the behavior is something that can occur only once denial is dispensed with and consequences are recognized. Once the force of the substance use is clearly seen, substituting with negative imagery can be started.

For example, if a client uses cocaine, the positive imagery may be that the drug will make him feel good and it will be better if he does use than if he doesn't. Negatively envisioning cocaine use would consist of the client learning to say and think, "If I use, I will lose control of my thoughts and feelings. It will cost a lot of money, which I don't have, and will put a bigger emotional and physical gap between me and my spouse." The cognitive aspect of this tool is to think only negative thoughts about the drug and its use. Replacement of positive imagery with negative imagery and repetition of the negative imagery are the key components to effective use of this technique. This may reduce the automatic positive associations over time and reduce the urge to use that drug.

Attribution Restructuring

Now that you know what attributions are, and you have some examples of how those attributions can be problematic, the work of attribution restructuring can begin. The heart of cognitive therapy lies in recognizing how we think and behave and in identifying problematic learning. The descriptions of thinking and behaving noted above point out some of the details in this process. People develop patterns of thinking over time. These patterns frequently occur without actively thinking it through; this is referred to as automatic thinking. Automatic thoughts can be developed into specific (and frequently solidly crystallized) sets of automatic thinking. It is important to realize that maladaptive automatic thoughts and attributions require detection prior to intervention.

Attribution restructuring means changing the meanings associated with people, places, and things. Change is the primary goal of attribution restructuring. Clever and articulate use of cognitive therapy concepts is needed to make these types of changes. Once detected, the process of altering and restructuring can begin with interventions focusing on cognitions. Much of what is in this chapter looks at options for making these changes.

Behavior Therapy

Behavior has an impact on feelings and thoughts. For example, an older woman who has a hearing deficit is living with her daughter and son-in-law. She wears a hearing aid, but to save on battery power she removes it and turns it off immediately after dinner every night. Even though they call to her and try to talk to her, she cannot hear. She complains to others that her daughter and son-in-law don't talk to her in the evening and aren't interested in interacting with her. Her behavior isolates her and she does not see the connection between behaving in a manner she identifies as thrifty and the feeling of being lonely.

The ways in which particular types of behavioral therapy can impact on a variety of situations is discussed below.

CLASSICAL CONDITIONING

Generally, behavior therapy is highly effective in reducing the production of problematic behaviors. Behavioral therapy is highly effective when used with a current problem that is relevant to the client's life (Gournay, Denford, Parr, & Newell, 2000). Behavioral therapy focuses on behavioral learning processes including *classical conditioning*. The principles of classical conditioning are:

1. People learn to associate a particular feeling state with a particular circumstance that then becomes a conditioned stimulus for this feeling.
2. Over time, this association is strengthened through repetition and rehearsal.

(See ■ Figure 30–2 on page 712 for an example of a behavior that responds very well to conditioning and intermittent reinforcement.) The therapist's goal in behavior therapy is to decrease or eliminate the association of a particular circumstance (the conditioned stimulus) with a particular feeling.

OPERANT CONDITIONING

Operant conditioning is another aspect of a behavioral learning process and is based on the ideas that:

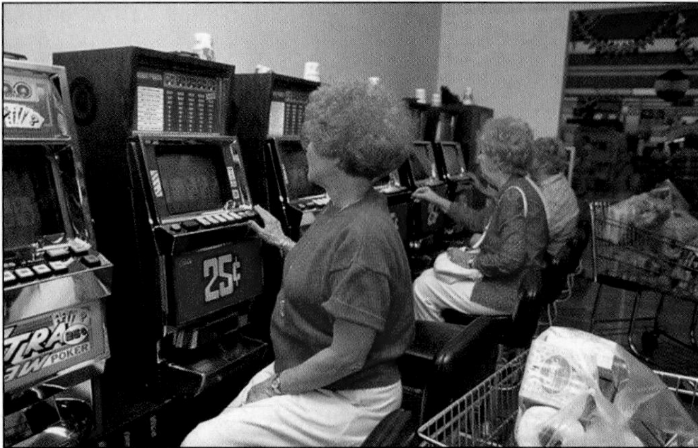

FIGURE 30–2 ■ *Intermittent reinforcement. Operant conditioning involves an association between a stimulus and a response. When people are rewarded for pulling the lever on a slot machine, they repeat the process.*

Source: Bonnie Kamin/Photoedit.

- People are positively reinforced for certain behaviors.
- People learn to seek further **positive reinforcement** (an environmental event that rewards, and thus increases the probability of, a behavioral response) by increasing that behavior.
- Positive reinforcement results from either getting something desirable or avoiding something unpleasant.

The therapist's goal in operant conditioning is to help the individual increase positive reinforcement through more adaptive and effective behavior. Behavioral contracts are ways in which a therapist and a client can plan for specific behavioral change. The effort to change health-related behavior could be facilitated with competent behavioral contracting. An effective behavioral contract must be tailored for the individual and a comprehensive behavioral assessment is necessary to formulate such a contract, as is the formulation of practical, measurable, and feasible objectives and goals. Behavioral contracting is covered in the nursing process section of this chapter.

RATIONAL EMOTIVE BEHAVIORAL THERAPY

Rational Emotive Therapy (RET) was originated by Albert Ellis (1975) and emphasizes cognitive causes of emotional problems along with the individual's taking personal responsibility for maintaining health-damaging thought habits and irrational beliefs. An irrational belief is a belief that lacks reason and sound judgment (Bond, Dryden, & Briscoe, 1999; Cowan & Brunero, 1997). Box 30–2 is a list of some common irrational thoughts that, when incorporated into an individual's belief system, are known to create unhealthy thoughts and feelings. The clinician skilled and expert in RET helps identify irrational thoughts structures with the client and then helps develop a plan to substitute more rational personal life philosophies and attitudes based on accurate and correctly perceived realities

BOX 30–2 Irrational Thoughts

- I need someone—often a specific person—to be with and lean on (I can't do everything by myself).
- It is easier for me to overlook or avoid thinking about tense situations than to face the problems and take the responsibility for correcting the situation.
- I should always be able, successful, and "on top of things" (if I'm not, I'm an inadequate, incompetent, hopeless failure).
- Everyone should love and approve of me (if they don't, I feel awful and unlovable).
- When the situation is scary or going badly, I should be—and can't keep from—worrying all the time.
- When things do not go the way I wanted and planned, it is terrible and I am, of course, going to get very disturbed. I can't stand it!
- Things have been this way so long, I can't do anything about these problems now.
- I know there is an answer to every problem. I should find it (if I don't, it will be awful).
- People who are evil and bad should be punished severely (and I have the right to get very upset if they aren't stopped and made to "pay the price").
- External events, such as other people, a screwed-up society, or bad luck, cause most of my unhappiness. Furthermore, I don't have any control over these external factors, so I can't do anything about my depression or other misery
- I don't like the way I'm feeling but I can't help it. I just have to accept it and go with my feelings.
- When my close friends and relatives have serious problems, it is only right and natural that I get very upset too

Source: Ellis, A. & Harper, R. (1975). *A new guide to rational living*. Albert Ellis Institute.

(Ellis, 1997). Healthy emotional consequences occur when rational thinking drives adequate functional behaviors.

Rational Emotive Behavior Therapy (REBT), as it is now known, identifies and corrects irrational beliefs. Rational and irrational beliefs, defined by REBT, form the basis of inferences derived to explain life experiences. Those inferences can be more or less functional, depending on the beliefs behind them. People who hold rational beliefs form inferences that are significantly more functional than those formed by people who hold irrational beliefs. The following Clinical Example illustrates how firmly held irrational beliefs can inhibit functioning.

CLINICAL EXAMPLE

Marvin, a 38-year-old forklift operator was injured on the job 4 years ago. Although his back injuries were treated and all tests indicate a complete recovery, he continues to complain of back pain and exhibits a reduced ability to function at work. His pain complaints have become chronic, and he is referred to a specialist in psychotherapy for chronic pain. In an REBT session he describes an early experience of observing his father's lengthy illness of cancer, during which his father was quite sedentary and his mother reacted catastrophically every time she saw Marvin's father attempt to be more active. In REBT it emerged that Marvin had acquired an irrational core belief that problems or fears are best responded to with rest, withdrawal, and being sedentary. Marvin's past pain symptoms were uncomfortable enough to trigger this response, consistent with his core belief. As he became more sedentary and less functional, his back became increasingly weak and prone to pain symptoms. His overfocus on the pain symptoms resulted in reduced activity levels, leading to a vicious cycle of increasing pain and withdrawal.

In REBT, Marvin learned to identify his irrational belief. This was accomplished through a Socratic question-and-answer format whereby Marvin was able to identify withdrawal and inactivity as leading to more problems rather than to fewer problems. The sources for this belief were clarified as well. This belief was reframed in a more rational direction—that many problems respond best to constructive and productive activity. Specifically, Marvin's chronic pain problem was likely to improve with exercise, physical therapy, and daily productive activity. Assignments were given between sessions for Marvin to develop his repertoire in these areas. As he successfully proceeded to do so, his pain symptoms diminished and his self-esteem increased.

The Socratic question-and-answer format is an important aspect of REBT. This method, illustrated in Box 30–3, allows the client to explore how a particular line of reasoning was allowed to develop and how it continues to exist. It focuses on a logical perspective of problems, which is an appealing and manageable therapeutic style to which many adults can relate. As with all therapeutic styles, though, there must be a fit between the client and the therapeutic intervention. Not all therapy will be useful, or even therapeutic, with all clients in all situations.

BOX 30–3 The Socratic Question-and-Answer Format

Marvin: "I spent the day in bed yesterday because my back hurt."

Therapist: "What did you hope that would accomplish?"

Marvin: "That my back would feel better."

Therapist: "Did it?"

Marvin: "No."

Therapist: "Can you ever remember a time when inactivity made your back feel better?"

Marvin: "No, it just gets worse."

Therapist: "So where and how did you come to believe that inactivity would make your back feel better?"

Marvin: "In my family we always rested when we were hurt."

Therapist: "Did that help your family?"

Marvin: "Come to think of it, not that I ever saw."

Therapist: "Maybe too much resting doesn't help?"

Marvin: "I never thought of it that way."

Therapist: "If too much resting doesn't help, what else might?"

Marvin: "Once when my back hurt I went to a chiropractor and did some exercises. I remember that helped."

Therapist: "What does that tell you about resting too much?"

Marvin: "Maybe it's not such a good idea."

BEHAVIOR MODIFICATION

Behavior modification frequently focuses on a target behavior that is somehow problematic for the individual (i.e., overeating) or problematic for the community (i.e., loud, verbal outbursts). The behavior is observed and tracked in objective and measurable terms, then addressed with a behavior modification plan. Both nonpharmacologic and pharmacologic interventions may be employed to assist in the modification of behavioral disturbances (Kolko, Bukstein, & Barron, 1999; Robinson, Smith, Miller, & Brownell, 1999). We will discuss nonpharmacologic behavioral modification interventions here. Pharmacologic interventions are discussed in Chapter 31.

A behavior modification program begins with the identification of a specific behavior that requires change. It is important to monitor the target behavior that requires the modification and develop a detailed database about that behavior. Observation of the problem behavior is carefully made, including:

- Antecedents (what came before).
- Precipitants (what appeared to cause or provoke the behavior).
- Particular expression of the behavior for that individual.
- Timing.
- Frequency.
- Duration.
- Individual strengths to be capitalized on in designing the plan.

To enable a client to modify behavior that is undesirable or unhealthy, support and involvement in a plan of action are required. One strategy for mobilizing a behavior modification program organizes the individual's hierarchy of difficulty with not performing the problem behavior. This hierarchy is established with the least distressing changes of the process at the low level of distress and the most distressing aspects at the highest hierarchical level. For example, scores from 0 to 100 would represent the level of distress as 0, or nothing, all the way to 100, or the highest level of difficulty they can imagine. Someone who overeats may have only slight distress, or a score of 15, when thinking about not eating at a movie or a sporting event. A much higher distress level at the top of one's hierarchy, a score of 85, might occur when considering what it would feel like to be in an unfamiliar or uncomfortable social environment and not be able to eat.

The individual is guided through imagining a situation at the lowest levels of distress initially and developing and rehearsing adaptive responses to the distress. This establishes a newly learned pattern that supplants the older, maladaptive responses. This is called **response prevention,** meaning the maladaptive responses, which were automatic, are being modified and replaced with adaptive behaviors. Gradually, the client advances through his or her hierarchy of distress learning to develop skills in responding competently at every step.

Desensitization, another behavioral modification treatment regimen, also uses a hierarchy to arrange treatment. Behaviors are identified and ordered according to how distressing they might be for the individual. The client imagines being in certain situations at various levels of distress and learns to cope before moving on to the next level of distress. See Box 30–4 for a desensitization hierarchy for a phobic fear of heights.

Assignments for graded exposures and response prevention are usually completed as homework accompanied by self-monitoring (through diaries and/or graphs) and clinical assessment of progress through the behavioral programming. The behavior modification plan requires a realistic appraisal of the difficulties facing someone who wants to make a change and includes a plan for those difficulties (Lindell & Reinke, 1999). A sample plan for someone wanting to quit smoking must include the following three steps:

1. An appreciation for triggering mechanisms urging one to smoke.
2. Activities prepared to substitute for the habit of smoking.
3. Recognizing what supports will promote success in unlearning the rituals of smoking behavior.

Under the circumstances of someone trying to quit smoking, the environment should be smoke free and all smoking materials and accoutrements must be disposed of in order to minimize relapses. There are psychopharmacologic supports for the smoking cessation process. See Chapter 31, Psychopharmacology, for more information. See Box 30–5 for behavior modification tips for smoking cessation.

THOUGHT STOPPING

Thought stopping is an example of a cognitive–behavioral psychotherapeutic technique that can be used to help a client change thinking processes. Changing thinking processes is important as cognitive–behaviorists maintain that a client's feelings can be strongly influenced by the pattern and process of thoughts (Tang & DeRubeis, 1999).

BOX 30–4 Desensitization Hierarchy for Phobic Fear of Heights

1. Develop 10 to 12 scenes of increasing approximation to the fear. *Example*: Tell the client to imagine:
   "You are going up a kitchen stepladder; step to the third rung, and look around."
   "Now you are going up to the top rung. You are up to the top. Look around at the cupboards. Look at the floor."
   "Now you are on the second floor of an office building. You walk toward the window and look out."
2. Continue in this manner, advancing the scene to nearer approximations of the fear each time the client is able to visualize without undue anxiety.
   "Now you go to the top of the Sears Tower. You go over to the guard rail and look straight down."
3. The final steps of the desensitization process include encouraging the client to try some of these behaviors in real life, after the simulations have been successful.

BOX 30–5 Smoking Cessation Behavior Modifications Guidance

Helping a Smoker to Quit

- Set up a grid indicating the typical smoking schedule.
- Develop a tracking mechanism for where the individual smoked.
- Use checklists for situations and interactions with others in which smoking is an element of the situation or interaction.
- Insert a set of behaviors to substitute for smoking.
- Provide self-help literature.
- Encourage those in the environment to also quit.
- Provide motivational material related to current health status.
- Problem-solve to enhance coping with stressors.
- Enhance skills for coping with stressors.
- Emphasize positive benefits.
- Provide individual support.
- Reinforce short-term success.
- Support through group therapy.

Clients sometimes have difficulty with repetitive, maladaptive thinking. Examples include:

- A client repeatedly thinks inaccurate negative thoughts about himself or herself.
- A client worries incessantly from thinking anxiety-evoking thoughts repeatedly.

For these clients the cognitive behavioral therapist may implement a procedure known as thought stopping. The client learns to stop negative or maladaptive thinking by visualizing or imagining an image, sensation, or circumstance associated with the stoppage of a particular thought process. Examples of thought stopping include these images or thinking by the client:

- Visualizing a traffic stop sign.
- Imagining hearing the word "stop" said loudly.
- Imagining the tactile sensation of leaning up against a closed door.

Thought stopping would be done whenever the identified negative or maladaptive thought occurred. Over time, the client learns to stop such thoughts in an almost reflexive manner. This technique would typically be used as part of a larger package of techniques that could also include developing alternative thoughts and mastering behavioral skills to alter outcomes in various problematic circumstances.

Cognitive–behavioral therapy (www.cognitive-behavior-therapy.org) is defined and explained on the Companion Website.

Cognitive–Behavioral Therapy

We learn from our experiences and the interpretation of those experiences. Cognitions and their behavioral sequelae determine how and what we learn. Labeling or assigning a certain meaning to an experience accompanies expectations about the outcome. Our behavior is usually consistent with those expectations while experiencing congruent feelings. The basic idea of cognitive–behavioral theory is that thoughts and behaviors lead to feelings.

MediaLink Cognitive–Behavioral Therapy

The goal in cognitive–behavioral treatment is to develop healthier labeling and an expectancy strategy that leads to more desirable feelings and an increase in a feeling of self-efficacy. Beck (1976) describes problem development as arising from relevant childhood learning of core beliefs and making associations (www.beckinstitute.org). ■ Figure 30–3 describes the basic premise of this formulation of human cognitive–behavioral problem development.

Following that early learning, labels and expectations influence the strategies the individual selects to compensate and cope. Situations are dealt with as they arise within the particular pattern that has been developed. ■ Figure 30–4 on page 716 displays the possible cognitive–behavioral model of problem development in panic disorder with agoraphobia. The following Clinical Example describes this problem development.

CLINICAL EXAMPLE

Webster is a traveling salesman who must drive long distances to meet with his clients. One day while having a meeting with a client, he experienced a panic attack. His symptoms included shortness of breath, rapid heartbeat, and thoughts of wanting to escape the situation. After this happened, he was very tired. He decided to stop work early and drive home. He noticed when he got home that he felt more relaxed and relieved. He hoped it was an isolated event that would not happen again.

In time, Webster began to have more panic attacks. He longed to be at home when these occurred because he experienced relief and more comfort there. Soon, he began to decrease his meetings with clients, trying to have telephone or Internet meetings with them instead. The more he succeeded in relieving himself of the burden of leaving his house, the more anxious he became when he was required to leave home. Eventually, he became almost completely unable to leave home whether it was for business, social, or any other purpose (such as an emergency with a friend). Even when thinking about stepping outside of his house, Webster had a panic attack. He had developed diagnosable panic disorder with agoraphobia at a severe level.

MediaLink Beck Institute

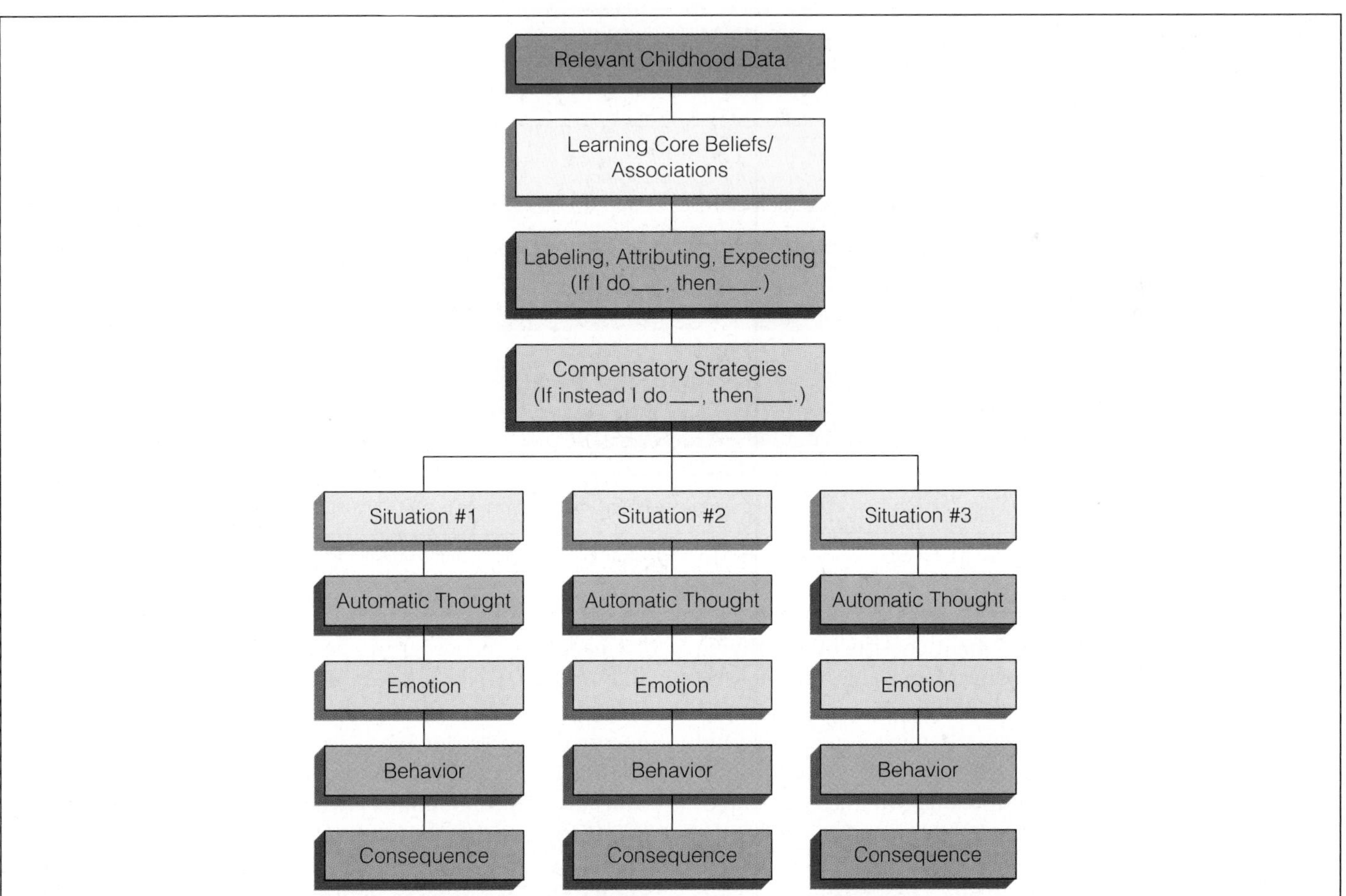

FIGURE 30–3 ■ *Cognitive-behavioral model of problem development.*

Source: Adapted from Cognitive Therapy and the Emotional Disorders by Beck, by permission of International Universities Press, Inc. Copyright 1976 by International Universities Press, Inc.

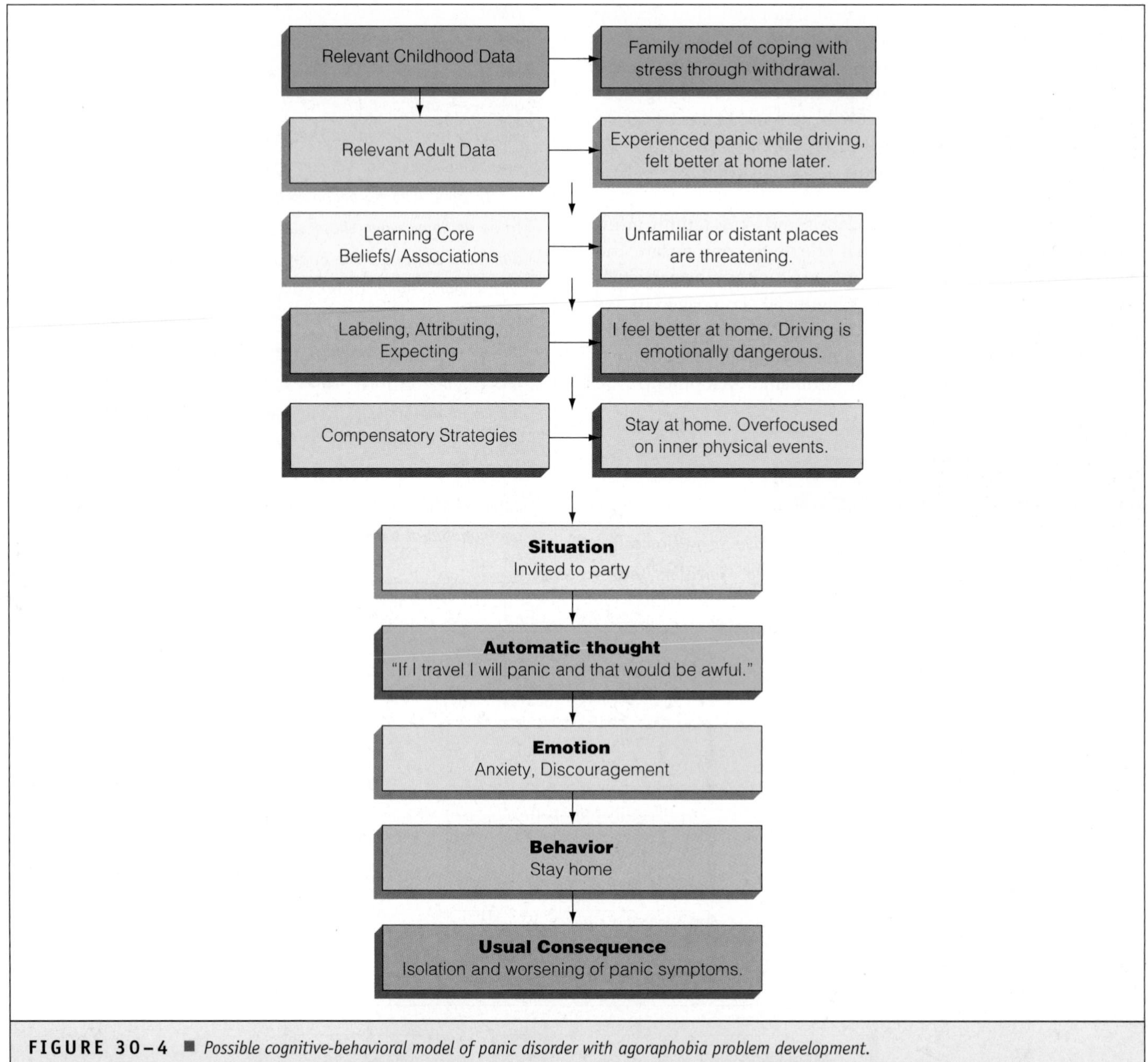

FIGURE 30–4 ■ *Possible cognitive-behavioral model of panic disorder with agoraphobia problem development.*

Source: Adapted from Cognitive Therapy and the Emotional Disorders by Beck, by permission of International Universities Press, Inc. Copyright 1976 by International Universities Press, Inc.

Cognitive and behavioral treatment consists of identifying and recognizing maladaptive thinking styles and working toward acquisition of new skills for managing stressors. Features of treatment include teaching, interpreting, reframing, and learning and practicing new behaviors (Kaas & Lewis, 1999). Once thoughts and behaviors are realistically and rationally framed and implemented, emotional reactions will be consistent with them. See the Using Research Evidence feature for a description of how these treatment features are incorporated into a group setting.

DIALECTICAL BEHAVIORAL THERAPY

Linehan specifically developed Dialectical Behavioral Therapy (DBT) for the outpatient treatment of chronically suicidal people with borderline personality disorder (Linehan et al., 1999). DBT is a specialized subset of the Cognitive–Behavioral treatment modalities. The client with borderline personality disorder tends to be crisis prone with intense relational episodes (Linehan, Heard, & Armstrong, 1993). In other words, interactions with others have the potential to disrupt the client powerfully. DBT is a biosocial behavioral model of treatment that assumes there is a disorder in the regulation of emotions and how the client tolerates stress (Bohus et al., 2000; Koerner & Linehan, 2000). The numerous dysfunctional patterns of behavior common in the diagnosis of borderline personality disorder, such as self-destructive behavior, inability to govern impulses, or severe dissociative

USING RESEARCH EVIDENCE

Mike Forbit, an 11-year-old boy, was brought to the clinic by his parents. He has always been an anxious child; however, lately he has not been functioning well in many areas. Mike's mother was especially concerned because she has anxiety disorder herself and worries that her son may not "grow out of it" as many of their friends keep saying. Your assessment of Mike verifies his heightened state of anxiety and you recommend a 10-session cognitive–behavioral group that incorporates children and parents into a treatment framework. The Forbits agree and begin treatment.

During this cognitive–behavioral oriented group intervention, relevant terms and definitions are discussed. The children are initially invited to describe cues of anxiety-provoking situations and the emotional, cognitive, and somatic components that accompany their experiences. You and your co-therapist employ several of the possible cognitive–behavioral foci throughout the group, such as:

- Relaxation techniques.
- The pros and cons of anxiety.
- Identifying automatic self-talk and identifying feelings accompanying anxiety-provoking situations.
- Identifying cognitive pitfalls.
- Recognizing triggers.
- Learning to make a hierarchy of anxiety provoking situations.
- Employing graded exposure.
- Cues for coping.
- Modifying anxious self-talk into coping self-talk.
- Building realistic self-evaluations.
- Developing self-reward strategies.

Exercises for rehearsal, problem solving, and creative thinking are also employed. Homework and assignments of all the above techniques are regularly given.

Mike and his parents attend each of the 10 weekly sessions, after which outcome evaluations are completed. You find that Mike's anxiety has decreased, he has fewer anxiety symptoms, and you set up a schedule for follow-up. You may note, however, that the anxiety level of Ms. Forbit, who is herself anxious, may not have changed. Mike is encouraged to continue with his cognitive–behavioral assignments in order to maintain the advances he has made.

These interventions were developed using cognitive–behavioral principles in conjunction with:

Toren, P., Wolmer, L., Rosenthal, B., Eldar, S., Koren, S., Lask, M., Weizman, R., & Laor, N. (2000). Case series: Brief parent–child group therapy for childhood anxiety disorders using a manual-based cognitive-behavioral technique. *Journal of the American Academy of Child and Adolescent Psychiatry, 39*, 1309–1312.

phenomena, are regarded within DBT as the client's attempts to problem solve.

DBT is a psychosocial treatment program with the focus on teaching clients four skills:

1. Mindfulness (attention to one's experience).
2. Interpersonal effectiveness.
3. Emotional regulation.
4. Distress tolerance.

DBT has cognitive as well as behavioral features. This concept of therapy focuses on the continuing balance between the necessity of accepting maladaptive behavior patterns (a cognitive feature) in both an intrapsychic and an interactional context while still working to change them (the behavioral feature). Improvements in rates of depression, dissociation, anxiety, and global stress occur with this method (Wiser & Telch, 1999).

DBT is a clearly structured therapy and integrates a wide choice of therapeutic strategies. It is a promising psychosocial intervention for improving interpersonal functioning among severely dysfunctional patients with borderline personality disorder (www.aabt.org).

CULTURAL ASPECTS OF COGNITIVE–BEHAVIORAL INTERVENTIONS

Cultural considerations involve more than an individual's race or ethnicity. Culture is an envelope that includes, among other characteristics, religion, spirituality, gender, disability, sexual orientation and expression, social status, and age. To be a competent provider of cognitive–behavioral interventions you must have an increased awareness of these variables at the minimum; you must be conscientious about who you are and how anyone different from who you are would be best addressed. See the Nursing Self-Awareness feature on page 718 to sensitize you to the forces of a dominant culture. How to implement this conscientiousness with a cognitive–behavioral intervention framework will be briefly stated here. Chapter 6, Cultural Competence and Psychiatric Epidemiology, explores cultural considerations in detail.

The individual is emphasized in cognitive–behavioral interventions (what the person thinks, feels, interprets, assigns meanings to, etc.); therefore, it can be the ideal venue to address multiculturalism in treatment. Consider the following clinical situation.

MediaLink 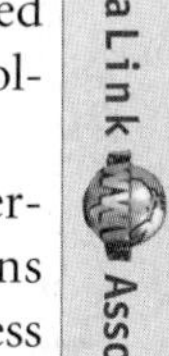 Association for Advancement of Behavior Therapy 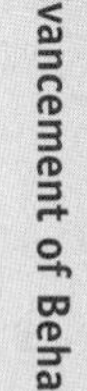

CLINICAL EXAMPLE

Rachel is very upset about being spoken to in a harsh and loud manner by her male supervisor at work. It seems to her that every day she feels demoralized after interacting with him. She is working with you within a cognitive–behavioral framework. Rachel is willing to make several changes in her thinking and behavior in order to feel and function better. She may require cognitive restructuring, mastery imagery, and assertiveness and communication assignments.

Now incorporate her cultural characteristics: She is young, has an untreated 20% hearing loss, and is Egyptian-American. You may change the overall structure of her plan (or not), but you would certainly shape your interventions around these specific issues in the direction dictated by the interventions mentioned above.

NURSING SELF-AWARENESS Forces of a Dominant Culture

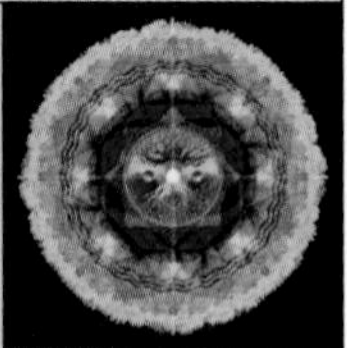

Are you able to see a difference between a member of a dominant cultural group, yourself, and a client? Listed below are some major characteristics. Fill in how you express these characteristics in your culture and define what the dominant group is for the situation. Is there a difference? Being a member of the dominant group in any of these characteristics shapes who you are, just as not being a member of the dominant group has the power to shape. Now see if there is a difference between you, your client, and the dominant culture on these characteristics. Make yourself aware on an ongoing basis of the influence this will have on your cognitive–behavioral interventions.

Characteristic	Your Characteristics	Dominant Group	Client's Characteristics
Religion			
Spirituality			
Gender			
Ability/Disability			
Sexual Orientation and Expression			
Social Status			
Age			
Race			
Ethnicity			

There is a further benefit to this combination of cognitive–behavioral interventions and multiculturalism. The value placed on the individual unlearning maladaptations, learning new skills, practicing them, and ultimately becoming independently proficient at implementing them is essentially an individual process. It empowers clients to use their cultural reality as opposed to negating cultural influences (Hays, 1995). It is also interesting to note how easily cognitive–behavioral interventions can be applied with clients whose primary language is not English because the concepts are concrete (specific thoughts, feelings, events, behaviors) and not abstract.

NURSING PROCESS

Behavioral Contracting

The effort to change health-related behavior may be facilitated with competent behavioral contracting. A behavioral contract is a behavior modification plan arranged as a more specific agreement between the individual and the caregivers who identify the behavior and design the plan as a team. An effective behavioral contract must be tailored for the individual client. A comprehensive behavioral assessment is necessary to form such a contract, as is the identification of practical and measurable objectives and goals that are feasible for the client. The components of a behavioral contract in the form of the nursing process follow.

Assessment

A comprehensive behavioral interview is the first step in developing a behavioral contract with the goal of client behavioral change. The purpose of the assessment interview is to assemble a complete picture of what the behavior is and what maintains it or keeps it going, so that ideas on how to change the behavior have the best chance of success. The interview process identifies problem behavior. It is useful to divide the problem behavior into four components to be explored in turn:

- *Behavioral* component asks what the client is doing.
- *Cognitive* component examines client thinking.
- *Affective* component identifies what the client is feeling.
- *Physiologic* component looks at the physical realities of the situation.

What precipitates or precedes this client's problem behavior? Try to identify when it occurs, such as only when the client is anxious, with certain people, or in certain places. What are the consequences of the problem behavior for this client? Assess whether the problem behavior endangers the client's life. Make a determination whether the problem behaviors make the client relax or get angry.

Other important assessments must be made as to the negative and positive reinforcements for the problem behavior. For example, with cigarette smoking, the **negative reinforcement** (alteration of an adverse stimulus to increase the probability that a behavioral response will occur) would be the health problems associated with smoking. There also could be family or societal disapproval of the behavior. Positive reinforcement with smoking behaviors could be the satisfaction of the nicotine craving or filling up time with an activity labeled by the client as enjoyable.

Environmental factors (family, economic, and social) may be influencing the problem behavior. The success of a behavioral contract can be traced to the awareness of the environment within which the contract is being implemented. If other family members or the client's friends smoke, or if social occasions are always in smoking areas, the behavioral contract needs to be sensitive to this aspect in order to be successful.

Assessing the intrapsychic factors influencing the problem behavior can be accomplished through the assessment interview. Catalog whether the client:

- Has assertiveness skills.
- Experiences stress when the client asserts physiologic needs with other people (such as stating to friends, "I have a lot of trouble staying away from cigarettes when others smoke around me.").
- Has fragile relationships or dependent or abusive relationships.

All of these factors would have to be taken into account in order to effectively develop a viable behavioral contract.

The thorough and comprehensive interview also includes any difficulties with depression, irritability, anxiety, psychotic symptomatology (hearing voices/seeing things or believing in unreal thoughts), substance or alcohol use/abuse, or addictive/compulsive behavior. Smoking would be a kind of addictive behavior, while refusing to adhere to bed rest instructions in order to do housework would be compulsive and self-destructive with, for example, cleaning compulsions.

Current psychosocial variables are essential features to be documented in a thorough interview and assessment. These variables include present employment, marital and family status, social and romantic functioning, and avocational pursuits. Hobbies can be quite powerful in their destructive as well as constructive impact, especially if the hobby revolves around a problematic set of behaviors (i.e., bowling and drinking beer while smoking).

Typical daily routines including eating, sleeping, and exercise habits contribute valuable information for the contract. If possible, observe the client in problem behavior activities to confirm or disconfirm self-reports of the behavior you are cataloging. Collateral information through family, work records, friends, colleagues, and other treatment providers can offer a perspective on the set of behaviors that the client may not be able to generate. Ultimately, the assessment interview seeks to identify how the client anticipates that this behavior change might alter his or her life.

Nursing Diagnosis: NANDA

Nursing diagnoses emerge from the comprehensive assessment. The individualized information you carefully acquired will be prioritized into the most relevant problem areas and addressed under the diagnostic category to which you have assigned the set of behaviors. The nature and intensity of the problem area determines whether it will be addressed immediately, or whether other issues are more pressing. Problems identified as needing less immediate intervention are monitored and addressed as prioritized issues are resolved.

Examples of nursing diagnoses that may arise from a cognitive behavioral assessment in preparation for the development of a behavioral contract include:

- Knowledge Deficit.
- Altered Family Processes.
- Impaired Social Interaction.
- Hopelessness.
- Ineffective Individual Coping.
- Ineffective Health Maintenance.

Outcome Identification: NOC

Evidence of a successful outcome for behavioral problems would be seen in the patterns of responses the client makes to circumstances that would previously have been distressing or difficult. Knowledge about one's disease process, medication, treatment regimen, or health behaviors would indicate a positive outcome for a knowledge deficit. If the client displayed hope, it would address the change in the diagnosed state of hopelessness. Altered Family Processes would be addressed with the outcome of family functioning and coping. When a client has behaviors that warrant the nursing diagnosis of Impulse Control, identification of harm and what triggers these behaviors, and then avoiding those high-risk situations, constitutes a successful outcome.

In general, outcomes for behavioral change are easily identified. Behaviors are objective criteria by which progress can be tracked. Behaviors can be compared to previous behaviors for similarities or differences. If less frequent than previously they may be considered to be changed.

Planning and Implementation: NIC

The planning phase of the nursing process with behavioral contracting requires observation of how the client interacted with you during the interview. These observations comprise components of the mental status exam such as appearance; facial expression; motor behavior; cooperativeness; quality of speech, including spontaneity, pace, volume, response time, coherence, and relevance; and goal directedness. Your observations on whether the client's affect was appropriate or inappropriate, along with notations on mood, lethality, delusions, hallucinations, and orientation to person-place-time-purpose contribute information necessary in planning to intervene. The client's immediate, short-term, and long-term memory abilities along with evidence of executive functioning (such as the ability to carry out several-step activities independently) give direction to how your client thinks. Each aspect of how someone thinks and reacts and remembers makes up their cognitive style—or the overall pattern of thought. A cognitive style is the way someone thinks best—verbal versus nonverbal; single versus multimedia preferences; independent functioning versus requiring support. For example, some people respond better to audiovisual rather than printed material, or they perform tasks more effectively with persistent encouragement versus occasional monitoring. These differences in cognitive style shape several components in your behavioral contract. This site, www.nacbt.org/, for the National Association of Cognitive–Behavioral Therapists is accessible through the Companion Website for the text. The site has information about cognitive–behavioral therapy and its uses in treatment.

MediaLink: Association: Cognitive–Behavioral Therapists

FORMING OF PRACTICAL AND MEASURABLE OBJECTIVES AND GOALS

Formulating practical and measurable objectives and goals is the next step in the behavioral contract. Objectives are small steps leading to goal attainment, while goals represent the overall desired outcomes. Prioritizing the behavioral objectives involves four main features:

1. The goal should be directly contributory to the desired result. In other words, how is this activity of tracking all cigarettes smoked and under what circumstances by the client going to help him or her stop smoking? (It will sensitize the client and you to what contributes to smoking behavior and will point out to the client just how much and when he or she smokes.)
2. The goal can objectively be monitored. (We know the objective is being reached when the client completes the tracking mechanism.)
3. The goal is easily understood by the client and all involved supportive significant others. (The client knows how to fill out the tracking mechanism and knows why he or she is tracking the behavior.)
4. The goal is not too difficult for the client to accomplish in the available time. (The client can fill out the form daily for 1 week.)

Behavioral goals should be objectively verifiable as contributing to positive treatment outcome. The change is required and relevant, not something outlandish (it is relevant to track how often one smokes through daily journaling; it is outlandish to set as a goal never having another craving to smoke). The goal is agreed upon and understood by the client, all significant others, and the treatment team, and is not likely to be contradictory to other important and unmodified aspects of the client's health and/or psychosocial, interpersonal, or intrapersonal functioning. Remember who you are formulating this contract with—you will not be asking a lifelong introvert to engage in sensitive self-disclosure in an intense support group.

NEGOTIATING A BEHAVIORAL CONTRACT

The basic rules for negotiating a behavioral contract include engaging the client as a colleague in the formulation of the contract, avoiding use of complex terminology or coercive formats, and making sure the client completely understands, agrees to, and, to the extent possible, feels comfortable with the contract. Potential problems can have a minimal impact if they are detected early in the process. If you anticipate and address them, the client does not have to experience failure simply because the contract was not designed well enough. Issues and problems include a lack of understanding, lack of commitment, lack of adequate follow-up monitoring, and a lack of a defined format or contingency plan for unforeseen problems. Poor design of the contract can happen when it is in conflict with important and unchangeable aspects of the client's psychosocial functioning. The Intervention box below summarizes the behavioral contracting process.

Adjustments to the contract to maximize success are regular evaluations and trouble-shooting meetings based on a sufficient collection of ongoing objective data describing contract compliance. Contracts can be adjusted in many ways including formal supports and prioritization of various objectives and appropriate revisions of goals. Creativity is an essential component in effective supervision of contract compliance.

Collecting data on contract compliance can be accomplished through client self-monitoring, client self-report at regular meetings, discussion in counseling sessions, and natural or scheduled observations of the client. Further information can be collected from relatives, friends, colleagues, and other treatment providers.

Optimizing the client's abilities to adhere to a behavioral contract requires careful assessment and determination of the client's barriers. Check for overall intellectual functioning as well as cognitive style. Emotional perspectives can influence performance and outcome. Does the client manifest depression, irritability, or anxiety that would interfere with contract adherence? It is important to design supports that will address these affective problems while promoting contract success. Motivational aspects of the individual can also play a large part in outcome (Burns & Spangler, 2000). Was the client poorly motivated to begin with and what was done to address this problem? If design features to address motivation were implemented, check to see how it is working. Is the client demonstrating a decline in motivation? If so, why (psychiatric, social, economic, or medical causation)? Address all underlying causative factors.

Physiology can affect outcome. Is the client experiencing side effects or is a main effect of a medication

INTERVENTION

Highlights of Developing a Behavioral Contract

Step	Purpose	Action	Strategy
1.	Comprehensive behavioral assessment	Interview	Interactions
2.	Formulating practical and measurable objectives and goals	Prioritizing	Evaluating abilities
3.	Negotiating a behavioral contract	Basic rules	Making adjustments
		Potential problems	Evaluating
4.	Optimizing the client's abilities to adhere to a behavioral contract	Barrier Determination • Intellectual • Emotional • Motivational • Physiologic	Constructive Catalysts • Psychotherapy • Relaxation Training • Biofeedback • Family Involvement

(such as mood stabilization for symptoms of mania) bothering the client? If the client perceives this behavioral change as threatening to an established lifestyle and interaction pattern or if the client becomes uncomfortable with the independence or responsibilities expected of him or her following the behavioral change, this could sabotage compliance.

Constructive catalysts are those tools that will enhance the process without interference. Some psychotherapeutic interventions are likely to be useful with most clients undergoing a stressor. These include general stress management, preparation for likely emotional consequences and adjustment difficulties that changing health behaviors can cause, the opportunity to ventilate and disclose feelings, and support. Relaxation training or biofeedback can be included for more specialized treatment and techniques (Davis, McKay, & Eshelman, 2000). Family Involvement, if there is involved family, is a powerful and useful catalyst for promoting and maintaining behavioral change. Significant others, particularly those with whom the client resides or will reside, are likely to provide important input mediating the level of contract adherence. It is therefore important to involve them as much as appropriate with formulation and implementation of behavioral contracts. If it doesn't fit for the involved family, it won't fit for the client.

■ Figure 30–5 is a sample behavioral contract format and outline and gives an overview of how the process of combining medications and behavioral change can be documented. Sections may be expanded or eliminated depending upon the targeted behavior and client need. Imagine a health behavior of your own that could be changed and walk yourself through this behavioral contract. If you can develop a plan to change your behavior, you may very well be successful helping others to change theirs.

MEDICATIONS

Often, clients will have anxiety when faced with making behavioral changes. This anxiety is best handled through supportive and instructive interactions. However, some individuals require physiologic support to prevent their anxiety from reaching panic levels. Anxiolytics, or antianxiety medications, could be administered in sufficient quantities to reduce that problematic affect yet leave

Sample Behavioral Contract Format

Client Name ______________________ Date __________

Problem behavior: ______________________

Problem Behavior Components

Behavioral	Affective
Cognitive	Physiological

Interview Findings

Depression	Anxiety	Substance or Alcohol Use/Abuse
Irritability	Psychotic Symptomatology	Addictive/Compulsive Behavior

Psychosocial Variables

Present Employment	Social/Romantic Functioning	Typical Daily Routines
Marital/Family Status	Avocational Pursuits	Eating/Sleeping/Exercise Habits
How the Client Anticipates That This Behavior Change Might Alter Any of the Above		

Collateral information ______________________

Cognitive Style

Which of the following apply for this contract?

- ☐ Psychotherapy for any current psychological problems.
- ☐ Relaxation Training/Biofeedback
- ☐ General stress management
- ☐ Preparation for likely emotional consequences and adjustment difficulties
- ☐ The opportunity to ventilate and disclose feelings
- ☐ Support

Contract Objectives and Goals

This Goal is agreed upon and understood by the client, all significant others, and the treatment team.

Signature ______________________

Signature ______________________

Signature ______________________

Signature ______________________

FIGURE 30–5 ■ *Sample behavioral contract format.*

the client with enough anxiety to be motivated to learn behavioral techniques for anxiety management where appropriate. Dosing anxiolytics such that there is no anxiety whatsoever is considered counter-therapeutic. Anxiety at low to moderate levels has been found in many circumstances to be motivating and healthful.

Evaluation

Evaluating client abilities and strengths, particularly with regard to learning and making changes, will help the design of the contract. Discover what other situations requiring behavioral change the client has mastered and how he or she accomplished that change. What specific personal or social strengths did the client employ in implementing that successful change? Evaluate client weaknesses with regard to learning and making changes as well. What has the client attempted to change without success? Try to ascertain what specific factors interfered with the success of that goal.

Formulated objectives and goals should draw upon strengths and prior patterns of successful change for the client. What the client is asked to do should mirror what the client has previously done successfully as closely as possible. This is because the best predictor of future behavior is past behavior.

In order for contracts to have successful outcomes, the contract needs to be carefully crafted. The components of a behavioral contract are to be framed in the success (i.e., maintain abstinence) rather than failure (i.e., will not relapse into use) mode.

Case Management

It is important to focus on the maintenance of the routines and schedules of cognitive–behavioral interventions once a plan of care has been established. The case manager can be helpful in sustaining that structure. The variety of interventions, such as group, individual therapy, behavior modification and self-study can all be promoted and supported through case management.

Community-Based Care and Home care

Each of the problems addressed with cognitive-behavioral interventions benefit from maintaining those interventions in the client's natural setting. Counseling, psychotherapy, and other treatments discussed in this chapter are frequently conducted in the community. The behavioral contract can be designed to address inpatient issues and community living, and enhance the transition from inpatient treatment to an outpatient setting. Additional supports can be built into the contract to assure the client's success when inpatient to outpatient care occurs. These interventions in the community maximize both the quality of life and management of symptoms.

Family psychoeducation can be an integral feature of community-based care and home care. Teaching about symptoms and how to address them with the planned interventions is supportive and reassuring. Involving significant others increases the likelihood that the plan of care is implemented and that frustrations and misunderstandings are minimized.

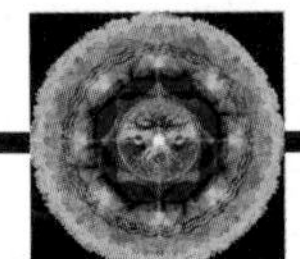

EXPLORE MediaLink

NCLEX review, case studies, and other interactive resources for this chapter can be found on the Companion Website at http://www.prenhall.com/kneisl. Click on Chapter 30 to select the activities for this chapter.

For animations, video tutorials, more NCLEX review questions, and an audio glossary, access the accompanying CD-ROM in this textbook.

BIBLIOGRAPHY

Beck, A. T. (1976). *Cognitive therapy and the emotional disorders.* New York: International Universities Press.

Beck, A. T., Freeman, A., & Associates. (1990). *Cognitive therapy of personality disorders*. New York: Guilford Press.

Bohus, M., Haaf, B., Stiglmayr, C., Pohl, U., Bohme, R., & Linehan, M. (2000). Evaluation of inpatient dialectical-behavioral therapy for borderline personality disorder—a prospective study. *Behaviour Research & Therapy 38,* 875–887.

Bond, F. W., Dryden, W., & Briscoe, R. (1999). Testing two mechanisms by which rational and irrational beliefs may affect the functionality of inferences. *British Journal of Medical Psychology, 72,* 557–566.

Burns, D. D., & Spangler, D. L. (2000). Does psychotherapy homework lead to improvements in depression in cognitive-behavioral therapy or does improvement lead to increased homework compliance? *Journal of Consulting and Clinical Psychology, 68,* 46–56.

Cowan, D., & Brunero, S. (1997). Group therapy for anxiety disorders using rational emotive behaviour therapy. *Australian & New Zealand Journal of Mental Health Nursing, 6,* 164–168.

Davis, M., McKay, M., & Eshelman, E. R., (2000). *The relaxation and stress reduction workbook*. Alcoa, TN: Fine Communications.

Ellis A. (1997). Albert Ellis on rational emotive behavior therapy. *American Journal of Psychotherapy, 51,* 309–316.

Ellis, A. (1975). *A new guide to rational living.* Upper Saddle River, NJ: Prentice Hall.

Gournay, K., Denford, L., Parr, A. M., & Newell, R. (2000). British nurses in behavioral psychotherapy: A 25 year follow-up. *Journal of Advanced Nursing, 32,* 343–351.

Hays, P. A. (1995). Multicultural applications of cognitive–behavioral therapy. *Professional Psychology: Research and Practice, 26,* 309–315.

Irvin, J. E., Bowers, C. A., Dunn, M. E., & Wang, M. C. (1999). Efficacy of relapse prevention: A meta-analytic review. *Journal of Consulting and Clinical Psychology, 67,* 563–570.

Kaas, M., & Lewis, M. L. (1999). Cognitive behavioral group therapy for residents in assisted living facilties. *Journal of Psychosocial Nursing, 37,* 9–15.

Kolko, D. J., Bukstein, O. G., & Barron, J. (1999). Methylphenidate and behavior modification in children with ADHD and comorbid ODD or CD: Main and incremental effects across settings. *Journal of the American Academy of Child & Adolescent Psychiatry, 38,* 578–586.

Kordacova, J. (1996). Irrational beliefs and mental health. *Ceska a Slovenska Psychiatrie, 92,* 75–82.

Koerner, K., & Linehan, M.M. (2000). Research on dialectical behavior therapy for patients with borderline personality disorder. *Psychiatric Clinics of North America, 23,* 151–167.

Lindell, K. O., & Reinke, L. F. (1999). Nursing strategies for smoking cessation. *Heart & Lung: The Journal of Acute and Critical Care, 28,* 295–302.

Linehan, M. M., Schmidt III, H., Dimeff, L. A., Craft, J. C., Kanter, J., & Comtois, K. A. (1999). Dialectical behavior therapy for patients with borderline personality disorder and drug-dependence. *American Journal on Addictions, 8,* 279–292.

Linehan, M. M., Heard, H. L., & Armstrong, H. E. (1993). Naturalistic follow-up of a behavioral treatment for chronically parasuicidal borderline patients. *Archives of General Psychiatry, 50,* 971–974.

Peden, A. R., Hall, L. A., Rayens, M. K., & Beebe, L. (2000). Negative thinking mediates the effect of self esteem on depressive symptoms in college women. *Nursing Research, 49,* 201–207.

Robinson, T. R., Smith, S. W., Miller, M. D., & Brownell, M. T. (1999). Cognitive behavioral modification of hyperactivity–impulsivity and aggression: A meta-analysis of school-based studies. *Journal of Educational Psychology, 91,* 195–203.

Skinner, B. F. (1989). The origins of cognitive thought. *American Psychologist, 44,* 12–18.

Skinner, B. F. (1984). The evolution of behavior. *Journal of the Experimental Analysis of Behavior, 41,* 217–221.

Skinner, B. F. (1974). *About behaviorism.* New York: Knopf.

Tang, T. Z., & DeRubeis, R. J. (1999). Sudden gains and critical sessions in cognitive–behavioral therapy for depression. *Journal of Consulting and Clinical Psychology, 67,* 894–904.

Wiser, S., & Telch, C. F. (1999). Dialectical behavior therapy for binge eating disorder. *Journal of Clinical Psychology, 55,* 755–768.

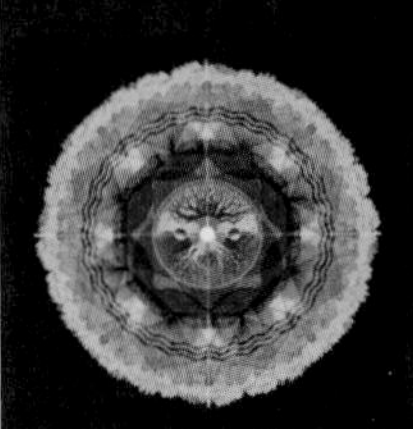

31

Chapter THIRTY-ONE

Psychopharmacology

EILEEN TRIGOBOFF

KEY TERMS

acetylcholinesterase inhibitors
akathisia
anticholinergic side effects
antidepressant medications
antipsychotic medications
anxiolytic medications
depot injection
disinhibition
extrapyramidal side effects (EPSEs)
hypertensive crisis
neuroleptic malignant syndrome (NMS)
parkinsonianism/parkinsonian syndrome
psychobiologic
tardive dyskinesia (TD)

FOCUS QUESTIONS

- **How would you define psychopharmacology based on the information in this chapter?**
- **How would you describe a psychopharmacologic problem that does not exist for nurses in other specialty areas?**
- **Would you be able to recognize the positive and negative impacts of psychiatric medications on behavior?**
- **Can you discuss three factors that affect the extent to which clients will comply with prescribed medication treatment regimens?**
- **How would you feel if you had to take these medications for an indefinite period of time?**
- **Can you describe major side effects associated with broad categories of psychotropic medications, and formulate nursing interventions to address them?**

MediaLink www.prenhall.com/kneisl

Additional resources for this chapter can be found on the Student CD-ROM accompanying this textbook, and on the Companion Website at www.prenhall.com/kneisl. Click on Chapter 31 to select the activities for this chapter.

CD-ROM
- Audio Glossary
- NCLEX Review
- EPSE: Parkinsonism Video
- Extrapyramidal Side Effects:
  Hands & Arms Tremor Video
  Grasping Tremor Video
  Lateral Tremor Video
  Akinesia & Pill Rolling Video
- EPSE: Dystonia/Akathisia Video
- EPSE: Akinesia Video
- Extrapyramidal Side Effects:
  Dystonia (Blepharospasm, Cervical Torticollolis) Video
  Bradykinesia (Shuffling Gait) Video
  Akathisia (Legs) Video
  Akinesia & Pill Rolling Video
  Tardive Dyskinesia (Mouth, Trunk, Ambulation) Video
- Neurological Synapse Animation
- Liver Enzyme (Cytochrome P450) Inhibition and Activation Animation
- Fluoxetine (Prozac) Drug Mechanism in Action Animation
- Methylphenidate (Ritalin) Drug Mechanism in Action Animation
- Diazepam (Valium) Drug Mechanism in Action Animation

Companion Website
- Additional NCLEX Review
- Case Study: Nurse's Role in Psychopharmacology

CHAPTER OUTLINE

CROSS REFERENCES

Other topics relevant to this content are: Alternative treatment, Chapter 32; Antianxiety medications, Chapter 16; Antipsychotic medications, Chapter 14; Biological aspects of psychiatric disorders, Chapter 4; Delirium, Chapter 12; Depression and bipolar disorders, Chapter 15; Interdisciplinary treatment, Chapter 2.

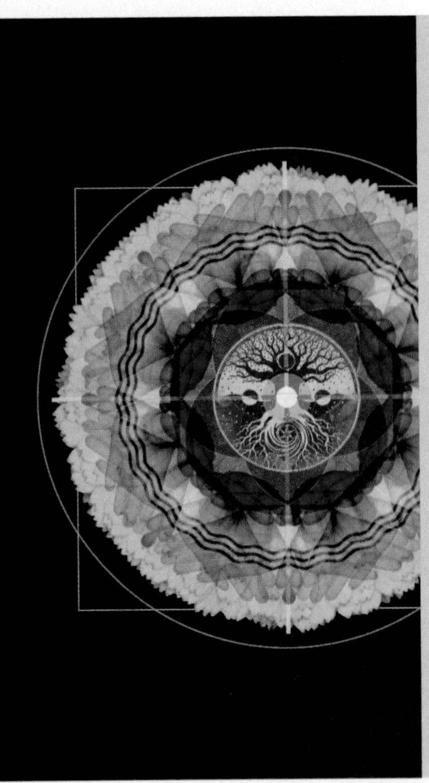

CRITICAL THINKING CHALLENGE

Medications in psychiatric treatment present an opportunity for the nurse to consider the definition of a competent and ethical treatment package. Consider the following situation with a schizophrenic client. Roberta has symptoms that cause her terrific difficulties that infiltrate her thinking, information processing, communication, and relationships. The discomfort she experiences is exceeded only by a sense of demoralization at the realization that she has a chronic and debilitating disease for which there is no cure. Roberta's antipsychotic medications cause extrapyramidal side effects (EPSEs) and the traditional antipsychotic medications she took for years cause tardive dyskinesia (TD) which can be permanent and disfiguring. Issues of adherence and the increased risk of TD (when frequent breaks in treatment occur) all contribute to ethical issues in treating schizophrenia and other psychotic disorders. Roberta sometimes has 6-month gaps between her menstruations. Up to 20% of women on traditional antipsychotics will have menstrual cycle changes due to prolactin level elevations. Rehabilitating or habilitating Roberta to a lifestyle with psychotic symptoms, or with less or no psychotic symptoms, requires a realistic view of her needs and abilities and specific training on how to cope with the mental illness and its impact on her life. How would you design a complete treatment protocol? ■

Psychiatric medications form the primary treatment for many psychiatric diagnoses. As can be seen in the Psychopharmacologic Timeline in Box 31–1, the years prior to the 1950s (when psychopharmacology became available and widely used) had to focus on behavioral interventions and sedative substances. More recently, the past six decades have shown us the beginning use, then enormous leaps of generations of compounds with major impacts, and even success, in treating many of the serious symptoms of mental illness. ■ Figure 31–1 on page 738 illustrates the drop in numbers of inpatients as a result of biologic and pharmacologic interventions. The impacts that psychopharmacology has had on serious mental illness indicates that the physiologic and behavioral responses are in answer to the physiologic impairment of the mental illness. Just like the symptoms of an endocrine disorder such as diabetes responds to treatment with insulin, mental illness is an imbalance of brain chemicals that can be addressed or corrected with medications.

Psychopharmacology is a primary treatment mode of psychiatric–mental health nursing care and requires nurses to monitor client response as well as identify problems or side effects. Ours is a holistic function, incorporating the client's life, likes, and activities along with symptomatology into a comprehensive focus of treatment. The aim of psychopharmacologic nursing interventions is to teach clients about their medications, including over-the-counter medications and supplements, and assist in problem solving (American Nurses Association [ANA], 2000).

Psychopharmacology and Nursing

The area of psychopharmacology has grown considerably in recent years. Psychiatric–mental health nursing has similarly grown, and our responsibilities to recipients of mental health care services involve, to a large degree, psychopharmacologic expertise. Our national professional organization, the American Nurses Association (ANA), examined this issue and the ANA's Task Force on Psychopharmacology set forth guidelines for this aspect of our nursing practice (ANA, 1994). The guidelines delineate three areas that unite the practice of psychiatric–mental health nursing with expertise in psychopharmacology. We must:

1. Integrate current data from the neurosciences.
2. Demonstrate knowledge of psychopharmacologic principles.
3. Provide safe and effective clinical management of clients taking these medications through assessment, diagnosis, and treatment.

Psychiatric–mental health nurses must understand current advances in psychobiology to maintain an updated knowledge base for clinical work. The goal of psychopharmacologic interventions is to promote clients' physiologic stability, so they can achieve psychologic, social, and spiritual growth. See Box 31–2 on page 728 for ANA guidelines regarding psychopharmacology.

The word *drugs* conjures up a variety of powerful positive and negative images. Media messages concerning the devastat-

BOX 31–1 Psychopharmacologic Timeline

164 BCE (Before the Common Era) to 1951 CE (Common Era)	Documentation of medicating "insane," "deranged," and mentally ill individuals describes administration of olive oil infused with narcotics, opium, morphine, other sedatives.
1948	Discovery of the hallucinogenic effects of lysergic acid diethylamide (LSD).
Antipsychotics	
1957	McGill University administers chlorpromazine (Thorazine) to treat psychosis.
1957	Trifluoperazine (Stelazine) developed and released.
1957	Perphenazine (Trilafon) developed and released.
1957	Thioridazine (Mellaril) developed and released.
1959	Fluphenazine (Prolixin) developed and released.
1967	Thiothixene (Navane) developed and released.
1967	Haloperidol (Haldol) developed and released.
1970	Mesoridazine (Serentil) developed and released.
1973	Loxapine (Loxitane) developed and released.
1990	Clozapine (Clozaril) re-released after extensive research to establish safety and use in North America.
1994	Risperidone (Risperdal) is an atypical antipsychotic developed and released.
1996	Olanzapine (Zyprexa) is an atypical antipsychotic developed and released.
1997	Quetiapine (Seroquel) is an atypical antipsychotic developed and released.
2001	Ziprasidone (Geodon) is an atypical antipsychotic developed and released.
2002	Aripiprazole (Abilify) is an atypical antipsychotic released in North America.
Antidepressants	
1952	Tuberculosis treatment with iproniazid caused energetic, even hypomanic and manic, responses. First monamine oxidase inhibitor.
1987	Fluoxetine (Prozac), the first selective serotonin reuptake inhibitor (SSRI) is developed and released.
2000	Fluoxetine (Prozac) indicated for Premenstrual Dysphoric Disorder (PMDD) and released as Sarafem.
2002	Escitalopram (Lexapro) is a single-isomer SSRI. Uses the "S" side (as opposed to the "R" side) of the citalopram molecule.
To Be Announced	Reboxetine (Vestra) is a norepinephrine-action antidepressant awaiting release in the United States.
Anxiolytics	
1960s	Meprobamate (Miltown, Equanil) is the first antianxiety agent to become popularly used.
1993	Zolpidem (Ambien), the first nonbenzodiazepine, is released.
1999	Zaleplon (Sonata) a nonbenzodiazepine, is released.
Acetylcholinesterase Inhibitors	
1993	Tacrine (Cognex) is the first acetylcholinesterase inhibitor released.
1997	Donepezil (Aricept) is released.
1999	Rivastigmine (Exelon) released, is the next generation of acetylcholinesterase inhibitor.
2001	Galantomine (Reminyl) is the latest in acetylcholinesterase inhibitors reported to cause fewer GI disturbances.

Sources: Rosner, F. (1978). *Julius Preuss' biblical and Talmudic medicine*. New York: Sanhedrin Press; Bernstein, J. G. (1995). *Handbook of drug therapy in psychiatry* (3rd ed.). St. Louis, MO: Mosby; and Conley, R. R. (Ed.). (2000). *Therapeutic advances in the treatment of schizophrenia*. Baltimore, MD: Excerpta Medica Office of Continuing Medical Education.

ing effects of IV drug use, alcoholism, and crack cocaine exemplify the negative image. Another image leaps from the pages of nursing and medical journals; pharmaceutical advertisements show people leading productive lives or smiling nurses, allegedly grateful for a medication that controls psychiatric symptoms. Yet another drug-related image is that of schoolchildren being inoculated against diphtheria, polio, and pertussis. All these images are powerful, and each is backed by truth.

THE CLIENT'S CULTURAL PERSPECTIVE

A vital aspect to competent care is accounting for the client's cultural perspective or meaning behind the behavior (Magnusson, Alexsson, Karlsson, & Oskarsson, 2000). Refusing to take medication may be more than paranoia or misunderstanding; it may be intrinsically representative of a cultural standard—for example, the belief that illness is caused by a supreme being, and that prayer and good wishes from others are the only acceptable routes to healing. Nurses often act as liaisons between the health care system and the culture of clients, making a bridge between the health care system and the client's belief system. This can be accomplished by being open and nonjudgmental about the cultural practice while promoting healthy aspects of its use. Psychiatric–mental health nurses may be especially challenged by certain cultural differences, however (Flaskerud & Nyamathi, 2000). A client's native language may provide a more detailed, or a more restricted, description of events than the English language. Nurses need to examine interventions and plans for care in light of the client's culture and commonly held views. For example, individualism is a dominant theme in the Western

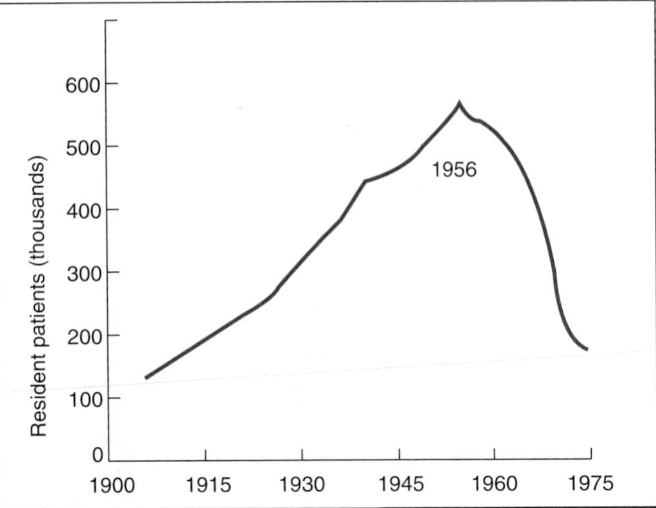

FIGURE 31–1 ■ *The greatest success story of biological psychiatry. This graph illustrates the dramatic lowering of numbers of inpatients since the advent of psychopharmacologic agents.*

Source: Smock, T. K. (1999). *Physiological psychology: A neuroscience approach*. Upper Saddle River, NJ: Prentice Hall.

world; however, this focus may not fit with people of a minority ethnicity who may hold values defining caretaking as a collective, rather than an individual, responsibility (Gerrish, 2000; Carrese & Rhodes, 2000).

It has been argued that it is difficult to incorporate non-Western sensibilities into our present psychiatric classification system. Your recognition of the validity of cultural backgrounds other than Western will promote client rights and afford clients legitimate entry into health care delivery systems (Perkins & Hazuda, 2000). An awareness of the issues relating to culture helps minimize the problem and is necessary for providing quality mental health care. See the Nursing Self-Awareness feature on page 729 to determine how your cultural inclinations influence your attitudes toward medications.

BOX 31–2 **ANA Guidelines on Psychopharmacology**

The psychiatric–mental health nurse can perform the following functions regarding psychopharmacology:

1. Describe psychopharmacologic agents.
2. Discuss the actions of psychopharmacologic agents, on a global scale down through cellular responses.
3. Differentiate psychiatric symptomatology from medication side effects.
4. Apply the basic principles of pharmacokinetics and pharmacodynamics.
5. Identify the appropriate use of psychopharmacologic agents in special populations.
6. Involve clients and their significant others.
7. Identify barriers to significant others' involvement.
8. Describe nonpsychopharmacologic interventions.
9. Demonstrate value of standardized rating scales.
10. Synthesize necessary information to develop psychopharmacologic education and treatment plans.

Source: Adapted with permission from American Nurses Association, *Psychiatric mental health nursing psychopharmacology project*, © 1994 American Nurses Publishing, American Nurses Association, Washington, DC.

Biologic Impact on Ethnically Distinct Groups

In addition to assessing for cultural impacts on behavior, you must also assess for the biologic impacts of medications on ethnically distinct groups. Factors such as benefits received from drug treatment, drug toxicity levels, and addiction liabilities are not the same for all groups of individuals (Dimsdale, 2000).

One important factor is the variation in metabolic rates among ethnic groups (an important point in evaluating the effectiveness of a medication). A high metabolic rate may produce effects below the optimal level, resulting in ineffective treatment. A low metabolic rate increases side effects. Because Asians have low metabolic rates, almost all Asians (95%) experience extrapyramidal side effects (EPSEs), as compared to European- and African-Americans, two-thirds of whom experience EPSE (Morita et al., 2000). Also because of metabolic differences, the therapeutic range for lithium differs among Asian, African-American, and Caucasian groups. The determination of effective lithium levels must take ethnicity into account.

The relationships between a client with a mental illness and the family have been examined for their **psychobiologic** (the study of the basics of psychiatry through biologic, chemical, and genetic impacts on thinking, mood, and behavior) impact. Typically, Mexican-Americans exude warmth and regard, which can positively affect a client's course of recovery. If a family is warm and they respond readily to a family member with schizophrenia, it is not as likely that the client will relapse as quickly as someone with schizophrenia staying in the midst of a family with low warmth (Lopez & Guarnaccia, 2000). Interestingly, the relapse rates of Anglo-Americans were unrelated to warmth.

Recognizing how ethnicity and phenotype determine response to drugs promotes the provision of culturally competent care. How ethnicity affects the expression of abnormal biologic processes is a growing field of study. Exploring the related literature will help you to incorporate this expanding knowledge base into your psychiatric–mental health nursing practice and promote your cultural competence.

ASSESSMENT OF THE CLIENT TAKING PSYCHIATRIC MEDICATIONS

Our responsibilities as nurses to clients receiving psychotropic medications are very different from the responsibilities of nurses in other settings. A nurse working with clients having cardiac difficulties, for example, may have clear physiologic indicators for the administration of drugs such as isosorbide dinitrate or nitroglycerin, but psychiatric nurses rarely have comparable consistent complexes of symptoms on which to base clinical judgments. In psychiatric work, nurses must often observe client behaviors closely to be aware of the sometimes subtle nature of the presenting symptom. Pacing, mild diaphoresis, slight increases in blood pressure or pulse, heightened muscle tone, and hypervigilant posture may be indicative of escalating anxiety, but they may also point to other problems such as caffeine toxicity, excessive use of tobacco, or side effects of psychopharmacologic agents. Accurate nursing assessment of client behavior is crucial if medications are to be given effectively and appropriately. Psychiatric nurses must also be attuned to the circumstances of adjunct pharmacotherapy (taking different medications at the same time).

Assessment is not a static process. It takes shape over time and includes a wide range of nursing knowledge. Similar behaviors indicating a wide array of vastly different sources often exist with psychiatric clients. A sleepy, isolated client with schizophrenia may be experiencing paranoid ideation, may have negative symptoms of the illness, may be having sedating side effects of the antipsychotic medication, or may be depressed as well as schizophrenic. Your assessment of this client and your clinical judgment will direct the nursing care. Whether you decide to administer a PRN antipsychotic, hold the next dose of antipsychotic, develop a treatment plan that includes motivational aspects, or discuss the possibility of depression with the other treatment team members depends upon your ongoing assessment of this client.

DRUG ADMINISTRATION

Administering psychiatric medications demands more than the six rights: the right medication, the right dose, the right route, the right time, to the right client, and using the right technology. These aspects of medication administration in psychiatry are confounded by the psychiatric illness. Knowing the side effects of the medication, in addition to the interactive effects with other psychiatric and medical–surgical medications, is another facet to psychiatric–mental health nursing.

Nursing SELF-AWARENESS

Your Psychopharmacology Views

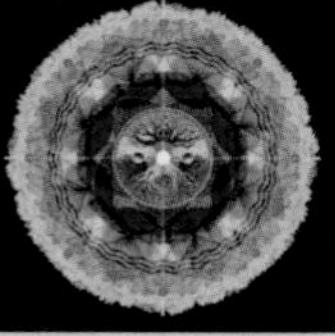

Your cultural inclinations have an influence on your attitudes toward medications. These attitudes have an impact on the major intervention in psychiatry—psychopharmacology.

Which of these views do you hold about medications? How will they affect the care you give clients?

- It'll make me healthier.
- This stuff will kill me.
- It's only for a short time.
- It's addictive.
- I'll take meds only if my life depends on it.
- Isn't modern pharmacology a wonderful thing?
- I take the right medication for the problem.
- Taking the meds will mean I'm a bad/weak person because I couldn't battle it on my own.
- Medicine is made from herbs—it's the same thing, so I'd rather take the herbs.
- I can't contaminate myself with these chemicals.
- It's a sign of my weakness that I need medication.

The right medication in a psychiatric setting depends on the nursing assessment skills of the nurse. The right medication may be one of a number of choices. A medication may be ordered by mouth (PO) for routine administration, but the client may refuse the medication. Assessment skills come into play here as well; you must determine whether the client needs a liquid or a pill, or whether a PRN injection is necessary. The right client, client identification regarding medication administration, is different than in medical–surgical settings because clients usually do not wear wristbands. They may be confused or have psychiatric symptoms that encourage them to spontaneously assume the identity of another client for any number of reasons including an effort to please the staff.

Documenting the rationale for the effect of medications is an important nursing responsibility. Follow-up documentation on a medication that was given as a PRN will simplify treatment decisions for the client. Did the PRN work? How did you determine the value of the PRN's effect? What behavioral indicators are you using in your evaluation of a medication's effectiveness?

CLIENT/FAMILY EDUCATION

Nursing responsibilities include educating clients about their medication. Adherence to medication regimens is often an issue for psychiatric clients, and nurses have explored the efficacy of teaching as a way of improving client adherence to medication regimens after discharge from inpatient settings. Variables related to adherence include socioeconomic status, marital status, number of concurrent medications, diagnosis, side effects, health benefits, and health values. Clients' individual differences must be addressed in the course of the teaching-learning process. See the Client/Family Teaching feature on page 730 "Strategies and Methods for Client Medication Teaching" for useful information.

An issue of great concern to many nurses is the planning of teaching-learning experiences for chronically mentally ill clients. Although this population has learning needs concerning care and treatment, teaching is often difficult, depending on the severity and chronicity of the illness. See Box 31–3 on page 730 for specific learning problems with different diagnostic groups.

Recidivism, the tendency to relapse into a previous mode of behavior requiring readmission to a treatment program, can be linked to a psychiatric client's psychoeducation. Helping a client change health-related behavior requires a thoughtful, comprehensive approach. See Designing a Behavioral Contract in Chapter 30 on pages 718–722. Interventions designed to match the client's learning, and teaching in the most relevant manner, can reduce recidivism and promote healthier behavior.

Another concern for nurses working with psychiatric clients is the need to assess their learning capacity at different points in their disorders. For example, when clients are first admitted to an inpatient unit, they may be too disorganized and symptomatic to focus on specific learning tasks. Depressed clients may be so psychomotorally slowed, because of hormonal shifts and dysfunctional neurotransmission, that they may be unable to learn. Given appropriate treatment and care, however, a client's

CLIENT / FAMILY TEACHING

Strategies and Methods for Client Medication Teaching

Discover effective learning methods already known to be successful for him or her. Identify those methods:

Repetition: Rehearsing or practicing the skill repeatedly can place it in a number of areas in the memory, thereby increasing the chances of retrieval.
Primacy: The first thing heard about or learned is the skill most easily retrieved and performed for these individuals.
Recency: The last, or most recent, thing heard about or learned is the skill most easily retrieved and performed for these individuals.
Association: Learning by hinging one memory to another.
Coding: Shaping the thought in your memory in a particular way to facilitate retrieval for skill performance.
Background information and explanation: Description of a skill with specific details can assist many to learn and perform reliably. Incorporating the client's value system into this method is most effective.
Reminder boxes: Physical prompts are helpful for clients who are concrete and need environmental hints.
Lists, notebooks: Making lists and keeping track of tasks and events in a notebook can be a powerful tool for clients with executive functioning deficits.
Videos: Visual learners can make use of a multimedia presentation of materials.
Positive transfer: If the client learned how to do Task A well, and it is similar enough to Task B, then Task B can be accomplished through transferring that learned behavior.
Positive reinforcement: Positive reinforcement is either getting something desirable or avoiding something unpleasant.

psychobiologic disequilibrium may be corrected, making learning possible.

Even when a nurse perceives that a client is ready to learn (cognitive abilities are intact), learning will not necessarily occur. Many nurses conduct medication groups on an acute psychiatric unit to not only address the importance of assessing cognitive abilities but also to explore affective and social issues that may contribute to effective learning experiences. After considering the client's readiness, knowledge, background, environment, beliefs, preferences, and lifestyle, involving the client and significant others in the design and implementation of the medication treatment plan will help ensure the client's active collaboration in his or her care.

In many ways, psychiatric clients are no different from other learners. When presented with material that is clearly beneficial to them, they are likely to be more interested in the learning process. An evaluation of teaching efforts is essential to completing the teaching–learning process. This part of the process can be as informal or formal as you choose or deem necessary to check the client's knowledge of information taught. You will not be able to evaluate a client's understanding of information unless, at minimum, the client verbally reiterates information or performs a return demonstration of the skill. A change in behavior over time is a powerful indication of learning. If you desire a more extensive evaluation you may consider using a "pretest/posttest" format. You can develop a written test to cover the content of the teaching and have the client complete the test *before* you begin teaching (a pretest). This provides a written measure of the client's learning needs and level of knowledge. After you implement and complete the teaching plan, the client completes the same examination (a posttest). Comparison of the pretest and posttest results yields a documented measure of how much learning has occurred as a result of your teaching intervention.

BOX 31-3 What Nurses Need to Know for Medication Teaching

Psychoses

- Cognitive difficulties secondary to thought disorder
- Motivational problems secondary to negative symptoms
- Unpleasant side effects from medication
- Persistance of positive symptoms (delusions) mitigating against adherence

Mood Disorders

- Persistent dysphoria leads to amotivation
- Self-destructiveness–lethality
- Manic irresponsibility
- Loss of manic or hypomanic egosyntonic excitement
- Unpleasant side effects from medications

Anxiety Disorders

- Addiction to antianxiety medication
- Quick action of many antianxiety agents leads to positive reinforcement of increasing dosages
- Lack of consistent provider knowledge of and expertise in application of effective nonmedication treatment strategies for anxiety problems

Personality Disorders

- Addictive or abusive use of medications
- Sensation seeking
- Manipulation

NEUROLEPTICS AND PSYCHOTROPICS

Recently, there has been significant change in the use of classes of medications for psychiatric symptomatology. In previous years, there were clear delineations between what was an antipsychotic and what was not. Empirical data and clinical expertise have led us to a less rigid application of chemical compounds. The complexities of psychiatric disorders and the desire to address the difficulties facing people who have these symptoms have resulted in a number of innovative medication regimens. Research further expanded our knowledge and a clearer vision of the capabilities of these compounds emerged. Now many medications have multiple indications beyond their original ones, which have necessitated more global terms to describe the medication. We still use classification names like "antipsychotic" and "antidepressant"; however, this is changing and some medications are labeled as being a "neuroleptic" or a "psychotropic" with the understanding that this medication can be used across some diagnostic groups. See ■ Table 31–1 for some examples of this changing psychopharmacologic landscape.

Examples of this phenomenon include fluoxetine (Prozac), an initial antidepressant, indicated as an antiobsessional drug and in premenstrual dysphoria disorder (PMDD); and risperidone (Risperdal), a newer antipsychotic, indicated for use in stabilizing the manic phase of bipolar disorder. There are also clinical applications of psychiatric medications to a different diagnostic group, or for a different set of psychiatric symptoms, than originally intended. There may not be a Food and Drug Administration (FDA) indication for the drug in those circumstances; however, clinical appropriateness has established the use pattern. This holds true for risperidone as treatment in dementia with agitation.

Clinical application of nonpsychiatric medications to treat a psychiatric diagnostic group or a set of psychiatric symptoms has also occurred. The most apparent example of a class of nonpsychiatric medications being used to treat psychiatric treatment is the anticonvulsant class. Valproic acid (Depakote), carbamazepine (Tegretol), and gabapentin (Neurontin) are all used as mood stabilizers as well as for their original indications.

The University of Iowa's Health Care Virtual Hospital Web site at www.vh.org/Providers/Conferences/CPS/contents.html can be accessed through the Companion Website for this text. The site has chapters on various psychopharmacologic topics that contain articles and information.

MediaLink Psychopharmacology Information

TABLE 31–1 Medications and Their Cross-Diagnostic Uses

	Psychosis	Dementia	Depression	Obsessions/ Compulsions	Mood Instability	PTSD	PMDD	Panic Disorder	Social Phobia	Convulsions	Cigarette Smoking	Migraine
Risperidone (Risperdal)	X	X			X							
Olanzapine (Zyprexa)	X				X							
Quetiapine (Seroquel)	X	X										
Tricyclic antidepressants			X					X				
SSRIs			X					X				
Fluoxetine (Prozac, Sarafem)			X	X			X	X				
Sertraline (Zoloft)			X	X		X		X				
Paroxetine (Paxil)			X					X	X			
Fluvoxamine (Luvox)			X	X				X				
Bupropion (Wellbutrin, Zyban)			X								X	
Divalproex (Depakote)		X			X					X		X
Carbamazepine (Tegretol)					X					X		

Antipsychotic Medications

The discovery of the first **antipsychotic drug**, chlorpromazine (Thorazine), is a prime example of the role chance has played in the history of psychopharmacology. Chlorpromazine was initially synthesized as an antihistamine and was not tried as a tranquilizer for clients with schizophrenia until 1952. Its effects on the behavior, thinking, affect, and perception of schizophrenic clients were so profound that knowledge of its properties was rapidly disseminated, and it became widely used within 3 to 4 years. Chlorpromazine's effects on the hospital practice of psychiatry were staggering. Its use contributed to reversing a steadily increasing population in U.S. mental institutions, and that population has progressively decreased ever since. One might say that chlorpromazine gave birth to the modern notions of psychiatric treatment—unlocked wards, milieu treatment, occupational and recreational therapy, and supervised living environments. The entire field of community mental health is ultimately linked to its discovery because it enabled clients to return to their homes or otherwise live outside an inpatient facility.

PSYCHOBIOLOGIC CONSIDERATIONS

Understanding the psychobiology of antipsychotic medications requires a basic knowledge of the functions of the central nervous system. An extended discussion of how these drugs work to reduce symptoms is beyond the scope of this chapter, but here is a brief overview of the basic mechanisms of action.

Generally, neuroleptics work by blocking a variety of CNS receptors. Drugs such as antipsychotics do not work only on the neurotransmitter system. Therefore, it is likely that several types of neurotransmitters and neuromodulators are affected by the administration of a single medication. While most neuroleptics have an affinity for several types of neurotransmitters, others are more specific and work more selectively. These differences account for the effects of the various neuroleptic medications. ■ Figure 31–2 shows the chemical structure of three neuroleptics.

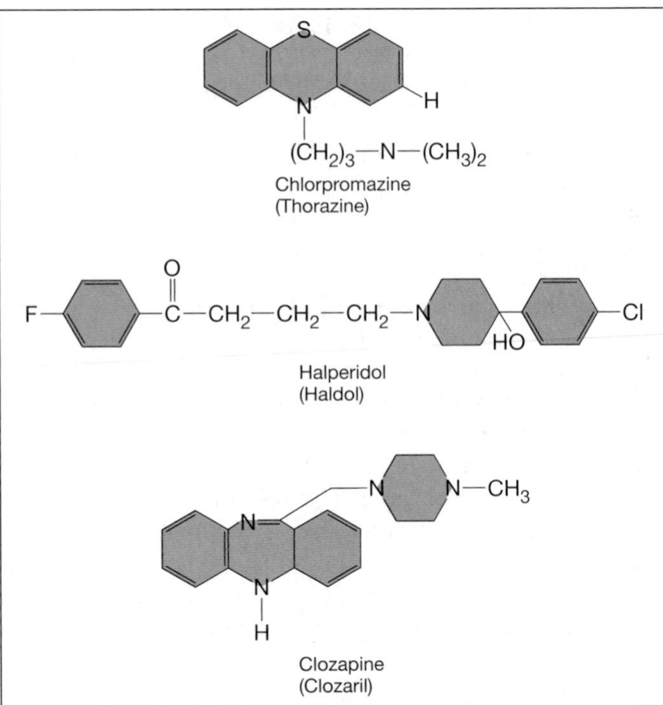

FIGURE 31–2 ■ *The chemical structure of three neuroleptic drugs. The antipsychotic efficacy of these medications is most likely related to the blockade of postsynaptic dopaminergic receptors, however, other neurotransmitter systems may be involved. Examples of adverse reactions to these medications include: parkinsonism, dry mouth, blurred vision, constipation, urinary retention.*

Source: Smock, T. K. (1999). *Physiological psychology: A neuroscience approach*. Upper Saddle River, NJ: Prentice Hall.

MAJOR EFFECTS

The beneficial effects of antipsychotic medications in all psychotic states have been demonstrated beyond question. Multiple and varied criteria have been used to measure improvement. These drugs have been used successfully in clients with delusional thinking, confusion, motor agitation, and motor retardation. Antipsychotic drug treatment also decreases formal thought disorder, blunted affect, bizarre behavior, social withdrawal, hallucinations, belligerence, and uncooperativeness.

The most common disintegrative condition treated with antipsychotic drugs is the group of symptoms traditionally labeled schizophrenia. (See Chapter 14 for information on evaluating schizophrenic clients and the diagnostic criteria in *DSM-IV-TR*.) The problem of assessment is complicated by the fact that many diseases can cause syndromes with features like those of schizophrenia. For example, delusions may indicate a variety of *DSM-IV-TR* conditions, including schizophrenia and dementia, Alzheimer's type, with delusions. The finer points of differentiation between these two conditions include cognitive functioning and the client's presenting history. (Chapter 12 provides a detailed discussion of delirium, dementia, and related disorders.) All clients manifesting psychotic symptoms should give a thorough medical history and take a physical examination, to rule out treatable medical illnesses, many of which are accompanied by behaviors considered psychotic or psychobiologic.

THE CHOICE OF A SPECIFIC DRUG

There are many antipsychotic medications on the market, and you may have noticed the recent expansion of this class of drugs. Drugs will have varying success rates with clients as individual responses frequently dictate use. The choice of a particular medication, then, depends on knowledge of the pharmacologic properties and side effects, the client's or a family member's history of drug response, and the prescriber's experience with various compounds. Important client variables are past successes with specific drugs, a history of allergies, and a history of serious or intolerable side effects. Some medications may have side effects with certain clients (sedation), which while not necessarily desired by the prescriber, may nevertheless prove to be helpful in treatment. Expect a certain amount of trial and error with each clinical application.

■ Table 31–2 summarizes the characteristics of the major antipsychotic medications. The list is extensive and growing, and it makes sense for each member of the treatment team to become familiar with just a few representative drugs, their predictable effects, and their common side effects. The characteristics covered in the table are discussed in the sections that follow.

There are now more than seven distinct chemical classes of antipsychotic medications commonly used in the United States. (One class, the phenothiazines, is subdivided into three different types of medications.) Thus, there is a broad choice in terms of side effects and potential client responsiveness. A client who is unresponsive to one class may well respond to another that circumvents a problem in absorption, accumulation at neurotransmitter receptor sites, or metabolism.

Table 31–2 also shows the wide range among these medications in milligram-per-milligram potency. This fact is most relevant when treating clients who require large doses. In such cases, a potent medication is best. Consumer issues and clinician concerns are addressed at www.FDA.gov, the Web site for the Food and Drug Administration in the United States. You can access the FDA through the Companion Website of this book.

NEWER ANTIPSYCHOTICS

The newer antipsychotics (they were called atypicals when they were first marketed) are those medications with a drastically different physiologic action than the traditional or conventional antipsychotics. The conventional antipsychotics primarily affected the positive symptoms of psychotic disorders, with little or no effect on the negative or cognitive symptoms. Their mechanism of action is thought to occur through nonselectively blocking the neurotransmitter dopamine D_2 receptors in the brain. To be clinically effective, these medications occupy between 70% and 90% of the D_2 receptors while the advent of EPSEs occurs at above 80% occupancy. The newer antipsychotics have a much reduced affinity for D_2 receptors, plus they all have an affinity for the serotonin receptors, a profile that appears to mitigate against EPSEs and has an impact on the negative symptoms of psychotic disorders (Conley, 2000).

These medications provide new options for the care and treatment of clients suffering from psychotic conditions. The search continues for psychopharmacologic treatments for psychoses. Medications are being researched and tested every day, and if they provide relief from symptoms without undue side effects, they will enhance our psychopharmacologic arsenal.

MediaLink FDA: Consumer Issues

TABLE 31–2 Antipsychotic Medications

Class	Generic Name	Trade Name	Usual Dosage Range (mg/day)	Side Effects		
				Sedative	Extrapyramidal*	Anticholinergic*
Phenothiazines						
Aliphatic	Chlorpromazine	Thorazine	150–1500	Very strong	Moderate	Strong
Piperidine	Thioridazine	Mellaril	150–800	Moderate	Minimal	Moderate
Piperazine	Trifluoperazine	Stelazine	10–60	Weak	Strong	Weak
	Fluphenazine	Prolixin	3–45	Weak	Strong	Weak
	Perphenazine	Trilafon	12–60	Weak	Strong	Weak
Butyrophenones	Haloperidol	Haldol	2–40	Weak	Strong	Weak
Thioxanthenes	Thiothixene	Navane	10–60	Weak	Strong	Weak
	Chlorprothixene	Taractan	40–600	Strong	Moderate	Strong
Dihydroindolones	Molindone	Moban	15–225	Weak	Moderate	Weak
Dibenzoxazepines	Loxapine	Loxitane	10–100	Moderate	Strong	Moderate
Dibenzodiazepines	Clozapine	Clozaril	12.5–900	Moderate	Weak	Strong
Benzisoxazole derivative	Risperidone	Risperdal	4–6	Weak	Weak	Weak
Thienobenzodiazepine	Olanzapine	Zyprexa	10–20	Moderate	Weak	Weak
Dibenzothiazepine derivative	Quetiapine	Seroquel	300–400	Moderate	Weak	Weak
Benzisothiazolyl piperazine derivative	Ziprazidone	Geodon	40–200	Moderate	Weak	Moderate

Extrapyramidal and anticholinergic side effects are discussed later in this chapter.

Clozapine (Clozaril)

The first on the market was clozapine (Clozaril). Clozapine is an antipsychotic drug with an unusual pharmacologic and clinical profile. It was used in Europe for several years and is now generally used in the U.S. with clients who cannot tolerate the EPSEs of other antipsychotics, or who have a treatment-resistant or treatment-refractory psychosis, as is the case with certain schizophrenic clients. Reviews of studies regarding the effectiveness of clozapine have demonstrated its decided impact on both negative and positive symptoms, with improvement evident on follow-up as well.

Serious Side Effects. Despite its capacity to ameliorate symptoms of some very recalcitrant clients, clozapine has some serious side effects. The most serious is agranulocytosis (a marked decrease in granulated white blood cells), which occurs in less than 1% of clients taking this medication. It is essential to monitor white blood cell (WBC) counts of clients taking clozapine. Immediately discontinuing the medication when agranulocytosis is detected and before signs of an infection develop will usually resolve the episode. If a client experiences agranulocytosis as a result of using clozapine, the drug cannot be reinstituted. There is a risk for agranulocytosis with a variety of other psychotropic medications (conventional antipsychotics, benzodiazepines); however, there is a higher risk with clozapine. This compound requires cautiously adjusting this rate to a lower level. There have been rates of agranulocytosis at significantly lower levels than the currently estimated 1% (i.e., 0.3%) (Kilian & Lawrence, 1999). One of the important questions for clozapine treatment remains, "Is there a specific risk period for agranulocytosis, and if there is, when does it occur?" The risk period establishes the frequency of blood monitoring that can be an impediment to clients' initial and continued use of the antipsychotic. Currently, it is estimated that agranulocytosis may occur up to a year following initial treatment with clozapine, although the vast majority of cases appear within 6 months. As a result of these data, blood monitoring for agranulocytosis is completed weekly for the first 6 months of therapy. If the WBC levels remain normal and regular use is not interrupted throughout those 6 months, then blood monitoring can be reduced to biweekly frequencies. Remember that blood monitoring must continue for 4 weeks following the discontinuation of clozapine.

Another serious side effect is the potential for seizure, which seems to be dose-related. Less acute but nonetheless important side effects include sedation, tachycardia, sialorrhea (drooling), weight gain, and hypotension. See the Intervention Box at right for guidelines to measuring orthostatic blood pressure.

INTERVENTION

Guidelines for Measuring Orthostatic Blood Pressure

1. Instruct the client to lie down for approximately 5 minutes. This allows for an equilibration of the blood pressure in the supine position and gives a precise supine reading. *Do not substitute a supine reading for a sitting reading!* Take the client's blood pressure and pulse.
2. Instruct the client to stand. Wait for approximately 30 seconds to 1 minute and retake the blood pressure and pulse. Waiting this brief period allows for a full evaluation of the initial orthostasis.
3. Wait 2 more minutes and retake the vital signs once again. This third set of measurements allows for an evaluation of the client's body mechanisms to compensate for the presence of any orthostasis that may be present.

Risperidone (Risperdal)

Risperidone was introduced in the United States in the spring of 1994. It is the first of a new class of antipsychotics, benzisoxazole derivatives, that does not clinically relate to any existing antipsychotic drug. Its unique feature is the relative absence of EPSE at the therapeutic dosing level. It addresses the positive, negative, and affective symptoms of schizophrenia and may also alleviate depression and anxiety. Risperidone has demonstrated an ability to suppress TD (discussed later in this chapter) without increasing parkinsonism (Jeste, Okamoto, Napolitano, Kane, & Martinez, 2000), somewhat like clozapine.

Dosage of this new medication has been described as "the 1-2-3" regimen, in which the client receives 1 mg BID, the next increase (slowly titrated according to client's tolerability and response) is to 2 mg BID, and the next increase after that is to 3 mg BID. This places the client at 6 mg/day, which is in the therapeutic window of 4 to 8 mg/day currently recommended. Doses less than 5 mg/day have been linked with a better outcome than those receiving higher doses (Conley, 2000). Risperidone can be administered up to 16 mg/day, but the absence of EPSEs fades over 10 mg/day. Response within 1 to 10 weeks gives the drug a fair trial. Dosage for older clients is lower, generally cutting the initial dosage in half (0.5 mg BID, 1 mg BID, and 1.5 mg BID) and taking at least a full week between dosage changes.

This medication has been very useful in the treatment of psychotic symptoms, and the clinical knowledge gained from using it regularly has been valuable. The opportunity to have risperidone available in a depot form is now being examined. Once the current trials have been completed, the additional administration mode for this medication will offer another choice in the array of treatments for psychotic symptoms. (See A Unique Route of Administration on page 735.)

DOSAGE

Dosage ranges of antipsychotic medications vary widely among clients. Medications must be titrated against the psychotic target symptoms and the appearance of side effects. Most clients are initially given a relatively low dose of an antipsychotic to test for adverse effects for 1 to 2 hours. Consider chlorpromazine, with an initial dose of 20 to 50 mg orally (PO) or 25 mg intramuscularly (IM). Then the medication is typically given in 300 to 400 mg (or IM equivalent) per day, and gradually increased by 25% to 50% each day until maximum improvement is noted or intolerable side effects are encountered. This type of progression is common with the various antipsychotic medications.

The treatment setting frequently influences the drug regimen. In a crowded hospital emergency room, for example, hourly doses of medication may be given until a client is sedated. In more completely staffed, private inpatient units, a client may be observed for several days before medication is given. However, in terms of long-term outcome and length of eventual remission, neither approach is superior to the other (Bowen, Garry, & Sajbel, 2000; Conley, 2000).

Clients who are extremely agitated, violent, severely withdrawn, or catatonic require significant doses during the first few days of treatment, delivered by injection to ensure rapid relief. Chlorpromazine, 50 to 100 mg IM, may be used, particularly if sedation is required. The nurse must be aware that this is an irritating drug; injections must be deeply intramuscular in either the buttocks or upper arms, and sites must be rotated. Substantial IM doses of the more potent antipsychotics, such as haloperidol 10 mg or trifluoperazine 10 mg, may be given to agitated clients. This approach frequently avoids some of the more troublesome side effects while ameliorating behavioral and cognitive symptoms.

Because antipsychotic medications have a rather long biologic half-life and many have significant sedative effects, there is little reason to give divided doses of medication after the initial days of treatment. It is recommended that the drugs, particularly the sedative ones such as chlorpromazine, be given in substantial doses at bedtime. In addition to promoting sleep, decreasing the chances the client will forget to take a dose after discharge, and saving nursing time in the hospital, this method saves money because large-dose capsules or tablets cost less than an equivalent amount of medication prepared in smaller doses.

After maximum clinical improvement has been obtained, antipsychotic medications are generally reduced gradually. Continuing to give a client modest doses of an antipsychotic following a psychotic episode lowers the chances of relapse and rehospitalization. Psychotherapy with schizophrenic clients may not be particularly effective without maintenance medications in conventional treatment settings, but it does improve psychosocial functioning in clients who are also taking maintenance medications. It is generally believed that clients should be kept on doses of antipsychotics sufficient to suppress symptoms for 3 months to 1 year following an acute episode. After such an interval, the client's course and life situation must be considered and treatment individualized. Some clients recover from a psychotic episode completely within 6 months. These clients, with schizophreniform disorder, should not receive long-term maintenance drug treatment. For individuals who have already experienced recurrent episodes of psychosis and demonstrate a deteriorating course, it is clearly advantageous to prevent relapses with drugs if possible.

THE DECISION TO USE A DRUG

Today, these general principles govern antipsychotic drug use:

- Drugs are given to treat target symptoms of schizophrenia or other psychotic disorders.
- Initial treatment may require parenteral doses. These are changed to oral pill or concentrate forms as the behavior disturbance subsides.
- Total dosages are tailored to individual needs; wide variations exist among clients.
- As soon as practical with drugs having sedating side effects, divided doses are changed to a single dose given at bedtime to maximize the drug's sedative properties.
- Most clients with a chronic course require maintenance doses for sustained improvement and to minimize the number of relapses.

Other considerations for using a particular medication include the use of adjunctive therapies (Bowen, Garry, & Sajbel, 2000). Do the medications needed to treat one problem blend well with any or all of the other medications the client may need? See ■ Table 31–3 on page 736 for antipsychotic drug interactions with other medications and substances to which your client may be exposed.

SPECIAL CONSIDERATIONS

These following special considerations apply to the use of antipsychotic medication.

A Unique Route of Administration

The phenothiazines fluphenazine (Prolixin) and haloperidol (Haldol) are available in long-acting intramuscular injectable forms that behave like timed-release capsules. These medications are gradually released over a long period of time, 2 to 3 weeks. Long-acting fluphenazine and haloperidol are available in decanoate (long-acting **depot injection**) preparations. The main advantage of decanoate forms is that they reduce clients' ambivalence about taking medication and eliminate the need for constant pill taking. The treatment team must also honor the clients' civil liberties; truly involuntary treatment can be performed only according to due process, as required by a particular state's mental hygiene laws.

The psychiatric–mental health nurse in a community setting may frequently have occasion to administer long-acting fluphenazine or haloperidol. With a client whose treatment will include a long-acting medication, a dose of regular fluphenazine or haloperidol is usually taken first to rule out the possibility of allergic reactions. Such reactions can be devastating if discovered after a 2- or 3-week supply of medicine has been given as a depot treatment. If no adverse reactions are noted within 1 hour, the long-acting form is injected, usually in the upper outer quadrant of the buttock or the vastus lateralis site.

The depot form of the newer antipsychotic risperidone, once available, will be useful for clients with positive symptomatology as well as problems with executive functioning, memory, or adherence. It is delivered IM via saline—as opposed to the sesame oil used in haloperidol and fluphenazine decanoate IM injections. A depot antipsychotic with considerably fewer side effects than haloperidol and fluphenazine has the potential to prolong antipsychotic med-

TABLE 31–3 Antipsychotic Drug Interactions

Combining One of These:	With One of These Antipsychotics:	Can Lead to These Problems:
Carbamazapine	Haloperidol	Decreased effect of either medication
Carbamazapine	Clozapine	Additive bone marrow suppression
Anticholinergics	Clozapine	Potentiate anticholinergic effect of clozapine
Benzodiazepines	Clozapine	Respiratory arrest, circulatory difficulties
Anticholinergic medication	Antipsychotic	Increased level of neuroleptic in the system with extrapyramidal side effects
Antacids	Phenothiazine antipsychotic	Decreased phenothiazine effect
Coffee, Tea, Milk, or Fruit juices	Phenothiazine antipsychotic	Decreased phenothiazine effect
CNS depressants such as: Narcotics, Anxiolytics, Alcohol, Barbiturates, or Antihistamines	Antipsychotic	Additive CNS depression

ication use and minimize dissatisfaction with and discontinuation of treatment.

Better routes for medication administration have been explored by various drug companies for years. As a result, there is yet another way to give olanzapine (Zyprexa) in a newly approved orally disintegrating tablet formulation. Called Zyprexa Zydis, these tablets begin disintegrating in the mouth within seconds. This allows them to be swallowed with or without liquid, thus limiting difficulties in swallowing and cheeking (hiding) behaviors. The Zydis form of medication is also being used with a variety of compounds in medical–surgical settings.

Medication Requirements of Certain Age Groups

In elderly clients, the agitation often associated with delirium, dementia, and related disorders is markedly responsive to antipsychotics. Other sedatives, such as barbiturates and benzodiazepines, may further compromise cerebral functioning, further depressing the level of awareness and concentration and thereby worsening the disorder. Doses of medications are generally reduced for older adults. Risperidone 1 mg/day, trifluoperazine (Stelazine) 5 to 20 mg/day, or haloperidol 1 to 6 mg/day might constitute adequate treatment.

Antipsychotic medications are effective in treating childhood psychoses and in managing the behavior problems associated with mental retardation. The general principle of reduced dosage is again applicable. The upper limit of the usual daily dosage for children under 12 might be 200 mg/day of chlorpromazine or thioridazine (Mellaril) or 20 mg/day per day of trifluoperazine. Amounts of individual IM injections of chlorpromazine must also be kept at 0.25 mg per pound of body weight every 6 to 8 hr, or not over 40 mg/day for up to 50 lb and not over 75 mg/day for children weighing 50 to 100 lb.

POTENTIAL SIDE EFFECTS OF ANTIPSYCHOTIC MEDICATIONS

Continuous contact with clients gives nurses an advantage over physicians and other professionals who may see a client only every other day or, at best, once a day. Both the dangerous and the more uncomfortable side effects frequently have a rapid onset and need attention promptly.

The side effects of antipsychotic medications that nurses must recognize can be divided into these classes:

- Autonomic nervous system
- Extrapyramidal
- Other central nervous system (CNS)
- Allergic
- Blood
- Skin
- Eye
- Endocrine
- Weight gain

■ Table 31–4 lists the side effects of various antipsychotic medications.

Autonomic Nervous System Effects

The antipsychotics all possess **anticholinergic side effects** and antiadrenergic side effects; that is, they interfere with the normal transmission of nerve impulses by acetylcholine and epinephrine, in both central and peripheral nerves. The most common side effects are the anticholinergic ones. These include dry mouth, blurred vision, constipation, urinary hesitance or retention, and, under rarer circumstances, paralytic ileus.

Orthostatic hypotension, also known as postural hypotension, is a common antiadrenergic effect. The primary danger here is injury from a fall. Clients receiving parenteral medications, such as chlorpromazine intramuscularly, must have their blood pressure monitored lying and standing before and a half hour after each dose. Clients should be advised to rise from a supine posi-

TABLE 31–4 Side Effects of Antipsychotic Medications

Effect	Chlorpromazine (Thorazine)	Haloperidol (Haldol)	Loxapine (Loxitane)	Molindone (Moban)	Risperidone (Risperdal)	Clozapine (Clozaril)
Akathisia	Occasional	Frequent	Occasional	Frequent	Occasional	Occasional
Allergic skin reactions	Occasional	Rare	Rare	Rare	Rare	Occasional
Anticholinergic effects	Frequent	Not reported	Rare	Occasional	Occasional	Rare
Blood dyscrasia	Occasional	Occasional	Not reported	Rare	Not reported	Occasional
Cholestatic jaundice	Occasional	Rare	Not reported	Not reported	Not reported	Not reported
Dystonias	Occasional	Frequent	Rare	Occasional	Rare	Occasional
Impotence	Occasional	Not reported	Not reported	Not reported	Rare	Rare
Parkinsonism	Occasional	Frequent	Frequent	Occasional	Rare	Rare
Photosensitivity	Occasional	Rare	Not reported	Not reported	Not reported	Not reported
Postural hypotension	Frequent	Occasional	Rare	Rare	Occasional	Frequent
Retinitis pigmentosa	Not reported	Not reported	Not reported	Not reported	Not reported	Not reported
Sedation	Frequent	Not reported	Occasional	Rare	Rare	Frequent

Effect	Thioridazine (Mellaril)	Thiothixene (Navane)	Trifluoperazine (Stelazine)	Fluphenazine (Prolixin)
Akathisia	Occasional	Occasional	Frequent	Frequent
Allergic skin reactions	Not reported	Rare	Rare	Rare
Anticholinergic effects	Frequent	Occasional	Frequent	Frequent
Blood dyscrasia	Rare	Rare	Rare	Rare
Cholestatic jaundice	Rare	Rare	Rare	Rare
Dystonias	Occasional	Occasional	Frequent	Frequent
Impotence	Occasional	Not reported	Occasional	Occasional
Parkinsonism	Occasional	Occasional	Frequent	Frequent
Photosensitivity	Occasional	Rare	Occasional	Occasional
Postural hypotension	Frequent	Occasional	Rare	Rare
Retinitis pigmentosa	Occasional	Not reported	Not reported	Not reported
Sedation	Frequent	Frequent	Not reported	Occasional

Effect	Olanzapine (Zyprexa)	Quetiapine (Seroquel)	Ziprasidone (Geodon)
Akathisia	Frequent	Rare	Occasional
Allergic Skin Reactions	Rare	Rare	Frequent
Anticholinergic Effects	Frequent	Not reported	Common
Blood Dyscrasia	Rare	Rare	Rare
Cholestatic Jaundice	Not reported	Not reported	Not reported
Dystonias	Not reported	Rare	Occasional
Impotence	Not reported	Not reported	Occasional
Parkinsonism	Not reported	Not reported	Occasional
Photosensitivity	Not reported	Not reported	Frequent
Postural Hypotension	Frequent	Occasional	Frequent
Retinitis Pigmentosa	Not reported	Not reported	Not reported
Sedation	Frequent	Occasional	Common

MediaLink Akinesia & Pill Rolling Video

MediaLink EPSE: Parkinsonism Animation/Tremor Videos

tion gradually and to sit down if they feel faint. Support stockings and a large intake of fluids may be indicated. This problem is much less significant with oral administration of the drug. However, nurses working with clients receiving oral antipsychotic medications should take both baseline and routine vital sign readings at regular intervals. This practice establishes the client's tolerance for medications without the untoward side effects of orthostatic hypotension and subsequent falls.

Extrapyramidal Side Effects

Another common and sometimes frightening group of adverse reactions results from the effects of antipsychotics on the extrapyramidal tracts of the central nervous system, which are involved in the production and control of involuntary movements. These **extrapyramidal side effects (EPSEs)** can be broken down into four types, each with distinguishing clinical characteristics and times of onset after the initiation of drug therapy as shown in the Assessment box below.

Types of EPSEs. The earliest and most dramatic reactions are the *acute dystonic reactions*, forms of dystonia. These occur in the first days of treatment, sometimes after a single dose of medication. They involve bizarre and severe muscle contractions. These reactions can be physically painful and are almost always frightening to the individual. They are readily reversible.

Parkinsonian syndrome so named because of its striking resemblance to true Parkinson's disease, commonly occurs after a week or two of the therapy. It is the result of dopamine blockade caused by the neuroleptic drugs. Treatment with oral medication is usually sufficient, since urgency is seldom a consideration in the management of this syndrome.

A third reversible extrapyramidal side effect is known as **akathisia.** This characteristically is a motor restlessness perceived subjectively by the client and experienced as an urge to pace, a need to shift weight from one foot to another, or an inability to sit or stand still. Akathisia is generally a later complication of drug treatment, occurring weeks to months into the course of therapy.

Accurate observation of the course of therapy by the psychiatric nurse can promote prompt recognition and proper interpretation of EPSEs. If care is not taken, the health care provider may misinterpret the increasing withdrawal, emotional blunting, apathy, and lack of spontaneity as increasing schizophrenic behavior. This error in interpretation may lead to a mistaken

ASSESSMENT Extrapyramidal Side Effects (EPSEs)

Dystonia

- Usually occurs within 48 hr after beginning treatment but may occur any time.
- Described by the client as "Sometimes my back tightens up," or "I get tongue-tied when I try to talk."
- Characterized by abnormal tonic contractions of muscle groups.
- Characterized by odd posturing and strange facial expressions. **Torticollis** (twisting of the neck), **opisthotonos** (spasms of the neck and back, forcing the back to arch and the neck to bend backward), and **oculogyric crisis** (a fixed gaze that cannot return to lateral once raised vertically.)
- More common in young males.
- Prophylactically treated by anticholinergics. Some clients may experience a "high" from this treatment.

Drug-Induced Parkinsonism

- Usually occurs after 3 or more weeks of treatment.
- Characterized by rigidity (cogwheeling), tremor, or regular rhythmic oscillations of the extremities, particularly the distal parts, and in the hands, by a pill-rolling movement of the fingers.
- Clients are more susceptible to aspiratation or to injury by falling.
- Treatment is decreasing the medication dosage or administering anticholinergics.

Akathisia

- From the Greek words "a" meaning "not," and "akathisia" meaning "able to sit."
- Usually occurs after 3 or more weeks of treatment.
- Described by the client as "My nerves are jumping," or "I feel like jumping out of my skin."
- A subjective need or desire to move, not a type of pattern or movement.
- *Mild akathisia:* vague feelings of apprehension and irritability.
- *Severe akathisia:* an inability to sit (or feels like he or she cannot sit) for more than a few seconds, resulting in running, rocking, or agitated dancing.
- Not always responsive to anticholinergics; it may necessitate lowering the medication dosage.
- There is an associated dysphoria not treated by anticholinergics or benzodiazepines.

Dopamine-Acetylcholine Imbalance in the Extrapyramidal System

- Characterized by hallucinations, dry mouth, blurred vision, decreased absorption of antipsychotics, decreased gastric motility, tachycardia, and urinary retention.

Tardive Dyskinesia (TD)

- Late onset during the course of treatment with antipsychotics, with frequently irreversible abnormal movements or a neurologic syndrome.
- Characterized by coordinated, arrhythmic, involuntary movements (lip smacking, tongue protrusion, rocking, foot tapping).
- Complications include an inability to wear dentures, impaired respirations, weight loss, and impaired gait and posture.
- Treatment is primary prevention through careful initial assessment of the client's needs, as well as continual evaluation of the course of treatment.
- Regular assessment for TD presence and severity.

increase in dosage of antipsychotic medication, which will aggravate the condition. Akathisia can also be confused with psychotic agitation, and this error also prompts an increase in medication. For a comparison of the two conditions, see the Assessment box on page 738. Clients with akathisia require a reduction in the dosage of offending agents and/or treatment with an antiparkinsonian drug. You can save the client many uncomfortable and worrisome days by being aware of the frequency with which these syndromes complicate treatment and by reporting any suspicious sign or symptom while reassuring the client of the reversibility of the syndrome in almost all cases.

Prophylactic Treatment. Whether clients should be treated prophylactically with antiparkinsonian agents, in view of the relatively high incidence of EPSEs, is open to debate. Some argue that the use of antiparkinsonian agents eventually leads to relatively higher antipsychotic doses, thereby increasing the probability of serious side effects. Another argument is that antiparkinsonian agents also pose risks and thus should be used only to counteract EPSEs, not to guard against their possible emergence. Moreover, a great many clients never develop the syndromes. If the likelihood of an extrapyramidal reaction is high (if, for example, the client has a history of them) and the possible consequences significant (the client may discontinue medication or drop out of treatment altogether), antipsychotic and antiparkinsonian agents are frequently initiated simultaneously.

Assessment of EPSEs. Nursing assessment of EPSEs is important to the quality care of clients receiving psychotropic medications (Weitzel, 2000). One difficulty is *consistency* of assessment among caregivers. For example, nurses usually assess for the presence of cogwheeling or muscle rigidity in clients receiving psychotropic drugs. However, the reliability among those assessments is sorely lacking; what one nurse may consider moderate to severe side effects may be assessed as mild to moderate by another nurse.

Two assessment tools are the Simpson Neurological Rating Scale for the assessment of extrapyramidal side effects and the Abnormal Involuntary Movement Scale (AIMS) for the assessment of iatrogenic movements resulting from particular psychotropic drugs. These assessment tools can be found on the Companion Website for this book (AIMS is discussed later in this chapter). They are helpful in quantifying EPSEs prior to administering a medication to counteract the side effect. Readministering the instruments after the medication is given helps you assess the amelioration of the side effect. These data chart the course of a client's side effects and the effectiveness of medications to decrease them. This information is critical to quality nursing care.

The last EPSE to emerge in the course of treatment is also the most severe because it can be largely irreversible. This is **tardive dyskinesia (TD)**, which frequently appears after years of antipsychotic drug treatment, although it can occur earlier. It usually appears after a maintenance dose is discontinued or reduced, and it can be masked—but not treated—by reinstituting the medication or the dosage or by switching to another drug (Ballesteros, Gonzalez-Pinto, & Bulbena, 2000).

Current estimates put the incidence of TD at 4% to 5% per year for young adults and as high as 25% after 1 year in elderly clients (Jeste et al., 2000). Early detection through regular examinations (at least every 6 months) is recommended.

There is no known cure for TD. The recommended intervention is to stop all medication to see if the syndrome resolves spontaneously. This course of action must be weighed against the client's need for medication and the likelihood of relapse into psychosis. Reserpine, deanol, and several other drugs have been used experimentally to treat tardive dyskinesia, with equivocal results (Sirota, Mosheva, Shabtay, Giladi, & Korczyn, 2000).

To properly assess the impacts psychopharmacology is having on your client, regular assessments must be completed, especially for evidence of TD. One commonly utilized tool to assess to the presence and the severity of TD is the Abnormal Involuntary Movement Scale or AIMS. See Box 31–4 on page 740 for an example of the AIMS tool. Directions on the assessment tool and the examination procedure guide you through a careful and complete TD screen. It is helpful to use a gooseneck lamp to enhance your abilities to see minute movements particularly in the oral/facial areas. Clinical practice dictates an AIMS be completed every 6 months during treatment. Use of a videocamera allows clinicians to record these observations and make multiple comparisons of the regular exams.

With the emergence of the newer antipsychotic medications such as clozapine and risperidone, which can have an effect on TD and are not likely to cause a significant number of TD cases, the choices in this area are expanding. As noted above, five of the newer antipsychotics have been known to reduce tardive dyskinesia. The sixth and most recent antipsychotic, aripiprazole, is currently being evaluated in this regard.

For an overview of EPSE, see the Assessment box on page 738. ■ Table 31–5 on page 741 lists the commonly used antiparkinsonian medications for addressing EPSEs.

MediaLink EPSE: Dystonia (Blepharospasm, Cervical Torticollolis Videos)

MediaLink EPSE: Akathisia

Other Central Nervous System Effects

CNS side effects of antipsychotic medications are sedation and reduction of the seizure threshold. Because antipsychotic drugs vary in their sedative effects, this side effect is troublesome, but it can be managed by changing to a less sedating agent. Seizures are not a contraindication for use of these drugs. However, their use requires close observation.

Allergic Effects

The principal allergic manifestation of the antipsychotics is cholestatic jaundice. This occurs much less frequently than in the early days of psychopharmacology, and it is usually a benign and self-limiting condition. Chlorpromazine, tricyclic antidepressants, and phenothiazines can all cause cholestatic jaundice, which is not universally thought to always be an allergic reaction. It is suggested that chlorpromazine exerts a direct toxic effect on the bile secretory mechanisms of the liver.

BOX 31-4 The Abnormal Involuntary Movement Scale

DEPARTMENT OF HEALTH AND HUMAN SERVICES
PUBLIC HEALTH SERVICE
Alcohol, Drug Abuse, and Mental Health Administration
NIMH Treatment Strategies in Schizophrenia Study

ABNORMAL INVOLUNTARY MOVEMENT SCALE (AIMS)

PATIENT NUMBER — — — —

DATA GROUP **aims**

EVALUATION DATE — — — — — —
M M D D Y Y

PATIENT NAME

RATER NAME

RATER NUMBER — — —

EVALUATION TYPE (*Circle*)

1 Baseline	4 Start double-blind	7 Start open meds	10 Early termination
2 2-Week minor	5 Major evaluation	8 During open meds	11 Study completion
3	6 Other	9 Stop open meds	

INSTRUCTIONS: Complete Examination Procedure before making ratings.
MOVEMENT RATINGS: Rate highest severity observed.

Code: 1 = None; 2 = Minimal, may be extreme normal; 3 = Mild; 4 = Moderate; 5 = Severe

	Item	(Circle One)				
FACIAL AND ORAL MOVEMENTS:	**1. Muscles of Facial Expression** e.g., movements of forehead, eyebrows, periorbital area, cheeks; include frowning, blinking, smiling, grimacing	1	2	3	4	5
	2. Lips and Perioral Area e.g., puckering, pouting, smacking	1	2	3	4	5
	3. Jaw e.g., biting, clenching, chewing, mouth opening, lateral movement	1	2	3	4	5
	4. Tongue Rate only increase in movement both in and out of mouth, NOT inability to sustain movement	1	2	3	4	5
EXTREMITY MOVEMENTS:	**5. Upper** *(arms, wrists, hands, fingers)* Include choreic movements, (i.e., rapid, objectively purposeless, irregular, spontaneous), athetoid movements (i.e., slow, irregular, complex, serpentine). Do NOT include tremor (i.e., repetitive, regular, rhythmic)	1	2	3	4	5
	6. Lower *(legs, knees, ankles, toes)* e.g., lateral knee movement, foot tapping, heel dropping, foot squirming, inversion and eversion of foot	1	2	3	4	5
TRUNK MOVEMENTS:	**7. Neck, shoulders, hips** e.g., rocking, twisting, squirming, pelvic gyrations	1	2	3	4	5

	Item	Response	Score
GLOBAL JUDGMENTS:	**8. Severity of abnormal movements**	None, normal	1
		Minimal	2
		Mild	3
		Moderate	4
		Severe	5
	9. Incapacitation due to abnormal movements	None, normal	1
		Minimal	2
		Mild	3
		Moderate	4
		Severe	5
	10. Patient's awareness of abnormal movements Rate only patient's report	No awareness	1
		Aware, no distress	2
		Aware, mild distress	3
		Aware, moderate distress	4
		Aware, severe distress	5
DENTAL STATUS:	**11. Current problems with teeth and/or dentures**	No	1
		Yes	2
	12. Does patient usually wear dentures?	No	1
		Yes	2

(continues)

BOX 31-4 The Abnormal Involuntary Movement Scale

Examination Procedure

Either before or after completing the Examination Procedure observe the patient unobtrusively, at rest (e.g., in waiting room.)
The chair to be used in this examination should be a hard, firm one without arms.

1. Ask patient to remove shoes and socks.
2. Ask patient whether there is anything in his/her mouth (e.g., gum, candy, etc.) and if there is, to remove it.
3. Ask patient about the current condition of his/her teeth. Ask patient if he/she wears dentures. Do teeth or dentures bother patient *now*?
4. Ask patient whether he/she notices any movements in mouth, face, hands, or feet. If yes, ask to describe and to what extent they *currently* bother patient or interfere with his/her activities.
5. Have patient sit in chair with hands on knees, legs slightly apart, and feet flat on floor. (Look at entire body for movements while in this position.)
6. Ask patient to sit with hands hanging unsupported. If male, between legs, if female and wearing a dress, hanging over knees. (Observe hands and other body areas.)
7. Ask patient to open mouth. (Observe tongue at rest within mouth.) Do this twice.
8. Ask patient to protrude tongue. (Observe abnormalities of tongue movement.) Do this twice.
9. Ask patient to tap thumb, with each finger, as rapidly as possible for 10–15 seconds; separately with right hand, then with left hand. (Observe facial and leg movements.)
10. Flex and extend patient's left and right arms (one at a time.) (Note any rigidity.)
11. Ask patient to stand up. (Observe in profile. Observe all body areas again, hips included.)
12. Ask patient to extend both arms outstretched in front with palms down. (Observe trunk, legs, and mouth.)
13. Have patient walk a few paces, turn, and walk back to chair. (Observe hands and gait.) Do this twice.

MediaLink EPSE: Bradykinesia/Akathisia Video

Many times, clients may have a record of an "allergic" reaction to a psychotropic medication without cholestatic jaundice or other evidence of allergic reactions documented. When these circumstances are clearly assessed, it may turn out that the client either experienced neuroleptic malignant syndrome (NMS) or a dystonic reaction. The dangers associated with NMS may have prompted an explanation to the client along the lines of the dangers associated with an allergic reaction. This communication may have been misinterpreted and was not detected or corrected.

The other false-positive report of an allergic reaction to a psychiatric medication is *dystonia*. A painful side effect such as dystonia is a negative experience to be avoided and may be communicated to caregivers as an allergy to assure avoidance of the compound at fault. Careful scrutiny of reports of allergies must be conducted regularly to determine true allergies so the client is protected from contact, but also to make sure no medications are removed from the array of effective treatments for that client.

Blood, Skin, and Eye Effects

Among the other side effects, agranulocytosis is the most serious. It is both potentially fatal and, fortunately, extremely rare. Usually the person gets an infection and deteriorates rapidly or begins to bleed spontaneously, requiring emergency medical attention. Many medications cause agranulocytosis, including benzodiazepines and antibiotics. (See the discussion on page 734.)

Skin eruptions, photosensitivity leading to severe sunburn, blue-gray metallic discolorations over the face and hands, and pigmentation changes in the eyes are all potential side effects. Clients are generally advised to avoid prolonged exposure to sunlight or to use a sunscreen agent when outdoors. These conditions usually remit.

One serious and permanent eye change is retinitis pigmentosa. This condition may occur in clients on dosages of thioridazine exceeding 800 mg/day. The condition may lead to blindness. Therefore, doses exceeding 800 mg per day are contraindicated.

MediaLink Dystonia Video

TABLE 31–5 Antiparkinsonian Medications

Generic Name	Trade Name	Maximum Daily Dosage	Available in Injectable Form
Amantadine	Symmetrel	300 mg	No
Benztropine	Cogentin	8 mg	Yes
Biperiden	Akineton	8 mg	Yes
Diphenhydramine	Benadryl	100 mg	Yes
Procyclidine	Kemadrin	15 mg	No
Trihexyphenidyl	Artane	15 mg	No

Endocrine Effects

Lactation in females and gynecomastia and impotence in males lead a list of endocrine changes that can occur with antipsychotic drug treatments. *Hyperprolactinemia* is a common side effect that will affect many aspects of the client's sex life. Difficulties with libido, arousal, excitation, orgasm, male ejaculatory volume, and overall performance can occur to a disturbing degree with hyperprolactinemia. You can imagine how these side effects would affect the regular or long-term use of the medication. Hyperprolactinemia is also responsible for oligomenorrhea or amenorrhea in women, galactorrhea in women and rarely in men, and, in cases of prolonged hyperprolactinemia, osteoporosis (Dickson & Glazer, 1999). Be alert to these endocrine changes, as a nurse will likely be the professional told about such problems.

Another endocrine problem surfacing recently is diabetes in people who have schizophrenia. The baseline occurrence of diabetes is elevated with schizophrenia (twice the rate of the general population), and seems to be further escalated by endocrine changes from psychotropics. While weight gain can certainly propel one into an increased diabetic risk, some studies show diabetes occurring in clients who have not gained significant weight. The particular medication used may be contributing. You should be alert to any changes in body functions reported by clients taking these medications.

Weight Gain

Weight gain is a significant side effect that affects self-esteem and poses health risks for the client. Antipsychotics, tricyclic antidepressants, lithium, anticonvulsants, and other classes of medications have individual compounds within the class that can cause an increase in weight. As mentioned above, an increase in weight can put an individual at risk for health problems such as diabetes, hypertension, and coronary artery disease. The impact of weight gain can be more disturbing than EPSEs to a client. Over time, this side effect can be a devastating force to long-term treatment and quality of life. Assiduous attention paid to the potential for weight gain issues from the inception of treatment can help minimize this particular side effect.

MediaLink Cytochrome P450 Actions Animation

Neuroleptic Malignant Syndrome

Neuroleptic malignant syndrome (NMS) is a severe and potentially life-threatening side effect of all psychotropic medications. This extreme condition is believed to be the result of dopamine blockade in the striatum of the brain or dopaminergic antagonism in the CNS. There are some interesting efforts to examine the genetic etiology of NMS; the search is on to discover phenotypes and genetic markers to this syndrome (Gurrera, 2000; Qureshi & Al-Habeeb, 2000). NMS occurs in 0.5 to 1% of clients taking neuroleptic medications. Men are affected more than women, approximately twice as much, and younger clients appear to be more susceptible than older ones (Silva, Munoz, Alpert, Perlmutter, & Diaz, 2000). NMS typically occurs within the first 2 weeks of treatment with a different medication or a dosage increase, but cases have been reported months after a new medication regimen has begun. Nurses are in the best position to assess for this condition because its symptoms are muscle rigidity, hyperpyrexia, altered consciousness, and diaphoresis. Because NMS often occurs in clients whose presentations are already complex, the nursing assessment can be difficult.

Treatment for NMS includes discontinuing all psychotropic medication immediately and supporting the client medically through the crisis. If cooling and rehydration are not achieved quickly, along with holding all psychotropics, the client may die. Caution in follow-up care is, of course, important. The pathology of NMS is complex and not completely understood at this time beyond the knowledge that the major symptoms of NMS are caused by the neuroleptic blockade of the dopamine receptors.

CLINICAL IMPLICATIONS

Nurses have many responsibilities to clients receiving neuroleptic drugs. To ensure the bioavailability and effectiveness of neuroleptic medications, it is important to understand the relationships between the medication and the liquid (or substance) you administer it with, as well as the relationships between medications. Some medications are not compatible with all substances. For an overview of the compatibility of drugs and typical liquids, see ■ Table 31–6 on page 744.

In addition to the liquid and drug compatibilities listed in Table 31–6, you need to be aware of other problematic combinations. Recent practice has shown a specific problem with the combination of grapefruit juice with several psychiatric medications. For example, two anxiolytic medications, triazolam (Halcion) and buspirone (BuSpar) are specifically called to your attention. Triazolam will not be metabolized efficiently and therefore remains at higher levels in the body, and buspirone can have a blood level nine times normal when taken with grapefruit juice. The explanation for this resides in grapefruit juice's furanocoumarins, compounds within grapefruit juice, and their ability to inhibit a liver enzyme (cytochrome P_{450}3A4 or CYP3A4) from metabolizing the medication out of the system. This inhibition of the enzyme allows the medication and its metabolites to remain in the system longer than usual, accumulating and causing higher blood levels, enhanced effects of the medication, and greater side effects (Koth & Cassavaugh, 2000).

The entire field of study on the cytochrome P_{450}s (or CYPs) is an extensive one, covering the intricacies of drug interactions, metabolism, and co-administration cautions. Although it may be difficult to envision a liver enzyme having a tremendous influence on psychiatric symptomatology, you will be able to see the impacts of these effects with your clients. The above paragraph talks about the impacts of inhibiting these enzymes, which determines whether the metabolism of a medication will be delayed. There is another cytochrome P_{450} action important to clinical practice called activating the enzyme. Activating the CYP enzyme, which means the compound will be moving through the system at an accelerated pace, has an entirely different clinical presentation. When a medication does not have enough time to exert its power, it will appear to not be addressing symptoms competently or it will appear to be considerably less effective than if it had the time to be fully utilized by the client's body.

Ultimately, either of these mechanisms of cytochrome P_{450} activation or inhibition can be accomplished through a variety of interactions among drugs, foods, liquids, or substances (e.g., nicotine). Being aware of the total picture of your clients and their medications in a holistic manner will alert you to drug–drug interactions as well as the dynamism of drug metabolism.

CLIENT/FAMILY EDUCATION

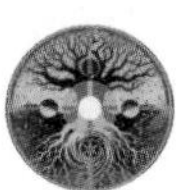

The Client/Family Teaching feature below points out the major areas to be addressed when educating clients and their family about antipsychotic medication treatments.

Antidepressant Medications

Like antipsychotic drugs, the original antidepressant medications were discovered accidentally. Four classes of antidepressants currently exist: tricyclic antidepressants (TCAs), monoamine oxidase inhibitors (MAOIs), selective serotonin reuptake inhibitors (SSRIs), and phenethylamine antidepressants. There are also atypical antidepressants, called so because of their variety of formulation and actions. In the case of imipramine (Tofranil), the first of the tricyclic antidepressants, investigators were actually searching for effective antipsychotics similar to chlorpromazine. Iproniazid, a MAOI, was discovered when tuberculous clients regularly treated with a similar drug, isoniazid, became less depressed. The antidepressants have shed considerable light on the biochemical mechanisms of the brain in both normal and abnormal emotional expression. See the Using Research Evidence feature on page 745 regarding psychopharmacology in the treatment of depression.

PSYCHOBIOLOGIC CONSIDERATIONS

Knowledge about the pharmacology of **antidepressant medications** has led to a theory of the biochemistry of depression. Basically, all the true antidepressants make the neuro-

MediaLink Case Study: Nurse's Role in Psychopharmacology

CLIENT / FAMILY TEACHING

Antipsychotics

Client and family education about antipsychotics centers upon the individual client's medications, responses to it (or them), side effects exhibited, and the client and family member's abilities and interests in learning.

This teaching plan points out the major areas to be addressed when educating clients and their family about antipsychotic medication treatments and must be individualized for the above issues.

What does this medication do?	"Antipsychotic medications help treat the emotional and thinking problems of schizophrenia or psychosis. It helps organize thinking, keep you in touch with reality, and reduce the symptoms of your illness. It is not a cure. When you stop taking this medication, the benefits wear off over time and you will have these problems again, possibly at a more disturbing level."
How should I take this medication?	"Take it as prescribed on a regular basis. If you feel that you cannot or do not want to continue, notify your therapist or prescriber before you take action."
What if I miss a dose?	"Take the dose as soon as you remember if it's only been a few hours. But if it is almost time for your next dose, do not take double or extra doses."
What other medicine does not mix with this antipsychotic?	Tailor this response to the specific medication prescribed. Mention the major drug interactions with prescribed medications, over-the-counter substances, alternative and complementary supplements, and, of course, alcohol and recreational drug use. There may even be interactions with caffeine, nicotine, and food items that need exploration in detail.
What side effects can I expect?	A discussion of the client's previous side effects with the substance drives this conversation. There is no need to overwhelm an individual with excess information, and there is a vital need for the client to know what actions to take when side effects occur. Delineate the ordinary and the extraordinary side effects with actions laid out for each. Some standard side effects are important to cover: dystonia, akathisia, agitation, confusion, sensitivity to sunlight, and changes to sexual expression.
Where can I keep my medication?	"In a safe place at room temperature. Do not keep it in the bathroom where there is a shower or bathtub, in the kitchen where there is a dishwasher, or above or right next to the kitchen sink. Medications should not be kept in a motor vehicle as temperatures can reach extreme levels within such an enclosed area. Moisture, light, and heat can affect your medication."
What do I do if I have a problem?	Give the names and numbers of who the client can reach for questions and for emergencies.

TABLE 31–6 Antipsychotic Medication and Lithium Compatibility with Liquids and Other Drugs

Liquid	Chlor-promazine	Flu-phenazine	Haloperidol	Lox-apine	Mesorid-azine	Thiori-dazine	Thio-thixene	Trifluo-perazine	Lithium Citrate
Water	C	C	C		C	C	C	C	C
Saline	C	C	X			C		C	C
Milk	C	C	X			X	C	C	C
Coffee	U	X	X	C		X	X	U	C
Tea	U	X	X			X	X	C	C
Apple juice/cider	X	X	C			X	X	X	X
Apricot juice	C	C				U	C	C	C
Cranberry juice	X			C	C	C	C		C
Grape juice	X		X		C	X		X	C
Grapefruit juice	C	C	X	C	C	C	C	C	C
Lemonade						C			C
Orange juice	C	C	C	C	C	C	C	C	C
Pineapple juice		C		C		X	C	C	C
Prune juice	U	C				X	C	C	C
Tang	X			C					C
Tomato juice	C	C	C			X	C	C	C
V-8	C	C				X	X	C	C
Cola	U	X	C	C		X	X	C	C
Ginger ale		C				C			
Mellow-Yellow		X				C		C	C
Orange soda	C	C				X		C	C
7-Up/Sprite	C	C		C		C		C	C
Soups/Pudding	C	C	C				C	C	C
Drug									
Chlorpromazine						X			X
Haloperidol									X
Lithium citrate	X	C	U	C	C	X	C	X	
Thioridazine	X	X	X	X	X		X		X
Trifluoperazine									X

C = compatible; X = incompatible; U = unconfirmed, conflicting data; blank = no data available.
Source: Department of Pharmacy, Buffalo Psychiatric Center, Buffalo, New York, 2000.

transmitters norepinephrine (NE) and serotonin (5-HT) more available to the synaptic receptors in the central nervous system. Tricyclics block the reuptake of these substances into the neuron after their release, thereby postponing their degradation. MAOIs interfere with the enzymes responsible for the actual breakdown of the neurotransmitter molecules. Since both are antidepressants, these observations have led to the theory that NE and 5-HT shortages in the brain cause depression, at least the type of depression that responds to drug therapy. The details of the dexamethasone suppression test (DST), an examination of psychoendocrine function in light of depressive behavior, can be found in Chapter 4, which provides an overview of the current psychobiologic theories of depression.

USING RESEARCH EVIDENCE

You are conducting an outpatient group consisting of seven people who are all in treatment for depression. This is a psychoeducational group with the goal of educating clients about symptoms of depression, available treatments, and prevention or minimalization of relapse. The group discovers that everyone has a different viewpoint about medications for their depressive symptoms. You are asked a number of questions about the latest information on these treatments as well as your clinical experience with antidepressants. You report that research indicates how well antidepressants work in treating the symptoms of major depression. Other group members wonder about criticisms they've heard about some studies. The popular media has stated from time to time that antidepressants are no better than placebo treatment, and results indicating otherwise are illusory.

The discussion centers around the most effective treatments and the research that drives competent practice. Overall, the literature shows that antidepressant response rates are approximately 50%, while placebo response rates hover at around 30%. Clinician bias has been raised as causing the discrepancy, implying that antidepressants are really no more effective than a placebo. Those clients wondering about whether their therapists could slant the interpretation of treatment outcomes discussed how the clients' self-ratings might resolve that problem. Research has shown, however, that the criticism that client self-ratings are more valid than clinician outcome ratings was not supported in any way.

The final aspect of care in depression talked about in the popular press exposed these clients to the assertion that psychotherapy could be superior to drugs in treating depression. You have seen journal articles regarding this very issue and are able to share how this has been examined in meta-analyses (studies that analyze the analyses of several studies) concerning studies with severely depressed individuals. It has not been supported that psychotherapy, while necessary in the treatment of depression, is superior to psychopharmacology in treatment efficacy.

Psychoeducational groups provide a very important function beyond giving facts about mental illness and treatment. Examining and discussing what the layman hears and reads allows correction to misconceptions and support to the scientific basis of care. There is a public health concern where definitive statements about the role of antidepressants and their relative benefit compared to psychotherapy can be misleading. Both clients and therapists may assume medications are unnecessary, leading to the institution of less than ideal treatment protocols. Keeping current with research and active in critical thinking skills gives your clients the benefit of psychiatric nursing expertise. Findings from antidepressant research, such as the reference cited below, are usually valid, meaning these medications are often specifically useful.

Quitkin, F. M., Rabkin, J. G., Gerald, J., Davis, J. M., & Klein, D. F. (2000). Validity of clinical trials of antidepressants. *American Journal of Psychiatry, 157*, 327–337.

The initial distinction to be understood in the psychopharmacology of depression is between true antidepressants and stimulants or euphoriants. TCAs and MAOIs are not stimulants and will not induce euphoria in healthy people. In a single dose, they have a sedative effect. Amphetamines and methylphenidate (Ritalin), on the other hand, are stimulants but not antidepressants in the pharmacologic sense. They can induce an increased sense of well-being in certain individuals, but do nothing to combat depression on a lasting basis.

Tricyclic antidepressants are the "first generation" of antidepressant medications. This means they were among the first medications identified as effective in the treatment of depression.

Since that time, a number of medications have been developed to treat the symptoms of major depression and the depressive features of schizoaffective disorder. Among these medications are the MAOIs, the SSRIs, and a number of atypical antidepressants with a variety of neurotransmittor actions.

Bupropion (Wellbutrin) is an oral antidepressant drug that is not a TCA and is unrelated to other known antidepressants. Bupropion has been well tolerated in people experiencing orthostatic hypotension with TCAs. This medication has a dose-related potential for causing seizures to a greater extent than other antidepressants. It has few anticholinergic side effects and essentially no important cardiovascular effects. Bupropion is also indicated for use as an aid to smoking cessation and supports the client through the process of quitting the habit of smoking. There are sustained-release formulations of this medication under two trade names (Wellbutrin SR and Zyban). For smoking cessation, the medication is used for up to 12 weeks.

Of note is the cross-diagnostic use of medications initially indicated for other conditions (discussed earlier in this chapter and referred to in Table 31–1). Fluoxetine (Prozac) is an antidepressant and was the first SSRI developed. This compound recently received an indication for yet another treatment regimen. Fluoxetine is formulated under the trade name Sarafem to treat the mood and physical symptoms of premenstrual dysphoric disorder (PMDD), which is differentiated from depression and other mental disorders. The dosing is flexible, with 10- or 20-mg pulvules available; 20 mg/day is the recommended dose.

As each new group of medications became available, practitioners initially used the new drugs to the partial exclusion of the old. When a client is not responding to a medication, it is helpful to have an array of choices from which to select further treatment. The side effect profiles of antidepressants remain one of the linchpins of successful care. If sedation is a side effect and the client is sleeping at a higher-than-preferred level, then a class of medications with less sedating side effects may be a better choice. Experience reinforces the truth that a number of treatment and medication options are necessary to effectively treat psychiatric disorders; therefore, all categories of antidepressants remain useful.

NURSING RESPONSIBILITIES WHEN CLIENTS RECEIVE UNCOMMON DRUG COMBINATIONS

As drug combinations and innovative psychobiologic therapies become more commonplace in the practice of psychiatry, psychiatric nurses must be observant for idiosyncratic responses among clients. Knowing the interactive effects of medications is an important feature of effective psychopharmacologic nursing. Planning and implementing care for this specialized client subpopulation are likely to be challenging, and you need to be aware of the underlying psychobiology to recognize potential drug-related behaviors among clients who are on multiple-drug regimens.

CLINICAL CONSIDERATIONS

The most important clinical consideration in the use of medications to treat depression is that antidepressant drugs are not effective in all cases of depressed mood. Evidence from research and clinical practice indicates that only a portion of depressive disorders respond to this category of drugs. For example, TCAs, MAOIs, and amphetamines are generally contraindicated in depression resulting from what commonly has been referred to as grief reaction or pathologic grief. Other types of depression, described in the DSM-IV-TR, may be more amenable to psychopharmacologic intervention. Thus, accurate diagnosis is necessary to ensure maximum effectiveness.

Clients for whom antidepressants are indicated usually suffer from characteristic symptoms: a severely depressed mood, loss of interest, an inability to respond to normally pleasurable events or situations, a depression that is worse in the morning and lessens slightly as the day goes on, early morning awakening (and an inability to fall asleep again), marked psychomotor retardation or agitation, appetite and weight changes, and excessive or inappropriate guilt. The DSM-IV-TR calls this melancholia. In fact, the symptoms of melancholia are the features that most reliably predict response to drug therapy (Schreiber, Stern, & Wilson, 2000). A significant, and commonly overlooked, clinical consideration is that antidepressants have a delayed-reaction onset. A client will not show lessening of depressed mood until 2 to 3 weeks after the institution of an adequate dose of TCAs, for example.

TRICYCLIC ANTIDEPRESSANTS (TCAs)

One of the most commonly used class of antidepressant drugs is TCAs. These compounds are close in chemical structure to phenothiazines and have many similar side effects, but they have profoundly different effects on mood, behavior, and cognition. TCAs are not antipsychotic agents when given to schizophrenic clients and may in fact aggravate a disintegrative pattern or precipitate overt symptoms in a client with latent disintegrative behavior. Imipramine (Tofranil) and amitriptyline (Elavil) are the two prime representative TCAs. Desipramine (Norpramin, Pertofrane), nortriptyline (Pamelor), and protriptyline (Vivactil) are compounds prepared in simpler forms (similar to the conversions made in normal metabolism) that are reported to reduce the incidence of side effects. (See ■ Figure 31–3).

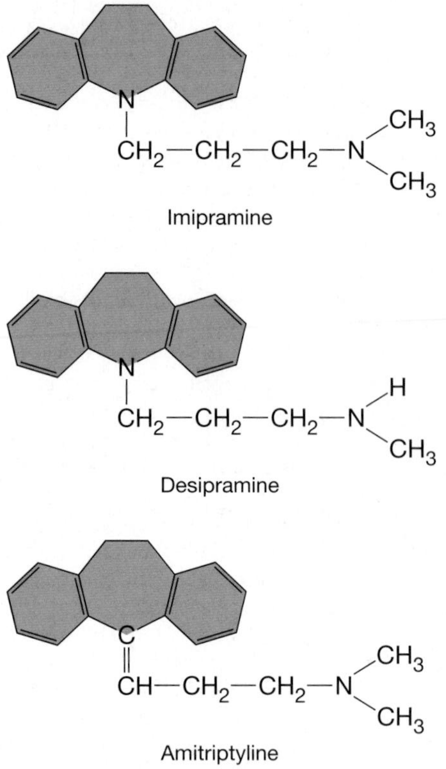

Imipramine

Desipramine

Amitriptyline

FIGURE 31–3 ■ *Chemical structures of three tricyclic antidepressants. Tricyclics, named for their consistent triple-ring structure, work through a host of neurochemical effects. Examples of adverse reactions to these medications include: blurred vision, dry mouth, constipation, cardiotoxicity.*

Source: Smock, T. K. (1999). *Physiological psychology: A neuroscience approach*. Upper Saddle River, NJ: Prentice Hall.

Dosage

What constitutes an adequate dose of tricyclics is a matter of debate. Using imipramine (considered the prototype TCA) as an example, most clinicians agree that most of the responsive clients with a major depression need doses of 50 to 300 mg/day. Dosages of other tricyclics, such as nortriptyline are not recommended above 150 mg/day.

After remission of the symptoms, clients who are put on a reduced maintenance dosage (perhaps 50% of the acute dosage) show less likelihood of relapse. Therefore, most clients are continued on treatment for 6 months to 1 year following a major depressive episode. Clients who have had repeated episodes may require longer drug maintenance or should be considered for treatment with a mood stabilizer because of the prophylactic effects on recurrent major depression and the depressive episodes of bipolar disorder.

Side Effects

Many of the common side effects of the tricyclic drugs are autonomic due to the anticholinergic characteristics of the medications. These side effects include dry mouth, blurred vision, constipation, palpitations, and urinary retention. Clients with glaucoma must be treated with caution. Some allergic skin reactions have been observed. TCAs also cause changes in the normal electrical conduction of the heart and are cardiotoxic, which is particularly significant in treating clients with a history of cardiovascular disease, especially heart block. Sudden death has occurred during tricyclic treatment. Clients with known heart disease and most elderly clients require electrocardiograms (ECGs) before, and periodically during, the course of tricyclic therapy. Several CNS effects may occur, including tremor, twitching, paresthesias, ataxia, and convulsions.

Overdose Effects

One aspect of TCA treatment that deserves attention is the consequences of an overdose. Significant overdoses may cause delirium; hyperthermia; convulsions; and even coma, shock, and respiratory failure. A lethal dose of an antidepressant such as amitriptyline is estimated at between ten and thirty times the usual daily therapeutic dose. Drug intake deserves close attention, because many clients treated with these drugs are severely suicidal. Serious overdosing is a medical emergency and may require resuscitative measures.

MONOAMINE OXIDASE INHIBITORS (MAOIs)

Clients who do not respond to tricyclic antidepressants may respond to another major class, MAOIs. These drugs generally are not as effective as tricyclics and are somewhat slower to act, sometimes requiring a month of treatment before improvement shows. Isocarboxazid (Marplan) is considered the most effective, with phenelzine (Nardil) and tranylcypromine (Parnate) slightly behind. Complicating the decision to use MAOIs is their association with several very severe side effects. Hepatic necrosis, commonly fatal, and **hypertensive crisis** leading to intracranial bleeding are among the most threatening. The latter reaction, heralded by severe headache, stiff neck, nausea, vomiting, and sharply increased blood pressure, follows the ingestion of foods that contain the amino acid tyramine and the ingestion of sympathomimetic medications.

Client/Family Education

The MAOI antidepressants require an especially strong, concerted teaching effort from nurses. These medications have many drawbacks that directly affect nursing intervention. For example, clients on MAOIs *must* avoid foods that contain even moderate amounts of tyramine; failure to do so will result in hypertensive crisis. The Client/Family Teaching feature on page 748 outlines the low-tyramine diet for clients taking MAOIs.

The principles guiding the use of MAOI and TCA medications are as follows:

- Drug treatment does not preclude psychotherapy, electroconvulsive therapy, or behavioral treatments if they are also indicated.
- Other antidepressant treatment should be given first unless there are contraindications, clinical indications for MAOI, or a past history of unresponsiveness to other antidepressants.
- Dosage may vary and may be limited by significant side effects.
- A response is seen 2 to 3 weeks after the therapeutic dose is reached.
- Clients with recurrent major depressive episodes with melancholia may require long-term maintenance treatment, although doses are usually lower than those needed in acute episodes.

SELECTIVE SEROTONIN REUPTAKE INHIBITORS (SSRIs)

Further development of antidepressants has been the result of a scientific search for drugs with fewer toxic side effects and greater biologic predictability in the treatment of depression. They are believed to be more neurotransmitter–specific and better able to treat conditions related to dopamine, serotonin, or norepinephrine dysfunctions.

There are disadvantages with the early antidepressants. Uncomfortable and sometimes intolerable side effects, and a number of use restrictions with certain populations, combined with the dietary restrictions of the MAOIs, make these drugs for depression inappropriate for many people.

The next class of antidepressant medications developed was the SSRIs. A profound difference with this group of drugs is their side effects. While all chemically different, SSRIs inhibit the reuptake (and thus the deactivation) of the neurotransmitter serotonin, allowing for the increased availability of serotonin at synapses. The first SSRI developed was fluoxetine. There are now a number of medications with this action. They are potent and highly specific reuptake blockers of serotonin.

The SSRIs opened our eyes to the mechanisms of synapses. For the first time, psychiatric–mental health nurses were able to see the direct impact of changing neurotransmitter concentrations. ■ Figure 31–4 on page 749 shows the structure of the synapse, and ■ Figure 31–5 on page 749 illustrates the chemical structure of three SSRI antidepressants. To see an animation of the synaptic action of these medications, see the text's CD-ROM.

MediaLink Fluoxetine in Action/Neurological Synapse Animation(s)

Side Effects

Although the side effects of SSRIs are less severe than those of other antidepressants, some may be intolerable for certain clients. See ■ Table 31–7 on page 750 for the SSRI side effect profile. Activation, a more energized state including decreased sleep and akathisia, is common. Special care must be taken with clients who have hypomania or mania in their histories. SSRIs may precipitate an emergence or a relapse.

See the Assessment boxes on pages 750 and 751 for SSRI discontinuation syndrome, serotonin syndrome, and the management and prevention of serotonin syndrome.

An important consideration with clients taking SSRIs is the proximity of the administration of MAOIs. Fluoxetine and a MAOI together may cause serious and fatal interactions. The half-life of fluoxetine is such that there must be a 5-week gap between taking fluoxetine and taking a MAOI, and vice versa. Sertraline (Zoloft), paroxetine (Paxil), citalopram (Celexa),

CLIENT / FAMILY TEACHING

Low-Tyramine Diet

The MAO inhibitors combine with certain foods and medications to produce a significant increase in blood pressure, which can be a health hazard. In general, foods that can cause this reaction are ones that have been *pickled, fermented, smoked,* or *aged*. The list below includes the main foods, fluids, and medications to avoid while taking an MAOI and for the 2 weeks after the MAOI is discontinued.

Foods and Beverages to Avoid Completely		Foods and Beverages to Avoid Taking in Large Amounts	
Meats and fish	Pickled herring, dried fish, unrefrigerated fermented fish, liver, caviar, fermented sausage (bologna, salami, pepperoni, summer sausage), hoisin sauce (fermented oyster sauce used in Oriental dishes)	Dairy products	Processed American cheese
		Fruits	Raisins, prunes, bananas, avocados, plums, canned figs
		Caffeine sources	Coffee, chocolate, colas
Vegetables	English broad peas, Chinese pea pods, Fava beans	Beverages	Domestic jug red wines;
Dairy products	Most cheeses (exceptions are listed under Allowed Foods), yogurt		domestic beers, ales, and stouts; sherry
Beverages	Chianti, aged wines, imported beers, aged beers		
Combination foods	Pizza, lasagna, souffles, macaroni and cheese, quiche, liver pate, caesar salads, eggplant parmesan		

All yeast products (such as Brewer's yeast) and yeast extracts (such as Marmite)

Medications to avoid	Cold medications, nasal decongestants (tablets, drops, sprays, etc.), hay fever and allergy medications, weight reduction preparations, "pep" pills, antiappetite medications, asthma inhalants

Foods and Beverages That May Be Taken Without Problems

Beverages	White wines
Any baked goods raised with yeast	
Dairy products	Cottage cheese, cream cheese, milk, cream, ice cream

Note: Although white wines are listed as having no tyramine, alcohol is a depressant and should not be ingested by individuals in treatment for depression.

Tyramine Content of Some Cheeses

English Stilton	17.3 mg/serving
Mozzarella	2.4 mg/serving
Grated Parmesan	0.2 mg/serving
Cream cheese	0

escitalopram (Lexapro) have shorter half-lives, and there must be a 1- or 2-week gap (both directions) with these medications and MAOIs.

■ Figure 31–6 on page 752 illustrates the process of serotonin neurotransmission, so important to the effectiveness of this new class of medications. Imagine the movement of the neurotransmitters back and forth across the synapse. This is the movement that SSRIs affect.

NEW GENERATION ANTIDEPRESSANTS

Venlafaxine (Effexor) is the first in a class of medications called phenethylamine antidepressants. It has two mechanisms of action: inhibiting the reuptake of both serotonin and norepinephrine.

Anticholinergic-like side effects may occur with venlafaxine. There are also reports of sustained increases in blood pressure with some clients. This last side effect seems to be dose-related, so nursing management of clients taking venlafaxine should include regular blood pressure monitoring. There is also a need for a time buffer regarding MAOIs: a 14-day gap after discontinuing an MAOI before starting venlafaxine, and at least a 7-day gap after discontinuing venlafaxine before starting an MAOI.

The side effects of this medication include nervousness and anorexia. Medications such as this one that have an activation component can cause nervous feelings. Anorexia may be a difficult side effect for underweight individuals. Other reported side effects include:

- Nausea
- Somnolence
- Dry mouth
- Dizziness
- Constipation
- Nervousness
- Sweating
- Asthenia
- Abnormal ejaculation/orgasm
- Anorexia

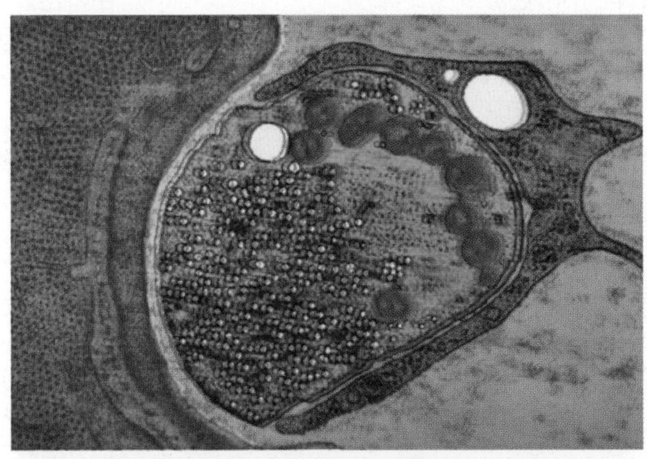

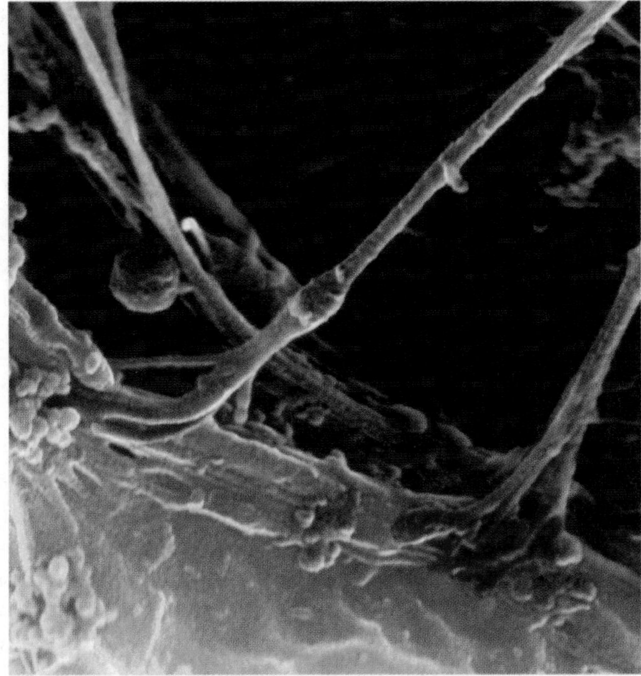

FIGURE 31–4 ■ *Structure of the synapse. The synapse at the top has many specialized characteristics. The electron micrograph shows the vesicles containing the synaptic transmitter, the abundance of mitochondria necessary for energy production and the abundance of protein in the presynaptic and postsynaptic densities. Above are incoming axons (purple) contacting dendrites (yellow) with non-neural cells nearby (green).*

Source: Smock, T. K. (1999). *Physiological psychology: A neuroscience approach*. Upper Saddle River, NJ: Prentice Hall.
Bottom photo source: Don W. Fawcett/Science Source, Photo Researchers, Inc.

F
O
CH_2
N
H
Paroxetine

F_3C — O — $CH(CH_2)_2NHCH_3$
Fluoxetine

$NHCH_3$
Cl
Cl
Sertraline

FIGURE 31–5 ■ *The chemical structures of three selective serotonin reuptake inhibitors (SSRIs). The antidepressant efficacy of these drugs is claimed to be related to their ability to block the reuptake of serotonin, thereby increasing the serotonin concentrations in the synaptic cleft. While this increase in concentration is almost immediate, the therapeutic benefits take 1 to 2 weeks to develop. The success rate of SSRIs is around 85%, and the SSRIs are generally better tolerated than traditional antidepressants. Some adverse reactions include anxiety, agitation, sleep disturbance, slight tremors, headaches, and sexual dysfunction (e.g., delayed ejaculation and impotence).*

Source: Smock, T. K. (1999). *Physiological psychology: A neuroscience approach*. Upper Saddle River, NJ: Prentice Hall.

The recommended starting dosage for venlafaxine is 75 mg/day, administered in divided doses and taken with food. The dose may be increased to 225 mg/day according to clinical needs, and even further increased to 375 mg/day. It is recommended that clients who have been taking venlafaxine for more than 1 week taper the dose when discontinuing the medication. Clients taking it for 6 weeks or more should time this taper over a 2-week period to minimize the risk of symptoms caused by discontinuing the medication.

Reboxetine (Vestra) is an antidepressant with a unique mechanism of action; the drug is the first in a new class of medications known as selective norepinephrine reuptake inhibitors (SNRIs). Reboxetine does not inhibit the reuptake of serotonin or dopamine nor does it inhibit monoamine oxidase. It has not been marketed as of this printing; however, it has received an FDA approval letter. Reboxetine is effective for moderate to severe depression and dysthymia. In addition, the medication is

TABLE 31–7 Side Effects of SSRIs

	Fluoxetine (Prozac)	Sertraline (Zoloft)	Paroxetine (Paxil)	Citalopram (Celexa)
Anticholinergic	0	1	1	1
Sedation	1–2	1–2	0–1	0–1
Activation	1–2	1–2	1–2	1–2
Hypotension	0	0	0	0–1
GI activation	1–2	1–2	1–2	1–2
Seizures	+	+	0	0
Compare this with a typical tricyclic antidepressant (amitriptyline [Elavil]):				
Anticholinergic	4			
Sedation	3			
Activation	0			
Hypotension	3			
GI activation	0			
Seizures	+			

0 = low; 4 = high; + = present

significantly more effective than placebo for relapse prevention, indicating long-term efficacy and tolerability. It is as effective as TCAs for major depression, and more effective than fluoxetine for depressive symptoms related to social functioning such as amotivation and negative self-perception. Onset of action may occur as early as 10 to 14 days after treatment initiation. Unlike the majority of SSRIs, reboxetine does not appreciably inhibit hepatic cytochrome isoenzymes, thereby lowering the potential for drug interactions. Reboxetine is currently available in the United Kingdom as Edronax but will be marketed in the United States under the trade name Vestra. For a look at the variety of antidepressant medications currently available from different classes with differing actions, see ■ Table 31–8 on page 752.

Issues of major concern to clinicians and recipients of psychopharmacologic treatments are drug interactions. With the wide range of medications available to treat each facet of psychiatric symptomatology comes the inevitable blending of incompatible agents. ■ Table 31–9 on page 753 demonstrates some of the interactions possible between antidepressants and other medications and substances.

OTHER DRUGS USED FOR DEPRESSION

Stimulants, such as amphetamines and methylphenidate (Ritalin), and the phenothiazines are less commonly used antidepressants. Stimulants are not a proven treatment. Phenothiazines may be particularly useful in the presence of agitation. Some clinicians and researchers believe that major depressive episodes with psychotic features (delusional depressions) respond better to a combination of an antidepressant and an antipsychotic agent or to electroconvulsive therapy (ECT) than to antidepressants alone. Others simply recommend higher-than-usual doses of antidepressants.

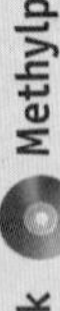
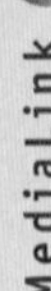
MediaLink Methylphenidate in Action Animation

ASSESSMENT — SSRI Discontinuation Syndrome

- Withdrawal from an SSRI will have symptoms including: dizziness, light-headedness, insomnia, fatigue, anxiety or agitation, nausea, headache, and sensory disturbances. It may also include hypomania, worsening of mood, aggressiveness, and suicidality.
- Symptoms have occurred in less than 5% of patients taking long-acting agents, compared to 86% in patients treated with fluvoxamine for panic disorder.
- A possible cause could be a hyposerotonergic state as long-term use of SSRI therapy may downregulate or desensitize postsynaptic serotonin receptors. Abrupt discontinuation may restore or even enhance serotonin reuptake resulting in a depletion of synaptic serotonin. May take 2 to 3 weeks for these systems to readapt.
- Mild, transient symptoms such as jitteriness, sleep disturbance, and heart palpitations have been reported in newborns whose mothers received SSRIs during pregnancy.
- Short-acting SSRIs cause more numerous symptoms that appear earlier after discontinuation and typically last up to 3 weeks.
- Abrupt discontinuation or "drug holidays" should be avoided with short-acting SSRIs.
- These agents should be tapered if discontinued.
- If symptoms appear, the taper needs to be more gradual.

ASSESSMENT Serotonin Syndrome

Definition

- Mental, autonomic, and neuromuscular changes.
- It is mild in most people, and with supportive care recovery is complete within 24–72 hours, although it can cause death under certain circumstances (11%).
- Seen in people taking 2 or more medications that increase the levels of serotonin in the CNS. This includes SSRIs, TCAs, and MAOIs.

Conditions of Diagnosis

- No antipsychotic medication used or increased in dose prior to onset of symptoms.
- No other obvious causes of confusion or fever.
- The client must have had a recent addition or increased dose of an agent that raises serotonin levels.

Symptoms

- Three of the following must be present:
  - Mental status changes (confusion, hypomania, anxiety, coma)
  - Agitation
  - Myoclonus
  - Shivering
  - Diarrhea
  - Hyperreflexia
  - Ataxia/Incoordination
  - Diaphoresis
  - Hyperpyrexia

Other Symptoms

Cardiovascular

- Sinus tachycardia
- Hypertension
- Hypotension

Gastrointestinal

- Nausea
- Abdominal pain
- Salivation

Motor Abnormalities

- Muscle rigidity
- Restlessness
- Tremor
- Nystagmus
- Seizures

Other

- Unreactive pupils
- Tachypnea

Management and Prevention of Serotonin Syndrome

- Supportive measures to reduce hypertension, tachycardia, hyperthermia, and respiratory distress.
- Suspected agent discontinued.
- OTCs that increase serotonin levels discontinued (dextromethorphan, pseudoephedrine, phenylpropanolamine).
- Benzodiazepines (lorazepam and diazepam) are used commonly to treat myoclonus and resultant hyperthermia.
- Severe cases not responding to benzodiazepines may respond to dantrolene (Dantrium) for relieving muscle rigidity and hyperthermia.
- Severe cases use antiserotonergic agents (cyproheptadine [Periactin], methylsergide [Sansert], propranolol [Inderal]).
- Reconsider using two or more serotonergic medications or consider switching to less serotonergic alternatives.

Note: Clonazepam is ineffective in treating serotonin syndrome.

Mood Stabilizers

The earliest medication discovery was made in 1949 by Australian physician John Cade. Cade found that lithium worked to subdue wild behavior in animals. To the astonishment of his colleagues, he went one step further and gave lithium to humans. Lithium was the drug of choice for the treatment of bipolar mood disorder for many years.

The psychopharmacologic treatment of conditions collectively labeled mania used to be virtually synonymous with lithium carbonate therapy in the United States. Many well-controlled clinical studies indicate unequivocally that lithium was initially the most effective agent for treating the vast majority of acute manic and hypomanic episodes. In addition, because of the absence of sedative side effects, the client felt much more related to the environment and able to function normally while under the influence of lithium.

In the last few years, several drugs have been added to the list of pharmacologic treatments for bipolar disorder. It started with the use of carbamazepine as a treatment to control bipolar symptoms in people who either could not take lithium or did not respond therapeutically to it.

Recognizing the potential effectiveness of carbamazepine in certain mood disorders, another seizure medication was prescribed, divalproex (Depakote), to treat clients with diagnoses of bipolar mood disorder or schizoaffective disorder.

The development of pharmacologic treatments for bipolar disorder has grown and is substantially improved from the clinically efficacious choices available even a decade ago. New guidelines for bipolar treatment have been created and have thus expanded our abilities to care for clients with bipolar disorders. The four main treatment guidelines for bipolar disorders (Expert Consensus Guideline Series, 2000) highlight these key recommendations:

1. A mood stabilizer is used in all phases of treatment.
2. Atypical, or newer, antipsychotics are preferable to conventionals (first-line use only when mania is accompanied by psychosis).

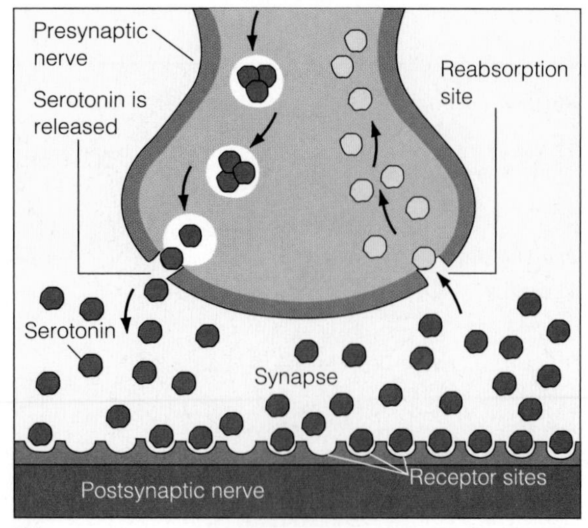

(A)

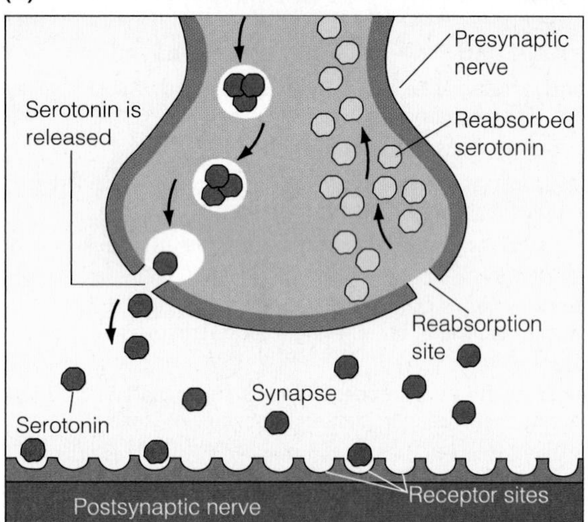

(B)

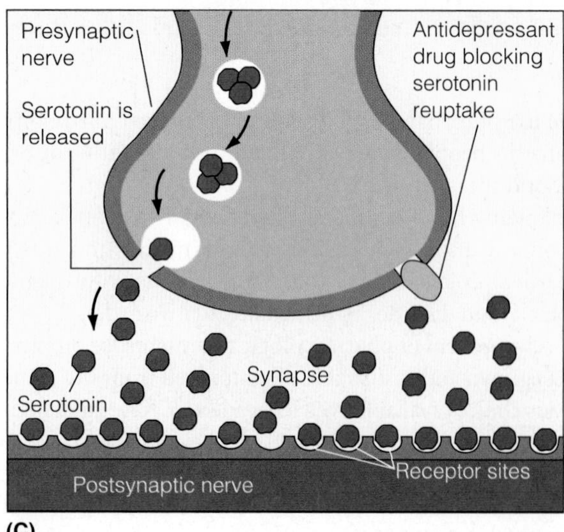

(C)

FIGURE 31–6 ■ *Serotonin neurotransmission. (A). A highly schematic model of normal serotonin (5-HT) neurotransmission. (B) In depression, there may be a shortage of 5-HT in the synapse. (C). The action of an antidepressant drug blocking 5-HT reabsorption (reuptake).*

TABLE 31–8 Antidepressant Medications

TCA	Other Antidepressants	SSRI
Imipramine (Tofranil)	Maprotiline (Ludiomil)	Fluoxetine (Prozac)
Amitriptyline (Elavil)	Amoxapine (Asendin)	Sertraline (Zoloft)
Desipramine (Norpramin)	Trazodone (Desyrel)	Paroxetine (Paxil)
Nortriptyline (Aventyl)	Bupropion (Wellbutrin)	Citalopram (Celexa)
Protriptyline (Vivactil)	Venlafaxine (Effexor)	Escitalopram (Lexapro)
	Mirtazepine (Remeron)	

3. Mild depression is treated initially with a mood stabilizer. Severe depression is treated from the beginning with an antidepressant plus a mood stabilizer.
4. Rapid cycling (mania or depression) is treated from the beginning with a mood stabilizer alone, preferably divalproex.

Treatment for mania consists of divalproex or lithium as the foundation of treatment for acute-phase and preventive treatment; alone or as adjunctive therapy with each other has been found to be desirable (Young et al., 2000). If the mania is accompanied by psychosis, the addition of an atypical antipsychotic is most effective. The Clinical Example of Chris on page 754 provides a description of a manic episode with psychotic features. The medications that were effective during the acute manic phase are also used for long-term prevention of mania. Bipolar depression usually necessitates lithium to stabilize clients in monotherapy for depression. If, for some reason, lithium is not used, divalproex or even lamotrigine (Lamictal) can be used.

The various treatments for bipolar disorder necessitate an in-depth view of drug interactions. See ■ Table 31–10 on page 754 for examples of the potential problems.

DOSAGE

The management of an acute manic episode involves rapid initiation of the selected mood stabilizer, increased to substantial doses during the first week of treatment. Lithium is available only in oral form in capsules and time-release tablets or as a liquid known as lithium citrate. Because lithium is an ion, its concentration can be measured in the blood. In the acute phase the blood level must usually attain a concentration of 1.0 to 1.5 mEq/L. After 1 week to 10 days, as the bipolar symptoms subside, the dosage of lithium can be decreased to 900 to 1,200 mg/day, with the blood level maintained in the range of 0.6 to 1.2 mEq/L for continuing control of symptoms.

The basic principles for lithium drug therapy are as follows:

TABLE 31–9 Antidepressant Drug Interactions

Combining One of These:	With One of These Antidepressants:	Can Lead to These Problems:
MAOI	SSRI	Serotonin syndrome, serious adverse reactions
St. John's Wort (herb)	SSRI	Sedative-hypnotic intoxication
MAOI	TCA	Hyperpyrexia, severe excitation
CNS depressants such as: Narcotics Anxiolytics Alcohol Barbiturates Antihistamines	TCA	Decreased TCA effect; additive CNS depression
Antihypertensive	TCA	Hypertensive crisis
Antipsychotic	TCA	Increased TCA effect, confusion, delirium, ileus
Anticholinergic medication	TCA	Additive anticholinergic effect
Antiarrhythmic	TCA	Additive antiarrhythmic effect, myocardial depression
SSRI	TCA	Increased TCA serum levels, elevated nortriptyline serum levels with adverse effects
Anticonvulsant	TCA	Decreased TCA effect, lower seizure threshold
Nicotine	TCA	Decreased TCA serum level
Foods or drugs containing tyramine	MAOI	Hypertensive crisis
Levodopa	MAOI	Hypertensive crisis

- Blood levels must be monitored after each dosage increase.
- Blood levels are checked every 2 to 3 months or when there is a behavioral reason to suspect a change.

For symptoms of breakthrough depression seen with bipolar depression, the dosing of divalproex or lithium must be maximized before other stabilizing or antidepressant agents are added to the regimen. After that episode resolves, the doses of the antidepressant medication are tapered slowly over the following 2 to 6 months. Special assessment skills are called into service during the tapering process to detect any resurgence of depressive symptomatology.

Length of treatment with medication for bipolar disorder is a debated issue. Clinical practice suggests prophylactic use of a mood stabilizer, preferably the compound effective during the acute phase of treatment, for at least 2 years. If the client has no intention of taking the medication that long, there may be a premature recurrence of the mania.

The following clinical example illustrates the appropriate use of medication in the case of a client suffering from bipolar disorder.

CLINICAL EXAMPLE

Chris, a 32-year-old legal aide, was brought to the clinic by her sister after she was fired from her position at a law firm. She had been arguing constantly with the lawyers and legal secretaries and stood on the conference room table, loudly telling people how to do their jobs. She had not slept in 3 days and was so irritable that she shoved a court clerk when approached about seeking care. Her sister stated that Chris was grandiose; spoke very quickly, moving from topic to topic in a rapid-fire style; and was belittling to everyone around her, and the family was worried about her. She had not taken any prescription or recreational compounds as far as the family knew. In the past 5 years she had been prescribed lithium, which seemed to help; however, Chris refuses to take it now because she experienced a metallic taste in her mouth.

On interview, Chris spoke about having special powers that involved being able to bring people back from the dead because she was a "sanctioned deity." Her episodes in the past did not include delusional thinking, and this was the first time her family could not contain her. Chris had some awareness that her behavior had frightened her family. She was told she had bipolar disorder with delusions. She was given divalproex sodium (Depakote) 250 mg tid and risperidone (Risperdal) 1 mg bid initially to control the mania and the psychosis. Chris was not hospitalized as her family agreed to supervise her care. After 1 week, the divalproex dosage was increased to 250 mg qid and Chris's behavior was under considerably better control.

TABLE 31–10 Mood Stabilizer Drug Interactions

Combining One of These:	With One of These Mood Stabilizers:	Can Lead to These Problems:
Carbamazapine	Lithium	Increased effect of lithium, lithium toxicity
MAOI	Lithium	Increased depressant and anticholinergic effects
SSRI	Lithium	Increased effect of lithium, lithium toxicity
NSAIDs	Lithium	Increased effect of lithium, lithium toxicity
Diuretics	Lithium	Increased lithium levels and potential lithium toxicity (monitor electrolytes, especially sodium)
Marijuana	Lithium	Increased lithium levels and potential lithium toxicity
Tetracyclines	Lithium	Lithium toxicity
Aminophylline	Lithium	Increased lithium secretion
Neuroleptics	Lithium	Encephalopathy
Thyroid hormones	Lithium	May induce hypothryoidism
Chlorpromazine	Valproic acid	Valproic acid toxicity
Lamotrigine	Valproic acid	Increased lamotrigine levels, decreased valproic levels
Benzodiazepines	Valproic acid	Excessive CNS depression
Clozapine	Carbamazapine	Additive bone marrow suppression
Haldol	Carbamazapine	Decreased effectiveness of either compound
Carbamazapine	Topamirate	Decreased topamirate level
CNS depressants	Topamirate	Possible topamirate-induced CNS depression as well as other adverse cognitive and neuropsychiatric effects

The use of anticonvulsants as mood stabilizers has its own unique set of effects and termination of treatment issues. Divalproex, carbamazapine, gabapentin, and lamotrigine all have sedation, gastrointestinal (GI) disturbances, and dizziness as side effects, along with others more specific to each compound. The body needs time to adapt to the medication; therefore, some side effects are temporary. However, dosage adjustments can minimize the impact of these side effects so that the quality of life is not shifted downward. An important client teaching aspect when using anticonvulsants as mood stabilizers is the inability for the body to handle abrupt discontinuation of these medications. Frank discussions must highlight the increased chance of having a seizure, even if the client has never had one, if the dose is not tapered slowly to discontinuation.

SIDE EFFECTS

Lithium has a significant number of side effects that can be troublesome and, in some cases, quite dangerous. Significant side effects are usually correlated with blood levels of lithium above 1.2 mEq/L. Common side effects include tremor, nausea, thirst, and polyuria. Thyroid goiter has also been seen as a side effect. Severe lithium poisoning is a potential medical emergency. Early signs include vomiting and diarrhea, lethargy, and muscle twitching. These may progress to ataxia and slurred speech. The client may become semiconscious or comatose; seizures may occur; and electrolyte imbalances may lead to cardiac arrest. This syndrome of severe toxicity ordinarily occurs only when the client has a blood lithium level of 2 to 3 mEq/L. The client may have overdosed or severely restricted food or salt intake (or taken diuretics) to induce this state.

Occasionally, very violent, agitated, or paranoid individuals with mania require adjunctive antipsychotic medications at the beginning of their treatment. These can be started simultaneously with the mood stabilizer, raised to whatever level is required to control the disintegrative behavior, then gradually reduced, and eliminated after therapeutic mood stabilizer levels have been effective for about 1 week.

CLIENT/FAMILY EDUCATION AND NURSING CONSIDERATIONS

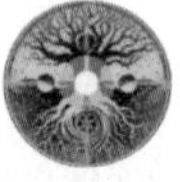

Box 31–5 on page 755 provides practical strategies for the client receiving lithium therapy.

PSYCHOBIOLOGY OF LITHIUM

Although the specifics of bipolar disorder are difficult to delineate, much can be said about the psychobiology of lithium.

BOX 31-5 Lithium Maintenance Toolbox

Keeping a Stable Lithium Level

1. Stabilize dosing schedule (through sustained release formula or divided doses).
2. If a dose is missed, take within 2 hours. If longer than 2 hours has elapsed, skip that one dose.
3. Ingest adequate dietary sodium.
4. Maintain hydration.
5. Replace fluids and electrolytes lost during exercise, exertion, GI illness.
6. Monitor for signs of side effects and lithium toxicity.

Watch for These Events to Cause Lithium Level Increases

1. Hydration status change
2. Increases in other medications
3. Marijuana use
4. Carbamazepine
5. Lithium overdose
6. Decreased sodium intake
7. Diuretic treatments
8. Medical illness
9. Nonsteroidal anti-inflammatory drug therapy
10. Tetracyclines
11. Fluid and electrolyte loss through fever, sweating, diarrhea, vomiting, dehydration

Lithium, not unlike the antidepressants, affects neurotransmitters, especially norepinephrine and serotonin. In short, lithium aids in the reduction of neurotransmitter release into the synapse and enhances its return, yielding a lower overall amount of the neurotransmitter in the synapse. Behaviorally, these biologic changes can be observed as an absence of mania or depression. What is unclear is why lithium takes up to a few weeks to be fully effective, when the drug's effects can be observed on synaptic activity almost immediately. Also, why do some people with bipolar disorder *not* respond at all to lithium therapy? Many psychobiologists believe that lithium's effects are likely to be based on neurocellular changes that occur over weeks or months after a client begins lithium therapy. A similar explanation may hold true concerning the effectiveness of other mood stabilizers.

Anxiolytic Medications

Medications in this class are used to treat a variety of problems from high levels of anxiety and panic to insomnia.

EFFECTS

The **anxiolytic medications** or antianxiety agents—sedatives and hypnotics—have very similar pharmacologic attributes. All can be used in small or moderate doses to relieve anxiety and in larger doses to induce sleep. Although they share the major clinical effect of tranquilization or **disinhibition** (loss or reduction of an inhibition) of fear-induced behavior, their side effects, including their addictive potentials and overdose sequelae, make certain representations of this category of medications more suitable for routine use and others better to reserve for limited, special circumstances.

Antianxiety medications are sometimes called *minor tranquilizers*, but this is a misleading term. Their effects on anxiety are qualitatively, not quantitatively, different from those of the "major tranquilizers" or antipsychotic medications.

DRUG CLASSIFICATION

The major categories of drug classification separate medications into groups according to their chemical composition and properties.

Meprobamate

Meprobamate (Miltown, Equanil) was the first antianxiety agent to gain popularity in the 1960s. The result of controlled studies of the effects of meprobamate compared to placebos are generally favorable but not overwhelmingly convincing. This, and the addictive and fatal overdose potentials of the drug, prompted investigators to develop more effective and safer medications that have all but made meprobamate obsolete.

Benzodiazepines and Nonbenzodiazepines

The major class of drugs today in the management of anxiety is the benzodiazepines and nonbenzodiazepines. This group, represented by alprazolam (Xanax), lorazepam (Ativan), and others, accounts for a very high percentage of all the psychoactive medications prescribed in the United States. This fact usually evokes a mixed response in professional circles. The easy distribution of drugs for such a ubiquitous human phenomenon as anxiety fosters the development of a pill-oriented and pill-dependent society, say critics. Sympathizers focus on the proven effectiveness of the drugs, which help people achieve higher levels of functioning, more pleasurable experiences, and even more productive psychotherapies in some instances.

The dosing and the timing of an antianxiety medication can be the difference between effective treatment of anxiety and interfering with a client's ability to learn and cope. Anxiety is a normal human response to threats of varying intensities and is not necessarily an experience to be avoided at all costs. At low to moderate levels, anxiety can be motivating and instructive and provide cues to the environment. But when anxiety passes these stages and proceeds to excess, panic can occur. Extreme feelings of anxiety such as panic are not motivating—in fact, they are immobilizing and learning is not possible. The clinical application and purpose of antianxiety medications is primarily to support clients through episodes of stress and anxiety at moderate to high levels. Medicating such that higher levels of anxiety are prevented allows the individual to have enough anxiety in a given situation to manage that anxiety with the coping skills taught by nurses, and to gauge their effectiveness. If antianxiety medications are given without regard to the actual anxiety level and the learning of the individual, it is possible to obliterate the need to learn to cope with stress. The client learns instead to rely on the medication to cope. An opportunity to promote stress management through psychopharmacology includes attention to these important issues.

New Drugs

In the last decade, anxiety-related research has expanded tremendously, and several new anxiolytic drugs have been introduced. The newer benzodiazepines give prescribers a wider range of therapies to target the often idiosyncratic manifestations of anxiety. Some of the new drugs have more rapid onsets and shorter half-lives (triazolam, quazepam [Doral]), while others have a usual benzodiazepine onset time and an extended half-life (clonazepam [Klonopin]).

With the psychobiologic knowledge explosion, a great variety of benzodiazepine drugs have been used in the treatment of a number of disorders. According to Chow, Tomlinson, and Chow (2000), benzodiazepines are used for many reasons:

- Anxiety disorders.
- Sleep disorders.
- Mood disorders.
- Anxiety associated with medical illness.
- Psychotic symptoms and disorders.
- Convulsive disorders.
- Involuntary movement disorders.
- Spastic disorders and acute muscle spasms.
- Intoxication and withdrawal from alcohol and other substances.
- Preanesthesia.
- Nausea and vomiting associated with chemotherapy.
- Anxiolytic, sedative, and amnestic effects in a wide range of stressful diagnostic procedures.

For a list of currently available benzodiazepines and nonbenzodiazepines, see ■ Table 31–11 at right.

New drugs and new uses for existing drugs are accompanied by new side effects and the need for new teaching plans developed by nurses for use in client education. The assessment skills of nurses must be finely tuned to detect unusual behaviors in relation to benzodiazepine therapy.

USES FOR ANXIOLYTICS

There is no question that benzodiazepines offer a rapid, effective, and safe treatment for the emotional state commonly known as anxiety. Caffeine interferes with the effectiveness of these drugs, both pharmacologically and as an irritant to client's mood and systems.

TABLE 31–11 Generic and Trade Names of Benzodiazepines and nonbenzodiazepines

Generic Name	Trade Names
Benzodiazepines	
Adinazolam	Deracyn
Alprazolam	Xanax
Bromazepam	Lexotan, Lexotanil, Lexomil
Brotizolam	Lendormin
Camazepam	Albego
Chlordiazepoxide	Librium, Libritabs, Elenium
Clobazam	Frisium
Clonazepam	Klonopin
Clorazepate	Tranxene
Clotiazepam	Clozan, Trecalmo
Cloxazolam	Enadel
Diazepam	Valium
Estazolam	ProSom, Nuctalm
Ethyl loflazepate	Meilax, Victan
Etizolam	Depas
Flunitrazepam	Rohypnol
Flurazepam	Dalmane, Dalmadorm
Halazepam	Paxipam
Ketazolam	Anxon, Unakalm
Loprazolam	Dormonoct
Lorazepam	Ativan
Lormetazepam	Loramet
Medazepam	Nobrium
Midazolam	Versed, Dormicum
Nitrazepam	Mogadon
Oxazepam	Serax
Oxazolam	Tranquit
Pinazepam	Domar
Prazepam	Centrax
Quazepam	Doral, Oniria, Dormalin, Quazium
Temazepam	Restoril
Tetrazepam	Musaril, Myolastan
Tofizopam (tofisopam)	Grandaxin, Seriel, Tavor
Triazolam	Halcion
Nonbenzodiazepines	
Buspirone	BuSpar
Meprobamate	Miltown, Equanil
Zaleplon	Sonata
Zolpidem	Ambien

These medications are absorbed much more rapidly and completely from the gastrointestinal tract than from intramuscular injection and are almost always administered orally. Exceptions are the intramuscular injections of lorazepam (Ativan) for extreme agitation and the use of intravenous diazepam (Valium) to induce sleep before anesthesia or to manage status epilepticus. Peak levels of chlordiazepoxide (Librium) are reached in the bloodstream 2 to 4 hours after oral ingestion, and peak levels of diazepam are reached in 1 to 2 hours.

The major side effects of benzodiazepines are related to their sedative qualities. Clients may complain of excessive drowsiness and must be cautioned against driving a car or operating other machinery.

Other drugs used to treat anxiety but generally less effective include the antihistamines diphenhydramine (Benadryl) and hydroxyzine (Vistaril, Atarax), the beta-blocker propranolol (Inderal), and methaqualone (Quaalude), a synthetic nonbarbiturate sedative. Methaqualone has been a much-abused drug, probably because of the intense euphoria associated with peak blood levels.

Another common use of benzodiazepines, especially diazepam and chlordiazepoxide, is in the detoxification of individuals addicted to alcohol. Given adequate doses of benzodiazepines to induce sedation (usually starting at 30 to 40 mg/day of diazepam or 150 to 350 mg/day of chlordiazepoxide), alcoholic clients can be smoothly withdrawn by stepwise reductions in chlordiazepoxide dose over a 1- to 2-week period, without encountering alcohol withdrawal delirium or grand mal seizures.

CLIENT/FAMILY EDUCATION AND NURSING CONSIDERATIONS

Client teaching is an especially important element in the care of clients taking antianxiety medications. As most people know, anxiety is a generally uncomfortable experience. Self-medication often becomes the relief-seeking behavior used by many with severe anxiety. Such a psychopharmacologic approach is *temporarily* helpful in the restoration of a person's capacities and internal comfort. When the client is able and ready to learn, however, other means of anxiety control *must* be taught. Many of the anxiolytic drugs (especially benzodiazepines) carry a potential for dependence and tolerance. Therefore, nurses have a responsibility to help clients control anxiety in the most effective and safest way possible.

PSYCHOBIOLOGY OF ANXIOLYTIC MEDICATIONS

Antianxiety drugs probably work through a process of synaptic activity involving the neurotransmitter gamma-aminobutyric acid (GABA) in the brain and spinal cord. Benzodiazepines most likely potentiate GABA, producing muscle relaxation. This mechanism involves a complex process of presynaptic and postsynaptic receptor activity. Recent research has yielded information about the presence of a postsynaptic receptor called the *benzodiazepine receptor*. As the term implies, benzodiazepines bind perfectly and with great specificity to these receptors, allowing for the sensation of relaxation. Two types of benzodiazepine receptors have been identified in the CNS. Type 1 receptors are located in parts of the brain responsible for sedation and nonbenzodiazepines bind exclusively to the Type 1 receptors. This makes the nonbenzodiazepines excellent choices for the treatment of sleep disturbances. Type 2 receptors are positioned in parts of the brain responsible for cognition, memory, and psychomotor functioning. Benzodiazepines bind with either Type 1 or Type 2 receptors. ■ Figure 31–7 on page 758 shows the chemical structure of four anxiolytics and ■ Table 31–12 on page 759 points out the potential drug interactions with anxiolytics and other medications and substances.

Treatment for Insomnia

The pharmacologic management of insomnia presents an interesting and challenging clinical problem. Many of the truly hypnotic drugs tend to have undesirable effects, including physiologic addiction, fatal overdose potential, and dangerous interactions with other medications because of liver enzyme induction. The first principle of treatment is to assess whether the insomnia is related to one of the major mental disorders, such as schizophrenia or major depression. If so, the insomnia can and should be treated as part of the larger problem, and sedative antipsychotics or antidepressants may be given at bedtime for this purpose.

In the management of simple insomnia without an associated major mental disorder, sedative–hypnotics are indicated for short-term treatment. Overall, the available sedative–hypnotics include certain antidepressants, benzodiazepines, nonbenzodiazepines, over-the-counter (OTC) medications, barbiturates, and some miscellaneous substances such as chloral hydrate and alcohol (Chow, Tomlinson, & Chow, 2000). Prescription medications have better effectiveness than the OTCs, while barbiturates are rarely, if ever, prescribed due to safety and addiction problems. The benzodiazepine compound flurazepam (Dalmane), 15 to 30 mg at bedtime, is an example of a commonly used historical insomnia treatment. This drug can be used on consecutive nights for about 1 month. Other benzodiazepine compounds that are used for their hypnotic qualities include triazolam and lorazepam. The rapid absorption, within 30 minutes, along with efficient elimination and the minimal hangover effects of sedation the following day with nonbenzodiazepines, make them the treatment of choice for insomnia (Skaer, 2000).

Zolpidem (Ambien) and zaleplon (Sonata) are two nonbenzodiazepines that are structurally very different from each other while being equally effective in the treatment of insomnia. Fast-acting, competent sleep-inducing, and quickly eliminated medications such as these can be used to our advantage without the difficulties associated with the other commonly used compounds. Clients using zolpidem may find it a little more difficult to fall asleep the first night without the medication, but zaleplon is not associated with any withdrawal or rebound effects.

MediaLink Diazepam in Action Animation

CLIENT/FAMILY EDUCATION AND NURSING CONSIDERATIONS

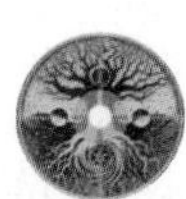

As with anxiolytics, insomnia preparations are generally intended for either occasional or short-term use.

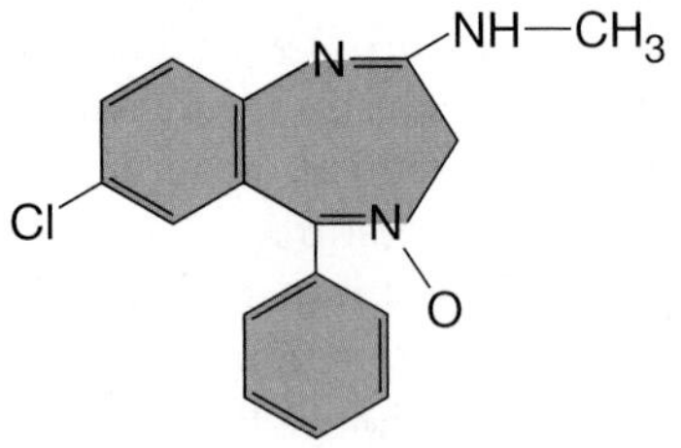

Chlordiazepoxide
(Librium)

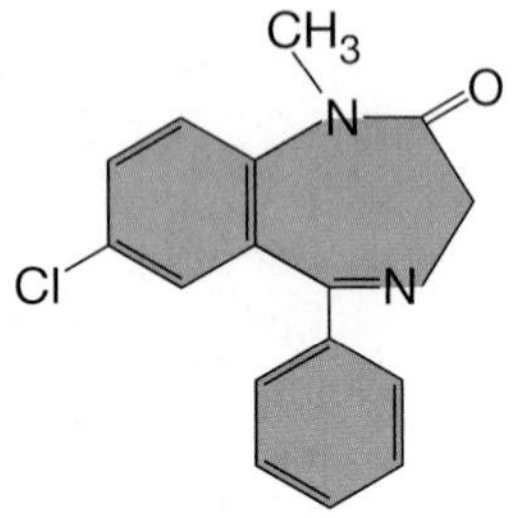

Diazepam
(Valium)

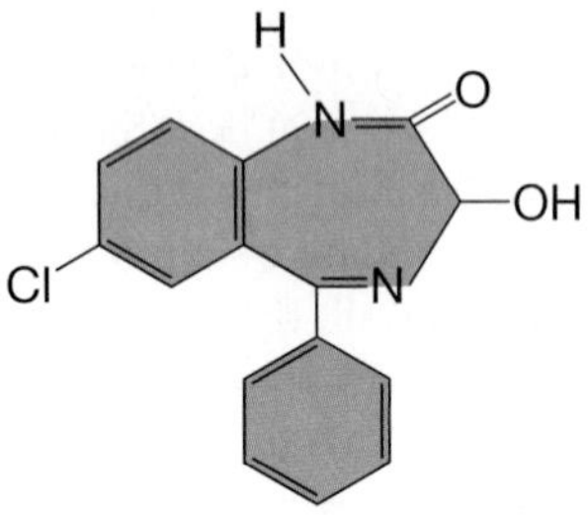

Oxazepam
(Serax)

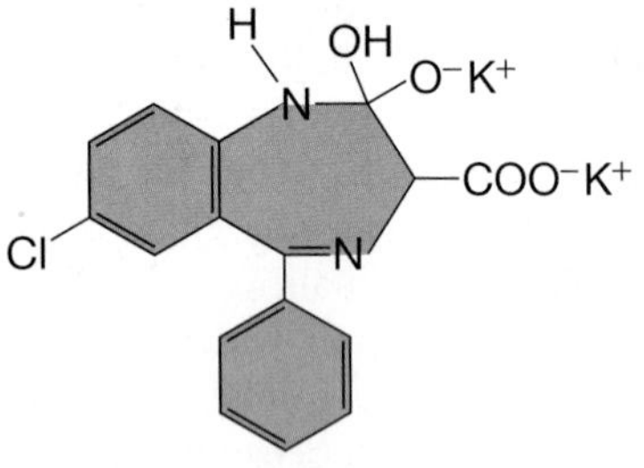

Clorazepate
(Tranxene)

FIGURE 31–7 ■ *The chemical structure of four anxiolytics. The antianxiety efficacy of these drugs is related to their impacts on GABA receptors. Adverse reactions that rarely require discontinuation of the medication, and can be managed via dose reduction, include: drowsiness, dizziness, disorientation.*

Source: Smock, T. K. (1999). *Physiological psychology: A neuroscience approach*. Upper Saddle River, NJ: Prentice Hall.

These medications are appropriate for clients newly admitted to a psychiatric inpatient unit or for clients in outpatient therapy who develop sleep disorders. As other medications (antidepressants, lithium, antipsychotics) start to yield a therapeutic effect, however, the need for sedative-hypnotic medication should almost, if not completely, abate.

Nurses working with clients in these situations need to help them regulate their sleep patterns. Here are some strategies to reinstitute regular sleep patterns:

- Avoid caffeine and nicotine.
- Exercise several hours before bedtime.
- Use relaxation techniques, including white noise.
- Avoid alcoholic beverages before bed.
- Eat tryptophan-rich foods.
- Follow a regular routine of retiring and rising.
- Avoid bright light before sleep.

It is essential that the nurse teaching relaxation techniques assess the client's sleep patterns and presleep routines, to prescribe the correct technique to meet the client's needs. Ongoing evaluation of the effectiveness of the relaxation intervention allows for a change in approach if necessary.

Acetylcholinesterase Inhibitors

A new class of medications with specific abilities has entered the dementia treatment realm: **acetylcholinesterase inhibitors.** The title of this class describes the work done by these compounds in the CNS. The enzyme responsible for the breakdown of a particular neurotransmitter is inhibited from acting by the medication. The enzyme is acetylcholinesterase, and the neurotransmitter it specifically works on is acetylcholine. The cholinergic system is involved in memory, abilities to logically progress from one step to the next in problem solving, and identification of objects and people in the environment, among other skills. Clients with dementia of the Alzheimer's type (DAT) have acetylcholine neurotransmitter deficits at the root of some of their problems. When the breakdown of acetylcholine is slowed, it allows more of the neurotransmitter to remain in the synapse, thus promoting acetylcholine's purpose—to transmit information from one cell to another. In mild to moderately affected individuals, when there is more acetylcholine in the CNS, cognitive functioning and memory improve (Cummings, 2000). This is essentially how these medications slow the progression of dementia in clients with early-stage DAT.

These medications are best utilized early in the dementing process when deficits are still only mild to moderate in scope. But the best time to institute treatment and the most effective use of the compounds are frequently thwarted by the realities of human nature. There are difficulties instituting treatment at early stages in that many people are not aware they are in the early stages of dementia. Frequently, there is an inability to grasp their own level of symptomatology combined with a general lack of information on the early signs, symptoms, or issues of dementia. Confabulation or denial prevent a client or loved ones from noting deficits or recognizing the implications of low-level difficulties. For example, a woman who is not able to tie her shoes may ask her husband to do that for her, while both of them attribute this situation to arthritis, musculoskeletal problems, or side effects from medications. Another example would be someone not balancing his checkbook anymore, stat-

TABLE 31–12 Anxiolytic Drug Interactions

Combining One of These:	With One of These Anxiolytics:	Can Lead to These Problems:
CNS depressants	Anxiolytics	Increased CNS depression, increased risk of apnea
Cimetidine	Alprazolam	Decreased alprazolam clearance
TCA	Alprazolam	Increased TCA plasma level
Kava (herb)	Alprazolam	May cause coma
MAOIs	Buspirone	Elevated blood pressure
Digoxin	Chlorazepate, lorazepam, oxazepam	May increase serum digoxin level, digoxin toxicity

ing the bank has always been correct, when in reality the simple math required to do so is a lost skill.

Think of this medication class as you would a similar psychopharmacologic class used to treat other psychiatric illnesses. It is a treatment for specific symptoms, not a cure. Acetylcholinesterase inhibitors do not alter the course of the underlying disease process or have an impact on the progressive nature of the disease. They are a way to temporarily improve neurotransmission and thus ameliorate memory deficits. The first of the acetylcholinesterase inhibitors was tacrine (Cognex). While not able to help all clients with DAT, it was the first step in the direction of active treatment for a major portion of people with dementing processes. There were problems with this medication in that it caused some liver toxicity, which could be controlled, and had several common side effects including GI disturbances and headache. From this beginning, subsequent compounds were developed. Donepezil (Aricept) and rivastigmine (Exelon) are newer acetylcholinesterase inhibitors with improved impacts on DAT and fewer difficulties from side effects (Rosenfeld & John, 2000). GI disturbances occur at a much lower level than the original compound, and headaches are reported at only a slightly higher level than clients taking placebo. There is even hope that these medications can somehow play a role in preventing individuals with cognitive deficits from converting to DAT.

See Chapter 12 for descriptions of the disorder DAT and its progression.

Herbal Medicines

Herbal medicines are widely used as an alternative or complementary therapy. (See Chapter 32 for an in-depth examination of these interventions.) One quarter of prescription drugs and hundreds of OTC drugs are derived from plants. Many herbal agents have powerful medicine-like actions and side effects. Herbs and plants generally take longer to act than pharmaceuticals, and few have the potency of a prescription.

One of the critical features of safe and effective nursing care is communication about alternative and complementary treatments. Keep in mind the variety of phrases used to describe alternative and complementary practices (complementary medicine, botanical, nutriceutical, herbal medicine, home remedy, natural remedy, health food, vitamin therapy, hemeopathic remedy, dietary supplement, phytomedicine, herbal tea).

The concomitant use of herbal medicines with psychiatric pharmaceuticals can be accomplished safely only when health providers know that their clients use them and their safety and effectiveness for the client's specific condition has been thoroughly appraised. Be sure to assess your clients for the use of herbal medicines.

There are many benefits to using alternative substances. For example:

- Self-treatment can be empowering.
- The very low concentrations of these substances could be helpful and might not be harmful.
- People feel safer using these "natural" products when distrust and fear is associated with chemical formulations.
- Standard labeling and dosing is possible.

However, there are potential problems with the use of alternative substances in psychiatry even though these alternative substances have lower potencies. Psychiatric indications for alternative substances currently exist only for St. John's wort for depression and ginkgo biloba for dementia, although alternative substances are frequently used for several other psychiatric symptoms and disorders. You may encounter clients using ma huang (ephedra) for general malaise, kava for anxiety and stress (see the FDA caution in Table 32–3 on page 778), and ginseng and SAMe for depression. Competent assessment and evaluation requires our awareness. of the potential for difficulties with alternative substances. Problems with using herbs may include:

- Contaminated product.
- Dosing inconsistencies.
- Delayed absorption of other coadministered medications.
- Worsening of high blood pressure, potassium imbalance, and coagulation problems.
- Side effects such as nerve damage, kidney damage, and liver damage.
- Advertising that makes unproven claims.
- Aggravation of allergic reactions.
- Interference with breast-feeding.
- Thinking that one is treating the problem, when in reality the symptoms could continue to worsen, making effective treatment much more difficult.

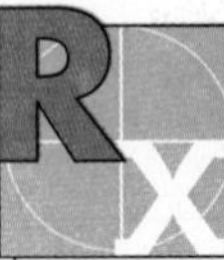

RX COMMUNICATION

Communicating with Your Client About Herbal Medicines

CLIENT: I don't like taking all these chemicals. It's not natural.

NURSE RESPONSE 1: Are you more comfortable taking medicine to help you when you know it is natural?

RATIONALE: This question gathers more data about what the client needs in order to feel better and raises the possibility of alternative substance use.

NURSE RESPONSE 2: Have you had bad experiences with anything in particular?

RATIONALE: This response makes the connection for the client between the idea and a possible result. It may also encourage discussion of recreational substance use.

ASSESSING HERB TAKING

Many clients do not tell health care providers about their herbal use for fear of being ridiculed or criticized. How do you find out what alternative therapies your clients are taking? Good interviewing skills will bring much of your client's life into the light for you. Use of these skills requires tolerance, a nonjudgmental stance, and some expressive questions. Questions such as "Do you do anything to improve your health?" or "What do you buy at the grocery store or health food store besides food?" can open the subject. See the Rx Communication feature above for examples of a conversation about this topic.

Be aware of the client's need to talk to a knowledgeable professional. The client may tell you about someone else who is taking alternatives while watching for your reaction. A nonjudgmental response to this information would include questions about what the client thinks about it, whether it has helped the individual, or whether the client would consider using this particular treatment. Not knowing about your client's use of botanicals risks dangerous drug interactions or costly/painful tests or treatments when an herb causes an unrecognized side effect.

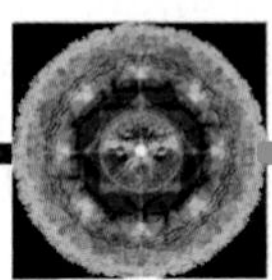

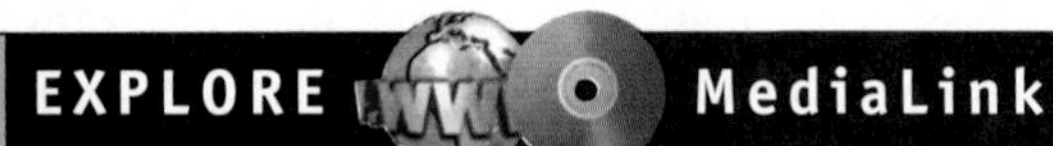

NCLEX review, case studies, and other interactive resources for this chapter can be found on the Companion Website at http://www.prenhall.com/kneisl. Click on Chapter 31 to select the activities for this chapter.

For animations, video tutorials, more NCLEX review questions, and an audio glossary, access the accompanying CD-ROM in this textbook.

BIBLIOGRAPHY

American Nurses Association. (2000). *Scope and standards of psychiatric–mental health nursing*. Washington, DC: Author.

American Nurses Association Task Force on Psychopharmacology. (1994). *Psychiatric–mental health nursing psychopharmacology project*. Washington, DC: American Nurses Association.

Ballesteros, J., Gonzalez-Pinto, A., & Bulbena, A. (2000). Tardive dyskinesia associated with higher mortality in psychiatric patients: Results of a meta-analysis of seven independent studies. *Journal of Clinical Psychopharmacology, 20*, 188–194.

Bernstein, J. G. (1995). *Handbook of drug therapy in psychiatry* (3rd ed.). St. Louis, MO: Mosby.

Bowen, G. T., Garry, M., & Sajbel, T. A. (2000). Guidelines for the use of combination antipsychotic medications in a psychiatric institutional setting. *Pharmacy & Therapeutics, 25*, 297–301.

Caroff, S. N., Mann, S. C., Keck, P. E., & Francis, A. (2000). Residual catatonic state following neuroleptic malignant syndrome. *Journal of Clinical Psychopharmacology, 20*, 257–259.

Carrese, J. A., & Rhodes, L. A. (2000). Bridging cultural differences in medical practice: The case of discussing negative information with Navajo patients. *Journal of General Internal Medicine, 15*, 92–96.

Chow, S. L., Tomlinson, B., & Chow, M. S. S. (2000). Pharmacologic management of insomnia: Assessing the nonbenzodiazepine hypnotics. *Formulary, 35*, 894–903.

Conley, R. R. (Ed.). (2000). *Therapeutic advances in the treatment of schizophrenia*. Baltimore, MD: Excerpta Medica Office of Continuing Medical Education.

Cummings, J. L. (2000). Cholinesterase inhibitors: A new class of psychotropic compounds. *American Journal of Psychiatry, 157*, 4–15.

Denvir, M. A., Sood, A., Dow, R., Brady, A. J., & Rankin, A. C. (1998). Thioridazine, diarrhea, and torsades de pointes. *Journal of Social Medicine, 91,* 145–147.

Dickson, R. A., & Glazer, W. M. (1999). Hyperprolactinemia and male sexual dysfunction, letter to editor. *Journal of Clinical Psychiatry, 60,* 125.

Dimsdale, J. E. (2000). Stalked by the past: The influence of ethnicity on health. *Psychosomatic Medicine, 62,* 161–170.

Expert Consensus Guideline Series. (2000). Updated guidelines for pharmacologic treatment of bipolar disorder. *Postgraduate Medicine, 108,* 43–47.

Flaskerud, J. H., & Nyamathi, A. M. (2000). Attaining gender and ethnic diversity in health intervention research: Cultural responsiveness versus resource provision. *Advances in Nursing Science, 22,* 1–15.

Flores, G. (2000). Culture and patient-physician relationship: Achieving cultural competency in health care. *The Journal of Pediatrics, 136,* 14–23.

Gerrish, K. (2000). Individualized care: Its conceptualization and practice within a multiethnic society. *Journal of Advanced Nursing, 32,* 91–99.

Gurrera, R. J. (2000). Sympathoadrenal hyperactivity and the etiology of neuroleptic malignant syndrome. *The American Journal of Psychiatry, 156,* 169–180.

Jeste, D. V., Okamoto, A., Napolitano, J., Kane, J. M., & Martinez, R. A. (2000). Low incidence of persistent tardive dyskinesia in elderly patients with dementia treated with risperidone. *The American Journal of Psychiatry, 157,* 1150–1155.

Jeste, D. V., Palmer, B. W., & Harris, M. J. (1999). Neuroleptic discontinuation in clinical and research settings: Scientific issues and ethical dilemmas. *Biological Psychiatry, 46,* 1050–1059.

Kilian, J. G. & Lawrence, C. (1999). Myocarditis and cardiomyopathy associated with clozapine. *Lancet, 354,* 1841–1845.

Lopez, S. R., & Guarnaccia, P. (2000). Cultural psychopathology: Uncovering the social world of mental illness. *Annual Review of Psychology, 51,* 571–598.

Magnusson, A., Axelsson, J., Karlsson, M. M., & Oskarsson, H. (2000). Lack of seasonal mood change in the Icelandic population: Results of a cross-sectional study. *American Journal of Psychiatry, 157,* 224–238.

Morita, S., Shimoda, K., Someya, T., Yoshimura, Y., Kamijima, K., & Kato, N. (2000). Steady-state plasma levels of nortriptyline and its hydroxylated metabolites in Japanese patients: Impact of CYP2D6 genotype on the hydroxylation of nortriptyline. *Journal of Clinical Psychopharmacology, 20,* 141–149.

Perkins, H. S., & Hazuda, H. P. (2000). Cross cultural medical ethics. *Journal of General Internal Medicine, 14,* 778.

Quitkin, F. M., Rabkin, J. G., Gerald, J., Davis, J. M., & Klein, D. F. (2000). Validity of clinical trials of antidepressants. *American Journal of Psychiatry, 157,* 327–337.

Qureshi, N. A., & Al-Habeeb, T. A. (2000). Sympathoadrenal hyperactivity and neuroleptic malignant syndrome. *American Journal of Psychiatry, 157,* 310–311.

Rosenfeld, V. & John, J. (2000). Rivastigmine: Selective cholinesterase inhibitor for the management of Alzheimer's disease. *Pharmacy & Therapeutics, 25,* 275–281.

Rosner, F. (1978). *Julius Preuss' biblical and Talmudic medicine*. New York: Sanhedrin Press.

Schreiber, R., Stern, P. N., & Wilson, C. (2000). Being strong: How black West-Indian Canadian women manage depression and its stigma. *Journal of Nursing Scholarship First Quarter*, 39–45.

Silva, R. R., Munoz, D. M., Alpert, M., Perlmutter, I. R., & Diaz, J. (2000). Neuroleptic malignant syndrome in children and adolescents. *Journal of the American Academy of Child and Adolescent Psychiatry, 38,* 184–194.

Sirota, P., Mosheva, T., Shabtay, H., Giladi, N., & Korczyn, A. (2000). Use of the selective serotonin 3 receptor antagonist ondansetron in the treatment of neuroleptic-induced tardive dyskinesia. *American Journal of Psychiatry, 157,* 287–289.

Skaer, T. L. (2000). Insomnia pharmacotherapy: Selecting a hypnotic agent. *Pharmacy & Therapeutics, 25,* 93–102.

Smock, T. K., (1999). *Physiological psychology: A neuroscience approach*. Upper Saddle River, NJ: Prentice Hall.

Terrill, K. R., Wheeler, M., Rollins, D. E., & Beckwith, M. C. (2000). Drug interactions reported with grapefruit juice. *Journal of Pharmaceutical Care in Pain & Symptom Control, 8,* 39–48.

Weitzel, C. A. (2000). Could you spot this psych emergency? *RN, 63,* 35–38.

Young, L. T., Joffe, R. T., Robb, J. C., MacQueen, G. M., Marriott, M., & Patelis-Siotis, I. (2000). Double-blind comparison of addition of a second mood stabilizer versus an antidepressant to an initial mood stabilizer for treatment of patients with bipolar depression. *American Journal of Psychiatry, 157,* 124–126.

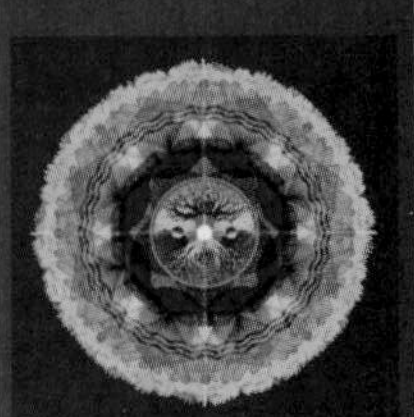

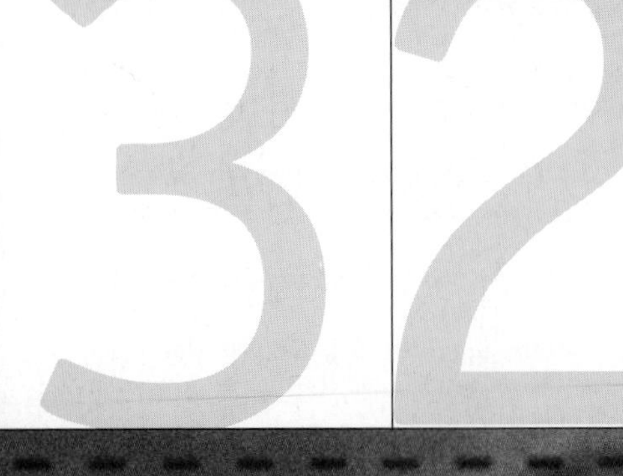

Complementary and Alternative Healing Practices

CAROL REN KNEISL

Chapter THIRTY-TWO

KEY TERMS

alternative therapies
biofeedback
complementary and alternative medicine (CAM)
complementary therapies
deep breathing
guided imagery
imagery
integrative therapies
mantra
medical meditation
meditation
progressive relaxation
visualization

FOCUS QUESTIONS

- **What are the therapeutic uses for each of the complementary and alternative medicine (CAM) techniques discussed in this chapter?**
- **If a client asked you to describe various CAM techniques, what important characteristics and functions would you include in the description?**
- **How can you apply CAM strategies in the care of clients in any health care or community setting?**
- **How can you personally use CAM strategies to enhance your personal and professional functioning?**
- **Which CAM techniques would you recommend to clients and their families for integration into a plan of care to promote, maintain, and restore emotional well-being?**
- **What cautions about CAM approaches would you give to clients and their families?**

MediaLink 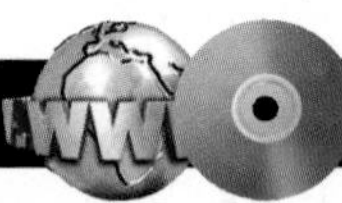 www.prenhall.com/kneisl

Additional resources for this chapter can be found on the Student CD-ROM accompanying this textbook, and on the Companion Website at www.prenhall.com/kneisl. Click on Chapter 32 to select the activities for this chapter.

CD-ROM
- Audio Glossary
- NCLEX Review

Companion Website
- Additional NCLEX Review
- Case Study: Teaching a Client About CAM

CHAPTER OUTLINE

CROSS REFERENCES

Other topics relevant to this content are: Assessment of stress and anxiety, Chapters 5 and 16; Insomnia and other sleep disorders, Chapter 19; Psychobiologic basis of mental disorder, Chapter 4; Psychotropic medications that decrease blood pressure, Chapter 31; Role of stress, anxiety, and coping, Chapter 5.

CRITICAL THINKING CHALLENGE

You and three of your classmates are discussing your most recent clinical experiences. Jenny tells the story of a toddler she was caring for on the pediatric oncology unit. Jamilla and Shi-An share what it's like to work in the intensive care unit. You discuss the events of your day in the psychiatric emergency room. The four of you agree that stress is, and will continue to be, a part of your nursing life regardless of your area of clinical practice. Living and working in a high-tech, stressful environment may cause you to feel apprehensive and to worry about your ability to live your life to its fullest potential. How can this chapter help you and your classmates cope with the stresses in your nursing life? ■

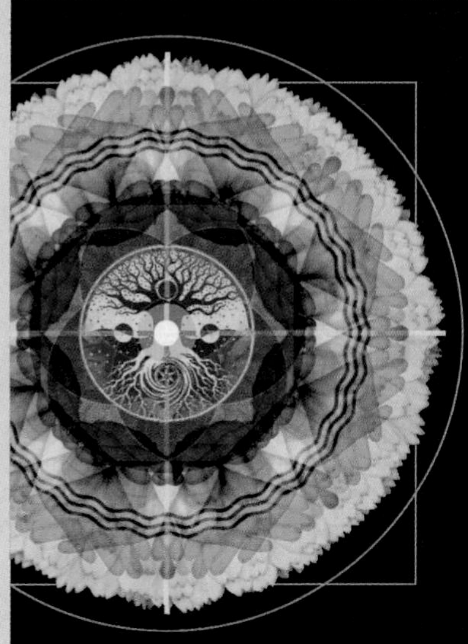

In many cultures around the world, health care and medical practices that are not currently an integral part of conventional Western medicine are used to relieve pain and cure illnesses. In Western culture they are referred to as **complementary and alternative medicine (CAM)**. **Complementary therapies** are those used in conjunction with conventional medical practices. **Alternative therapies** are those that are used instead of conventional medicine. The term **integrative therapies** is being used more often in hospitals, medical centers, and universities in North America as increasing numbers of contemporary Western health care providers are incorporating the most appropriate, safe, and effective of these ancient traditions and healing approaches into their practice. Programs in integrative medicine and CAM centers are in existence in several settings such as the University of Arizona in Tucson, Beth Israel Deaconess Medical Center and Harvard University in Boston, University of Maryland, University of Toronto in Canada, and many other centers in North America.

Nursing, with its tradition of holistic care—providing care for the whole person (mind, body, and spirit) in all its uniqueness—is especially well suited to deliver integrative therapy. Florence Nightingale herself encouraged holistic care by recognizing the importance of the environment, touch, light, aromatics, music, and quiet reflection to the healing process. Holistic nursing is described in Box 32–1.

Integrative complementary and alternative approaches such as those described in this chapter provide nurses with yet another way to promote clients' well-being.

Move Toward CAM and Integrative Therapies

Ancient traditions and healing practices are being rediscovered by consumers and providers of health care in Western culture. Increasing numbers of consumers are seeking out CAM on their own, asking questions of their health care providers, and requesting that CAM be added to their plan of care.

NATIONAL CENTER FOR CAM

In 1992, the Office of Alternative Medicine was established at the National Institutes of Health in response to increasing interest in CAM among the general population. This office funded and studied a wide range of CAM therapies. Before this time, most studies of CAM had serious methodologic problems and their lack of scientific validity was justly criticized. The results of the office's scientifically designed and implemented studies resulted in greater acceptance by the medical community and increased credibility for CAM. As a result, the office was upgraded in 1998 to a fully recognized national center at the National Institutes of Health (NIH) and is now called the National Center of Complementary and Alternative Medicine (NCCAM). Much of the research in CAM today is funded by the NCCAM.

Five major domains of complementary and alternative medicine have been identified by the NCCAM. They are explained, with examples, in ■ Table 32–1.

CONSUMERS OF CAM

In a national survey, 67.6% of respondents had used at least one CAM therapy in their lifetime (Kessler et al., 2001a). Research studies show that half or more of study participants use CAM at the following rates:

- 53% of people with anxiety attacks (Kessler et al., 2001b).
- 57% of people with severe depression (Kessler et al., 2001b).
- 61% of persons with gastroesophageal reflux (Hayden et al., 2002).
- 41% of children and young adults with inflammatory bowel disease (Heuschkel et al., 2002).
- 49% of colorectal cancer patients in Alberta, Canada (Tough, Johnston, Verhoef, Arthur, & Bryant, 2002).
- 64% of participants older than 65 from an urban academic hospital's ambulatory geriatrics practice (Cohen, Ek, & Pan, 2002).
- 49.6% of women with gynecologic cancer (Swisher et al., 2002).

BOX 32–1 What Is Holistic Nursing?

Holistic nursing embraces all nursing, which has as its goal the enhancement of healing the whole person from birth to death. Holistic nursing recognizes that there are two views regarding holism: holism involves identifying the interrelationships of the bio-psycho-social-spiritual dimensions of the person, recoznizing that the whole is greater than the sum of its parts; and holism involves understanding the individual as a unitary whole in mutual process with the environment. Holistic nursing responds to both views, believing that the goals of nursing can be achieved within either framework.

The holistic nurse is an instrument of healing and a facilitator in the healing process. Holistic nurses honor the individual's subjective experience about health, health beliefs, and values. To become therapeutic partners with individuals, families, and communities, holistic nursing practice draws on nursing knowledge, theories, research, expertise, intuition, and creativity. Holistic nursing practice encourages peer review of professional practice in various clinical settings and integrates knowledge of current professional standards, laws, and regulations governing nursing practice.

Practicing holistic nursing requires nurses to integrate self-care, self-responsibility, spirituality, and reflection in their lives. This may lead the nurse to greater awareness of the interconnectedness with self, others, nature, and God/Life Force/Absolute/Transcendent. This awareness may further enhance the nurses' understanding of all individuals and their relationships to the human and global community, and permits nurses to use this awareness to facilitate the healing process.

Source: American Holistic Nurses' Association. (2002). *What is holistic nursing?* Retrieved June 2, 2002, from the World Wide Web, www.ahna.org/about/whatis.html.

TABLE 32–1 NCCAM's Major Domains of Complementary and Alternative Therapies

Alternative Medical Systems	Mind–Body Interventions	Biological-Based Therapies	Manipulative and Body-Based Methods	Energy Therapies
• Acupuncture • Chinese herbal medicine • Qi Gong • Ayurveda • Homeopathy • Naturopathy	• Meditation • Relaxation • Hypnosis • Art, music, and dance therapy • Prayer	• Herbs • Special diet therapies • Megadoses of vitamins or minerals • Substances such as bee pollen or shark cartilage	• Chiropractic • Tai chi • Yoga • Massage • Rolfing	• Therapeutic touch • Reiki • Electromagnetic therapy

Note: This list represents the major CAM therapies in use. It is not all-inclusive.

Source: Adapted from *Major domains of complementary and alternative medicine*, National Center for Complementary and Alternative Medicine, National Institutes of Health, Bethesda, MD.

► 67% of HIV-infected persons (Duggan, Peterson, Schutz, Khuder, & Charkraborty, 2001).

Similar results are found in studies of persons with stress, allergies, neurologic problems, diabetes, chronic sinusitis, and other physical and emotional problems.

People use CAM methods for several reasons. The most common reasons are listed in Box 32–2. There is no question that the move toward CAM reflects a consumer-driven health care environment.

Nursing Role in CAM

Nurses have several imporant roles in relationship to CAM approaches and integrative therapies. We are often in a position of being able to identify the need for CAM; suggest CAM therapies to treatment team members and to clients, their family members, or their friends; encourage clients to consider using a CAM therapy if appropriate; enlist the support of the treatment team, family members, and friends; and help clients to find providers.

Second, we may be CAM practitioners ourselves. Nurses may be practitioners of CAM therapies in a variety of settings—hospital, outpatient clinic, home, community, private practice office, and so on. The most common CAM therapies that nurses provide are relaxation techniques (such as deep breathing, active progressive relaxation, visualization, and meditation), bodywork techniques (such as massage), and energy therapies (such as therapeutic touch and Reiki). Some of these therapies, such as the relaxation techniques, visualization, meditation, and therapeutic touch are discussed in detail in this chapter. CAM therapies that require further training or equipment or are usually provided by others are discussed briefly.

Third, we are teachers of CAM therapies. Nurses play a significant role in making clients and their families aware of these methods and teaching them how to use them effectively. As health care educators, we have an important role in encouraging clients to be informed health consumers. And fourth, we can coordinate the integration of CAM services into a client's plan of care. See the Using Research Evidence feature on page 766.

BOX 32–2 Reasons Why People Seek CAM Therapies

- Wanting greater control over their lives
- Having a sense of responsibility for their own health care
- Wanting a more holistic orientation in health care so that body, mind, and spirit are addressed
- Concern over the side effects of conventional therapies
- Finding the results of conventional treatments to be inadequate
- Identifying with a particular philosophy or practice because of cultural background

HELPING CLIENTS BECOME INFORMED HEALTH CONSUMERS

Integrative CAM approaches are creative and powerful tools under the following circumstances:

1. The approach used has been demonstrated to be safe and effective.
2. The method is appropriate for that particular client.
3. The client learns to use the method properly.

The appropriateness of individual CAM methods and guidelines for proper use are identified later in this chapter in the discussion of techniques. Safety and effectiveness, the expertise of the practitioner, quality of service delivery, integrating CAM into a treatment plan, and quackery and fraud are discussed below.

Safety and Effectiveness

Many CAM therapies are not well regulated and researched. You can determine the safety and effectiveness of CAM methods and read any consumer advisories and news releases of the most recent research by accessing NCCAM's Web site at www.nccam.nih.gov.

MediaLink Case Study: Teaching a Client About CAM

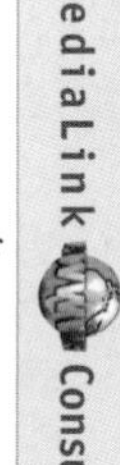

MediaLink Consumer Advisories

USING RESEARCH EVIDENCE

Judy Krasinski is a psychiatric–mental health nurse who is a member of the treatment team in the wellness center of a large urban medical center. Jay, a new client, has recently been referred to the wellness center for evaluation of anxiety and depression, as well as an evaluation of the herbs and other natural medicines he is taking. Jay has HIV, and is on an HAART (highly active antiretroviral therapy) regimen to treat his symptoms.

Jay has been on edge, worries about his future constantly, and has been moody and feeling blue. The results of the Beck Depression Inventory indicated that Jay is moderately depressed. Jay's depression has not improved despite treatment with Paxil and then Celexa. When Judy found that Jay has been taking garlic supplements, she became even more concerned, knowing that garlic supplements have been found to inhibit the effectiveness of saquinavir, one of the protease inhibitors in Jay's medication protocol. Judy also learned that Jay has not informed his prescriber of the herbs and other products he takes because he felt it wasn't important for his doctor to know and that, in addition, he probably wouldn't understand.

In addition to providing Jay with information about the effects of garlic supplements on protease inhibitors, Judy met with the other members of the team to discuss the possibility of CAM therapies to supplement and enhance his treatment for anxiety and depression. The team has suggested two programs based on the following research to augment his treatment: massage therapy and a mindfulness meditation program.

Henrickson, M. (2001). Clinical outcomes and patient perceptions of acupuncture and/or massage therapies in HIV-infected individuals. *AIDS Care, 13*(6), 743–748.

Williams, K. A., Kolar, M. M., Reger, B. E., & Pearson, J. C. (2001). Evaluation of a wellness-based mindfulness stress reduction intervention: A controlled trial. *American Journal of Health Promotion, 15*(6), 422–432.

MediaLink CAM Research

Another source is the current literature. The National Library of Medicine (NLM) and NCCAM have jointly developed a means of easy access to the literature on CAM from 1966 to the present. Over 11 million CAM journal citations can be found on NLM's PubMed at www.ncbi.nlm.nih.gov/entrez. Information on dietary supplements can be obtained through the NIH Office of Dietary Supplements (www.dietary-supplements.info.nih.gov). You can also access these resources through a direct link on the Companion Website for this book.

Encourage your clients to become informed health consumers. Help them to gather the following information about CAM:

- Advantages and disadvantages
- Risks
- Side effects
- Expected results
- Length of treatment
- Interaction with conventional Western medications

Clients can also gather information in informal ways such as testimonials by others. However, while testimonials from others who are or have been clients may be helpful, they should not be the sole criterion in selecting a therapy. Informed health care consumers and health care practitioners will seek information on controlled scientific trials such as those summarized on the Web sites listed above.

By helping clients become informed health consumers, you also help them to avoid fraudulently marketed products that are:

- Useless (such as electronic devices that claim to cure serious illnesses by sending electrical energy into the body).
- Have serious drug-interaction risks (such as those which may cause a reduction in the therapeutic effect of oral contraceptives and the therapeutic effect of drugs used to treat HIV or prevent transplant rejection).

Tips on avoiding fraudulently marketed products are listed in the Client/Family Teaching feature below. A guide to fraud, quackery, and informed decision making is available on www.quackwatch.com, a Web site maintained by a physician. This data can be accessed on the Companion Website for this text.

MediaLink Guide to Fraudulent Products

CLIENT / FAMILY TEACHING

Tips for Avoiding Fraudulent Health Claims

- Be suspicious of claims for a "miracle cure," an "exclusive product," or a "magical discovery."
- Check out claims on the Internet and in advertisements on television and radio and in newspapers and magazines.
- Understand that claiming to be "natural" doesn't necessarily mean that the product is safe.
- Impressive sounding terminology may be a way to disguise the lack of good science.
- Be skeptical about claims that the government, research scientists, or the medical profession have conspired to suppress a product. Cures for serious disease are widely reported in the media. They are not hidden in obscure magazine ads, paid television advertisements, or Web site promotions.
- "Quick relief" or "quick cure" claims are unreliable, especially if the disease is serious.
- Beware of products that claim to treat a wide spectrum of unrelated illnesses.

Practitioner Expertise

Encourage clients to examine the background, qualifications, and competence of a potential CAM practitioner. If there is licensure or certification for the particular CAM practice, is the practitioner licensed or certified? National organizations of CAM practitioners can provide referrals as well as information on legislation and state registration or licensing. Health regulatory bodies can provide information on state licensure or registration and any complaints lodged against specific practitioners.

Encourage clients to also talk with other health care providers or former clients, who may be able to address the question of competence and the quality of the services the practitioner provides. Clients should actually interview the CAM practitioner, asking about education, licensure, certification, treatment approach, and possible side effects or problems with the specific technique. Nurses who practice CAM methods can be credentialed by any one of several specialty bodies and/or the American Holistic Nurses' Association (Frisch, Keegan, Guzzetta, & Quinn, 2000) or licensed to practice specific CAM therapies in states where their use is governmentally regulated.

Quality and Costs of Service Delivery

Clients should visit the practitioner's office, clinic, or hospital to personally see the conditions under which treatment will be given. Are conditions safe and clean? Are regulated standards for medical care and safety adhered to?

Costs may also be an important consideration for clients. Although increasing numbers of insurers are covering costs of CAM services, not all do. Clients may have to pay directly for CAM services. Practitioners and health insurers should be able to tell clients which services are reimbursable.

INTEGRATING CAM INTO A TREATMENT PLAN

Integrating CAM into a treatment plan can take place only when clients discuss all CAM treatments and therapies with their primary physical or mental health care providers. Some CAM treatments affect physical or mental functioning, and certain herbs can interfere with or potentiate treatment with conventional medications.

Selecting Appropriate Clients

Most CAM techniques require that a client is motivated to participate in the interventions, is able to concentrate, and can follow directions, some of which may be quite complex. Assess clients to see if they meet these criteria.

Techniques that are lengthy and introspective or meditative should probably not be used with clients who are severely depressed, hallucinating, delusional, or have loss of contact with reality. Introspective techniques may lead to an increased loss of contact with reality, withdrawal, or increased rumination. Brief and externally focused techniques would be better for these clients. Clients who have multiple problems or are in extremely stressful situations may not have the time or energy to focus on or learn complex CAM techniques. Avoid adding another stressor to these clients' lives. Mental health problems that often respond well to CAM therapies are identified in Box 32–3.

BOX 32–3 **Mental Health Problems and Related CAM Therapies**

Alcohol Abuse

- Acupuncture
- Herbal therapy (kudzu)
- Meditation/medical meditation
- Yoga

Alzheimer's Dementia

- Herbal therapy (gingko)
- Massage
- Medical meditation (see the Caring for the Spirit feature on pages 774 and 775)

Anxiety

- Acupressure
- Biofeedback
- Breathing and relaxation techniques
- Guided imagery
- Healing touch/therapeutic touch
- Self-hypnosis
- Massage
- Meditation/medical meditation

Attention Deficit Hyperactivity Disorder

- Biofeedback

Depression

- Acupuncture
- Healing touch/therapeutic touch
- Herbal therapy (St. John's wort)
- Meditation/medical meditation
- Transcranial magnetic stimulation

Insomnia

- Breathing and relaxation techniques
- Herbal therapy (valerian)
- Meditation

Obsessive–Compulsive Disorder

- Acupuncture
- Medical meditation

Stress

- Breathing and relaxation exercises
- Healing touch/therapeutic touch
- Massage
- Meditation/medical meditation

Monitoring Health Problems

Clients participating in a CAM program should first discuss the program with their health care provider. Because many of these techniques lower blood pressure, decrease heart rate, and reduce pain and anxiety, clients' medications should be closely monitored. Monitoring is particularly important for psychiatric clients receiving psychotropic medications that may cause hypotension. Clients with cardiac problems may be at increased risk for cardiac arrhythmia because of vasovagal stimulation with certain techniques such as active progressive relaxation.

Experimenting with What Works

It is not necessary to use every suggestion or technique in this chapter. If one particular CAM technique doesn't seem to help, encourage the client to move on to another one. What is important is to give each a fair trial and to experiment to find out what works in each person's individual situation. As Mahatma Gandhi once said, "As long as you derive inner help and comfort from anything, keep it."

> **Nursing SELF-AWARENESS**
>
> **Body Scanning to Assess Body Tension**
>
> 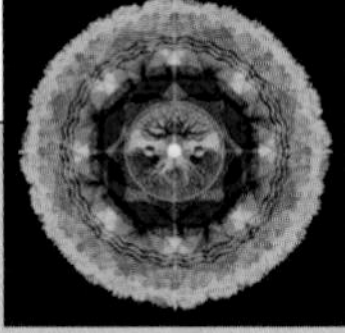
>
> In order to help others become aware of their own body tension, you must first become aware of where you carry tension in your own body. Use the following step-by-step guide to perform a self-assessment. You can follow these same guidelines when teaching clients and their families.
>
> - Make sure that the spine is straight before beginning body scanning or any of the other exercises described in this chapter. Stand, sit, or lie on the floor, whichever is most comfortable, while maintaining good posture.
> - Begin by closing your eyes and turning your attention to your own internal world, focusing on your body.
> - Focus on your toes and move up slowly.
> - As you do this, ask yourself: "Where am I tense?"
> - Become aware of all of the muscles in your body and especially the parts of your body that feel tense or tight.
> - Notice the location of the tenseness and talk to yourself about it, reminding yourself that muscular tension is self-induced. Perhaps you might say: "The muscles in the back of my neck feel tight. This means that I'm creating tension in my body. Tension causes me problems."

Deep Breathing and Relaxation Exercises

Unfortunately, many clients do not reduce the stresses in their lives because they do not realize that they are at the mercy of involuntary fight-or-flight responses (such as those discussed in Chapter 5). Many fail to identify environmental, physiologic, or cognitive sources of stress. Like clients in any other health care setting, psychiatric clients must endure time pressures, weather, noise, crowds, interpersonal demands, job performance demands, and various threats to security and self-esteem. And, perhaps more than clients in many of the other settings in which nurses practice, psychiatric clients experience cognitive stress because of how they interpret and label their experiences. For instance, a client might interpret the boss's facial expression as amused rather than pleased or as disgruntled rather than quizzical. This interpretation is likely to provoke anxiety. Dwelling on one's concerns and anxieties causes physical tension in the body, which in turn creates the subjective feeling of uneasiness and leads to more anxious thoughts.

The deep breathing and relaxation exercises that follow are based on the belief that mind and body are interrelated and that the condition of one will eventually affect the condition of the other. A relaxed body is incompatible with anxiety. If the body is relaxed, the mind will feel relaxed as well.

BODY SCANNING TO ASSESS BODY TENSION

The importance of body states and their relationship to stress have been emphasized by Eastern philosophies such as yoga and Zen. Because stress and body tension are simultaneous, one of the first steps in recognizing stress and anxiety is recognizing tension in the body. Body scanning helps you to become aware of where tension collects in your body and is an effective way to begin any of the relaxation techniques that follow. Use the step-by-step guide in the Nursing Self-Awareness feature above to help yourself become aware of the tension you carry in your body. You can use the same step-by-step guide to teach body scanning to your clients.

ENHANCING RELAXATION WITH MUSIC

Many people find that listening to soothing music is relaxing. Music, on audiotape, compact disc (CD), videotape, or digital video disc (DVD) can help clients reduce anxiety and achieve relaxation and can also be a substitute for, or adjunct to, pain medication and tranquilizers. Recorded music may be used before or during surgery, dental work, chemotherapy, kidney dialysis, and during recovery from spinal injury or burns (Gagner-Tjelleson, Yurkovich, & Gragert, 2001). You can teach clients to lower their blood pressure 10 to 20 points by using a combination of visual imagery and music. Music with 60 beats per minute can help those with cardiac arrhythmias achieve a better-regulated heart rate.

How does music achieve its relaxing effect? Soothing music produces endorphins in the brain, the same "feel-good" chemicals that running and meditation produce. These natural opiates, secreted by the hypothalamus, reduce the intensity with which pain is felt. Because people vary in their response to music, encourage clients to experiment with different kinds of music to discover which has positive effects and then to develop their own personal library. Tapes, CDs, and DVDs specifically for stress reduction are sold in bookstores and through catalogs. They are often available through local public libraries.

Recommend that clients pay attention to their breathing as they listen to music. Slow and deep breathing enhances the relaxing effect of music.

BREATHING EXERCISES

Under most circumstances, people take breathing for granted as an automatic body function. They usually become aware of their pattern of breathing only when it has gone awry, such as when they are out of breath. Breathing properly can, by itself, reduce stress. Breathing calmly and deeply keeps the blood well oxygenated and purified. It helps remove waste materials from the blood and clears thinking. Poorly oxygenated blood may contribute to fatigue, mental confusion, anxiety, muscular tension, and feelings of depression. The following exercises are designed to facilitate proper breathing.

Awareness of Breathing

Do you breathe properly, or does your breathing actually deprive you of oxygen? Take time to pay attention to your own breathing. Begin by placing one hand just below your rib cage and taking a deep breath. Notice what happens when you inhale. Does your hand move in? Does your hand move out? Does your hand move at all? If your hand moves out, you are breathing properly. But if your hand moves in or doesn't move at all, it's probably because you learned, as most did, to hold your stomach in and push your chest out while breathing. People who breathe this way do not fill the lungs to full capacity; they fill only the top third or top half.

Deep Breathing

During **deep breathing**, you move the diaphragm downward and fill the lower part of the lungs with air. The chest expands as the middle part fills with air, and the shoulders move upward as the upper part fills. To teach yourself or a client how to take deep, healthful breaths, follow the directions in the Client/Family Teaching feature below.

Deep breathing becomes easier with practice. It may become almost automatic. This is an exercise few resist—it's easy to do, it's inconspicuous, and it yields fast results.

Ten-to-One Count

This exercise is also quick and simple. To teach yourself or a client how to perform the ten-to-one exercise, follow the directions in the Client/Family Teaching feature below. Some people use an abbreviated version and begin counting at the number 5; others require the full count of 10 to feel calm.

Alternate-Nostril Breathing

Although somewhat more difficult, alternate-nostril breathing, which stems from the practice of yoga, also helps reduce tension and sinus headaches. To teach yourself or a client how to take deep, healthful breaths, follow the directions in the Client/Family Teaching feature below.

CLIENT / FAMILY TEACHING

Guidelines for Deep-Breathing Exercises

Deep-Breathing

- Sit, stand, or lie with your spine straight.
- Scan your body for tension.
- Place one hand on your chest and the other on your abdomen.
- Inhale slowly and deeply so that your abdomen pushes your hand up.
- Visualize your lungs slowly filling with air. Your chest should move only slightly as you inhale, but you should be aware of the movement of your abdomen.
- Exhale through your moouth, making a soft, whooshing sound by blowing gently. Keep your face, mouth, and jaw relaxed.
- Be aware of what it feels like and what you sound like when you breathe properly.
- Continue to take long, slow, deep breaths for at least 10 minutes at a time, once or twice a day.
- Increase the frequency if you wish, once you have mastered the technique.
- Scan your body for tension again, comparing the tension to what it was like before you began the deep-breathing exercise.

Ten-to-One Count

- Sit, stand, or lie with your spine straight.
- Scan your body for tension.
- Incorporate the guidelines in the deep breathing exercise above.
- Inhale, taking a deep breath, while saying the number 10 to yourself.
- Then exhale slowly, letting out all the air in your lungs.
- Inhale again, saying the number 9 to yourself.
- As you exhale, tell yourself: "I feel more relaxed than I did at number 10."
- With your next breath, say the number 8 to yourself.
- As you exhale, remind yourself: "I feel more relaxed than I did at number 9."
- Continue counting down and experience increasing calmness as you approach number 1.
- Scan your body for tension again, comparing the tension to what it was like before you began the deep-breathing exercise.

Alternate-Nostril Breathing

- Sit, stand, or lie with your spine straight.
- Scan your body for tension.
- Close off your right nostril by lightly pressing it with your right thumb.
- Then inhale through your left nostril as slowly and quietly as possible.
- Remove your thumb from the right nostril and use your forefinger to close off the left nostril.
- Exhale slowly through your right nostril.
- Inhale through your right nostril as slowly and quietly as possible.
- Follow the procedure outlined above, closing your right nostril with your right thumb while exhaling through your left nostril.
- The basic cycle is 10 breaths; this can be increased up to 25 breaths.
- Scan your body for tension again, comparing the tension to what it was like before you began the deep-breathing exercise.

It may be easier to breathe through the right nostril at certain times of the day and through the left nostril at other times. The reason is that people breathe primarily through one nostril for approximately 4 hours and then breathe primarily through the other for the next 4 hours.

PROGRESSIVE RELAXATION

The technique of **progressive relaxation** is based on the premise that muscle tension is the body's physiologic response to anxiety-provoking thoughts. Muscular tension increases the feeling of anxiety and reinforces it. Deep muscle relaxation, by contrast, decreases physiologic tension and blocks anxiety.

Progressive relaxation decreases pulse and respiratory rates, blood pressure, and perspiration. In addition, it helps reduce anxiety. Clients with muscle spasms, lower-back pain, tension headaches, insomnia, anxiety, depression, fatigue, irritable bowel syndrome, hypertension, or mild phobias are among those who can achieve positive results using this technique. Some clients report feeling less alert after either active or passive progressive relaxation. When alertness is important, one of the other deep breathing exercises is probably better.

It may take longer to master progressive relaxation than the deep-breathing techniques discussed earlier. With practice, however, one can learn to relax faster and easier.

Active Progressive Relaxation

Active progressive relaxation helps people identify which muscles or muscle groups are chronically tense by distinguishing between sensations of tension (purposeful muscle tensing) and deep relaxation (a conscious relaxing of the muscles). You can teach yourself or your clients active progressive relaxation by implementing the procedure outlined in the Client/Family Teaching feature "Guidelines for Active Progressive Relaxation" below.

Passive Progressive Relaxation

In *passive progressive relaxation*, the muscles are not tensed. The goal is to relax the muscles without first tightening them. The sequence in which body parts are relaxed differs from that of the active progressive method. Begin with muscles easiest to relax (in the toes) and progress to muscles most difficult to relax (in the head). The sequence is as follows: feet, lower legs, knees and upper legs, hips and buttocks, lower back, lower arms and hands, chest and diaphragm, abdomen, pelvis and genitals, neck, forehead and upper face, mouth and jaw.

Visualization and Imagery

Emil Coue, a French pharmacist, began to use the power of imagination with clients around the turn of the century. Carl Jung used it in his psychiatric practice during the early part of the century. Most recently, contemporary clinicians and individual clients have had remarkable success in the use of visualization to achieve control over serious physical illness and emotional discomfort.

Positive **visualization**, or **imagery**, uses the healing power of a person's own imagination and positive thinking to create powerful mental pictures or images to reduce stress or promote healing. Because of the vivid mental images that can be created, imagery has been considered by some to be a form of hypnosis (see the following section on hypnotherapy and self-hypnosis). Visualization should be used in conjunction with the body-scanning and deep-breathing exercises discussed earlier.

Not everyone finds using the imagination in this way easy, and the technique may not work for everyone. Constructing a detailed, effective visualization requires time, patience, and practice. Some people find that **guided imagery**—using an outside resource such as an actual person who guides the

---

CLIENT / FAMILY TEACHING

Guidelines for Active Progressive Relaxation

In active progressive relaxation, each muscle or muscle grouping is tensed for 5 to 7 seconds and then relaxed for 20 to 30 seconds. Repeat the cycle.

Four major muscle groups are covered in this order: (1) hands, forearms, and biceps; (2) head, face, throat, and shoulders; (3) chest, abdomen, and lower back; (4) thighs, buttocks, calves, and feet using this procedure:

- Practice progressive relaxation while lying down or seated in a chair with feet firmly on the floor.
- Begin active progressive relaxation by tightening the right fist (5 to 7 seconds) and paying attention to the tension. Allow the muscles of the right fist to relax (20 to 30 seconds), while noticing the pleasant difference.
- Do the same with the left fist—tensing, relaxing, and noticing the difference.
- Follow the same procedure for the forearms (tensing and relaxing as explained above), and then for the biceps, remembering to compare the difference in sensation between tensed and relaxed muscles.
- Progress through the next major muscle group—head, face, throat, and shoulders.
- Move to the third major muscle group—chest, abdomen, and lower back.
- End with the fourth major muscle group—thighs, buttocks, calves, and feet.
- Remember to return to muscle groups that are only partially relaxed to bring about deeper relaxation.

Caution: Counsel clients to observe some cautions while carrying out this technique. To avoid soft tissue and spinal injury, the muscles of the neck and back should not be excessively tightened. Tightening the muscles of the toes and feet too vigorously could also result in uncomfortable muscle cramps. Clients with cardiac arrhythmias should be cautioned against vasovagal stimulation by tensing muscles too tightly. Postoperative clients should probably avoid active progressive relaxation, a practice that could increase pain in the postoperative period. Teach these clients passive progressive relaxation instead.

imagery process or a voice on an audiotape or CD—helps to create a series of images. Implement the guidelines in the Client/Family Teaching feature "Guidelines for Constructing a Visualization" below with soft background music to record your own guided imagery experience for relaxation, guidance, or symptom control or healing or to assist clients with guided imagery.

Nurses interested in gaining expertise in incorporating guided imagery into their practice might consider a certification program. Both the American Holistic Nurses Association (www.ahna.org) and the Academy for Guided Imagery (www.ncpii@aol.com) provide continuing education and certification programs. Such data can be accessed through a direct resource link on the Companion Website for this book.

VISUALIZATION FOR RELAXATION

Relaxing through visualization is enhanced by constructing in one's own mind a relaxing environment. Some people find the soothing sounds of the seashore calming; others prefer to imagine themselves floating above the world on a soft cloud or a magic carpet. Still others relax as they imagine themselves descending on a slow-moving escalator into a calmer and more relaxed state. If visualization seems difficult (and if a warm bath, hot tub, or swimming pool is relaxing), try constructing a visualization while in warm water, combining the physiologic effects of the warm water with the products of the imagination.

VISUALIZATION FOR GUIDANCE

Visualization can also be useful when seeking guidance, direction, or help with decision making. Upon reaching a special soothing place, visualize an "inner advisor" or "wise person." You can ask for an image to appear or use someone you know—a valued teacher, a historical figure (Florence Nightingale, Martin Luther King, Jr., Mother Theresa), a beloved grandparent (see the Client/Family Teaching feature "Guidelines for Constructing a Visualization" below).

VISUALIZATION FOR SYMPTOM CONTROL OR HEALING

Visualization techniques for symptom control or healing can be part of a well-rounded health program. For example, visualization can be used with conventional medical treatment for cancer clients and with preoperative clients to control postoperative pain and enhance tissue healing. Clients with vascular problems: migraine headache, hypertension, or Raynaud's disease benefit from visualization. Allergies, asthma, rheumatoid arthritis, gastritis, colitis, peptic ulcer, insomnia, anxiety, depression, and chronic pain all respond to visualization. Two suggestions for visualizations are given in the Client/Family Teaching feature "Guidelines for Constructing a Visualization" below.

MediaLink Continuing Education/Certification

Hypnotherapy and Self-Hypnosis

Hypnotherapy is the therapeutic use of suggestion during an altered state of consciousness to effect positive changes in a person's behavior and to treat a range of health conditions. It has been used as an adjunct to anesthesia or in place of anesthesia, to decrease pain, to treat tension and migraine headaches, to decrease dependence on tobacco, for weight control, in dentistry, and in trance-like states to access the deepest levels of the mind. Although hypnotherapy has been practiced in many cultures for thousands of years, its use in health care became more common in the mid-twentieth century when the American Medical Association approved its use as a valid medical intervention (Goldberg, 1999). In hospitals today, it is not uncommon to find anesthesiologists, nurses, surgeons, psychologists, and social workers who use hypnosis in their therapeutic work.

Nurses who wish to use hypnosis in their clinical practice must recognize this as an advanced intervention that requires specialized training in hypnotherapy. It is also important to be aware of whether your state board of nursing identifies hypnosis as within the scope of practice of nurses.

People practice self-hypnosis—hypnosis accomplished by oneself without the help of a second party as hypnotist—to

CLIENT / FAMILY **TEACHING**

Guidelines for Constructing a Visualization

- Assume a position of comfort—either lying down or sitting up.
- Take five cleansing deep breaths. With each inhalation, imagine that you are taking in calmness and peacefulness. With each exhalation imagine that you are releasing tension, discomfort, and worry.
- Allow your body to become increasingly relaxed with each deep breath.
- Use all your senses—seeing, hearing, touching, smelling, tasting—as you imagine yourself to be in an especially beautiful and wonderful place for you. What are the colors, shapes, and living things in your special place? What do you hear and smell? What objects and shapes do you feel? What do you usually taste in this place?
- If constructing a visualization for guidance, put your wise person into your special place. Use all your senses to imagine this person. What color hair, eyes, and skin does your wise person have? What are the textures of that person's clothes? What smells do you associate? What does it feel like to grasp that person's hand?
- If constructing a visualization for pain or symptom relief, the goal would be to change the orange or red lights associated with the pain to blue lights that signify a change to pain-free or calm areas. Another visualization involves attaching a symbolic visual image to the pain (a lump in the throat, a hammer pounding the head, a dog gnawing on a bone) and then imagining the symbol becoming weakened as the pain or symptom lessens.
- When you're ready, allow the images to fade. Take whatever time you need to bring yourself back to your outer world by slowly opening your eyes and stretching.

achieve significant relaxation, to make positive suggestions for change (to lose weight, to stop smoking, to overcome fear of the dark or insomnia), and to increase learning and remembering. ■ Table 32–2 gives examples of some life problems and hypnotic suggestions that can be used to overcome them.

Most people can achieve significant relaxation within 2 days with self-hypnosis. Self-hypnosis can be self-taught through books on the subject. Community adult education programs and holistic health centers often offer courses on self-hypnosis. Self-hypnosis is clinically effective in relieving insomnia, low to moderate levels of chronic pain, tics and tremors, and low to moderate levels of anxiety. It is a well-established treatment for chronic fatigue.

Meditation

The increased use of meditation in North America owes much to Herbert Benson, a Harvard physician, who identified and promoted the scientific benefits of meditation as a relaxation response almost 30 years ago (Benson & Klipper, 2000). **Meditation** is a kind of self-discipline that helps one achieve inner peace and harmony by focusing uncritically on one thing at a time. Meditation has been associated with various religious practices and philosophies for thousands of years. It is seen as a way of becoming one with a higher power or the universe, finding enlightenment, and achieving such virtues as selflessness. However, the person who practices meditation need not associate it with religion or philosophy. It can be practiced as a means of reducing inner discord and increasing self-knowledge.

EFFECTS OF MEDITATION

The state of meditation is equivalent to a state of deep rest. The heart rate slows, the body uses less oxygen, and blood lactate—a waste product of metabolism—decreases sharply. There are beneficial effects on cardiovascular functioning at rest and during acute stress situations (Barnes, Treiber, & Davis, 2001). Vitality is increased, and body pain, anxiety, and depression are decreased (Williams, Kolar, Reger, & Pearson, 2001). Flatulence, belching, bloating, and diarrhea were all decreased in subjects with irritable bowel syndrome who meditated twice a day for 15 minutes over a 6-week period (Keefer & Blanchard, 2001). Meditation was also found to be effective in decreasing mood disturbance and stress symptoms in both males and females of various ages with a wide variety of cancer diagnoses, stages of illness, and educational backgrounds (Carlson, Ursuliak, Goodey, Angen, & Speca, 2001). Alpha brain waves, present during states of calm alertness, increase as does the secretion of dopamine (Kjaer et al., 2002).

STEPS IN MEDITATING

Meditation exercises can be relatively easy to learn. Some people experience immediate relief and pleasure in only one session. To experience deeper effects, the person needs to practice

TABLE 32–2 Life Problems and Related Hypnotic Suggestions

Life Problem	Hypnotic Suggestion
Fear of coming into a dark house at night	I can come in tonight feeling relaxed and glad to be home.
Anxiety that prevents working or studying to meet deadlines	I can work steadily and calmly. My concentration is improving as I become more relaxed.
Insomnia	I will gradually become more and more drowsy. In just a few minutes, I will be able to fall asleep and will sleep peacefully all night.
Chronic fatigue	I can wake up feeling refreshed and relaxed.
Minor chronic headache or backache	As I become more relaxed, my headache (backache) lessens. In just a few minutes, it will go away. Soon, my head will be cool and relaxed. Gradually I will feel the muscles in my back loosen, and in an hour, they will be completely relaxed. Whenever these symptoms come back, I will simply turn my ring a quarter of a turn to the right and the pain will relax away.
Feelings of inferiority	The next time I see __________, I can feel secure in myself. I can feel relaxed and at ease because I am perfectly all right.
Anxiety about an upcoming evaluation or test	Whenever I feel nervous, I can say to myself . . . (insert your special key word or phrase here) . . . and relax.
Chronic anger or chronic guilt	I can turn off anger (guilt) because I am the one who turns it on. I will relax my body and breathe deeply.
Worry about interpersonal rejection	Whenever I lace my fingers together, I will feel confidence flowing through me.
Chronic tension or discomfort in a particular part of the body.	I will think about my _____ every hour and let it relax.

Source: Copied with permission from Davis, M., Eshelman, E. R., & McKay, M. (2000). *The relaxation and stress reduction handbook* (5th ed.). Oakland, CA: New Harbinger Publications (www.newharbinger.com).

meditation regularly for at least a month. There are four major requirements for successful meditation. They are discussed in Box 32–4.

Many people who meditate prefer to use a **mantra,** a syllable, word, or name that is repeatedly chanted aloud. Some teachers of meditation insist that each person have a special mantra with a specific meaning and vibration to achieve individual effects. Others recommend the use of any word or phrase the individual is drawn to, such as love or calm. Some popular mantras are *om* (I am), *so-ham* (I am he), *sa-ham* (I am she), *Shalom* (peace), and *The Lord Is My Shepherd.*

Avoid chanting too loudly or too vigorously. After about 5 minutes, shift to whispering the mantra as you relax more deeply. When it is not possible to chant aloud, you can chant silently.

MEDICAL MEDITATION

More recently, scientific research has demonstrated that one of the newest and most cutting-edge advances in CAM is medical meditation. **Medical meditation**—meditation combined with adaptations of kundalini yoga (one of several forms of yoga)—as developed by a physician, Darma Singh Khalsa, has specific physiologic effects that can target such disorders as arthritis, anxiety disorder, Alzheimer's, diabetes, depression, hypertension, and many other physical and mental conditions (Khalsa & Stauth, 2001). Yoga is "a journey of the body, mind, and spirit on a path toward unity" (Fontaine, 2000). Thus, it is much more than simply a fitness-oriented practice.

Medical meditations unite the body, mind, and spirit by amplifying the energy system of the body that is, according to Hindu tradition, located in the seven major *chakras.* Chakras are concentrated areas of energy vertically aligned through the center of the body from the crown of the head to the pelvis (see ■ Figure 32–1). The chakras influence the physical body, the emotions, and the spirit. Each chakra corresponds to specific body structures and organs and has specific functions. The three lower chakras are primarily involved with basic elements of life such as survival, power, financial security, and procreation. The four higher chakras are involved with the higher, more advanced elements of life such as intellect, intuition, compassion, and spirituality.

BOX 32–4 The Four Major Requirements for Successful Meditation

1. **A quiet place.** The environment for meditation should be one that minimizes distractions—a quiet place set aside as a haven from the urgencies of everyday life.
2. **A comfortable position.** A comfortable position that can be held for 20 minutes without stress facilitates meditation.
3. **An object or thought to focus on.** A repeated word, an object or symbol to look at or think about, or a specific thought or feeling helps keep distracting thoughts from entering the mind.
4. **A passive attitude.** A passive attitude requires understanding that thoughts and distractions will occur and can be cleared from the mind. If they occur, they should be noted and released without concern about their interference. It is counterproductive to worry about how well you are doing at meditating.

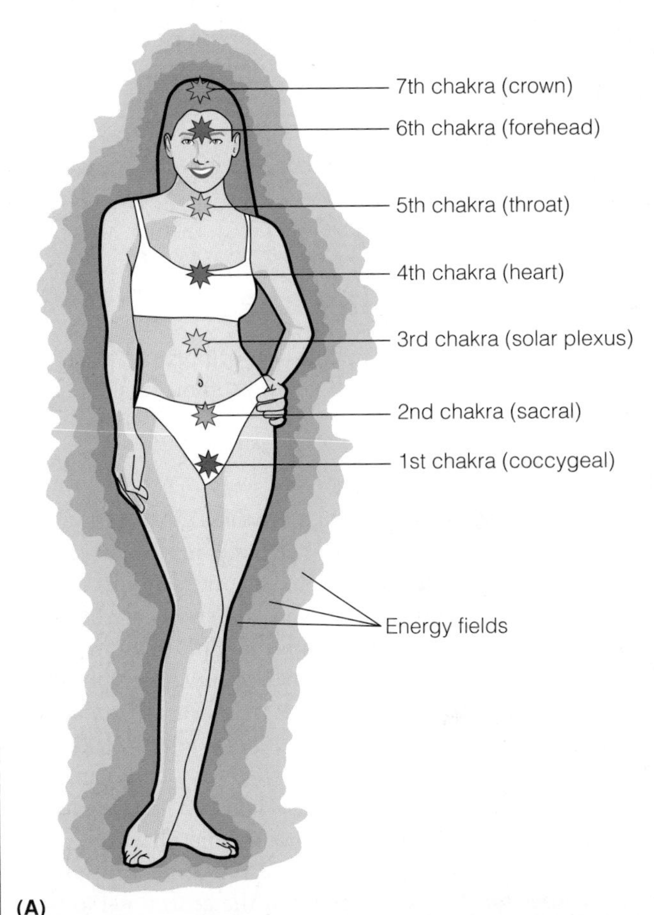

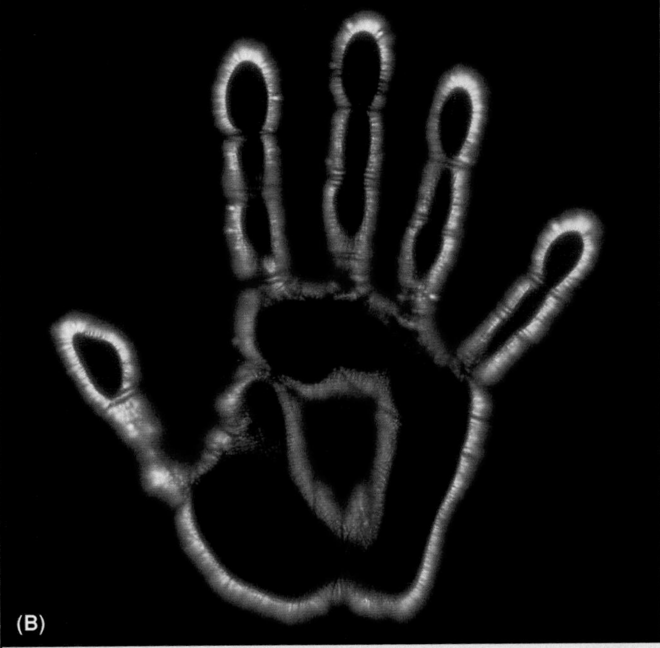

FIGURE 32–1 ■ *Energy fields of the body. (A) The seven major chakras, according to Hindu tradition, are concentrated areas of energy. (B) Kirlian photography captures the auras or biofields in the human body.*

Photo Source (B): Nigel Garion-Hutchings/FullSpectrum.

Medical meditations are very specific. They involve special postures and movements, exact positioning of the hands and fingers, specific mantras, and specific breathing patterns in order to activate specific chakras. Examples of medical meditations for stress relief and resolving issues from the past, preventing heart attack, and improving cognitive function are discussed and illustrated in the Caring for the Spirit feature on pages 775 and 776.

Pressure Point Therapies

Several approaches use the application of pressure or stimulation to specific points on the body to promote healing, relieve pain, or promote wellness.

ACUPUNCTURE

MediaLink Acupuncture Certification

Acupuncture originated in China more than 2,000 years ago and has grown in popularity in the United States for the past 20 years as more anesthesiologists, neurologists, nurses, specialists in physical medicine, and specialists in addictions are becoming trained and certified by the National Commission for the Certification of Acupuncturists (www.nccaom.org) as practitioners. *Acupuncture* is based on the belief that the vital life energy of the body (qi, pronounced chee) circulates along 12 major and 8 secondary pathways, called meridians. These pathways are linked to specific organs and organ systems. Hair-thin needles placed at acupuncture sites are used to stimulate the meridians.

According to the NIH (1997), stimulating acupuncture points causes biochemical changes in the central nervous system that either change the experience of pain or release other chemicals, such as hormones, that influence the body's self-regulating systems. The biochemical changes may stimulate the body's natural healing abilities and promote physical and emotional well-being. Promising results have emerged in treating postoperative and chemotherapy nausea and vomiting, nausea and vomiting associated with pregnancy, and for relieving dental pain (Kaptchuk, 2002). The data are equivocal or contradictory for conditions such as chronic pain, back pain, headache, chronic and acute pain, circulatory functions, mood-related mental disorders, and schizophrenia.

MediaLink American Massage Therapy Association

Acupuncture, specifically auricular acupuncture (see ■ Figure 32–3), is widely used to ease withdrawal and treat addiction in alcoholics, drug addicts, and smokers in North America and in Europe.

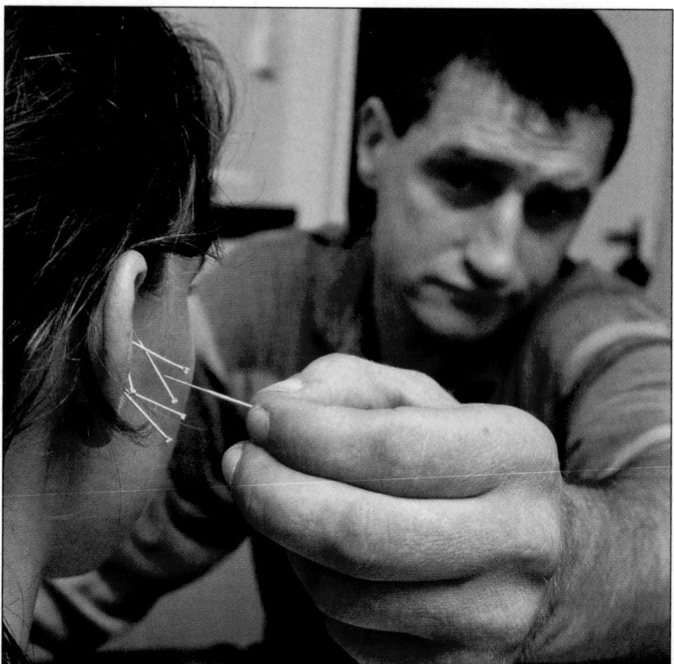

FIGURE 32–3 ■ *Auricular acupuncture.*

Source: Andrew Errington/Getty Images Inc.-Stone.

Evidence from controlled studies regarding its effectiveness as a treatment has been inconclusive. A recent study did not support the use of acupuncture as a stand-alone treatment for cocaine addiction or in situations in which clients receive only minimal concurrent psychosocial treatment (Margolin et al., 2002). Further research into the effectiveness of acupuncture as an ancillary therapy in addiction treatment is needed.

ACUPRESSURE

Acupressure is based on the same principles as acupuncture, but does not use needles; it stimulates the meridians by using finger pressure or implements. Shiatsu massage, Jin Shin Jyutsu, and Jin Shin Do are forms of acupressure that stem from the Japanese tradition. Reflexology is the practice of acupressure on particular points of the feet, hands, and ears. Foot reflexology points are illustrated in ■ Figure 32–4.

While these practices involve advanced training, you can incorporate noninvasive hand, foot, or ear massages into your clinical practice (Fontaine, 2000). The Client/Family Teaching feature "Self-Help Pressure Point and Finger Holding Techniques" on page 776 discusses pressure points and finger holds that you can teach others as a self-help process.

Touch Therapies for Healing

Touch therapies for healing or the "laying on of hands" to help heal is as old as history. There are several CAM modalities that involve the use of touch for healing. Massage is one of the best known. Massage has been helpful for persons with cancer (Gecsedi, 2002), autistic children (Escalona, Field, Singer-Strunck, Cullen, & Hartshorn, 2001), people who are depressed or addicted (Field, 2002), and, in combination with aromatherapy, for persons with dementia (Smallwood, Brown, Coulter, Irvine, & Copland, 2001). Nurses have traditionally used massage to ease a client's discomfort and to develop a connection with the client. Increasing numbers of nurses focus on this CAM modality as licensed massage therapists in private practice and are affiliated with the American Massage Therapy Association (AMTA) (www.amta.org). This Web site can be accessed through the Companion Website for this book. Another is Reiki, a gentle laying on of hands corre-

CARING FOR THE SPIRIT

Medical Meditation as an Example of Integrative Medicine

Medical meditation—a coming together of meditation and yoga—balances and regenerates spiritual and physical energies, thus forging a healing alliance in which the spirit nurtures body and mind. According to Dr. Dharma Singh Khalsa, medical meditation will "spark the spirit, and unite the mutually supportive energies of the spirit, mind, and body" (Khalsa & Stauth, 2001, p. 275).

There are five unique attributes of medical meditation that make it more powerful than standard meditation:

1. Special postures and movements.
2. Exact positioning of the hands and fingers.
3. Specific mantras.
4. Specific breathing patterns.
5. A unique focus of concentration.

Three medical meditations, with their five unique attributes, accompanied by illustrations, are presented as examples.

Medical Meditation 1: For Stress Relief and Resolving Issues from the Past

- Tune in and center yourself by chanting "Ong Namo,Guru Dev Namo" three times
- Position your body as shown, keeping your spine straight. You can sit on the floor or in a chair.
- Focus your eyes at the tip of your nose.
- Take four complete breaths per minute, through the nose, in this order: inhale for 5 seconds, hold for 5 seconds, exhale for 5 seconds.
- This medical meditation is done without a mantra.
- Your hands should be at the center of your chest. Point your fingers upward. The tips of your thumbs should touch each other, and each of your fingertips should touch the corresponding fingertip on the other hand. Keep a space between your palms.
- Take 11 minutes to do this meditation.
- End by inhaling deeply and holding your breath for 10 seconds, then exhale. Repeat 2 more times.

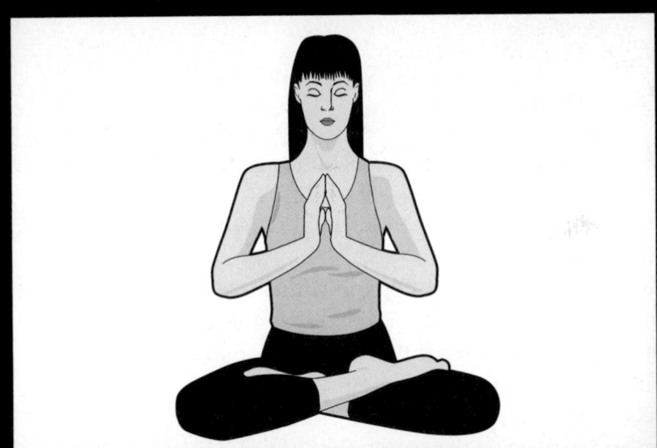

Figure 32–2(A)

Medical Meditation 2: To Prevent Heart Attacks by Keeping the Arteries Open

- Tune in and center yourself by chanting "Ong Namo,Guru Dev Namo" three times.
- Keeping your spine straight, sit with your left heel at the perineum while your right knee is at the chest and your right foot is flat on the floor. Keep your forearms parallel to the floor.
- Use any mantra you wish, such as "Ong," repeated mentally as you inhale, and "Sohung," repeated mentally as you exhale. This is an empowering and heart-opening mantra that means "The Creator is within me."
- Keep your hands flat and facing down. The right palm should rest on top of the left hand. The tips of the thumbs should touch.
- Take 7 minutes to do this meditation. Add 5 minutes per session for each week of practice until you work up to 31 minutes per session.
- End by inhaling deeply, holding your breath for 10 seconds, then exhale. Repeat two more times.

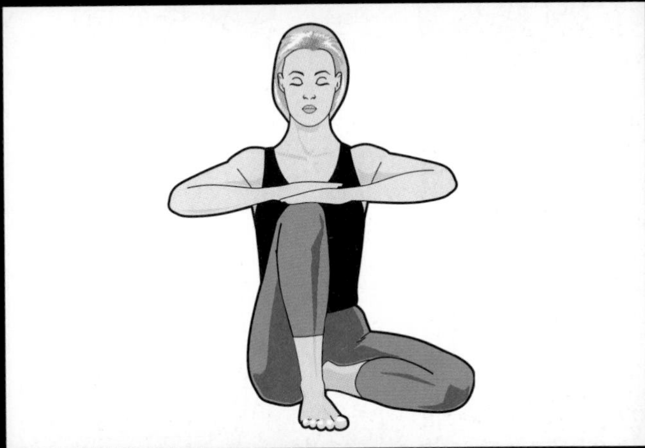

Figure 32–2(B)

(continues)

CARING FOR THE SPIRIT

Medical Meditation 3: For Improving Cognitive Function, Focus, and Coordination

- Tune in and center yourself by chanting "Ong Namo, Guru Dev Namo" three times.
- Position your body as shown, keeping your spine straight. You can sit on the floor or in a chair.
- Close your eyes and focus at the third eye point (between the eyebrows at the root of the nose).
- Breathe only through your nose, one complete breath per circle.
- This medical meditation is done without a mantra.
- Bend your elbows with your hands at shoulder level and your palms facing forward. Make fast, circular motions to the outside. Your thumbs should touch slightly as your hands pass the center of your chest. Move as quickly as possible.
- Take 3 to 11 minutes to do this meditation.
- End by inhaling, holding your breath for 10 seconds, and then exhale. Repeat two more times.

Source: Courtesy of Dharma Singh Khalsa, MD. Author of *Meditation as Medicine*.

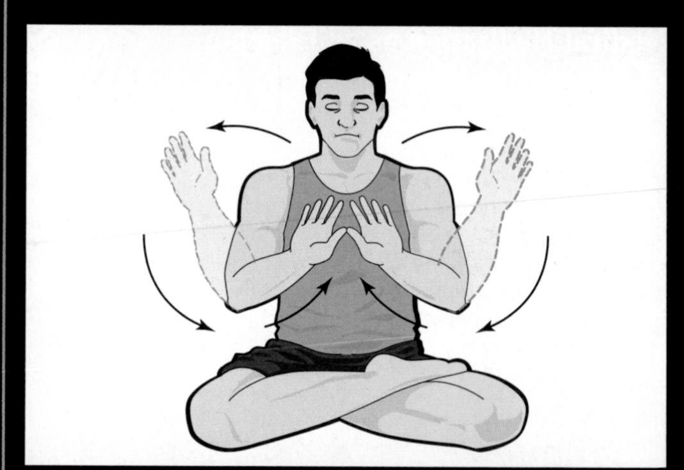

Figure 32–2(C)

sponding to the seven main chakras (Nield-Anderson & Ameling, 2001).

Most laying on of hands modalities are involved with the transfer of energy (see the earlier discussion of chakras). Nurses around the globe are using touch therapies for healing with their clients to assist in easing pain and anxiety, promoting relaxation, accelerating wound healing, diminishing depression, and increasing the sense of well-being (Umbreit, 2000).

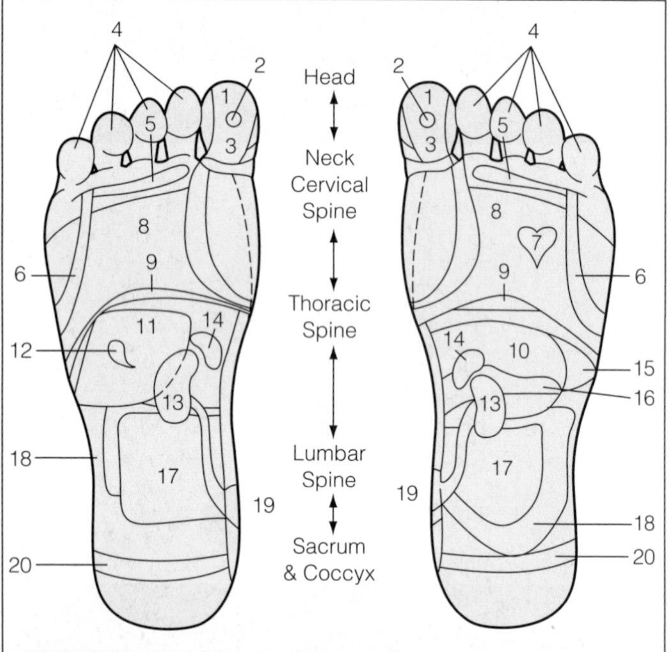

FIGURE 32–4 ■ *Foot reflexology points.*

Source: Fontaine, K. L. (2000). *Healing practices: Alternative therapies for nursing*. Upper Saddle River, NJ: Prentice Hall.

THERAPEUTIC TOUCH

Therapeutic touch (TT) was developed by Dolores Krieger (1979, 1993), a nursing professor, as a nursing activity. TT is defined as an intentionally directed process of energy exchange during which the TT practitioner uses the hands as a focus to facilitate the healing process. During this process, the therapist may direct energy from a universal source, or energy is transferred from one place to another within the body of the client. TT has one of the strongest research bases of the CAM modalities, probably due to the large number of nursing studies devoted to TT. For this reason, *energy field disturbance* has become an NANDA diagnosis. Nurse practitioners of TT can be found across North America. In the United States, you can contact nurse practitioners of TT at www.therapeutic-touch.org. In Canada, there are TT groups in Ontario (www.therapeutictouchnetwork.com), British Columbia, Alberta, and the Canadian Atlantic Coast. These resources can be found on the Companion Website for this text.

PHASES IN THERAPEUTIC TOUCH

TT is a conscious, deliberate act composed of four phases: Centering, Assessing/Scanning, Intervention, and Evaluation/Closure. Although the phases are described sequentially below, they are dynamic and often performed concurrently and repeated as often as necessary by experienced practitioners:

1. *Centering:* Centering is a process of bringing the body, mind, and emotions to a quiet, focused state of consciousness in order to find an inner sense of equilibrium and connect with the inner core of wholeness and stillness. This phase serves to gather and focus the healer's energies on the client and exclude extraneous thoughts from the mind, a process akin to meditation. This state of centeredness is maintained throughout the TT process.

MediaLink American/Canadian TT Nurses

CLIENT / FAMILY TEACHING

Self-Help Pressure Point and Finger Holding Techniques

Pressure Point Therapy to Ease Tension and Restore Energy

- Hold your left palm in front of you, fingers together.
- Using your right thumb, massage the fleshy spot between your thumb and index finger for a slow count of 15 (this spot is a key pressure point).
- Then switch hands, and repeat the process.

Finger Holds to Improve General Well-Being

- Gently hold the appropriate finger on either hand while imagining negative emotions melting away and physical symptoms easing.
- *Thumb*. Corresponds to worrying, depression, and anxiety. Physical symptoms may be stomachaches, headaches, skin problems, and nervousness.
- *Index finger*. Corresponds to fear, mental confusion, and frustration. Physical symptoms are digestive problems and muscular problems such as backaches.
- *Middle finger*. Corresponds to anger, irritability, and indecisiveness. Physical symptoms are eye or vision problems, fatigue, and circulation problems.
- *Ring finger*. Corresponds to sadness, fear of rejection, grief, and negativity. Physical symptoms are digestive, breathing, or serious skin problems.
- *Little finger*. Corresponds to insecurity, effort, overdoing it, and nervousness. Physical symptoms are sore throat and bone or nerve problems.

Source: Fontaine, K. L. (2000). *Healing practices: Alternative therapies for nursing* (p. 214) Upper Saddle River, NJ: Prentice Hall.

2. *Assessing/Scanning:* Holding the hands two to six inches away from the client's body, as in ■ Figure 32–5, the TT practitioner moves the hands from the head to the feet in a rhythmic and symmetric manner to determine the nature of the dynamic energy field. Sensory cues such as warmth, coolness, static, blockage, pulling, and tingling are described by some practitioners. These areas indicate a static condition, an imbalance, or congestion in the client's energy field that extends beyond the person's physical body.
3. *Intervention: Clearing,* also called *unruffling,* is an intentional intervention process of facilitating the flow of energy through the field. Clearing is achieved by using sweeping hand movements, with the palms facing toward the client, from the midline to the outer edge of the body while continuing to move in a rhythmic and symmetric manner from the head to the feet. The intent of this process is *balancing* and *rebalancing* the bioenergetic field. It involves the transfer of energy through the TT practitioner to the client with

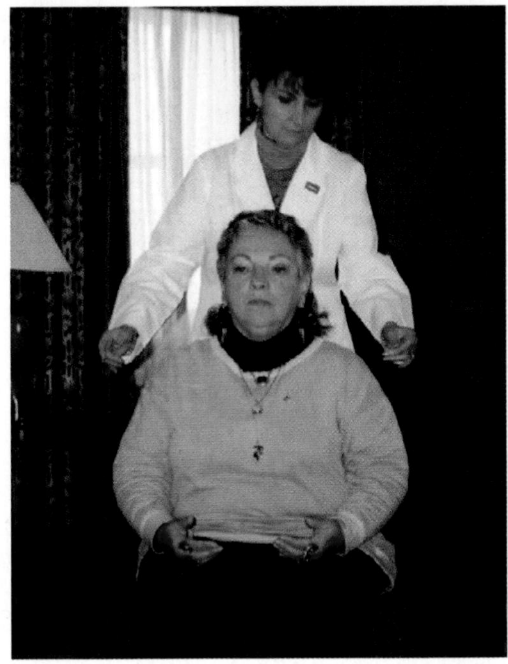

(a)

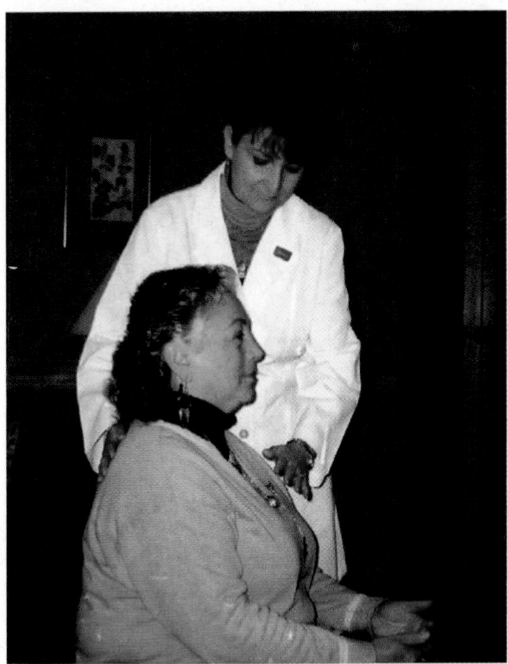

(b)

FIGURE 32–5 ■ *The process of healing touch.*

Source: Nurse Healers–Professional Associates International (The official organization for Therapeutic Touch), 3760 South Highland Drive #429, Salt Lake City, Utah 84106, 801-273-3399, www.therapeutic-touch.org.

the intent of bringing balance to areas of imbalance. The TT practitioner projects, directs, and modulates energy to reestablish order in the system.

4. *Evaluation/Closure:* Reassessment of the bioenergy field completes the session. The TT practitioner uses professional, informed, and intuitive judgment to determine when to end the session and elicits feedback from the client. Evaluation is an ongoing process that guides the responses, intention, and knowledgeable interaction of the practitioner.

EFFECTIVENESS OF THERAPEUTIC TOUCH

Clients report a sense of relaxation and relief from pain. Krieger's early research (1979) demonstrated experimentally that TT has produced a significant change in the hemoglobin component of red blood cells. Advocates of TT have found that, although the freeing of bound energy varies with each recipient, it does seem to facilitate the repatterning of energy necessary for healing. Research indicates that TT can reduce pain, accelerate the healing process, decrease anxiety, and result in a person's emotional and spiritual growth.

Herbal Therapy

Natural herbs have been used as medicines across the ages and across all cultures. Their use has grown tremendously within the past 10 years. There are thousands of natural herbal products that are used for symptom relief in a variety of conditions. Fewer herbs are used for treatment of emotional symptoms or mental disorder. ■ Table 32–3 lists the natural medicines that are likely to be effective and safe for clients with psychiatric-related symptoms.

However, be aware that there may be insufficient reliable information available to judge the effectiveness or safety

TABLE 32–3 Natural Medicines Used for Psychiatric Symptoms

Psychiatric Symptom	Natural Medicine	Effectiveness and Safety[a]
Anxiety/restlessness	Kava[b]	Comparable to low-dose benzodiazepines for short-term treatment of anxiety.
		Likely safe when used orally and short term.
		Possibly unsafe over the long term or in high doses (severe adverse effects including liver toxicity).
Dementia	Ginkgo leaf extract	Likely effective; effect is similar to donezepil (Aricept).
		Likely safe when used orally.
		Likely unsafe when used intravenously (IV).
	SAMe (S-Adenosylmethionine)[c]	Likely safe orally, IV, and intramuscularly (IM).
Depression	St. John's wort	Possibly as effective as fluoxetine (Prozac) and sertraline (Zoloft).
		Likely safe when used orally and short term.
		Possibly unsafe in large doses (1,800 mg or more per day).
	SAMe	Possibly as effective as oral tricyclic antidepressants.
Encephalopathy (alcoholic) or peripheral neuropathy	Thiamine (Vitamin B_1)	Likely safe when taken orally.
		Rare hypersensitivity when taken IM or IV.
Sleep disturbance/insomnia	Melatonin	Likely effective for jet lag and insomnia.
		Likely ineffective for work shift change adjustment.
		Possibly safe when used orally or parenterally.

[a]According to the sources listed, these natural medicines are thought likely to be effective and safe when used appropriately. It is important to validate safety and effectiveness with the most up-to-date sources.

[b]NCCAM has placed studies of Kava on hold, pending further guidance from the Federal Food and Drug Administration (FDA). To view the FDA advisory, go to www.cfsan.fda.gov/.

[c]Available studies are limited by small numbers of subjects, inconsistent diagnostic criteria, and short treatment periods.

Sources: Brunner, R., Azbel, V., Madhusoodanan, S., et al. (2000). Comparison of an extract of hypericum (LI 160) and sertraline in the treatment of depression: A double-blind, randomized pilot study. *Clinical Therapies, 22,* 411–419; Jellin, J. M., Gregory, P. J., Batz, F., & Bonakdar, K. (2002). *Pharmacist's letter/prescriber's letter natural medicines comprehensive database* (4th ed.). Stockton, CA: Therapeutic Research Faculty; and Wettstein, A. (2000). Cholinesterase inhibitors and ginkgo extracts—are they comparable in the treatment of dementia? Comparison of published placebo-controlled efficacy studies of at least six months' duration. *PhytoMedicine, 6,* 393–401.

TABLE 32–4 Commonly Used Natural Medicines That Should Not Be Taken in Combination with Psychotropic Drugs[a]

Psychotropic Drug	Natural Medicine
Anticonvulsants	Sage
Carbamazepine (Tegretol)	Grapefruit juice/psyllium
Antidepressants	European mistletoe/SAMe/St. John's wort
Clomipramine (Anafranil)	Grapefruit juice
Monoamine oxidase inhibitors (MAOIs)	American ginseng/black tea/brewer's yeast/caffeine/cocoa/coffee/cola nut/ephedra/fenugreek/ginkgo leaf extract/green tea/guarana/panax ginseng/passionflower/phenylalanine/wine/yohimbe
Serotonin Agonists	5-HTP
Serotonin Antagonists	5-HTP
SSRIs	St. John's wort/SAMe
Fluoxetine (Prozac)	Melatonin
Fluvoxamine (Luvox)	Melatonin
Tricyclics	Belladonna/St. John's wort/SAMe/yohimbe
Antipsychotics	American ginseng/coffee/panax ginseng/Siberian ginseng (*Eleutherococcus*)
Clozapine (Clozaril)	Black tea/caffeine/cocoa/coffee/cola nut/green tea/guarana
Central Nervous System Depressants	German chamomile/hawthorn/kava/melatonin/stinging nettle (above ground parts)/wine
Alcohol	Gamma hydroxybutyrate (GHB)/kava/Siberian ginseng/valerian
Central Nervous System Stimulants	American ginseng/panax ginseng
Caffeine	cocoa/black tea/ephedra/green tea/guarana/panax ginseng
Fenfluramine	St. John's wort
Lithium	Black tea/caffeine/cocoa/coffee/green tea/guarana/psyllium
Phenothiazines	Evening primrose oil/yohimbe
Sedatives	Goldenseal/gotu kola/kava/passionflower/Siberian ginseng/valerian
Barbiturates	Ginger/goldenseal/kava/passionflower/Siberian ginseng/St. John's wort/valerian
Benzodiazepines	Kava/melatonin/valerian
Alprazolam (Xanax)	Kava
Midazolam (Versed), Triazolam (Halcion)	Grapefruit juice
Buspirone (BuSpar)	Grapefruit juice

[a]These combinations result in either canceling out the therapeutic effect of the psychotropic drug, potentiating the effects above and beyond what is therapeutically intended, or causing untoward side effects. This table contains only those combinations that are likely to be clinically significant. It does not include all possible problematic combinations nor does it include all incidents of case reports.

Source: Blumenthal, M., Goldberg, A., & Brinkman, J. (2000). *Expanded commission E monographs*. Newton, MA: Integrative Medicine Communications; and Jellin, J. M., Gregory, P. J., Batz, F., & Bonakdar, K. (2002). *Pharmacist's letter/prescriber's letter natural medicines comprehensive database* (4th ed.). Stockton, CA: Therapeutic Research Faculty.

of many herbs. Testing in clinical trials is relatively recent, and little long-term random testing has been conducted. Misconceptions also abound. For example, one common misconception is that the herb goldenseal can be used to mask the results of laboratory tests for illicit drug use. Goldenseal has been found to be ineffective for this purpose.

Encourage clients to discuss with their health care provider all natural remedies that they ingest. Some may potentiate the effects of psychotropic medications; others may block the effects. Others may increase the extent of adverse side effects. The psychotropic medications and the herbs that affect them are listed in ■ Table 32–4.

Safety and effectiveness of herbs can be validated at the following Web sites:

1. U.S. Food and Drug Administration: www.fda.gov.
2. National Center for Complementary and Alternative Medicine: www.nccam.nih.gov.
3. University of Washington Medicinal Herb Garden: www.nnlm.nlm.hig.gov.

These data can also be found as resource links on the Companion Website for this book.

Biofeedback

Visceral learning, known as **biofeedback,** is a technique for gaining conscious control over involuntary body functions such as blood pressure and heart rate, which are mediated by the autonomic nervous system. It has been shown, for example, that migraine headaches can be relieved by increasing blood flow to the hands (Scharff, Marcus, & Masek, 2002). Biofeedback has also been found to be useful in treating tension headaches, insomnia, muscle or colon spasm, pain, hypertension, asthma, stuttering, bruxism (grinding of the teeth), and epilepsy. The psychological states achieved through biofeedback can be beneficial in decreasing anxiety and phobic reactions.

The technique is based on giving continuous feedback about the results of each attempt at control. In a typical session, a person might be given this feedback by equipment that amplifies body signals and translates them into a flashing light or a steady tone. Once people can "see" a heartbeat, for instance, and observe when it slows down or speeds up, they have the information they need to control their heart rate by slowing a flashing light or altering a tone. Inexpensive equipment for home use is available.

Repetitive Transcranial Magnetic Stimulation (rTMS)

In repetitive transcranial magnetic stimulation, a powerful electrical current is sent through an insulated coil of wire, which is placed on the client's head generating a magnetic field, which creates an electrical current that causes neurochemical changes in specifically targeted structures of the brain. As a therapy, rTMS is still experimental. The most promising beneficial effects of this experimental treatment are in clients with depression (McNamara, Ray, Arthurs, & Boniface, 2001). A study of persons with schizophrenia also showed significant improvement in medication-resistant hallucinating clients after 10 days of treatment (d'Alfonso et al., 2002). A longitudinal study at 3- and 6-month intervals suggests that rTMS could replace electroconvulsive therapy (ECT) as a treatment for major depression (Dannon, Dolberg, Schreiber, & Grunhaus, 2002). There is no pain involved with rTMS, and no anesthesia is required.

Eye Movement Desensitization Reprocessing (EMDR)

Eye movement desensitization reprocessing is a controversial intervention suggested for posttraumatic stress disorder and dissociative identity disorder, which asks clients to recall traumatic memories or a feared stimulus while making a series of rapid lateral eye movements. There is no definitive theoretical explanation of how EMDR might work other than the suggestion by Stickgold (2002) that it is the repetitive redirection of attention in EMDR that induces a neurobiologic state, similar to that of rapid eye movement (REM) sleep, which assists in the integration of traumatic memories into the cortex of the brain. The research into EMDR is contradictory. Perkins and Rouanzoin (2002) note several factors that may account for confusion in the literature—the lack of a convincing explanation of exactly how EMDR works, inaccurate and selective reporting of research, inadequately designed studies, and biased or inaccurate reviews by various groups. This is clearly an area in which well-designed empirical studies are needed.

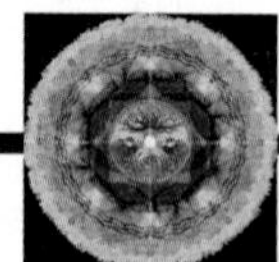

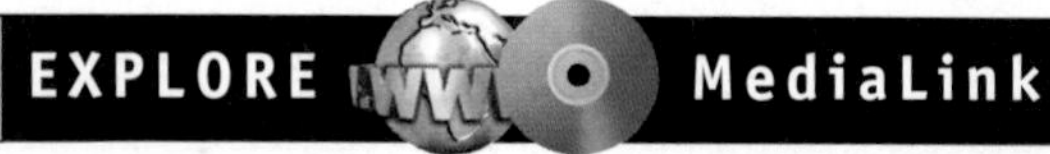

NCLEX review, case studies, and other interactive resources for this chapter can be found on the Companion Website at http://www.prenhall.com/kneisl. Click on Chapter 32 to select the activities for this chapter.

For animations, video tutorials, more NCLEX review questions, and an audio glossary, access the accompanying CD-ROM in this textbook.

BIBLIOGRAPHY

Barnes, V. S., Treiber, F. A., & Davis, H. (2001). Impact of transcendental meditation on cardiovascular function at rest and during acute stress in adolescents with high normal blood pressure. *Journal of Psychosomatic Research, 51*(4), 597–605.

Benson, H., & Klipper, M. Z. (2000). *The relaxation response*. New York: William Morrow & Co.

Carlson, L. E., Ursuliak, Z., Goodey, E., Angen, M., & Speca, M. (2001). The effects of a mindfulness meditation-based stress reduction program on mood and symptoms in cancer outpatients: 6-month follow-up. *Support Care Cancer, 9*(2), 112–123.

Cohen, R. J., Ek, K., & Pan, C. X. (2002). Complementary and alternative medicine (CAM) use by older adults: A comparison of self-report and physician chart documentation. *Journal of Gerontological Alternative Biologic Science and Medical Science, 57*(4), M223–227.

d'Alfonso, A. A., Aleman, A., Kessels, R. P., Schouten, E. A., Postma, A., vanDerLinden, J. A., et al. (2002). Transcranial magnetic stimulation of left auditory cortex in patients with schizophrenia: Effects on hallucinations and neurocognition. *Journal of Neuropsychiatry and Clinical Neuroscience, 14*(1), 77–79.

Dannon, P. N., Dolberg, O. T., Schreiber, S., & Grunhaus, L. (2002). Three and six-month outcome following courses of either ECT or rTMS in a population of severely depressed individuals—preliminary report. *Biological Psychiatry, 51*(8), 687–690.

Duggan, J., Peterson, W. S., Schutz, M., Khuder, S., & Charkraborty, J. (2001). Use of complementary and alternative therapies in HIV-infected patients. *AIDS Patient Care and STDs, 15*(3), 159–167.

Escalona, A., Field, T., Singer-Strunck, R., Cullen, C. & Hartshorn, K. (2001). Improvements in the behavior of children with autism following massage therapy. *Journal of Autism and Developmental Disorders, 31*(5), 513–516.

Field, T. (2002). Massage therapy. *Medical Clinics of North America, 86*(1), 163–171.

Fontaine, K. L. (2000). *Healing practices: Alternative therapies for nursing*. Upper Saddle River, NJ: Prentice Hall.

Frisch, N. C., Keegan, L., Guzzetta, C. E., & Quinn, J. A. (2000). *AHNA standards of holistic nursing: Guidelines for caring and healing*. Gaithersburg, MD: Aspen.

Gagner-Tjellesen, D., Yurkovich, E. E., & Gragert, M. (2001). Use of music therapy and other ITNIs in acute care. *Journal of Psychosocial Nursing and Mental Health Services, 39*(10), 26–37.

Gecsedi, R. A. (2002). Massage therapy for patients with cancer. *Clinical Journal of Oncological Nursing, 6*(1), 52–54.

Goldberg, B. (1999). *Alternative medicine: The definitive guide*. Tiburon, CA: Future Medicine Publishing.

Hayden, C. W., Bernstein, C. N., Hall, R. A., Vakil, N., Garewal, H. S., & Fass, R. (2002). Usage of supplemental alternative medicine by community-based patients with gastroesophageal reflux disease (GERD). *Digestive Disorders Science, 47*(1), 1–8.

Heuschkel, R., Afzal, N., Wuerth, A., Zurakowski, D., Leichtner, A., Kemper, D., et al. (2002). Complementary medicine use in children and young adults with inflammatory bowel disease. *American Journal of Gastroenterology, 97*(2), 382–388.

Jellin, J. M., Gregory, P.J., Batz, F., & Bonakdar, K. (2002). *Pharmacist's letter/prescriber's letter natural medicines comprehensive database* (4th ed.). Stockton, CA: Therapeutic Research Faculty.

Kaptchuk, T. J. (2002). Acupuncture: Theory, efficacy, and practice. *Annals of Internal Medicine, 136*(5), 374–383.

Keefer, L., & Blanchard, E. B. (2001). The effects of relaxation response meditation on the symptoms of irritable bowel syndrome: Results of a controlled treatment study. *Behavioral Research and Therapy, 39*(7), 801–811.

Kessler, R. C., Davis, R. B., Foster, D. F., Van Rompay, M. I., Walters, E. E., Wilkey, S. A., et al. (2001a). Long-term trends in the use of complementary and alternative medical therapies in the United States. *Annals of Internal Medicine, 135*(4), 262–268.

Kessler, R. C., Soukup, J., Davis, R. B., Foster, D. F., Wilkey, S. A., Van Rompey, M. I., et. al. (2001b). The use of complementary and alternative therapies to treat anxiety and depression in the United States. *American Journal of Psychiatry, 158*(2), 289–294.

Khalsa, D. S., & Stauth, C. (2001). *Meditation as medicine: Activate the power of your natural healing force*. New York: Simon & Schuster.

Kjaer, T. W., Bertelsen, C., Piccini, P., Brooks, D., Alving, J., & Lou, H. C. (2002). Increased dopamine tone during meditation-induced change of consciousness. *Brain Research and Cognitive Brain Research, 13*(2), 255–259.

Krieger, D. (1993). *Accepting your power to heal.* Sante Fe, MN: Bear & Co.

Krieger, D. (1979). *The therapeutic touch*. Upper Saddle River, NJ: Prentice Hall.

Margolin, A., Kleber, H. D., Avants, S. K., Konefal, J., Gawin, F., Stark, E., et al. (2002). Acupuncture for the treatment of cocaine addiction: A randomized controlled trial. *Journal of the American Medical Association, 287*(1), 55–63.

McNamara, B., Ray, J. L., Arthurs, J., & Boniface, S. (2001). Transcranial magnetic stimulation for depression and other psychiatric disorders. *Psychological Medicine, 31*(7), 1141–1146.

National Institutes of Health Consensus Panel. (1997). *Acupuncture: National Institutes of Health consensus development statement*. Bethesda, MD: National Institutes of Health.

Nield-Anderson, L., & Ameling, A. (2001). Reiki: A complementary therapy for nursing practice. *Journal of Psychosocial Nursing and Mental Health Services, 39*(4), 42–49.

Perkins, B. R., & Rouanzoin, C. C. (2002). A critical evaluation of current views regarding eye movement desensitization and reprocessing (EMDR): Clarifying points of confusion. *Journal of Clinical Psychology, 58*(1), 77–97.

Scharff, L., Marcus, D. A., & Masek, B. J. (2002). A controlled study of minimal contact thermal biofeedback treatment in children with migraine. *Journal of Pediatric Psychology, 27*(2), 109–119.

Smallwood, J., Brown, R., Coulter, F., Irvine, E., & Copland, C. (2001). Aromatherapy and behavior disturbances in dementia: A randomized controlled trial. *International Journal of Geriatric Psychiatry, 16*(10), 1010–1013.

Stickgold, R. (2002). EMDR: A putative neurobiological mechanism of action. *Journal of Clinical Psychology, 58*(1), 61–75.

Swisher, E. M., Coh, D. E., Goff, B. A., Parham, J., Herzog, T. J., Rader, J. S., et al. (2002). Use of complementary and alternative medicine among women with gynecologic cancers. *Gynecologic Oncology, 84*(3), 363–367.

Tough, S. C., Johnston, D. W., Verhoef, M. J., Arthur, K., & Bryant, H. (2002). Complementary and alternative medicine use among colorectal cancer patients in Alberta, Canada. *Alternative Therapies in Health and Medicine, 8*(2), 54–56, 58–60, 62–64.

Umbreit, A. W. (2000). Healing touch: Applications in the acute care setting. *AACN Clinical Issues, 11*(1), 105–119.

Williams, K. A., Kolar, M. M., Reger, B. E., & Pearson, J. C. (2001). Evaluation of a wellness-based mindfulness stress reduction intervention: A controlled trial. *American Journal of Health Promotion, 15*(6), 422–432.

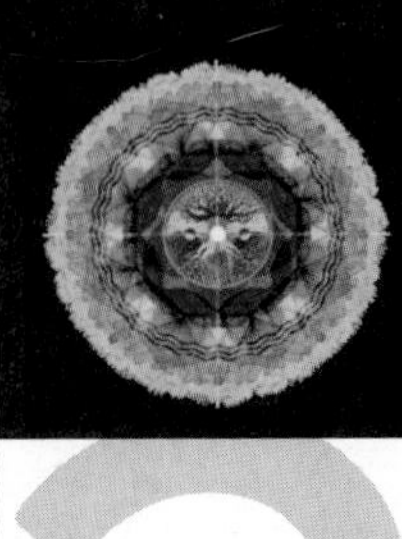

33

Chapter THIRTY-THREE

Crisis Intervention

CAROL REN KNEISL
ELIZABETH A. RILEY

KEY TERMS

anticipatory guidance
crisis
crisis intervention
maturational crisis
situational crisis
vicarious traumatization

FOCUS QUESTIONS

- **What types of crises can a person experience?**
- **How would you trace the sequence of a crisis and determine its significance for the nursing care of clients in crisis?**
- **Why is an understanding of the origins of a crisis and balancing factors important in the assessment phase of crisis management?**
- **What are three possible crisis intervention modalities for a person in crisis?**
- **Why might you feel overwhelmed in caring for clients experiencing a crisis?**

MediaLink 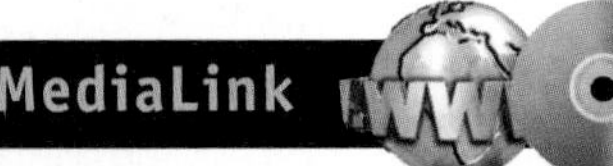 www.prenhall.com/kneisl

Additional resources for this chapter can be found on the Student CD-ROM accompanying this textbook, and on the Companion Website at www.prenhall.com/kneisl. Click on Chapter 33 to select the activities for this chapter.

CD-ROM

- Audio Glossary
- NCLEX Review

Companion Website

- Additional NCLEX Review
- Care Plan: Client in Crisis
- Case Study: Crisis Intervention Principles

CHAPTER OUTLINE

CROSS REFERENCES

Other topics relevant to this content are: Anxiety, fight-or-flight response to stress, coping with stress, and defense mechanisms, Chapter 5; Cognitive therapy techniques, Chapter 30; Nursing intervention in anxiety, panic, acute stress disorder, and posttraumatic stress disorder, Chapter 16; Physical effects of stress, Chapter 5; Relaxation techniques and other strategies for managing stress, Chapter 32; Suicide and lethality assessment, Chapter 22; Violence and abuse in families, Chapter 23; Violence in the psychiatric setting, Chapter 34.

CRITICAL THINKING CHALLENGE

Katrinka V., a 43-year-old nurse, is a survivor of domestic violence. She and John, her husband of 15 years, have two children. Last night after a long period of drinking, John threatened Katrinka and the children with a gun. Katrinka managed to get herself and the children out of the house and into her car where they spent the night. In the morning, Katrinka, distraught and highly anxious, arrived at the psychiatric emergency room. She said: "I can't think of what to do. I've got to get to my job and the kids have to go to school. It's not safe for any of us at either place. What should I do?"

Katrinka is in crisis. How do you understand her current situation? What critical areas do you need to assess? What interventions would be helpful? ■

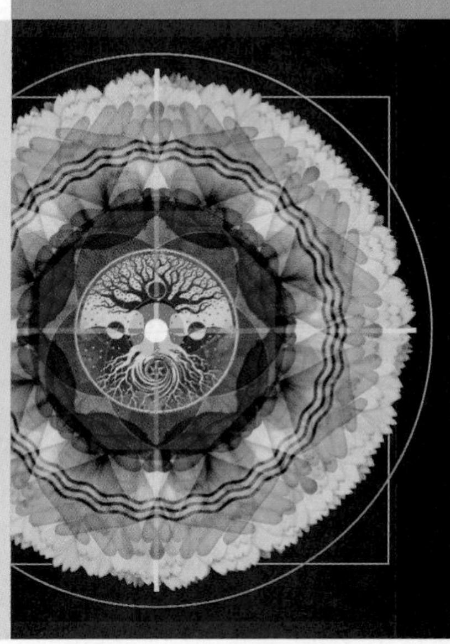

In the most devastating terrorist onslaught ever waged against the United States, knife-wielding hijackers crashed two airliners into New York City's World Trade Center, toppling its twin 110-story towers.

The deadly calamity was witnessed on television screens across the world as a third plane slammed into the Pentagon, and a fourth crashed outside Pittsburgh. The death toll, thought to number almost 3,000, also included firefighters, police officers, and medical personnel killed while attempting to rescue victims. The impact on New York City was horrific. Many people lost their jobs because businesses were demolished and tourists stayed away. Even the usual winter holiday festivities for which New York City is famous were conducted with an air of great sadness. The impact on the rest of the country—survivors, citizens, and visitors alike—and in fact, around the world, was tremendous, as these examples illustrate.

CLINICAL EXAMPLE

Nguyen, a visitor from Malaysia, was walking across the Brooklyn Bridge, admiring the view of Lower Manhattan, when he saw the plane hit the first tower. He stood on the bridge in horror, watching the fireball as people jumped from the buildings. Although he has long since returned to Malaysia, he has nightmares in which he relives the experience over and over.

Two teenagers were at home in Arizona watching TV while getting ready for school when they saw the news. First, they experienced sadness, then disbelief, confusion, anger, and, finally, fear. One said, "Now I know that terrorism isn't just something you see on the evening news that happens on the other side of the world. My life has been changed forever."

Alistair works at an airport outside of Liverpool, England. People were gathered around him, chatting about the disaster, crying, and praying. Alistair left work sick that day. He told his supervisor that he felt nauseated and weak in the knees at the thought that airplanes at his airport could be targeted and that life was so fragile.

Do you remember how you felt on Tuesday, September 11, 2001? Did you feel helpless? Did you know what to do or say to others? Did you believe that you were in danger? Did you call anyone? Did you talk about the event with others? Did you want it all to go away? If you answered "yes" to any of these questions, you know what a crisis feels like. Chances are that you, your family, and your community were in crisis, along with many other individuals, families, and communities.

A **crisis** occurs when an individual is in a situation in which usual problem-solving or adapting methods are inadequate to resolve a problem or conflict, causing a state of disequilibrium. People involved in these incidents may be unable to effectively manage stressful events or environmental changes. They may be unable to function and feel paralyzed and powerless.

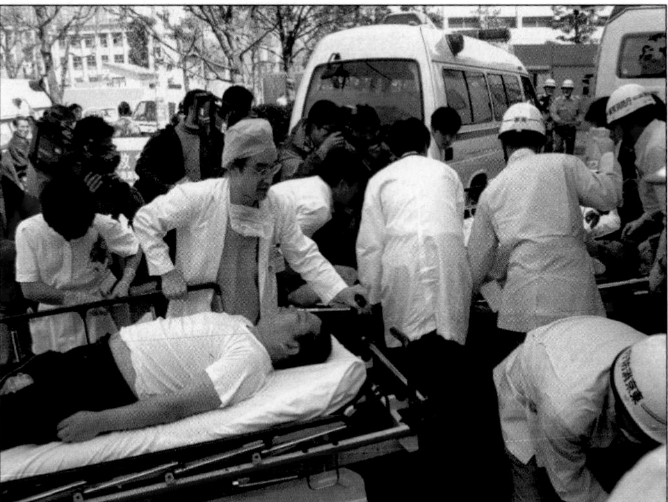

FIGURE 33–1 ■ *Threats to physical and mental well-being cause crises around the world. Here, rescue workers attend to victims of a poison gas attack in Tokyo.*

Source: AP/WorldWide Photos/Chiaki Tsukumo.

It is likely that this crisis will continue to have effects far into the future. For example, it is believed that these terrorist attacks have increased the risks of substance abuse and mental illness for United States children (Baker, 2002). In the 5 to 8 weeks after the attacks, Vlahov et al. (2002) found a substantial increase in cigarette smoking, alcohol consumption, and marijuana use in Manhattan adults and adolescents.

Other examples of situations that have caused a crisis on a more limited scale are discussed in the following Clinical Example.

CLINICAL EXAMPLE

An ex-employee comes into an office building and shoots 15 people; a tragic school bus accident claims five 6-year-olds and their teacher; two teenagers from the same high school commit suicide the same week; a 66-year-old man retires and feels useless and considers suicide; a 23-year-old woman finds out that she has a fatal illness; a premature baby is born; a 12-year-old is kidnapped while walking home from school.

Nurses are intimately connected with crises. We often interact with people who are faced with new, frightening, and troublesome situations such as that in ■ Figure 33–1. Because of who we are, where we work, and our accessibility to individuals and families, we are in a position to offer supportive and therapeutic interventions that can change people's lives. You can help if you understand how to effectively intervene, that is, if you understand how to implement crisis intervention skills. **Crisis intervention** is a conceptual framework for intervention that calls for short-term, action-oriented assistance focused on problem solving, with a goal of restoring the individual's equilibrium. Effective crisis intervention will call for all the skills that a well-prepared nurse can muster.

Crisis intervention is not the specialty of any one professional group, however. People who intervene in crises come from the fields of nursing, medicine, psychology, social work, and theology. Police officers, teachers, school guidance counselors, rescue workers, and bartenders, among others, are often on the spot in moments of crisis. Crisis intervention can be the business of many different people. The Association of Traumatic Stress Specialists provides training programs and board certification for qualified intervenors. The association represents those who serve victims of crime, veterans, refugees, natural disasters, holocaust survivors, terrorist attacks, line-of-duty-related injuries and deaths, victims of school and workplace violence, victims of political persecution, and others who have experienced traumatic stress. The association can be reached at www.atss-hq.com through the Companion Website of this book.

Crisis as Disequilibrium

The word *crisis* stems from the Greek krinein, "to decide." In Chinese, two characters are used to write the word; one is the character for danger and the other the character for opportunity. A crisis is an acute, time-limited state of disequilibrium resulting from situational, developmental, or societal sources of stress. The interaction between *danger* and *opportunity* will become clearer as you read this chapter.

CRISIS AS A TURNING POINT

Crisis situations are turning points or junctures in a person's life that result in a new equilibrium. The new equilibrium may be close to that of the precrisis state, or it may be a more positive or more negative state. If the new equilibrium is more positive, the person experiences personal growth, increased competence, a better social network, newfound problem-solving abilities, or an improved self-image. If the new equilibrium is more negative, it is possible that the individual may lose skills, adopt a regressive stance, develop socially unacceptable behaviors, or develop a mental disorder. Unsuccessful negotiation of a crisis leaves the person feeling anxious, threatened, and ineffective. Individuals may also respond to a crisis event with disturbed personal coping or with frankly psychotic behavior. This process is illustrated in ■ Figure 33–2.

Because a state of disequilibrium is so uncomfortable, a crisis is self-limiting. That is, even without intervention, a crisis will resolve itself with either a favorable or an unfavorable conclusion. However, a person experiencing a crisis alone is more vulnerable to unsuccessful negotiation than a person working through a crisis with help. Working with another person increases the likelihood that the person in crisis will resolve it in a positive way. This is why crisis intervention is sometimes referred to as primary prevention for posttraumatic stress disorder (PTSD; refer to Chapter 16). See also the Using Research Evidence feature on page 786, which discusses the effects on a client of experiencing a crisis alone.

MediaLink Trauma Specialists Association

COMMON CHARACTERISTICS OF CRISES

To understand the concept of crisis fully and to appreciate the interaction of risk factors, we must differentiate among levels of distress to illustrate what a crisis is not. Stress is not crisis. Everyone feels stress at various times, in a variety of forms. Stress is pressure and tension. Stressful situations may demand our attention and may be exhausting, but they are not crises. An

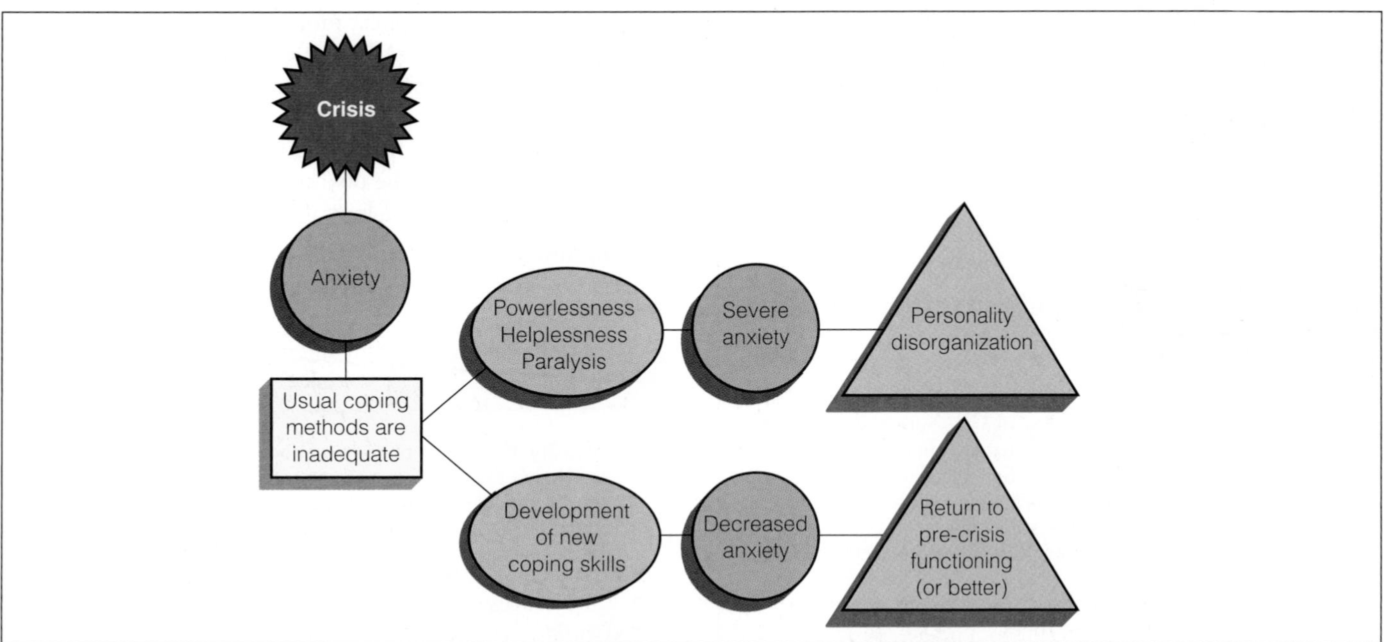

FIGURE 33–2 ■ *The progression of a crisis to either successful or unsuccessful resolution depends on what people do when they discover that their usual coping mechanisms are ineffective.*

USING RESEARCH EVIDENCE

Mrs. Blankenship, a middle-aged African-American woman, has been admitted for a crisis evaluation and brief stay at the private psychiatric hospital in which you work. She has requested that a female do her admission interview. In reviewing her records, you note that she has had multiple hospitalizations for crisis-type episodes, severe anxiety, and obsessive–compulsive disorder.

She is tearful and anxious, as well as depressed, and asks you to leave the door open and not to sit in front of it. Mrs. Blankenship connects most of her anxiety to the fact that she lives in a housing project in which stealing and drugs run rampant. Her greatest fear is for her own safety and the safety of her grandchildren. She is articulate and without ideas of suicide or homicide. She is not psychotic.

You are working the full week, and Mrs. Blankenship will be your client for the next five days. On the third day she tells you of a time when she was held captive for six hours and brutally raped, sharing her fear that she is "going crazy." You implement the following interventions: Your interventions are based on your understanding of the research studies cited below that indicate that many individuals who seek psychiatric help have been traumatized and the trauma has not been recognized or adequately treated:

- Explaining to Mrs. Blankenship that many of her problems could be related to the attack
- Exploring with Mrs. Blankenship the coping styles that emerged from this event
- Encouraging Mrs. Blankenship to make connections between the event and her current situation
- Helping her select an outpatient therapist who is competent to treat trauma victims
- Arranging for Mrs. Blankenship to meet the therapist while she is still in the hospital.

Cooke, A. L., & Shear, K. W. (2001). Treatment of a 50-year-old African-American woman whose chronic posttraumatic stress disorder went undiagnosed for over 20 years. *American Journal of Psychiatry, 158*(6), 866–870.

Ormel, J., Oldehinkle, A. J., & Brilman, E. I. (2001). The interplay and etiological continuity of neuroticism, difficulties, and life events in the etiology of major and subsyndromal, first and recurrent depressive episodes in later life. *American Journal of Psychiatry, 158*(6), 885–891.

emergency is a situation that often demands an immediate response to ensure the survival of an individual. Although neither stress nor an emergency are themselves a crisis, stress or an emergency can ultimately precipitate a crisis. A crisis is not a mental disorder. A crisis can happen to someone who never had a mental disorder or to someone who is currently experiencing a mental disorder. Common characteristics of crises are discussed in Box 33–1.

RISK FACTORS AND BALANCING FACTORS

Why do some people effectively manage disequilibrium while others go into crisis? There are several risk factors, in addition to the nature of the trauma or experience, that place individuals at high risk for crisis. These factors are identified in Box 33–2.

In addition to these risk factors, Aguilera (1998) indicates that these three balancing factors are important to the successful resolution of disequilibrium:

1. *Perception of the event:* How individuals perceive and understand the event/crisis in their lives. Are they being punished? Is this happening only to them and never to anyone else? How will the event affect their future? Do they see the situation realistically, or is it distorted?
2. *Situational supports:* The availability of people who can help individuals in crisis solve the problem. Meaningful relationships with others give support and assistance during the crisis. Individuals with inadequate support are likely to experience a decrease in self-esteem. In turn, lowered self-esteem may make an event appear more threatening.
3. *Coping mechanisms:* All people use mechanisms to cope with anxiety and tension. Because the individual has used these coping mechanisms with success in the past, they become part of the coping repertoire. These tension-relieving mechanisms can be obvious or subtle (see the discussion in Chapter 5).

If all these balancing factors are present when an individual experiences a state of disequilibrium, it is unlikely that a crisis

BOX 33–1 Common Characteristics of Crises

- Many situational crises are experienced as sudden. The person is usually not aware of a warning signal, whether or not others could "see it coming." The individual or family may feel that they have had little or no preparation for the event or trauma.
- The crisis may be experienced as ultimately life threatening, whether this perception is realistic or not.
- Communication with significant others is often decreased or cut off.
- There may be perceived or real displacement from familiar surroundings or significant loved ones.
- All crises have an aspect of loss, whether actual or perceived. The losses can include an object, a person, a hope, a dream, or any significant factor for that individual.

BOX 33–2 Risk Factors for Crisis

- Intensity of exposure to the situation
- Preexisting psychiatric symptoms and diagnosis
- Prior history of traumatic exposure
- Family history of psychiatric problems, anxiety, and/or antisocial behavior
- Early separation from parents
- Childhood abuse
- Poverty
- Cultural expectations that prohibit asking others for help
- Degree of threat to life (being on a plane that crashes versus watching a plane crash from a distance)

will result. ■ Figure 33–3 illustrates how these balancing factors affect the outcome of a stressful event.

Biopsychosocial Theories of Crisis

The recognition of crisis has a long history. Roberts (2000) notes that as long ago as 400 BC, physicians of the time understood that a crisis was a hazardous life event. It was not until the twentieth century, however, that strategies for helping people to cope with crisis were developed. Theories of crisis and crisis intervention resulted from early research studies that are now classics, as well as more recent events in the field of mental health. Some of these are:

- Lindemann's (1944) landmark study of the survivors of the tragic Coconut Grove nightclub fire in Boston that identified symptoms common to individuals experiencing acute grief. Lindemann determined that if grieving was delayed or absent, the crisis resulted in negative outcomes.
- The observations of, and treatment by, military psychiatrists of battle-weary and emotionally upset soldiers at the front lines that allowed the soldiers to return to duty rather than having to be sent to inpatient psychiatric facilities.
- Tyhurst's (1957) studies of the stages individuals go through when experiencing transition states such as migration, retirement, and civilian disasters, led to the identification of three phases—a period of impact, a period of recoil, and a posttraumatic period of recovery. Tyhurst's stages are discussed later in this section.
- Federal funding was made available in 1961 for community-based mental health programs such as suicide prevention and crisis services, including crisis telephone counseling services, known popularly as hot lines.

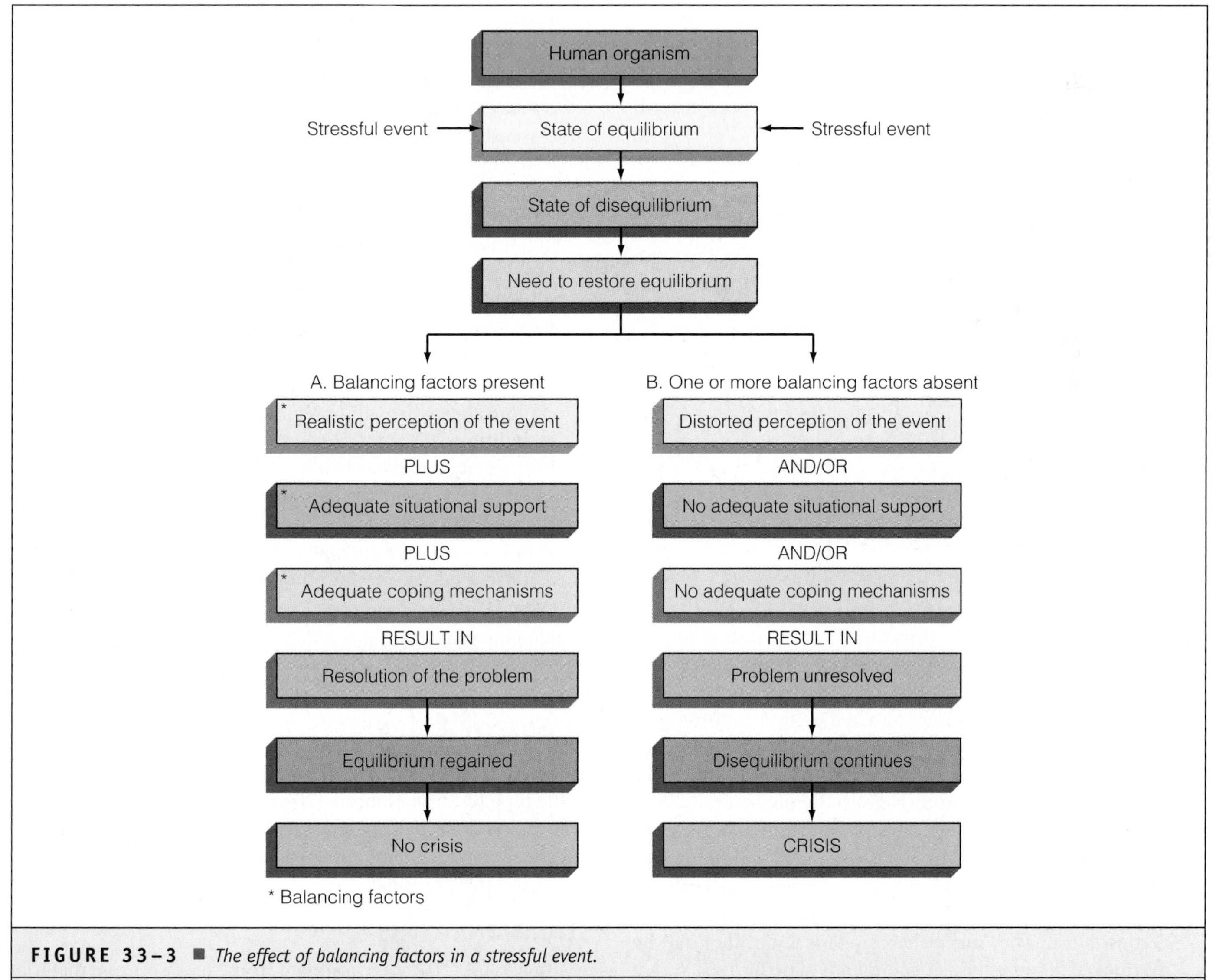

FIGURE 33–3 ■ *The effect of balancing factors in a stressful event.*

Source: Aguilera, D. C. *Crisis intervention: Theory and methodology,* 8th ed. St. Louis: C. V. Mosby. Copyright 1998, with permission from Elsevier Science.

- Caplan's (1964) work in preventive psychiatry and anticipatory guidance in the early days of the Peace Corps expanded on Lindemann's earlier work. Caplan studied developmental crises and accidental crises. He determined that successfully navigating the stages of a crisis required using new coping skills.
- The publication by the American Psychiatric Association of the *Diagnostic and Statistical Manual of Mental Disorders* in 1980 provided, for the first time, a system to measure the severity of psychosocial stressors and to reflect that severity with the psychiatric diagnosis via Axis IV (see Chapter 9).
- The development of more contemporary methods of crisis intervention such as Roberts' seven-stage crisis intervention model for frontline crisis workers (Roberts, 2000).

The etiology, psychobiology, epidemiology, comorbidity, and treatment of crisis and its sequelae are complicated. Some theories that attempt to explain what happens in a crisis and how to intervene in crisis are described below.

MediaLink Case Study: Crisis Intervention Principles

CAPLAN'S STAGES OF A CRISIS REACTION

Caplan (1964) studied various developmental crisis reactions to premature births, infancy, childhood, and adolescence, as well as accidental crises such as illness and death. According to Caplan, the four stages of a crisis reaction are:

1. *Phase 1:* An initial increase in tension that comes from the emotionally hazardous crisis-precipitating event.
2. *Phase 2:* When the individual is unable to resolve the crisis quickly, tension and disruption of daily living increase.
3. *Phase 3:* If the individual attempts but fails to resolve the crisis by usual problem-solving techniques, tension increases to such a level that the individual may become depressed
4. *Phase 4:* At the final stage, the person may partly resolve the crisis by using new coping skills. Mental disruption or disorder may occur if the person does not develop new coping skills to manage the crisis.

TYHURST'S STAGES OF DISASTER

Tyhurst (1957) identified three overlapping stages in response to a disaster.

1. The first stage, *impact,* is stimulated by the catastrophe. The victims recognize what is happening to them and are concerned mainly with the present. During this acute phase, the victim's major concern may be staying alive. According to Tyhurst, about 75% of the victims experience shock and confusion. Although they appear dazed, they also exhibit the physical signs of fear. Another group of people, up to 25%, remain coherent. They logically and rationally assess the situation and develop and implement a plan for dealing with the immediate problems brought on by the catastrophe. A third group, also up to 25%, may panic or become immobilized with fear. They may behave hysterically, or they may be overlooked because they sit and silently stare into space.
2. In *recoil,* the second stage, the initial stress of the disaster has passed, and victims may no longer find their lives in immediate danger, although injuries and other discomforts come to their awareness. Emergency shelter, food, and clothing become available. Their behavior is usually dependent—they want to be taken care of. Weeping is common as survivors begin to realize all that has happened to them.
3. The full impact of the losses the victims have experienced comes in the third, or *posttrauma,* period. Grief is a predominant response to the losses in their lives. Disturbed and psychotic responses may occur.

These stages are as relevant today as they were then, and helped mental health care workers understand the experiences of the victims of the World Trade Center terrorist attack—workers in the towers, visitors, survivors, rescuers and medical personnel, and those who experienced the disaster by watching it at home on their television sets.

ROBERTS' MODEL OF CRISIS INTERVENTION

Roberts' seven-stage model of crisis intervention (2000) has been used to help people in acute psychologic crisis and acute situational crisis, and persons diagnosed with acute stress disorder. The seven stages are:

1. Plan and conduct a thorough assessment (including lethality assessment, assessment of dangerousness to self or others, and assessment of immediate psychosocial needs).
2. Make interpersonal contact, establish rapport, and rapidly establish the relationship (conveying genuine regard and respect for the client, acceptance, reassurance, and a nonjudgmental attitude; refer to Chapter 28).
3. Examine the dimensions of the problem in order to define it (including the "last straw" of the precipitating event).
4. Encourage an exploration of feelings and emotions through active listening (refer to Chapter 8).
5. Explore and assess past coping attempts and generate and explore alternatives and previously untried coping methods or solutions.
6. Restore cognitive functioning through the implementation of an action plan based on cognitive mastery (refer to Chapter 30).
7. Follow up with the client and leave the door open for future contact, especially around the time of the anniversary of the event (exactly 1 month or 1 year after the victimization).

■ Figure 33–4 illustrates Roberts' seven-step model.

Types of Crises

In the contemporary view, the origin of a crisis is as important as the type of crisis. Roberts (2000) points out that if we know how the crisis began, we have a better opportunity to intervene effectively. Two general categories of crisis origins are situational and maturational.

SITUATIONAL CRISIS

A **situational crisis** can originate from three sources: material or environmental (fire or natural disaster); personal or physical (heart attack, diagnosis of fatal illness, bodily disfigurement);

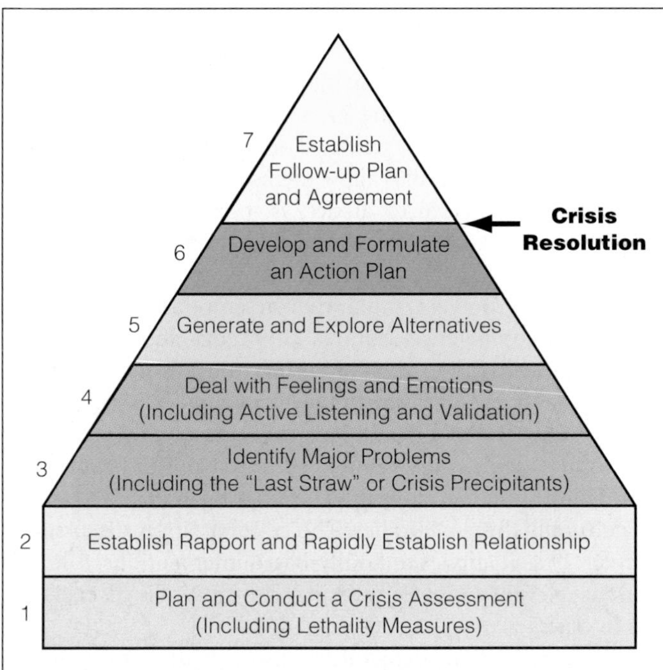

FIGURE 33–4 ■ *Roberts' seven stage model of crisis intervention.*

Source: Roberts, A. R. (Ed.). (2000). *Crisis intervention handbook: Assessment, treatment, and research* (2nd ed.). New York: Oxford University Press. Used by permission of Oxford University Press, Inc.

and interpersonal or social (death of a loved one or divorce). Often, these life-threatening events motivated people to take significant action in their close relationships that altered their life course (Cohan & Cole, 2002).

Because the event leading to the situational crisis is usually unanticipated, one generally cannot do anything directly to prevent it. In a more indirect sense, an individual can attempt to keep healthy and focus on the most effective methods of interacting with others. However, the complexity of the experience influences the ability of the individual to resolve the trauma. For instance, a person coping with one traumatic incident is more likely to resolve the experience than someone faced with multiple traumas or factors (Maes, Mylle, Delmeire, & Janca, 2001). An example of a situational crisis (in which the origin of the crisis is the husband's diagnosis of terminal cancer) follows.

CLINICAL EXAMPLE

Sally, age 52, is a social worker at a local mental health clinic, who is feeling increasingly less able to function since she learned that her husband has a terminal form of cancer that is inoperable. Many arrangements need to be made, including finding adequate medical treatment and doing appropriate evaluations of her husband. Sally has been unable to work for 2 to 3 days and now tells a psychiatric–mental health nurse that she can no longer function—she has been unable to make any of the required phone calls, despite knowing she is the person who must coordinate everything. Sally speaks of feeling overwhelmed, shakes her head, and says, "Can you believe it? I do this all the time for others, but I can't do it now. Isn't that a joke?"

MATURATIONAL CRISIS

A **maturational crisis** involves life cycle changes or normal transitions of human development. These are the traditional stages of human development that include infancy, childhood, puberty, adolescence, adulthood, middle age, and old age. During each stage, the individual is subject to unique stressors. Each stage of development is characterized by developmental tasks the individual must accomplish in order to progress to the next level. A failure at any one level compromises the next stage of development.

Maturational crises also include such changes as marriage, retirement, and the transition from student to worker. Crises associated with these states arise when the individual enters a new area of development or functioning and cannot adapt to functioning at that level. If the person experiences additional trauma or change, the risk for experiencing a crisis increases. Whenever people experience more than two life changes or traumatic events, their coping capacity may be strained, and the potential for crisis becomes greater.

An example of a maturational crisis (wherein the origin of the crisis is a decision to divorce complicated by multiple stressors) follows.

CLINICAL EXAMPLE

Bernie is a 62-year-old man who has had several hospitalizations for paranoid schizophrenia over the past 40 years. Bernie's wife Alice moved out of their apartment and told Bernie that she has decided to seek a divorce. After Alice moved out, the apartment caught fire and burned. Bernie moved to a boarding house and has become depressed and stopped taking his medication. He began to have auditory hallucinations. Bernie has come to the crisis center accompanied by the police, who found him crying, sobbing, and mumbling incoherently.

NURSING PROCESS

Clients in Crisis

Crisis intervention as a therapeutic strategy is strongly humanistic. People are viewed as capable of personal growth and as having the ability to influence and control their own lives. According to these concepts, the task of the person who intervenes in the crisis is to help the individual understand what combination of events led to the crisis, and guide the individual, prior to a maladaptive response, toward a resolution that will meet the person's unique needs and foster future growth and strength. Especially during the acute phase, the goal of crisis intervention is to restore the person to the pretrauma level of functioning as quickly as possible.

In addition to the interventions discussed in this section, other strategies that are employed with clients in crisis can be found in other chapters. They are cognitive therapy interventions (Chapter 30), pharmacologic interventions (Chapter 31), and stress management techniques (Chapter 32).

MediaLink Care Plan: Client in Crisis

Assessment

Assessment takes place on three levels: individual, family, and sociocultural.

INDIVIDUAL ASSESSMENT

Assessment of the individual is the first phase of crisis intervention. The nurse or helper must focus on assessing the following elements that relate to the person and the problem. Collect data about:

- The client's coping style.
- The precipitating event.
- The situational supports.
- The client's perception of the crisis.
- Any guilt a disaster survivor may feel about having survived or about the client's own behavior that helped the client survive.
- The client's ability to handle the problem.

Assessment is an essential and critical step of crisis intervention and the basis for later decisions about how and when to intervene, and whom to call (the first step of Roberts' model).

Also assess and evaluate the client's suicide potential. (See Chapter 22 for lethality assessment.) During this time, a client may need to be hospitalized to ensure safety, and a referral to a therapist or emergency room of the local hospital may be necessary. Part of the overall assessment is to determine what is necessary to return this client to a state of equilibrium; this may be different from what is necessary to solve the problem.

MediaLink Disaster Responder Training

FAMILY ASSESSMENT

Meet with as many family members as possible to assess family resources, coping skills, and interpersonal styles. Crises often accompany role changes in families or increased stresses in families that do not have the resources to meet the challenge.

Some common family crises are the death of a family member, the terminal illness of a family member, single parenting, divorce, drug/alcohol dependence, family violence, infidelity, remarriage, mental illness, incest, and "empty nest syndrome."

SOCIOCULTURAL ASSESSMENT

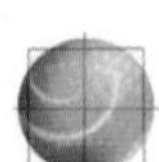

A critically important source of the meaning of an individual's response to stress or trauma is the broader sociocultural context in which the person lives. A client's culture influences the sources of distress a client experiences, as well as the client's symptomatology, interpretation of symptoms, and methods of coping. How one is raised influences how one experiences distress, whether or not one seeks help, and whether or not individuals allow themselves to be disabled. For example, in some cultures, anxiety is considered a problem of individual strength or moral code, as opposed to a mental health problem. In some cultures it may be more appropriate to have a physical problem, rather than an emotional problem.

Cultural competence requires knowledge about other cultures and sensitivity to the culture of your clients in order to select the interventions that will likely be most helpful (see also Chapter 6). Cultural sensitivity involves much more than simply identifying a family's ethnic origins or health practices. Think about developing a culturagram as an aid to assessing culturally diverse families. The culturagram is discussed in Chapter 29 as it applies to family-based interventions. It is just as relevant a tool for working with culturally diverse families in crisis.

To be effective in sociocultural assessment, you must also become aware of the influences and beliefs from your own experiences. If you are not familiar with a client's culture, ask respectful questions to help the client to fully express his or her distress. For example, "I want to understand how all of this might affect you. Can you tell me more about how you feel about this situation? Tell me how your neighbors (your friends/your family) might feel about it."

DISASTER ASSESSMENT

Nurses as citizens are often at the scene of natural disasters or may be called on to help. Nurses can be particularly helpful during the initial stage of a disaster because, in addition to having the ability to provide care to the injured, they have the skills needed to perform physical assessments and assess psychologic distress. The Red Cross trains health care professionals as responders in disasters. Accessing the Web site (www.redcross.org/services/nursing), which can found on a direct link on the Companion Website for this book, will provide information on the different training programs available.

Nursing Diagnosis: NANDA

People in crisis may have a variety of problems and symptoms. They may appear overwhelmed, calm, or agitated. They may speak clearly or they may ramble. Some appear rational, others psychotic. An individual's personal response as well as his or her perception of the event will guide you toward determining the nursing diagnoses. The most common nursing diagnoses for people in crisis are:

- Ineffective Coping.
- Interrupted Family Processes.
- Risk for Self-Directed Violence.
- Anxiety.
- Acute Confusion.
- Spiritual Distress.

- Sleep Deprivation.
- Risk for Post-Trauma Syndrome.
- Dysfunctional Grieving.
- Impaired Social Interaction.

Outcome Identification: NOC

Outcome criteria for clients in crisis should be determined in collaboration with the client to avoid irrelevant goals and unworkable solutions. Consider the following as possible outcome criteria for a client in crisis:

- The client will be able to identify effective, as well as ineffective, coping patterns.
- The client will be able to employ effective coping strategies.
- The client will ask for help when necessary.
- The client will use available social support.
- The client will report an increase in psychological comfort and a decrease in negative feelings.

Planning and Implementation: NIC

Effective planning for crisis intervention must be:

- Based on careful assessment.
- Developed in active collaboration with the person in crisis and the significant people in that person's life.
- Focused on immediate, concrete, contributing problems.
- Based on an understanding of human dependence needs.
- Appropriate to the person's level of thinking, feeling, and behaving.
- Consistent with the person's lifestyle and culture.
- Time limited, concrete, and realistic.
- Mutually negotiated and renegotiated.
- Organized to provide for follow-up.

Many of these principles form the basis for the therapeutic communication strategies in the Rx Communication feature below.

Effective intervention is based on the ability to implement the second step of Roberts' model—make interpersonal contact, establish rapport, and rapidly establish the relationship (conveying genuine regard and respect for the client, acceptance, reassurance, and a nonjudgmental attitude). One-to-one interventions to make interpersonal contact, establish rapport, and establish the relationship are important to an individual in crisis. However, nurses who work with people in crisis often need to use many nontraditional interventions, which can be as important as any verbal interventions. Working successfully with people in crisis is based on having a flexible, open view of what may be therapeutic with different individuals. You must have a full repertoire of skills and interventions that can be individualized to help all types of clients in crisis including the ability to assist with spiritual needs. The Caring for the Spirit feature on page 792 offers suggestions that integrate body, mind, and spirit.

Several different types of crisis intervention that can be used are discussed below. Burgess and Roberts (2000) have identified modalities that have been found to be most useful with persons with a diagnosed mental disorder who is also in crisis. These modalities are discussed in ■ Figure 33–5 on page 793.

CRISIS COUNSELING

Crisis counseling is a type of brief, solution-focused therapy. Unlike therapies that focus on bringing about major personality changes, crisis counseling focuses on solving immediate problems. It lasts five or six sessions and involves individuals, groups, or families. The following techniques are used:

- Listening actively and with concern. (See Box 33–3 on page 794 for communication strategies specific to working with a person in crisis.)
- Exploring the dimension of the problem, including the "last straw," in order to define it (Roberts' third step).
- Encouraging the open expression of feelings (Roberts' fourth step).
- Helping the client gradually accept reality.
- Assessing past coping attempts and helping the client explore new ways of coping with problems (Roberts' fifth step).
- Linking the client to a social network.

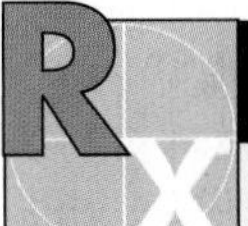

COMMUNICATION

Client in Crisis

Client: How will I ever be able to get my son back from the foster home that child services put him in? I can never seem to be able to do anything right with him.

NURSE RESPONSE 1: Jim, if you could rank yourself as a Dad on a scale of 1 to 10, with 10 meaning always doing everything "right" and 1 meaning never doing anything "right," where would you rank yourself?

RATIONALE: Using a scaling question will open the door to discussing with Jim the skills and competencies that are within Jim's control and that need to be worked on.

NURSE RESPONSE 2: Let's talk about what you have been doing with Jimmy that is "right."

RATIONALE: This intervention has two goals: Attempting to elicit a behavioral description of the interaction between father and son and helping the client identify his parenting strengths.

CARING FOR THE SPIRIT

Helping Clients to Recuperate from Crisis

It is important for people who have experienced a crisis or trauma to stay grounded. Suggest the following exercises to someone who is feeling confused, upset, in disbelief, or hopeless.

1. Sit on a chair, feel your feet on the ground, press on your thighs, feel your behind on the seat, and your back supported by the chair; look around you and pick six objects that have red or blue in them. This should allow you to feel in the present, more grounded, and in your body. Notice how your breath gets deeper and calmer. You may want to go outdoors and find a peaceful place to sit on the grass. As you do, feel how your body is held and supported by the ground.
2. Gently pat the different parts of your body with your hand, with a loose wrist. Your body may feel more tingling, more alive, sharp, and you may feel more connected to your feelings.
3. Tense your muscles, each group at a time. Hold your shoulders with your arms across your chest, tighten your grip, and pat your arms up and down. Do the same with your legs, tighten them and hold them from the outside, patting through their length. Tighten your back, tighten your front, then gently release the tension. This may help you to feel more balanced.
4. If you believe in prayer or in a greater power, pray for the rest of the souls of the dead, for the healing of the wounded, and for the consolation of the grieving. Pray for peace, understanding, wisdom, and for the forces of good to prevail. Do not give up faith in the ultimate goodness of being and keep your trust in humanity.

Take comfort in knowing that we humans are extremely resilient and have been able to recuperate from the most horrendous tragedies.

Source: Adapted from USDHHS Substance Abuse and Mental Health Services Administration. (2002). *After a disaster: Self-care tips for dealing with stress*. Retrieved August 9, 2002, from the World Wide Web, www.mentalhealth.org.

- Engaging in decision counseling or problem solving with the client, thus restoring cognitive mastery (Roberts' sixth step).
- Reinforcing newly learned coping devices.
- Following up the case after resolution of the crisis and leaving the door open for future contact, especially around the time of the anniversary of the event (Roberts' seventh step).

Box 33–4 on page 794 summarizes the ABCs of crisis counseling.

TELEPHONE COUNSELING

MediaLink NAMI

Suicide prevention and crisis intervention centers rely heavily on telephone counseling by volunteers who have professional consultation available to them. Also known as hot lines and often available around the clock, they allow callers to remain anonymous and test what it feels like to ask for assistance. No appointment, travel time, or money is necessary, and help is immediately available. The volunteers usually work within a protocol that indicates what information they need from the client to assess the crisis. Their goal is to plan steps to provide immediate relief and then long-term follow-up if necessary.

The calls made to a hot line usually fall into one of four categories: crisis calls, ventilation calls, combinations of ventilation and information calls, or information-only calls. Calls that request information and ventilation are handled by supportive listening and the giving of information. Crisis calls need special techniques. Workers in crisis intervention centers generally follow a step-by-step agency protocol.

ASSISTING WITH ENVIRONMENTAL CHANGES

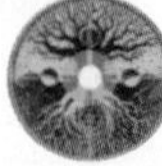

Working with an individual or a family in crisis may require taking steps to provide shelter. It may be necessary to find shelter for a homeless person, to obtain shelter in a safe house for an abused woman and her children, or to arrange for in-home health care.

ANTICIPATORY GUIDANCE

Anticipatory guidance is providing assistance in anticipation of the potential for crisis, thus averting it. These are some examples of anticipatory guidance: discussing methods of contraception with adolescents or young adults, preparing a child and the family for a tonsillectomy, arranging for a volunteer from the Reach for Recovery Program to visit a woman who has had a mastectomy, preparing a list of helpful phone numbers for the newly discharged schizophrenic client.

HELPING DEVELOP SOCIAL SUPPORTS

Immediate social support is crucial for clients in crisis because it may counteract or negate long-term adverse effects (Davidhizar & Shearer, 2002). Many people in crisis have limited social supports and are not always sure about how to access supports or develop them. You can help a client develop social supports by: introducing a woman whose husband is an alcoholic to Al-Anon groups in her community, referring a family with a terminally ill member to a local hospice, giving a rape victim the telephone number of the rape crisis hot line, informing the newly discharged client with bipolar disorder and his family of the National Alliance for the Mentally Ill (NAMI) local group or national Web site (www.nami.org).

CRITICAL INCIDENT STRESS DEBRIEFING (CISD)

A specific model of group crisis intervention, built on (1) the historical tenets of one-to-one crisis intervention and (2) the interactive group psychotherapy of Yalom (featured in Chapter 29), has been formulated by Mitchell and Everly (1996). Known as Critical Incident Stress Debriefing (CISD), this

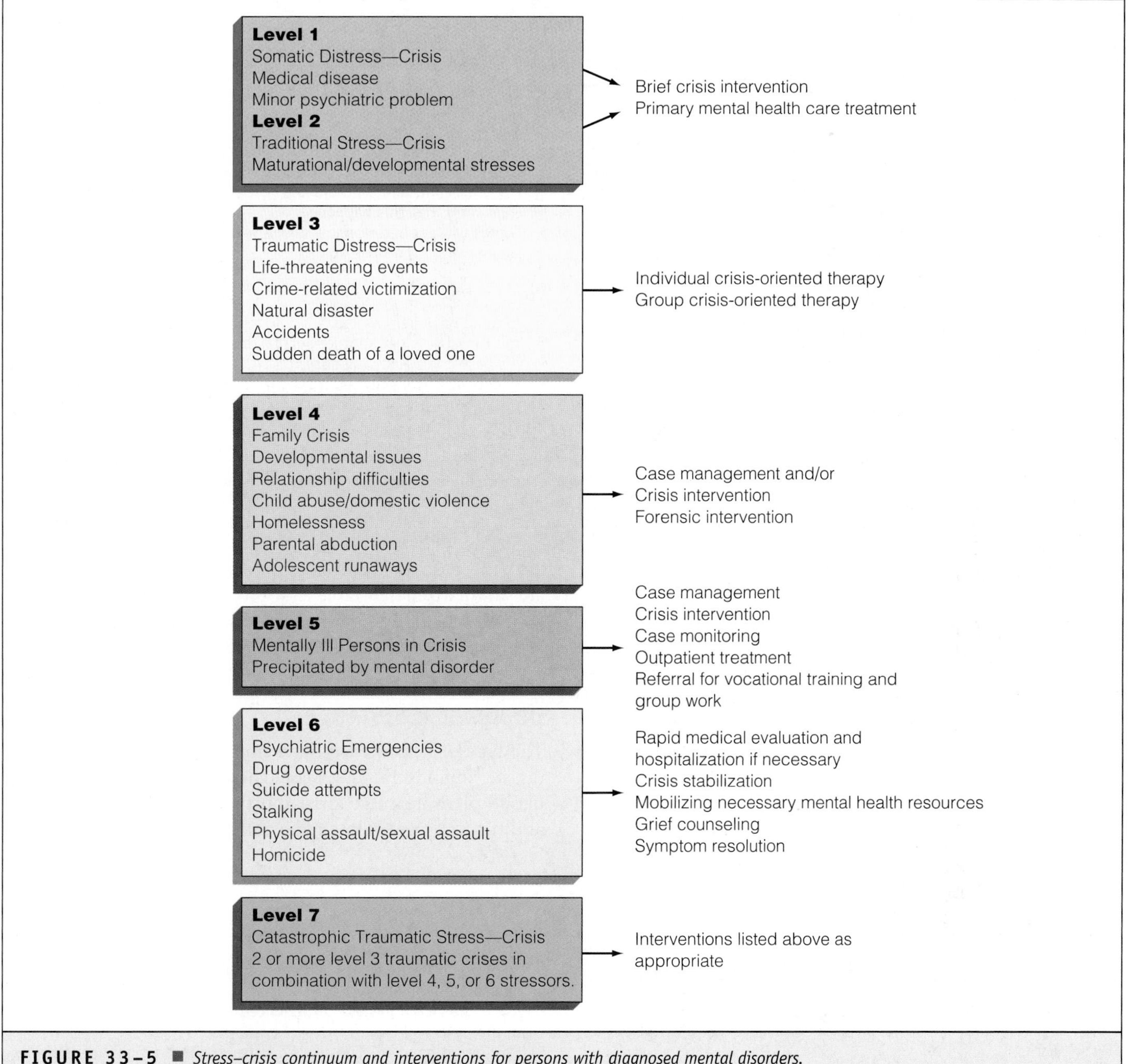

FIGURE 33–5 ■ *Stress–crisis continuum and interventions for persons with diagnosed mental disorders.*

Source: Based on data from Burgess, A. W., & Roberts, A. R. (2000). Crisis intervention for persons diagnosed with clinical disorders based on the stress–crisis continuum. In A. R. Roberts (Ed.), *Crisis intervention handbook: Assessment, treatment, and research* (2nd ed.) (pp. 56–76). New York: Oxford University Press. Used by permission of Oxford University Press, Inc.

seven-phase group meeting has both psychologic and psychoeducation elements, but should not be considered psychotherapy (Everly, Lating, & Mitchell, 2000). The debriefing process offers an opportunity for individuals affected by a traumatic event to share their thoughts and feelings in a safe and controlled environment. It has been used effectively in many different settings; to debrief staff on an inpatient unit after a suicide, to debrief inmates after a murder in a jail (Stoll & Edwards, 2001), to debrief crisis line volunteers (Kinzel & Nanson, 2000), to debrief school children and school personnel after a multiple shooting in a school, as well as to debrief rescue and health care workers after the World Trade Center attack (Hammond & Brooks, 2001). The Intervention Box on page 795 reviews the formal stages of CISD.

CISD is an important component of effective group crisis intervention. A multifaceted approach to group crisis intervention that includes CISD principles is Critical Incident Stress Management, discussed next.

CRITICAL INCIDENT STRESS MANAGEMENT

Critical incident stress management (CISM) is a comprehensive, integrative, and multifaceted approach to crisis intervention

BOX 33–3 Communication Strategies in Crisis Work

- Using silence—gives the person time to reflect and become more aware of feelings. Silence can prompt elaboration. Simply being with the person is supportive.
- Using nonverbal communication—maintaining eye contact, head nodding, caring facial expressions, and occasional "uh-huhs" lets the person know that you are in tune
- Paraphrasing—understanding, empathy, and interest are conveyed by repeating portions of what the person said. Paraphrasing also checks for accuracy, clarifies misunderstandings, and lets people know they have been heard. You could say, "So, you are saying that . . .", or "I have heard you say that . . ."
- Reflecting feelings—helps the person identify and articulate emotions. You could say, "You sound angry, scared, etc., does that fit for you?"
- Allowing the expression of emotions—is an important part of healing. Venting often helps the person work through feelings in order to better engage in constructive problem solving.

Some Do's and Don't's

Do Say:

- These are normal reactions to an abnormal situation.
- It is understandable that you feel this way.
- It wasn't your fault; you did the best you could.
- I am sorry that this happened.
- Things will get better, and you will feel better, although they may never be the same again.

Don't Say:

- It could have been worse.
- You can always get another pet/car/house or have another child.
- It's best if you just stay busy.
- I know just how you feel.
- You need to get on with your life.

Source: Adapted from USDHHS Substance Abuse and Mental Health Services Administration. *Disaster counseling*. Retrieved August 9, 2002, from the World Wide Web, www.mentalhealth.org.

based on the notion that no single intervention alone is effective in crisis work. CISM consists of multiple components that span the time sequence of a crisis, and can be applied to individuals, families, small groups, large groups, communities, and organizations. Note that CISM is often used with health care staff who have been assaulted (Flannery, 2001), emergency personnel (D'Andrea & Waters, 2000), in occupational health settings (Lim, Childs, & Gonsalves, 2000), and in incidents involving terrorism, violence, disasters, and other crises (Everly, 2000).

According to Everly and Mitchell (1999), who founded the International Critical Incident Stress Foundation (www.icisf.org), there are seven core components or stages of CISM, which are summarized in ■ Table 33–1 on page 796. As you familiarize yourself with these core components, note that they encompass all of the interventions discussed previously in this section.

MediaLink Critical Incident Stress Foundation

DISASTER ASSISTANCE

The type of help needed by victims of disaster changes as the disaster unfolds. Initially, people need information about evacuation plans, rescue efforts, and the location of food, shelter, and medical care. The media can provide this information,

BOX 33–4 ABCs of Crisis Counseling

Achieve Contact (Safety and Security)

- Introduce yourself, name, role, and purpose.
- Assure or provide for the physical and emotional safety of the victim.
- Ask the victim how he or she would like to be addressed.
- As appropriate, collect information regarding residency and health conditions for contacting family members, any support systems, or friends.
- Assess if the victim takes or needs medication.
- Identify the victim's feelings, reactions, and perceptions of the event.

Boil Down the Problem (Ventilate and Validate)

- Ask the victim to briefly describe what has just happened.
- Encourage the victim to talk about the present.
- Ask what is the most pressing problem (one at a time).
- Review and clarify what you heard as the primary and most immediate problem.
- Ask if the victim has ever experienced a similar situation or crisis in the past.
- How was it handled? Consider how the victim can regain control.

Cope with the Problem (Predict and Prepare)

- What does the victim want to happen? (Give additional options that may be more realistic.)
- What is the most important need?
- Explore what the victim feels is the best solution.
- Help the victim formulate a plan of action with resources, activities, and a timeline for accomplishing the plan.
- Reaffirm the future and talk in hopeful terms of a "new normal" or a "new reality."
- Arrange for follow-up contact or visit with the victim.
- Connect the victim to resources that offer longer-term support.

Source: ABCD tip card was developed by the Association of Traumatic Stress Specialists, *"Recognizing Standards of Excellence in Response, Treatment & Service"*, PO Box 2747 • Georgetown TX USA • 78627 • 512-868-3677 • 512-868-3678 fax • admin@atss-hq.com • www.atss-hq.com © 2002 ATSS • The ABCD Model of Crisis Intervention was created by Romaine Edwards and Warren Jones; revisions by David Lowenberg, Paul Forgach, Carol Hacker, PhD, Jayne Crisp, CTS, CVAS, Paul Hamilton, MDiv.

INTERVENTION

Phases of Critical Incident Stress Debriefing (CISD)

Introduction Phase (Sets the Tone for the Subsequent Phases)

- Explain the purpose of the meeting.
- Explain and give an overview of the process.
- Motivate the participants.
- Assure confidentiality.
- Explain the guidelines.
- Identify the team members.
- Answer questions or concerns.

Fact Phase (Imparting Power to the Participants Through Giving Information)

- Assist in discussing the facts of the incident.
- Ask participants to tell who they are.
- Ask participants to tell how they were involved in the incident.
- Ask participants to tell what happened from their perspective.

Thought Phase (Transition Between Impersonal Outside Facts and That Which Is Internal, Close, and Personal)

- Ask each participant to discuss his or her first thoughts or most prominent thoughts about the traumatic event.
- Expect to hear emotional comments.

Reaction Phase (Cathartic Ventilation with a Potential for Emotional Abreaction)

- Most of the discussing is done by the participants.
- Discussion is freewheeling.
- Ask participants what the worst thing was about the situation, what they would choose to erase, and what aspect of the situation causes the most pain.

Symptom Phase (Consensual Normalization and Attacking the Myth of Unique Weakness or Vulnerability)

- Move the group toward more cognitively oriented material.
- Ask participants to describe any cognitive, physical, emotional, or behavioral experiences they encountered at the scene of the incident.
- Ask about any symptoms that followed subsequently.

Teaching Phase (Moving Further Away from Emotional Content of the Reaction Phase)

- Acknowledge symptoms described in the symptom phase.
- Reaffirm that symptoms are normal, typical, or predictable after what they've been through.
- Forewarn the group about possible symptoms they might experience in the future.
- Involve participants in stress management activities (see Chapter 32).

Reentry Phase (Identification of Homogenizing Themes That May Be Used to Facilitate Closure and Provide a Psychological Uplift)

Participant Roles

- Introduce any new material they wish to discuss.
- Review old material already discussed.
- Ask any questions.
- Discuss whatever would help them to bring closure to the debriefing.

Debriefing Team Roles

- Answer any questions.
- Inform and reassure.
- Provide appropriate handouts and other written material.
- Provide referral sources for assessment, therapy, and so on.
- Summarize the debriefing experience with words of respect, encouragement, appreciation, support, and direction.

Source: Based on data from Everly, G. S., Jr., Lating, J. M., & Mitchell, J. T. (2000). Innovations in group crisis intervention. In A. R. Roberts (Ed.), *Crisis intervention handbook: Assessment, treatment, and research* (pp. 83–86). New York: Oxford University Press.

especially when there is time to plan and anticipate need (as with floods or hurricanes).

After acute needs are met at the disaster scene, in makeshift hospitals, or in emergency rooms, morgues, and shelters, more far-reaching interventions are necessary. People need housing, jobs, and help in reconstructing their emotional lives. Two federal agencies assist with meeting the needs of both survivors and responders. The Federal Emergency Management Agency (FEMA) has a crisis counseling assistance and training program that provides mental health services to all individuals affected by a disaster (www.fema.gov). The Substance Abuse and Mental Health Services Administration (SAMHSA) of the Department of Health and Human Services also meets the mental health needs of survivors and responders (www.mentalhealth.org). Such data can be accessed on the Companion Website for this book.

These are the psychologic needs of victims both during and after a disaster:

- Talking about the experience and expressing their feelings of fear, panic, loss, and grief.
- Becoming fully aware and accepting of what has happened to them.
- Resuming concrete activities and reconstructing their lives with the social, physical, and emotional resources available.

To guide victims and their families through the crisis, crisis workers should:

- Listen with concern and sympathy, and ease the way for them to tell their tragic story, weep, express feelings of anger, loss, frustration, and despair.
- Help them accept in small doses the tragic reality of what has happened. This means staying with them during the initial stages of shock and denial. It also may mean accompanying them back to the scene of the tragedy and being available for support when they are faced with the full impact of their loss.

MediaLink Crisis Training Resources

TABLE 33–1 Critical Incident Stress Management (CISM): The Seven Core Components

Intervention	Timing	Activation	Goals	Format
1. Precrisis preparation	Precrisis phase	Anticipation of crisis	Set expectations; improve coping	Groups; organizations
2. Individual crisis intervention	Anytime, anywhere	Symptom driven	Symptom mitigation; return to function, if possible; referral if needed; stress management	Individuals; large groups
Large groups:				
3a. Demobilizations and staff consultation (rescuers) 3b. Group briefing for schools, businesses, and large civilian groups	Shift disengagement or anytime postcrisis	Event driven	To inform and consult; to allow for psychological decompression; stress management	Large groups; organizations
4. Critical incident stress debriefing (CISD)	Postcrisis (1–10 days); at 3–4 weeks for mass disasters	Usually symptom driven; can be event driven	Facilitate psychological closure; symptom mitigation; triage	Small groups
5. Defusing	Postcrisis (within 12 hours)	Usually symptom driven	Symptom mitigation; possible closure; triage	Small groups
Systems:				
6a. Family CISM; 6b. Organizational consultation	Anytime	Either symptom driven or event driven	Foster support; communications; symptom mitigation; closure, if possible; referral, if needed	Families; organizations
7. Follow-up; referral	Anytime	Usually symptom driven	Assess mental status; access higher level of care	Individual; family

Source: Everly, G., & Mitchell, J. (1999). *Critical incident stress management (CISM): A new era and standard of care in crisis intervention* (2nd ed.). Ellicott City, MD: Chevron Publishing. Used with permission.

- Help them make contact with relatives, friends, and other resources required for beginning the process of social and physical reconstruction. This could mean making telephone calls to locate relatives, accompanying someone to apply for financial aid, or giving information about social and mental health care agencies for follow-up services.

People who are panicked should receive prompt attention to minimize the potential for contagious panic that sometimes occurs in large groups. One strategy to help a panic-stricken person is to give the person a small, structured task that focuses energies constructively. Remember, however, that assigning tasks beyond the person's capabilities will add to the person's anxiety and feeling of helplessness. When in a disaster situation, remember to also incorporate concepts and intervention strategies related to death and loss.

The effects of a disaster are felt long after the disaster is over. Provide anticipatory guidance that includes self-care tips to victims and their families so that they can mange their post-disaster experiences. Self-care tips are in the Client/Family Teaching feature on page 797.

Evaluation

Nurses in acute care or short-term settings may not see the long-term effects of their interventions. Typically, nurses in these settings need to evaluate the crisis, set up the plan, and begin implementing it.

In long-term settings, you can evaluate the client or family response to the intervention by determining whether clients have resumed their precrisis level of functioning, or show evidence of increased functioning (growth). A nurse in either a long-term or short-term setting may also have an opportunity to evaluate whether a similar problem might lead to another crisis for the client.

It is difficult to evaluate the effectiveness of disaster intervention because of the large numbers of people involved and the disruptive nature of a disaster. Evaluation can take place at many different levels. Nurses can evaluate their work with individual clients; mental health care agencies can monitor statistics on groups of clients; government agencies can assess the numbers of unemployed and homeless; public health departments can measure the extent of disease and disability.

CLIENT / FAMILY **TEACHING**

Self-Care Tips After a Disaster

Things to Remember When Trying to Understand Disaster Events

- No one who sees a disaster is untouched by it.
- It is normal to feel anxious about your and your family's safety.
- Profound sadness, grief, and anger are normal reactions to an abnormal event.
- Acknowledging your feelings helps you to recover.
- Focusing on your strengths and abilities will help you to heal.
- Accepting help from community programs and resources is healthy.
- Everyone has different needs and different ways of coping.
- It is common to want to strike back at people who have caused great pain. However, nothing good is accomplished by hateful language or actions.

Signs that Adults Need Stress Management Assistance

- Difficulty communicating thoughts
- Difficulty sleeping
- Difficulty maintaining balance
- Easily frustrated
- Increased use of drugs/alcohol
- Limited attention span
- Poor work performance
- Headaches/stomach problems
- Tunnel vision/muffled hearing
- Colds or flulike symptoms
- Disorientation or confusion
- Difficulty concentrating
- Reluctance to leave home
- Depression, sadness
- Feelings of hopelessness
- Mood swings
- Crying easily
- Overwhelming guilt and self-doubt
- Fear of crowds, strangers, or being alone

Ways to Ease the Stress

- Talk with someone about your feelings—anger, sorrow, and other emotions—even though it may be difficult.
- Encourage others, as well as yourself, not to tell your stories in a repetitive way—this ultimately deepens the trauma. Instead, support and hear one another, but with breaks and interruptions of the story from beginning to end.
- Don't hold yourself directly responsible for the disastrous event or be frustrated because you feel that you cannot help directly in the rescue work.
- Take steps to promote your own physical and emotional healing by staying active in your daily life patterns or by adjusting them. This healthy outlook will help you and your family (i.e., healthy eating, rest, exercise, relaxation, meditation).
- Maintain a normal household and daily routine, limiting demanding responsibilities for yourself and your family.
- Spend time with family and friends.
- Participate in memorials, rituals, and use of symbols as a way to express feelings.
- Use existing support groups of family, friends, and house of worship.
- Establish a family emergency plan—this can be very comforting.
- Seek outside professional assistance if these self-help strategies are not helping you or you find that you are using drugs/alcohol in order to cope.

Source: Adapted from USDHHS Substance Abuse and Mental Health Services Administration. (2002). *After a disaster: Self-care tips for dealing with stress.* Retrieved August 9, 2002, from the World Wide Web, www.mentalhealth.org.

In evaluating the aftereffects of a disaster, it is important to note that there may be an impact on those who are not direct victims of the disaster.

CLINICAL EXAMPLE

Matilda worked as a short-order cook in a restaurant in the World Trade Center. The morning of September 11, Matilda decided to call in sick, although she was well. Matilda's fiancé, a waiter at the same restaurant, was killed. Matilda now has vivid nightmares. She alternates between feeling sad and angry. Matilda refuses to attend church anymore, asking God, over and over, why He spared her and not the others.

Janelle frantically tried to reach her mother, who worked in Tower 2 of the World Trade Center, on her cell phone, but was not successful. After 3 hours of frantic activity, Janelle, exhausted, sat down on a curb and sobbed. When her cell phone finally rang, it was Janelle's mother calling from a tugboat that had evacuated survivors. She was dirty and scared, but okay. Despite this good news, Janelle couldn't stop crying. Months later, she still feels anxious.

A disaster can affect the mental health of various groups—a condition known as vicarious traumatization (discussed later in this chapter). The groups most commonly at increased risk are identified in the list below. Those individuals who are most affected are listed first:

1. Next-of-kin
2. Injured survivors and their close ones
3. Uninjured survivors
4. Onlookers (the helpless helpers, who are at particularly high risk)
5. Rescuers
6. Body handlers
7. Health personnel (many mass injury situations may demand difficult prioritizing)
8. People responsible for the disaster
9. Coworkers in workplace disasters
10. Evacuees

The most important aspect of evaluation is to review how the interventions were implemented and the effectiveness of the relief work. Disaster preparedness is needed to effectively intervene when the unthinkable—a disaster—occurs. Many hospitals and clinics have ongoing drills to prepare for the possibility of a disaster. It is important that you understand your role and the tasks and functions for which you are responsible.

Case Management, Community-Based Care, and Home Care

Crisis intervention often takes place in the home or the community at large through home crisis visits and mobile crisis teams.

HOME CRISIS VISITS

Home visits are made when telephone counseling does not suffice or when the crisis workers need to obtain additional information by direct observation or to reach a client who is unobtainable by telephone. Home visits are appropriate when crisis workers need to initiate contacts rather than waiting for clients to come to them—for example, when a telephone caller is assessed to be highly suicidal or when a concerned family member, neighbor, physician, or clergyman informs the agency of clients in potential crisis. Home crisis visits are also an effective intervention for persons with serious mental illnesses (Joy, Adams, & Rice, 2000), helping to keep them functioning in the community. Often, clients in crisis are too disorganized or distraught to seek help by themselves. The police may arrange for a home crisis visit to avoid imprisoning or hospitalizing a client. Problems for which home crisis visits are usually instituted are spousal abuse, child abuse, psychiatric emergencies (such as drug overdose, suicide attempt or other life-threatening self-abuse, stalking, assault, rape, and homicide), and medical emergencies.

Psychiatric emergencies are considered to be difficult to manage for the following reasons:

- There may be incomplete information about the situation.
- The client may be disruptive or only minimally helpful.
- There is a sense of urgency in order to initiate effective intervention (Burgess & Roberts, 2000).

In many agencies, the crisis team often consists of a man and a woman who are highly skilled and experienced in crisis intervention. The male–female team is generally perceived as less threatening than two men, two women, or a single person. Their goal is to defuse the situation with as little disruption and violence as possible and to engage the clients in longer-term treatment. They may also be members of mobile crisis units (discussed later in this section).

There are others who intervene in community crises as well. The public health nurse is in an excellent position to identify, assess, and intervene with clients experiencing a life crisis. Public health nurses often have access to community resources as well as informal communication lines, and they usually maintain contact with families and clients for longer periods of time than nurses in other settings. They are often recognized by the community as knowledgeable experts who are available for immediate assistance as in the following example.

CLINICAL EXAMPLE

Emily, age 78, and her sister Frances, age 84, lived in a run-down part of town. Frances became seriously ill with pneumonia and became progressively weaker. Emily became more anxious about Frances's health when her sister refused to see a doctor. Emily feared that her sister would die or need to go to a nursing home. Emily felt paralyzed and didn't know what to do. When the visiting nurse came by to visit Emily's neighbor, Emily asked the nurse to see Frances. Together, they were able to persuade Frances to get medical care so that she could stay home.

MOBILE CRISIS UNITS

Mobile crisis units (MCUs) are community-based programs that are designed to be able to deliver crisis services to any location in the community. MCUs are staffed by teams that may include psychiatrists, psychiatric–mental health nurses, substance abuse counselors, psychologists, psychiatric social workers, child welfare workers, or other trained professionals.

The specific functions of MCUs vary by community. The typical advantages that MCUs provide are:

- Intervening in crisis situations without delay.
- Providing increased community access to services.
- Assessing clients in their own community environment.
- Avoiding unnecessary hospitalizations.
- Facilitating hospitalization or detoxification when needed.
- Avoiding unnecessary arrests.
- Consultation to law enforcement.

MCUs are thought to reduce the costs of mental health treatment as well as the number of inpatient admissions to psychiatric facilities. In fact, community-based mobile crisis services resulted in 8% fewer hospitalizations than hospital-based interventions (Guo, Biegel, Johnsen, & Dyches, 2001). The use of MCUs has also decreased psychiatric symptomatology, reduced homelessness, and increased global functioning in a population of homeless severely mentally ill persons (Morris & Warnock, 2001).

Vicarious Traumatization of Crisis Workers

Disasters and traumatic experiences shake the foundations of our beliefs about how other people behave toward one another, and can shatter our assumption that the world is a safe place. Nurses and other crisis workers are routinely exposed to victim suffering and to the aftereffects of inhumane acts (see ■ Figure 33–6). They are at risk for becoming what Means (2002) calls "a wounded healer."

Vicarious traumatization, also known as secondary trauma response, is a condition in which psychological aftereffects are experienced by those who assist victims of traumatic events.

CLINICAL EXAMPLE

Brian is a police officer from Buffalo, New York, who volunteered to assist the New York City Police Department in the days immediately after the terrorist attack at the World Trade Center. He was on a team looking for people who still might be alive in the rubble. Although Brian considered himself "tough" and had a macho image among his fellow officers, he burst into tears and had to be led away from the site to meet with a mental health counselor. Brian acts tougher than ever, but still bursts into tears and has difficulty controlling his emotions.

Sheila was a mental health nurse at a hospital located only a few blocks from the World Trade Center. She was also a volunteer who assisted survivors and first responders (firefighters, police officers, paramedics) and counseled them for several weeks. Sheila became preoccupied with the stories of her clients. Her insomnia and angry outbursts at home prompted Sheila to seek counseling for herself.

You should expect that you are vulnerable to this condition if you work with clients in the highly disorganized crisis period, or with those who are victims of sexual assault (Ghahramanlou & Brodbeck, 2000), violence, or disaster. Vicarious traumatization can also affect your own physical health by inducing gastrointestinal problems (such as gastritis or peptic ulcer), hypertension, and fatigue (Badger, 2001). In the home or the workplace, you could experience:

- An increase in the number of sick days.
- Indecision or difficulty with problem solving.
- Isolation or withdrawal.
- Behavioral outbursts.

Should this happen, seek additional supports, supervision, and referral for professional assistance.

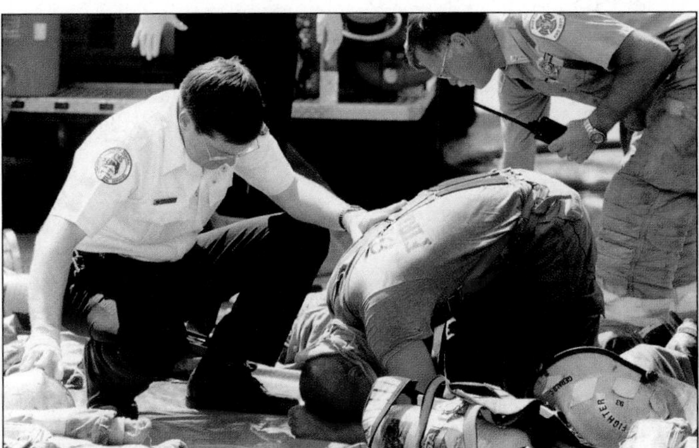

FIGURE 33–6 ■ *Exhausted nurses and other crisis workers.*

Source: T. Mack/In the Dark Photography.

Nursing Self-Awareness

It is important that you develop increased awareness of yourself and are able to handle your feelings so that you can intervene in a tense situation. It will help you to reflect upon your answers to the following questions:

- Do I believe that people who are in crisis are helpless?
- Can I contain my own anxiety when I am working with someone who is severely anxious?
- How do I feel when I'm not in control in certain situations?
- How do I react to people who are frightened? Angry? Threaten me?
- Do I have ideas that will hinder my ability to help others? For example, do I believe any of the following: Women who are raped are asking for it; men should be strong and not show emotions; children should be seen and not heard?

To remain effective in crisis work, and to continue to grow personally and professionally, you should pay attention to these important behaviors:

- Respect and believe in a person's capacity to grow and change.
- Be aware of the impact on yourself of repeatedly listening to horrible stories.
- Formulate your own outlets for stress, frustration, and anger.
- Deal with your own fears about violence and your own vulnerability to stress and conflict.
- Develop realistic expectations about what you can do for others.
- Respect each person's own unique timetable for crisis resolution.
- Collaborate with other crisis intervenors and community groups.

You will become more skilled as you incorporate each of these behaviors into your professional repertoire.

Some additional activities that you can undertake to take care of yourself and lessen the personal impact of disaster and crises has to do with self-nurturance. Focus on what you did right every day, monitor your own reactions, keep a journal in which you write your own personal thoughts and feelings, and practice the self-care tips in the Nursing Self-Awareness feature on page 800. People in crisis will expect you to help them regain control of themselves, not to control them. Being self-assured and composed will help your clients to regain control.

Nursing SELF-AWARENESS — Self-Care Tips for Emergency and Disaster Response Workers

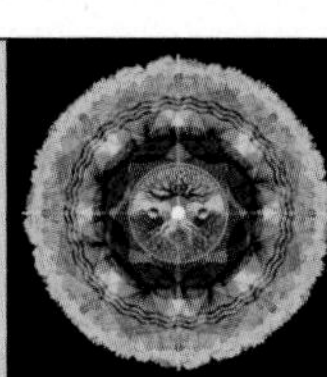

Normal Reactions to a Disaster Event

- No one who responds to a mass casualty event is untouched by it.
- Profound sadness, grief, and anger are normal reactions to an abnormal event.
- You may not want to leave the scene until the work is finished.
- You will likely try to override stress and fatigue with dedication and commitment.
- You may deny the need for rest and recovery time.

Signs That You May Need Stress Management Assistance

- Difficulty communicating thoughts
- Difficulty remembering instructions
- Difficulty maintaining balance
- Uncharacteristically argumentative
- Difficulty making decisions
- Limited attention span
- Unnecessary risk taking
- Tremors/headaches/nausea
- Tunnel vision/muffled hearing
- Colds or flulike symptoms
- Disorientation or confusion
- Difficulty concentrating
- Loss of objectivity
- Easily frustrated
- Unable to engage in problem solving
- Unable to let down when off duty
- Refusal to follow orders
- Refusal to leave the scene
- Increased use of drugs/alcohol
- Unusual clumsiness

Ways to Help Manage Your Stress

- Limit on-duty work hours to no more than 12 hours per day.
- Make work rotations from high-stress to lower-stress functions.
- Make work rotations from the scene to routine assignments as practicable.
- Use counseling assistance programs available through your agency.
- Drink plenty of water and eat healthy snacks like fresh fruit or dried fruit, nuts, trail mix, whole grain breads, and other energy foods at the scene.
- Keep yourself hydrated with water, mineral water, decaffeinated coffee or tea, juice, and electrolyte supplements.
- If you are able to, take calcium supplements, which can counteract high levels of lactic acid produced by tension, and vitamin C, which may help you to maintain alertness.
- Take frequent, brief breaks from the scene as practicable.
- Talk about your emotions to process what you have seen and done.
- Stay in touch with your family and friends.
- Participate in memorials, rituals, and use of symbols as a way to express feelings.
- Pair up with a responder so that you may monitor one another's stress.

Source: Adapted from USDHHS Substance Abuse and Mental Health Services Administration. (2002). *Self-care tips for emergency and disaster response workers*. Retrieved August 9, 2002, from the World Wide Web, www.mentalhealth.org.

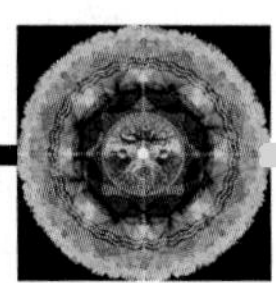

EXPLORE MediaLink

NCLEX review, case studies, and other interactive resources for this chapter can be found on the Companion Website at http://www.prenhall.com/kneisl. Click on Chapter 33 to select the activities for this chapter.

For animations, video tutorials, more NCLEX review questions, and an audio glossary, access the accompanying CD-ROM in this textbook.

BIBLIOGRAPHY

Aguilera, D. C. (1998). *Crisis intervention: Theory and methodology*. St. Louis, MO: Mosby.

Badger, J. M. (2001). Understanding secondary traumatic stress. *American Journal of Nursing, 101*(7), 26–32.

Baker, D. R. (2002). A public health approach to the needs of children affected by terrorism. *Journal of the American Medical Women's Association, 57*(2), 117–118, 121.

Burgess, A. W., & Roberts, A. R. (2000). Crisis intervention for persons diagnosed with clinical disorders based on the stress–crisis continuum. In A. R. Roberts (Ed.), *Crisis intervention handbook: Assessment, treatment, and research* (2nd ed.) (pp. 56–76). New York: Oxford University Press.

Caplan, G. (1964). *Principles of preventive psychiatry*. New York: Basic Books.

Cohan, C. L., & Cole, S. W. (2002). Life course transitions and natural disaster: Marriage, birth, and divorce following Hurricane Hugo. *Journal of Family Psychology, 16*(1), 14–25.

Cooke, A. L., & Shear, K. W. (2001). Treatment of a 50-year-old African-American woman whose chronic posttraumatic stress disorder went undiagnosed for over 20 years. *American Journal of Psychiatry, 158*(6), 866–870.

D'Andrea, L. M., & Waters, C. (2000). Predicting post-incident stress in emergency personnel: A guide for mental health professionals on critical incident stress management teams. *International Journal of Emergency Mental Health, 2*(1), 33–41.

Davidhizar, R., & Shearer, R. (2002). Helping children cope with public disasters: Support given immediately after a traumatic event can counteract or even negate long-term adverse effects. *American Journal of Nursing, 102*(3), 26–33.

Everly, G. S., Jr. (2000). Crisis management briefings (CMB): Large group crisis intervention in response to terrorism, disasters, and violence. *International Journal of Emergency Mental Health, 2*(1), 53–57.

Everly, G. S., Jr., Lating, J. M., & Mitchell, J. T. (2000). Innovations in group crisis intervention: Critical incident stress debriefing (CISD) and critical incident stress management (CISM). In: Roberts, A. R. (2000). *Crisis intervention handbook: Assessment, treatment, and research* (2nd ed.) (pp. 77–100). New York: Oxford University Press.

Everly, G. S., Jr., & Mitchell, J. T. (1999). *Critical incident stress management (CISM): A new era and standard of care in crisis intervention* (2nd ed.). Ellicott City, MD: Chevron Publishing.

Fernando, L. (2002). The World Trade Center disaster. *Canadian Journal of Psychiatry, 47*(3), 284–291.

Flannery, R. B., Jr. (2001). The assaulted staff action program (ASAP): Ten year empirical support for critical incident stress management (CISM). *International Journal of Emergency Mental Health, 3*(1), 5–10.

Ghahramanlou, M., & Brodbeck, C. (2000). Predictors of secondary trauma in sexual assault trauma counselors. *International Journal of Emergency Mental Health, 2*(4), 229–240.

Glass, T. A., & Schoch-Spana, M. (2002). Bioterrorism and the people: How to vaccinate a city against panic. *Clinics for Infectious Disorders, 34*(2), 217–223.

Guo, S., Biegel, D. E., Johnsen, J. A. & Dyches, H. (2001). Assessing the impact of community-based mobile crisis services on preventing hospitalization. *Psychiatric Services, 52*(2), 223–228.

Hammond, J., & Brooks, J. (2001). The world trade center attack. Helping the helpers: The role of critical incident stress management. *Critical Care, 5*(6), 315–317.

Herman, R., Kaplan, M. & LeMelle, S. (2002). Psychoeducational debriefings after the September 11 disaster. *Psychiatric Services, 53*(4), 479–485.

Kinzel, A., & Nanson, J. (2000). Education and debriefing: Strategies for preventing crises in crisis-line volunteers. *Crisis, 21*(3), 126–134.

Joy, C. B., Adams, C. E., & Rice, K. (2000). Crisis intervention for people with severe mental illnesses. *Cochrane Database Systems Review, 2*, CD001087.

Lim, J. J., Childs, J., & Gonsalves, K. (2000). Critical incident stress management. *AAOHN Journal, 48*(10), 487–497.

Lindemann, E. (1944). Symptomatology and management of acute grief. *American Journal of Psychiatry, 101*, 141–148.

Lipkin, M. (2002). Medical ground zero: An early experience of the World Trade Center disaster. *Annals of Internal Medicine, 136*(9), 704–707.

Maes, M., Mylle, J., Delmeire, L., & Janca, A. (2001). Pre- and post-disaster negative life events in relation to the incidence and severity of post-traumatic stress disorder. *Psychiatry Research, 105*(1–2), 1–12.

Means, J. J. (2002). Mighty prophet/wounded healer. *Journal of Pastoral Care, 56*(1), 41–49.

Mitchell, J. T., & Everly, G. S., Jr. (1996). *Critical incident stress debriefing: An operations manual.* Ellicott City, MD: Chevron Publishing.

Morris, D. W., & Warnock, J. K. (2001). Effectiveness of a mobile outreach and crisis services unit in reducing psychiatric symptoms in a population of homeless persons with severe mental illness. *Journal of the Oklahoma State Medical Association, 94*(8), 343–346.

Ormel, J., Oldehinkel, A. J., & Brilman, E. I. (2001). The interplay and etiological continuity of neuroticism, difficulties, and life events in the etiology of major and subsyndromal, first and recurrent depressive episodes in later life. *American Journal of Psychiatry, 158*(6), 885–891.

Roberts, A. R. (Ed.). (2000). *Crisis intervention handbook: Assessment, treatment, and research* (2nd ed.). New York: Oxford University Press.

Stoll, B., & Edwards, L. A. (2001). Critical incident stress management with inmates: An atypical application. *International Journal of Emergency Mental Health, 3*(4), 245–247.

Tyhurst, J.S. (1957). The role of transition states—including disasters—in mental illness. In *Symposium on preventive and social psychiatry* (pp. 1–23). Washington, DC: Walter Reed Army Institute of Research.

Vlahov, D., Galea, S., Resnick, H., Ahern, J., Boscarino, J. A., Bucuvalas, M., et al. (2002). Increased use of cigarettes, alcohol, and marijuana among Manhattan, New York, residents after the September 11th terrorist attacks. *American Journal of Epidemiology, 155*(11), 988–996.

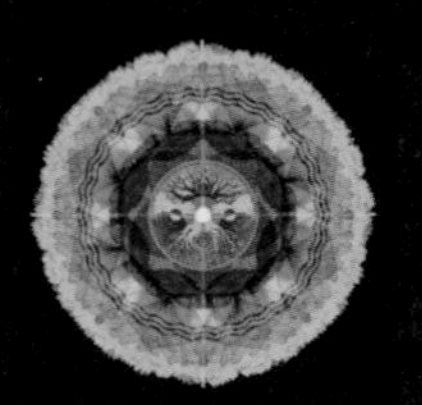

34

Chapter THIRTY-FOUR

Intervening in Violence in the Psychiatric Setting

SUE C. DELAUNE

FOCUS QUESTIONS

- **What theoretical perspectives are useful in understanding violence?**
- **Which risk factors contribute to violent behavior?**
- **How would you deescalate potentially violent behavior?**
- **What strategies for intervening with violent clients would you be willing to implement?**
- **What are some common staff responses to violence?**

KEY TERMS

critical incident stress debriefing (CISD) model
dangerousness
restraint
seclusion

MediaLink 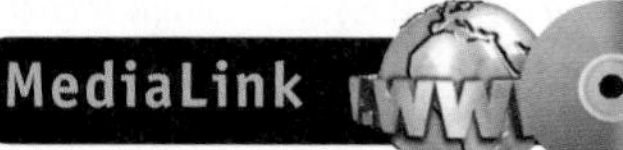 www.prenhall.com/kneisl

Additional resources for this chapter can be found on the Student CD-ROM accompanying this textbook, and on the Companion Website at www.prenhall.com/kneisl. Click on Chapter 34 to select the activities for this chapter.

CD-ROM
- Audio Glossary
- NCLEX Review

Companion Website
- Additional NCLEX Review
- Care Plan: Impulse Control Disorder
- Case Study: Pervasive Developmental Disorders

CHAPTER OUTLINE

CROSS REFERENCES

Other topics relevant to this content are: Anger and aggression in the adolescent, Chapter 26; Cognitive and behavioral techniques for anger management, Chapter 30; Critical incident stress debriefing, Chapter 33; Family violence, Chapter 23; Forensic nursing, Chapter 35; Rights of clients and the concept of the least restrictive environment, Chapter 10; Suicide as violence against the self, Chapter 22.

CRITICAL THINKING CHALLENGE

Harold, an 80-year-old retired jeweler, was admitted to the inpatient unit after striking a nurse's aide at the extended care facility where he has resided for 10 years. On admission he is mute, does not eat, wanders in and out of other clients' rooms, and is easily frustrated. He has started to strike out at the nursing staff when they attempt to assist him with routine self-care activities. The staff has requested a case conference to develop a new approach to his care.

How do you rate Harold's potential for violence? What primary need should Harold's treatment team address? Think of some specific measures staff members could implement to increase safety for Harold, other clients, and care providers. ■

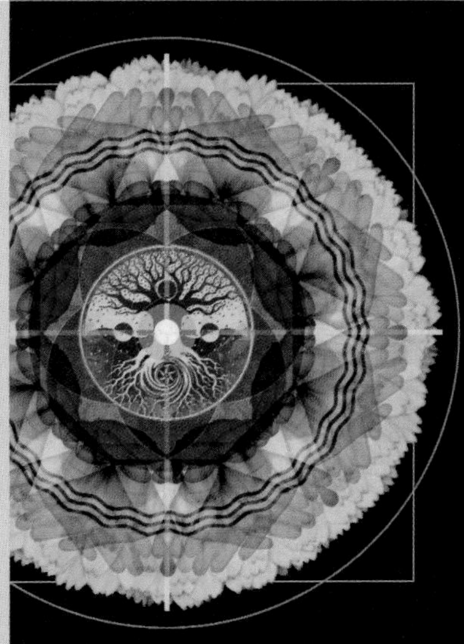

MediaLink Data on Workplace Assault

There is increasing recognition in society and in nursing that violence is a significant health problem. Violence is also an ever-increasing problem in health care environments. According to the Occupational Safety and Health Administration (OSHA) (2000), the highest number of nonfatal assaults in the work-place were on nursing staff in health care institutions. The majority of nonfatal assaults occurred in service industries, such as nursing homes, hospitals, and facilities providing residential care and other social services, such as halfway homes (OSHA, 2000). However, health care providers in every setting—psychiatric–mental health, emergency departments, surgical suites, pediatric units, long-term care facilities, and home health—are potential targets of violent behavior. Additional OSHA data can be accessed through a direct resource link on the Companion Website for this book (www.osha.gov).

Nurses are physically assaulted, threatened, and verbally abused more often than other professionals (Carlsson, Dahlberg, & Drew, 2000). In a survey by the American Nurses Association (2001), 25% of nurses were fearful of sustaining an on-the-job assault, and 17% reported that they had been physically assaulted in the past year. Psychiatric–mental health nursing staff in public sector facilities are at greater risk of occupational injury than workers who are engaged in industries that have been traditionally considered to be high risk, such as mining, heavy construction, and manufacturing (Echternacht, 1999). The epidemic of violence in the health care environment is a global problem. For example, in the United Kingdom, health care workers are at four times the normal risk of experiencing work-related violence than the general population (Beech, 2001).

MediaLink Case Study: Pervasive Developmental Disorder

Psychiatric–mental health nurses play an essential role in assessing clients for the risk of violence and initiating preventive measures (Gilmore-Hall, 2001). Factors that have contributed to the increasing violence in health care facilities include:

- Downsizing of staff.
- Change in skill level of staff members, which includes increased numbers of paraprofessionals.
- Severity of psychiatric symptoms among a small group of very aggressive clients.

These trends, and the fact that nurses are the most frequent victims of assault, magnify the need for psychiatric–mental health nurses to learn to accurately assess and intervene with clients in order to maintain safety.

This chapter provides theoretic perspectives for understanding aggressive and violent behavior. It also describes successful preventive measures such as exploring potential causative factors, recognizing warning signs of violence, nursing interventions, and client/staff education.

Biopsychosocial Theories

The ongoing debate in psychiatry of "nature vs. nurture" (what we are born with versus what we learn) extends into the study of the causes of violence. The expression of aggressive behavior is affected by a complex interaction of biologic and psychosocial factors. Therefore, there is no simple answer for the etiology of violent behavior, and no single theoretic framework can sufficiently explain or predict violence. According to the Centers for Disease Control & Prevention (CDC) (2001), the following factors may be related to violence:

- Neurobiology
- Hormones
- Neurochemistry
- Early childhood experiences
- Mental illness

There is wide diversity among individuals and the situations in which they live. It is, therefore, more valuable to consider violence from a variety of perspectives.

BIOLOGIC FACTORS

Current research is exploring the biologic basis of aggression. While it is likely that violence may be influenced by many biologic variables—genetic factors, hormonal factors, neurotransmitters, and neurophysiologic factors—the relationship between these factors and violent behaviors remains uncertain.

Physiologic changes within the brain may result in violent behavior. Trauma and other disturbances that produce anoxia (e.g., cardiorespiratory arrest) are likely culprits in the development of aggression in some individuals. For example, some people who experience brain tumors or cerebral vascular accidents (strokes) demonstrate violent behavior. Physiologic disorders such as severe hypoglycemia and other metabolic disorders, encephalitis, and dementia may also lead to violence.

In order to understand the underpinnings of violence, it is important for nurses to understand the structures of the brain and their effects on emotion and behavior; see ■ Figure 34–1 and the points listed below:

- The frontal lobe is the area in which reason and emotion interact; it regulates the ability to problem solve, plan ahead, and restrain impulses. This structure mediates both purposeful behavior and thought and affects limbic system functioning. Damage to the frontal lobe (which often occurs with head trauma) impairs judgment and can cause personality changes and aggressive outbursts (Brower & Price, 2001). These outbursts may be triggered by minor environmental stimuli.
- The amygdala, located in the lateral temporal lobe, directs emotional responses including the aggressive expression of anger.
- The hippocampus regulates the recall of recent experiences and new information. Impairment in this area interferes with learning from past experiences, as is often demonstrated by individuals with impulsive behavior.
- The hypothalamus, which serves as a relay between the cerebral cortex and the lower autonomic centers and the spinal cord somatic centers, is the route through which the mind influences bodily function.
- Temporal lobe dysfunction (occurring with seizures) may cause some people to become aggressive. It is not unusual for some individuals to become violent in the postictal phase of a seizure.

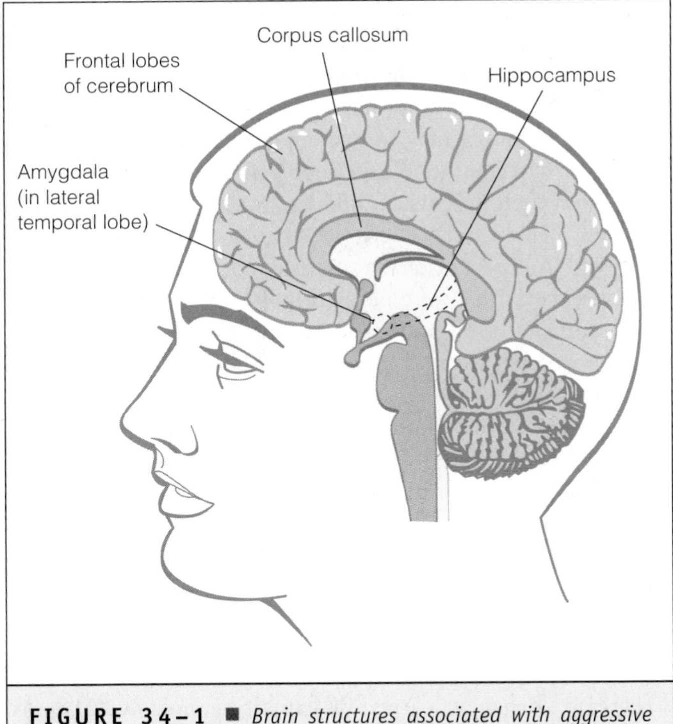

FIGURE 34–1 ■ *Brain structures associated with aggressive behavior.*

- The limbic system (neurons that form a ring around the corpus callosum) mediates primitive emotions and basic drives, such as appetite, sexual urges, and aggression. Dysfunction of the limbic system may result in an increase or decrease in aggressive behavior.

One research study analyzed data from electroencephalograms (EEGs) to identify any brain wave variances in children and adolescents who demonstrated out-of-control, explosive behaviors. The findings suggest that an innate characteristic of the central nervous system (CNS) of certain individuals may predispose them to violent behavior (Bars, Heyrend, Simpson, & Munger, 2001).

Numerous research studies substantiate that neurotransmitters, hormones, enzymes, and signaling molecules influence aggression (Lee & Coccaro, 2001; Nelson & Chiavegatto, 2001; Mitsis, Halperin, & Newcorn, 2000). In addition to reading the information in ■ Table 34–1, consider the following factors related to the physiologic basis for aggression:

- Aggressive impulsivity has been linked to abnormal functioning of the serotonin and noradrenergic systems (Oquendo & Mann, 2000).
- The link between serotonin and aggression and impulsivity is supported by the calming effect of paroxetine (Paxil), which inhibits serotonin reuptake (Cherek, Lane, Pietras, & Steinberg, 2002).

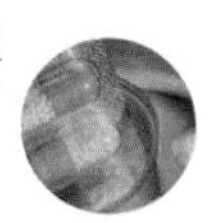

- Low gamma-aminobutyric acid (GABA) levels may correlate with some aspects of aggressiveness and may be genetically regulated. Medications such as benzodiazepines and anticonvulsants, which increase plasma GABA, improve symptoms of mood disorders and can decrease aggression (Bjork et al., 2001).

These psychopharmacologic agents are discussed later in this chapter on pages 812–813 and also in Chapter 31.

GENETIC THEORIES

No one gene or variant thereof has yet been identified as the causative factor of aggressive behavior. However, genes that encode various components of the serotonin system are being studied as risk factors in aggression (Veenstra-VanderWeele, Anderson, & Cook, 2000). A study of twins conducted by Hudziak, Rudiger, Neale, Heath, & Todd (2000) concludes that genetic factors exerted much influence on attention problems and aggression in children. Lesch & Merschdorf (2000) agree

TABLE 34–1 Role of Neurotransmitters in Aggression

Transmitter	Function	Description
Acetylcholine	Exerts excitatory effect. Facilitates transmission of nerve impulses across myoneural junction.	A deficiency (such as occurring in Alzheimer's disease) may increase aggressive behavior by lowering the threshold for confusion and impairing memory.
Dopamine	Regulation of emotional responses and movement.	Increased levels heighten sexual activity, aggressive behavior, and vigilance.
Gamma-aminobutyric acid (GABA)	Exerts inhibitory response on brain activity.	Exerts a regulatory effect on violence.
Norepinephrine	Exerts excitatory response. Is inactivated by monoamine oxidase (MAO).	May increase vigilance and aggression
Serotonin (5-HT)	Influences the processing of information. Modulates sleep, sensory responses, and mood.	Variations in 5-HT levels lead to misperception of stimuli, which may result in aggressive behavior.

Sources: Data from Kaplan, H. I., & Sadock, B. J. (2000). *Kaplan & Sadock's synopsis of psychiatry and study guide*. Philadelphia, PA: Lippincott; and Kuhn, M. (1998). *Pharmacotherapeutics: A nursing process approach* (4th ed.). Philadelphia: Davis.

BOX 34–1 Mental Disorders in Which Aggressiveness Often Occurs

- Antisocial personality disorder
- Borderline personality disorder
- Conduct disorder
- Delusional disorder
- Dementia of the Alzheimer's type
- Intermittent explosive disorder
- Schizophrenia
- Substance-related disorders

that inappropriately aggressive behavior is influenced by serotonergic gene expression. The genetic study of violence is continuing at a rapid pace and is focusing on specific molecular genetic markers for aggressiveness.

PSYCHOSOCIAL THEORIES

The psychoanalytic, psychological, and sociocultural theories that contribute to our understanding of the complex behavior of aggression are described below.

Psychoanalytic Theory

Freud (1961) theorized that aggression is one of the two innate drives, the other being the pleasure principle. This viewpoint states that it is instinctive for humans to express anger in aggressive ways. When aggression is directed inward, depression results.

MediaLink CDC Data on Violence

Psychological Theory

Aggression may be viewed as a direct result of unmet needs and wants. Whenever an individual's basic needs are unmet, the resulting threat to one's existence may cause the person to respond in an aggressive manner. The frustration that arises from unmet needs may escalate to aggressiveness.

There are some mental disorders in which aggressiveness is more likely to occur. Box 34–1 lists some of the disorders, as defined by the American Psychiatric Association (2000), in which aggressive behavior is prominent; note that the list is not inclusive.

It is also important to note that the diagnosis alone does not make the client violence prone. Rather, clients who have these disorders are likely to experience impairments in impulse control, sensory–perceptual functioning, cognitive functioning, and social skills. Individuals who have poor coping skills and feelings of helplessness and powerlessness are at high risk of exhibiting violent behavior.

Sociocultural Theory

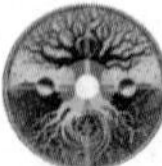

There are numerous psychosocial variables that influence the development and expression of violent behavior. Current research is examining the effects of child abuse, emotional rejection in childhood, and parenting styles as precursors to the development of violence (Barnow, Lucht, & Freyberger, 2001; Gupta, Nwosa, Nadel, & Inamdar, 2001). Dysfunctional family dynamics and negative factors in the childhood home may contribute to violence. Many violent individuals had childhood experiences of poor parenting, separation from their parents as children, or physical and/or sexual abuse and neglect (CDC, 2001). A study conducted at the University of Montreal in Canada suggested that childhood negative experiences were negated by parental supervision and maternal and paternal caregiving styles characterized by warmth (Brendgen, Vitaro, Tremblay, & Lavoie, 2001).

It is critical to be culturally sensitive when interacting with clients, especially those demonstrating the potential for violence. The expression of aggressive behavior is significantly influenced by culture. There is a real potential for gender and racial discrimination to occur unless the nurse is culturally sensitive when assessing the onset of violence.

BEHAVIORAL THEORY

Is aggressive behavior learned by witnessing violence? There is ongoing debate about the impact on children of viewing violence as portrayed in media such as television, movies, music, and video games. The American Academy of Pediatrics (2001) recognizes exposure to media violence as a significant risk to the health of children and adolescents. Their statement is based on research indicating that media violence may contribute to aggressive behavior and desensitization to violence.

According to the CDC (2001), witnessing violence has far-reaching consequences on children's development. For example, inner-city youth both witness violence and are victims of violence at very high rates. Children who witness domestic violence are at risk for developing numerous problems, such as depression, anxiety, and violence directed at peers. Such children are also more likely than children who have not been exposed to domestic violence to attempt suicide, abuse alcohol and other drugs, and commit sexual assault crimes (CDC, 2001). Additional CDC data can be accessed through a direct resource link on the Companion Website for this book (www.cdc.gov).

HUMANISTIC THEORIES

Being valued as a person and judged as worthy affects one's self-esteem, a basic need (Maslow, 1970). Valuing oneself as a significant person with something to contribute is part of self-esteem. If a person feels undervalued, unneeded, or insignificant, self-esteem becomes threatened. One response to such an existential threat may be aggressiveness. Acting out in an aggressive manner may be an individual's attempt to communicate self-importance. When individuals feel they are inadequate, they begin to feel hopeless—for themselves and the future. Those who have such a nihilistic perspective may indeed be more likely to demonstrate violence toward self and others.

NURSING PROCESS

Clients Who Are Violent

Using the nursing process as the framework for delivery of care to violent clients results in:

- Quality delivery of care.
- Continuity of care.
- Compliance with professional standards.

ASSESSMENT

Assessing psychiatric clients for their violence potential is an ongoing process and occurs across the continuum of care (in both inpatient and community-based settings). The prediction of who in a given setting poses a risk for violence, and the perception that someone is more likely to be violent, is known as **dangerousness.** An assessment that someone is dangerous determines fundamental decisions about the need for hospitalization, special supervision, emergency psychopharmacologic intervention, and community placement options (see ■ Figure 34–2 on pages 808–809). The prediction of danger is the result of an assessment and is essential for guiding treatment decisions.

An increased risk for violence among acutely disturbed clients is associated with the following variables:

- History of violence.
- Severity of psychopathology.
- Higher levels of hostility–suspiciousness, thinking disturbance, and agitation–excitement (as measured on the Brief Psychiatric Rating Scale [BPRS]).
- Length of time in the hospital.
- Early age of onset of psychiatric symptoms.
- Frequency of admission to psychiatric hospitals.

A clinical example of a client who meets almost all of these criteria follows.

CLINICAL EXAMPLE

Gaetano, a 40-year-old single man, was brought to the psychiatric emergency room by the police in response to a call from Gaetano's mother. He had been pounding on the door of his mother's home, screaming obscenities and wielding a knife, and she was terrified. The staff recognized Gaetano immediately—he had been hospitalized there more than 20 times over the past several years. He was diagnosed with paranoid schizophrenia at age 18. Early in his illness, he responded well to the supportive hospital environment and medications but did not follow up with day treatment, residential care, or medication when released from the inpatient setting.

It is important to begin your assessment by taking comprehensive violence histories on admission. The goal of history taking is to find patterns or trends in violent behaviors in order to identify the conditions under which an individual is likely to act violently.

Clients and significant others are important sources of information. Interview questions about the violent client's history should be open and direct, as if you were questioning a suicidal individual. Ask, "How much have you thought about violence?" "What have you done about it?" "What is the most violent thing you have done?" Do not, however, rely on client responses as the sole basis for your assessment. Also review the client's history and past records.

Managing and reducing the risk of violence is based on careful assessment of client behaviors. In addition to interviewing, observation is a tool most useful for gathering data about escalation of client aggressiveness. See the Assessment box below for a listing of behavioral and verbal clues that indicate violence. Predicting the potential for violence helps one to anticipate and prevent aggressive outbursts.

There is increased potential for aggressive behavior with substance abuse. Determine whether the client is under the influence of drugs including CNS depressants (e.g., alcohol, benzodiazepines), stimulants (e.g., cocaine, amphetamines), hallucinogens (e.g., PCP, LSD), and narcotics (e.g., morphine, oxycontin). In addition to substance abuse, other risk factors for violence are listed in the Assessment box on page 810.

A thorough assessment also collects data about the client's sleep pattern, nutritional status, and history of medical problems such as temporal lobe epilepsy. The client's ability to solve problems and cope with stressors should also be noted.

MediaLink Care Plan: Impulse Control Disorder

Nursing Diagnosis: NANDA

Clients who are violent usually have numerous problems, including poor impulse control, low self-esteem, and dysfunctional interpersonal relationships. The relevant nursing diagnoses for clients exhibiting violence are:

- Risk for Violence: Directed at Others.
- Risk for Violence: Self-Directed.
- Anxiety.

ASSESSMENT

Indicators of Impending Violence

Verbal	Behavioral
Threats of harm	Clenched jaws
Loud, demanding voice tone	Frowning, glaring
Abrupt silence	Intense staring
Sarcastic remarks	Flushing of face and neck
Pressured speech	Smirking grin
Illogical responses	Dilated pupils
Yelling, screaming	Pacing
Statements of fear and/or suspicion	Pounding fists
	Heightened vigilance

I. Clinical history

A. Diagnosis at discharge
Axis I: ______________
____
Axis II: ______________
____

B. Age: ______________

C. Sex: ____ M ____ F

D. Admitting status
____ 72-HR hold ____ Vol.
____ 14-DAY cert. ____ Other
____ Noncontested

E. Use of self-soothers (e.g., comfort wrap)?
Time out or quiet time?
____
____
____
____ Yes ____ No

F. Age at onset: ______________

G. Psychotropic medications:
___ Taking prior to admission
___ Not taking prior to admission

Medications:
____
____
____
____

H. Previous criminal history
____ Yes ____ No
____
____

I. Use of ETOH/street drugs
____ Yes ____ No
____
____
____

II. Violence history

A. Previous institutional violence ____ Yes ____ No

Type of institution: ______________ Date(s): ______ ______
Number of incidents: ______________ ______ ______

Type of violence:				
	Against person	____ Yes	____ No	Date ______
	Family	____ Yes	____ No	Date ______
	Stranger	____ Yes	____ No	Date ______
	Inmate/client	____ Yes	____ No	Date ______
	RN/LPT/MD	____ Yes	____ No	Date ______
	Other	____ Yes	____ No	Date ______
				Who ______
	Weapon used	____ Yes	____ No	Date ______
	Against property	____ Yes	____ No	Date ______
	Type	______________		
	Verbal threat (only)	____ Yes	____ No	Date ______
Situational factors:	Time of day	______		
	Location	______		
	Engaged in therapeutic activity	____ Yes	____ No	
	Type of activity	______		

Other factors ______________
____
____
____

Interactional factors: Engaged in interaction with victim:
Type of interaction ______________
____
With whom: ______________
Content of conversation, request:
____
____

FIGURE 34–2 ■ *A violence assessment tool.* *(continues)*

- Individual Ineffective Coping.
- Self-Esteem Disturbance.

Outcome Identification: NOC

Clients who demonstrate violent behaviors challenge the entire treatment team. It is imperative that team members agree on the expected client outcomes. Listed below are some outcomes that apply to clients with aggressive behavior:

- Identify precipitating events prior to losing control.
- Refrain from self-injury and from injuring others.
- Identify alternative methods for expressing anger.
- Refrain from impulsive behavior.

Response to violence: Medications ____ Yes ____ No
Type and dose: ______________________

Seclusion only ____ Yes ____ No
Seclusion/restraint ____ Yes ____ No
Milieu management ____ Yes ____ No
Combination ____ Yes ____ No
(list) ______________________

Client's response to intervention(s): ______________________

B. Community violence
Previous violence: ____ Yes ____ No
Number of incidents: ______ Date(s): ______ ______

Type of violence:				
	Against person	____ Yes	____ No	Date ______
	Family	____ Yes	____ No	Date ______
	Stranger	____ Yes	____ No	Date ______
	Inmate/client	____ Yes	____ No	Date ______
	RN/LPT/MD	____ Yes	____ No	Date ______
	Other	____ Yes	____ No	Date ______
				Who ______
	Weapon used	____ Yes	____ No	Date ______
	Against property	____ Yes	____ No	Date ______
	Type	______		
	Verbal threat (only)	____ Yes	____ No	Date ______
Situational factors:	ETOH	____ Yes	____ No	Amount ______
	Street drugs	____ Yes	____ No	
	Type	______		

Time of day ______ Activity ______

Location ______ ______
Other factors ______

Interactional factors: Engaged in interaction with victim: ____ Yes ____ No
Type of interaction: ______________________

Others present: ______________________

Content of conversation, request, argument, or dispute: ______________________

FIGURE 34–2 ■ *A violence assessment tool.*

Even though there is a list of suggested outcomes provided above, remember that each client, violent or not, is an individual who has unique needs.

Planning and Implementation: NIC

The major goal for all clients is maintenance of safety; this is especially true for those who are at risk for violence. Protecting the client and others from harm is the primary goal for all health care providers in every setting. Balance the issue of safety maintenance with the need for assuring individual freedom of the violent client. Providing treatment in the least restrictive environment, while maintaining safety, is of paramount importance. Refer to Chapter 10 for a discussion of the legal and ethical ramifications of the least restrictive environment.

Working successfully with clients who demonstrate violence, or the potential for violence, calls for teamwork, critical thinking, and creativity on the part of the entire treatment team. ■ Figure 34–3 on page 811 provides a model for analyzing the risks versus the benefits of several different interventions for a violent client. You may employ a variety of methods, including developing a therapeutic relationship, milieu management, limit setting, pharmacologic agents, behavioral interventions, restrictive measures, and client education.

THERAPEUTIC RELATIONSHIP

Establishing rapport with the client helps reduce suspiciousness by building trust. When clients feel they are in a supportive, trusting relationship, there is less need to "prove" their superiority. Safety maintenance is a key element of a therapeutic relationship. Safety refers not only to physical but also to psychological factors; the environment must be one in which the client feels safe to express feelings and risk learning new behaviors.

A therapeutic nurse–client relationship also involves the nurse's demonstration of compassion and caring, which is actualized through presence, or therapeutic use of self. Be aware of the need to help clients learn to enhance self-esteem. Avoid labeling aggressive behavior as "attention-seeking" without doing a complete assessment to determine the precipitating events that led to the aggressive outburst.

Active listening is essential when working with violent clients or those who are at risk for becoming violent. Listen for the expression of unmet needs (such as control and dependency) and for the expression of the ability to regain/maintain control.

MILIEU MANAGEMENT

Be aware that the mental health care environment may be dehumanizing and depersonalizing. When clients feel devalued, aggressiveness usually escalates. Environmental elements contributing to violence on inpatient psychiatric units include space and location, time of day, architectural design, staffing patterns, activity levels, and client population composition.

Space and Location. Space and location factors include territoriality, privacy, and overcrowding. The concept of territoriality involves defending physical objects or the space a client has identified or "staked out" as personal space. For example, a client often "claims" a special chair on the unit, and a new client comes along and sits in it. The resulting conflicts over special territory also raise the issue of privacy.

Overcrowding is also related to the issue of privacy. Clients who are suspicious or have been abused as children often have difficulty tolerating people near them or touching them.

Architectural Design. Architectural designs that create blind spots and opportunities for nonobservation can also increase the risk of violence. Mirrors have been used effectively to cope with particular architectural design problems in psychiatric units.

How a unit and staff choose to handle potentially dangerous items such as glass, belts, and matches is complex and is related not only to institutional policy and unit philosophy but also to individual clinical judgment. On many units, staff monitors these items, by using sign-up procedures or by locking them up and distributing them at the discretion of the staff or a member of the client government. The significant issue is developing an awareness that location of these items often creates areas where violence occurs. Sometimes the simple installation of one additional client telephone or a minor structural alteration on a unit can significantly reduce the number of violent incidents.

Staffing Patterns. The relationship between staffing patterns and violence is not well understood. Optimal staffing, often cited as a prerequisite for achieving treatment objectives, is being rigorously studied by the American Nurses Association and other professional groups. Whether a given hospital environment has sufficient staff to manage potentially violent clients depends on the amount of care required by the total client population at that period of time.

Activity Level. Activity level refers to the participation of clients in therapeutic activities. Peak times for violent incidents tend to be mealtimes and periods of concentrated treatment programming. In both situations, there is a high concentration of clients, and performance and participation are demanded. Ways of handling the problems suggested by activity level include scheduling, coordinating, and withdrawing. Scheduling staff breaks and mealtimes during client meals can create a situation of temporary understaffing on the unit. Staggering mealtimes for clients and staff is a simple mechanism that may prevent violent behavior. Coordinating client activities with the nursing staff schedule is an important consideration.

Staff who attempt to cajole or coerce clients into participation often create a situation in which the client feels trapped, and striking out becomes the only defense. Sometimes the most valuable intervention with any client—but particularly with one who is agitated, angry, or frightened—is temporary with-

ASSESSMENT

Risk Factors for Violence

- Availability of and/or possession of weapons
- Cognitive impairment
- Cruelty to animals
- Fire setting
- History of childhood abuse
- History of drug/alcohol abuse
- History of violence directed toward others
- History of witnessing family violence
- Impulsivity
- Psychotic symptoms (e.g., hallucinations, delusions)
- Suicidal behavior

Jason is a voluntary client hospitalized on an open unit who punched another client, fracturing his jaw. You assess Jason after he hit his peer and find him very calm. You place him on 1:1 supervision with staff until you can decide on a course of action. You review his record and discover that he has been in prison for assault and battery. While hospitalized he has not engaged in any violence before today. You call the doctor, the nursing supervisor, the social worker and security; you also call in extra staff to maintain safety.

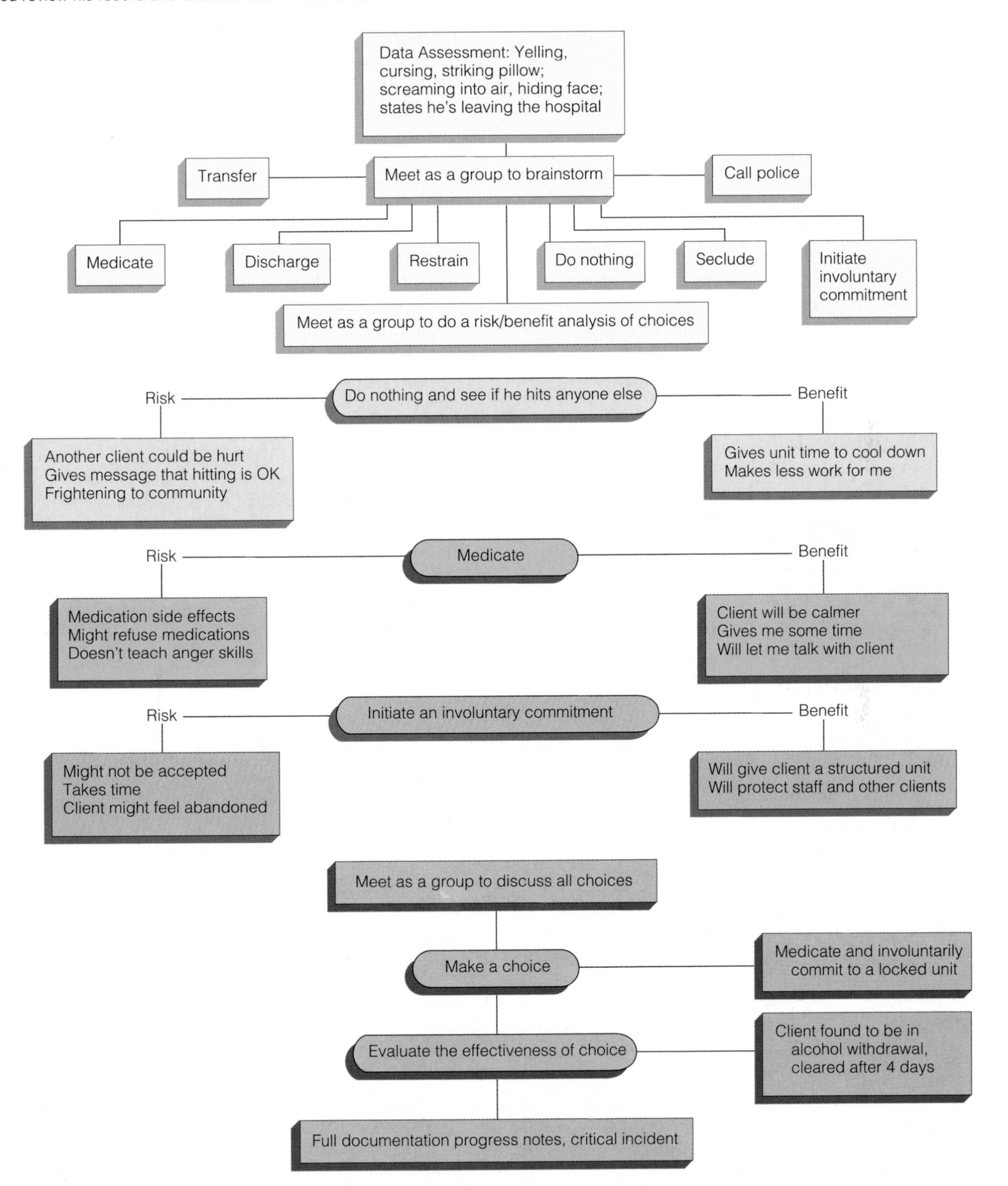

FIGURE 34–3 ■ *Risk/benefit analysis as a means of making decisions about the treatment of a violent client.*

drawal. This allows the client quiet time free from the anxiety of interpersonal demands. Making frequent, short, individualized contact with the client is more reassuring and does more to deescalate a situation than forcing the client to attend a community meeting or other activity where the client's behavior is likely to be the focal point of discussion. Individualizing the milieu activities of clients may be as important to advancing their treatment and preventing violence as the proper medication regimen.

LIMIT SETTING

Setting limits on inappropriate behavior is necessary when the client becomes increasingly agitated and aggressive. But remember to use limit setting as a therapeutic intervention, not as a punitive tool. The intent of limit setting is not to control the client but rather to provide consistent expectations and guidelines for self-control. Setting limits must be viewed as a temporary process to protect the client and others. Limits are implemented only until the client demonstrates, either verbally or behaviorally, the ability to establish and maintain self-control. The Intervention box below lists recommendations for setting limits.

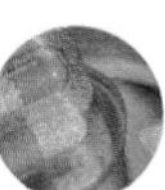

Pharmacologic Interventions. Many pharmacologic agents are currently used to reduce aggressiveness. The selective serotonin reuptake inhibitors (SSRIs) such as fluoxetine (Prozac) and paroxetine (Paxil) are being studied to determine why they are effective in decreasing aggressive behaviors in some clients. Several studies indicate that inhibition of serotonin is the mechanism for reduction of aggressive behaviors (Cherek et al., 2002; Goodman & New, 2000).

Other medications frequently used are haloperidol (Haldol) and thiothixene (Navane). Long-acting injectable fluphenazine (Prolixin) and haloperidol are used with clients discharged to the community to be followed as outpatients, as well as with clients who have histories of noncompliance. The second-generation antipsychotic agents such as clozapine (Clozaril) and risperidone (Risperdal) have been demonstrated to reduce the symptoms of agitation and aggression while producing fewer extrapyramidal side effects than the conventional antipsychotics (Chengappa et al., 2002; Tune, 2001). An anticonvulsant agent, valproic acid (Depakene), potentiates GABA-induced inhibition and thus leads to decreased aggressiveness in many individuals (Kaplan & Sadock, 2000). ■ Table 34–2 lists pharmacologic agents used in reducing aggression.

Current medication practice involves the combination of antianxiety and antipsychotic medications. The benzodiazepine lorazepam (Ativan) is commonly prescribed with an antipsychotic to reduce anxiety and to decrease aggressiveness (Currier & Trenton, 2002). This combination reduces anxiety and permits the use of a lower dose of the neuroleptic, thereby reducing the potential of developing tardive dyskinesia. Although use of medication is the most widely used treatment for the control of vio-

INTERVENTION

Limit Setting

Nursing Intervention	Rationale
State limits in specific and direct language.	Decreases possibility of misunderstanding.
Use a calm, unhurried approach.	Promotes a sense of security.
Offer time-out periods/one-to-one sessions in a quiet area.	Diminishes sensory stimuli.
Explain the limits and consequences during initial interactions (i.e., tell the client what is expected with the related outcomes).	People tend to behave according to expectations.
Assure client that the staff will not allow client to hurt self and/or others.	Promotes a sense of safety and conveys external controls.
Expect all staff to consistently reinforce limits.	Consistency promotes behavior shaping.
Accept the client while rejecting the inappropriate behavior.	Protects self-esteem and reinforces behavioral limits.
Reward the desirable behavior(s).	Promotes continued demonstration of expected behavior(s).
Continuously evaluate the need for limits; discontinue external limits as soon as the client is able to self-regulate.	Empowers client to exercise self-control.

TABLE 34–2 Psychopharmacologic Agents Used to Reduce Aggression

Classification	Generic Name	Trade Name
Neuroleptic	Haloperidol	Haldol
	Fluphenazine	Prolixin
	Loxapine	Loxitane
	Clozapine	Clozaril
	Risperidone	Risperdal
Selective serotonin reuptake inhibitor (SSRI)	Paroxetine	Paxil
	Fluoxetine	Prozac
Benzodiazepine	Lorazepam	Ativan
	Clonazepam	Klonopin
Anxiolytic	Buspirone	BuSpar
Anticonvulsant	Carbamazepine	Tegretol
	Valproic acid	Depakene
Mood stablizer	Lithium	Eskalith, Lithane, Lithobid
Beta blocker	Propranolol	Inderal

lent behavior in institutional settings, it is important to recognize that pharmacologic agents alone are not the answer to violence.

CLIENT EDUCATION

Education is an important intervention for clients who have a history of violence or for those who are at risk of becoming violent. Client teaching focuses on empowering the client: providing the client with tools for increasing self-responsibility. Some specific topics appropriate for teaching aggressive clients are:

- Anger management.
- Social skills training.
- Problem solving.
- Communication skills training.
- Assertiveness training.
- Relaxation skills (see Chapter 32).

The Client and Family Teaching feature provides an outline for a five-session class on anger management; it can be modified as needed.

CALMING THE ESCALATING CLIENT

Avoiding client injury that can occur with the use of seclusion and restraints requires an attempt to use alternative methods to calm clients who are escalating. A study designed to determine what expert psychiatric–mental health nurses do to deescalate an escalating client revealed that these nurses were skilled at:

- Noticing the client.
- Reading the situation and the client.
- Determining where the client was on the continuum of aggressive behavior.
- Understanding the meaning of the client's behavior.
- Knowing the intervention the client needed.
- Connecting interpersonally with the client.
- Matching the intervention to the client's needs (Johnson & Hauser, 2001).

Some strategies for reducing escalation and averting a crisis are given in Box 34–2. The techniques listed are directed at deescalating behavior and should be used before the client becomes out of control.

BOX 34–2 Deescalation Strategies for Aggressive Clients

- Diversion
- Exercise
- Change of surroundings
- Release from schedule or "demands"
- Relaxation
- Music
- Quiet periods
- Being read to or talked to by employees
- A quiet walk
- Reciting phrases or counting
- Thought stopping (a cognitive-behavioral technique in which the client examines angry thoughts and feelings that drive action; see Chapter 30)

RESTRICTIVE MEASURES: VERBAL INTERVENTIONS

All interventions must be considered within the context of the principle of least restrictiveness. This principle requires staff to use less restrictive measures of control before resorting to more restrictive interventions. Staff members must document their efforts to intervene with a client using verbal strategies before they intervene physically.

Forming a therapeutic relationship with the potentially violent client is often the first step to containing the violent behavior. It is important to convey control in the situation by using clear, calm statements (see the Rx Communication feature) and a confident physical stance rather than through remarks or cues that can be interpreted as challenging. A confrontational, aggressive, or threatening manner or a tendency to overidentify with the client's experience can make the staff member a target of violence and actually precipitate violence.

Several strategies are suggested as guidelines for establishing quick rapport and an alliance with the potentially violent client.

CLIENT / FAMILY TEACHING

Anger Management Class

Session 1: What Is Anger?

- Signs and symptoms
- Causes: Just or unjust anger
- Responses: Thoughts, feelings, and actions

Session 2: Managing Anger Through Relaxation

- Importance and advantages
- The Relaxation Response
- Demonstration and practice

Session 3: Managing Anger Through Communication

- Importance and advantages
- Communication process
- Assertive communication
- Demonstration, role play, practice

Session 4: Problem Solving

- Importance and advantages
- Process of problem solving
- Demonstration and practice

Session 5: Closure: Putting It All Together

- Review of processes
- Exercise: Responding to a situation
- Self-evaluation

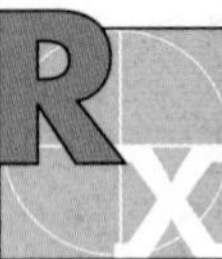

COMMUNICATION

Angry, Nonverbal Client

CLIENT: Flares his nostrils and glares at the nurse.

NURSE RESPONSE 1: "Steven, you look angry today."

RATIONALE: Stating an observation such as how the client appears, as well as using a feeling word, encourages communication.

NURSE RESPONSE 2: "Steven, I can tell that you are upset. Tell me why you are upset."

RATIONALE: When you know a client is upset, this direct approach creates an opportunity for the client to discuss the feelings and thoughts with you.

Clinical judgment and the situation itself must dictate the appropriateness of their use. Some violent behavior occurs impulsively and without warning. Most episodes, however, involve an escalation of behavior and are therefore more appropriate for verbal intervention. Examples of verbal interventions and positional strategies for working with potentially violent clients are provided in the Intervention box below. The overall goal is to protect the client's already damaged self-esteem as much as possible in order to decrease the potential for violent behavior.

Sometimes verbal interventions are insufficient to contain the situation, particularly when the violent behavior occurs impulsively. In these instances, additional interventions—including medications, behavioral techniques, and seclusion and restraint—can be used with or instead of the verbal strategies.

RESTRICTIVE MEASURES: SECLUSION AND RESTRAINT

Various behavioral strategies established around the principle of progressive isolation are often attempted before initiation of seclusion and restraint. The therapeutic intent is to reduce disruptive stimulation and provide the client with a contained, well-defined space for reassurance and protection. Depending on unit construction, the client can be encouraged to seek quiet refuge at the back of the unit or in a private room. Isolation can progress from the back of the unit to the client's room to open seclusion or a quiet room as indicated. These strategies are typically used in conjunction with the medications previously mentioned and to avoid the more restrictive procedures of seclusion and restraint.

When efforts to contain the client's behavior using verbal techniques or the administration of medications and behav-

INTERVENTION

Verbal Interventions and Positional Strategies

Technique	Rationale
Approach the client from the side. Do not stand face-to-face with a potentially violent person.	Decreases the tendency of the violent person to project and externalize the assault.
Leave plenty of space between yourself and the client.	Reduces anxiety and the opportunity for assault.
Speak slowly, directly, in a normal tone of voice, using simple statements like, "Mr. Jones, put the chair down," or "Mrs. Clark, let's sit down and talk about what's bothering you." Encourage the client to sit down. If the client is pacing and can't sit down, pace with the client.	Reduces anxiety, communicates control, increases the client's self-esteem, and models negotiation.
Center your statements on the issues concerning the client. For example, if the client states, "The nurse said I'm too sick to leave the hospital," a response such as, "You're upset at this big disappointment" will likely be more effective than "I can see how you must be upset by that."	Deflects attention away from the staff member who has become the target for the violent behavior.
When responding to the client's anger at not being allowed to leave, try saying, "I'm interested in understanding how terrible that is for you, Mr. Lewis."	Avoids challenging the client and expresses interest in the client's perspective.
Express clear expectations of control. For example, "I expect you can control yourself."	Communicates clarity and emphasizes the client's ability to control own behavior.
It is probably best to not touch clients when they are upset and posing an immediate danger.	Communicates respect for the client and maintains a comfortable distance, thereby reducing the client's sense of threat.
Acknowledge nonviolent behavior. When the client sits down to talk, try stating, "Thank you for sitting with me, I can listen better this way."	Focuses on the client's strength and maintains the client's self-esteem.

ioral techniques do not prevent the violent behavior, or if an assault occurs without warning, staff must intervene to restrain the client in order to protect the client and others.

Client Rights. In the past few years, there has been a concerted effort by federal agencies, professional associations, and health care facilities to reduce the use of seclusion and restraint. Client safety is the primary reason for the trend toward eliminating seclusion and restraint in health care settings. According to the National Mental Health Association (NMHA) (2000), as many as 150 Americans die every year from the improper use of restraints. Asphyxiation and cardiac arrest are the cause of most deaths associated with psychiatric restraints.

The NMHA supports proposed federal legislation requiring improved staff training in crisis deescalation techniques and advocates for improved access to medication and community-based treatment for individuals with severe mental illness. The Children's Health Act of 2000 enacted by the 104th Congress requires any public or health care facility that receives federal funding to protect and promote the rights of each resident with regard to restraints or involuntary seclusion. This act also mandates that restraints and seclusion may be imposed only to ensure physical safety and only on the written order of a physician or other licensed practitioner. Another significant part of this legislation is the implementation of regulations for appropriate staffing levels and training.

In 1999, the Health Care Financing Administration (HCFA) (which is now called the Center for Medicare & Medicaid Services) disseminated the following definitions to health care facilities:

- Seclusion: "The involuntary confinement of a person in a room or an area where the person is physically prevented from leaving."
- Restraint: "Any manual method or physical or mechanical device, material or equipment attached or adjacent to the client's body that he or she cannot easily remove that restricts freedom of movement or normal access to one's body."

The movement toward a restraint-free environment of care is the exemplification of least restrictive measures. *Seclusion and restraint are to be used only in the case of behavioral emergency.*

CLINICAL EXAMPLE

Upon Gaetano's admission to the psychiatric emergency room, he is disheveled, unable to cooperate with the staff, and is screaming and flailing. He is tormented with delusions and hallucinations that frighten him and lead him to strike out at others in the belief that they are trying to hurt him. He has a history of assaults toward his mother and the nursing staff. The staff assess Gaetano's risk for imminent violence to be high and administer haloperidol IM and place him in a seclusion room where they hope he will rest and feel safer.

Box 34–3 provides an overview of the American Psychiatric Nurses Association's (APNA's) principles for using seclusion and restraint (APNA, 2000).

Additional APNA (http://apna.org), NMHA (www.nmha.org), HCFA (www.cms.hhs.gov), and Joint Commission on Accreditation of Health Care Organizations (JCAHO) (www.jcaho.org) data can be accessed through direct resource links on the Companion Website for this book.

Facilities using seclusion and restraint require staff attendance at assault training programs. These programs teach policies and procedures for dealing with assaultive clients, including assessment, prevention of escalating aggressiveness, and legal and clinical documentation requirements, as well as appropriate physical contact for use with violent clients.

At no time should students or other untrained personnel intervene using these techniques, because they involve actual physical contact with clients, thereby increasing the risk of personal injury.

Care of the Client in Seclusion and Restraint. Psychiatric–mental health nurses have a major responsibility in the decision to isolate and restrain as well as in caring for the client while in seclusion and restraints. Once the decision has been made to seclude and restrain a potentially violent client, a leader is chosen from among the available staff. The leader is responsible for designating roles to be performed by the remaining staff and for directing the steps in the seclusion and restraint procedure. Choice of the leader is important and can be based on various factors, including familiarity with the client. Remember that the goal is to gain maximum cooperation from the client and minimize violence.

After a leader is chosen, a sufficient number of personnel must be gathered. This support staff should convey confidence and calm, reflecting a detached, professional approach to a familiar procedure. Staff members should avoid intimidating language and physical stances, since these behaviors may provoke the client's potential for violence. It is often sufficient to have the support staff gather around the leader the first time the

BOX 34–3 American Psychiatric Nurses Association Position Statement on the Use of Seclusion and Restraint

- Emphasizes prevention and reduction of the use of these restrictive methods
- Calls for their use only in behavioral emergencies that pose an immediate risk of harm to a client or others
- Calls on psychiatric–mental health nurses to provide leadership in establishing a treatment environment that is client focused and noncoercive
- Urges working within a collaborative relationship with the client and family
- Focuses on the need for an individualized treatment plan that promotes the client's self-management

Source: Seclusion and restraint: Position statement & standards of practice. A publication of the American Psychiatric Nurses Association, 2001, Arlington, VA. Retrieved January 11, 2002, from the World Wide Web, www.apna.org.

MediaLink Seclusion and Restraint Resources

client is approached. This show of force may be enough, and the client may comply without further intervention.

One staff member is assigned responsibility for managing the unit environment and other clients. This person is responsible for supporting and calming the other clients, who may become anxious during the procedure. In addition, the area near the seclusion room must be cleared of clients or physical obstructions to minimize the potential for injury.

Once the unit environment is safe, the team approaches the violent client. The leader offers a clear, brief statement of the purpose and rationale for seclusion or restraint. For example, the client is told that his or her behavior is out of control and that time in seclusion is required to help him or her regain control. The other team members position themselves around the client for easy access to the client's limbs. The leader then asks the client to walk into the seclusion room accompanied by staff. At this point, further discussion or negotiation should be avoided as it frequently aggravates the situation. The behavioral options given to the client must be kept simple, clear, and minimal.

Once a client is placed in seclusion or restraint, nursing observations of the client's behavior are required every 15 minutes. These checks include a description of the client's behavior, as well as routine care activities, including meals, circulation checks, and toileting. These observations should be conducted by nursing staff entering the seclusion room and participating in a verbal exchange with the client. Document content of these dialogues, paying particular attention to a reduction in the client's symptoms, responsiveness to limits, capacity to discuss options, and increased capacity to tolerate frustration. Documentation of these behavioral checks and routine physical care activities is required.

Release from Seclusion and Restraint. Clients may be released from seclusion and restraint when the client's behavior is under control and no longer poses a danger to self or others. The decision to release from seclusion or remove restraint is based on an assessment of data gathered while the client is in seclusion. The ability of the client to control his or her behavior has been observed many times during the course of seclusion or restraint and is the basis for the decision to release.

PROFESSIONAL EDUCATION

Educational opportunities about the reduction of violence in the workplace should be ongoing. Essential information to be taught is the process of deescalation. The focus of the staff must be on the prevention, rather than the management, of aggressive behavior. The educational programs are designed to help nurses:

- Understand ways in which they increase their vulnerability to assault.
- Develop provocation profiles (recognizing one's own personal triggers for aggression) of themselves to increase their sensitivity and awareness.
- Role-play conversations with violent clients.
- Practice teamwork for physical restraint procedures.
- Promote a safe, nonblaming environment to discuss their experiences of working with violent clients.
- Develop sensitivity to the effects their own experiences of violence have in their daily work.

COLLEGIAL SUPPORT

Nurses who have been assaulted by clients need the support of their coworkers. An initial approach is to encourage nurses who have been attacked to discuss their feelings. Staff victims of violence need a safe, supportive environment. The critical incident stress debriefing (CISD) model is often used to help staff members come to terms with the attack (Flannery, 2001). CISD is a group interaction facilitated by mental health clinicians to allow personnel to talk about their thoughts, feelings, and reactions to a stressful event. Refer to Chapter 33 for a complete explanation of CISD. Providing supportive crisis intervention for the staff may decrease the potential for retaliation and long-term negative consequences.

Evaluation

There are many elements to consider in evaluating the effectiveness of strategies for violence management. Individual characteristics, biologic factors, conditions in the social environment, and the interpersonal styles of both clients and staff contribute to violent behavior. In spite of our theoretic understandings of violent behavior and efforts to implement management strategies to decrease the likelihood of its occurrence, we are not yet able to predict with certainty when someone will act in a violent manner. The fact is that violence occurs in health care settings and that psychiatric–mental health nurses are victims of assault from psychiatric clients.

Specific evaluative criteria to be considered for violent clients are listed below. The client will:

- Refrain from verbal outbursts.
- Refrain from striking others.
- Refrain from violating other's personal space.
- Identify factors that precipitate violent behaviors.
- Identify feelings when angry or frustrated.
- Vent negative feelings appropriately.
- Identify alternative ways to cope with problems.

Case Management, Community-Based Care, and Home Care

The concept of least restrictive environment is used to guide the planning of nursing care for all clients. However, when aggressive behavior begins to intensify, the safety of everyone involved—client, staff, and others in the community—overrides the client's right to freedom.

In order to assist aggressive clients to function in the community, it may be helpful to teach family members, friends, and

***Nursing* SELF-AWARENESS**

Factors That Influence Your Response to Violence

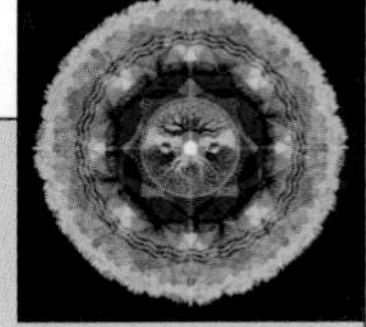

Nurses working with violent clients need to monitor themselves regarding the following:

- Their ability to use anger constructively and not to take clients' anger personally.
- Their capacity for clear verbal communication.
- Their capacity for self-analysis.
- Their capacity to listen.
- Their capacity to both establish and maintain empathic linkages with clients and to disengage.
- Their capacity to understand their fears and anxieties about violence.
- Their belief that violent clients are amenable to treatment.

significant others specific techniques for defusing violence. Refer back to Box 34–2 on page 813 for suggestions. Also teach family members, friends, and significant others the indicators for impending violence (see the Client/Family Teaching feature on page 813).

Milieu management is not limited to inpatient treatment settings. When working in outpatient areas, such as clinics and offices, be aware of the relationship between the physical environment and the potential for violence. For example, a safe office arrangement calls for the furniture to be arranged in such a way that you can exit without being trapped. Having easy access to an emergency call system is also essential in maintaining the safety of both staff and clients.

Nursing Self-Awareness

Not every nurse can work with violent mentally ill clients. Since such work can be frightening and upsetting, it is important to take the time for self-reflection and to examine your reactions to others. This is particularly important when working with violent clients, since your own stress and anxiety can greatly interfere with your ability to attend to subtle cues and to initiate sensitive interventions in a timely manner.

Self-awareness is a process that helps you to avoid personalizing client comments and behaviors. Whenever we "take it personally," objectivity is lost and therapeutic effectiveness decreases. Often our responses to client aggressiveness reflect the beliefs that we incorporated as children. For example, as young children, some of us learned that anger was something to be feared and avoided at all costs. Others of us may have learned that aggressive expression of anger is powerful. These beliefs adopted in childhood often govern the behavior of adults. Self-reflection helps us to determine how our own beliefs influence our responses to clients. The Nursing Self-Awareness feature on this page lists some areas for you to consider when you work with violent clients.

USING RESEARCH EVIDENCE

Marty, a client on an inpatient unit, is becoming more aggressive toward staff and other clients. In an attempt to avoid using seclusion and restraints, the nursing staff decides to use the following interventions in an attempt to deescalate the client's behavior:

- Identify the intensity of the client's behavior.
- Make a personal connection with the client by having a one-to-one interaction.
- Determine the meaning of the client's behavior (i.e., understand what the client needs).

Other approaches that may be useful in helping Marty calm down are deep breathing and the therapeutic use of music.

Gagner-Tjellesen, D. Yurkovich, E. E., & Gragert, M. (2001). Use of music therapy and other ITNIs in acute care. *Journal of Psychosocial Nursing and Mental Health Services, 39,* 26–37.

Johnson, M. E., & Hauser, P. M. (2001). The practices of expert psychiatric nurses: Accompanying the patient to a calmer personal space. *Issues in Mental Health Nursing, 22,* 651–668.

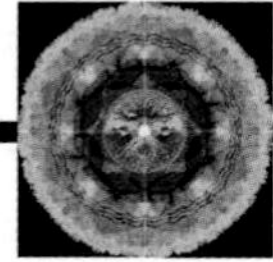

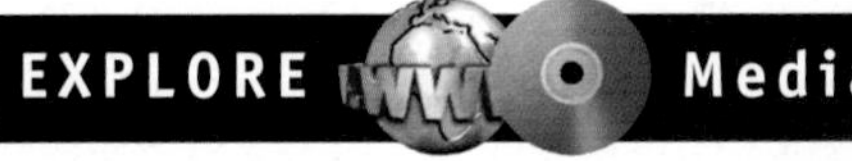

NCLEX review, case studies, and other interactive resources for this chapter can be found on the Companion Website at http://www.prenhall.com/kneisl. Click on Chapter 34 to select the activities for this chapter.

For animations, video tutorials, more NCLEX review questions, and an audio glossary, access the accompanying CD-ROM in this textbook.

BIBLIOGRAPHY

American Academy of Pediatrics Committee on Public Education. (2001). Media violence. *Pediatrics, 108,* 1222–1226.

American Nurses Association. (2001). *Nurses say health and safety concerns play major role in employment decisions.* Retrieved January 11, 2002, from the World Wide Web, www.NursingWorld.org.

American Psychiatric Association. (2000). *Diagnostic and statistical manual of mental disorders* (4th ed., Text Revision). Washington, DC: Author.

American Psychiatric Nurses Association. (2000). *Position statement on the use of seclusion and restraint.* Retrieved January 11, 2002, from the World Wide Web, www.apna.org.

Barnow, S., Lucht, M., & Freyberger, H. J. (2001). Influence of punishment, emotional rejection, child abuse, and broken homes on aggression in adolescence: An examination of aggressive adolescents in Germany. *Psychopathology, 34,* 167–173.

Bars, D. R., Heyrend, F. L., Simpson, C. D., & Munger, J. C. (2001). Use of visual evoked-potential studies of EEG data to classify aggressive, explosive behavior of youths. *Psychiatric Services, 52,* 81–86.

Beech, B. (2001). Sign of the times or the shape of things to come? A 3-day unit of instruction on "aggression and violence in health settings for all students during preregistration nurse training." *Accident & Emergency Nursing, 9,* 204–211.

Bjork, J. M., Moeller, F. G., Kramer, G. I., Kram, M., Suris, A., Rush, A. J., et al. (2001). Plasma GABA levels correlate with aggressiveness in relatives of patients with unipolar depressive disorder. *Psychiatry Research, 101,* 131–136.

Brendgen, M., Vitaro, R., Tremblay, R. E., & Lavoie, F. (2001). Reactive and proactive aggression: Predictions to physical violence in different contexts and moderating effects of parental monitoring and caregiving behavior. *Journal of Abnormal Child Psychology, 29,* 292–304.

Brower, M. C., & Price, B. H. (2001). Neuropsychiatry of frontal lobe dysfunction in violent and criminal behavior: a critical review. *Journal of Neurology & Neurosurgery in Psychiatry, 71,* 6, 720–726.

Carlsson, G., Dahlberg, K. & Drew, N. (2000). Encountering violence and aggression in mental health nursing: a phenomenological study of tacit caring knowledge. *Issues in Mental Health Nursing, 21,* 533–545.

Centers for Disease Control & Prevention. (2001). *National youth violence prevention center.* Retrieved March 2, 2002, from the World Wide Web, www.safeyouth.org.

Chengappa, K. N., Vasile, J., Levine, J., Ulrich, R., Baker, R., Gopalani, A., et al. (2002). Clozapine: its impact on aggressive behavior among patients in a state psychiatric hospital. *Schizophrenia Research, 53,* 1–6.

Cherek, D. R., Lane, S. D., Pietras, C. J., & Steinberg, J. L. (2002). Effects of chronic paroxetine administration on measures of aggressive and impulsive responses of adult males with a history of conduct disorder. *Psychopharmacology, 159,* 266–274.

Currier G. W., & Trenton, A. (2002). Pharmacological treatment of psychotic agitation. *CNS Drugs, 16,* 219–228.

Echternacht, M. R. (1999). Potential for violence toward psychiatric nursing students: Risk reduction techniques. *Journal of Psychosocial Nursing, 37,* 36–39.

Flannery, R. B., Jr. (2001). The assaulted staff action program (ASAP): Ten year empirical support for critical incident stress management (CISM). *International Journal of Emergency Mental Health, 3*(1), 5–10.

Freud, S. (1961). *Civilization and its discontents.* New York: Norton.

Gagner-Tjellesen, D., Yurkovich, E. E., & Gragert, M. (2001). Use of music therapy and other ITNIs in acute care. *Journal of Psychosocial Nursing and Mental Health Services, 39,* 26–37.

Gilmore-Hall, A. (2001). Violence in the workplace: Are you prepared? *American Journal of Nursing, 101,* 55–56.

Goodman, M., & New, A. (2000). Impulsive aggression in borderline personality disorder. *Current Psychiatry Reports, 2,* 56–61.

Gupta, V. B., Nwosa, N. M., Nadel, T. A., & Inamdar, S. (2001). Externalizing behaviors and television viewing in children of low-income minority parents. *Clinical Pediatrics, 40,* 337–341.

Health Care Financing Administration; Medicare and Medicaid Programs. (1999). *Hospital conditions of patient's rights: Interim final rule.* Washington, DC: Author.

Hudziak, J. J., Rudiger, L. P., Neale, M. C., Heath, A. C., & Todd, R. D. (2000). A twin study of inattentive, aggressive, and anxious/depressed behaviors. *Journal of American Academy of Child & Adolescent Psychiatry, 39,* 469–476.

Johnson, M. E., & Hauser, P. M. (2001). The practices of expert psychiatric nurses: Accompanying the patient to a calmer personal space. *Issues in Mental Health Nursing, 22,* 651–668.

Kaplan, H. I., & Sadock, B. J. (2000). *Kaplan & Sadock's synopsis of psychiatry and study guide.* Philadelphia, PA: Lippincott.

Kuhn, M. (1998). *Pharmacotherapeutics: A nursing process approach* (4th ed.). Philadelphia: Davis.

Lee, R., & Coccaro, E. (2001). The neuropsychopharmacology of criminality and aggression. *Canadian Journal of Psychiatry, 46,* 24–25.

Lesch, K. P., & Merschdorf, Y. (2000). Impulsivity, aggression, and serotonin: A molecular psychobiological perspective. *Behavioral Science & Law, 18,* 581–604.

Maslow, A. (1970). *Motivation and personality* (2nd ed.). New York: Harper & Row.

Mitsis, E. M., Halperin, J. M., & Newcorn, J. H. (2000). Serotonin and aggression in children. *Current Psychiatry Reports, 2,* 95–101.

National Mental Health Association. (2000). NMHA news release. Retrieved January 11, 2002, from the World Wide Web, www.nmha.org/newsroom/ system/news).

Nelson, R. J., & Chiavegatto, S. (2001). Molecular basis of aggression. *Trends in Neuroscience, 24,* 713–719.

Occupational Safety and Health Administration. (2000). *Guidelines for workplace violence prevention programs for health care and social service workers.* Washington, DC: U.S Department of Labor.

Oquendo, M. A., & Mann, J. J. (2000). The biology of impulsivity and suicidality. *Psychiatric Clinics of North America, 23,* 11–25.

Tune, L. E. (2001). Risperidone for the treatment of behavioral and psychological symptoms of dementia. *Journal of Clinical Psychiatry, Suppl 21,* 29–32.

Veenstra-VanderWeele, J., Anderson, G. M., & Cook, E. H. (2000). Pharmacogenetics and the serotonin system: Initial studies and future directions. *European Journal of Pharmacology, 41,* 165–181.

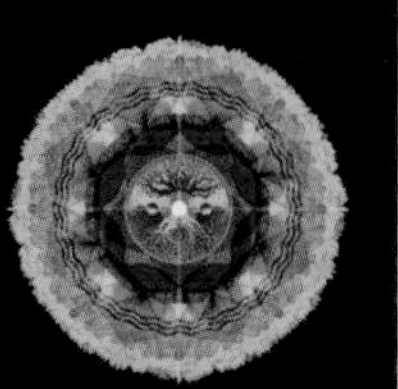

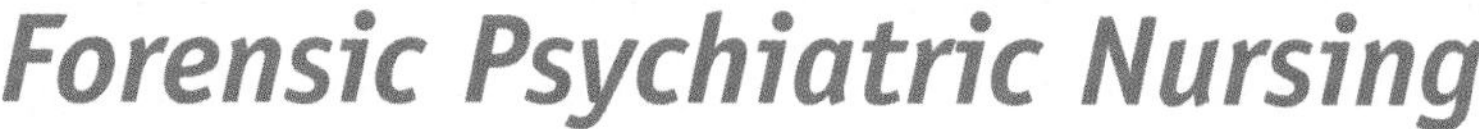

Forensic Psychiatric Nursing

JUDITH CORAM

35

Chapter THIRTY-FIVE

FOCUS QUESTIONS

- If asked to describe the role functions of the psychiatric forensic nurse, what would you say?
- What are the differences between the therapeutic nurse–client relationship and the forensic relationship?
- Why is the determination of legal sanity a complicated process?
- What does a competency therapist do?
- What do fact witnesses and expert witnesses do?
- What personal and professional qualities are essential in order to be an effective psychiatric forensic nurse?

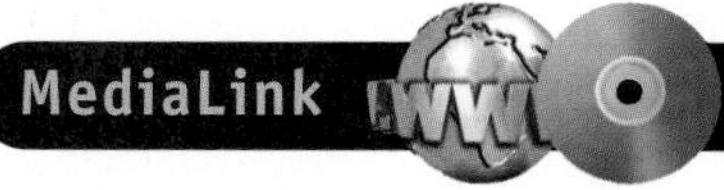

Additional resources for this chapter can be found on the Student CD-ROM accompanying this textbook, and on the Companion Website at www.prenhall.com/kneisl. Click on Chapter 35 to select the activities for this chapter.

CD-ROM
- Audio Glossary
- NCLEX Review

Companion Website
- Additional NCLEX Review
- Care Plan: Competency Therapy
- Case Study: Psychiatric Forensic Examiner

KEY TERMS

competence to proceed
diminished capacity
expert witness
fact witness
forensic examiner
forensic nursing
legal sanity
malingering
psychiatric forensic nursing
victimology

CHAPTER OUTLINE

CROSS REFERENCES

Other topics relevant to this content are: Battering of women and child abuse, Chapter 23; Elder abuse, Chapter 27; Ethical and legal aspects, Chapter 10; Munchausen by proxy, Chapter 20; Violence in the psychiatric setting, Chapter 34.

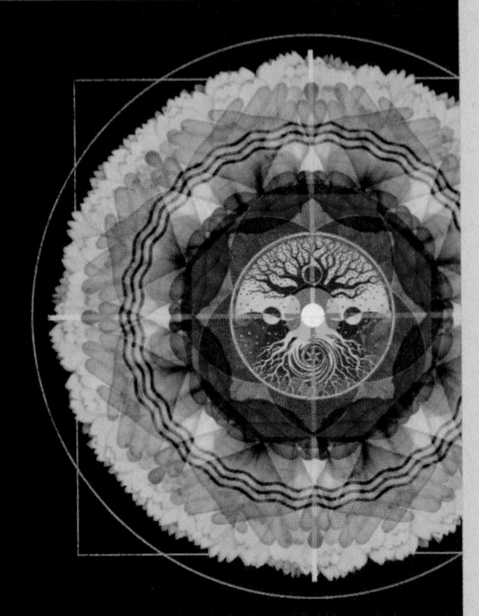

CRITICAL THINKING CHALLENGE

You are the forensic examiner ordered by the court to evaluate David B. for legal sanity and competence on his charge of child murder. David is accused of battering his girlfriend's 18-month-old son while babysitting him. When you meet with David in jail, he tells you he has been diagnosed as schizophrenic. He also tells you that he has not taken medications since his last release from prison, and that voices told him to harm the child.

What information would be important to have before completing your formal report to the court? What is your opinion regarding David's legal sanity? What is your opinion regarding David's competence to proceed? How do you handle your personal feelings about David and what he has done? ■

Interpersonal violence and other criminal behaviors have been studied for decades with an eye to understanding the causes. Recently, television programs and novels with forensic themes have generated great popular interest in forensic science. More people than ever before are seeking information about forensics and enrolling in courses related to forensic science. And growing numbers of nurses are considering careers in this specialty field. Forensic nursing seeks to examine and understand criminal behaviors and the incidents related to them on an individual level.

Our legal system in the United States is based on the assumption that the majority of criminal offenders choose to commit crimes for rational reasons, of their own free will, and deserve to be punished. A minority of mentally disturbed offenders are so irrational and/or unable to control their behavior that criminal culpability (responsibility) is difficult to impose. Fewer than 4% of criminal defendants pursue a defense of legal insanity. Even fewer, less than 1%, are eventually acquitted by reason of insanity.

While most defendants are not mentally ill, we still seek to understand their behavior and thinking at the time of the act. This may be done on-scene prior to arrest, as part of a court-ordered evaluation, during criminal profiling, or as part of an evaluation prior to release into the community. If a pattern of violence is identified in the examination of a victim, the forensic nurse uses the information in an attempt to interrupt the pattern, hoping to prevent future violence and injury. During an evaluation with a perpetrator, the psychiatric forensic nurse attempts to comprehend the event by understanding the perpetrator's background, values, and motivation. Motivation is partly determined by examining the perpetrator's mental state at the time of the crime.

Forensic Nursing as an Emerging Specialty Area

The term *forensic nursing* was officially coined in 1992 when about 70 nurses, whose practice combined the science of nursing with elements of forensic science within the health care and criminal justice systems, gathered in Minneapolis for the first national convention for sexual assault nurses. The following year, the group expanded to include nurses working in death investigation and legal nurse consulting, and organized the International Association of Forensic Nurses in recognition of the need for a nursing response to people identified as the victims of violence. Their goals included the identification and interruption of the cycle of violence, especially toward women, the elderly, and children. The American Nurses Association (ANA) officially recognized forensic nursing as a specialty practice area in 1995. A combined effort between these two groups produced a set of standards for the practice of forensic nursing (ANA & International Association of Forensic Nurses, 1997).

Forensic nursing is a growing specialty in other countries around the globe, especially in the United Kingdom, Australia, Germany, the Netherlands, Japan, and Canada. In all of these countries there is great diversity in the definitions of and roles for forensic nurses. In the United States, the forensic nursing role is evolving mainly as an advanced practice role (Hufft, 2000) as we continue to strive to answer the questions pertaining to the place of forensic practice in nursing. Canadian nurses are dealing with similar questions. The Canadian Nurses Association is working collaboratively with the Correctional Service of Canada to develop a special interest group in forensic nursing (Peternelj-Taylor, 2000).

NURSING ROLE FUNCTIONS

Forensic nursing is an expanded scope of practice. That is, **forensic nursing** is a new specialty area of practice that combines elements of nursing science, forensic science, and the criminal justice system. Intersections lie within other disciplines (forensic science, criminal science), rather than within other specialty areas of nursing.

Forensic nursing is not determined by where it is practiced (as are critical care nursing, perioperative nursing, or flight nursing), or by the type of client (as in pediatric nursing or hospice nursing). It is determined by the nature of the nurse–client relationship and the nursing role functions being performed. Role functions are the nursing acts, behaviors, and skills related to a particular category of practice. For example, the nursing role functions required in the intensive care unit are very different from those required in the school setting. In forensic nursing, the role functions concentrate on four areas:

1. Identification of evidence.
2. Collection of evidence.
3. Documentation of evidence.
4. Preservation of evidence.

In forensic nursing, the nurse–client relationship is predicated on the possibility that a crime has been committed. The forensic nurse contributes data toward answering the question of whether or not a crime has been committed. There is an investigative quality to the nursing assessment that does not exist in other areas of practice.

Elsewhere, a nurse may be expected to describe and report findings, but not to interpret them. For example, a school nurse may observe and document the design of marks on a child's back, but the forensic child abuse specialist would make an assessment of "patterned injury" that includes speculation about the type of weapon used in the suspected battering. Where the school nurse treats the immediate injury, the forensic nurse sees the possibility that a crime has been committed and collects evidence that will help to determine if that is true. Similarly, while a pediatric nurse without forensic training takes a history of repeated apnea spells, the forensic nurse may look further for suspected Munchausen syndrome by proxy (MSP). MSP is a factitious disorder in which one person persistently fabricates symptoms in another person for the purpose of indirectly assuming the sick role. A common presentation is in reports of interrupted breathing (Naegele & Clarke, 2001). MSP is further discussed in Chapter 20.

UNDERSTANDING BOTH VICTIM AND PERPETRATOR

Forensic nurses understand that there are two sides to any criminal act, brought together at a point in time by the perpetrator's motivation, background, and value system and by the characteristics of the victim: the victimology. Forensic nurses who work with either the victim or the perpetrator know that having an understanding of both enhances their evidence collection. For example, a forensic nurse completing a rape exam might use the Comprehensive Sexual Assault Assessment Tool (CSAAT) in her interview. The CSAAT provides law enforcement with a detailed description of the perpetrator's sexual and postoffense behavior. Likewise, because of the possibility of victim selection, the professional assembling a criminal profile will include victimology factors in the data collection.

SUBSPECIALTIES IN FORENSIC NURSING

Forensic nursing is comprised of several subspecialty areas of practice (Saunders, 2000). They all share the same medicolegal aspects of forensic nursing, but the nature of the nurse–client relationship differs. *Physiologic forensic nurses* focus on the alleged victim. *Psychiatric forensic nurses* work with the alleged perpetrator, and the needs of the court become the focus of the interaction.

Physiologic Forensic Nursing

Physiologic forensic nurses focus on the application of forensic aspects of health care in the scientific investigation and treatment of trauma and/or medicolegal issues (Goll-McGee, 1999). Their client is the alleged victim, either living or dead. Role functions in physiologic forensic nursing include:

- Forensic photography.
- Bite mark identification.
- Identification of sharp or blunt trauma.
- Assessment of sexual assault trauma.
- Identification of patterned injury.
- Establishment of chain of custody.
- Assessment of pattern of injury in abuse.

Physiologic forensic nurses work as coroners or death investigators, sexual assault nurse examiners (Girardin, 2001), child abuse specialists or elder abuse specialists (Fulton, 2000), battered woman specialists, or legal nurse consultants (Lorenzo, 2000).

Psychiatric Forensic Nursing

Psychiatric forensic nursing can be defined as the psychiatric nursing assessment, evaluation, and treatment of individuals pending a criminal hearing or trial. The defendant is the client, and the client's thinking and behavior prior to, and during, the commission of the crime are the primary focus of the nurse–client relationship. Psychiatric forensic nurses work as forensic examiners, competency therapists, and consultants to attorneys or law enforcement. The wide range of possible psychiatric forensic nursing roles functions are listed in Box 35–1.

> **BOX 35–1 Psychiatric Forensic Nursing Role Functions**
>
> - Forensic evaluation for legal sanity or competence to proceed
> - Assessment of capacity to formulate intent
> - Assessment of potential for violence or to reoffend
> - Parole/probation considerations
> - Assessment of racial/cultural factors during crime
> - Consultation on countermeasures to violence
> - Assisting in jury selection
> - Investigation of criminal history
> - Sexual predator screening and assessment
> - Courtroom consultation to attorneys
> - Competency therapy
> - Formal written reports to court
> - Expert witness services
> - Police training
> - Review of police reports
> - On-scene consultation to law enforcement

The dimensions of practice in psychiatric forensic nursing are affected both by the nature of the client and the client's current involvement with the criminal justice system. The core of practice is psychiatric–mental health nursing. However, the relationship between client and nurse is markedly different from that in a psychiatric–mental health nursing role because of the alternative social context of the situation that precipitates their interaction. In addition, the setting—a crime scene, a courtroom, a psychiatric hospital, or a correctional facility—influences the forensic nurse's practice.

Recall that evidence collection is central to the role of all forensic nurses. One way evidence collection is performed within psychiatric forensic nursing is in the finding of intent or diminished capacity in the perpetrator's thinking at the time of the crime. This finding aids in determining the level of degree of crime and may later influence the perpetrator's sentence. Psychiatric forensic nurses who work as competency therapists collect evidence by spending many hours with a defendant and carefully documenting the dialogue.

Literature defining the characteristics of psychiatric–mental health nurses who overlap into forensic areas did not exist prior to 1993. Nor was there written work describing the expanded role of the clinical nurse specialist who chooses to practice in an area that contains elements of physiologic forensic nursing, psychiatric–mental health nursing, correctional nursing, law enforcement, and the criminal justice system. A national study, undertaken as part of a master's thesis to collect data on the number of registered nurses providing psychiatric forensic nursing services in the United States and their forensic role functions, brought to light the confusion between the terms *forensic* and *correctional* (Coram, 1993). It can be argued that the expansion of this new area of practice will be better served by regulating definitive roles in both areas.

Correctional Nursing. Many correctional nurses claim identification as forensic nurses because their client is incarcerated. However, the nature of their nurse–client relationship is not investigative. *Correctional nursing* is defined by the location of the work or the legal status of the client, rather than the nursing role functions being performed. Correctional nurses treat the inmate's present medical or mental health needs. They often care for inmates without knowing the nature of their crimes, because it is believed it would prejudice the level of care. They do not play a role in determining future dangerousness or release. Role functions in correctional nursing include determining the need for restraint, assessing risk for custodial suicide, and administering wound care, among several others. A correctional nurse working in a jail or a prison may perform a forensic nursing role function, such as a male rape exam, or collection of DNA specimens. However, many correctional nurses decline these tasks because they believe it interferes with their advocacy role with the inmate.

Correctional Mental Health Nursing. *Correctional mental health nurses* care for inmates housed in a jail or prison's psychiatric unit, or in a forensic psychiatric hospital's long-term ward where persons adjudicated as "not guilty by reason of insanity" are treated. However, the nature of their relationship with the client remains focused on the client's present needs, rather than his or her thinking or behavior in the past (at the time of the crime). An examination of the nursing role functions being performed will point out that correctional mental health nurses perform psychiatric nursing skills, rather than forensic nursing skills. ■ Table 35–1 illustrates the differences in forensic psychiatric nursing, correctional nursing, and correctional mental health nursing.

Correctional mental health nurses make substantial and valued contributions to the care, treatment, rehabilitation, and management of individuals in secure facilities who are deemed legally insane. It is a difficult and challenging client population to work with (Rayel, 2000), and personal safety is an issue during every shift. The dedication of correctional mental health nurses has significantly increased the quality of care for their clients. There are high expectations for this specialized area of practice that continues to contribute to the growing fund of nursing knowledge.

Roles Within Psychiatric Forensic Nursing

Roles within psychiatric forensic nursing include forensic examiner, competency therapist, and consultant to law enforcement or the criminal justice system.

FORENSIC EXAMINER

The **forensic examiner** conducts court-ordered evaluations of legal sanity or competency to proceed, answers any specific medicolegal questions as directed by the court, and renders an expert opinion in a written report or courtroom testimony. Court-ordered sanity or competency evaluations can be requested by the defense, prosecution, or the court. They are usually initiated because of the defendant's history or behavior at the scene, in jail, or in the courtroom. A thorough and complete forensic examination includes:

1. Face-to-face interview.
2. Review of police reports.
3. Thorough psychosocial history.

The ethical forensic examiner will decline a request for an examination or expert opinion if denied any of the three.

MediaLink Case Study: Psychiatric Forensic Examiner

TABLE 35–1 Differentiating Psychiatric Forensic Nursing

Variables	Correctional Nursing	Correctional Mental Health Nursing	Psychiatric Forensic Nursing
Who is the client?	Jail/prison inmate	Jail/prison inmate Client committed to forensic hospital following "not guilty by reason of insanity" plea	Attorney The court
Mindset of nurse	Supportive Accepting Empathic	Supportive Accepting Empathic	Objective Neutral Detached
Focus of the nurse–client relationship	Inmate's current physical or mental health needs	Inmate or client's current and future needs with eye to reintegration into community	Defendant's behavior and thinking at time of crime
Location	Cell or secured unit Inmate may be escorted to a centralized clinic	Psychiatric unit within a jail/prison Long-term unit within a forensic hospital	Community Jail or prison Hospital ward
Primary purpose of relationship	Nursing care of inmate's present physical or mental health needs	Psychiatric nursing care of client's (inmate's) present mental health needs	Pretrial completion of court-ordered sanity/competency evaluation
Examples of nursing role functions	Treatment of injury Suicide assessment	Medication teaching Therapeutic groups One-to-one counseling	Evidence collection Report to court Court testimony
Timing	During incarceration	Length of court-ordered commitment, after adjudication	Pretrial

The ethical forensic examiner's expert opinion is based on the scientific processing of:

- Collected pertinent clinical data.
- Observed client behavior.
- Forensic evidence in police reports and laboratory reports.
- Results of psychological testing.
- Thorough psychosocial history.

Some experts prefer to review background information before interviewing the defendant. Some prefer to do the interview "cold." A skilled interviewer will note clinical findings, including symptoms of mental disorder, behavior, past diagnoses, personality traits, emotions, cognitive abilities, and the psychodynamics of interpersonal relationships (Emiley, 2002). It is valuable to include the observations of other staff who interact with the defendant, since it is not unusual for the defendant to attempt to mislead the interviewer.

Differences Between Forensic and Therapeutic Relationships

There are marked differences between therapeutic and forensic relationships. They are discussed below and summarized in ■ Table 35–2.

Cognitive Set. The cognitive set of the forensic examiner differs from that of treatment personnel. While treatment staff strive to be supportive, accepting, and empathic, the forensic examiner strives to remain neutral, objective, and detached. For example, a mental health treatment intake interview is usually client structured (nonconfronting or nonprobing), based mostly on information from the client, and for the purpose of treatment. The purpose of the forensic evaluation, on the other hand, is legal adjudication. The forensic examiner controls the interview, which is frequently adversarial. While mental health personnel advocate for the client, the forensic examiner advocates for the issues or the completed evaluation. Further, mental health personnel tend to trust information given by the client because it is the client who sought treatment. The forensic examiner confirms the accuracy of all information. In fact, forensic nursing is characterized by intuitive suspiciousness and critical thinking (Winfrey & Smith, 1999). The differences between therapeutic and forensic relationships are also illustrated in the following Clinical Example.

CLINICAL EXAMPLE

Jeb explains to the intake staff at the community mental health center that he recently moved from Oklahoma, where he was diagnosed with paranoid schizophrenia and treated with olanzapine and clonazepam. At first, he refuses to give the names of his family, explaining that he believes they are trying to kill him. The intake staff route the information to an available counselor, who notes the diagnosis, opens a case file, assigns him a case manager, and orders a 30-day supply of his regular medications. She also initiates a request for subsidized housing and welfare benefits.

A few days later, Jeb is arrested for attempted burglary and sent to a forensic hospital for evaluation of legal sanity and competence. He gives the same history at the forensic hospital that he did at the community mental health center. However, the forensic evaluator halts the administration of medication in order to observe for symptoms, and requests validation of the diagnosis from the mental health facility in Oklahoma.

TABLE 35–2 Differences Between Therapeutic and Forensic Relationships

In Role as Mental Health Practitioner	In Role as Forensic Examiner
Individual is a client of the practitioner.	Individual is a client of the attorney requesting the evaluation.
Nature of the privilege is "therapist-client" and includes confidentiality	Nature of the privilege is "attorney–client" or "attorney–work product." Client is informed that anything he discusses can be discussed with the attorney.
Mindset of practitioner is supportive, accepting, and empathic.	Mindset of the examiner is neutral, objective, and detached.
Expertise area of practitioner is selected therapeutic techniques.	Expertise area of examiner is psycholegal evaluation standards.
Standards of practice dictated by diagnostic criteria and accepted treatment.	Standards of practice dictated by legal criteria for adjudication of case.
Interview loosely structured by client.	Interview more structured, led by examiner.
Evaluation deemed complete based on information provided by the client.	Evaluation deemed complete by checking accuracy of sources.
Nature of the interview is rarely adversarial.	Nature of the interview is frequently adversarial.
Practitioner advocates for the client.	Examiner advocates for the issues or results of the evaluation.
Outcome of relationship to benefit client.	Outcome of relationship to aid the legal process.

The state hospital in Oklahoma replies that Jeb has never been a client there. His family reports that Jeb has never been treated for mental illness, but that he does have a history of substance abuse that includes illegal drugs as well as prescription medications, and an extensive criminal record.

Reconstructing the Defendant's Mental State. Since the issue of legal sanity is based on the client's thinking and behavior in the past at the moment of the crime, it is necessary to reconstruct the mental state of the defendant. This requires an evaluation of the evidence at the scene, witness statements of the symptoms or behavior they observed, and the defendant's self-report of symptoms and disclosed motivation. An assessment of the defendant's affect at the time is based on:

- Whether the defendant was able to use cognitive processing and reasoning ability.
- Whether the defendant was using drugs.
- The presence of a medical condition.
- The social context of the crime.
- Any causation explanation offered by the defendant.

After the collection of data and the interview, the forensic examiner applies legal standards to the data. This includes local jurisdiction statutes and state law, as well as definitions of mental state, legal sanity, and competency.

Professional Qualities of a Forensic Examiner

As a forensic examiner, you must be able to verbalize an exceptional understanding of major mental illnesses and personality disorders. You must keep abreast of theories being developed on social deviancy and interpersonal violence, and keep current on social trends (for example, changes in drug use, growth of gang activity, or cult participation) both nationally and in your own jurisdiction.

The successful forensic examiner is able to:

- Separate personal opinion from professional opinion. *Personal opinion is based on your background, upbringing, education, and values. Professional opinion is based on scientific principle, advanced education in a specific field of endeavor, and the unbiased standards set by research in that area.*
- Isolate personal feelings in dealing with cases of criminal violence. *Sexual deviance, ethnic norms, or cultural behaviors that may not reflect your own personal value system may be integral to the questioning.*

Determining Legal Sanity

Legal sanity differs from *clinical sanity,* which is the absence of a major mental disorder. **Legal sanity** is defined as an individual's ability to know right from wrong with reference to the act charged, the capacity to know the nature and quality of the act charged, and the capacity to form the intent to commit the crime. Legal sanity is determined for the specific time of the act, as determined by the court order. It may be the brief period of a physical assault or the length of a crime spree over several days.

In most states, the presence of a major mental disorder is a prerequisite for a finding of legal insanity. State insanity laws may have wording variations, but will cite the "presence of mental disorder or defect." Either can be used toward a finding of legal insanity. The term *mental disorder* usually refers to a major mental illness, while *mental defect* usually refers to developmental disability or some physiologic condition affecting cognition, such as a head injury, brain tumor, or dementia. Examples of mental disorders that may trigger an insanity defense include schizophrenia, mania, delusional disorders, posttraumatic stress disorder, amnesia or dissociation, and addiction.

The forensic examiner must be alert for possible malingering of a mental illness. **Malingering** a mental illness (intentionally producing false or exaggerated psychological symptoms) is not uncommon. *The Diagnostic and Statistical Manual of Mental Disorders*, published by the American Psychiatric Association (APA), states that facing a forensic evaluation is a strong indicator for suspecting the malingering of a mental illness (APA, 2000).

The burden of proving legal insanity is on the defense. Proof of criminal guilt must be determined "beyond a reasonable doubt" (i.e., it is about 90% to 95% likely that the defendant committed the act). The need for civil commitment in mental health law is based on "clear, cogent, and convincing" evidence (somewhere between 51 and 90%, usually around 75%). Legal insanity is determined by "a preponderance of the evidence" (at least 51%).

It is extremely important that the forensic nurse specialist have a clear knowledge of which legal standard is being used in the jurisdiction where the case is being heard, and be able to articulate its meaning in the courtroom. The legal standards most commonly used are discussed below.

M'Naghten Rule. In most jurisdictions, the determination of legal sanity is based on the *M'Naghten Rule,* which was the result of a famous case in England.

CLINICAL EXAMPLE

Daniel M'Naghten was a Scottish carpenter who believed that Jesuits and Tories were tormenting him. He told his family that spies for the government were following him and laughing at him. He was evicted from his boarding house because of his bizarre behavior. In 1843 he stalked Prime Minister Sir Robert Peel, eventually shot Peel's secretary, and was charged with the death. Nine psychiatrists testified at the trial (three for the defense, three for the prosecution, and three who listened to the evidence and observed M'Naghten's behavior in the courtroom). All nine agreed M'Naghten suffered from monomania (probably paranoid schizophrenia today) and was not legally sane, according to the legal tests at the time. The jury huddled in the courtroom for two minutes and then found him to be legally insane. He was sent to the local mental institution, Bethlehem Hospital. The public was outraged, believing hospitalization to be too lenient. The queen ordered a task force in the House of Lords to review the case and come up with a new legal standard.

Although the M'Naghten Rule was not applied in this famous case, it was a result of its conclusion.

Irresistible Impulse. A volitional component was added to the cognitive component of the M'Naghten Rule in 1929. This became known as the Irresistible Impulse test, which holds that a defendant is exculpated (freed from blame) even if the defendant knew the criminal act was wrong but could not restrain his conduct because of mental disease or defect. A modern interpretation of the standard is known as *The Policeman at the Elbow Test.* That is, would the defendant have committed the act had he known he was being observed by a police officer?

American Law Institute Model Penal Code. The Model Penal Code was approved in 1962 to serve as a guide for states wishing to reform their criminal law. It suggests that a person is not responsible for criminal conduct if, at the time of such conduct, the person, because of mental disease or mental defect, lacked substantial capacity either to appreciate the criminality (wrongfulness) of his conduct or to conform his conduct to the requirements of the law. The code specifies that the terms *mental disease* and *mental defect* do not include abnormal thinking that is manifested by only repeated criminal or otherwise antisocial conduct. The intent of the wording was to preclude the use of personality or character disorders in an insanity defense.

Guilty But Mentally Ill. The insanity defense periodically comes under fire from a public who believes that it is too lenient a response to violence. Some states have opted to use another option—guilty but mentally ill—in which the defendant's psychotic state is acknowledged, and the defendant receives court-ordered treatment. Once stable, the defendant is transferred to a prison for the remainder of the sentence.

Legal Insanity Defense

A legal insanity defense is a choice. The following are examples of the many reasons why an insanity defense is raised:

1. Presence of or history of mental illness

CLINICAL EXAMPLE

Carolyn has a 12-year history of bipolar disorder and noncompliance with medication after discharge from a hospital. Two weeks prior to the alleged offense, she began having difficulty sleeping, her behavior became erratic, and she spent most nights walking up and down the streets in her neighborhood. Two nights ago she was observed removing items from garages and painting driveways with colorful rainbows. She has been charged with burglary and malicious mischief.

2. Depression with suicidality

CLINICAL EXAMPLE

Martin became despondent over his loss of employment when the plant in which he worked closed. Financial stress led to marital problems, and his wife left him last month. Upon receiving notice that she had filed for divorce and custody of their two children, he began drinking heavily and firing random rifle shots over the neighbor's house. He ruminates on how he would rather be dead than alive without his children. He curses his own cowardice for not committing suicide. When the police arrive, Martin fires at them in an attempt to force them to shoot him. He is later charged with six counts of first-degree assault (Mohandie & Meloy, 2000).

3. Developmental disability

CLINICAL EXAMPLE

Zoë has been tested and determined to have an IQ of 64. At age 38, she still lives in her elderly parents' basement. One day, Zoë walked upstairs to find her mother nonresponsive on the couch and attempted to care for her by swaddling her in warm blankets. Her mother died of asphyxia, and the prosecutor charged Zoë with negligent homicide.

4. Sexual deviancy

CLINICAL EXAMPLE

Hank estimates that he has molested approximately 250 children prior to this, his first arrest. He recounts his own abuse history beginning at age eight.

5. Dissociative states, including a claim of multiple personality

CLINICAL EXAMPLE

Kathy entered the interview room clutching a small stuffed animal and a palm-size Bible. She explained that she had 34 personalities, and that any "bad acts" were committed by an evil personality, Mordred.

6. Medical issues

CLINICAL EXAMPLE

The lone gunman climbed the tower in the center of the university campus and systematically began shooting at students below. He was finally shot by a police sniper. On autopsy, it was discovered that he had a small brain tumor.

7. Munchausen syndrome by proxy

CLINICAL EXAMPLE

Unbeknownst to Diana, her infant had been placed in a special hospital room outfitted with microcameras. Videotape caught Diana attempting to smother the baby for up to a minute before nurses entered the room and intervened. Diana was later charged with attempted homicide. Her attorney explained that Diana was overwhelmed with a need for attention (Morrision, 1999).

8. Medication

CLINICAL EXAMPLE

Eight members of the high school wrestling team were arrested on charges of sexual assault following the gang-rape of a 14-year-old female. Two of the boys reported that the coach had pressured them into taking steroids.

9. Personality disorder

CLINICAL EXAMPLE

Recently released from prison on parole, John contacts his old friend Paul for a place to stay. To celebrate his release, John and Paul get drunk and high, then decide to steal a convertible for an overnight joyride to Seattle. "I just don't understand it," John explained, "Every time I get out of prison, I get into trouble."

Diminished Capacity

Diminished capacity is an element of the insanity law that refers to the defendant's capacity to form the intent to commit a specific act. There are four levels of intent—purposely, knowingly, recklessly, or negligently—and a court may order an evaluation specific to one level, depending on the degree of crime charged. A finding of diminished capacity is based on legal criteria in each state. In Washington State the cause of the inability to form intent must be a mental disorder, not amounting to insanity, and not emotions like jealousy, fear, anger, or hatred. The mental disorder must be causally connected to the lack of specific intent, not just reduced perception, awareness, understanding, or overreaction.

It is not uncommon for a defendant who is intoxicated on drugs or alcohol at the time of the offense to enter a plea of diminished capacity, especially if a blackout occurred. However, having a blackout implies that one cannot remember, not that one was unable to make decisions at the time. While it is true that a person's sensibilities are numbed and judgment impaired while intoxicated, altering one's own cognition voluntarily with drugs or alcohol does not excuse criminal behavior. Many states have case law stipulating that voluntary consumption or intoxication precludes this defense. However, should a person be drugged involuntarily and commit a criminal act while under the influence, the behavior may be excused. The following clinical examples illustrate this difference in two different scenarios:

CLINICAL EXAMPLE

Scenario 1

Wayne was invited to the first party of the year and wanted to make a charming impression on the new woman in town. He decided that a couple of drinks at home before he left would help loosen him up. At the party he took part in several of the drinking contests, hoping to catch her eye. Three hours later, he was not sure where he was, but he felt very sure that he had been insulted. He became angry. Undaunted by cries for him to stop, Wayne began breaking furniture to prove how he had been wronged. Waking up in jail to find he had been arrested for $5,000 worth of damage, Wayne blurted out, "How can they hold me responsible for something I don't remember doing?"

Scenario 2

The new woman invited Wayne to the first party of the year. He didn't really know most of the people who would be going, but he *wanted to be part of her crowd. Wayne was not aware that someone had laced the punch with several hits of acid, and he would not have had any punch had he known. Wayne did not use drugs and had no inclination to begin. After drinking several glasses, Wayne began to panic. He believed himself to be under attack and began breaking furniture apart to protect himself. Several hours later he awoke in jail. His attorney later explained why he would not be found criminally responsible for the $5,000 worth of damage.*

MediaLink Care Plan: Competency Therapy

COMPETENCY THERAPIST

No person may be tried if he is incompetent. The conviction of an incompetent defendant is a violation of the Fourteenth Amendment—the right to due process. Therefore, a court will remand the incompetent defendant to a "suitable facility" (usually a locked unit in a mental hospital) for treatment to regain competency. Since courts have held that defendants cannot be hospitalized or incarcerated indefinitely, court orders will stipulate a specific period of time in which the defendant is given treatment (*Jackson v. Indiana*, 1972).

Traditionally, treatment for incompetence meant little more than the prescribing of antipsychotic or other medications. With registered nurses moving into this role, a more holistic approach is being taken—one that encompasses the client's physical, emotional, and spiritual needs. Psychiatric forensic nursing role functions for the competency therapist include:

- Administration of assessment tools.
- Assessment of competence and mental disorder.
- Forensic interview.
- Documentation of client's progress toward competence.
- Completion of formal report to court.
- Expert witness testimony.

The Using Research Evidence feature demonstrates the application of the competency therapist role.

Competency therapists work with the defendant on one-to-one and group levels. An initial assessment of problem areas, based on the 13 items in the McGarry checklist, discussed later in the chapter, will identify the barriers to the defendant's competence. It is important that the competency therapist retains objectivity and does not confuse this type of education/training with psychotherapy. The focus of the relationship needs to be on the defendant's thinking and behavior at the time of the crime, not, for instance, the defendant's history of abuse or failed interpersonal relationships. Competency therapists realize that their client is still the court and that the product is a competent defendant and completed report. Competency therapists who advocate for the defendant, rather than for the process, need to reassess their ability to keep boundaries clear

USING RESEARCH EVIDENCE

Ramon is a 22-year-old male from Malaysia here on a student visa. He has been admitted to the forensic unit for evaluation of competence to proceed following his arrest on charges of unlawful imprisonment and second-degree assault. He has been accused of stalking and harassing a female coed for several weeks, then breaking into her apartment with a gun and not allowing her to leave. Her roommate called the police and a standoff ensued, during which Ramon threatened to shoot himself.

During the evaluation period, Ramon secluded himself in his room and socialized little with others. He placed several long-distance calls to his father in Malaysia and expressed regret and sorrow over losing his government-sponsored scholarship and the inevitability of deportation. Although he has denied feeling depressed, staff members noted that Ramon has missed several meals, claiming to be fasting.

Davilla, the nurse providing competency therapy, notes that Ramon has refused to attend classes and groups, stating that the outcome of his case was predetermined and there was no reason to discuss his legal options. When Davilla suggests speaking to the psychiatrist about antidepressant medication, Ramon states that he is not willing to take any medication. There has been some indication that Ramon would prefer not to be assigned to female staff members.

Davilla agrees to meet with Ramon individually, but sets the expectation that he attend competency classes, even if he chooses not to participate. She establishes that it will be necessary that he speak to her because of the court order. She explains the law committing him to the forensic unit, and what will need to be accomplished before he can be returned to court.

Davilla contacts the hospital chaplain to request an inservice program for the staff on Islam and the annual tradition of Ramadan. She differentiates the symptoms of depression from his cultural and religious practices and understands stalking as pathology of attachment, the core issue of which is "a poor style" of attachment by the stalker.

During their sessions together, she explores Ramon's perception of his relationship with the alleged victim. Davilla allows him to discuss "the relationship" through his point of view and value system. He recounts, "We were friends since we were children. When we were seven, our parents agreed that we would marry. I had other college choices, but I came here to be with her. In the beginning, everything was fine. We continued to see each other in Malaysian student group activities. Then she started having American friends. She let the men touch her in public. She forgot that she was to be married to me. I didn't want to hurt her, but I had to make her see that she had to follow our families' wishes. What I did was my right."

As communication and understanding grow, Davilla is able to discuss with Ramon the cultural differences in his upbringing and the law. With the guidance of his attorney, he is able to cooperate and is returned to court as competent to proceed.

Davilla's evaluation was based on the following studies:

Del Ben, K., Fremouw, W. (2002). Stalking: Developing an empirical typology to classify stalkers. *Journal of Forensic Sciences, 47*(1), 152–158.

Fisher B. S., Cullen F. T, & Turner, M. G. (2002). Being pursued: Stalking victimization in a national study of college women. *Criminology & Public Policy, 1*(2), 257–308.

(Jacobson, 2002) and should perform some introspection and seek supervision for countertransference issues (see Chapter 28).

Competence to Proceed

While legal insanity is a test of culpability, competence to proceed, that is, to stand trial, is an issue of triability. It is defined as having the capacity to assist one's attorney and to understand the proceedings. Forensic psychology has described competency as the most important mental health inquiry pursued in the criminal law system. An estimated 24,000 to 60,000 defendants are evaluated annually in the United States (Poythress, Hoge, Bonnie, Monahan, & Eisenberg, 2001). The legal standard for most jurisdictions is based on the federal case of *Dusky v. United States* (1960), which decided competence on the basis of whether or not the defendant has "sufficient present ability to consult with his lawyer with a reasonable degree of rational understanding and whether he has a rational and factual understanding of the proceedings against him."

Not only does legal sanity differ from competence to proceed in definition (see ■ Table 35–3), but also in time frame:

1. Legal sanity is determined for a point in time in the *past,* at the moment of the crime.
2. Competence is a determination for the *future,* at the time of the defendant's hearing or trial.

Since competence to stand trial is a determination of mental state in the future, the defendant's competency must be determined anew each time he goes to court. A prior finding of incompetence, even when due to developmental disability, does not preclude a subsequent finding of competency in a later, unrelated case.

Developmental disability does not preclude competence to stand trial. There are many forms of disability affecting different cognitive functions: attention span, ability to read and comprehend, memory, and abstract reasoning. Each function would be addressed in the evaluation and the weight given to each determined by the court.

A history of chronic mental illness also does not preclude competence to stand trial (*Feuger v. United States,* 1962), and neither does the existence of mental illness symptoms at the time of the trial. The presence of delusions may or may not have an impact. It depends on whether the delusion is related to the courtroom, the crime, or the proceedings. The specific content of the delusion, and the degree to which the symptoms affect the abilities and skills needed to be competent, are what are important.

The 13 criteria of the McGarry Checklist, identified in the Assessment box on page 830, are the national standard for determining competence to proceed. The court may weigh each item differently, or selectively weigh items differently for individual defendants. It is the responsibility of the forensic examiner or competency therapist to assess the defendant on all the issues and report to the court with substantiated data, not "just a gut feeling."

Occasionally, the court will request an evaluation on a specific competency issue, such as whether a defendant is competent to act as his or her own attorney. To waive the right to representation requires a higher level of competence than that required to stand trial. Other specific evaluations include whether a defendant is competent to give the confession, competent to be sentenced, or competent to receive the death penalty.

EXPERT WITNESS

By license, any registered nurse can be subpoenaed to court as a fact witness. In this role, you testify as to what you personally saw, heard, performed, or documented related to a particular client's care. You are questioned as to these firsthand experiences, and then excused from the courtroom.

An expert witness is recognized by the court as having a high level of skill or expertise in a designated area in order to render an opinion on a legal matter in court. As an expert witness, you will be subpoenaed to court to testify on your involvement with the defendant. You will testify as to the role functions you performed and to your documentation. At this point, the court will allow you to give additional testimony in the form of your professional opinion, based on your conclusions, as to the defendant's legal sanity, competence to proceed, future dangerousness, or likelihood of committing future felonious acts. It is an expansion of the nurse's scope of practice to function as an expert in a court of law alongside surgeons, clinical psychologists, psychiatrists, and others.

Once you take the stand, you will undergo a three-step process before being allowed to testify as an expert. The attorney will ask you questions regarding your training, education, and specialized knowledge. You answer the questions, and the judge concludes your acceptability as an expert. It is valuable to have your curriculum vitae prepared in advance. Copies for the attorneys or court should be available.

TABLE 35–3 Legal Sanity and Competence to Proceed

Elements	Legal Sanity	Competence to Proceed
Legal test	Culpability	Triability
Time frame	In the past, at the time of the act	In the future, at the time of the hearing/trial
Definition	The capacity to assist one's attorney, to understand the proceedings	Ability to know right from wrong, capacity to form intent to commit the crime

ASSESSMENT McGarry Checklist of Competency Issues

1. **Appraisal of available legal defenses:** The defendant's awareness of possible legal defenses and how consistent these are with the reality of the defendant's circumstances.
2. **Unmanageable behavior:** The appropriateness of the current motor and verbal behavior of the defendant and the degree to which this behavior would disrupt the conduct of a trial.
3. **Quality of relating to attorney.** Interpersonal capacity of the defendant to relate to the average attorney.
4. **Planning of legal strategy including guilty pleas to lesser charges where pertinent:** Degree to which the defendant can understand, participate, and cooperate with counsel in planning a strategy for the defense that is consistent with the reality of the circumstances.
5. **Appraisal of role of principals in the courtroom:** The defendant's understanding of the role of the defense counsel, prosecuting attorney, judge, jury, defendant, and witnesses.
6. **Understanding of court procedure:** Degree to which the defendant understands the basic sequence of events in a trial and their import.
7. **Appreciation of charges:** The defendant's understanding of the charges and their seriousness.
8. **Appreciation of range and nature of possible penalties:** The defendant's understanding of restrictions which could be imposed and their possible duration.
9. **Appraisal of likely outcome:** How realistically the defendant perceives the likely outcome and the degree to which impaired understanding contributes to a less adequate or inadequate participation in own defense.
10. **Capacity to disclose to attorney available pertinent facts surrounding the offense:** The defendant's capacity to give a basically consistent, rational, and relevant account of the motivational and external facts.
11. **Capacity to realistically challenge prosecution witnesses:** The defendant's capacity to recognize distortions in prosecution testimony.
12. **Capacity to testify relevantly:** The defendant's ability to testify with coherence, relevance, and independence of judgment.
13. **Self-defeating vs. Self-serving motivation:** The defendant's motivation to adequately protect self and appropriately utilize legal safeguards to this end.

Source: Adapted from Ackerman, M. (1999). *Essentials of forensic psychological assessment*. New York: John Wiley & Sons. This material is used by permission of John Wiley & Sons, Inc.

To establish credibility as an expert and to have one's opinion given equal weight in court opposite a psychiatrist, the forensic nurse specialist must have expertise, trustworthiness, and presentational style. These characteristics are described in Box 35–2.

Expertise is established by your credentials. Trustworthiness is the degree of honesty exuded in your demeanor and opinion, as perceived by the judge or jury. Presentation style is how you come across to others. You may be credible, trustworthy, and an authority in a specialty area, but without the ability to communicate in a concise and convincing fashion, the value of your testimony is limited.

BOX 35–2 Establishing Credibility as an Expert Witness

Credentials

- Academic background
- Professional training
- Experience
- Membership in professional associations

Trustworthiness

- Honesty
- Objectivity

Presentation Style

- Dress and demeanor
- Ability to communicate to a jury

CONSULTANT TO ATTORNEYS

Psychiatric forensic nurses may be used as a resource for education and information about mental illness by either side of the courtroom. Or you may be asked to attend the hearing as a courtroom observer who listens to other witness testimony for the purpose of guiding further cross-examination. You may also be asked to assist in preparation for trial by giving information about mental illness, personality disorders, or paraphilias. You may be asked to testify regarding mental health treatment options, medications, and community resources.

CONSULTANT TO LAW ENFORCEMENT

Interagency cooperation between mental health agencies and law enforcement has increased over the last decades, partly due to community need caused by deinstitutionalization. The mental health personnel summoned in those situations function as advocates for the defendant, whose well-being is the focus of the interaction that may result in civil detention and admission to a hospital. Community mental health nurses have traditionally acted in this role.

Psychiatric forensic nurses are expanding their scope of practice by working as consultants to law enforcement in hostage negotiation and criminal profiling. These roles differ from that described above in purpose and philosophy.

Hostage Negotiation

In the late 1970s, the Federal Bureau of Investigation began expanding hostage negotiation team structure by recommending the use of consultants who could address the mental state of the perpetrator and recommend appropriate negotiation strategies. In the next decade, local police agencies began to develop specialized teams and use consultants. Police agencies that use a consultant in hostage incidents reported significantly more negotiated surrenders, significantly fewer incidents ending with tactical team assaults, and fewer incidents in which the perpetrator killed or seriously injured a hostage (Slatkin, 2000).

When functioning as a behavioral sciences expert, the role of the psychiatric forensic nurse on a hostage negotiation team differs markedly from that of the community mental health nurse. You are not an advocate of the perpetrator, but of the process of hostage negotiation. Duties within this role are listed in Box 35–3.

Over half of all hostage incidents involve hostage-takers who are classified in law enforcement as mentally disturbed. This includes persons with thought, mood, or personality disorders. While it is essential for the consultant to be knowledgeable about mental illness, it is more important to have a clear understanding of the purpose of the negotiation process. The successful consultant needs to be able to:

- Think clearly while under stress.
- Possess emotional maturity.
- Have the ability to communicate with persons from all socioeconomic classes.
- Demonstrate common sense and be "streetwise."
- Cope with uncertainty (time, location, weather, outcome).
- Be willing to accept responsibility with no authority.
- Express commitment to the negotiation process.

It is essential to clearly understand the potential role in any plan to assault during a rescue. It is also essential that the consultant receives the same negotiator training as the officers.

Criminal Profiling

Psychiatric forensic nurses working with law enforcement may be asked to participate in the part of an investigation now formally known as Criminal Investigative Analysis. This will occur only after you have established your credibility as a forensic practitioner in your specialty area. Formerly known as criminal profiling, it is no substitute for a thorough and well-planned investigation and is only one tool among many that law enforcement uses to eliminate suspects or to narrow leads. Criminal profiling is an educated attempt to provide law enforcement with specific information on the type of individual who would have committed a certain crime after studying behavioral and psychological indicators left at a violent crime scene (O'Toole, 1999).

Profilers come from a variety of backgrounds—law enforcement, psychology, psychiatry, criminal justice, sociology, and now, forensic nursing. While a background in behavioral science is fundamental, and an understanding of psychopathology necessary, other specialized education is not as important as having investigative experience.

The profiler will collect all of the data, attempt to reconstruct the situation, formulate a hypothesis, develop a profile, test it, and check for results. As ■ Figure 35–1 illustrates, the method of developing a profile is similar to the nursing process. In testing the hypothesis, skilled profilers isolate their own emotions and attempt to reconstruct the crime using the criminal's reasoning process (Fintzy, 2000). If you attempt to analyze the situation based on your own values or logic, you will misinterpret the criminal's behavior. A skilled profiler is patient. By not jumping to conclusions, your opinion is slowly formed based on an examination of the data.

In addition to consulting during an investigation, the psychiatric forensic nurse may be asked by law enforcement for suggestions on how to interview a subject. A prosecutor may ask for suggestions in cross-examining a defendant.

BOX 35–3 Duties of Consultant to Hostage Negotiation Team

- Availability for 24-hour response with a Special Weapons and Tactics team (SWAT), tactical teams, or patrol officers on the scene
- Consultation regarding negotiation techniques
- Assessment of perpetrator's mental status
- Liaison with mental health agencies
- Participation in postincident critique
- Assessment of released hostages
- Assessment of hostage negotiator stress
- Communication skill training of law enforcement officers

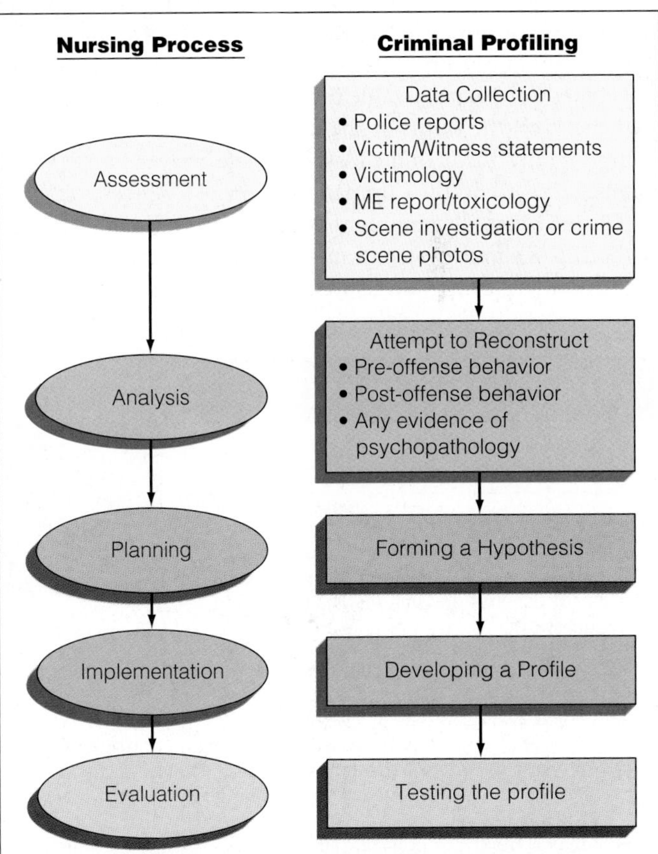

FIGURE 35–1 ■ *Criminal profiling process compared with the nursing process.*

MediaLink Forensic Associations

MediaLink International Association of Forensic Nurses

Professionalism in the Role

The psychiatric forensic nurse must be highly skilled in interpersonal relations and communication. Developing collegial relationships with other disciplines is central to the role because of the intersections of practice that overlap with the domain of other disciplines.

You should not practice in this area if you hold a narrow conceptualization of the issues facing clients, if you are motivated by punishment (Evans, 2000), or if you perceive motivation primarily within a cause-and-effect framework. You must be accepting of others' values and not attempt to supplant your own in your interactions with the defendant. Answering the questions in the Nursing Self-Awareness feature below will help you to determine whether you can maintain the high standards necessary for ethical forensic psychiatric nursing practice.

PROFESSIONAL CREDIBILITY

Traditionally, the role of forensic examiner has been confined to the scope of practice of the psychiatrist or psychologist. The prerequisite to the expanded role of a forensic examiner by a forensic nurse specialist is educational preparation and experience. A graduate degree, with additional training in forensic nursing, will add professional credibility. Several colleges and universities offer degree programs as well as certification courses in forensic subspecialities. The International Association of Forensic Nurses (IAFN) is at work on certification examinations for forensic nurses. To date, testing has been developed for sexual assault nurse examiner certification. You can check on the status of the development of other certification programs through the IAFN Web site, www.iafn.org, which can be accessed on the Companion Website for this book.

Clinical role development requires not only skill in data gathering in a multisystem framework, but also critical thinking skills in interpreting and using information for problem solving. Credibility is substantiated by membership or certification in such organizations as the IAFN, the American Academy of Forensic Sciences (www.aafs.org), and the American College of Forensic Examiners (www.acfe.org) which has a board of forensic nurse examiners. The forensic nurse specialist is encouraged to seek board certification in areas previously represented only by psychiatrists or psychologists. Such data can be found on the Companion Website for this text.

Forensic nursing is predicated on a search for truth. The search for justice is left to the court. Because forensic nurses are not tools for the prosecution, it is very important that psychiatric forensic nurses hold firmly to professional ethics. Those that provide expert witness services should never be viewed as "hired guns"—individuals who provide agreed-upon testimony for a price. You will find pride in the integrity of your professional opinion when you do not sacrifice truth for the sake of persuasion.

> ***Nursing* SELF-AWARENESS**
>
> **Ethical Forensic Psychiatric Nursing Practice**
>
> 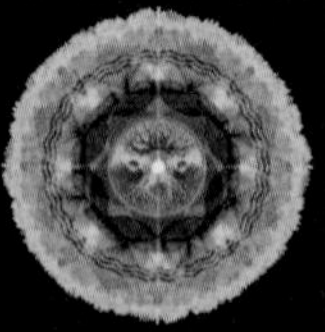
>
> Maintaining the high standards of a forensic professional in order to provide accurate and objective court-ordered evaluations, while protecting yourself, depends on your answers to the following questions.
>
> - Are your professional opinions based on scientific principle, knowledge, education, training, and experience?
> - Do you avoid conflicts of interest and advocacies?
> - Is continuing your professional development a priority for you?
> - Do you understand that establishing clear boundaries creates an atmosphere of safety and predictability within which treatment can thrive?
> - Are you cognizant of when self-disclosure may reverse the roles?
> - Do you acknowledge feelings of countertransference and seek out clinical supervision?

PERSONAL SAFETY

You must attend to your personal safety. The interactions you will have with perpetrators or defendants are usually involuntary on their part. They most likely did not seek out your services and will not be happy to see you. While it may be true that all of us are capable of committing a crime given the right circumstances and that not all criminals are dangerous people, you will meet some who are.

In working with violent perpetrators, predators, and those who are just mean for the sake of continuing a lifetime of threatening, intimidating, harassing behavior, it will be a natural occurrence to be fearful—for yourself, for your family, for your property. You need to acknowledge this feeling when it occurs and be willing to talk about it.

Victim–Witness Notification

State departments of corrections provide victim–witness notification programs. These programs notify involved and interested parties when a violent offender, sex offender, or serious drug offender moves through the system. The forensic nurse specialist who has been a witness for the prosecution becomes eligible if the offender was found guilty. You are notified when the offender is approved for furlough from prison or work-release, approved for parole, completes the sentence, transfers from prison to work release or community supervision, escapes from custody, or is recaptured.

COMMUNITY ACTIVISM

Psychiatric forensic nurses strive to expand the influence of these pioneering roles by participating in public forums that address violence as a health care issue. You can become a catalyst and effect social change by participating on local, statewide, or national task forces examining needed changes in law. Examples of community activities in which you could participate include interagency work on a diversion program for mentally ill misdemeanants, drafting legislation toward changes in legal sanity commitment, and proposing legislation to allow prosecution of psychiatric inpatients for serious assault on staff.

There are also entrepreneurial opportunities available to psychiatric forensic nurses. Private businesses, schools, and medical facilities often request education or training or assessment for circumstances such as the potential for workplace or school violence.

CHALLENGES OF FORENSIC PSYCHIATRIC NURSING

Nursing is still a career predominantly held by females. Psychiatric forensic nursing overlaps into areas that are not only new for nursing, but also for women. Traits necessary to succeed in this area are autonomy and assertiveness. To work in forensic psychiatry, you must confront obstacles imposed by predominantly male systems and offenders and defendants, and learn to cope with dangerous situations and hostile environments. The challenges in this new area of forensic nursing are:

- Being identified as professional.
- Finding mentors.
- Breaking into traditionally male networks.
- Being viewed as having expert power.
- Working in a predominantly male atmosphere.
- Communicating in an effective manner.
- Understanding the potential for danger and threat of violence.

Psychiatric forensic nursing appeals to a particular type of nurse, male or female, who thrives on the opportunity to work in a stimulating intellectual environment, and who seeks out the opportunity to apply clinical skills to complex legal problems. An expanded role is as much a way of thinking as it is a set of role functions. Because nursing places such high value on tradition, challenges are made to those who push the boundaries. Individuals who meet the challenge are characteristically confident in their own knowledge and abilities and have strong convictions about the value of the far-reaching effects their practice can have on the profession of nursing.

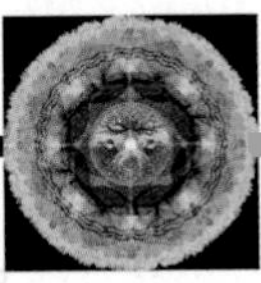

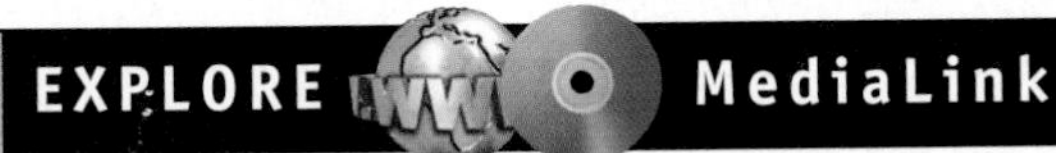

NCLEX review, case studies, and other interactive resources for this chapter can be found on the Companion Website at http://www.prenhall.com/kneisl. Click on Chapter 35 to select the activities for this chapter.

For animations, video tutorials, more NCLEX review questions, and an audio glossary, access the accompanying CD-ROM in this textbook.

BIBLIOGRAPHY

Ackerman, M. (1999). *Essentials of forensic psychological assessment*. New York: John Wiley & Sons.

American Nurses Association & International Association of Forensic Nurses. (1997). *Scope and standards of forensic nursing practice*. Washington, DC: American Nurses Publishing.

American Nurses Association. (1995). *Scope and standards of nursing practice in correctional facilities*. Washington, DC: Author.

American Psychiatric Association. (2000). *Diagnostic and statistical manual of mental disorders* (4th ed., Text Revision). Washington, DC: Author.

Coram, J. W. (1993). *Role development within a new subspecialty: Forensic nursing*. Thesis submitted for master's degree. Washington State University.

Del Ben, K., & Fremouw, W. (2002). Stalking: Developing an empirical typology to classify stalkers. *Journal of Forensic Sciences, 47*(1), 152–158.

Dusky v. United States, 362 U.S. 402 (1960).

Emiley, S. F. (2002). Forensic psychological evaluations: Back to basics. *The Forensic Examiner, 11*(1&2), 31–35.

Evans, M. (2000). Re-visioning nurses' punitive attitudes within forensic psychiatric and correctional nursing: The significance of ethical sophistication. *Journal of Psychosocial Nursing, 38*(4), 8–13.

Feuger v. United States, 302 F.2d 214 (1962).

Fintzy, R. T. (2000). Clinical profiling: An introduction to behavioral evidence analysis. *American Journal of Psychiatry, 157*(9), 1532–1555.

Fulton, D. R. (2000). Recognition and documentation of domestic violence in the clinical setting. *Critical Care Nursing Quarterly, 23*(2), 26–34.

Girardin, B. (2001). Is this forensic specialty for you? *RN, 64*(12), 37–41.

Goll-McGee, B. (1999). The role of the clinical forensic nurse in critical care, *Critical Care Nursing Quarterly, 22*(1), 8–18.

Hufft, A. (2000). The role of the forensic nurse in the USA. In Robinson, D., Kettles, A. (Eds.), *Forensic nursing and multidisciplinary care of the mentally disordered offender* (pp. 213–226). London: Jessica Kingsley Publishers.

Jackson v. Indiana, 406 U. S. 715 (1972).

Jacobson, G. A. (2002). Maintaining professional boundaries: Preparing nursing students for the challenge. *Journal of Nursing Education, 41*(6), 279–281.

Koss, M., & Hoffman, K. (2000). Survivors of violence by male partners: Gender and cultural considerations. In R. M. Eisler & M. Hersen (Eds.), *Handbook of gender, culture, and health* (pp. 471–490). Mahwah, NJ: Lawrence Erlbaum Associates.

Lorenzo, P. (2000). Distinguishing the legal nurse consultant. *Legal Assistant Today, 18*(1), 12–13.

Mohandie, K., & Meloy, J. R. (2000). Clinical and forensic indicators of "suicide by cop." *Journal of Forensic Sciences, 45*(2), 384–389.

Morrision, C. A. (1999). Cameras in hospital rooms: The fourth amendment to the constitution and Munchausen syndrome by proxy. *Critical Care Nursing Quarterly, 22*(1), 65–68.

Naegele T., & Clark, A. (2001). Forensic Munchausen syndrome by proxy: An emerging subspecies of child sexual abuse. *Forensic Examiner, 10*(3&4), 21–23.

O'Toole, M. E. (1999). Criminal profiling: The FBI uses criminal investigative analysis to solve crimes. *Corrections Today, 61*(1), 44–46.

Parrott, H. J. (2000). Stalking: evil, illness, or both? *International Journal of Clinical Practice, 54*(4), 239–242.

Peternelj-Taylor, C. (2000). The role of the forensic nurse in Canada. In Robinson, D., Kettles, A. (Eds.), *Forensic nursing and multidisciplinary care of the mentally disordered offender* (pp. 192–212). London: Jessica Kingsley Publishers.

Poythress, N., Hoge, S. K., Bonnie, R. J., Monahan, J., & Eisenberg, M. (2001). The MacArthur adjudicative competence study: Executive summary. *Behavioral Sciences and the Law, 15,* 329–345.

Rayel, M. G. (2000). Clinical and demographic characteristics of elderly offenders at a maximum-security forensic hospital. *Journal of Forensic Sciences, 45*(6), 1193–1196.

Saunders, L. (2000). Forensic nursing. *Australian Nursing Journal, 8*(3), 49–50.

Slatkin, A. A. (2000). The role of the mental health consultant in hostage negotiations: Questions to ask during the incident phase. *The Police Chief, 67*(7), 64.

Smoyak, S. A. (2000). Stalking: Ambiguous language can mask a crime. *Journal of Psychosocial Nursing and Mental Health Services, 38*(4), 6–7.

White, S. W. (2000). Elder abuse: Critical care nurse role in detection. *Critical Care Nursing Quarterly, 23*(2), 20–25.

Winfrey, M. E., & Smith, A. R. (1999). The suspiciousness factor: Critical care nursing and forensics. *Critical Care Nursing Quarterly, 22*(1), 1–7.

APPENDIX A

DSM-IV-TR CLASSIFICATION

NOS = Not Otherwise Specified

An *x* appearing in a diagnostic code indicates that a specific code number is required.

An ellipsis (. . .) is used in the names of certain disorders to indicate that the name of a specific mental disorder or general medical condition should be inserted when recording the name (e.g., 293.0 Delirium Due to Hypothyroidism).

If criteria are currently met, one of the following severity specifiers may be noted after the diagnosis:

Mild

Moderate

Severe

If criteria are no longer met, one of the following specifiers may be noted:

In Partial Remission

In Full Remission

Prior History

DISORDERS USUALLY FIRST DIAGNOSED IN INFANCY, CHILDHOOD, OR ADOLESCENCE

Mental Retardation

Note: *These are coded on Axis II.*
317 Mild Mental Retardation
318.0 Moderate Mental Retardation
318.1 Severe Mental Retardation
318.2 Profound Mental Retardation
319 Mental Retardation, Severity Unspecified

Learning Disorders

315.00 Reading Disorder
315.1 Mathematics Disorder
315.2 Disorder of Written Expression
315.9 Learning Disorder NOS

Motor Skills Disorder

315.4 Developmental Coordination Disorder

Communication Disorders

315.31 Expressive Language Disorder
315.32 Mixed Receptive-Expressive Language Disorder
315.39 Phonological Disorder
307.0 Stuttering
307.9 Communication Disorder NOS

Pervasive Developmental Disorders

299.00 Autistic Disorder
299.80 Rett's Disorder
299.10 Childhood Disintegrative Disorder
299.80 Asperger's Disorder
299.80 Pervasive Developmental Disorder NOS

Attention-Deficit and Disruptive Behavior Disorders

314.xx Attention-Deficit/Hyperactivity Disorder
.01 Combined Type
.00 Predominantly Inattentive Type
.01 Predominantly Hyperactive-Impulsive Type
314.9 Attention-Deficit/Hyperactivity Disorder NOS
312.xx Conduct Disorder
.81 Childhood-Onset Type
.82 Adolescent-Onset Type
.89 Unspecified Onset
313.81 Oppositional Defiant Disorder
312.9 Disruptive Behavior Disorder NOS

Feeding and Eating Disorders of Infancy or Early Childhood

307.52 Pica
307.53 Rumination Disorder
307.59 Feeding Disorder of Infancy or Early Childhood

Tic Disorders

307.23 Tourette's Disorder
307.22 Chronic Motor or Vocal Tic Disorder
307.21 Transient Tic Disorder
Specify if: Single Episode/Recurrent
307.20 Tic Disorder NOS

Elimination Disorders

_____.__ Encopresis
787.6 With Constipation and Overflow Incontinence
307.7 Without Constipation and Overflow Incontinence
307.6 Enuresis (Not Due to a General Medical Condition)
Specify type: Nocturnal Only/Diurnal Only/Nocturnal and Diurnal

Other Disorders of Infancy, Childhood, or Adolescence

309.21 Separation Anxiety Disorder
Specify if: Early Onset
313.23 Selective Mutism
313.89 Reactive Attachment Disorder of Infancy or Early Childhood
Specify type: Inhibited Type/Disinhibited Type
307.3 Stereotypic Movement Disorder
Specify if: With Self-Injurious Behavior
313.9 Disorder of Infancy, Childhood, or Adolescence NOS

DELIRIUM, DEMENTIA, AND AMNESTIC AND OTHER COGNITIVE DISORDERS

Delirium

293.0 Delirium Due to . . . *[Indicate the General Medical Condition]*
____.__ Substance Intoxication Delirium *(refer to Substance-Related Disorders for substance-specific codes)*
____.__ Substance Withdrawal Delirium *(refer to Substance-Related Disorders for substance-specific codes)*
____.__ Delirium Due to Multiple Etiologies *(code each of the specific etiologies)*
780.09 Delirium NOS

Dementia

294.xx* Dementia of the Alzheimer's Type, With Early Onset *(also code 331.0 Alzheimer's disease on Axis III)*
.10 Without Behavioral Disturbance
.11 With Behavioral Disturbance
294.xx* Dementia of the Alzheimer's Type, With Late Onset *(also code 331.0 Alzheimer's disease on Axis III)*
.10 Without Behavioral Disturbance
.11 With Behavioral Disturbance
290.xx Vascular Dementia
.40 Uncomplicated
.41 With Delirium
.42 With Delusions
.43 With Depressed Mood
Specify if: With Behavioral Disturbance
Code presence or absence of a behavioral disturbance in the fifth digit for Dementia Due to a General Medical Condition:
0 = Without Behavioral Disturbance
1 = With Behavioral Disturbance
294.1x* Dementia Due to HIV Disease *(also code 042 HIV on Axis III)*
294.1x* Dementia Due to Head Trauma *(also code 042 HIV on Axis III)*
294.1x* Dementia Due to Head Trauma *(also code 854.00 head injury on Axis III)*
294.1x* Dementia Due to Parkinson's Disease *(also code 332.0 Parkinson's disease on Axis III)*
294.1x* Dementia Due to Huntington's Disease *(also code 333.4 Huntington's disease on Axis III)*
294.1x* Dementia Due to Pick's Disease *(also code 331.1 Pick's disease on Axis III)*
294.1x* Dementia Due to Creutzfeldt–Jakob Disease *(also code 046.1 Creutzfeldt–Jakob disease on Axis III)*
294.1x* Dementia Due to . . . *[Indicate the General Medical Condition not listed above] (also code the general medical condition on Axis III)*
____.__ Substance-Induced Persisting Dementia *(refer to Substance-Related Disorders for substance-specific codes)*
____.__ Dementia Due to Multiple Etiologies *(code each of the specific etiologies)*
294.8 Dementia NOS

Amnestic Disorders

294.0 Amnestic Disorder Due to . . . *[Indicate the General Medical Condition]*
Specify if: Transient/Chronic
____.__ Substance-Induced Persisting Amnestic Disorder *(refer to Substance-Related Disorders for substance-specific codes)*
294.8 Amnestic Disorder NOS

Other Cognitive Disorders

294.9 Cognitive Disorder NOS

MENTAL DISORDERS DUE TO A GENERAL MEDICAL CONDITION NOT ELSEWHERE CLASSIFIED

293.89 Catatonic Disorder Due to . . . *[Indicate the General Medical Condition]*
310.1 Personality Change Due to . . . *[Indicate the General Medical Condition]*
Specify type: Labile Type/Disinhibited Type/Aggressive Type/Apathetic Type/Paranoid Type/Other Type/Combined Type/Unspecified Type
293.9 Mental Disorder NOS Due to . . . *[Indicate the General Medical Condition]*

SUBSTANCE-RELATED DISORDERS

The following specifiers apply to Substance Dependence as noted:
[a]With Physiological Dependence/Without Physiological Dependence
[b]Early Full Remission/Early Partial Remission/Sustained Full Remission/Sustained Partial Remission
[c]In a Controlled Environment
[d]On Agonist Therapy
The following specifiers apply to Substance-Induced Disorders as noted:
[I]With Onset During Intoxication/[W]With Onset During Withdrawal

Alcohol-Related Disorders

ALCOHOL USE DISORDERS

303.90 Alcohol Dependence[a,b,c]
305.00 Alcohol Abuse

ICD-9-CM code valid after October 1, 2000.

Alcohol-Induced Disorders

303.00 Alcohol Intoxication
291.81 Alcohol Withdrawal
Specify if: With Perceptual Disturbances
291.0 Alcohol Intoxication Delirium
291.0 Alcohol Withdrawal Delirium
291.2 Alcohol-Induced Persisting Dementia
291.1 Alcohol-Induced Persisting Amnestic Disorder
291.x Alcohol-Induced Psychotic Disorder
.5 With Delusions[I,W]
.3 With Hallucinations[I,W]
291.89 Alcohol-Induced Mood Disorder[I,W]
291.89 Alcohol-Induced Anxiety Disorder[I,W]
291.89 Alcohol-Induced Sexual Dysfunction[I]
291.89 Alcohol-Induced Sleep Disorder[I,W]
291.9 Alcohol-Related Disorder NOS

Amphetamine (or Amphetamine-Like)–Related Disorders

Amphetamine Use Disorders

304.40 Amphetamine Dependence[a,b,c]
305.70 Amphetamine Abuse

Amphetamine-Induced Disorders

292.89 Amphetamine Intoxication
Specify if: With Perceptual Disturbances
292.0 Amphetamine Withdrawal
292.81 Amphetamine Intoxication Delirium
292.xx Amphetamine-Induced Psychotic Disorder
.11 With Delusions[I]
.12 With Hallucinations[I]
292.84 Amphetamine-Induced Mood Disorder[I,W]
292.89 Amphetamine-Induced Anxiety Disorder[I]
292.89 Amphetamine-Induced Sexual Dysfunction[I]
292.89 Amphetamine-Induced Sleep Disorder[I,W]
292.9 Amphetamine-Related Disorder NOS

Caffeine-Related Disorders

Caffeine-Induced Disorders

305.90 Caffeine Intoxication
292.89 Caffeine-Induced Anxiety Disorder[I]
292.89 Caffeine-Induced Sleep Disorder[I]
292.9 Caffeine-Related Disorder NOS

Cannabis-Related Disorders

Cannabis Use Disorders

304.30 Cannabis Dependence[a,b,c]
305.20 Cannabis Abuse

Cannabis-Induced Disorders

292.89 Cannabis Intoxication
Specify if: With Perceptual Disturbance
292.81 Cannabis Intoxication Delirium
292.xx Cannabis-Induced Psychotic Disorder
.11 With Delusions[I]
.12 With Hallucinations[I]
292.89 Cannabis-Induced Anxiety Disorder[I]
292.9 Cannabis-Related Disorder NOS

Cocaine-Related Disorders

Cocaine Use Disorders

304.20 Cocaine Dependence[a,b,c]
305.60 Cocaine Abuse

Cocaine-Induced Disorders

292.89 Cocaine Intoxication
Specify if: With Perceptual Disturbances
292.0 Cocaine Withdrawal
292.81 Cocaine Intoxication Delirium
292.xx Cocaine-Induced Psychotic Disorder
.11 With Delusions[I]
.12 With Hallucinations[I]
292.84 Cocaine-Induced Mood Disorder[I,W]
292.89 Cocaine-Induced Anxiety Disorder[I,W]
292.89 Cocaine-Induced Sexual Dysfunction[I]
292.89 Cocaine-Induced Sleep Disorder[I,W]
292.9 Cocaine-Related Disorder NOS

Hallucinogen-Related Disorders

Hallucinogen Use Disorders

304.50 Hallucinogen Dependence[b,c]
305.30 Hallucinogen Abuse

Hallucinogen-Induced Disorders

292.89 Hallucinogen Intoxication
292.89 Hallucinogen Persisting Perception Disorder (Flashbacks)
292.81 Hallucinogen Intoxication Delirium
292.xx Hallucinogen-Induced Psychotic Disorder
.11 With Delusions[I]
.12 With Hallucinations[I]
292.84 Hallucinogen-Induced Mood Disorder[I]
292.89 Hallucinogen-Induced Anxiety Disorder[I]
292.9 Hallucinogen-Related Disorder NOS

Inhalant-Related Disorders

Inhalant Use Disorders

304.60 Inhalant Dependence[b,c]
305.90 Inhalant Abuse

Inhalant-Induced Disorders

292.89 Inhalant Intoxication
292.81 Inhalant Intoxication Delirium
292.82 Inhalant-Induced Persisting Dementia
292.xx Inhalant-Induced Psychotic Disorder
.11 With Delusions[I]
.12 With Hallucinations[I]
292.84 Inhalant-Induced Mood Disorder[I]
292.89 Inhalant-Induced Anxiety Disorder[I]
292.9 Inhalant-Related Disorder NOS

Nicotine-Related Disorders

Nicotine Use Disorder

305.1 Nicotine Dependence[a,b]

Nicotine-Induced Disorder

292.0 Nicotine Withdrawal
292.9 Nicotine-Related Disorder NOS

Opioid-Related Disorders

Opioid Use Disorders

304.00 Opioid Dependence[a,b,c,d]
305.50 Opioid Abuse

Opioid-Induced Disorders

292.89 Opioid Intoxication
Specify if: With Perceptual Disturbances
292.0 Opioid Withdrawal
292.81 Opioid Intoxication Delirium
292.xx Opioid-Induced Psychotic Disorder
.11 With Delusions[I]
.12 With Hallucinations[I]
292.84 Opioid-Induced Mood Disorder[I]
292.89 Opioid-Induced Sexual Dysfunction[I]
292.89 Opioid-Induced Sleep Disorder[I,W]
292.9 Opioid-Related Disorder NOS

Phencyclidine (or Phencyclidine-Like)–Related Disorders

Phencyclidine Use Disorders

304.60 Phencyclidine Dependence[b,c]
305.90 Phencyclidine Abuse

Phencyclidine-Induced Disorders

292.89 Phencyclidine Intoxication
Specify if: With Perceptual Disturbances
292.81 Phencyclidine Intoxication Delirium
292.xx Phencyclidine-Induced Psychotic Disorder
.11 With Delusions[I]
.12 With Hallucinations[I]
292.84 Phencyclidine-Induced Mood Disorder[I]
292.89 Phencyclidine-Induced Anxiety Disorder[I]
292.9 Phencyclidine-Related Disorder NOS

Sedative-, Hypnotic-, or Anxiolytic-Related Disorders

Sedative, Hypnotic, or Anxiolytic Use Disorders

304.10 Sedative, Hypnotic, or Anxiolytic Dependence[a,b,c]
305.40 Sedative, Hypnotic, or Anxiolytic Abuse

Sedative-, Hypnotic-, or Anxiolytic-Induced Disorders

292.89 Sedative, Hypnotic, or Anxiolytic Intoxication
292.0 Sedative, Hypnotic, or Anxiolytic Withdrawal
Specify if: With Perceptual Disturbances
292.81 Sedative, Hypnotic, or Anxiolytic Intoxication Delirium
292.81 Sedative, Hypnotic, or Anxiolytic Withdrawal Delirium
292.82 Sedative, Hypnotic, or Anxiolytic-Induced Persisting Dementia
292.83 Sedative-, Hypnotic-, or Anxiolytic-Induced Persisting Amnestic Disorder
292.xx Sedative-, Hypnotic-, or Anxiolytic-Induced Psychotic Disorder
.11 With Delusions[I,W]
.12 With Hallucinations[I,W]
292.84 Sedative-, Hypnotic-, or Anxiolytic-Induced Mood Disorder[I,W]
292.89 Sedative-, Hypnotic-, or Anxiolytic-Induced Anxiety Disorder[W]
292.89 Sedative-, Hypnotic-, or Anxiolytic-Induced Sexual Dysfunction[I]
292.89 Sedative-, Hypnotic, or Anxiolytic-Induced Sleep Disorder[I,W]
292.9 Sedative-, Hypnotic, or Anxiolytic-Related Disorder NOS

Polysubstance-Related Disorder

304.80 Polysubstance Dependence[a,b,c,d]

Other (or Unknown) Substance-Related Disorders

Other (or Unknown) Substance Use Disorders

304.90 Other (or Unknown) Substance Dependence[a,b,c,d]
305.90 Other (or Unknown) Substance Abuse

Other (or Unknown) Substance-Induced Disorders

292.89 Other (or Unknown) Substance Intoxication
Specify if: With Perceptual Disturbances
292.0 Other (or Unknown) Substance Withdrawal
Specify if: With Perceptual Disturbances
292.81 Other (or Unknown) Substance-Induced Delirium
292.82 Other (or Unknown) Substance-Induced Persisting Dementia
292.83 Other (or Unknown) Substance-Induced Persisting Amnestic Disorder
292.xx Other (or Unknown) Substance-Induced Psychotic Disorder
.11 With Delusions[I,W]
.12 With Hallucinations[I,W]
292.84 Other (or Unknown) Substance-Induced Mood Disorder[I,W]
292.89 Other (or Unknown) Substance-Induced Anxiety Disorder[I,W]
292.89 Other (or Unknown) Substance-Induced Sexual Dysfunction[I]
292.89 Other (or Unknown) Substance-Induced Sleep Disorder[I,W]
292.9 Other (or Unknown) Substance-Related Disorder NOS

Polysubstance-Related Disorder

304.80 Polysubstance Dependence[a,b,c,d]

Other (or Unknown) Substance-Related Disorders

Other (or Unknown) Substance Use Disorders

304.90 Other (or Unknown) Substance Dependence[a,b,c,d]
305.90 Other (or Unknown) Substance Abuse

Other (or Unknown) Substance-Induced Disorders

292.89 Other (or Unknown) Substance Intoxication
Specify if: With Perceptual Disturbances
292.0 Other (or Unknown) Substance Withdrawal
Specify if: With Perceptual Disturbances
292.81 Other (or Unknown) Substance-Induced Delirium
292.82 Other (or Unknown) Substance-Induced Persisting Dementia
292.83 Other (or Unknown) Substance-Induced Persisting Amnestic Disorder
292.xx Other (or Unknown) Substance-Induced Psychotic Disorder
.11 With Delusions[I,W]
.12 With Hallucinations[I,W]
292.84 Other (or Unknown) Substance-Induced Mood Disorder[I,W]
292.89 Other (or Unknown) Substance-Induced Anxiety Disorder[I,W]
292.89 Other (or Unknown) Substance-Induced Sexual Dysfunction[I]
292.89 Other (or Unknown) Substance-Induced Sleep Disorder[I,W]
292.9 Other (or Unknown) Substance-Related Disorder NOS

SCHIZOPHRENIA AND OTHER PSYCHOTIC DISORDERS

295.xx Schizophrenia
The following Classification of Longitudinal Course applies to all subtypes of Schizophrenia:
Episodic With Interepisode Residual Symptoms (*Specify if:* With Prominent Negative Symptoms)/Episodic With No Interepisode Residual Symptoms
Continuous (*Specify if:* With Prominent Negative Symptoms)
Single Episode in Partial Remission (*Specify if:* With Prominent Negative Symptoms)/Single Episode in Full Remission
Other or Unspecified Pattern
.30 Paranoid Type
.10 Disorganized Type
.20 Catatonic Type
.90 Undifferentiated Type
.60 Residual Type
295.40 Schizophreniform Disorder
Specify if: Without Good Prognostic Features/With Good Prognostic Features
295.70 Schizoaffective Disorder
Specify type: Bipolar Type/Depressive Type
297.1 Delusional Disorder
Specify type: Erotomanic Type/Grandiose Type/Jealous Type/Persecutory Type/Somatic Type/Mixed Type/Unspecified Type
298.8 Brief Psychotic Disorder
Specify if: With Marked Stressor(s)/Without Marked Stressor(s)/With Postpartum Onset
297.3 Shared Psychotic Disorder
293.xx Psychotic Disorder Due to . . . *[Indicate the General Medical Condition]*
.81 With Delusions
.82 With Hallucinations
_____.__ Substance-Induced Psychotic Disorder *(refer to Substance-Related Disorders for substance-specific codes)*
Specify if: With Onset During Intoxication/With Onset During Withdrawal
298.9 Psychotic Disorder NOS

MOOD DISORDERS

Code current state of Major Depressive Disorder or Bipolar I Disorder in fifth digit:
1 = Mild
2 = Moderate
3 = Severe Without Psychotic Features
4 = Severe With Psychotic Features
Specify: Mood-Congruent Psychotic Features/Mood-Incongruent Psychotic Features
5 = In Partial Remission
6 = In Full Remission
0 = Unspecified
The following specifiers apply (for current or most recent episode) to Mood Disorders as noted:
[a]Severity/Psychotic/Remission Specifiers/[b]Chronic/[c]With Catatonic Features/[d]With Melancholic Features/[e]With Atypical Features/[f]With Postpartum Onset
The following specifiers apply to Mood Disorders as noted:
[g]With or Without Full Interepisode Recovery/[h]With Seasonal Pattern/[i]With Rapid Cycling

Depressive Disorders

296.xx Major Depressive Disorder
.2x Single Episode[a,b,c,d,e,f]
.3x Recurrent[a,b,c,d,e,f,g,h]
300.4 Dysthymic Disorder
Specify if: Early Onset/Late Onset
Specify if: With Atypical Features
311 Depressive Disorder NOS

Bipolar Disorders

296.xx Bipolar I Disorder
.0x Single Manic Episode[a,c,f]
Specify if: Mixed
.40 Most Recent Episode Hypomanic[g,h,i]
.4x Most Recent Episode Manic[a,c,f,g,h,i]
.6x Most Recent Episode Mixed[a,c,f,g,h,i]
.5x Most Recent Episode Depressed[a,b,c,d,e,f,g,h,i]
.7 Most Recent Episode Unspecified[g,h,i]
296.89 Bipolar II Disorder[a,b,c,d,e,f,g,h,i]
Specify (current or most recent episode):
Hypomanic/Depressed
301.13 Cyclothymic Disorder
296.80 Bipolar Disorder NOS
293.83 Mood Disorder Due to . . . *[Indicate the General Medical Condition]*

Specify type: With Depressive Features/With Major Depressive-Like Episode/With Manic Features/With Mixed Features
_____.__ Substance-Induced Mood Disorder *(refer to Substance-Related Disorders for substance-specific codes)*
Specify type: With Depressive Features/With Manic Features/With Mixed Features
Specify if: With Onset During Intoxication/With Onset During Withdrawal
296.90 Mood Disorder NOS

Anxiety Disorders

300.01 Panic Disorder Without Agoraphobia
300.21 Panic Disorder With Agoraphobia
300.22 Agoraphobia Without History of Panic Disorder
300.29 Specific Phobia
Specify type: Animal Type/Natural Environment Type/Blood-Injection-Injury Type/Situational Type/Other Type
300.23 Social Phobia
Specify if: Generalized
300.3 Obsessive-Compulsive Disorder
Specify if: With Poor Insight
309.81 Posttraumatic Stress Disorder
Specify if: Acute/Chronic
Specify if: With Delayed Onset
308.3 Acute Stress Disorder
300.02 Generalized Anxiety Disorder
293.84 Anxiety Disorder Due to . . . *[Indicate the General Medical Condition]*
Specify if: With Generalized Anxiety/With Panic Attacks/With Obsessive-Compulsive Symptoms
_____.__ Substance-Induced Anxiety Disorder *(refer to Substance-Related Disorders for substance-specific codes)*
Specify if: With Generalized Anxiety/With Panic Attacks/With Obsessive-Compulsive Symptoms/With Phobic Symptoms
Specify if: With Onset During Intoxication/With Onset During Withdrawal
300.00 Anxiety Disorder NOS

SOMATOFORM DISORDERS

300.81 Somatization Disorder
300.82 Undifferentiated Somatoform Disorder
300.11 Conversion Disorder
Specify type: With Motor Symptom or Deficit/With Sensory Symptom or Deficit/With Seizures or Convulsions/With Mixed Presentation
307.xx Pain Disorder
.80 Associated With Psychological Factors
.89 Associated With Both Psychological Factors and a General Medical Condition
Specify if: Acute/Chronic
300.7 Hypochondriasis
Specify if: With Poor Insight
300.7 Body Dysmorphic Disorder
300.82 Somatoform Disorder NOS

Factitious Disorders

300.xx Factitious Disorder
.16 With Predominantly Psychological Signs and Symptoms
.19 With Predominantly Physical Signs and Symptoms
.19 With Combined Psychological and Physical Signs and Symptoms
300.19 Factitious Disorder NOS

Dissociative Disorders

300.12 Dissociative Amnesia
300.13 Dissociative Fugue
300.14 Dissociative Identity Disorder
300.6 Depersonalization Disorder
300.15 Dissociative Disorder NOS

Sexual and Gender Identity Disorders

Sexual Dysfunctions

The following specifiers apply to all primary Sexual Dysfunctions:
Lifelong Type/Acquired Type
Generalized Type/Situational Type
Due to Psychological Factors/Due to Combined Factors

Sexual Desire Disorders

302.71 Hypoactive Sexual Desire Disorder
302.79 Sexual Aversion Disorder

Sexual Arousal Disorders

302.72 Female Sexual Arousal Disorder
302.72 Male Erectile Disorder

Orgasmic Disorders

302.73 Female Orgasmic Disorder
302.74 Male Orgasmic Disorder
302.75 Premature Ejaculation

Sexual Pain Disorders

302.76 Dyspareunia (Not Due to a General Medical Condition)
306.51 Vaginismus (Not Due to a General Medical Condition)

Sexual Dysfunction Due to a General Medical Condition

625.8 Female Hypoactive Sexual Desire Disorder Due to . . . *[Indicate the General Medical Condition]*
608.89 Male Hypoactive Sexual Desire Disorder Due to . . . *[Indicate the General Medical Condition]*
607.84 Male Erectile Disorder Due to . . . *[Indicate the General Medical Condition]*
625.0 Female Dyspareunia Due to . . . *[Indicate the General Medical Condition]*
608.89 Male Dyspareunia Due to . . . *[Indicate the General Medical Condition]*
625.8 Other Female Sexual Dysfunction Due to . . . *[Indicate the General Medical Condition]*
608.89 Other Male Sexual Dysfunction Due to . . . *[Indicate the General Medical Condition]*

_____.__ Substance-Induced Sexual Dysfunction *(refer to Substance-Related Disorders for substance-specific codes)*
Specify if: With Impaired Desire/With Impaired Arousal/With Impaired Orgasm/With Sexual Pain
Specify if: With Onset During Intoxication
302.70 Sexual Dysfunction NOS

Paraphilias

302.4 Exhibitionism
302.81 Fetishism
302.89 Frotteurism
302.2 Pedophilia
Specify if: Sexually Attracted to Males/Sexually Attracted to Females/Sexually Attracted to Both
Specify if: Limited to Incest
Specify type: Exclusive Type/Nonexclusive Type
302.83 Sexual Masochism
302.84 Sexual Sadism
302.3 Transvestic Fetishism
Specify if: With Gender Dysphoria
302.82 Voyeurism
302.9 Paraphilia NOS

Gender Identity Disorders

302.xx Gender Identity Disorder
.6 in Children
.85 in Adolescents or Adults
Specify if: Sexually Attracted to Males/Sexually Attracted to Females/Sexually Attracted to Both/Sexually Attracted to Neither
302.6 Gender Identity Disorder NOS
302.9 Sexual Disorder NOS

EATING DISORDERS

307.1 Anorexia Nervosa
Specify type: Restricting Type; Binge-Eating/Purging Type
307.51 Bulimia Nervosa
Specify type: Purging Type/Nonpurging Type
307.50 Eating Disorder NOS

SLEEP DISORDERS

Primary Sleep Disorders

Dyssomnias

307.42 Primary Insomnia
307.44 Primary Hypersomnia
Specify if: Recurrent
347 Narcolepsy
780.59 Breathing-Related Sleep Disorder
307.45 Circadian Rhythm Sleep Disorder
Specify type: Delayed Sleep Phase Type/Jet Lag Type/Shift Work Type/Unspecified Type
307.47 Dyssomnia NOS

Parasomnias

307.47 Nightmare Disorder
307.46 Sleep Terror Disorder
307.46 Sleepwalking Disorder
307.47 Parasomnia NOS

Sleep Disorders Related to Another Mental Disorder

307.42 Insomnia Related to . . . *[Indicate the Axis I or Axis II Disorder]*
307.44 Hypersomnia Related to . . . *[Indicate the Axis I or Axis II Disorder]*

Other Sleep Disorders

780.xx Sleep Disorder Due to . . . *[Indicate the General Medical Condition]*
.52 Insomnia Type
.54 Hypersomnia Type
.59 Parasomnia Type
.59 Mixed Type
_____.__ Substance-Induced Sleep Disorder *(refer to Substance-Related Disorders for substance-specific codes)*
Specify type: Insomnia Type/Hypersomnia Type/Parasomnia Type/Mixed Type
Specify if: With Onset During Intoxication/With Onset During Withdrawal

IMPULSE-CONTROL DISORDERS NOT ELSEWHERE CLASSIFIED

312.34 Intermittent Explosive Disorder
312.32 Kleptomania
312.33 Pyromania
312.31 Pathological Gambling
312.39 Trichotillomania
312.30 Impulse-Control Disorder NOS

ADJUSTMENT DISORDERS

309.xx Adjustment Disorder
.0 With Depressed Mood
.24 With Anxiety
.28 With Mixed Anxiety and Depressed Mood
.3 With Disturbance of Conduct
.4 With Mixed Disturbance of Emotions and Conduct
.9 Unspecified
Specify if: Acute/Chronic

PERSONALITY DISORDERS

Note: *These are coded on Axis II.*
301.0 Paranoid Personality Disorder
301.20 Schizoid Personality Disorder
301.22 Schizotypal Personality Disorder
301.7 Antisocial Personality Disorder
301.83 Borderline Personality Disorder
301.50 Histrionic Personality Disorder
301.81 Narcissistic Personality Disorder
301.82 Avoidant Personality Disorder
301.6 Dependent Personality Disorder
301.4 Obsessive–Compulsive Personality Disorder
301.9 Personality Disorder NOS

OTHER CONDITIONS THAT MAY BE A FOCUS OF CLINICAL ATTENTION

Psychological Factors Affecting Medical Condition

316 . . . *[Specified Psychological Factor] Affecting . . . [Indicate the General Medical Condition]*
Choose name based on nature of factors:
Mental Disorder Affecting Medical Condition
Psychological Symptoms Affecting Medical Condition
Personality Traits or Coping Style Affecting Medical Condition
Maladaptive Health Behaviors Affecting Medical Condition
Stress-Related Physiological Response Affecting Medical Condition
Other or Unspecified Psychological Factors Affecting Medical Condition

Medication-Induced Movement Disorders

332.1 Neuroleptic-Induced Parkinsonism
333.92 Neuroleptic Malignant Syndrome
333.7 Neuroleptic-Induced Acute Dystonia
333.99 Neuroleptic-Induced Acute Akathisia
333.82 Neuroleptic-Induced Tardive Dyskinesia
333.1 Medication-Induced Postural Tremor
333.90 Medication-Induced Movement Disorder NOS

Other Medication-Induced Disorder

995.2 Adverse Effects of Medication NOS

Relational Problems

V61.9 Relational Problem Related to a Mental Disorder or General Medical Condition
V61.20 Parent–Child Relational Problem
V61.10 Partner Relational Problem
V61.8 Sibling Relational Problem
V62.81 Relational Problem NOS

Problems Related to Abuse or Neglect

V61.21 Physical Abuse of Child
(code 995.54 if focus of attention is on victim)
V61.21 Sexual Abuse of Child
(code 995.53 if focus of attention is on victim)
V61.21 Neglect of Child
(code 995.52 if focus of attention is on victim)
_____.__ Physical Abuse of Adult
V61.12 (if by partner)
V62.83 (if by person other than partner) *(code 995.81 if focus of attention is on victim)*
_____.__ Sexual Abuse of Adult
V61.12 (if by partner)
V62.83 (if by person other than partner) *(code 995.83 if focus of attention is on victim)*

Additional Conditions That May Be a Focus of Clinical Attention

V15.81 Noncomplicance With Treatment
V65.2 Malingering
V71.01 Adult Antisocial Behavior
V71.02 Child or Adolescent Antisocial Behavior
V62.89 Borderline Intellectual Functioning
Note: *This is coded on Axis II.*
780.9 Age-Related Cognitive Decline
V62.82 Bereavement
V62.3 Academic Problem
V62.2 Occupational Problem
313.82 Identity Problem
V62.89 Religious or Spiritual Problem
V62.4 Acculturation Problem
V62.89 Phase of Life Problem

ADDITIONAL CODES

300.9 Unspecified Mental Disorder (nonpsychotic)
V71.09 No Diagnosis or Condition on Axis I
799.9 Diagnosis or Condition Deferred on Axis I
V71.09 No Diagnosis on Axis II
799.9 Diagnosis Deferred on Axis II

MULTIAXIAL SYSTEM

Axis I Clinical Disorders
Other Conditions That May Be a Focus of Clinical Attention
Axis II Personality Disorders
Mental Retardation
Axis III General Medical Conditions
Axis IV Psychosocial and Environmental Problems
Axis V Global Assessment of Functioning

MULTIAXIAL ASSESSMENT

A multiaxial system involves an assessment on several axes, each of which refers to a different domain of information that may help the clinician plan treatment and predict outcome. There are five axes included in the DSM-IV multiaxial classification:

Axis I	Clinical Disorders Other Conditions That May Be a Focus of Clinical Attention
Axis II	Personality Disorders Mental Retardation
Axis III	General Medical Conditions
Axis IV	Psychosocial and Environmental Problems
Axis V	Global Assessment of Functioning

The use of the multiaxial system facilitates comprehensive and systematic evaluation with attention to the various mental disorders and general medical conditions, psychosocial and environmental problems, and level of functioning that might be overlooked if the focus were on assessing a single presenting problem. A multiaxial system provides a convenient format for organizing and communicating clinical information, for capturing the complexity of clinical situations, and for describing the heterogeneity of individuals presenting with the same diagnosis. In addition, the multiaxial system promotes the application of the biopsychosocial model in clinical, educational, and research settings.

The rest of this section provides a description of each of the DSM-IV axes. In some settings or situations, clinicians may prefer not to use the multiaxial system. For this reason, guidelines for reporting the results of a DSM-IV assessment without applying the formal multiaxial system are provided at the end of this section.

AXIS I | **Clinical Disorders**

Other Conditions That May Be a Focus of Clinical Attention

Disorders Usually First Diagnosed in Infancy, Childhood, or Adolescence (*excluding Mental Retardation, which is diagnosed on Axis II*)

Delirium, Dementia, and Amnestic and Other Cognitive Disorders

Mental Disorders Due to a General Medical Condition

Substance-Related Disorders

Schizophrenia and Other Psychotic Disorders

Mood Disorders

Anxiety Disorders

Somatoform Disorders

Factitious Disorders

Dissociative Disorders

Sexual and Gender Identity Disorders

Eating Disorders

Sleep Disorders

Impulse-Control Disorders Not Elsewhere Classified

Adjustment Disorders

Other Conditions That May Be a Focus of Clinical Attention

AXIS I: CLINICAL DISORDERS—OTHER CONDITIONS THAT MAY BE A FOCUS OF CLINICAL ATTENTION

Axis I is for reporting all the various disorders or conditions in the Classification except for the Personality Disorders and Mental Retardation (which are reported on Axis II). The major groups of disorders to be reported on Axis I are listed in the box at the top of the page. Also reported on Axis I are Other Conditions That May Be a Focus of Clinical Attention.

When an individual has more than one Axis I disorder, all of these should be reported. If more than one Axis I disorder is present, the principal diagnosis or the reason for visit should be indicated by listing it first. When an individual has both an Axis I and an Axis II disorder, the principal diagnosis or the reason for visit will be assumed to be on Axis I unless the Axis II diagnosis is followed by the qualifying phrase "(Principal Diagnosis)" or "(Reason for Visit)." If no Axis I disorder is present, this should be coded as V71.09. If an Axis I diagnosis is deferred, pending the gathering of additional information, this should be coded as 799.9.

AXIS II: PERSONALITY DISORDERS AND MENTAL RETARDATION

Axis II is for reporting Personality Disorders and Mental Retardation. It may also be used for noting prominent maladaptive personality features and defense mechanisms. The listing of Personality Disorders and Mental Retardation on a separate axis ensures that consideration will be given to the possible presence of Personality Disorders and Mental Retardation that might otherwise be overlooked when attention is directed to the usually more florid Axis I disorders. The coding of Personality Disorders on Axis II should not be taken to imply that their pathogenesis or range of appropriate treatment is fundamentally different from that for the disorders coded on Axis I. The disorders to be reported on Axis II are listed in the box on the next page.

In the common situation in which an individual has more than one Axis II diagnosis, all should be reported. When an individual has both an Axis I and an Axis II diagnosis and the Axis II diagnosis is the principal diagnosis or the reason for visit, this should be indicated by adding the qualifying phrase

AXIS II	Personality Disorders
Mental Retardation	
Paranoid Personality Disorder	Narcissistic Personality Disorder
Schizoid Personality Disorder	Avoidant Personality Disorder
Schizotypal Personality Disorder	Dependent Personality Disorder
Antisocial Personality Disorder	Obsessive-Compulsive Personality Disorder
Borderline Personality Disorder	Personality Disorder Not Otherwise Specified
Histrionic Personality Disorder	Mental Retardation

"(Principal Diagnosis)" or "(Reason for Visit)" after the Axis II diagnosis. If no Axis II disorder is present, this should be coded as V71.09. If an Axis II diagnosis is deferred, pending the gathering of additional information, this should be coded as 799.9.

Axis II may also be used to indicate prominent maladaptive personality features that do not meet the threshold for a Personality Disorder (in such instances, no code number should be used). The habitual use of maladaptive defense mechanisms may also be indicated on Axis II.

AXIS III: GENERAL MEDICAL CONDITIONS

Axis III is for reporting current general medical conditions that are potentially relevant to the understanding or management of the individual's mental disorder. These conditions are classified outside the "Mental Disorders" chapter of ICD-9-CM (and outside Chapter V of ICD-10). A listing of the broad categories of general medical conditions is given in the box to the right.

As discussed in the "Introduction," the multiaxial distinction among Axis I, Axis II, and Axis III disorders does not imply that there are fundamental differences in their conceptualization, that mental disorders are unrelated to physical or biological factors or processes, or that general medical conditions are unrelated to behavioral or psychosocial factors or processes. The purpose of distinguishing general medical conditions is to encourage thoroughness in evaluation and to enhance communication among health care providers.

General medical conditions can be related to mental disorders in a variety of ways. In some cases it is clear that the general medical condition is directly etiological to the development or worsening of mental symptoms and that the mechanism for this effect is physiological. When a mental disorder is judged to be a direct physiological consequence of the general medical condition, a Mental Disorder Due to a General Medical Condition should be diagnosed on Axis I and the general medical condition should be recorded on both Axis I and Axis III. For example, when hypothyroidism is a direct cause of depressive symptoms, the designation on Axis I is 293.83 Mood Disorder Due to Hypothyroidism, With Depressive Features, and the hypothyroidism is listed again and coded on Axis III as 244.9.

In those instances in which the etiological relationship between the general medical condition and the mental symptoms is insufficiently clear to warrant an Axis I diagnosis of Mental Disorder Due to a General Medical Condition, the appropriate mental disorder (e.g., Major Depressive Disorder) should be listed and coded on Axis I; the general medical condition should be coded only on Axis III.

There are other situations in which general medical conditions are recorded on Axis III because of their importance to the overall understanding or treatment of the individual with the mental disorder. An Axis I disorder may be a psychological reaction to an Axis III general medical condition (e.g., the development of 309.0 Adjustment Disorder With Depressed Mood as a reaction to the diagnosis of carcinoma of the breast). Some general medical conditions may not be directly related to the mental disorder but nonetheless have important prognostic or treatment implications (e.g., when the diagnosis on Axis I is 296.30 Major Depressive Disorder, Recurrent, and on Axis III is 427.9 arrhythmia, the choice of pharmacotherapy is influenced by the general medical condition; or when a person with diabetes mellitus is admitted to the hospital for an exacerbation of Schizophrenia and insulin management must be monitored).

When an individual has more than one clinically relevant Axis III diagnosis, all should be reported. If no Axis III disorder is present, this should be indicated by the notation "Axis III: None." If an Axis III diagnosis is deferred, pending the gathering of additional information, this should be indicated by the notation "Axis III: Deferred."

AXIS III	General Medical Conditions (with ICD-9-CM codes)
Infectious and Parasitic Diseases (001–139)	
Neoplasms (140–239)	
Endocrine, Nutritional, and Metabolic Diseases and Immunity Disorders (240–279)	
Diseases of the Blood and Blood-Forming Organs (280–289)	
Diseases of the Nervous System and Sense Organs (320–389)	
Diseases of the Circulatory System (390–459)	
Diseases of the Respiratory System (460–519)	
Diseases of the Digestive System (520–579)	
Diseases of the Genitourinary System (580–629)	
Complications of Pregnancy, Childbirth, and the Puerperium (630–676)	
Diseases of the Skin and Subcutaneous Tissue (680–709)	
Diseases of the Musculoskeletal System and Connective Tissue (710–739)	
Congenital Anomalies (740–759)	
Certain Conditions Originating in the Perinatal Period (760–779)	
Symptoms, Signs, and Ill-Defined Conditions (780–799)	
Injury and Poisoning (800–999)	

AXIS IV: PSYCHOSOCIAL AND ENVIRONMENTAL PROBLEMS

Axis IV is for reporting psychosocial and environmental problems that may affect the diagnosis, treatment, and prognosis of mental disorders (Axes I and II). A psychosocial or environmental problem may be a negative life event, an environmental difficulty or deficiency, a familial or other interpersonal stress, an inadequacy of social support or personal resources, or other problem relating to the context in which a person's difficulties have developed. So-called positive stressors, such as job promotion, should be listed only if they constitute or lead to a problem, as when a person has difficulty adapting to the new situation. In addition to playing a role in the initiation or exacerbation of a mental disorder, psychosocial problems may also develop as a consequence of a person's psychopathology or may constitute problems that should be considered in the overall management plan.

When an individual has multiple psychosocial or environmental problems, the clinician may note as many as are judged to be relevant. In general, the clinician should note only those psychosocial and environmental problems that have been present during the year preceding the current evaluation. However, the clinician may choose to note psychosocial and environmental problems occurring prior to the previous year if these clearly contribute to the mental disorder or have become a focus of treatment—for example, previous combat experiences leading to Posttraumatic Stress Disorder.

In practice, most psychosocial and environmental problems will be indicated on Axis IV. However, when a psychosocial or environmental problem is the primary focus of clinical attention, it should also be recorded on Axis I, with a code derived from the section "Other Conditions That May Be a Focus of Clinical Attention."

For convenience, the problems are grouped together in the following categories:

- **Problems with primary support group**—e.g., death of a family member; health problems in family; disruption of family by separation, divorce, or estrangement; removal from the home; remarriage of parent; sexual or physical abuse; parental overprotection; neglect of child; inadequate discipline; discord with siblings; birth of a sibling
- **Problems related to the social environment**—e.g., death or loss of friend; inadequate social support; living alone; difficulty with acculturation; discrimination; adjustment of life-cycle transition (such as retirement)
- **Educational problems**—e.g., illiteracy; academic problems; discord with teachers or classmates; inadequate school environment
- **Occupational problems**—e.g., unemployment; threat of job loss; stressful work schedule; difficult work conditions; job dissatisfaction; job change; discord with boss or co-workers
- **Housing problems**—e.g., homelessness; inadequate housing; unsafe neighborhood; discord with neighbors or landlord
- **Economic problems**—e.g., extreme poverty; inadequate finances; insufficient welfare support

AXIS IV	Psychosocial and Environmental Problems
Problems with primary support group	
Problems related to the social environment	
Educational problems	
Occupational problems	
Housing problems	
Economic problems	
Problems with access to health care services	
Problems related to interaction with the legal system/crime	
Other psychosocial and environmental problems	

- **Problems with access to health care services**—e.g., inadequate health care services; transportation to health care facilities unavailable; inadequate health insurance
- **Problems related to interaction with the legal system/crime**—e.g., arrest; incarceration; litigation; victim of crime
- **Other psychosocial and environmental problems**—e.g., exposure to disasters, war, other hostilities; discord with nonfamily caregivers such as counselor, social worker, or physician; unavailability of social service agencies

When using the Multiaxial Evaluation Report Form, the clinician should identify the relevant categories of psychosocial and environmental problems and indicate the specific factors involved. If a recording form with a checklist of problem categories is not used, the clinician may simply list the specific problems on Axis IV.

AXIS V: GLOBAL ASSESSMENT OF FUNCTIONING

Axis V is for reporting the clinician's judgment of the individual's overall level of functioning. This information is useful in planning treatment and measuring its impact, and in predicting outcome.

The reporting of overall functioning on Axis V can be done using the Global Assessment of Functioning (GAF) Scale. The GAF Scale may be particularly useful in tracking the clinical progress of individuals in global terms, using a single measure. The GAF Scale is to be rated with respect only to psychological, social, and occupational functioning. The instructions specify, "Do not include impairment in functioning due to physical (or environmental) limitations."

The GAF scale is divided into 10 ranges of functioning. Making a GAF rating involves picking a single value that best reflects the individual's overall level of functioning. The description of each 10-point range in the GAF scale has two components: the first part covers symptom severity, and the second part covers functioning. The GAF rating is within a particular decile if **either** the symptom severity **or** the level of functioning falls within the range. For example, the first part of the range 41–50 describes "serious symptoms (e.g., suicidal ideation, severe obsessional rituals, frequent shoplifting)" and the second part includes "any serious impairment in social, occupational, or school functioning (e.g., no friends, unable to keep a job)." It should be noted that in situations where the individual's symptom severity and level of functioning are discordant, the final GAF rating always reflects the worse of the two. For example, the GAF rating for an individual who is a significant danger to self but is otherwise functioning well would be below 20. Similarly, the GAF rating for an individual with minimal psychological symptomatology but significant impairment in functioning (e.g., an individual whose excessive preoccupation with substance use has resulted in loss of job and friends but no other psychopathology) would be 40 or lower.

In most instances, ratings on the GAF Scale should be for the current period (i.e., the level of functioning at the time of the evaluation) because ratings of current functioning will generally reflect the need for treatment or care. In order to account for day-to-day variability in functioning, the GAF rating for the "current period" is sometimes operationalized as the lowest level of functioning for the past week. In some settings, it may be useful to note the GAF Scale rating both at time of admission and at time of discharge. The GAF Scale may also be rated for other time periods (e.g., the highest level of functioning for at least a few months during the past year). The GAF Scale is reported on Axis V as follows: "GAF =," followed by the GAF rating from 0 to 100, followed by the time period reflected by the rating in parentheses—for example, "(current)," "(highest level in past year)," "(at discharge)."

In order to ensure that no elements of the GAF Scale are overlooked when a GAF rating is being made, the following method for determining a GAF rating may be applied:

STEP 1: Starting at the top level, evaluate each range by asking "is either the individual's symptom severity OR level of functioning worse than what is indicated in the range description?"

Global Assessment of Functioning (GAF) Scale

Code	(Note: Use intermediate codes when appropriate, e.g., 45, 68, 72.)
100/91	Superior functioning in a wide range of activities, life's problems never seem to get out of hand, is sought out by others because of his or her many positive qualities. No symptoms.
90/81	Absent or minimal symptoms (e.g., mild anxiety before an exam), good functioning in all areas, interested and involved in a wide range of activities, socially effective, generally satisfied with life, no more than everyday problems or concerns (e.g., an occasional argument with family members).
80/71	If symptoms are present, they are transient and expectable reactions to psychosocial stressors (e.g., difficulty concentrating after family argument), no more than slight impairment in social, occupational, or school functioning (e.g., temporarily falling behind in schoolwork).
70/61	Some mild symptoms (e.g., depressed mood and mild insomnia) OR some difficulty in social, occupational, or school functioning (e.g., occasional truancy, or theft within the household), but generally functioning pretty well, has some meaningful interpersonal relationships.
60/51	Moderate symptoms (e.g., flat affect and circumstantial speech, occasional panic attacks) OR moderate difficulty in social, occupational, or school functioning (e.g., few friends, conflicts with peers or co-workers).
50/41	Serious symptoms (e.g., suicidal ideation; severe obsessional rituals, frequent shoplifting) OR any serious impairment in social, occupational, or school functioning (e.g., no friends, unable to keep a job).
40/31	Some impairment in reality testing or communication (e.g., speech is at times illogical, obscure, or irrelevant) OR major impairment in several areas, such as work or school, family relations, judgment, thinking, or mood (e.g., depressed man avoids friends, neglects family, and is unable to work; child frequently beats up younger children, is defiant at home, and is failing at school).
30/21	Behavior is considerably influenced by delusions or hallucinations OR serious impairment in communication or judgment (e.g., sometimes incoherent, acts grossly inappropriately, suicidal preoccupation) OR inability to function in almost all areas (e.g., stays in bed all day; no job, home, or friends).
20/11	Some danger of hurting self or others (e.g., suicide attempts without clear expectation of death; frequently violent; manic excitement) OR occasionally fails to maintain minimal personal hygiene (e.g., smears feces) OR gross impairment in communication (e.g., largely incoherent or mute).
10/1	Persistent danger of severely hurting self or others (e.g., recurrent violence) OR persistent inability to maintain minimal personal hygiene OR serious suicidal act with clear expectation of death.
0	Inadequate information.

The rating of overall psychological functioning on a scale of 0–100 was operationalized by Luborsky in the Health-Sickness Rating Scale (Luborsky L: "Clinicians' Judgments of Mental Health." *Archives of General Psychiatry* 7:407–417, 1962). Spitzer and colleagues developed a revision of the Health-Sickness Rating Scale called the Global Assessment Scale (GAS) (Endicott J, Spitzer RL, Fleiss JL, Cohen J: "The Global Assessment Scale: A Procedure for Measuring Overall Severity of Psychiatric Disturbance." *Archives of General Psychiatry* 33:766–771, 1976). A modified version of the GAS was included in DSM-ILL-R as the Global Assessment of Functioning (GAF) Scale.

STEP 2: Keep moving down the scale until the range that best matches the individual's symptom severity OR the level of functioning is reached, **whichever is worse.**

STEP 3: Look at the next lower range as a double-check against having stopped prematurely. This range should be too severe on **both** symptom severity **and** level of functioning. If it is, the appropriate range has been reached (continue with step 4). If not, go back to step 2 and continue moving down the scale.

STEP 4: To determine the specific GAF rating within the selected 10-point range, consider whether the individual is functioning at the higher or lower end of the 10-point range. For example, consider an individual who hears voices that do not influence his behavior (e.g., someone with long-standing Schizophrenia who accepts his hallucinations as part of his illness). If the voices occur relatively infrequently (once a week or less), a rating of 39 or 40 might be most appropriate. In contrast, if the individual hears voices almost continuously, a rating of 31 or 32 would be more appropriate.

In some settings, it may be useful to assess social and occupational disability and to track progress in rehabilitation independent of the severity of the psychological symptoms.

GLOBAL ASSESSMENT OF FUNCTIONING (GAF) SCALE

Consider psychological, social, and occupational functioning on a hypothetical continuum of mental health illness. Do not include impairment in functioning due to physical (or environmental) limitations.

APPENDIX B

2003–2004 NANDA-APPROVED NURSING DIAGNOSES

Activity Intolerance
Activity Intolerance, Risk for
Adaptive Capacity: Intracranial, Decreased
Adjustment, Impaired
Airway Clearance, Ineffective
Anxiety
Anxiety, Death
Aspiration, Risk for
Attachment, Parent/Infant/Child, Risk for Impaired
Body Image, Disturbed
Body Temperature: Imbalanced, Risk for
Bowel Incontinence
Breastfeeding, Effective
Breastfeeding, Ineffective
Breastfeeding, Interrupted
Breathing Pattern, Ineffective
Cardiac Output, Decreased
Caregiver Role Strain
Caregiver Role Strain, Risk for
Communication, Readiness for Enhanced
Communication: Verbal, Impaired
Confusion, Acute
Confusion, Chronic
Constipation
Constipation, Perceived
Constipation, Risk for
Coping: Community, Ineffective
Coping: Community, Readiness for Enhanced
Coping, Defensive
Coping: Family, Compromised
Coping: Family, Disabled
Coping: Family, Readiness for Enhanced
Coping (Individual), Readiness for Enhanced
Coping, Ineffective
Decisional Conflict (Specify)
Denial, Ineffective
Dentition, Impaired
Development: Delayed, Risk for
Diarrhea
Disuse Syndrome, Risk for
Diversional Activity, Deficient
Dysreflexia, Autonomic
Dysreflexia, Autonomic, Risk for
Energy Field, Disturbed
Environmental Interpretation Syndrome, Impaired
Failure to Thrive, Adult
Falls, Risk for
Family Processes, Dysfunctional: Alcoholism
Family Processes, Interrupted
Family Processes, Readiness for Enhanced
Fatigue
Fear
Fluid Balance, Readiness for Enhanced
Fluid Volume, Deficient
Fluid Volume, Deficient, Risk for
Fluid Volume, Excess
Fluid Volume, Imbalanced, Risk for
Gas Exchange, Impaired
Grieving, Anticipatory
Grieving, Dysfunctional
Growth, Disproportionate, Risk for
Growth and Development, Delayed
Health Maintenance, Ineffective
Health Seeking Behaviors (Specify)
Home Maintenance, Impaired
Hopelessness
Hyperthermia
Hypothermia
Identity: Personal, Disturbed
Infant Behavior, Disorganized
Infant Behavior: Disorganized, Risk for
Infant Behavior: Organized, Readiness for Enhanced
Infant Feeding Pattern, Ineffective
Infection, Risk for
Injury, Risk for
Knowledge, Deficient (Specify)
Knowledge (specify), Readiness for Enhanced
Latex Allergy Response
Latex Allergy Response, Risk for
Loneliness, Risk for
Memory, Impaired
Mobility: Bed, Impaired
Mobility: Physical, Impaired
Mobility: Wheelchair, Impaired
Nausea
Neurovascular Dysfunction: Peripheral, Risk for
Noncompliance (Specify)
Nutrition, Imbalanced: Less than Body Requirements
Nutrition, Imbalanced: More than Body Requirements
Nutrition, Imbalanced: More than Body Requirements, Risk for
Nutrition, Readiness for Enhanced
Oral Mucous Membrane, Impaired
Pain, Acute
Pain, Chronic
Parenting, Impaired
Parenting, Readiness for Enhanced
Parenting, Risk for Impaired
Perioperative Positioning Injury, Risk for
Poisoning, Risk for

Source: NANDA Nursing Diagnoses: Definitions and Classification, 2003-2004. Philadelphia: North American Nursing Diagnosis Association. Used with permission.

Post-Trauma Syndrome
Post-Trauma Syndrome, Risk for
Powerlessness
Powerlessness, Risk for
Protection, Ineffective
Rape-Trauma Syndrome
Rape-Trauma Syndrome: Compound Reaction
Rape-Trauma Syndrome: Silent Reaction
Relocation Stress Syndrome
Relocation Stress Syndrome, Risk for
Role Conflict, Parental
Role Performance, Ineffective
Self-Care Deficit: Bathing/Hygiene
Self-Care Deficit: Dressing/Grooming
Self-Care Deficit: Feeding
Self-Care Deficit: Toileting
Self-Concept, Readiness for Enhanced
Self-Esteem, Chronic Low
Self-Esteem, Situational Low
Self-Esteem, Risk for Situational Low
Self-Mutilation
Self-Mutilation, Risk for
Sensory Perception, Disturbed (Specify: Visual, Auditory, Kinesthetic, Gustatory, Tactile, Olfactory)
Sexual Dysfunction
Sexuality Patterns, Ineffective
Skin Integrity, Impaired
Skin Integrity, Risk for Impaired
Sleep Deprivation
Sleep Pattern Disturbed
Sleep, Readiness for Enhanced
Social Interaction, Impaired
Social Isolation
Sorrow, Chronic
Spiritual Distress
Spiritual Distress, Risk for
Spiritual Well-Being, Readiness for Enhanced
Spontaneous Ventilation, Impaired
Sudden Infant Death Syndrome, Risk for
Suffocation, Risk for
Suicide, Risk for
Surgical Recovery, Delayed
Swallowing, Impaired
Therapeutic Regimen Management: Community, Ineffective
Therapeutic Regimen Management, Effective
Therapeutic Regimen Management: Family, Ineffective
Therapeutic Regimen Management, Ineffective
Therapeutic Regimen Management, Readiness for Enhanced
Thermoregulation, Ineffective
Thought Processes, Disturbed
Tissue Integrity, Impaired
Tissue Perfusion, Ineffective (Specify type: renal, cerebral, cardiopulmonary, gastrointestinal, peripheral)
Tissue Perfusion, Ineffective (Peripheral)
Transfer Ability, Impaired
Trauma, Risk for
Unilateral Neglect
Urinary Elimination, Impaired
Urinary Elimination, Readiness for Enhanced
Urinary Incontinence, Functional
Urinary Incontinence, Reflex
Urinary Incontinence, Stress
Urinary Incontinence, Total
Urinary Incontinence, Urge
Urinary Incontinence, Risk for Urge
Urinary Retention
Ventilatory Weaning Response, Dysfunctional
Violence: Other-Directed, risk for
Violence: Self-Directed, risk for
Walking, Impaired
Wandering

INDEX

Note: *t* following a page number indicates a table,
i following a page number indicates an illustration.

B

C

E

G

I

J

K

L

M

SINGLE PC LICENSE AGREEMENT AND LIMITED WARRANTY

READ THIS LICENSE CAREFULLY BEFORE OPENING THIS PACKAGE. BY OPENING THIS PACKAGE, YOU ARE AGREEING TO THE TERMS AND CONDITIONS OF THIS LICENSE. IF YOU DO NOT AGREE, DO NOT OPEN THE PACKAGE. PROMPTLY RETURN THE UNOPENED PACKAGE AND ALL ACCOMPANYING ITEMS TO THE PLACE YOU OBTAINED THEM. ***THESE TERMS APPLY TO ALL LICENSED SOFTWARE ON THE DISK EXCEPT THAT THE TERMS FOR USE OF ANY SHAREWARE OR FREEWARE ON THE DISKETTES ARE AS SET FORTH IN THE ELECTRONIC LICENSE LOCATED ON THE DISK:***

1. GRANT OF LICENSE and OWNERSHIP: The enclosed computer programs and data ("Software") are licensed, not sold, to you by Pearson Education, Inc. ("We" or the "Company") and in consideration of your purchase or adoption of the accompanying Company textbooks and/or other materials, and your agreement to these terms. We reserve any rights not granted to you. You own only the disk(s) but we and/or our licensors own the Software itself. This license allows you to use and display your copy of the Software on a single computer (i.e., with a single CPU) at a single location for academic use only, so long as you comply with the terms of this Agreement. You may make one copy for back up, or transfer your copy to another CPU, provided that the Software is usable on only one computer.

2. RESTRICTIONS: You may not transfer or distribute the Software or documentation to anyone else. Except for backup, you may not copy the documentation or the Software. You may not network the Software or otherwise use it on more than one computer or computer terminal at the same time. You may not reverse engineer, disassemble, decompile, modify, adapt, translate, or create derivative works based on the Software or the Documentation. You may be held legally responsible for any copying or copyright infringement which is caused by your failure to abide by the terms of these restrictions.

3. TERMINATION: This license is effective until terminated. This license will terminate automatically without notice from the Company if you fail to comply with any provisions or limitations of this license. Upon termination, you shall destroy the Documentation and all copies of the Software. All provisions of this Agreement as to limitation and disclaimer of warranties, limitation of liability, remedies or damages, and our ownership rights shall survive termination.

4. LIMITED WARRANTY AND DISCLAIMER OF WARRANTY: Company warrants that for a period of 60 days from the date you purchase this SOFTWARE (or purchase or adopt the accompanying textbook), the Software, when properly installed and used in accordance with the Documentation, will operate in substantial conformity with the description of the Software set forth in the Documentation, and that for a period of 30 days the disk(s) on which the Software is delivered shall be free from defects in materials and workmanship under normal use. The Company does not warrant that the Software will meet your requirements or that the operation of the Software will be uninterrupted or error-free. Your only remedy and the Company's only obligation under these limited warranties is, at the Company's option, return of the disk for a refund of any amounts paid for it by you or replacement of the disk. THIS LIMITED WARRANTY IS THE ONLY WARRANTY PROVIDED BY THE COMPANY AND ITS LICENSORS, AND THE COMPANY AND ITS LICENSORS DISCLAIM ALL OTHER WARRANTIES, EXPRESS OR IMPLIED, INCLUDING WITHOUT LIMITATION, THE IMPLIED WARRANTIES OF MERCHANTABILITY AND FITNESS FOR A PARTICULAR PURPOSE. THE COMPANY DOES NOT WARRANT, GUARANTEE OR MAKE ANY REPRESENTATION REGARDING THE ACCURACY, RELIABILITY, CURRENTNESS, USE, OR RESULTS OF USE, OF THE SOFTWARE.

5. LIMITATION OF REMEDIES AND DAMAGES: IN NO EVENT, SHALL THE COMPANY OR ITS EMPLOYEES, AGENTS, LICENSORS, OR CONTRACTORS BE LIABLE FOR ANY INCIDENTAL, INDIRECT, SPECIAL, OR CONSEQUENTIAL DAMAGES ARISING OUT OF OR IN CONNECTION WITH THIS LICENSE OR THE SOFTWARE, INCLUDING FOR LOSS OF USE, LOSS OF DATA, LOSS OF INCOME OR PROFIT, OR OTHER LOSSES, SUSTAINED AS A RESULT OF INJURY TO ANY PERSON, OR LOSS OF OR DAMAGE TO PROPERTY, OR CLAIMS OF THIRD PARTIES, EVEN IF THE COMPANY OR AN AUTHORIZED REPRESENTATIVE OF THE COMPANY HAS BEEN ADVISED OF THE POSSIBILITY OF SUCH DAMAGES. IN NO EVENT SHALL THE LIABILITY OF THE COMPANY FOR DAMAGES WITH RESPECT TO THE SOFTWARE EXCEED THE AMOUNTS ACTUALLY PAID BY YOU, IF ANY, FOR THE SOFTWARE OR THE ACCOMPANYING TEXTBOOK. BECAUSE SOME JURISDICTIONS DO NOT ALLOW THE LIMITATION OF LIABILITY IN CERTAIN CIRCUMSTANCES, THE ABOVE LIMITATIONS MAY NOT ALWAYS APPLY TO YOU.

6. GENERAL: THIS AGREEMENT SHALL BE CONSTRUED IN ACCORDANCE WITH THE LAWS OF THE UNITED STATES OF AMERICA AND THE STATE OF NEW YORK, APPLICABLE TO CONTRACTS MADE IN NEW YORK, AND SHALL BENEFIT THE COMPANY, ITS AFFILIATES AND ASSIGNEES. HIS AGREEMENT IS THE COMPLETE AND EXCLUSIVE STATEMENT OF THE AGREEMENT BETWEEN YOU AND THE COMPANY AND SUPERSEDES ALL PROPOSALS OR PRIOR AGREEMENTS, ORAL, OR WRITTEN, AND ANY OTHER COMMUNICATIONS BETWEEN YOU AND THE COMPANY OR ANY REPRESENTATIVE OF THE COMPANY RELATING TO THE SUBJECT MATTER OF THIS AGREEMENT. If you are a U.S. Government user, this Software is licensed with "restricted rights" as set forth in subparagraphs (a)-(d) of the Commercial Computer-Restricted Rights clause at FAR 52.227-19 or in subparagraphs (c)(1)(ii) of the Rights in Technical Data and Computer Software clause at DFARS 252.227-7013, and similar clauses, as applicable.

Should you have any questions concerning this agreement or if you wish to contact the Company for any reason, please contact in writing: Prentice-Hall, New Media Department, One Lake Street, Upper Saddle River, NJ 07458.